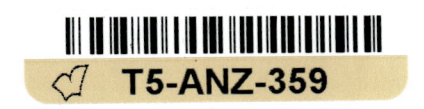

Reggie Zhan, M.D.
Kaiser Permanente
Dept. of Pathology
6111 Executive Blvd.
Rockville, MD 20852

Dermatopathology

Content Strategist: Russell Gabbedy
Content Development Specialist: Joanne Scott
Senior Project Manager: Beula Christopher
Design: Christian J. Bilbow
Illustration Manager: Jennifer Rose
Marketing Manager(s) (UK/USA): Gaynor Jones / Abigail Swartz

Dermatopathology
Second Edition

Edited by

Dirk M. Elston, MD

Director, Ackerman Academy of Dermatopathology;
Clinical Professor of Dermatology, Rutgers Robert Wood Johnson School of Medicine;
Clinical Professor of Medicine (Dermatology), New York College of Osteopathic Medicine
New York, NY, USA

Tammie Ferringer, MD

Section Head and Fellowship Director of Dermatopathology
Departments of Dermatology and Laboratory Medicine
Geisinger Medical Center
Danville, PA, USA

with

Christine J. Ko, MD
Steven Peckham, MD
Whitney A. High, MD, JD, MEng
David J. DiCaudo, MD
Sunita Bhuta, MD

For additional online content visit the expertconsult.com

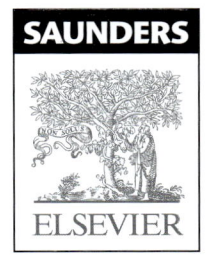

SAUNDERS
ELSEVIER

ELSEVIER
SAUNDERS

SAUNDERS an imprint of Elsevier Limited

© 2014, Elsevier Limited. All rights reserved.

First edition 2009
Second edition 2014
 Reprinted 2014 (twice), 2015, 2016

The right of Dirk M. Elston and Tammie Ferringer to be identified as authors of this work has been asserted by them in accordance with the Copyright, Designs and Patents Act 1988.

No part of this publication may be reproduced or transmitted in any form or by any means, electronic or mechanical, including photocopying, recording, or any information storage and retrieval system, without permission in writing from the publisher. Details on how to seek permission, further information about the Publisher's permissions policies and our arrangements with organizations such as the Copyright Clearance Center and the Copyright Licensing Agency, can be found at our website: www.elsevier.com/permissions.

This book and the individual contributions contained in it are protected under copyright by the Publisher (other than as may be noted herein).

Some of the images in this book are in the public domain.

Notices
Knowledge and best practice in this field are constantly changing. As new research and experience broaden our understanding, changes in research methods, professional practices, or medical treatment may become necessary.

Practitioners and researchers must always rely on their own experience and knowledge in evaluating and using any information, methods, compounds, or experiments described herein. In using such information or methods they should be mindful of their own safety and the safety of others, including parties for whom they have a professional responsibility.

With respect to any drug or pharmaceutical products identified, readers are advised to check the most current information provided (i) on procedures featured or (ii) by the manufacturer of each product to be administered, to verify the recommended dose or formula, the method and duration of administration, and contraindications. It is the responsibility of practitioners, relying on their own experience and knowledge of their patients, to make diagnoses, to determine dosages and the best treatment for each individual patient, and to take all appropriate safety precautions.

To the fullest extent of the law, neither the Publisher nor the authors, contributors, or editors, assume any liability for any injury and/or damage to persons or property as a matter of products liability, negligence or otherwise, or from any use or operation of any methods, products, instructions, or ideas contained in the material herein.

ISBN: 978-0-7020-5527-0
E-ISBN: 978-0-7020-5528-7

ELSEVIER your source for books, journals and multimedia in the health sciences
www.elsevierhealth.com

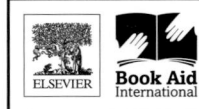

Working together to grow libraries in developing countries
www.elsevier.com • www.bookaid.org

The publisher's policy is to use paper manufactured from sustainable forests

Printed in China

Last digit is the print number: 9 8 7 6 5

Contents

Online Lectures and Atlas Materials — vi
Preface — vii
List of Contributors — viii
Acknowledgments — ix
Dedications — x

Chapter 1: The basics: diagnostic terms, skin anatomy, and stains — 1
Tammie Ferringer and Christine J. Ko

Chapter 2: Benign tumors and cysts of the epidermis — 37
Dirk M. Elston

Chapter 3: Malignant tumors of the epidermis — 56
Dirk M. Elston

Chapter 4: Pilar and sebaceous neoplasms — 71
Dirk M. Elston

Chapter 5: Sweat gland neoplasms — 86
Dirk M. Elston

Chapter 6: Melanocytic neoplasms — 105
Dirk M. Elston

Chapter 7: Interface dermatitis — 134
Dirk M. Elston

Chapter 8: Psoriasiform and spongiotic dermatitis — 150
Dirk M. Elston

Chapter 9: Blistering diseases — 161
Whitney A. High

Chapter 10: Granulomatous and histiocytic diseases — 172
Tammie Ferringer

Chapter 11: Inflammatory vascular diseases — 183
Dirk M. Elston

Chapter 12: Genodermatoses — 208
Tammie Ferringer

Chapter 13: Alterations in collagen and elastin — 213
Tammie Ferringer

Chapter 14: Metabolic disorders — 224
Tammie Ferringer

Chapter 15: Disorders of skin appendages — 234
Dirk M. Elston

Chapter 16: Panniculitis — 249
Dirk M. Elston

Chapter 17: Bacterial, spirochete, and protozoan infections — 257
Dirk M. Elston

Chapter 18: Fungal infections — 270
Dirk M. Elston

Chapter 19: Viral infections, helminths, and arthropods — 286
Dirk M. Elston

Chapter 20: Fibrous tumors — 309
Dirk M. Elston

Chapter 20a: Key diagnostic features of additional soft tissue neoplasms (Online only)
Christine J. Ko and Tammie Ferringer

Chapter 21: Tumors of fat, muscle, cartilage, and bone — 341
Tammie Ferringer

Chapter 22: Neural tumors — 354
Tammie Ferringer

Chapter 23: Vascular tumors — 366
Dirk M. Elston

Chapter 24: Cutaneous T-cell lymphoma, NK-cell lymphoma, and myeloid leukemia — 390
David J. DiCaudo

Chapter 25: B-cell lymphoma and lymphocytic leukemia — 404
Steven Peckham

Chapter 26: Metastatic tumors and simulators — 416
Christine J. Ko

Appendix 1: Dermatopathology mnemonics — 425

Appendix 2: Skin ultrastructure — 426
Sunita Bhuta

Appendix 3: External agents and artifacts — 428
Tammie Ferringer

Index — 432

Indicates additional online material

Online Lectures and Atlas Materials

1. **Author narrated lectures – 27 presentations with approximately 2,000 slides and over 8 hours running time.**
2. **Clinical image atlas – with approximately 600 images.**
3. **Histopathology atlas – with approximately 500 images.**
4. **Infectious disease atlas – with approximately 2,500 histopathologic images.**
5. **Soft tissue tumor atlas – with approximately 300 histopathologic images.**

Access the complete contents online at www.expertconsult.com

Preface

This text is designed to cover the essentials of dermatopathology in a style that is enjoyable and easily understood. **Please note that you are holding only a portion of the book in your hands! Much of it is online in the form of online lectures and extensive digital image atlases. For this edition, we have added updated online lectures with many new entities, a high quality clinical image atlas, extensive infectious disease atlas, soft tissue tumor atlas, lymphoma atlas and more. Be sure to check out all the online features at www.expertconsult.com** For students of dermatopathology, we hope the book and lectures make your way a little easier. For those in practice, we hope the book becomes one of your favorite references and one that your reach for often.

Dirk M. Elston

List of Contributors

With contributions by Patricia Malerich, MD; Lindsay Sewell, MD; Nektarios Lountzis, MD; David Adams, MD; Martie Jewell, MD; Chad Thomas, MD; Sasha Kramer, MD; Eric Hossler, MD; Morgan Wilson, MD; Puja Puri, MD; Michael Conroy, MD; Seth Forman, MD, and Carly Elston.

Monkey Pox slides courtesy of Erik Stratman, MD.

Chancroid and granuloma inguinale slides courtesy of Brooke Army Medical Center teaching file.

Lucio phenomenon slide courtesy of David M. Scollard, MD.

Kimura's disease slide courtesy of Jim Fitzpatrick, MD.

Contributing authors

Sunita Bhuta, MD
Chief, Head and Neck Pathology;
Professor, Pathology and Laboratory Medicine;
Director, Transmission Electron Microscopy Laboratory
David Geffen School of Medicine, UCLA
Los Angeles, CA, USA

David J. DiCaudo, MD
Head, Dermatopathology Division;
Associate Professor, Dermatology and Laboratory Medicine/Pathology
Department of Dermatology
Mayo Clinic College of Medicine
Scottsdale, AZ, USA

Dirk M. Elston, MD
Director, Ackerman Academy of Dermatopathology;
Clinical Professor of Dermatology, Rutgers Robert Wood Johnson School of Medicine;
Clinical Professor of Medicine (Dermatology), New York College of Osteopathic Medicine
New York, NY, USA

Tammie Ferringer, MD
Section Head and Fellowship Director of Dermatopathology
Departments of Dermatology and Laboratory Medicine
Geisinger Medical Center
Danville, PA, USA

Whitney A. High, MD, JD, MEng
Associate Professor, Dermatology and Pathology;
Director, Dermatopathology Laboratory (Dermatology)
University of Colorado School of Medicine
Denver, CO, USA

Christine J. Ko, MD
Associate Professor of Dermatology and Pathology
Departments of Dermatology and Pathology
Yale University
New Haven, CT, USA

Steven Peckham, MD
Director, Surgical Pathology
Wilford Hall USAF Ambulatory Surgical Center
San Antonio, TX, USA

Acknowledgments

I would like to thank my fellow authors as well as the residents and fellows of Geisinger Medical Center, The Ackerman Academy of Dermatopathology, Brooke Army Medical Center, and Wilford Hall Medical Center. They were the testing ground for many of the ideas in the book as well as the style of presentation.

Special thanks are due to David Adams, Martie Jewell, Sasha Kramer, Chad Thomas, Pattie Malerich, Lindsay Sewell, Nick Lountzis, Jake Bauer, Marjan Yousefi, Morgan Wilson, Eric Hossler, and Greg Jacobsen who helped to organize and review lecture notes so that no topic would be forgotten.

This text would not have been possible without the help and support of Dr Bill Tyler, who remains the backbone of the Geisinger dermatopathology service, and Tammie Ferringer, who is always there for the residents and fellows. She quietly and elegantly makes everything possible. Thank you both for your help and support.

The tremendous teaching resources of the Ackerman Academy of Dermatopathology, Geisinger Medical Center, and Brooke Army Medical Center made this book and all of the additional online resources possible. Special thanks are also due to Tammy Rodenhaver for her willingness to pitch in and do whatever is necessary to support academics at Geisinger. We would also like to acknowledge the faculty, nurses, secretaries, histology techs, librarians, and front desk personnel at the Ackerman Academy of Dermatopathology and Geisinger Medical Center, who support one another and make each a truly special place for learning and patient care.

The editors and authors would like to thank the editorial and publication team at Elsevier, without whom these texts would not have been possible.

Dedications

This book is dedicated to my wife and best friend Kathy, my children Carly and Nate who make me so proud, and to all of those students of dermatopathology, young and old, who make it such a pleasure to teach.

This book would not have been possible without my teachers Dean Pearson, Tim Berger, Jim Graham, George Lupton, and Wilma Bergfeld. It has also been my privilege to work with, and learn from, Martha McCollough, Tom Davis, Karen Warschaw, Les Libow, Bill Tyler and Tim Gardner. Thank you for your friendship and for all you have taught me.

Dirk M. Elston

This work is dedicated to my daughter Emily who has filled holes in my life that I did not know I had, my husband Jim and mother Judy for their patience, understanding and support and to the memory of my father Elzie. None of this would be possible without the incredible guidance and tutelage of Dirk M. Elston and would lack purpose without the curiosity and eagerness of the residents and fellows that go on to become my colleagues and friends.

Tammie Ferringer

To Peter, Dylan, and Owen.

Christine J. Ko

To my Ms, old and new …

Whitney A. High

To my parents, James and Hilda, who have always encouraged me to do my best.

Steven Peckham

To my wife Valerie, our children Matthew and Gianna, and all the dermatology residents, past and present, whom I have had the pleasure to teach.

David J. DiCaudo

The basics: diagnostic terms, skin anatomy, and stains

Tammie Ferringer, Christine J. Ko

Glossary of terms

Acantholysis
- Loss of cell–cell adhesion

Acanthosis
- Increase in thickness of the epidermis
- Regular (all rete pegs descend to the same level) or irregular (rete pegs descend to different levels in the papillary dermis)

Anaplasia
- Atypical nuclei (abnormal size, shape, staining) and pleomorphism (variation in nuclear characteristics)

Apoptosis (pronounced apohtosis)
- "Programmed cell death"
- "Dead red" keratinocytes with pyknotic nuclei
  - *Although the term is often applied to any necrotic or dyskeratotic keratinocyte, it is best reserved for physiologic programmed cell death or pathologic processes that produce death through a similar pathway*

Arborizing
- Branching, often refers to rete or vasculature

Asteroid body
- Collections of eosinophilic material seen in sporotrichosis
- Also refers to star-shaped intracytoplasmic inclusions seen in giant cells of sarcoidosis or berylliosis or other granulomatous processes

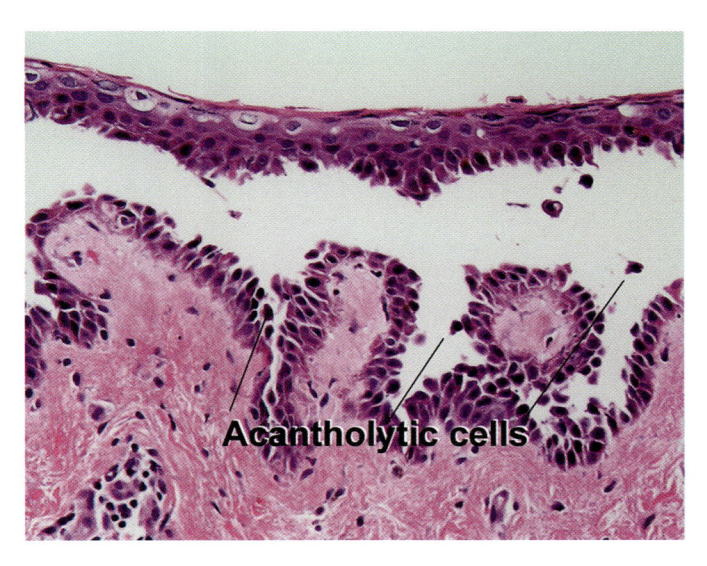

Fig 1-1 Acantholysis, pemphigus vulgaris

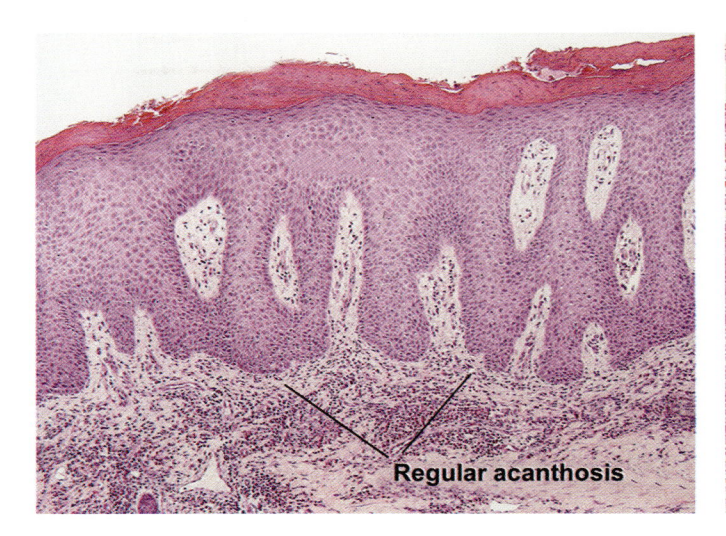

Fig 1-2 Acanthosis, psoriasis

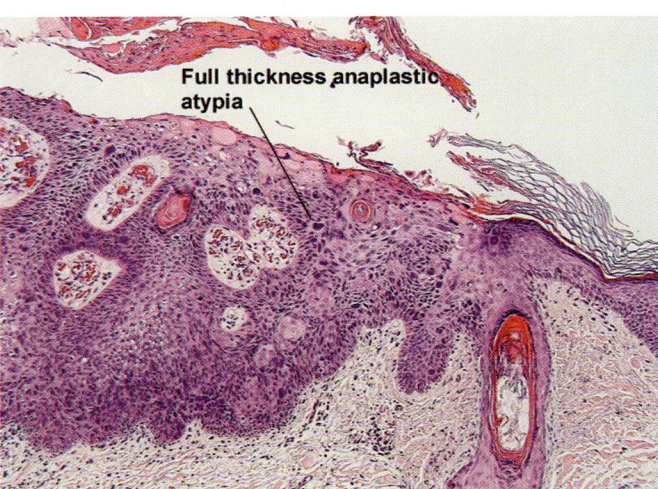

Fig 1-3 Anaplasia, Bowen's disease

Dermatopathology

Atrophy
- Decrease in thickness of epidermis

Ballooning degeneration
- Destruction of epidermis by dissolution of cell attachments and intracellular edema

Caterpillar body
- Pale pink linear basement membrane material within epidermis, seen in porphyria cutanea tarda
- Represents degenerated type IV collagen

Civatte/colloid bodies
- Pink, globular remnants of keratinocytes

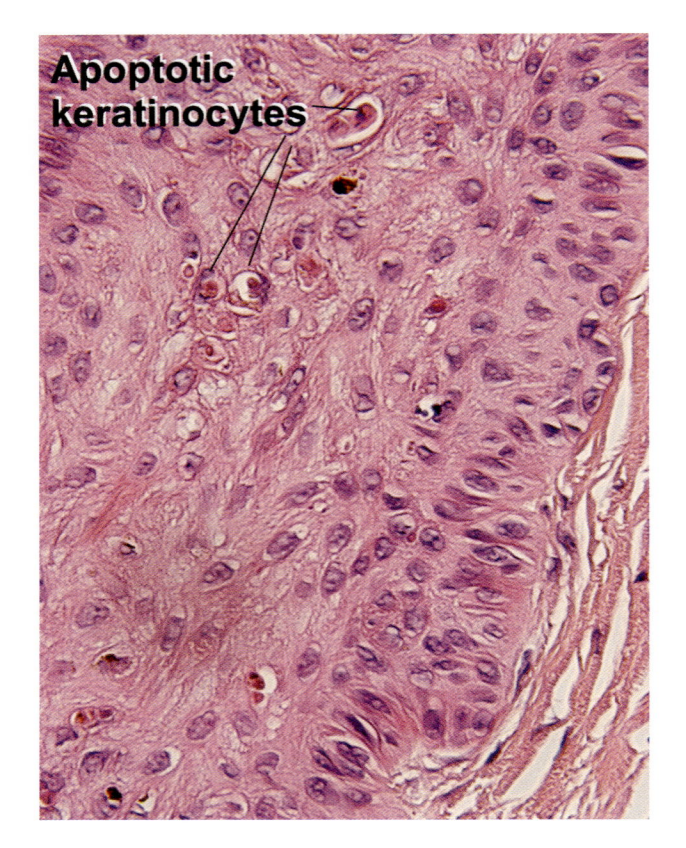

Fig 1-4 Apoptosis, outer root sheath, catagen follicle

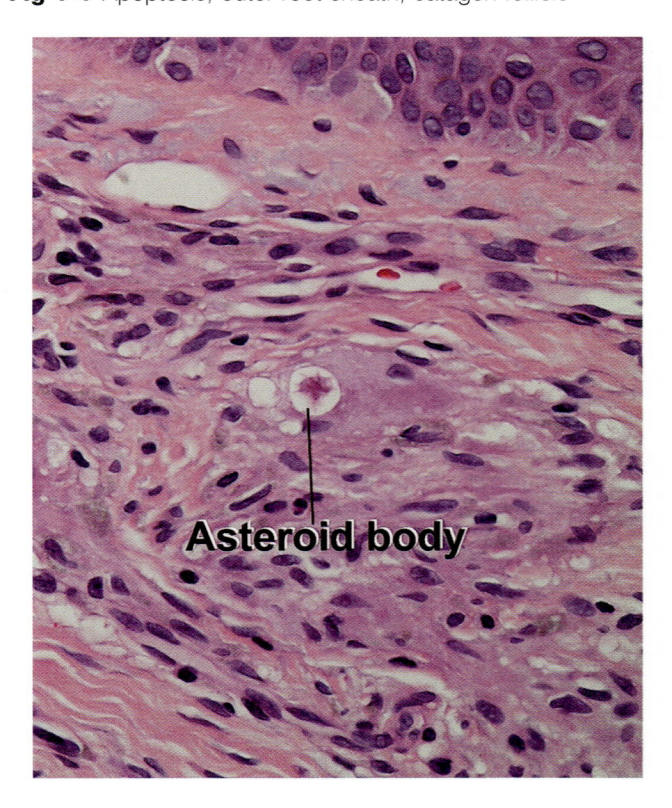

Fig 1-5 Asteroid body, sarcoidosis

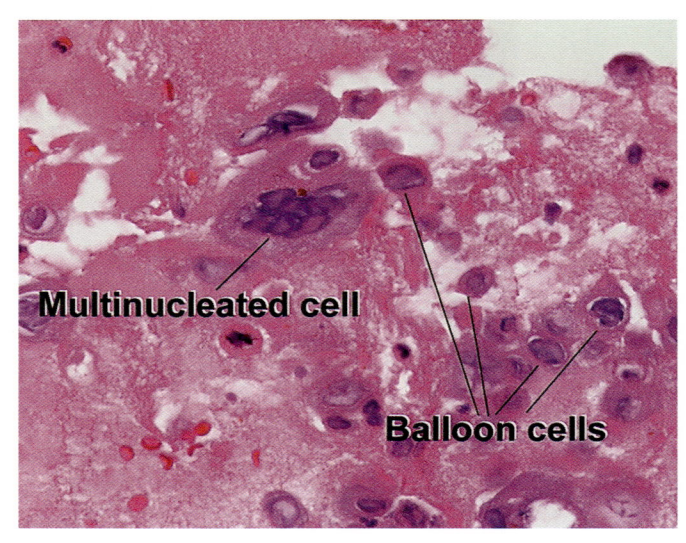

Fig 1-6 Ballooning degeneration, herpes simplex

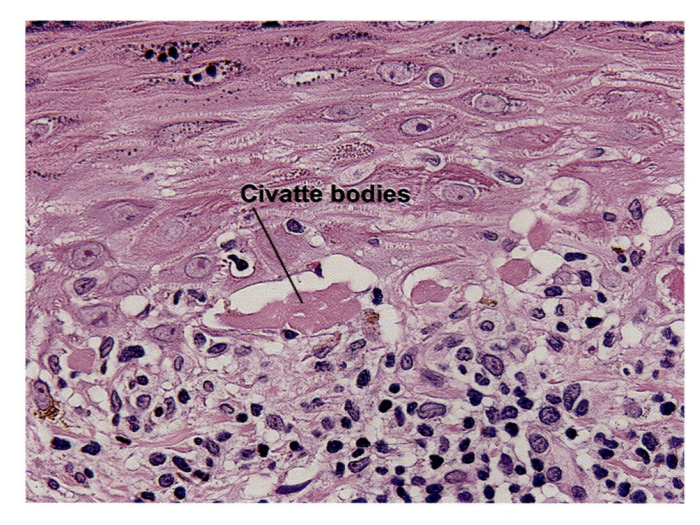

Fig 1-7 Civatte bodies, lichen planus

Collagen entrapment
- Collagen fibers surrounded by histiocytes/spindle cells (collagen balls)

Cornoid lamellae
- 45° angle parakeratosis in a column above a focus with a diminished granular layer and underlying dyskeratotic cells

Corps ronds/grains/dyskeratosis
- Corps ronds = rounded nucleus with halo of pale to pink dyskeratotic cytoplasm
- Grain = dark blue flattened nucleus surrounded by minimal cytoplasm
- Dyskeratosis = abnormal, individual-cell keratinization

Cowdry A body
- Also known as the Lipshutz body
- Intranuclear pink inclusions of herpesvirus infection

Cowdry B body
- Intranuclear pink inclusions of adenovirus and poliovirus infection

Crust
- Serum/fluid with inflammatory cells/debris in stratum corneum

Donovan body
- Intracytoplasmic collections of bacteria seen in granuloma inguinale

Dutcher body
- Intracytoplasmic pink masses of immunoglobulin that invaginate into the nucleus of plasma cells and appear to be intranuclear

Effacement
- Loss of normal rete pattern

Eosinophilic spongiosis
- Spongiosis with eosinophils in the epidermis

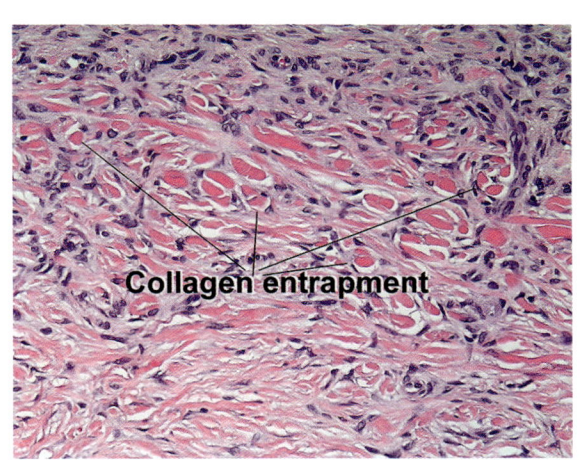

Fig 1-8 Collagen entrapment, dermatofibroma

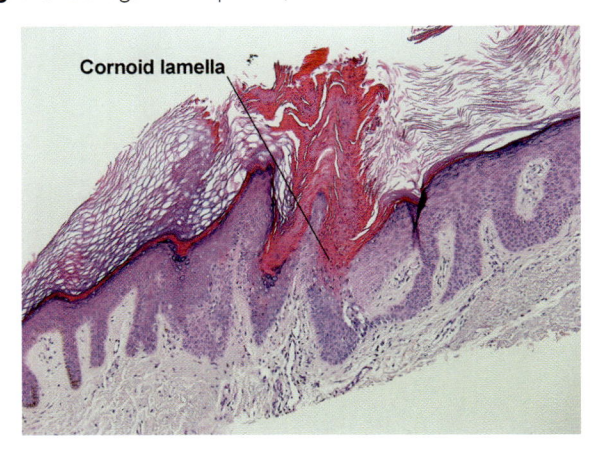

Fig 1-9 Cornoid lamellae, porokeratosis

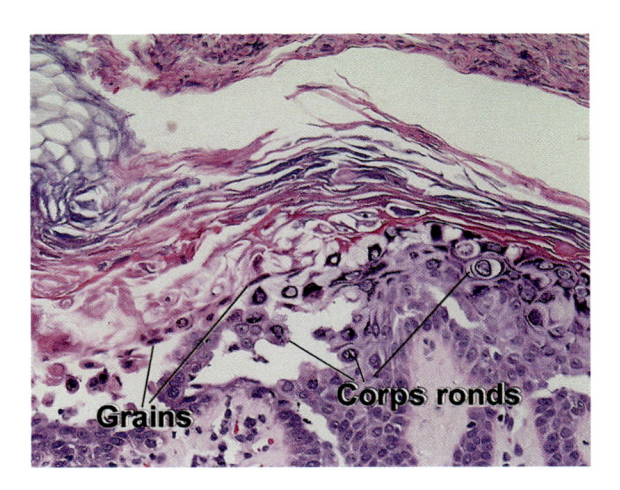

Fig 1-10 Corps ronds/grains, Darier's disease

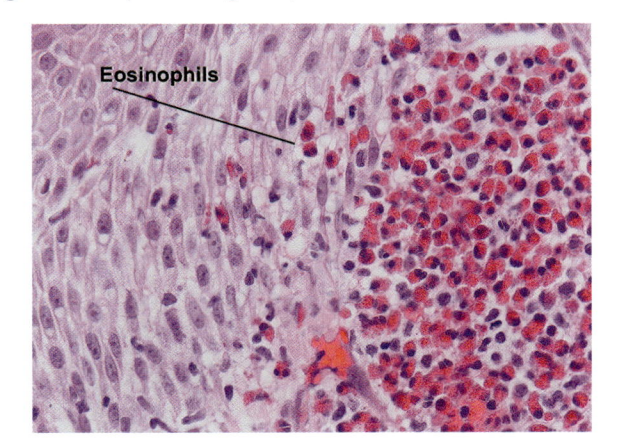

Fig 1-11 Eosinophilic spongiosis, incontinentia pigmenti

Epidermolytic hyperkeratosis

- Coarse, irregular hypergranulosis associated with disruption of cell membranes
- Associated with keratin 1 and 10 mutations

Epidermotropism

- Lymphocytes in epidermis with relative absence of spongiosis: term usually reserved for mycosis fungoides

Erosion

- Partial loss of epidermis

Exocytosis

- Lymphocytes in the epidermis with associated spongiosis: term usually used when discussing spongiotic dermatitis

Festooning

- Papillary dermis retains an undulating pattern (often used to describe porphyria cutanea tarda)

Flame figure

- Collagen encrusted with major basic protein from eosinophils

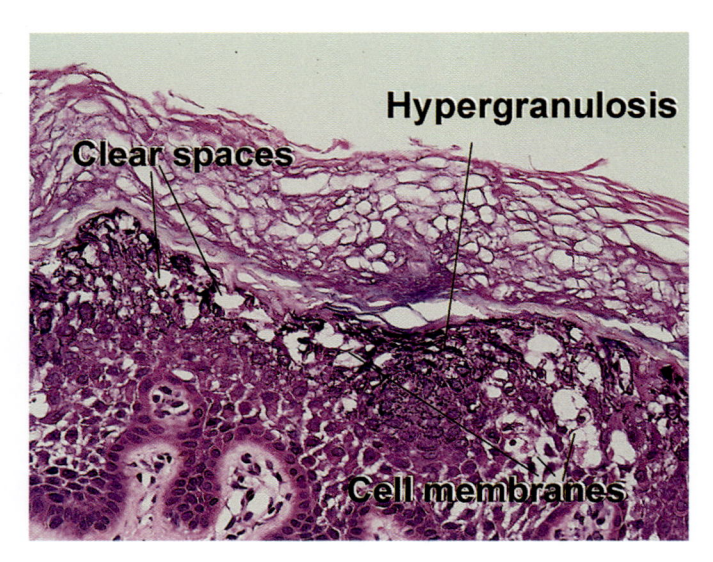

Fig 1-12 Epidermolytic hyperkeratosis

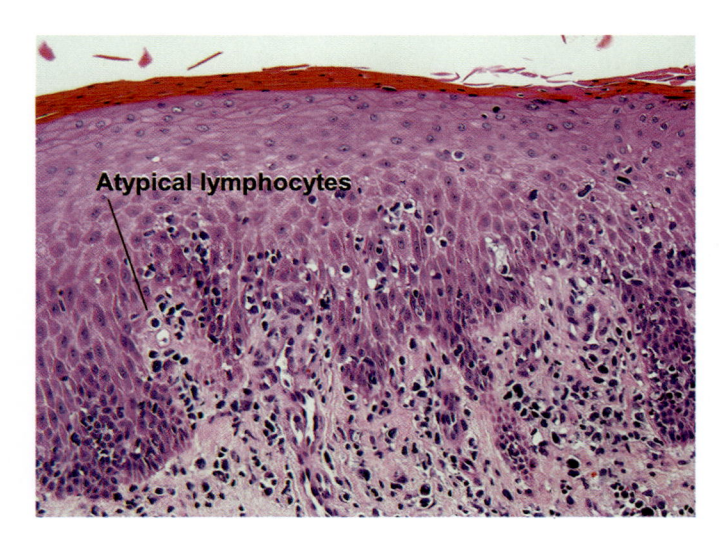

Fig 1-13 Epidermotropism, mycosis fungoides

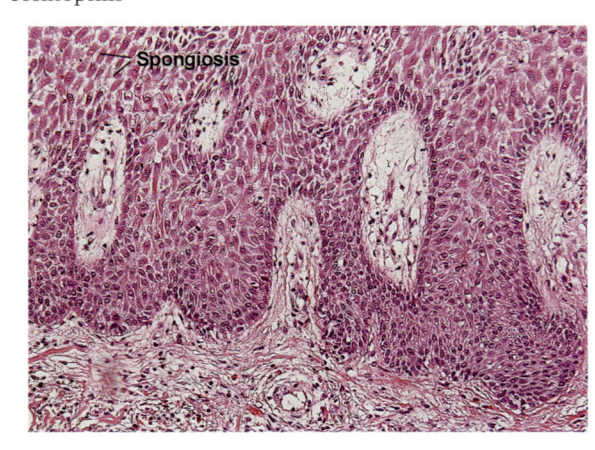

Fig 1-14 Lymphocyte exocytosis, subacute spongiotic dermatitis

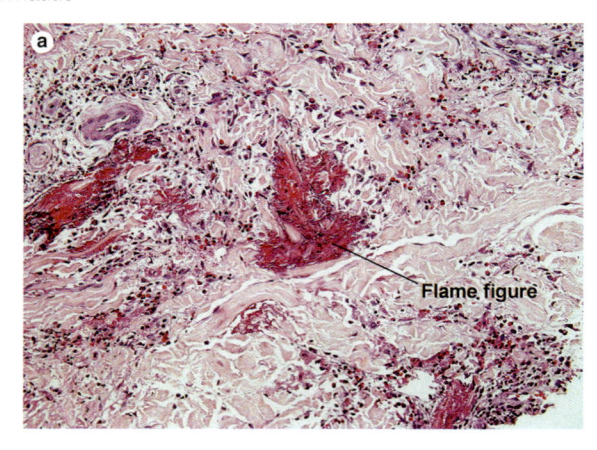

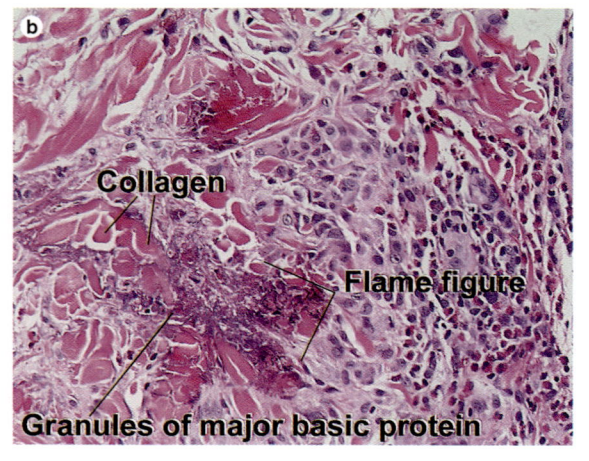

Fig 1-15 Flame figure, Wells' syndrome

Foam cell
- Lipid-laden histiocyte

Follicular mucinosis
- Alteration of hair sheath anatomy by pools of mucin

Granulomatous
- Composed of granulomas (collections of histiocytes)

Grenz zone
- Uninvolved area of dermis beneath the epidermis or adjacent to a hair follicle (border zone)

Guarnieri body
- Eosinophilic inclusions of smallpox

Henderson–Paterson body
- Intracytoplasmic oval, pink inclusions of molluscum infection

Hyper-/hypogranulosis
- Increased/decreased granular layer

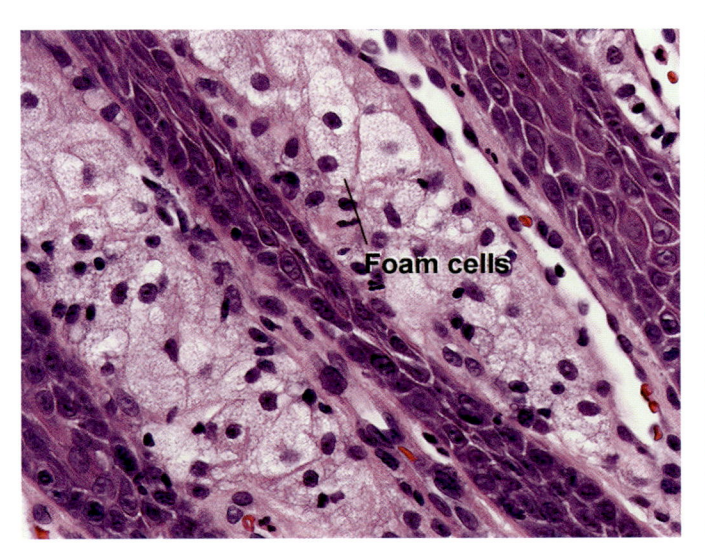

Fig 1-16 Foam cells, verruciform xanthoma

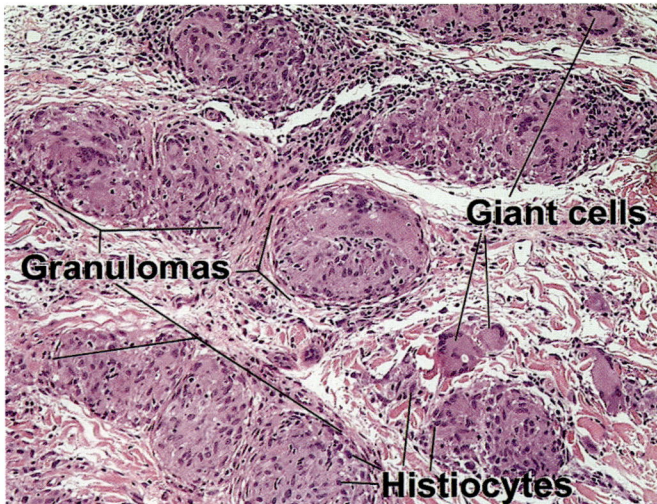

Fig 1-18 Granulomas, sarcoid

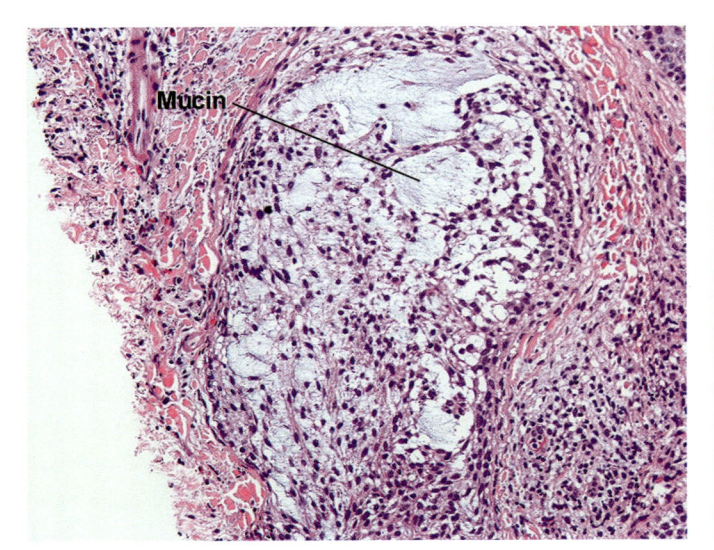

Fig 1-17 Follicular mucinosis, alopecia mucinosis

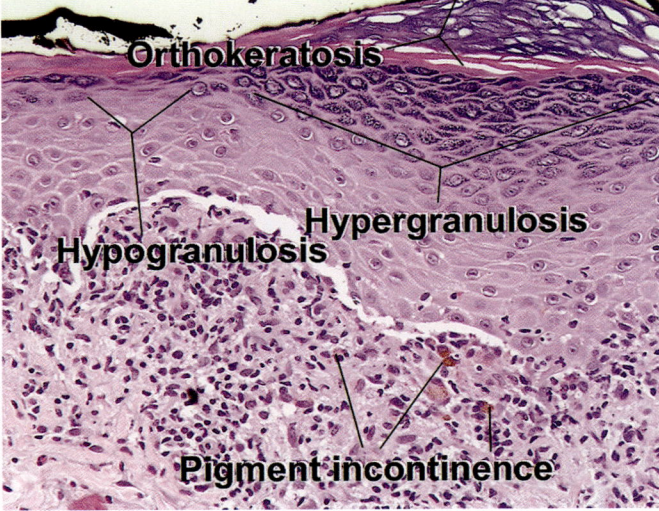

Fig 1-19 Hyper-hypogranulosis, lichen planus

Hyper-/hypopigmentation
- Increased/decreased melanin pigment

Interface
- Generally refers to the dermoepidermal junction

Kamino body
- Dull pink to amphophilic basement membrane material within the epidermis in a Spitz nevus

Karyorrhexis
- Fragmentation of neutrophils (leukocytoclasis). (If neutrophils resemble ants with segmented bodies, then karyorrhexis resembles dismembered ants and scattered ant heads)

Koilocytes
- Keratinocytes with clear cytoplasm and shrunken "raisin-like" pyknotic nuclei

Leishman–Donovan body
- Intracytoplasmic collections of amastigotes in leishmaniasis

Lentiginous epidermal hyperplasia
- Elongated bulbous rete

Lentiginous melanocytic growth pattern
- Proliferation predominantly along the dermoepidermal junction

Leukocytoclasia
- Fragmentation of neutrophils, also referred to as karyorrhexis

Lichenoid dermatitis
- Interface dermatitis with destruction of the basal layer and Civatte body formation (Figure 1.7)

Lichenoid infiltrate
- A band-like infiltrate, generally composed predominantly of lymphocytes, located at the dermoepidermal junction

Medlar body
- Brown, round structure resembling overlapping copper pennies
- Divide by septation, resembling a hot-cross bun

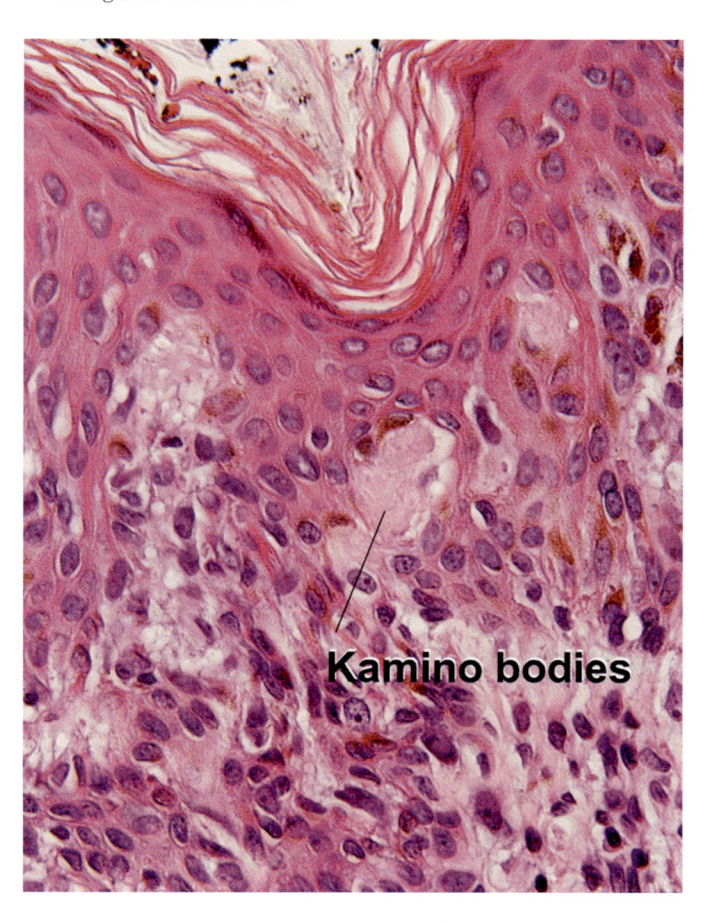

Fig 1-20 Kamino bodies, Spitz nevus

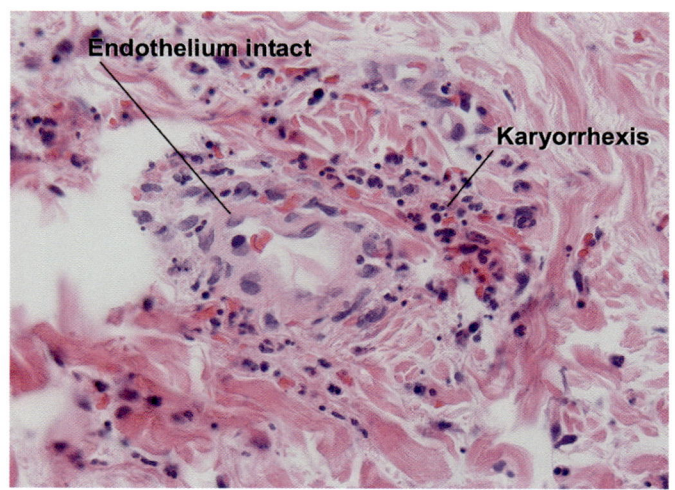

Fig 1-21 Karyorrhexis, leukocytoclastic vasculitis

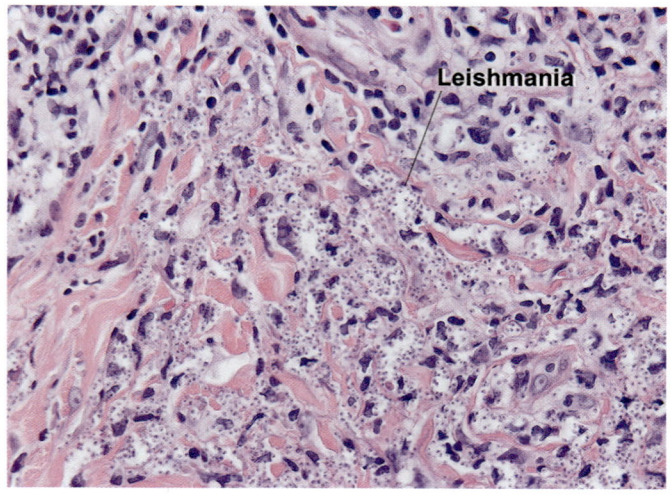

Fig 1-22 Leishman–Donovan bodies, leishmaniasis

Metachromasia
- The property of staining a different color from the stain itself (i.e., the purple color of mast cell granules with the blue stain methylene blue)

Michaelis–Gutman body
- Intra- and extracellular calcified, concentric circular structures, seen in malakoplakia

Munro microabscess
- Collection of neutrophils in the stratum corneum, as seen in psoriasis

Necrobiosis
- Pale-staining smudged necrotic collagen

Negri body
- Inclusions within neurons seen in rabies infection

Orthokeratosis
- Stratum corneum without retained nuclei

Pagetoid cells
- Large cells with abundant cytoplasm within the epidermis

Pagetoid scatter
- Buckshot scatter of atypical cells within the epidermis

Palisading
- Picket fence-like arrangement at the periphery

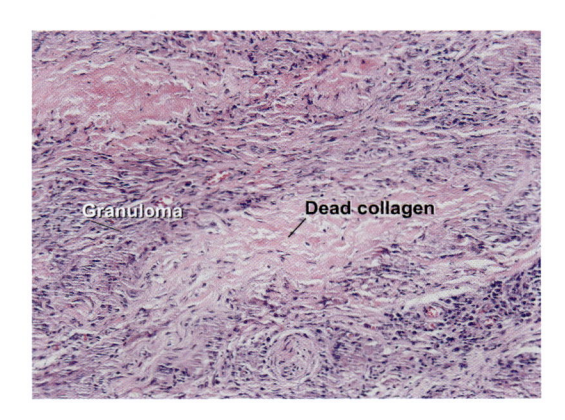

Fig 1-25 Necrobiosis, necrobiosis lipoidica

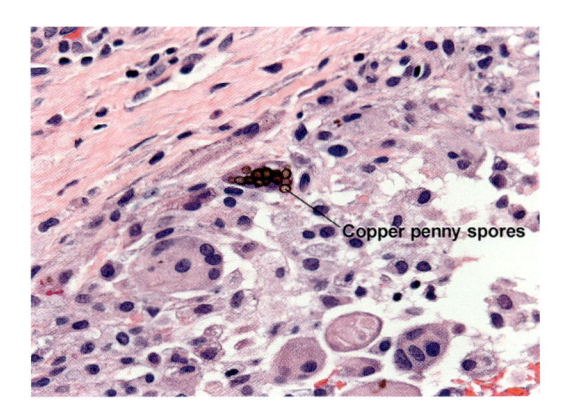

Fig 1-23 Medlar bodies, chromomycosis

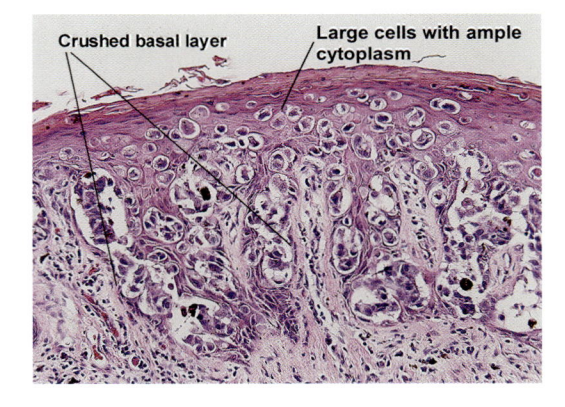

Fig 1-26 Pagetoid cells and pagetoid scatter, Paget's disease

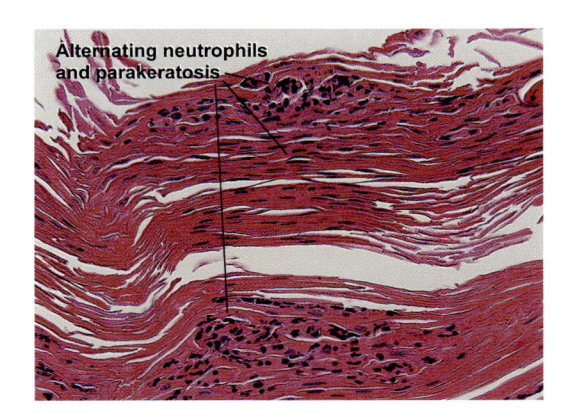

Fig 1-24 Munro microabscess, psoriasis

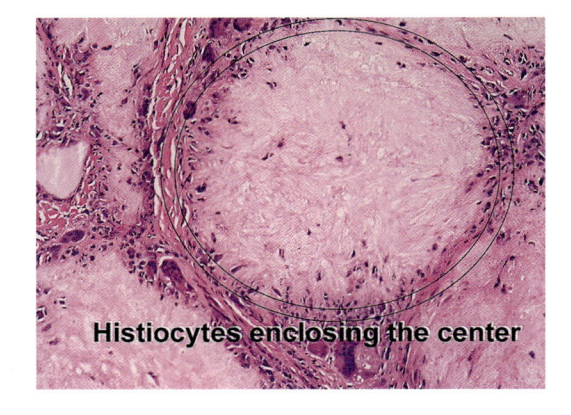

Fig 1-27 Palisading, gout

Papillary mesenchymal body
- Structure that resembles the whorl of plump mesenchymal cells normally present in the hair papilla (seen in trichoblastoma and trichoepithelioma)

Papillomatosis
- Exophytic finger-like projections

Parakeratosis
- Stratum corneum with retained nuclei

Pigment incontinence
- Melanin within dermal macrophages and free within the dermis

Pleomorphism
- Variation in nuclear size/shape

Psammoma body
- Extracellular laminated, calcified structures seen in meningioma, papillary thyroid carcinoma, ovarian carcinoma

Pseudoepitheliomatous hyperplasia (PEH)
- Prominent acanthosis of the adnexal epithelium and epidermis, mimics squamous cell carcinoma
- Often associated with trapping of elastic fibers

Pseudohorn cyst
- Keratin-filled cystic structure that is the result of cutting through invaginations of the stratum corneum (similar to a horn cyst, but connects to the surface)

Reticular degeneration
- Destruction of epidermis with cell membranes remaining in a net-like pattern

Reticulated
- Network of interconnecting strands (net-like)

Russell body
- Intracytoplasmic pink collections of immunoglobulins in plasma cells, seen in rhinoscleroma and other conditions with many plasma cells

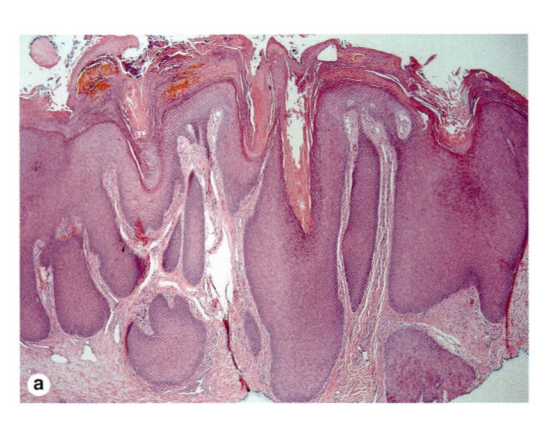

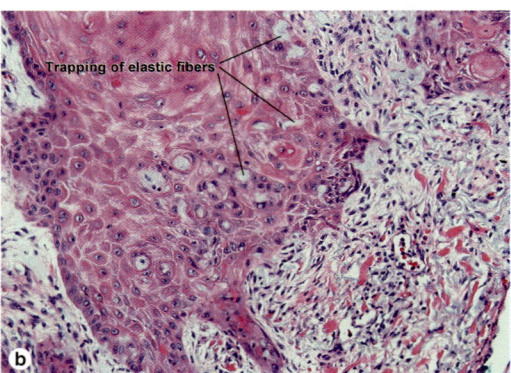

Fig 1-29 (a) PEH, syringosquamous metaplasia following trauma. (b) Elastic fiber trapping in PEH

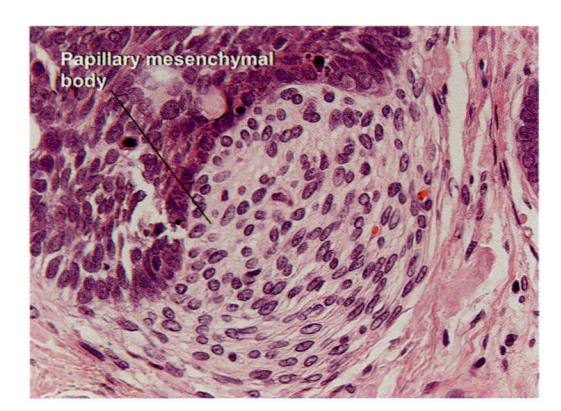

Fig 1-28 Papillary mesenchymal body, trichoepithelioma

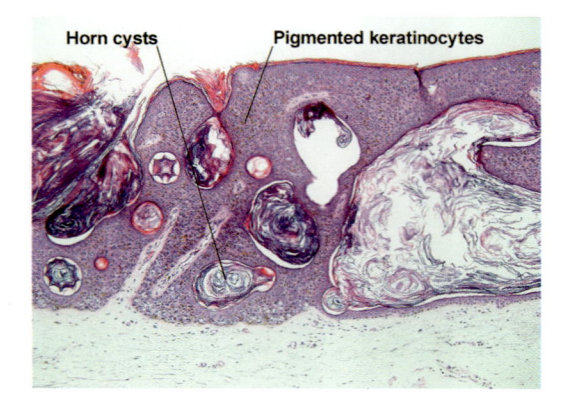

Fig 1-30 Pseudohorn cyst, seborrheic keratosis

Schaumann body
- Laminated calcified structure seen in sarcoidosis

Shadow cells
- Cells with barely visible outlines of nuclei

Spongiform pustule of Kogoj
- Neutrophils in the stratum spinosum, associated with spongiosis at periphery (typical of psoriasis)

Spongiosis
- Intercellular edema in epidermis with stretching of cell–cell junctions

Squamotization (or squamatization)
- Loss of cuboidal/columnar basal cells, with deepest layer now being polyhedral, pink squamous cells

Squamous eddies
- Circular whorls of squamous cells

Storiform
- Cartwheel or basket-weave pattern

Vacuolar change
- Formation of clear spaces within the basal layer

Verocay body
- Structure composed of two nuclear palisades enclosing pink cytoplasmic processes, seen in schwannoma

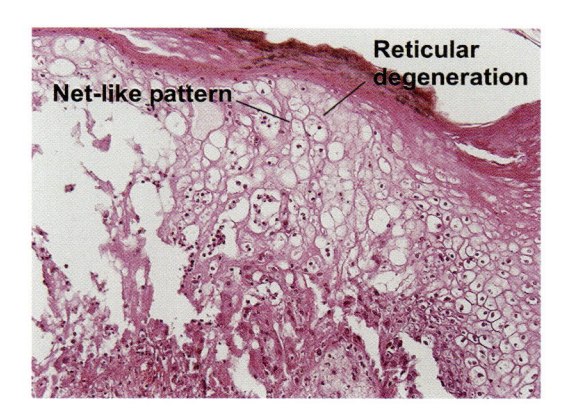

Fig 1-31 Reticular degeneration, variola

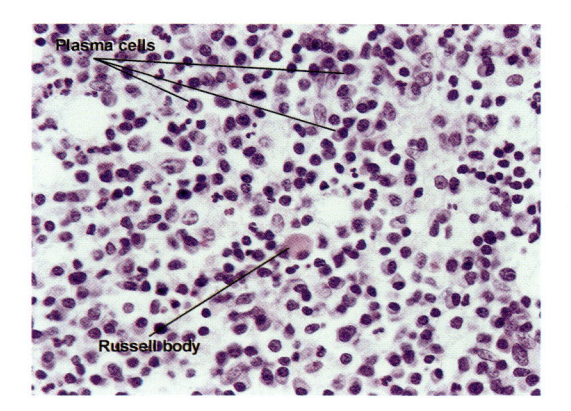

Fig 1-32 Russell body, rhinoscleroma

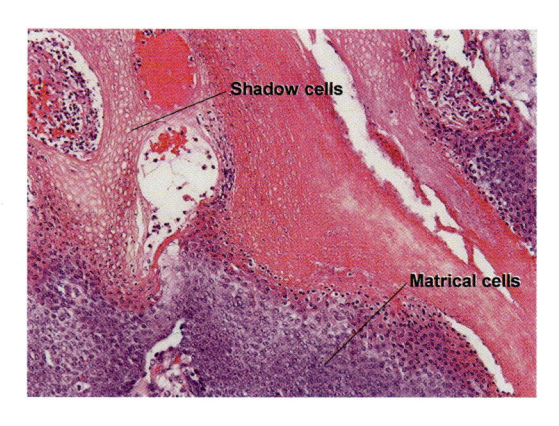

Fig 1-33 Shadow cells, pilomatricoma

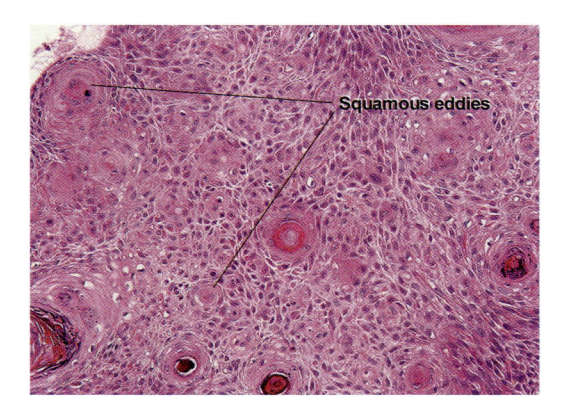

Fig 1-34 Squamous eddies, irritated seborrheic keratosis

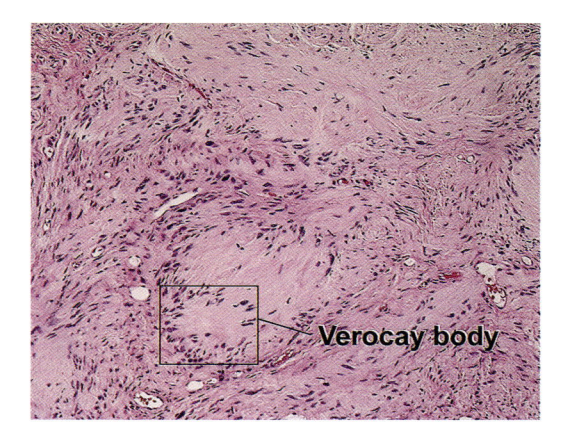

Fig 1-35 Verocay body, schwannoma

Villus

- Projection of papillary dermis covered by a layer of epidermal cells into a cavity

Normal skin anatomy

Scalp skin

Key features

- Numerous follicles that extend down into the panniculus
- Associated sebaceous glands, arrector pili muscles

Facial skin

Key features

- Thin epidermis
- Basket-weave stratum corneum
- Hair follicles and sebaceous glands numerous in the dermis
- *Demodex* mites common
- Eyelid and ear skin have many vellus hair follicles
- In the upper dermis of eyelid skin, skeletal muscle bundles are present
- On the conjunctival surface of the eyelid, stratum corneum and hair follicles are absent, but goblet cells are present

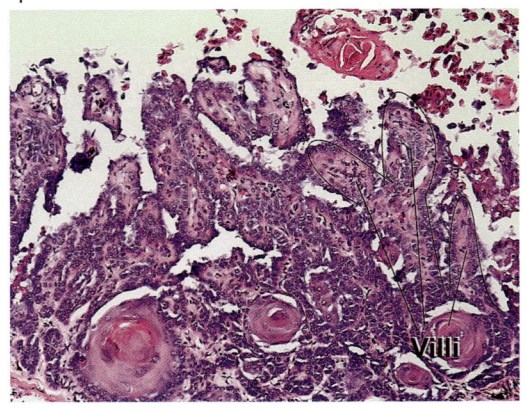

Fig 1-36 Villi, warty dyskeratoma

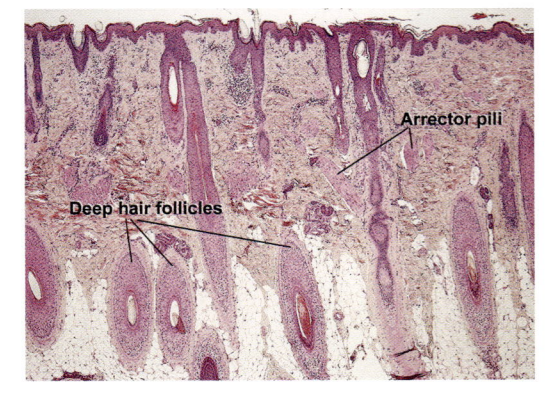

Fig 1-37 Normal scalp with follicles rooted in the fat

Skin of the trunk

Key features

- Very thick dermis, especially in skin from the back
- Scattered hair follicles and sebaceous glands
- Projections of fat extend upward to envelop adnexae

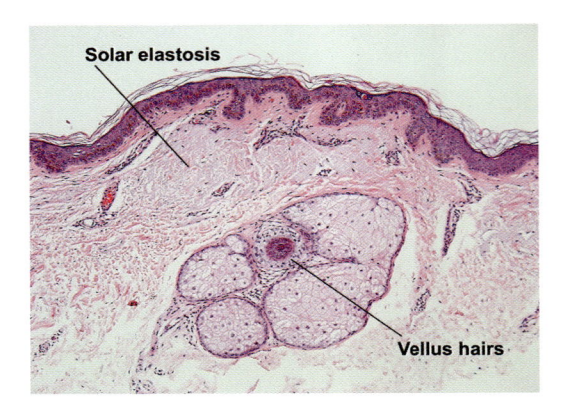

Fig 1-38 Sun-damaged facial skin

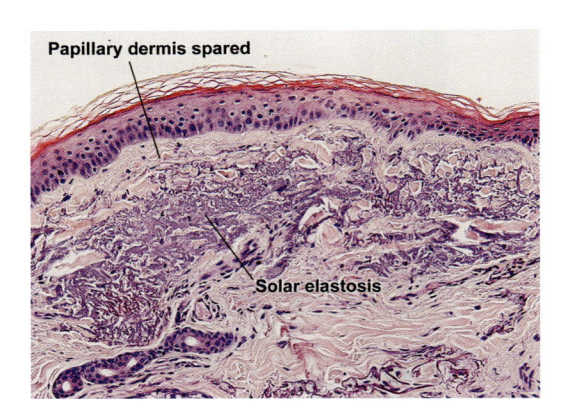

Fig 1-39 Sun-damaged skin. Solar elastosis spares papillary dermis

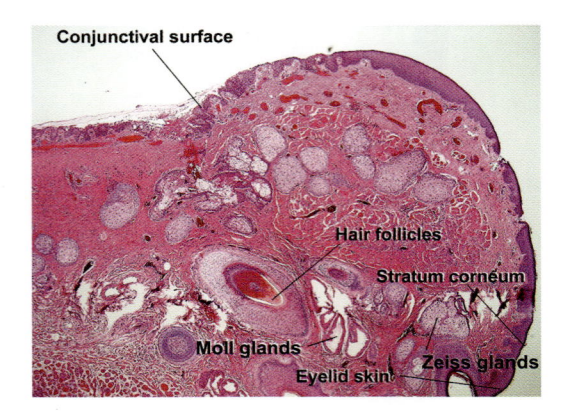

Fig 1-40 Eyelid

Areolar skin

Key features

- Slight acanthosis of the epidermis with basilar hyperpigmentation
- Sometimes there is a central invagination of the epidermis that leads to a follicle and sebaceous glands
- Smooth muscle bundles in the mid–deep dermis
- Apocrine glands in the reticular dermis

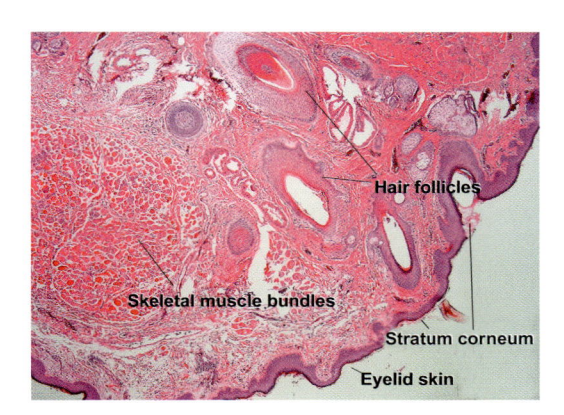

Fig 1-41 Eyelid

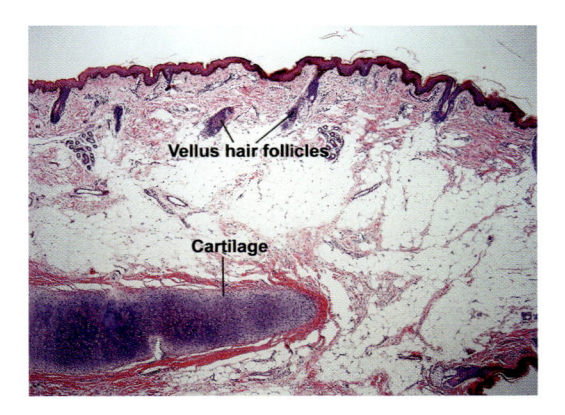

Fig 1-42 Ear

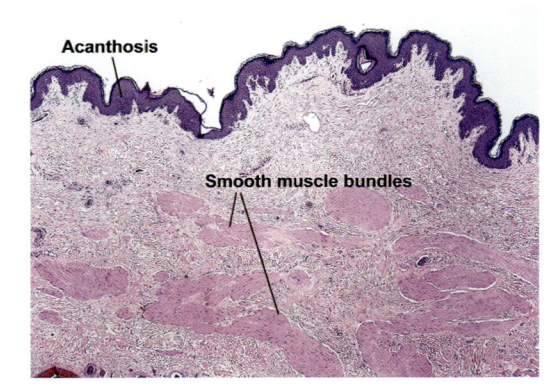

Fig 1-43 Areolar skin, smooth muscle bundles

Acral skin

Key features

- Compact eosinophilic stratum corneum
- Slight papillomatosis present on dorsal surfaces

Volar skin

Key features

- Compact eosinophilic hyperkeratosis with underlying stratum lucidum
- No hair follicles or sebaceous glands
- Eccrine glands numerous
- Meissner and Pacinian corpuscles may be seen

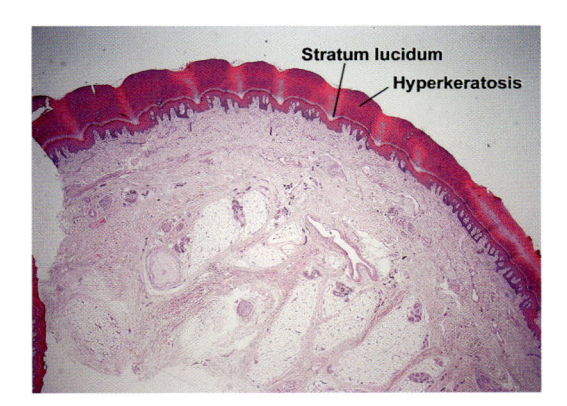

Fig 1-44 Volar skin, thick stratum corneum and deep Pacinian corpuscles

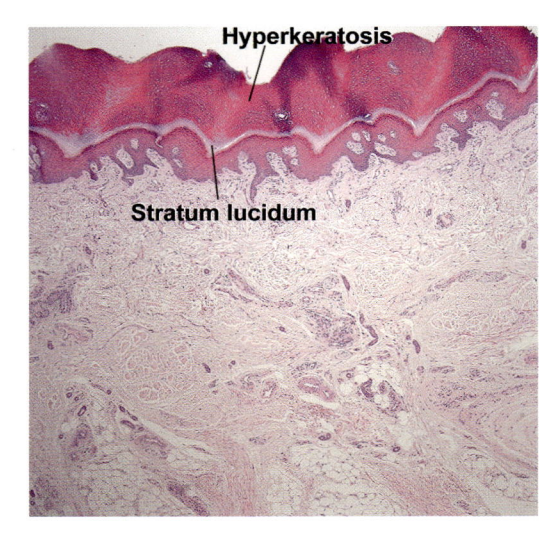

Fig 1-45 Volar skin, stratum lucidum

12   Dermatopathology

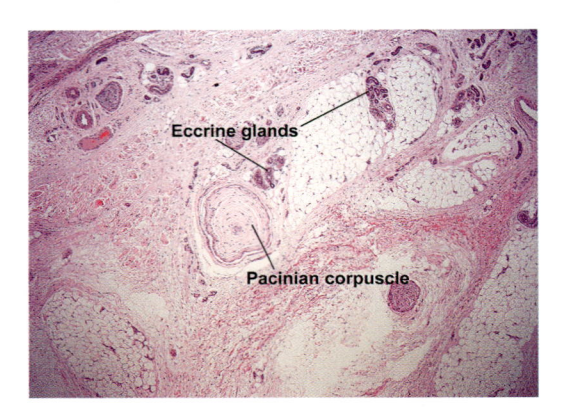

Fig 1-46 Volar skin, eccrine glands and Pacinian corpuscle

Mucosa

Key features
- Absent granular layer
- Keratinocytes are large and pale (filled with glycogen)
- Dilated vessels in the submucosa
- Smooth muscle bundles may be present

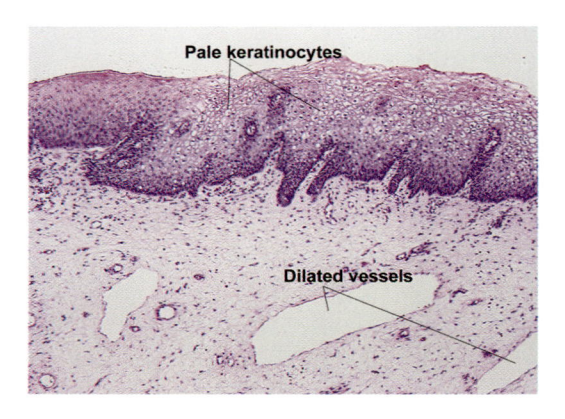

Fig 1-47 Mucosa

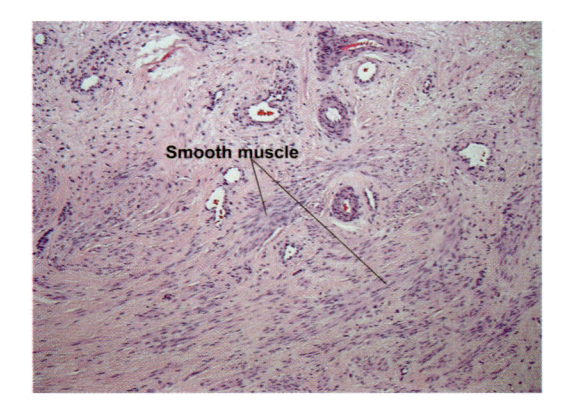

Fig 1-48 Smooth muscle in submucosa

Nasal turbinate

Key features
- Erectile tissue with fibrous septa and vascular sinusoids
- Mucous glands

Fetal skin

Key features
- Stellate and spindled fibroblasts (mesenchyme)
- Densely cellular

Hair anatomy

Infundibulum

Key features
- From epidermis down to insertion of sebaceous gland
- Intraepidermal portion = acrotrichium
- Keratinizes in the pattern of the normal epidermis with a granular layer (keratohyaline granules)

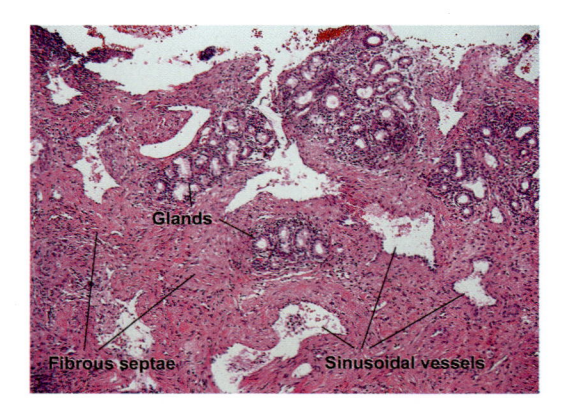

Fig 1-49 Nasal turbinate mucosa: erectile tissue with mucous glands

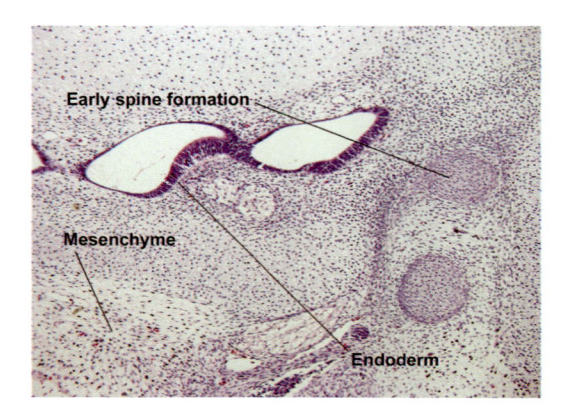

Fig 1-50 Fetal mesenchyme

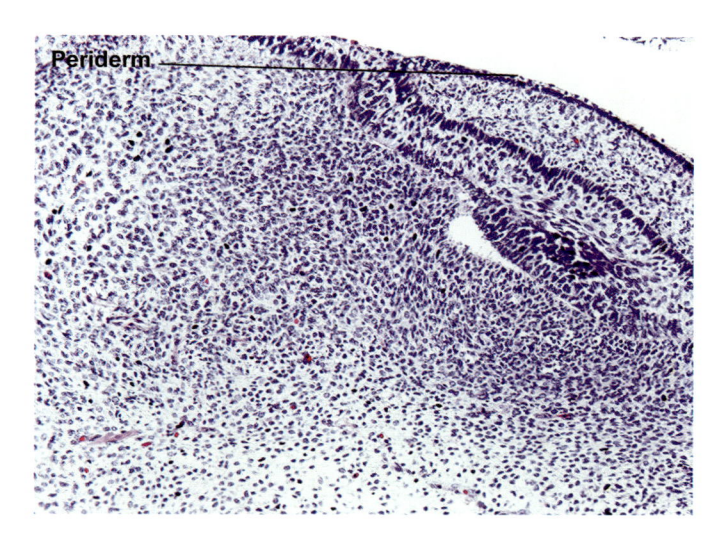

Fig 1-51 Fetal periderm

Isthmus

Key features

- From the insertion of the sebaceous gland to the insertion of the arrector pili muscle (bulge)
- Keratin is formed in the absence of a granular layer = trichilemmal keratinization
- The inner root sheath is lost at this level and the outer root sheath develops an inner corrugated, dense pink cornified layer; peripheral palisading of the outer root sheath is seen

Stem

Key features

- From the insertion of the arrector pili muscle (bulge) to Adamson's fringe
- Only present in anagen hairs

Adamson's fringe
- The point above which hair cornifies
- Dermatophytes only infect cornified hair above Adamson's fringe
- Above Adamson's fringe, Huxley's layer of the inner root sheath no longer has trichohyalin granules
- Hair tends to retract from the inner root sheath above Adamson's fringe
  - *The inner root sheath is fused and blue-gray at this level and trichohyalin granules are not seen*
  - *The outer root sheath is composed of pink cells with peripheral palisading*

Bulb

Key features

- Below the stem portion of the anagen hair follicle
- From Adamson's fringe to the base of the follicle
- The bulb has three zones: matrix, supramatrix, keratogenous zone
  - *Matrix: from base to critical line (widest point of the bulb and papillae)*
  - *Supramatrix: from critical line to B-fringe (point at which the outer root sheath becomes multilayered and Henle's layer no longer has trichohyalin granules)*
  - *Keratogenous zone: from B-fringe to Adamson's fringe*
- Layers of the hair follicle that can be seen:
  - *Fibrous root sheath*
  - *Vitreous basement membrane zone*
  - *Outer root sheath*
  - *Inner root sheath*
    - *Henle's layer*
    - *Huxley's layer*
    - *Cuticle of the inner root sheath*
  - *Hair shaft*
    - *Cuticle of the hair shaft*
    - *Cortex*
  - *Medulla*

Anagen hairs have a stem and a bulb which produces the hair shaft, whereas telogen hairs lack an inferior segment. Telogen hairs are easily recognized in vertical sections, as the club hair and surrounding trichilemmal keratin give the impression of a flame thrower.

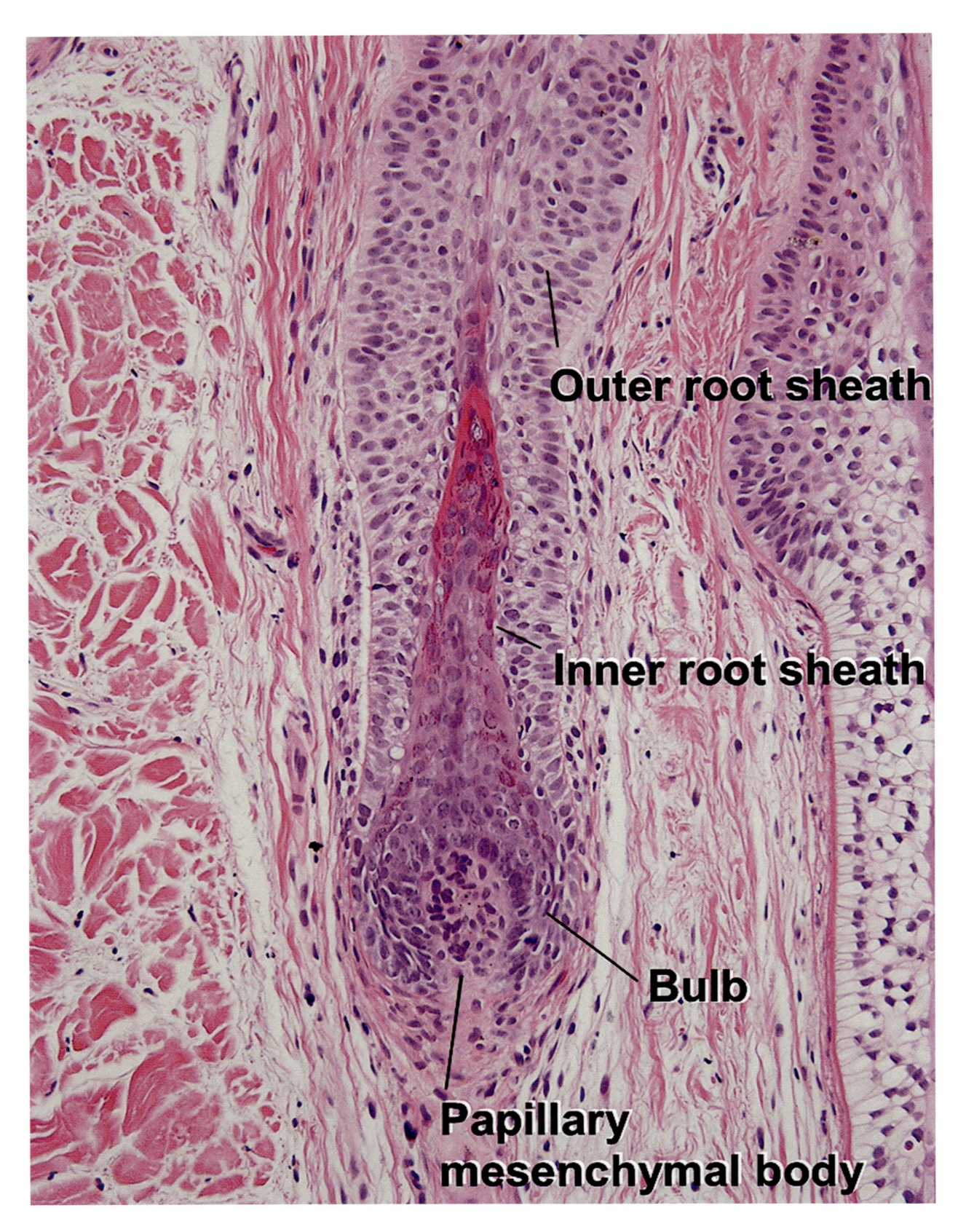

Fig 1-52 Hair, vertical section

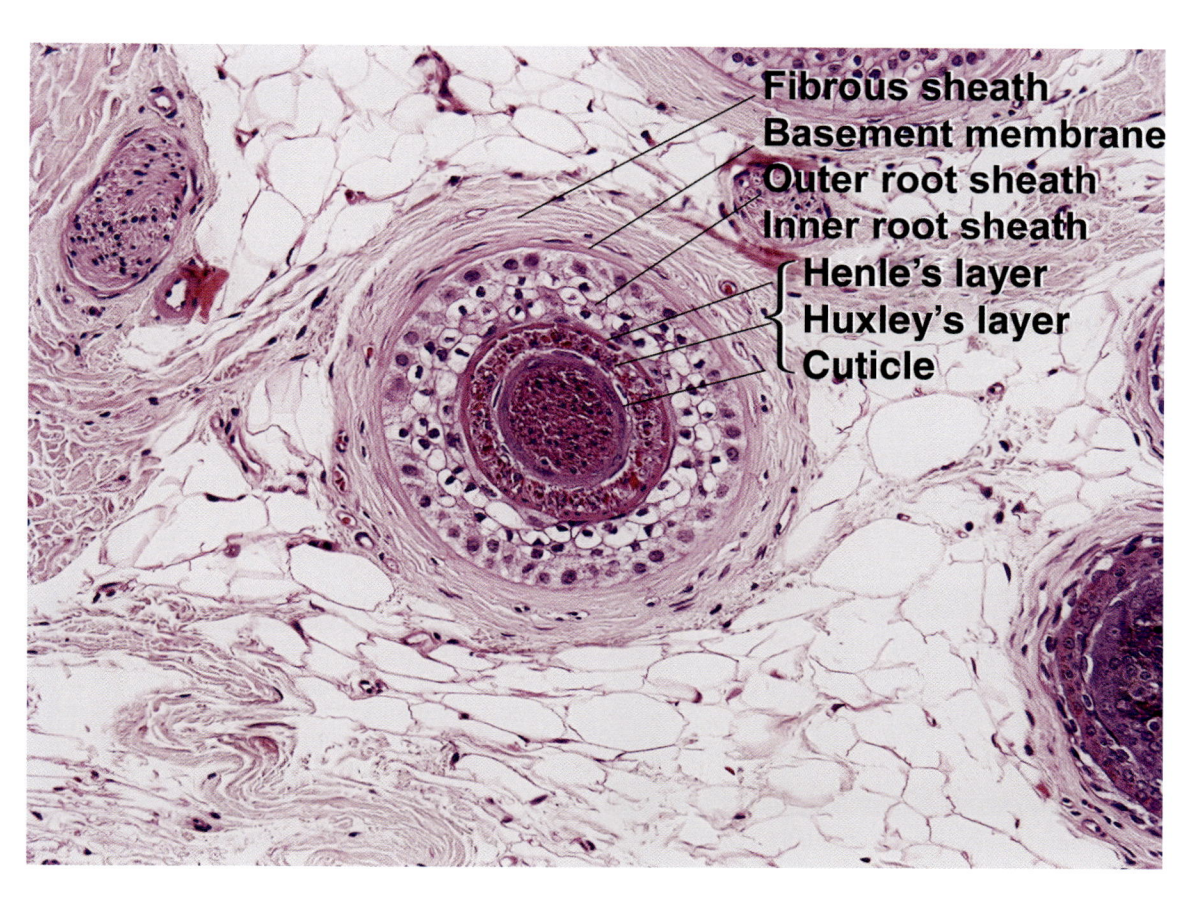

Fig 1-53 Hair, transverse section

Labels: Fibrous sheath, Basement membrane, Outer root sheath, Inner root sheath, Henle's layer, Huxley's layer, Cuticle

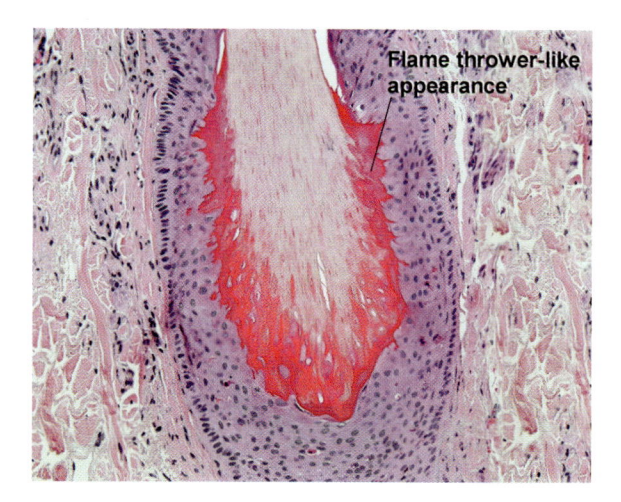

Fig 1-54 Telogen hair

Label: Flame thrower-like appearance

Nail anatomy

Key features

- Nail plate
- Nail bed: between distal edge of lunula and the proximal edge of onychodermal band
- Framing portion: proximal nail fold, lateral nail folds, distal nail fold
- Ensheathing portion: "cuticle," *aka* eponychium, hyponychium, solehorn, bed horny layer

Cuticle

- "Visible" cuticle (*aka* eponychium) is the thick keratinous material that borders the proximal nail fold and adheres to the nail plate
- "True" cuticle is located beneath the "visible" portion and is derived from the ventral part of the proximal nail fold
- The true cuticle is generally not seen, but it is sometimes visible as "flakes" of keratinous material parallel to the proximal nail fold

Hyponychium

- The space, epithelium, keratinous material ventral to the nail plate

Solehorn

- Subungual white to colorless keratin, extends from the distal nail bed underneath the onychodermal band to below the free, distal edge of the nail plate

Nail matrix

- Proximal part makes the surface of the nail; distal part makes the ventral nail plate

Dermatopathology

Lunula
- Visible portion of nail matrix
- Anchoring portion (mesenchyme)

Types of keratinization of the nail

Onychokeratinization (no granular layer)
- Hard keratin of nail plate

Onycholemmal keratinization
- Ventral part of proximal nail fold (+ granular layer), bed epithelium (the cuticle, bed horny layer, solehorn) (no granular layer)

Epidermoid keratinization
- Dorsal proximal nail fold, lateral folds, hyponychium

Types of inflammatory cells

Dermal dendrocyte

Key features
- Macrophage-type cells located in the dermis
- Many are factor XIIIa+, some are S100+
- Likely serve as antigen-presenting cells

Giant cell

Key features
- Cell with multiple nuclei, usually abundant cytoplasm

Types
- Foreign-body: nuclei are arranged haphazardly
- Langerhans: nuclei are arranged in a wreath shape
- Osteoclast-like: nuclei are arranged haphazardly and eccentrically; cytoplasm is deep pink with a scalloped border that molds to adjacent structures
- Touton: nuclei are arranged in a wreath with foamy cytoplasm peripherally
- Ringed siderophage: Touton giant cell with hemosiderin (characteristic of the fibrous histiocytoma type of dermatofibroma)

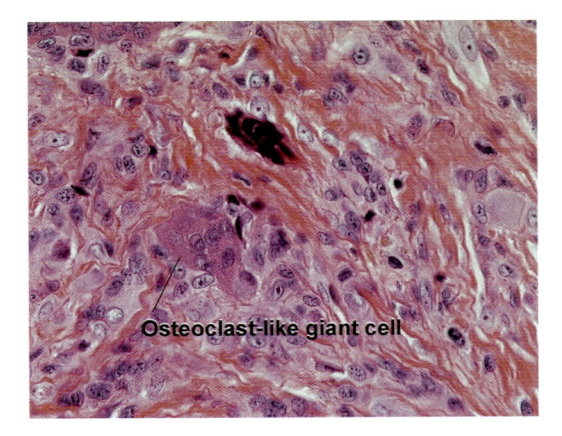

Fig 1-55 Osteoclast-like giant cell

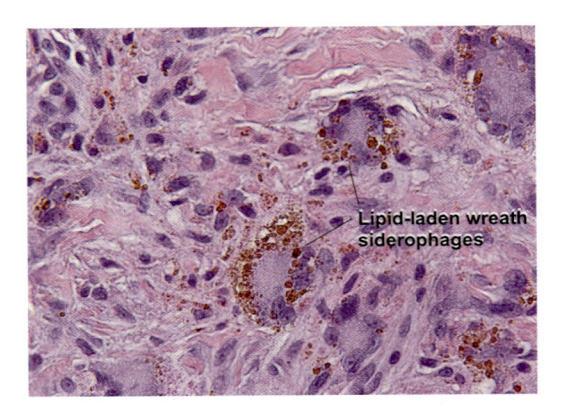

Fig 1-56 Ringed lipidized siderophage (Touton giant cell with hemosiderin) in dermatofibroma

Histiocyte

Key features
- Epithelioid cell with a central, round/oval nucleus and surrounding cytoplasm
- Most are derived from a monocyte that takes up residence in tissue
- Functions include phagocytosis and antigen presentation
- Tend to coalesce in tissue with no intervening connective tissue

Langerhans cell

Key features
- Dendritic cells in epidermis and dermis
- CD1a+, S100+, peanut agglutinin, langerin+
- Nucleus is typically eccentric and may be reniform (kidney-shaped)
- Originate in bone marrow and function in presenting antigens to T cells
- Contain Birbeck granules, tennis racket-shaped rod and oval bodies seen on electron microscopy

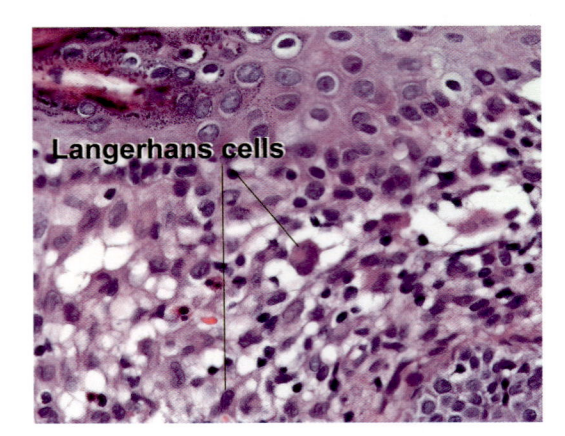

Fig 1-57 Langerhans cell histiocytosis

Lymphocyte

Key features

- Round, dark nucleus, generally with no visible cytoplasm
- B-cell lymphocytes produce antibodies and are important for humoral immunity
- Natural killer (NK) cells are part of the innate immune system
- T-cell lymphocytes mature in the thymus and are important in cell-mediated immunity
- TH1 cells produce interleukin-1 (IL-1), IL-2, IL-12, and interferon-gamma (IFN-γ) and are important for cell-mediated immunity and function in activating macrophages
- TH2 cells produce IL-4, IL-5, and IL-10 and are important for humoral immunity

Mast cell

Key features

- "Fried-egg" appearance with central round nucleus and surrounding oval, bluish cytoplasm
- Contain metachromatic granules composed of heparin, histamine, tryptase, carboxypeptidase, leukotrienes
- Important in immediate-type hypersensitivity reactions

Neutrophil

Key features

- Predominant cell in acute infection
- Multilobulated nucleus

Eosinophil

Key features

- IL-5 induces eosinophil production
- Bilobed nucleus with granular cytoplasm containing major basic protein, eosinophil cationic protein, catalase, and other proteins

Plasma cell

Key features

- Eccentric nucleus with "clock face"
- Perinuclear pale space corresponding to rough endoplasmic reticulum (described by Hopf)
- Pink cytoplasm

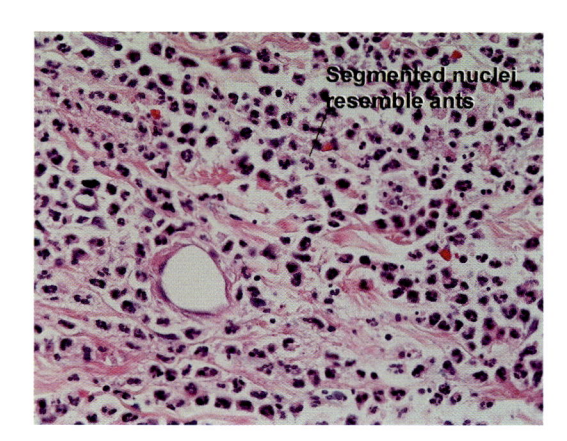

Fig 1-59 Neutrophils in Sweet's syndrome

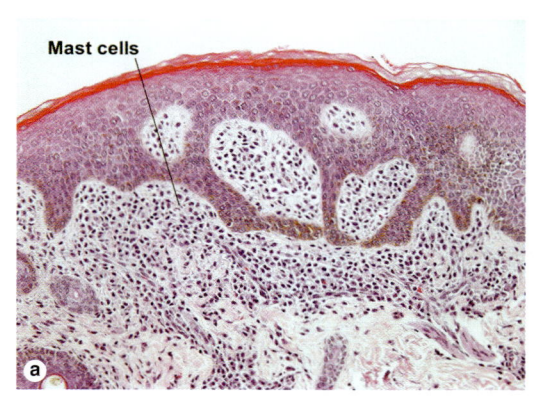

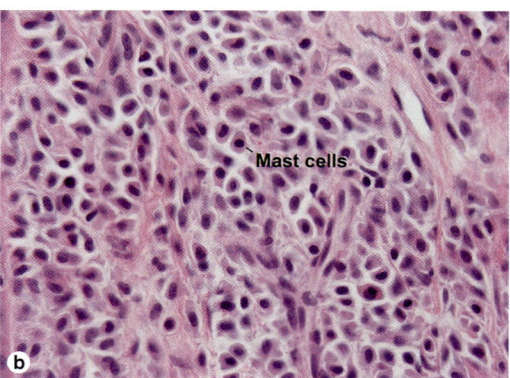

Fig 1-58 Mastocytoma

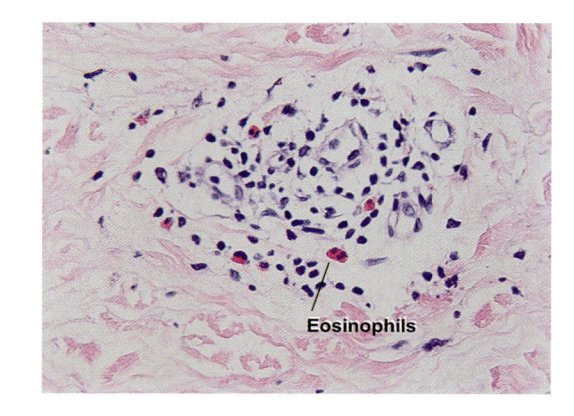

Fig 1-60 Eosinophils in dermal hypersensitivity response

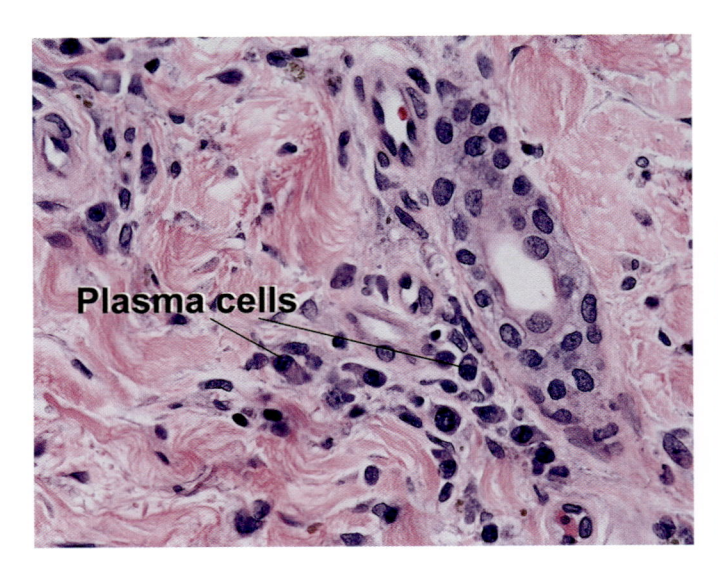

Fig 1-61 Plasma cells

Histochemical stains

The affinities of various dyes have been exploited as histochemical "special" stains to aid in identification of cell type, mucopolysaccharides, muscle, lipid, iron, melanin, calcium, elastin, collagen, amyloid, and infectious organisms. Hematoxylin and eosin (H&E) is the routine staining choice for microscopic interpretation resulting in blue nuclei and pink cytoplasm.

Connective tissue stains

Masson's trichrome stain

- Differentiates collagen (blue-green) from smooth muscle (red)
- Example: scar versus leiomyoma

Important pitfall: Very young collagen can stain red

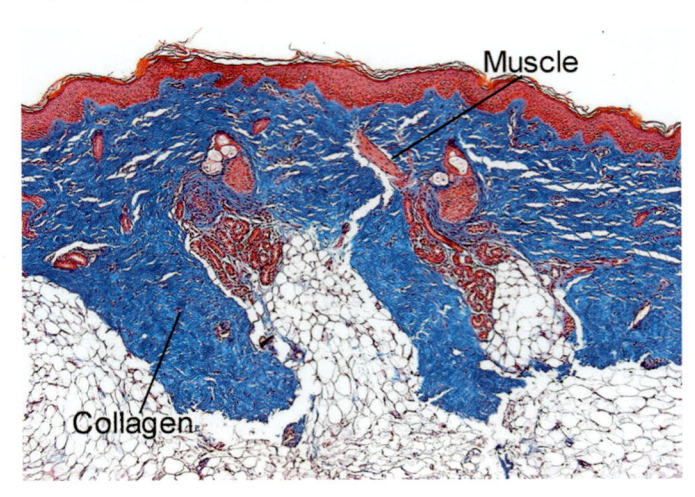

Fig 1-62 Normal skin with Masson's trichrome

Verhoeff–Van Gieson stain

- Elastic fibers are black
- Examples: absence or reduction in scar, mid-dermal elastolysis, anetoderma, cutis laxa
- Example: distorted fibers in pseudoxanthoma elasticum

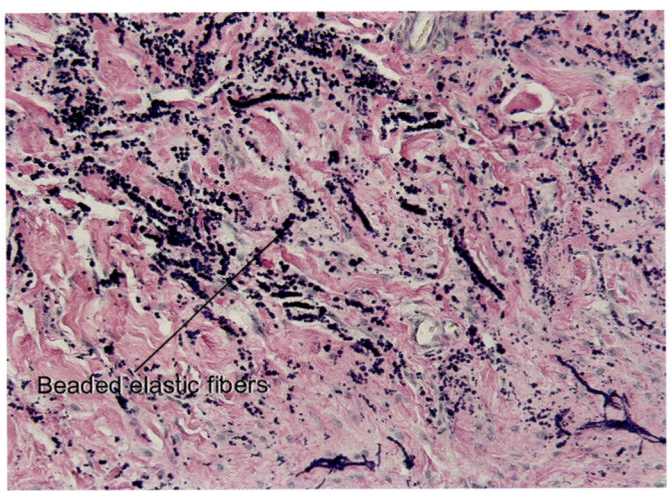

Fig 1-63 Beaded elastic fibers in elastofibroma dorsi (Verhoeff–Van Gieson)

Mast cell stains

Toluidine blue

- Stains mast cell granules metachromatically (i.e. the dye is blue but the granules stain purple)
- Also stains mucin (see below)

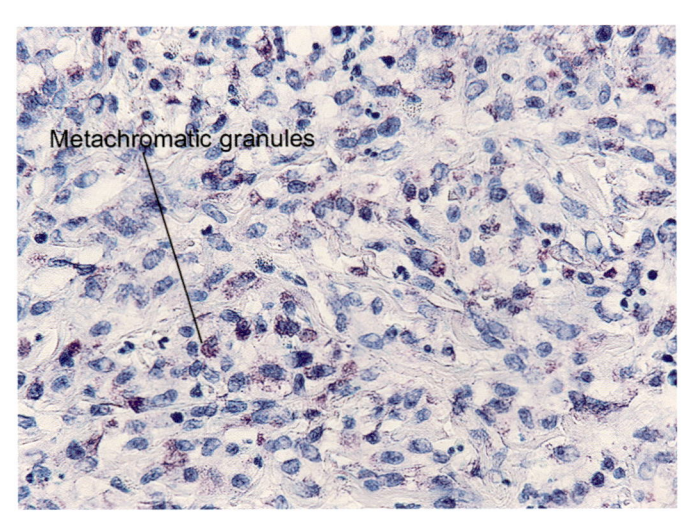

Fig 1-64 Metachromatic staining of mast cells in urticaria pigmentosa (toluidine blue)

Leder stain (naphthol ASD chloroacetate esterase)

- Mast cell cytoplasm stains red (not dependent on presence of granules)
- Also stains myeloid cells (example: leukemia cutis)

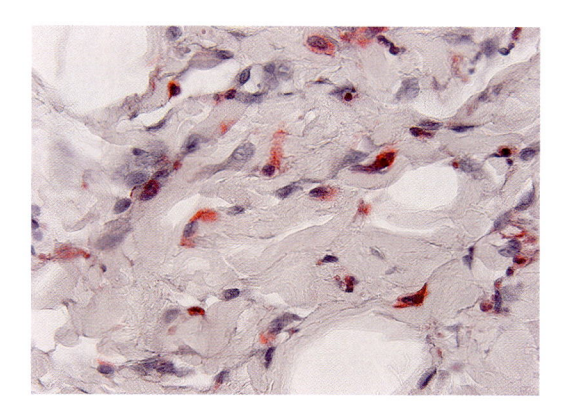

Fig 1-65 Mast cells in urticaria pigmentosa (Leder)

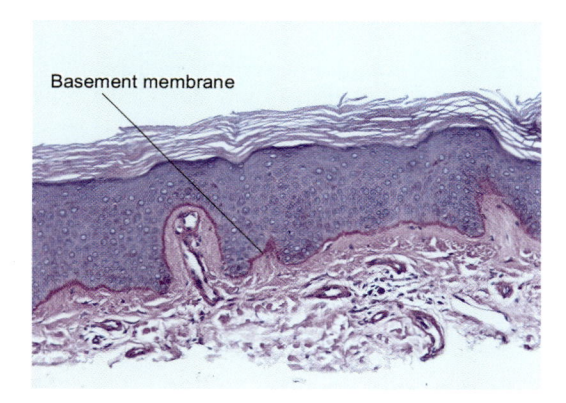

Fig 1-66 PAS-positive basement membrane

Carbohydrate stains

PAS (Periodic acid-Schiff)

- Stains glycogen, neutral mucopolysaccharides (such as basement membrane), and fungi red
  - *Glycogen is diastase labile, i.e. sections exposed to diastase before staining do not stain red with PAS reaction*
- Useful in clear cell acanthoma, trichilemmoma
  - *Fungi and neutral mucopolysaccharides (basement membrane) are diastase resistant, i.e. stain red with PAS after diastase exposure*
- Useful in tinea corporis, tinea versicolor, candida, basement membrane thickening of lupus erythematosus, thickened vessel walls in porphyria
- Acid mucopolysaccharides, such as hyaluronic acid, do not stain with PAS

Alcian blue

- Demonstrates acid mucopolysaccharides by staining them blue
- In normal skin, most mucin is sulfated acid mucopolysaccharide (heparin, chondroitin, and dermatan sulfates). In most pathologic states with increased dermal mucin, the mucin is predominantly non-sulfated hyaluronic acid
  - *Non-sulfated acid mucopolysaccharides (hyaluronic acid) stain with Alcian blue at pH 2.5 but not at pH 0.5*
    - Examples: follicular mucinosis, granuloma annulare, myxoid cyst, dermal mucin in lupus erythematosus
  - *Sulfated acid mucopolysaccharides stain with Alcian blue at both pH 2.5 and pH 0.5*
- Alcian blue can be used with and without hyaluronidase to differentiate hyaluronic acid from other mucopolysaccharides

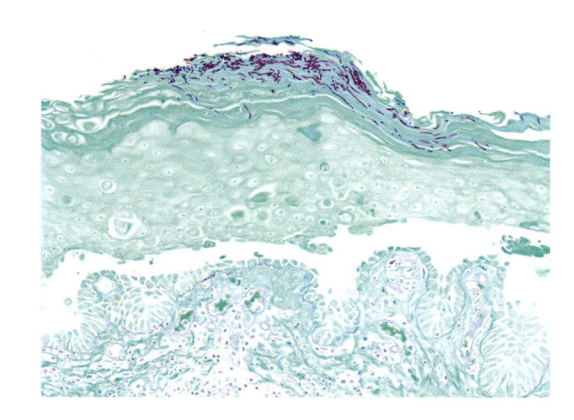

Fig 1-67 PAS-positive fungi within the stratum corneum of tinea versicolor (PAS with light green counterstain)

Colloidal iron

- Blue color indicates acid mucopolysaccharides
- As with Alcian blue, hyaluronidase digestion can be combined with colloidal iron to differentiate between hyaluronic acid and other mucosubstances

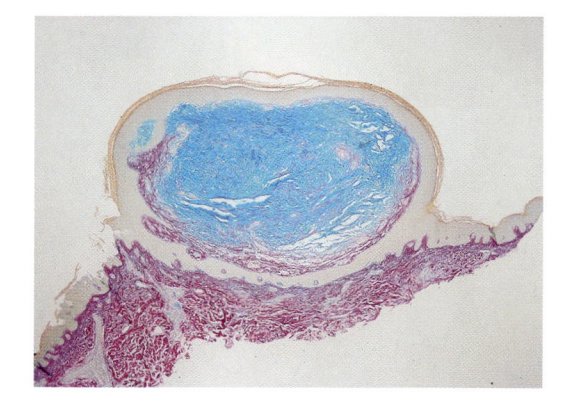

Fig 1-68 Focal mucinosis with colloidal iron

Dermatopathology

Toluidine blue
- Similar staining pattern as Alcian blue for acid mucopolysaccharides but metachromatic (reddish purple)
- Technically more complicated than Alcian blue and is used less often
- Metachromatically stains mast cells (see above)

Mucicarmine
- Stains acid mucopolysaccharides pink to red
- Stains the mucinous capsule of *Cryptococcus neoformans* pink to red

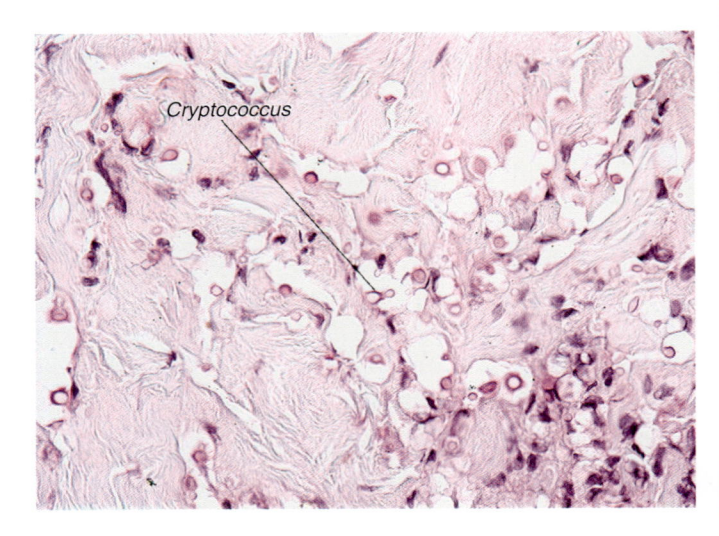

Fig 1-69 Pink capsule of *Cryptococcus* with mucicarmine

Amyloid

Congo red
- Amyloid stains brick red and displays "apple green" birefringence with polarized light

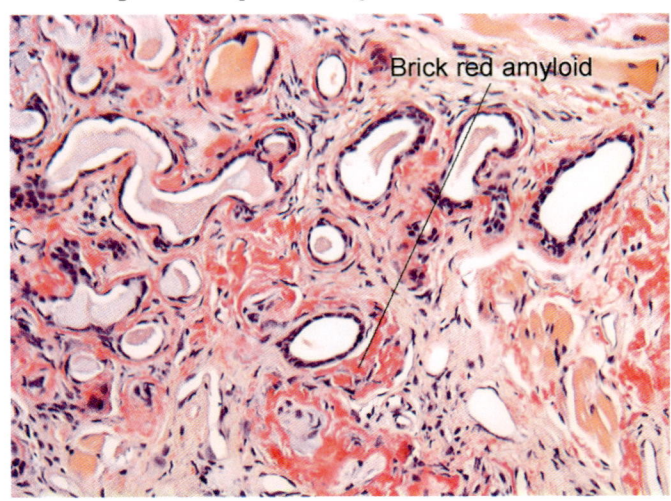

Fig 1-70 Congo red-stained amyloid in a salivary gland viewed with light microscopy

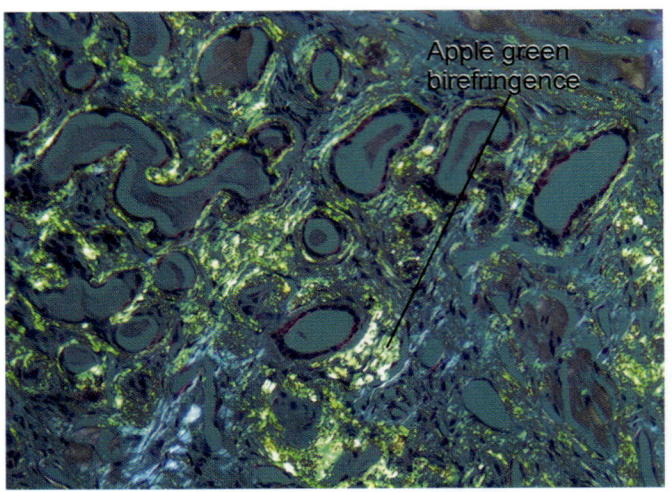

Fig 1-71 Congo red-stained amyloid in a salivary gland viewed with polarized light

Thioflavin T
- Sections must be examined with a fluorescent microscope causing amyloid to have a yellow to yellow-green appearance

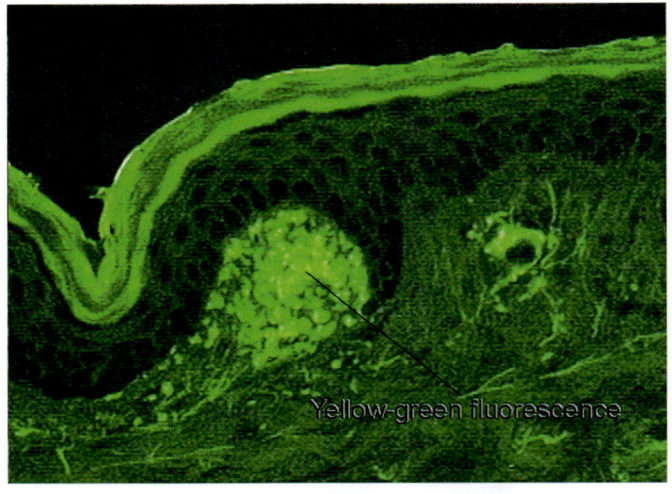

Fig 1-72 Lichen amyloid with thioflavin T

Crystal violet
- Metachromatically results in a red-purple color of amyloid

Iron

Prussian blue (Perls stain)
- Ferric ions react to form a deep blue color
- Useful to distinguish melanin from hemosiderin
- Example: hemosiderin in pigmented purpuric dermatosis
- Does not demonstrate iron in intact red blood cells

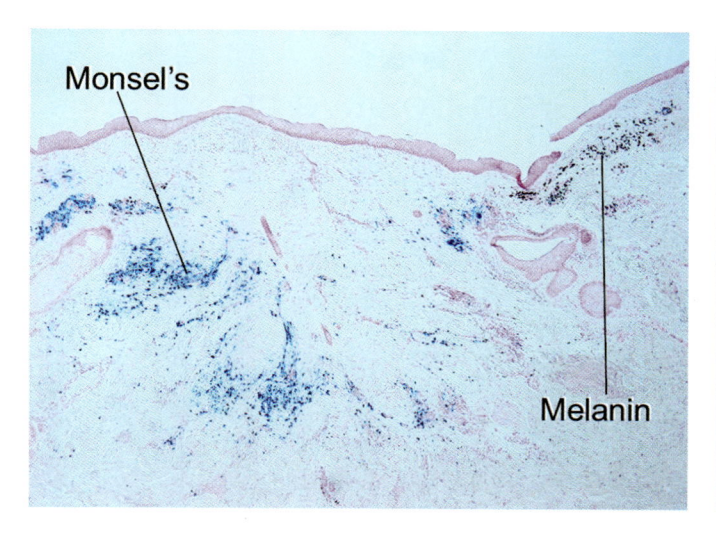

Fig 1-73 Blue iron deposition from Monsel's (ferric subsulfate) tattoo with Perls iron stain

Melanin

Fontana–Masson

- A silver stain that results in a black precipitate with melanin

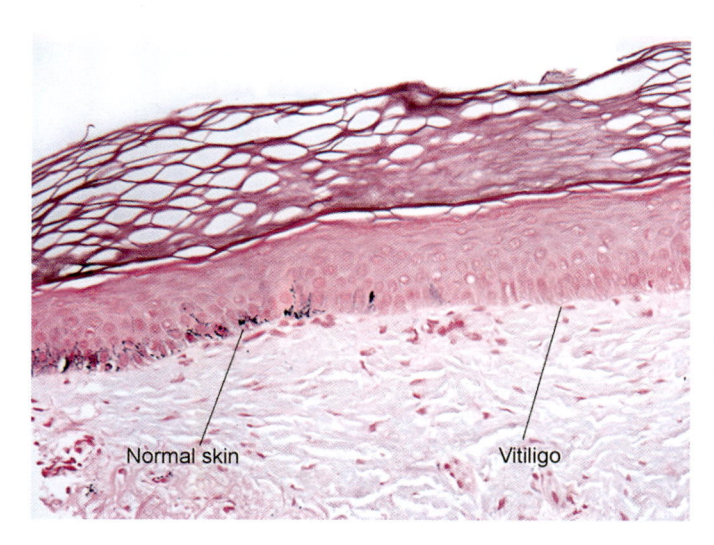

Fig 1-74 Absence of melanin in vitiligo is contrasted with adjacent normal skin (Fontana–Masson)

Calcium

Von Kossa

- A silver stain that stains calcium salts black
- Examples: pseudoxanthoma elasticum, calcinosis cutis, calciphylaxis

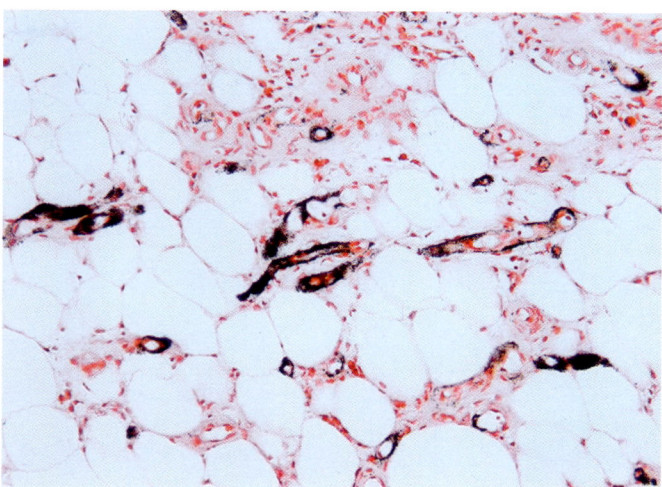

Fig 1-75 Calcium deposition in the small vessels of the subcutaneous fat in calciphylaxis (Von Kossa)

Alizarin red

- Binds directly to calcium ions resulting in an orange-red color

Lipids

Oil red O

- Requires fresh frozen tissue, as lipid is removed during routine processing

Sudan black

- Requires fresh tissue

Osmium tetroxide

- Requires fresh tissue

Bacteria

Brown–Hopps

- A modification of the Brown–Brenn technique
- Gram-positive organisms stain blue and Gram-negative organisms stain red

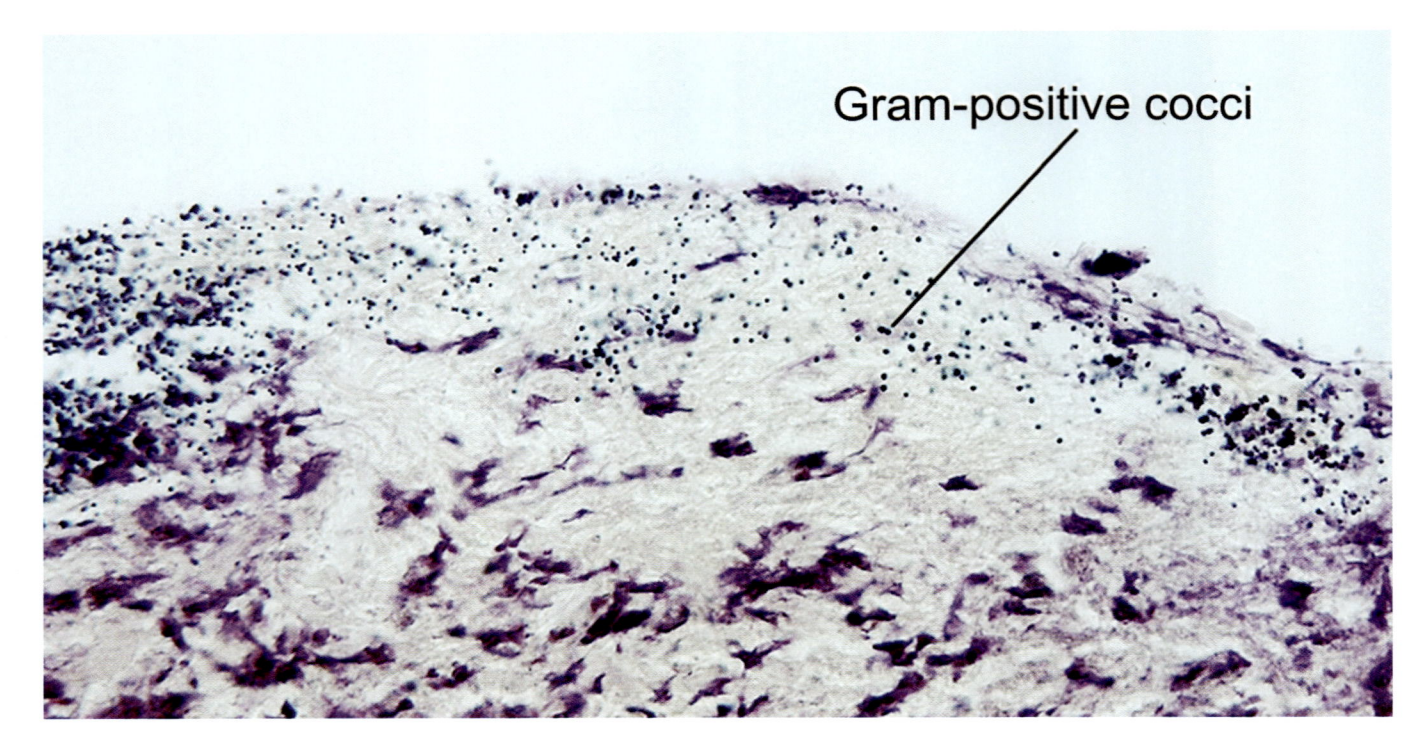

Fig 1-76 Gram-positive cocci in an ulcer bed

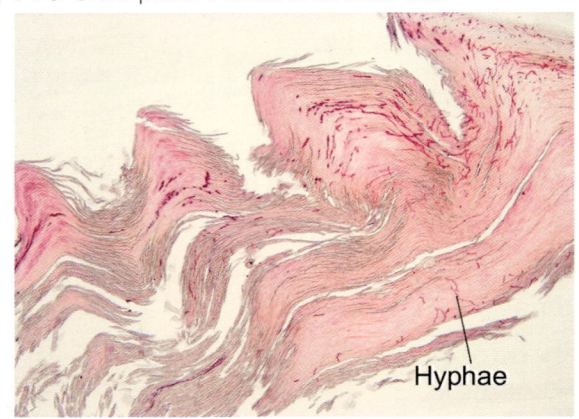

Fig 1-77 PAS-positive hyphae of onychomycosis

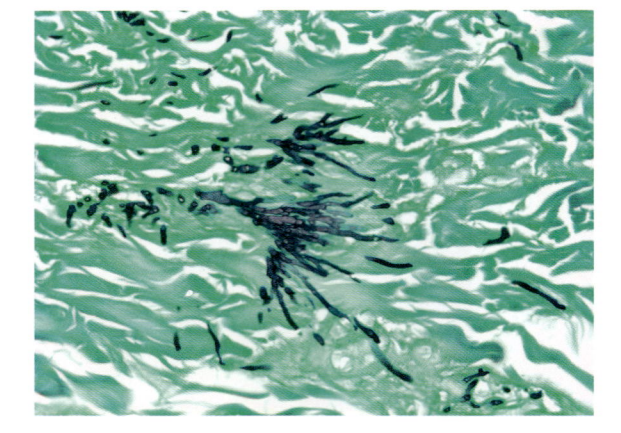

Fig 1-78 *Aspergillus* with GMS

Fungi

PAS (Periodic acid–Schiff)
- Fungi are PAS positive and diastase resistant (see above)

GMS (Grocott's methenamine silver)
- Gray-black reaction with fungal wall
- Also stains *Nocardia* and *Actinomyces*

Mycobacteria

Ziehl–Neelsen acid-fast stain; Fite acid-fast stain; Kinyoun's acid-fast stain
- Mycobacteria appear bright red
- Fite is preferred for "partially acid-fast" organisms such as lepra bacilli, atypical mycobacteria, and *Nocardia*. Fite preserves color due to use of peanut oil before staining and gentle decolorization

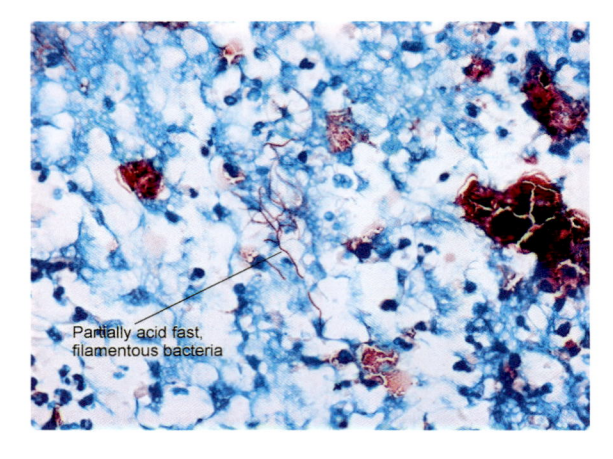

Fig 1-79 *Nocardia* with Fite stain

Auramine–rhodamine

- Requires a fluorescent microscope
- Mycobacteria fluoresce reddish yellow

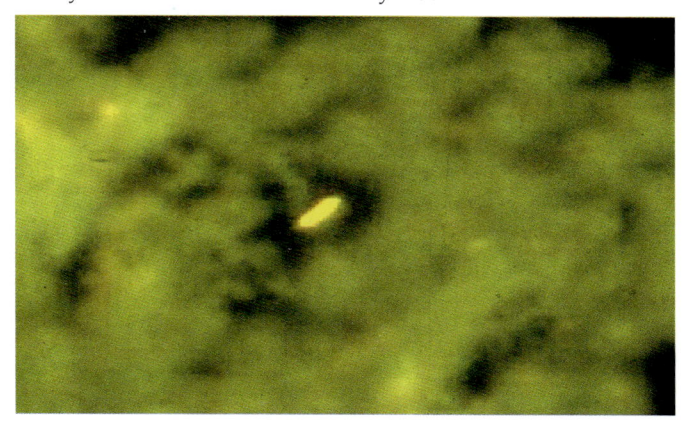

Fig 1-80 *Mycobacterium* with auramine–rhodamine as viewed with a fluorescent scope

Spirochetes

Warthin–Starry (technically more difficult than the others, so sometimes referred to as the "worthless Starry")

Dieterle

Steiner (modified Dieterle stain)

- Silver stains resulting in black spirochetes
- Examples: Lyme disease (around vessels and in dermal papillae), syphilis (in lower epidermis)
- Also stains *Legionella*, *Bartonella*, and Donovan bodies of granuloma inguinale

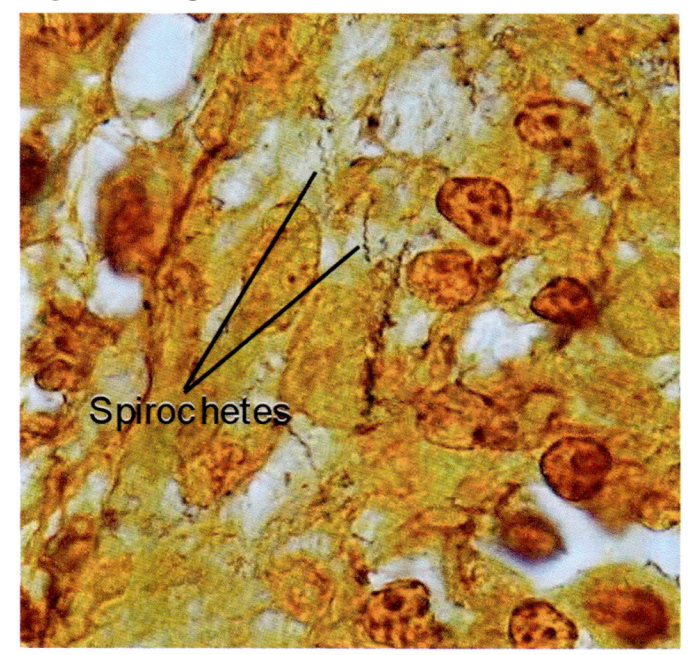

Fig 1-81 Spirochetes with Steiner stain

Other "special" stains

Giemsa

- Giemsa has many uses including highlighting myeloid and mast cell granules purplish blue
- Giemsa also stains many types of organisms including bacteria, *Leishmania* and *Histoplasma*

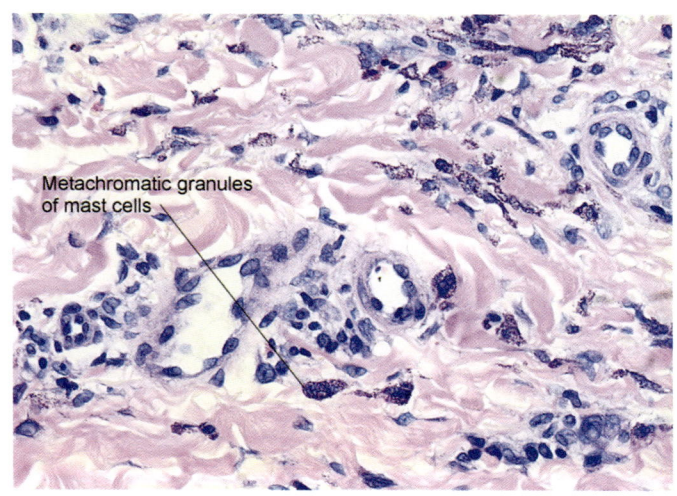

Fig 1-82 Metachromatic granules within mast cells of urticaria pigmentosa (Giemsa)

Immunohistochemical stains

Histochemical stains are now being supplemented by immunohistochemical techniques in fixed, paraffin-embedded tissue. Antibodies directed towards the antigen of interest are conjugated to peroxidases. Enzyme histochemical reactions for the peroxidase, such as diaminobenzidine method (DAB), are used to visualize the presence of enzyme–antibody–antigen complex fixed to tissue as a stable brown product. 3-amino-9-ethylcarbazole (AEC) can alternatively be used giving a red reaction, but does not archive as well.

Immunopathologic antibodies are used in dermatopathology to differentiate carcinoma, melanoma, sarcoma, neural neoplasms, and lymphomas. A panel of antibodies is generally recommended rather than a single stain because aberrant staining is common in neoplasms. Independent and internal controls should be assessed to assure proper reactivity.

Epithelial markers

AE1/AE3

- Cocktail of high- and low-molecular-weight monoclonal cytokeratin antibodies
- Expressed in the epidermis and adnexal epithelium
- Stains all epithelial tumors (squamous cell carcinoma and adnexal tumors) and generally excludes mesenchymal, melanocytic, and hematopoietic tumors
- Also stains epithelioid sarcoma, synovial sarcoma and mesothelioma

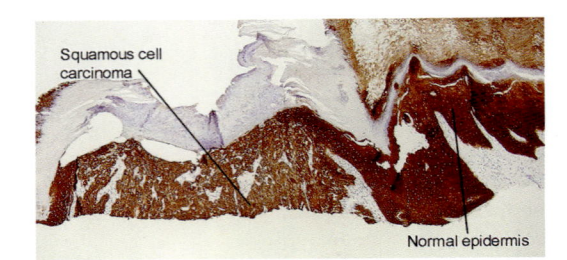

Fig 1-83 AE1/AE3 positivity of squamous cell carcinoma

CK polyclonal keratin (pankeratin)

- Polyclonal cocktail that offers greater sensitivity than AE1/AE3

p63

- Expressed in basal and spinous cells of the epidermis, germinative cells of sebaceous glands, and myoepithelial cells of the sweat glands
- Lack of reactivity in metastatic carcinoma assists in differentiation from primary cutaneous adnexal neoplasms
- Useful in identification of cutaneous spindle cell squamous cell carcinoma from other spindle cell neoplasms

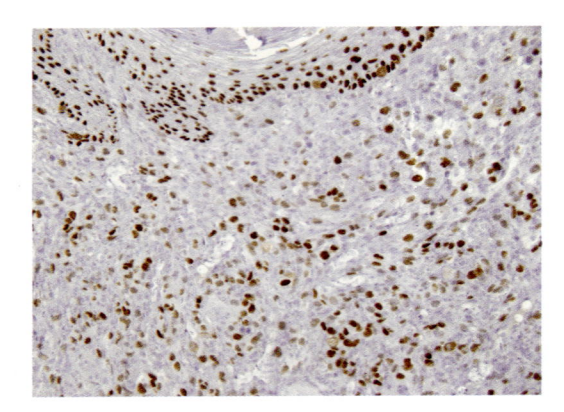

Fig 1-84 p63 in spindle cell squamous cell carcinoma

CAM5.2

- CAM5.2 detects low-molecular-weight cytokeratins present in most glandular neoplasms without staining the epidermis or stratified squamous epithelium
- Marks Paget's disease and extramammary Paget's disease

CK7

- Used in determining the origin of metastatic carcinoma
- In general a marker of non-gastrointestinal adenocarcinoma (see Table 1.1)
- Marks Paget's disease and extramammary Paget's disease

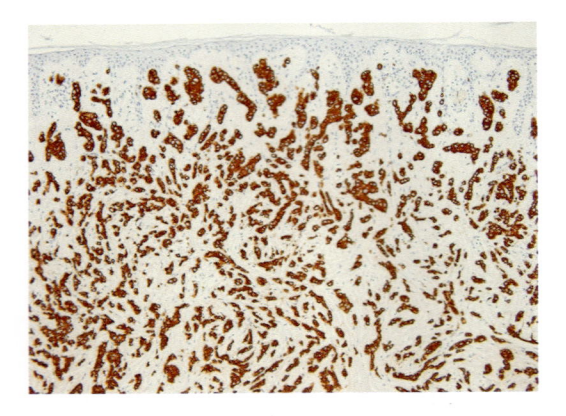

Fig 1-85 CK7 reactivity of metastatic breast carcinoma

CK20

- Marks Merkel cell carcinoma predominantly in a paranuclear pattern and distinguishes from metastatic oat cell carcinoma of the lung that is typically negative
- Used in determining the origin of metastatic carcinoma (see Table 1.1)
- Marker of gastrointestinal adenocarcinoma
- Highlights sparse Merkel cells within the basaloid islands of desmoplastic trichoepithelioma but not basal cell carcinoma

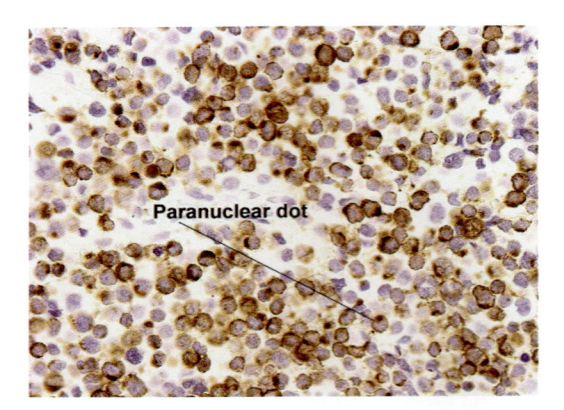

Fig 1-86 Paranuclear dot with CK20 in Merkel cell carcinoma

Table 1-1 Metastatic carcinoma of unknown origin

	CK20–	CK20+
CK7+	Breast, lung, mesothelioma	Bladder, pancreatic
CK7–	Hepatocellular, prostate, renal, neuroendocrine and squamous carcinoma of lung	Colon

CDX2

- Marker of intestinal adenocarcinoma
- Useful for diagnosis of cutaneous metastatic colon adenocarcinoma and extramammary Paget's disease associated with an underlying colorectal tumor

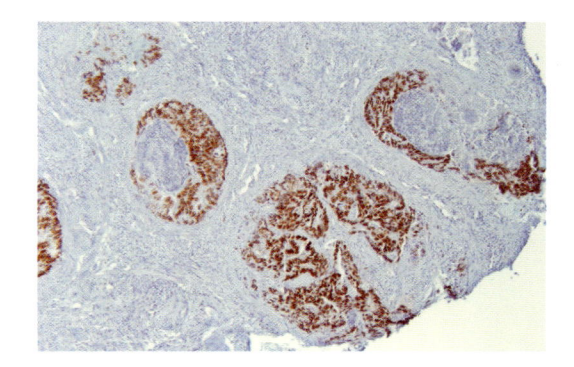

Fig 1-87 Metastatic colon carcinoma with CDX2

Renal cell carcinoma (RCC)

- Positive in most cutaneous metastases from renal cell carcinoma and negative in other clear cell tumors of the skin

Thyroid transcription factor (TTF-1)

- Useful in the small blue cell tumor differential diagnosis
- Reactive in metastatic small cell lung carcinoma and negative in Merkel cell carcinoma

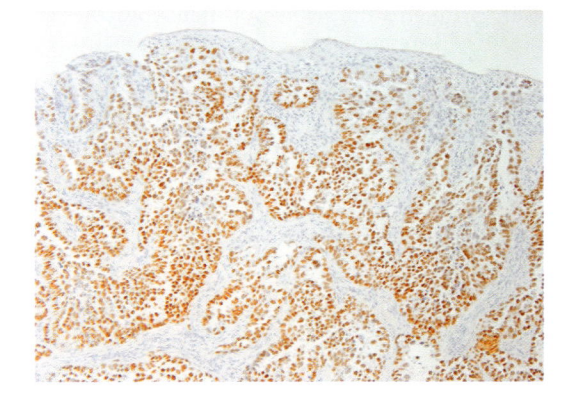

Fig 1-88 TTF-1 in metastatic adenocarcinoma of the lung

Epithelial membrane antigen (EMA)

- Highlights normal sebaceous and sweat glands
- Positive in sebaceous carcinoma, Paget's and extramammary Paget's
- Positive in squamous cell carcinoma but negative in basal cell carcinoma

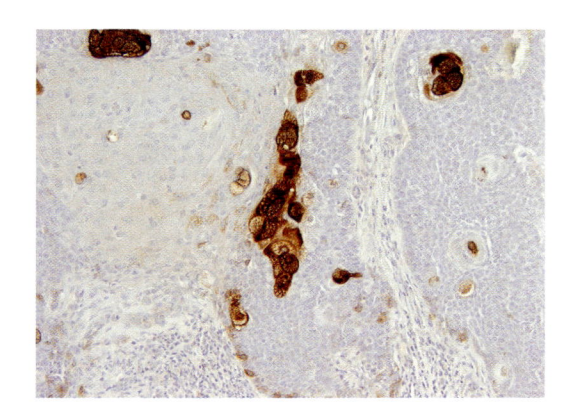

Fig 1-89 EMA positivity in sebaceous epithelioma

Carcinoembryonic antigen (CEA)

- Sweat glands are immunoreactive
- Positive in sweat gland neoplasms, Paget's, extramammary Paget's, and most adenocarcinomas

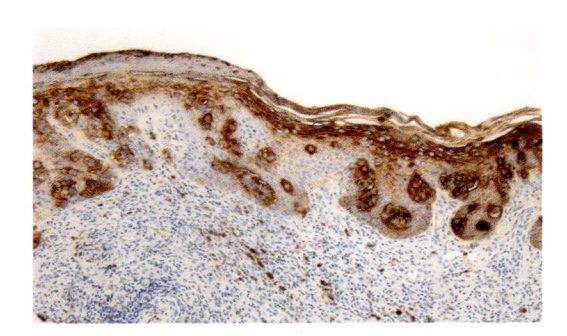

Fig 1-90 CEA-positive pagetoid cells of Paget's disease

Adipophilin

- Expressed in lipid droplets of sebaceous and xanthomatous lesions
- Can help distinguish sebaceous carcinoma from squamous cell carcinoma and basal cell carcinoma

Ber-EP4

- Marks most epithelial cells, but not those undergoing squamous differentiation
- Positive in basal cell carcinoma and negative in squamous cell carcinoma

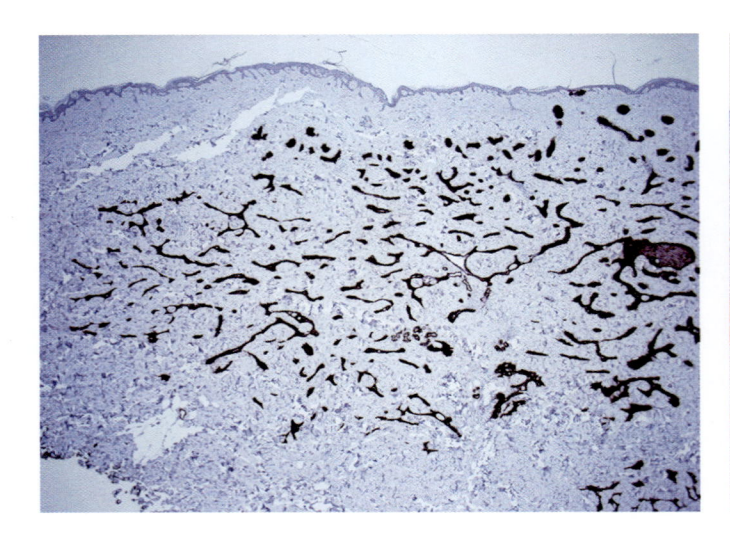

Fig 1-91 Infiltrating basal cell carcinoma with Ber-EP4

Mesenchymal markers

Desmin

- Positive staining in skeletal and most smooth muscle
- Generally negative in vascular smooth muscle (including glomus cells)

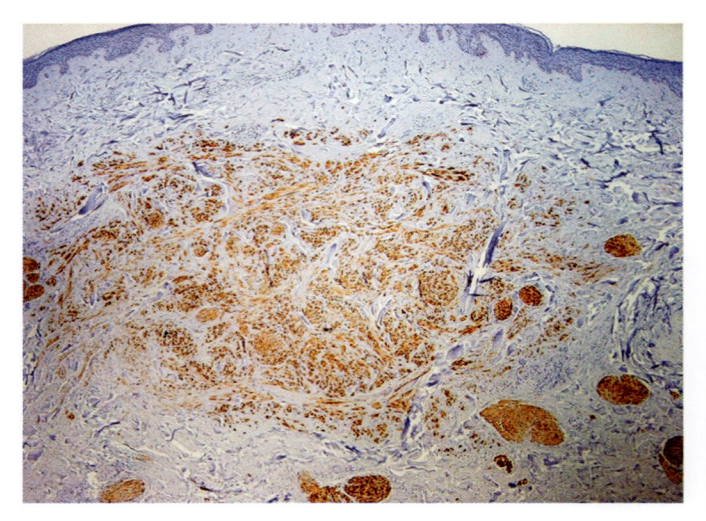

Fig 1-92 Desmin-positive piloleiomyoma

Smooth muscle actin (SMA)

- Positive in smooth muscle, including vascular smooth muscle
- Examples: glomus tumor, leiomyosarcoma

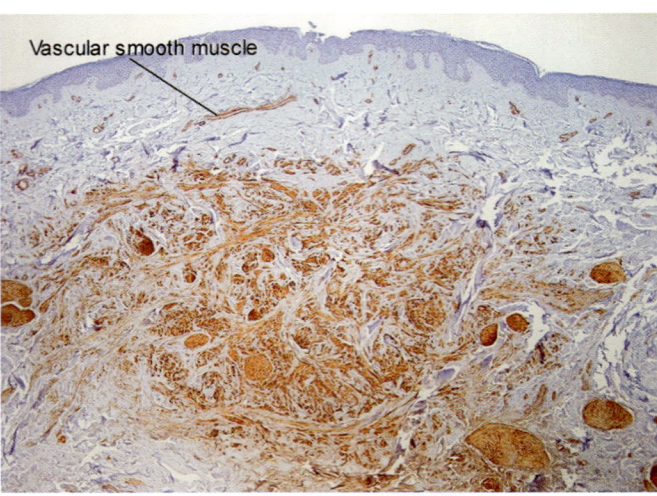

Fig 1-93 Piloleiomyoma with SMA. Note positive staining of normal surrounding vascular smooth muscle in contrast to the absence of reactivity with desmin in Figure 1.92

CD34

- Marker of vascular endothelium and hematopoietic progenitor cells
- Positive in dermatofibrosarcoma protuberans and negative in dermatofibroma
- Positive in spindle cell lipoma, sclerotic fibroma, solitary fibrous tumor, superficial acral fibromyxoma, pleomorphic fibroma, and pleomorphic hyalinizing angiectatic tumor
- Decreased staining in morphea
- Increased staining in nephrogenic systemic fibrosis
- Stains connective tissue around normal hair follicles
- Typically highlights the stroma of trichoepitheliomas but not basal cell carcinomas

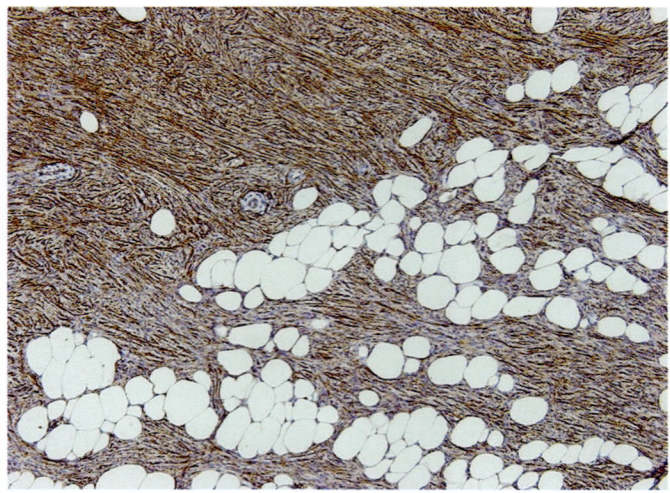

Fig 1-94 Dermatofibrosarcoma protuberans with CD34

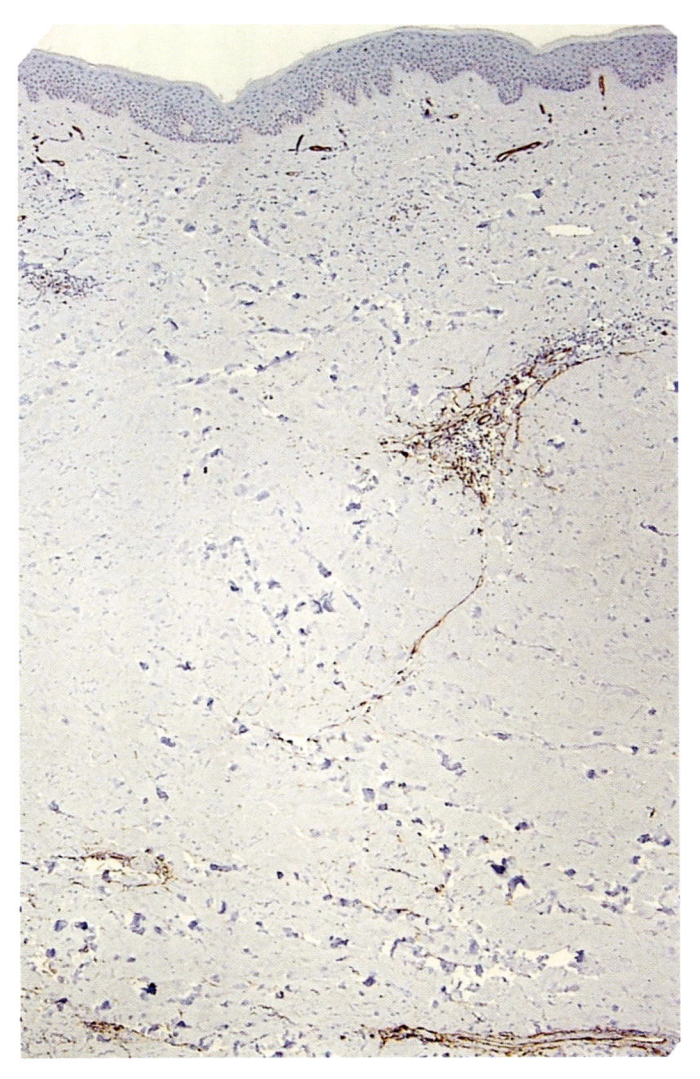

Fig 1-95 Decreased CD34 expression in the interstitial dermis of morphea

Factor XIIIa

- Highlights a population of dermal dendritic cells
- Positive in dermatofibroma and negative in dermatofibrosarcoma protuberans
- Positive in fibrous papule of the face

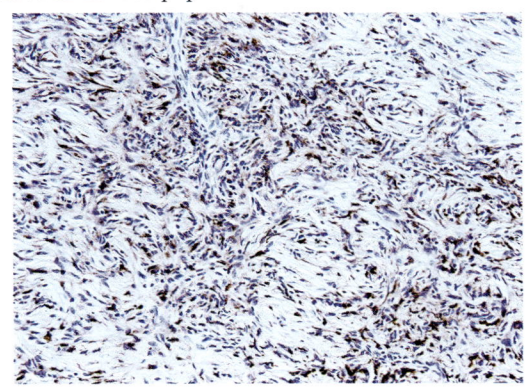

Fig 1-96 Dermatofibroma with factor XIIIa

CD31

- Helpful in confirming vascular origin of tumors
- More specific vascular marker than CD34

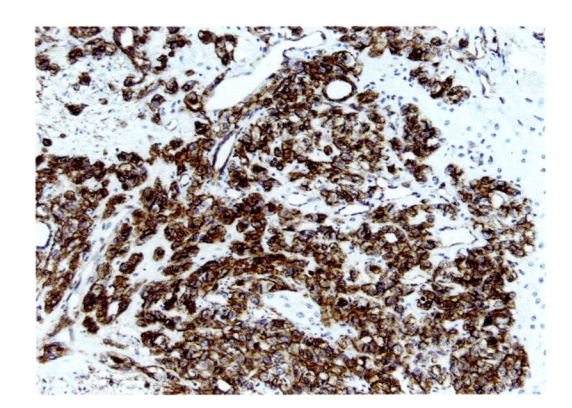

Fig 1-97 CD31-positive angiosarcoma

D2-40 (podoplanin)

- Lymphatic endothelial marker
- Increases detection of lymphovascular invasion
- Lack of reactivity in metastatic carcinoma assists in differentiation from primary cutaneous adnexal neoplasms

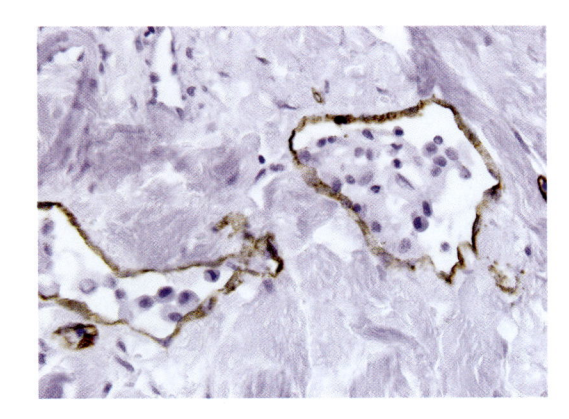

Fig 1-98 Intralymphatic invasion of melanoma with D2-40

UEA-1 (Ulex europeus agglutinin)

- Binds vascular endothelium

GLUT1 (glucose transporter)

- Expressed in endothelial cells with blood–tissue barrier function as in placenta
- Positive in infantile hemangiomas (except RICH and NICH) and negative in vascular malformations
- Also stains perineurial cells and perineurioma

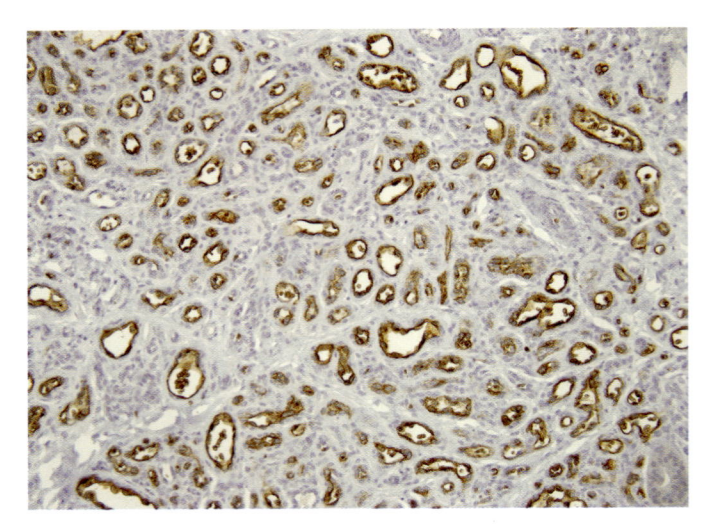

Fig 1-99 GLUT1 in infantile hemangioma

Vimentin

- Stains mesenchymal cells, endothelial cells, fibroblasts, melanocytes, lymphocytes, macrophages but does not react with keratinocytes or other epithelium
- General marker of sarcomas
- Excludes most carcinomas except rare spindle cell carcinomas and synovial sarcoma

Neuroectodermal markers

S100

- Reactivity is observed for neural crest-derived cells and some mesenchymal lines
- Stains melanocytes, Langerhans cells, sweat glands, nerves, schwann cells, myoepithelial cells, fat, muscle, and chondrocytes
- Useful in differential diagnosis of spindle cell neoplasms
- Examples: desmoplastic melanoma, Langerhans cell histiocytosis, granular cell tumor, Rosai–Dorfman disease

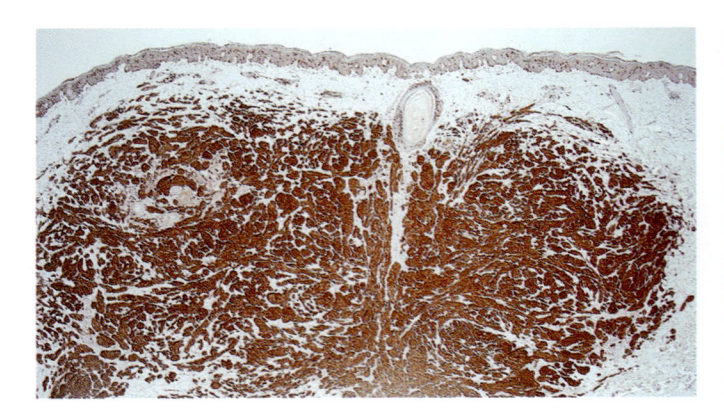

Fig 1-100 Granular cell tumor with S100

S100A6 (calcyclin)

- Member of the S100 protein superfamily
- Stains melanocytes, Schwann cells, Langerhans cells, and dermal dendrocytes thus expressed in nevi, particularly those with type C Schwann cell-like features, and some neural and fibrohistiocytic tumors
- Positive in cellular neurothekeoma while S100 is negative
- Reactive in most atypical fibroxanthomas but is not specific and also stains other entities in the cutaneous spindle cell tumor differential diagnosis
- Has been reported to stain Spitz nevi strongly and diffusely but spitzoid melanomas have weak or patchy staining in the dermis only

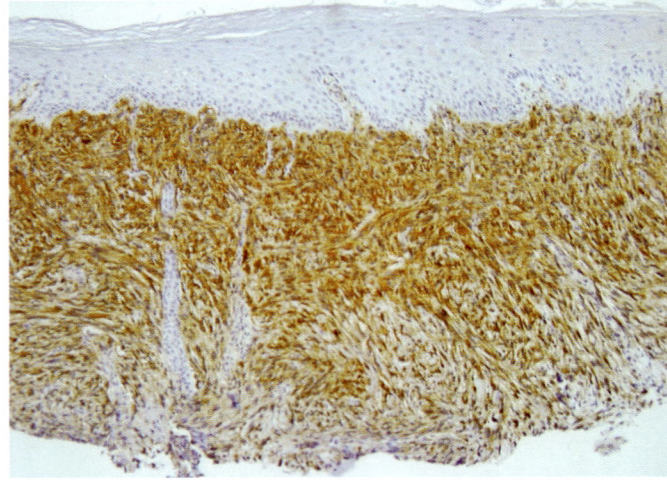

Fig 1-101 S100A6 in atypical fibroxanthoma

HMB-45

- Premelanosome marker
- Loss of staining of melanocytes with descent into the dermis is a manifestation of loss of premelanosomes. As such, it serves as a marker of normal maturation
- Loss of staining in deep dermal component of most benign nevi, but uniform staining of blue nevi
- Does not stain desmoplastic melanoma reliably

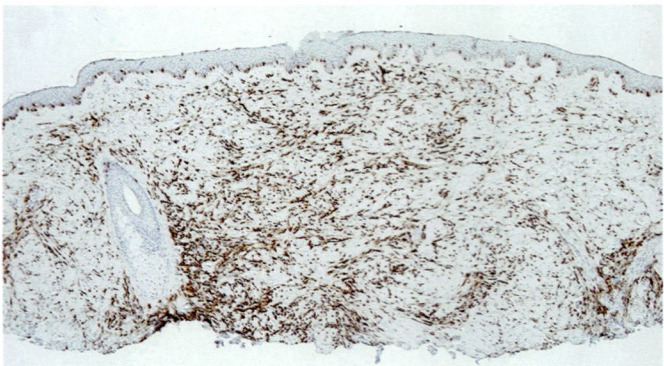

Fig 1-102 HMB-45-positive staining throughout a blue nevus

Melan-A and Mart-1

- Two different antibodies that stain the same epitope
- Stain melanocytic lesions
- Do not stain desmoplastic melanoma reliably

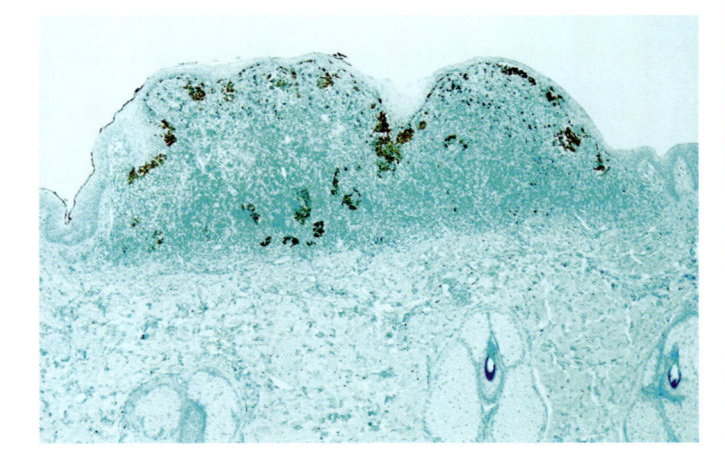

Fig 1-103 Obscured nevus cells in the lymphocytic infiltrate of halo nevus with Mart-1

p75 (nerve growth factor receptor)

- Early neural crest marker
- Expressed in type C (spindled) melanocytes and schwann cells
- Sensitive marker for spindle cell and desmoplastic melanoma

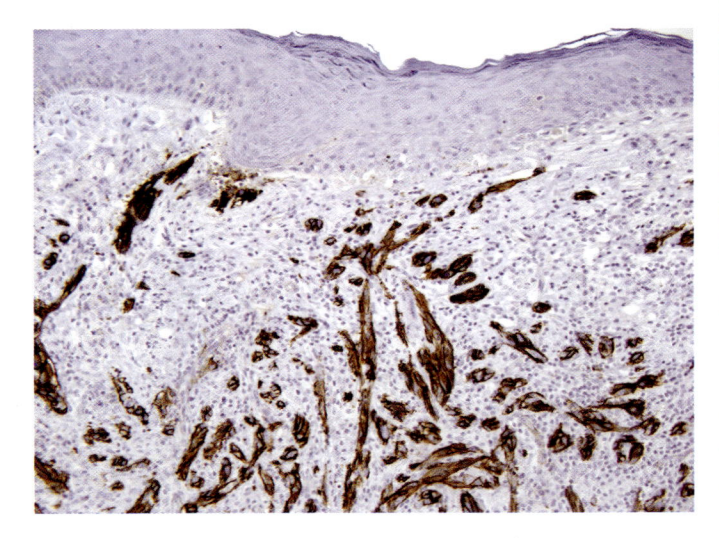

Fig 1-104 p75 in desmoplastic melanoma

Microphthalmia-associated transcription factor (MITF)

- Essential in development and survival of melanocytes
- Nuclear melanocytic marker
- Positive in cellular neurothekeomas

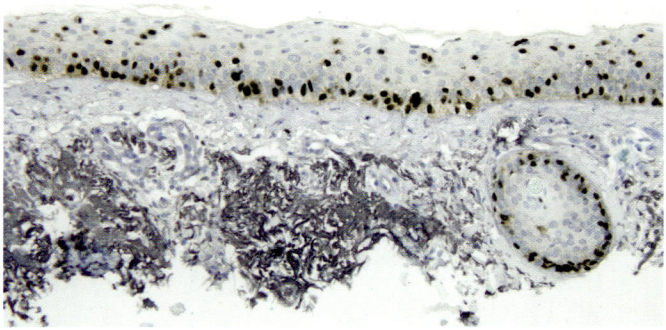

Fig 1-105 Nuclear reactivity of melanocytes in melanoma *in situ* with MITF

Sox-10

- Nuclear marker of Schwann cells and melanocytes
- Sensitive marker of melanoma, including conventional, spindled, and desmoplastic types

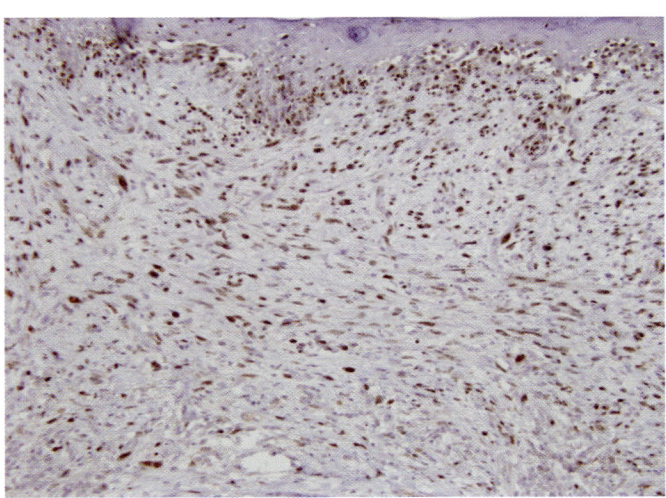

Fig 1-106 Nuclear reactivity of melanocytes in desmoplastic melanoma with Sox-10

Neuroendocrine markers

Neuron-specific enolase (NSE)

- Positive in neuroendocrine cells, neurons, and tumors derived from them
- Positive in so many other cell lines that it is sometimes referred to as "non-specific enolase"

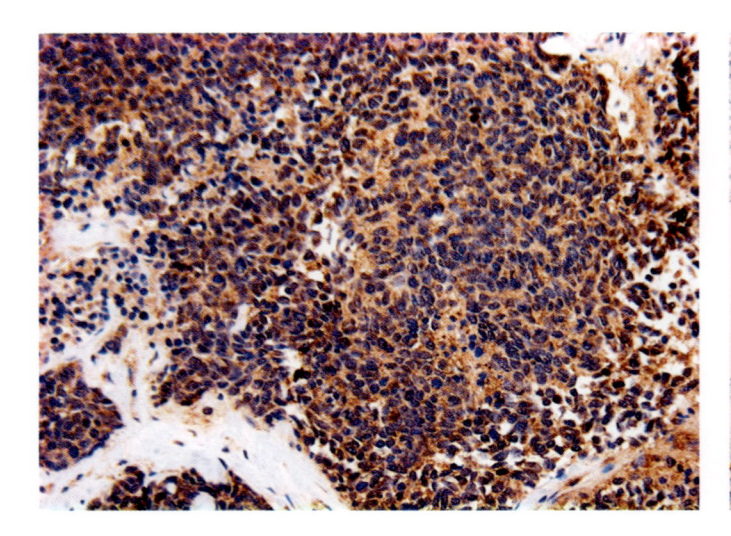

Fig 1-107 NSE in Merkel cell carcinoma

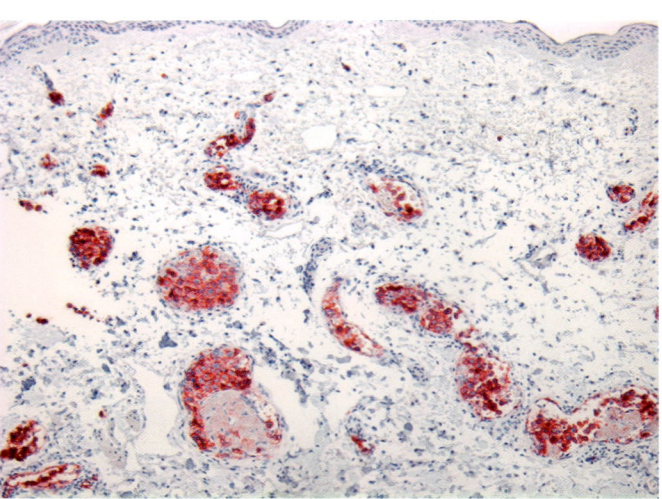

Fig 1-108 CD20 positivity in intravascular lymphoma using amino-9-ethylcarbazole (AEC) as the enzyme in the enzyme–antibody–antigen complex, resulting in a red product

Chromogranin
- Positive in Merkel cell carcinoma

Synaptophysin
- Positive in Merkel cell carcinoma

Hematopoietic markers

CD45Ra (LCA)
- Leukocyte common antigen (LCA) is a general marker of hematolymphoid differentiation
- LCA is present on all hematopoietic cells and their precursors with the exception of maturing erythroids and megakeratocytes

CD45Ro (UCHL-1)
- Mature T cells

CD20
- B-cell antigen (often absent in plasma cells)
- Positive in B-cell lymphomas and negative in T-cell lymphomas
- Target for rituximab. Loss correlates with rituximab resistance

CD10 (CALLA)
- Common acute lymphoblastic leukemia antigen (CALLA) is an early marker of B-cell differentiation
- Useful in differential diagnosis of B-cell lymphoproliferative disorders (see Table 1.2)
- Positive in periadnexal mesenchymal cells, staining only the stroma of trichoblastomas but the epithelial cells of basal cell carcinoma
- Expressed in most atypical fibroxanthomas but not uncommonly seen in the other tumors in the differential diagnosis of cutaneous spindle cell tumors
- Marker of renal cell carcinoma but also expressed in other cutaneous clear cell lesions including: balloon cell nevi, clear cell hidradenoma, and sebaceous tumors

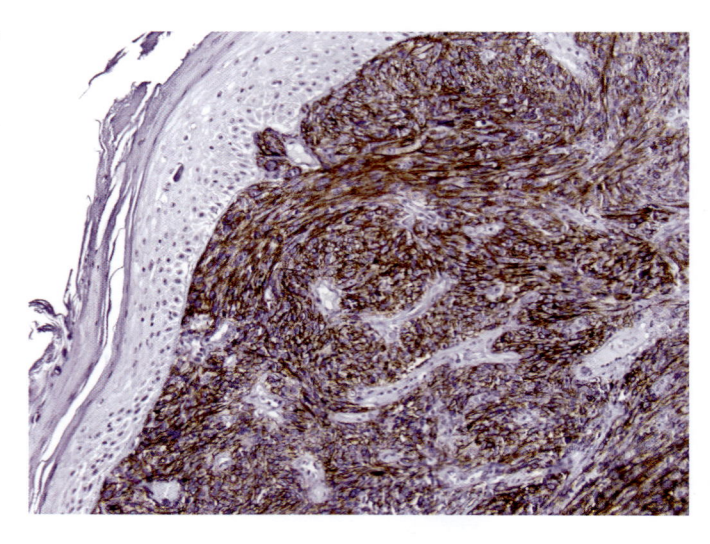

Fig 1-109 CD10 in atypical fibroxanthoma

CD79a

- Plasma cell and B-cell marker

CD138 (syndecan-1)

- Plasma cell marker

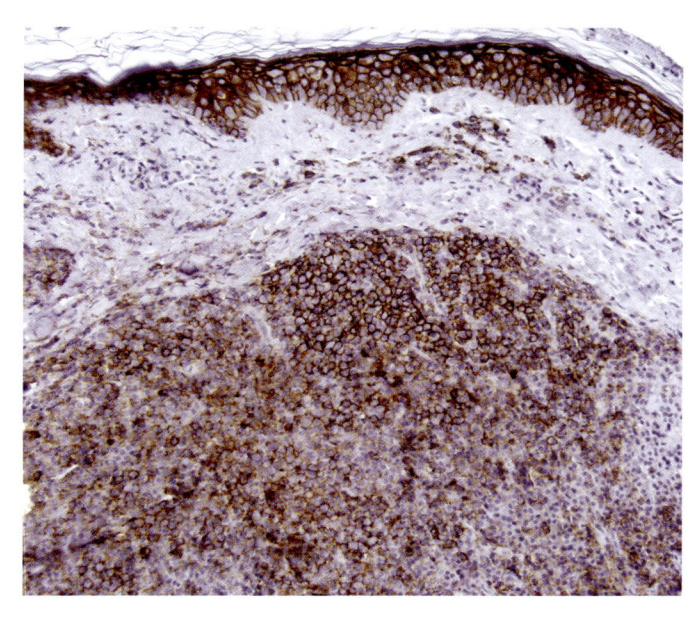

Fig 1-110 CD138 in plasmacytoma

CD3

- Pan-T-cell marker
- Positive in T-cell lymphomas but negative in B-cell lymphomas

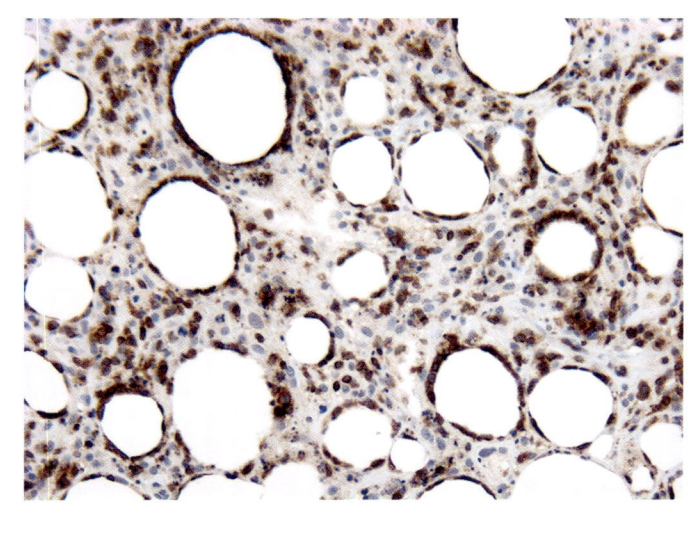

Fig 1-111 CD3-positive lymphocytes of subcutaneous T-cell lymphoma

CD4

- T-helper lymphocytic marker

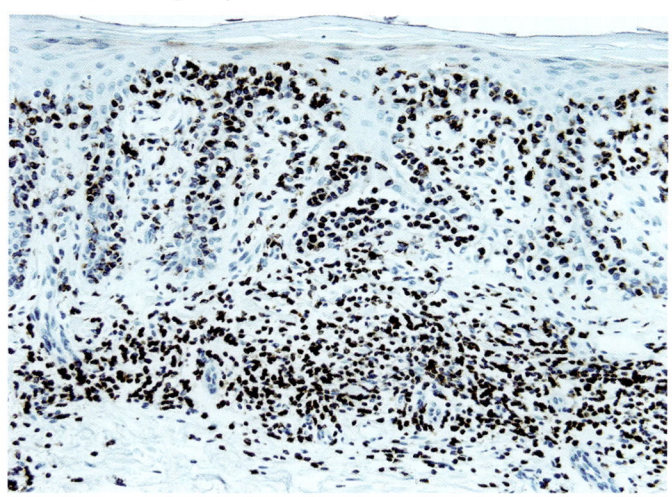

Fig 1-112 CD4-positive epidermotropic cells of mycosis fungoides

CD8

- T-cell cytotoxic/suppressor marker

CD5

- Pan-T-cell marker like CD3 but aberrant loss in CTCL is common
- Positive in mantle cell lymphoma and infiltrates of chronic lymphocytic leukemia

CD30 (Ki-1, BERH2)

- Originally identified on Reed–Sternberg cells of Hodgkin's disease
- Positive in activated lymphocytes of anaplastic large cell lymphoma and lymphomatoid papulosis
- Many positive cells may be seen in scabies nodules and chronic tick bites

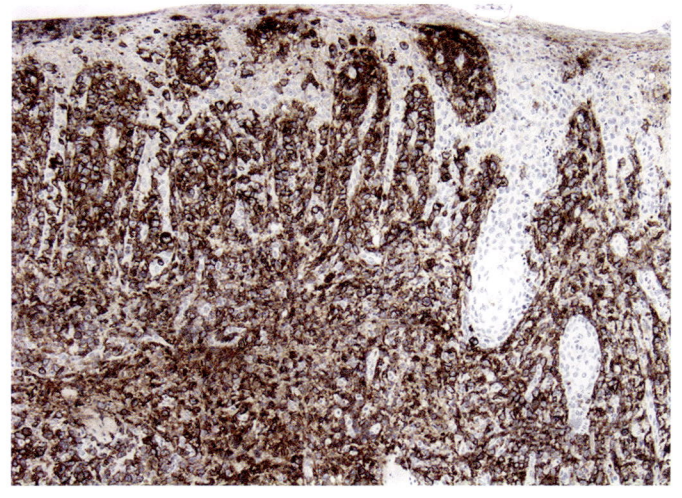

Fig 1-113 CD30-positive anaplastic large cell lymphoma

CD7
- Immature T-lymphocyte antigen
- Most commonly lost antigen in T-cell lymphoma

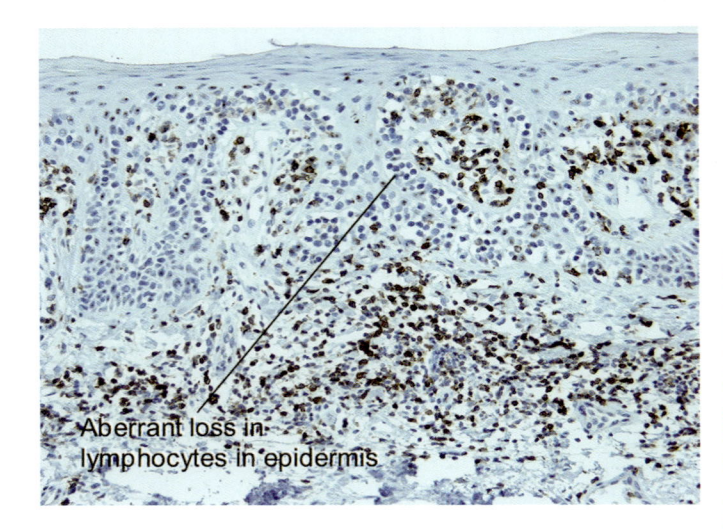

Fig 1-114 Aberrant loss of CD7 in epidermotropic cells of mycosis fungoides (compare with Figure 1.112)

CD56
- Marker of NK cells and subsets of T cells
- Stains blastic plasmacytoid dendritic cell neoplasm (formerly known as blastic NK/T-cell lymphoma or CD4+/CD56+ hematodermic neoplasm)

CD68 (KP-1)
- Reactive in virtually all monocyte/macrophage cells

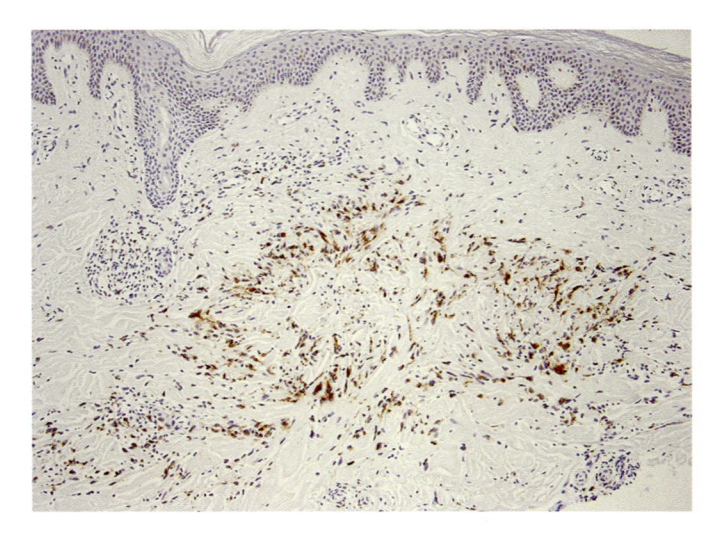

Fig 1-115 CD68-positive histiocytes of granuloma annulare

CD163
- Reactive in monocytes and macrophages

CD123
- Marker of plasmacytoid dendritic cells
- Positive in blastic plasmacytoid dendritic cell neoplasm

Myeloperoxidase
- Major constituent of granules of neutrophilic myeloid cells
- Marker for acute myeloid leukemia

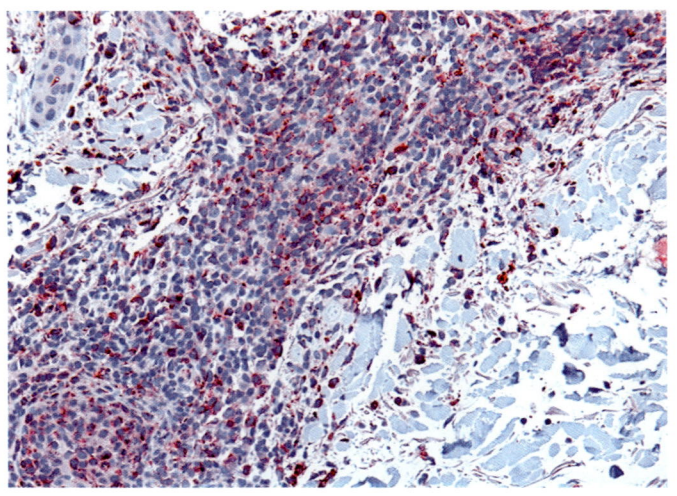

Fig 1-116 Myeloperoxidase reactivity in leukemia cutis using amino-9-ethylcarbazole (AEC) as the enzyme in the enzyme–antibody–antigen complex, resulting in a red product

ALK-1
- Anaplastic lymphoma kinase expressing chromosomal translocation t (2,5)
- Positive in most systemic anaplastic large cell lymphoma and negative in primary cutaneous anaplastic large cell lymphoma
- Those few patients with ALK-1-negative systemic anaplastic large cell lymphoma have a poor prognosis

Kappa/lambda
- Normally expressed in a ratio of two-thirds kappa to one-third lambda
- 10-fold deviation from this ratio suggests a clonal B-cell proliferation

CD117 (c-Kit)
- Expressed in mast cells and melanocytes
- In nevi and primary melanoma there is a decrease in expression in the dermal component
- Typically lost in metastatic cutaneous melanoma

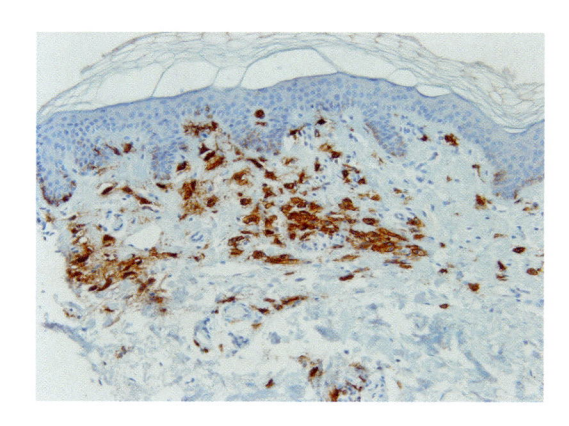

The basics: diagnostic terms, skin anatomy, and stains

Fig 1-117 CD117 in urticaria pigmentosa

CD1a

- Stains Langerhans cells
- Examples: Langerhans cell histiocytosis

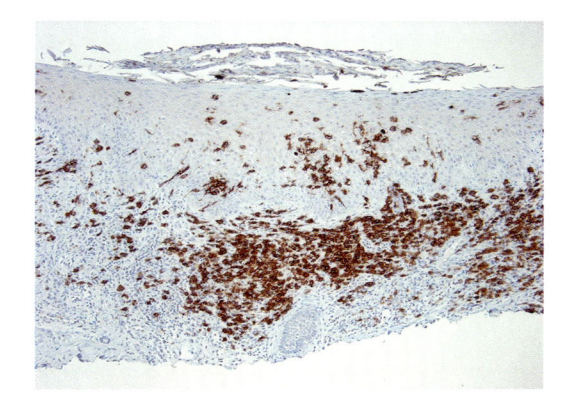

Fig 1-118 CD1a in Langerhans cell histiocytosis

Langerin (CD207)

- Surrogate marker for presence of Birbeck granules in Langerhans cells

CD43 (Leu-22)

- Pan-T-cell marker
- Aberrant coexpression with B-cell marker CD20 is strongly suggestive of B-cell lymphoma

BCL2

- An oncogene that inhibits apoptosis
- Useful in differential diagnosis of B-cell lymphoproliferative disorders (see Table 1.2)
- Most basal cell carcinomas reveal diffuse BCL2 staining, whereas trichoepitheliomas only show staining of the outermost epithelial layers of the tumor islands

Table 1-2 Cutaneous B-cell lymphoproliferative disorders

	BCL2	CD10	BCL6	MUM-1
Reactive germinal centers in pseudo B-cell lymphoma	–	+	+	–
PCMZL	+	–	–	–[a]
PCFCL	–[b]	–[c]	+[d]	–
2° CFL	+	+	+	–
PCLBCL-leg	+	–	+/–	+

PCMZL, primary cutaneous marginal zone lymphoma
PCFCL, primary cutaneous follicle center lymphoma
2° CFL, secondary cutaneous follicular lymphoma
PCLBCL-leg, primary cutaneous large B-cell lymphoma, leg type
NOTES: Immunoreactivity refers to the malignant cells in all cases except the reactive germinal center. BCL2 also stains background normal T cells.
[a]Plasma cells are positive with MUM-1 but the neoplastic B cells are negative in PCMZL.
[b]Only 10–20% of PCFCL are BCL-2 positive.
[c]Most PCFCL have a diffuse histologic pattern and are CD10 negative but cases with a follicular pattern are CD10 positive.
[d]The BCL6-positive malignant cells are outside the follicle.

Multiple myeloma oncogene-1 (MUM-1)

- Expressed in plasma cells, activated T cells, and subset of germinal center cells
- Distinguishes primary cutaneous diffuse large B-cell lymphoma, leg type from diffuse follicle center lymphoma
- Reactivity reported in anaplastic large cell lymphoma, lymphomatoid papulosis, and blastic plasmacytoid dendritic cell neoplasm
- Also expressed in benign and malignant melanocytic cells

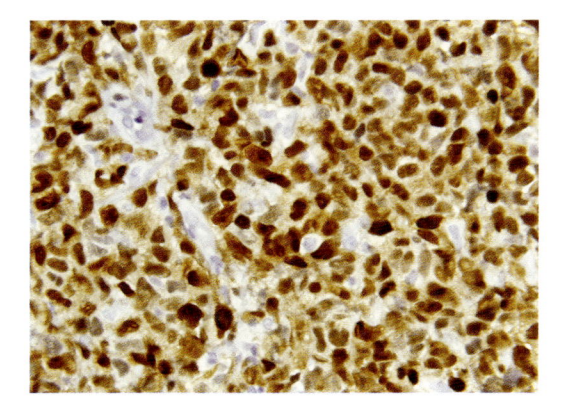

Fig 1-119 MUM-1 in diffuse large B-cell lymphoma, leg type

CD21
- Follicular dendritic cell marker
- Highlights residual follicle in lymphoma
- CD23 has a similar staining pattern

BetaF1
- Identifies αβ T cells

Table 1-3 Spindle cell neoplasms

	AE1/AE3	CD10	S100/Sox-10	Desmin
Squamous cell carcinoma	+	–/+	–	–
Atypical fibroxanthoma	–	+	–	–
Malignant melanoma	–	–/+	+	–
Leiomyosarcoma	–	–/+	–	+

Table 1-4 Small blue cell tumor

	S100	Synaptophysin	LCA	TTF-1	CK20
Lymphoma	–	–	+	–/+	–
Merkel cell carcinoma	–/+	+	–	–	+
Malignant melanoma	+	–	–	–	–
Metastatic small cell carcinoma of the lung	–	+/–	–	+	–

Table 1-5 Tumors with intraepidermal buckshot scatter (pagetoid spread)

	CK7	CEA	S100
Paget's disease	+	+	–
Bowens disease	–/+	–	–
Malignant melanoma	–	–	+

Infectious disease markers

Specific immunohistochemical antibodies to viral, bacterial, fungal, and parasitic antigens are available for detection and identification of the causative agents in many infectious diseases including HHV8, HSV, VZV, CMV, EBV, *Bartonella*, *Rickettsia*, *Treponema*, *Borrelia*, *Aspergillus*, *Leishmania*, and others.

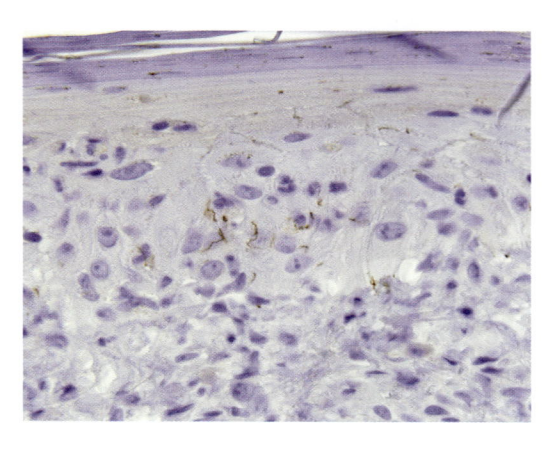

Fig 1-120 Immunohistochemical identification of *Treponema pallidum* in syphilis

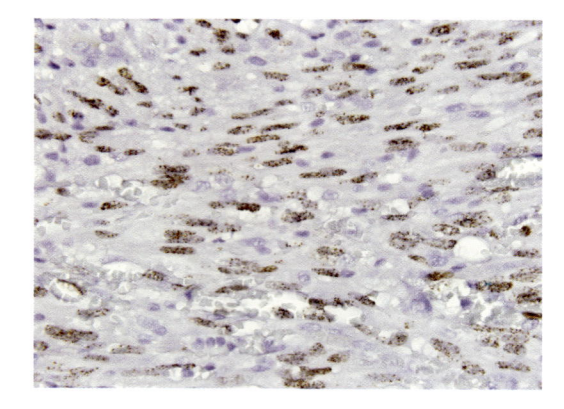

Fig 1-121 Immunohistochemical identification of HHV8 in Kaposi sarcoma

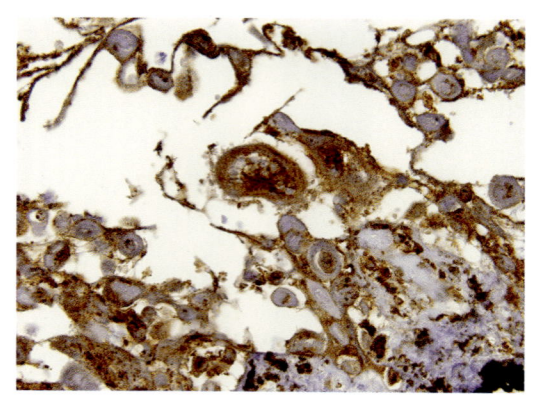

Fig 1-122 Immunohistochemical identification of VZV in multinucleate giant cell

Proliferation markers

Mib-1 (Ki-67)

- Nuclear proliferation marker
- Not cell type specific
- Expressed in all active phases of the cell cycle (G1, M, G2, and S)
- Pattern and number of reactive melanocytes can be helpful in diagnosing melanocytic lesions

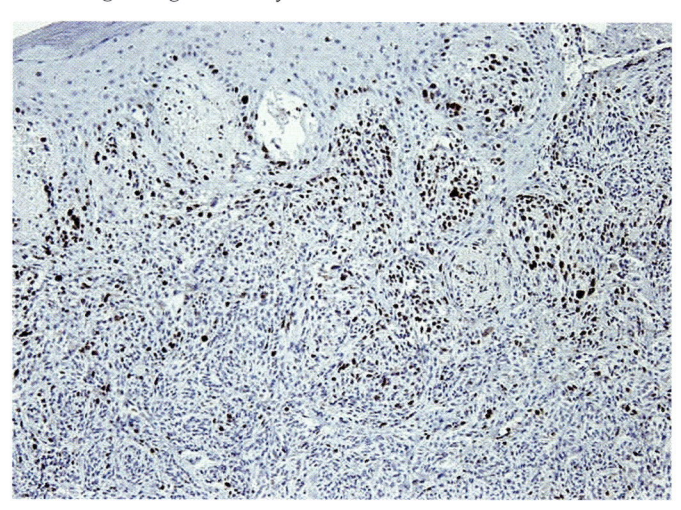

Fig 1-123 Mib-1 positivity in malignant melanoma. Positive background reactive lymphocytes must be distinguished from Mib-1-positive melanocytes by cytology or double staining technique

pHH3

- Mitotic marker that only stains cells in the M phase of the cell cycle
- Helps differentiate mitoses from apoptotic or hyperchromatic nuclei

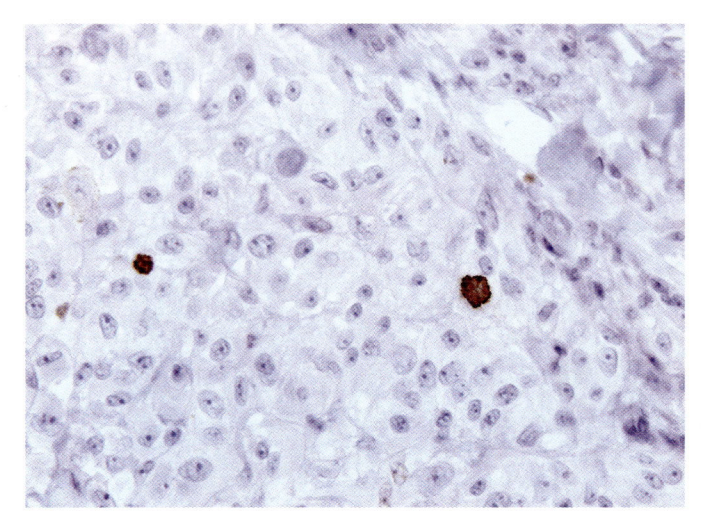

Fig 1-124 pHH3-positive mitotic figures in malignant melanoma

Transport media

Routine

For most purposes, 10% buffered formalin is the recommended fixative. The length of time for fixation depends on the specimen size: 1–2 h per mm of thickness is required.

Electron microscopy

Glutaraldehyde is the preferred fixative for electron microscopy.

Immunofluorescence

For tissue that is not flash-frozen, Michel's medium (ammonium sulfate) is the preferred transport media for immunofluorescence. Normal saline also performs well.

Further reading

Alcaraz I, Cerroni L, Rütten A, et al. Cutaneous metastases from internal malignancies: a clinicopathologic and immunohistochemical review. Am J Dermatopathol 2012;34(4):347–393.

Anstey A, Cerio R, Ramnarain N, et al. Desmoplastic malignant melanoma. An immunocytochemical study of 25 cases. Am J Dermatopathol 1994;16(1):14–22.

Bahrami S, Malone JC, Lear S, et al. CD10 expression in cutaneous adnexal neoplasms and a potential role for differentiating cutaneous metastatic renal cell carcinoma. Arch Pathol Lab Med 2006;130(9):1315–1319.

Benner MF, Jansen PM, Meijer CJ, et al. Diagnostic and prognostic evaluation of phenotypic markers TRAF1, MUM1, BCL2 and CD15 in cutaneous CD30-positive lymphoproliferative disorders. Br J Dermatol 2009;161(1):121–127.

Buonaccorsi JN, Plaza JA. Role of CD10, wide-spectrum keratin, p63, and podoplanin in the distinction of epithelioid and spindle cell tumors of the skin: an immunohistochemical study of 81 cases. Am J Dermatopathol 2012;34(4):404–411.

Córdoba A, Guerrero D, Larrinaga B, et al. Bcl-2 and CD10 expression in the differential diagnosis of trichoblastoma, basal cell carcinoma, and basal cell carcinoma with follicular differentiation. Int J Dermatol 2009;48(7):713–717.

Cota C, Vale E, Viana I, et al. Cutaneous manifestations of blastic plasmacytoid dendritic cell neoplasm-morphologic and phenotypic variability in a series of 33 patients. Am J Surg Pathol 2010;34(1):75–87.

Elston DM, Gibson LE, Kutzner H. Infectious diseases. In: Lin F, Prichard J, eds. Handbook of Practical Immunohistochemistry. New York: Springer; 2011, Ch. 29.

Eyzaguirre E, Haque AK. Application of immunohistochemistry to infections. Arch Pathol Lab Med 2008;132(3):424–431.

Fox MD, Billings SD, Gleason BC, et al. Expression of MiTF may be helpful in differentiating cellular neurothekeoma from plexiform fibrohistiocytic tumor (histiocytoid predominant) in a partial biopsy specimen. Am J Dermatopathol 2012;34(2):157–160.

Fullen DR, Lowe L, Su LD. Antibody to S100a6 protein is a sensitive immunohistochemical marker for neurothekeoma. J Cutan Pathol 2003;30(2):118–122.

Fullen DR, Reed JA, Finnerty B, et al. S100A6 expression in fibrohistiocytic lesions. J Cutan Pathol 2001;28(5):229–234.

Helm KF. Immunohistochemistry of skin tumors. In: Dabbs DJ, ed. Diagnostic Immunohistochemistry. Philadelphia: Churchill Livingstone; 2002, 313–327.

Hoefnagel JJ, Vermeer MH, Jansen PM, et al. Bcl-2, Bcl-6 and CD10 expression in cutaneous B-cell lymphoma: further support for a follicle centre cell origin and differential diagnostic significance. Br J Dermatol 2003;149(6):1183–1191.

Hudson AR, Smoller BR. Immunohistochemistry in diagnostic dermatopathology. Dermatol Clin 1999;17(3):667–680.

Kucher C, Xu X, Pasha T, et al. Histopathologic comparison of nephrogenic fibrosing dermopathy and scleromyxedema. J Cutan Pathol 2005;32(7):484–490.

Lau SK, Chu PG, Weiss LM. Immunohistochemical expression of Langerin in Langerhans cell histiocytosis and non-Langerhans cell histiocytic disorders. Am J Surg Pathol 2008;32(4):615–619.

Lazova R, Tantcheva-Poor I, Sigal AC. P75 nerve growth factor receptor staining is superior to S100 in identifying spindle cell and desmoplastic melanoma. J Am Acad Dermatol 2010;63(5):852–858.

Lora V, Kanitakis J. CDX2 expression in cutaneous metastatic carcinomas and extramammary Paget's Disease. Anticancer Res 2009;29(12):5033–5037.

Macarenco RS, Ellinger F, Oliveira AM. Perineurioma: a distinctive and underrecognized peripheral nerve sheath neoplasm. Arch Pathol Lab Med 2007;131(4):625–636.

Mohamed A, Gonzalez RS, Lawson D, et al. SOX10 expression in malignant melanoma, carcinoma, and normal tissues. Appl Immunohistochem Mol Morphol 2012; Nov 28:Epub.

Murphy M, Fullen D, Carlson JA. Low CD7 expression in benign and malignant cutaneous lymphocytic infiltrates: experience with an antibody reactive with paraffin-embedded tissue. Am J Dermatopathol 2002;24(1):6–16.

North PE, Waner M, Mizeracki A, et al. GLUT1: a newly discovered immunohistochemical marker for juvenile hemangioma. Hum Pathol 2000;31(1):11–22.

Ostler DA, Prieto VG, Reed JA, et al. Adipophilin expression in sebaceous tumors and other cutaneous lesions with clear cell histology: an immunohistochemical study of 117 cases. Mod Pathol 2010;23(4):567–573.

Perna AG, Smith MJ, Krishnan B, et al. CD10 is expressed in cutaneous clear cell lesions of different histogenesis. J Cutan Pathol 2005;32(5):348–351.

Pilloni L, Bianco P, Difelice E, et al. The usefulness of c-Kit in the immunohistochemical assessment of melanocytic lesions. Eur J Histochem 2011;55(2):e20.

Plaza JA, Ortega PF, Stockman DL, et al. Value of p63 and podoplanin (D2-40) immunoreactivity in the distinction between primary cutaneous tumors and adenocarcinomas metastatic to the skin: a clinicopathologic and immunohistochemical study of 79 cases. J Cutan Pathol 2010;37(4):403–410.

Poniecka AW, Alexis JB. An immunohistochemical study of basal cell carcinoma and trichoepithelioma. Am J Dermatopathol 1999;21(4):332–336.

Pouryazdanparast P, Yu L, Cutlan JE, et al. Diagnostic value of CD163 in cutaneous spindle cell lesions. J Cutan Pathol 2009;36(8):859–864.

Ribé A, McNutt NS. S100A6 protein expression is different in Spitz nevi and melanomas. Mod Pathol 2003;16(5):505–511.

Rose AE, Christos PJ, Lackaye D, et al. Clinical relevance of detection of lymphovascular invasion in primary melanoma using endothelial markers D2-40 and CD34. Am J Surg Pathol 2011;35(10):1441–1449.

Roullet M, Gheith SM, Mauger J, et al. Percentage of γδ T cells in panniculitis by paraffin immunohistochemical analysis. Am J Clin Pathol 2009;131(6):820–826.

Sachdev R, Robbins J, Kohler S, et al. CD163 expression is present in cutaneous histiocytomas but not in atypical fibroxanthomas. Am J Clin Pathol 2010;133(6):915–921.

Saglam A, Uner AH. Immunohistochemical expression of Mum-1, Oct-2 and Bcl-6 in systemic anaplastic large cell lymphomas. Tumori 2011;97(5):634–638.

Schach CP, Smoller BR, Hudson AR, et al. Immunohistochemical stains in dermatopathology. J Am Acad Dermatol 2000;43:1094–1100.

Schimming TT, Grabellus F, Roner M, et al. pHH3 immunostaining improves interobserver agreement of mitotic index in thin melanomas. Am J Dermatopathol 2012;34(3):266–269.

Shin J, Vincent JG, Cuda JD, et al. Sox10 is expressed in primary melanocytic neoplasms of various histologies but not in fibrohistiocytic proliferations and histiocytoses. J Am Acad Dermatol 2012;67(4):717–726.

Skobieranda K, Helm KF. Decreased expression of the human progenitor cell antigen (CD34) in morphea. Am J Dermatopathol 1995;17(5):471–475.

Smith KJ, Tuur S, Corvette D, et al. Cytokeratin 7 staining in mammary and extramammary Paget's disease. Mod Pathol 1997;10(11):1069–1074.

Su LD, Schnitzer B, Ross CW, et al. The t(2; 5)-associated p80 NPM/ALK fusion protein in nodal and cutaneous CD30+ lymphoproliferative disorders. J Cutan Pathol 1997;24(10):597–603.

Tellechea O, Reis JP, Domingues JC, et al. Monoclonal antibody Ber EP4 distinguishes basal-cell carcinoma from squamous-cell carcinoma of the skin. Am J Dermatopathol 1993;15(5):452–455.

Vitte F, Fabiani B, Bénet C, et al. Specific skin lesions in chronic myelomonocytic leukemia: a spectrum of myelomonocytic and dendritic cell proliferations: a study of 42 cases. Am J Surg Pathol 2012;36(9):1302–1316.

White WL. Immunomicroscopy in diagnostic dermatopathology: an update on cutaneous neoplasms. Adv Dermatol 1999;14:359–397.

Wood WS, Tron VA. Analysis of HMB-45 immunoreactivity in common and cellular blue nevi. J Cutan Pathol 1991;18(4):261–263.

Benign tumors and cysts of the epidermis

Dirk M. Elston

A clinical image atlas for entities throughout the text can be found in the on-line content for this book.

Benign acanthomas

Acanthomas are benign cutaneous neoplasms characterized by an expansion of the epidermis. The acanthoma may be composed of clones of cells that displace or compress the preexisting epidermis. In contrast to the reactive acanthosis seen in inflammatory disorders, the rete ridge pattern is commonly ablated by the neoplastic tissue of an acanthoma.

Seborrheic keratoses

Seborrheic keratoses are acanthomas composed of small polygonal keratinocytes about the size of acrosyringeal keratinocytes (the cells that make up the intraepidermal portion of the eccrine duct). The cells are typically smaller than the cells of the surrounding epidermis, and they are commonly pigmented. Architectural subtypes of seborrheic keratoses include acanthotic, hyperkeratotic, reticulated, and clonal. Any of these subtypes may be pigmented, irritated (spindling of cells and squamous eddy formation), or inflamed (usually lymphoid inflammation). Melanoacanthoma is a distinct subtype of seborrheic keratosis composed of small keratinocytes and dendritic melanocytes.

Seborrheic keratoses produce a characteristic loose lamellar "shredded-wheat" stratum corneum. Exceptions include irritated or inflamed seborrheic keratosis. Instead of the characteristic loose lamellar horn, irritated or inflamed seborrheic keratoses produce a compact brightly eosinophilic parakeratotic stratum corneum. Adjacent unaffected areas of the seborrheic keratosis still produce the characteristic loose lamellar stratum corneum, and it is common to see remnants of loose stratum corneum above areas of compact stratum corneum. Melanoacanthomas produce a deeply eosinophilic compact parakeratotic stratum corneum, even when they are not irritated or inflamed.

Seborrheic keratoses may express BCL-2, a marker associated with resistance to programmed cell death (apoptosis). Activating point mutations in the gene encoding fibroblast growth factor receptor 3, a tyrosine kinase receptor, are also common in seborrheic keratoses.

Acanthotic seborrheic keratosis

Key features

- Broad sheets of small polygonal keratinocytes with intervening horn cysts
- Loose lamellar "shredded-wheat" or "onion-skin" keratin
- Commonly pigmented

Acanthotic seborrheic keratoses are composed of broad sheets of cells with intervening horn cysts or pseudohorn cysts. Horn cysts are completely encased within the acanthoma, whereas pseudohorn cysts open to the surface. Like other seborrheic keratoses, they may become irritated or inflamed.

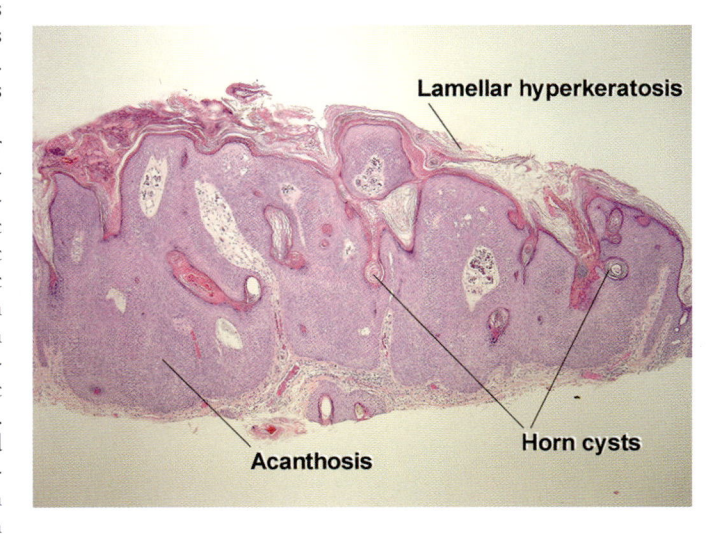

Fig 2-1 Acanthotic seborrheic keratosis

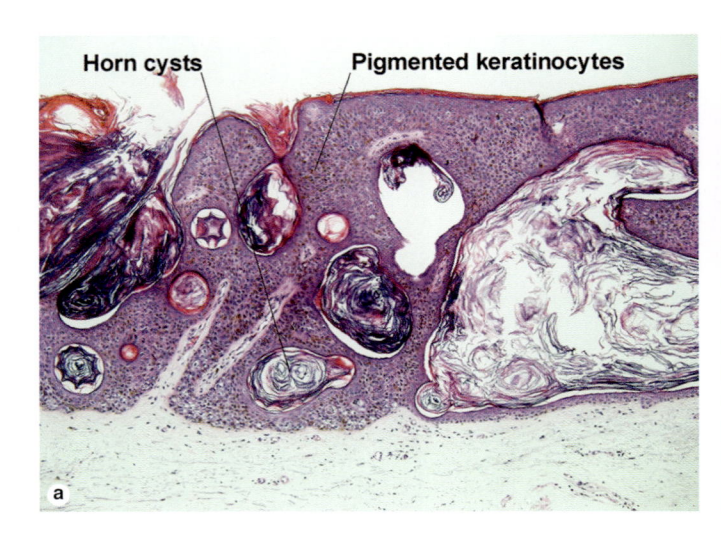

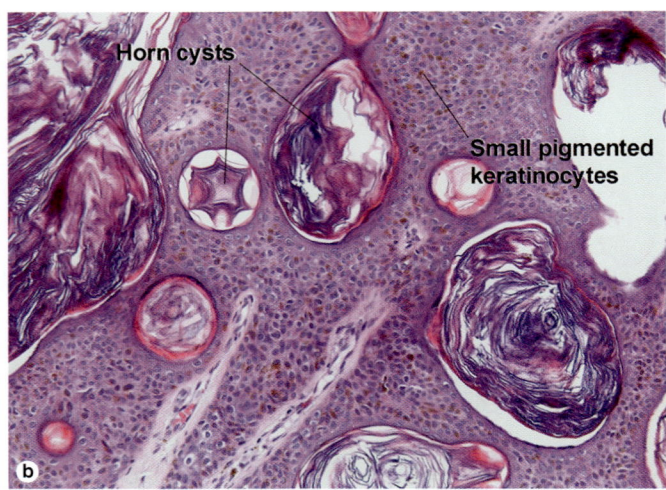

Fig 2-2 Pigmented acanthotic seborrheic keratosis

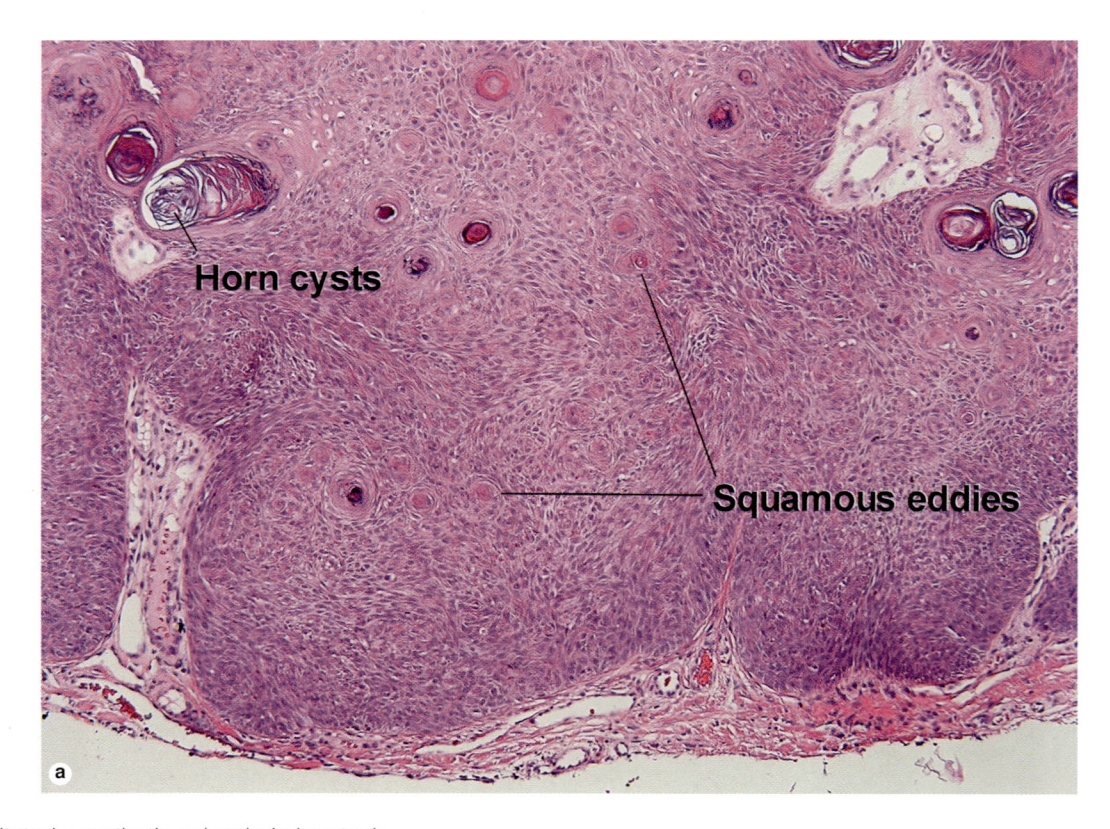

Fig 2-3 Irritated acanthotic seborrheic keratosis

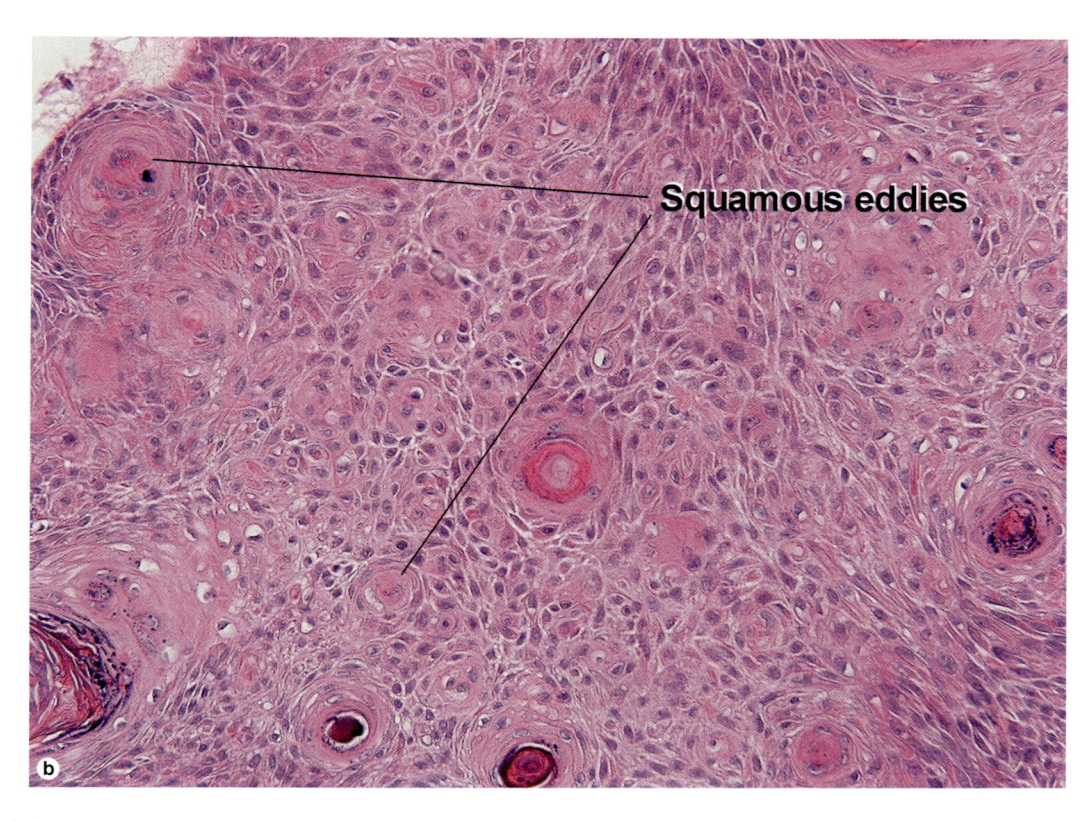

Benign tumors and cysts of the epidermis Chapter 2   39

Fig 2-3, cont'd

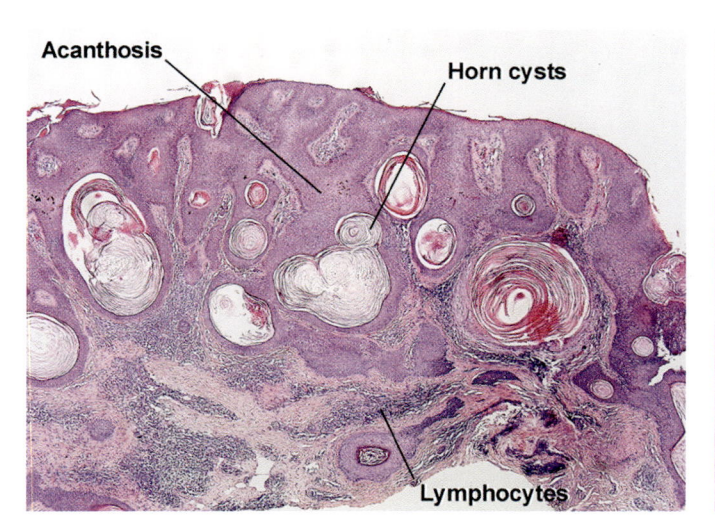

Fig 2-4 Inflamed acanthotic seborrheic keratosis

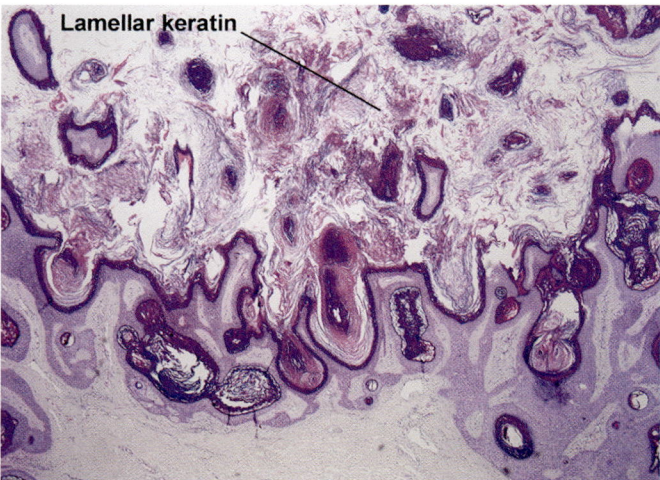

Fig 2-5 Hyperkeratotic seborrheic keratosis

Hyperkeratotic seborrheic keratosis

Key features

- Tall stacks of loose lamellar "shredded-wheat" keratin
- Papillomatosis – hills and dales that may produce a "church-spire" appearance

The tall stacked stratum corneum is typically much thicker than the epidermis. As in other forms of seborrheic keratosis, the keratin has a loose lamellar "shredded-wheat" appearance unless the lesion has become irritated or inflamed. Papillomatosis is characteristic, but variable in degree. Horn cysts are inconspicuous or absent.

40 Dermatopathology

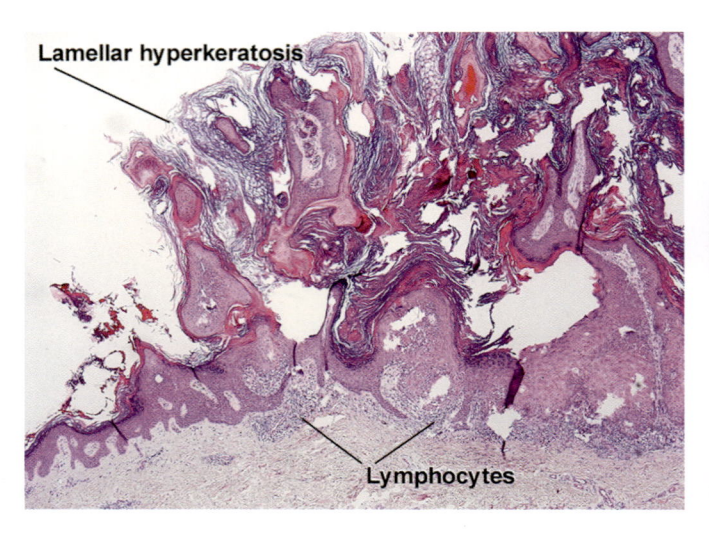

Fig 2-6 Inflamed hyperkeratotic seborrheic keratosis

Reticulated seborrheic keratosis (adenoid seborrheic keratosis)

Key features

- Thin pigmented interlacing downward extensions of the epidermis
- Reticular (lace-like) configuration of epidermis interspersed with horn cysts

The lesion is composed of thin interlacing strands of epidermis, typically two cells thick. These strands are generally pigmented.

Differential Diagnosis

Solar lentigo

Key features

- Shares thin pigmented interlacing extension of the epidermis
- These are shorter and more bulbous than those in reticulated seborrheic keratosis
- Lacks horn cysts

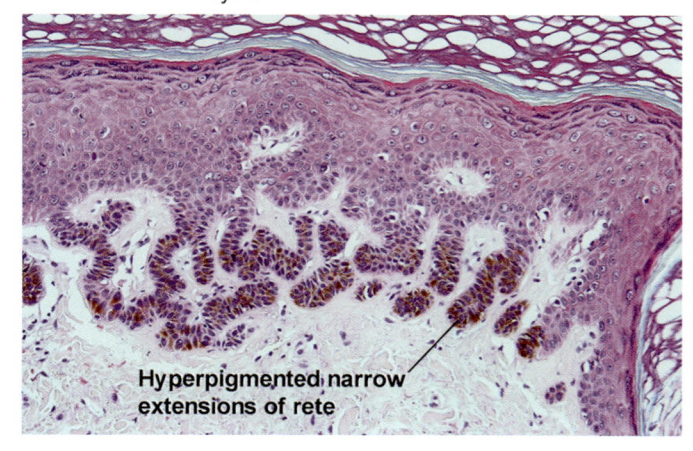

Fig 2-8 Solar lentigo

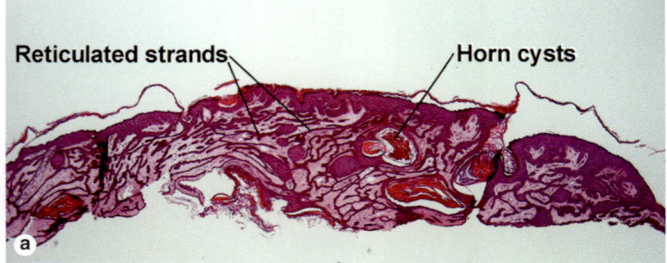

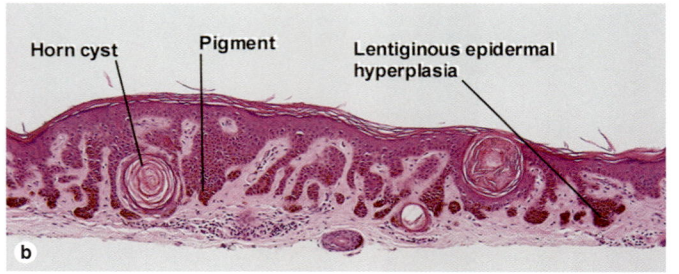

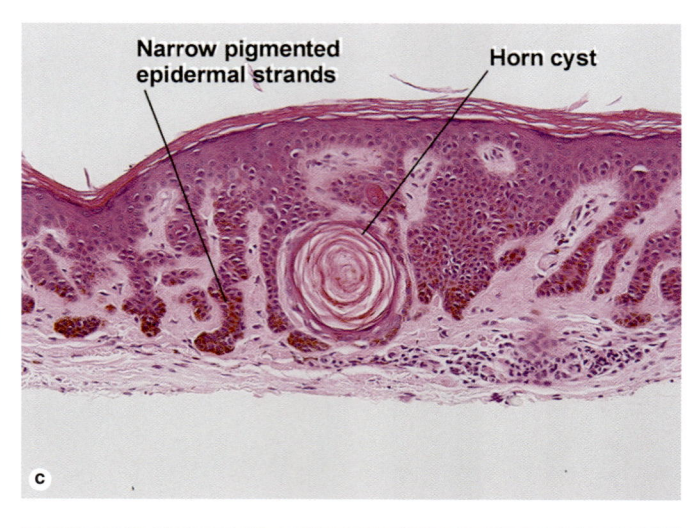

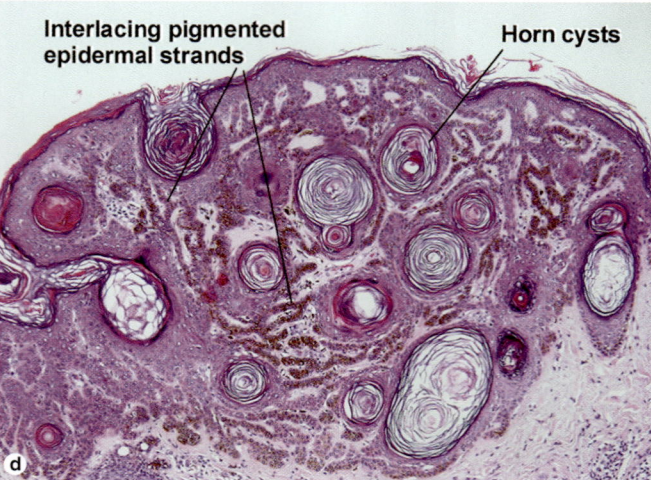

Fig 2-7 Reticulated seborrheic keratosis

Dowling–Degos disease/reticulated pigmented anomaly of the flexures

Key features

- Resembles multiple foci of reticulated seborrheic keratosis "hanging off" hair follicles
- Comedo-like dilated keratin-filled follicular infundibula

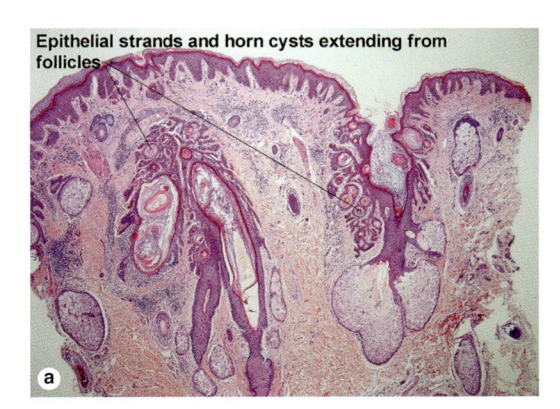

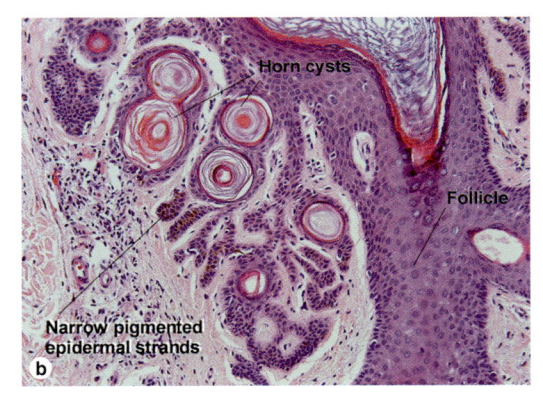

Fig 2-9 Dowling–Degos disease

Clonal seborrheic keratosis

Key features

- Clonal islands of small keratinocytes within the epidermis
- Bland uniform nuclei
- Absence of duct differentiation within clonal nests

Clonal seborrheic keratosis is characterized by islands of small keratinocytes with uniform bland nuclei. The nests are embedded within the epidermis. Sometimes, the nests are large enough that the normal epidermis is reduced to thin strands separating the large nests. Horn cysts are usually absent. The nests may demonstrate pigment. There may be squamous eddies (irritated seborrheic keratosis), lymphocytes (inflamed seborrheic keratosis), or both. In contrast to Bowen's disease, the cells are uniform and atypia is absent. In contrast to hidroacanthoma simplex, no ducts are present within the clones.

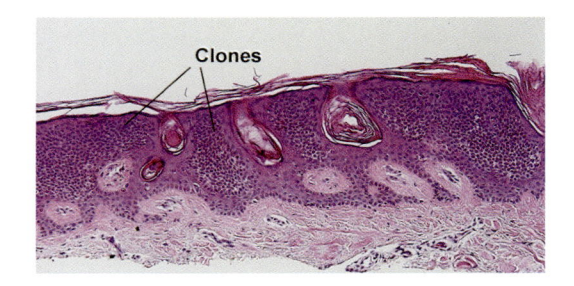

Fig 2-10 Clonal seborrheic keratosis

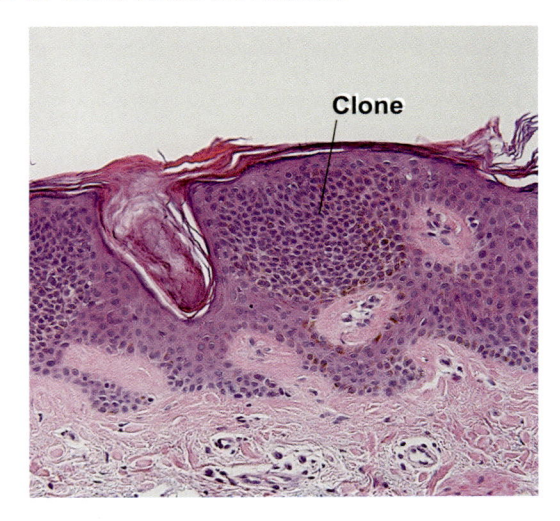

Fig 2-11 Pigmented clonal seborrheic keratosis

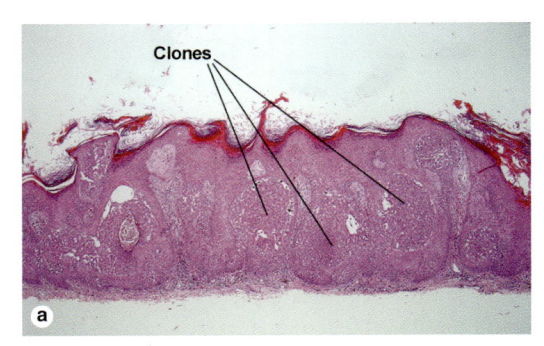

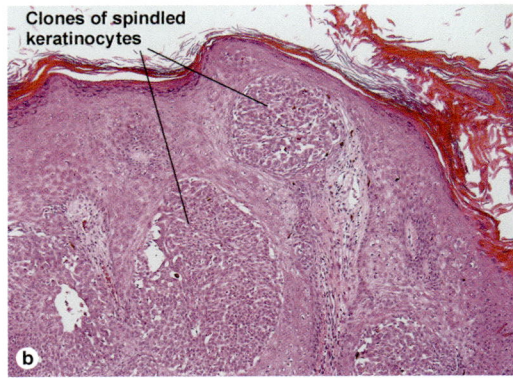

Fig 2-12 Irritated clonal seborrheic keratosis

Dermatopathology

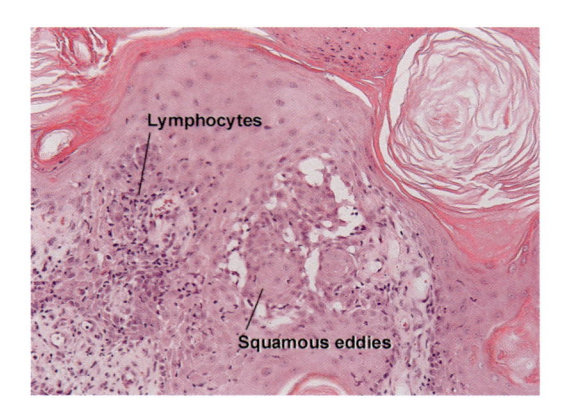

Fig 2-13 Irritated and inflamed clonal seborrheic keratosis

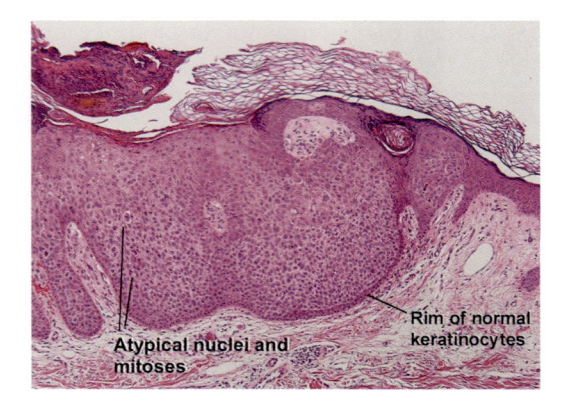

Fig 2-15 Clonal Bowen's disease

Differential Diagnosis

Hidroacanthoma simplex

Key features

- Clonal islands of small keratinocytes similar in appearance to those of clonal seborrheic keratosis
- Ducts present focally within the clonal islands

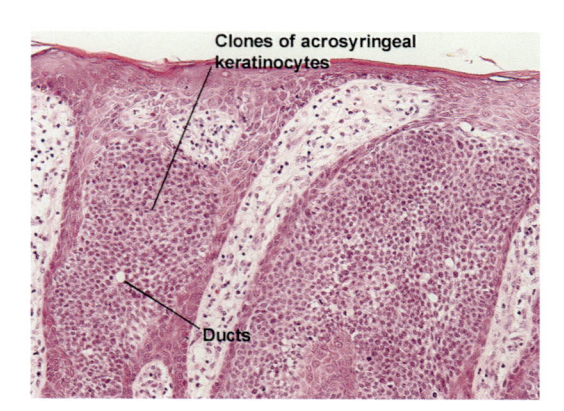

Fig 2-14 Hidroacanthoma simplex

Bowen's disease

Key features

- Clonal islands of atypical keratinocytes within the epidermis
- Cells may be anaplastic or glassy and eosinophilic
- Buckshot scatter of cells may be present focally
- Apoptotic keratinocytes commonly scattered within nests
- Overlying stratum corneum becomes compact and parakeratotic where clones touch surface
- More typical Bowen's disease may be present in the adjacent skin

Pigmented seborrheic keratosis

Key features

- Pigment within keratinocytes
- May be acanthotic, hyperkeratotic, reticulated, or clonal
- When clonal, the pigment is restricted to the clonal islands

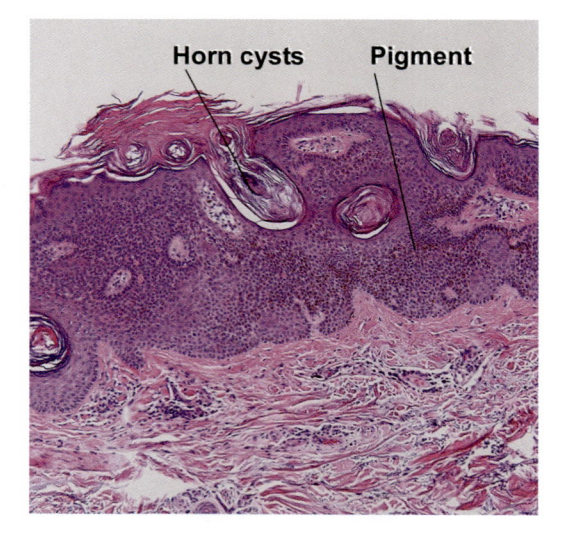

Fig 2-16 Pigmented seborrheic keratosis

Irritated seborrheic keratosis

Key features

- Squamous eddies
- Spindled keratinocytes
- Horn cysts common
- Keratin commonly becomes compact, eosinophilic, and parakeratotic
- Keratin often retains a loose lamellar pattern in some areas

Benign tumors and cysts of the epidermis   Chapter 2   43

Irritated seborrheic keratosis is characterized by the formation of squamous eddies within the epidermis and the presence of spindled keratinocytes. Some areas of the tumor typically still produce a loose lamellar "shredded-wheat" pattern of keratin, and horn cysts composed of loose lamellar keratin are often present. In areas, the keratin becomes compact, eosinophilic, and parakeratotic. A zone of loose lamellar keratin may be seen above the dense eosinophilic keratin. This was produced before the lesion became irritated. It has since been pushed upward.

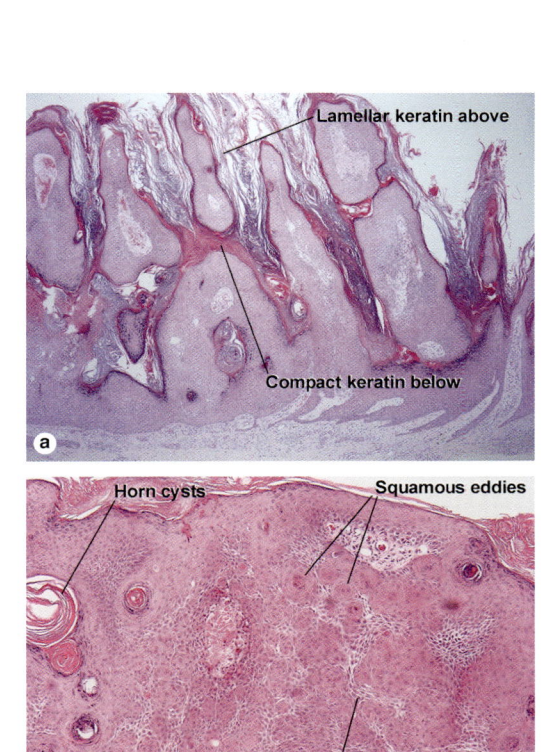

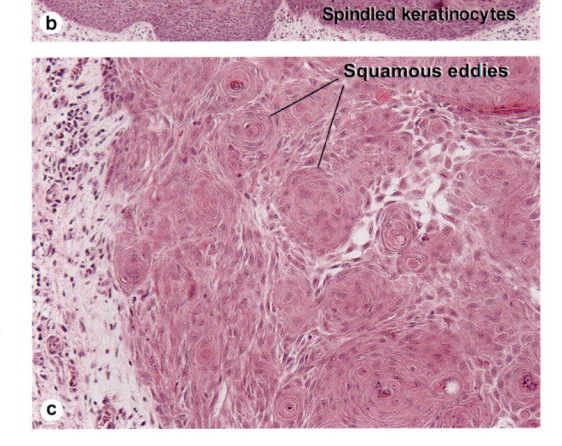

Fig 2-17 Irritated seborrheic keratosis with prominent squamous eddies

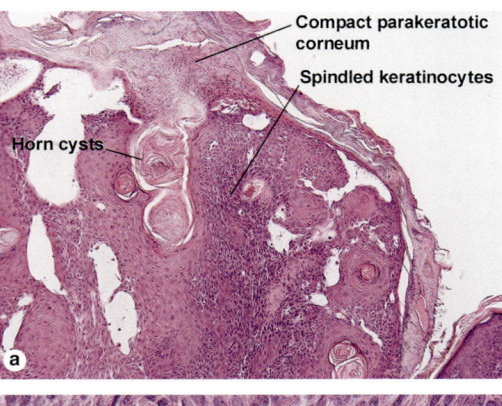

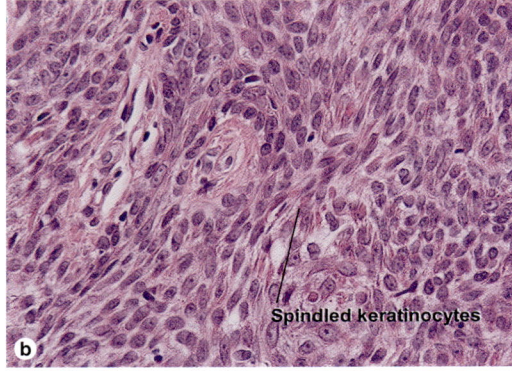

Fig 2-18 Irritated seborrheic keratosis with prominent spindling of keratinocytes

Inflamed seborrheic keratosis

Key features

- Lymphocytes and spongiosis
- In areas, the stratum corneum becomes compact, eosinophilic, and parakeratotic
- Loose lamellar keratin is commonly retained in other areas
- Horn cysts are common
- Lichenoid interface dermatitis may be present
- An overlying crust may be present

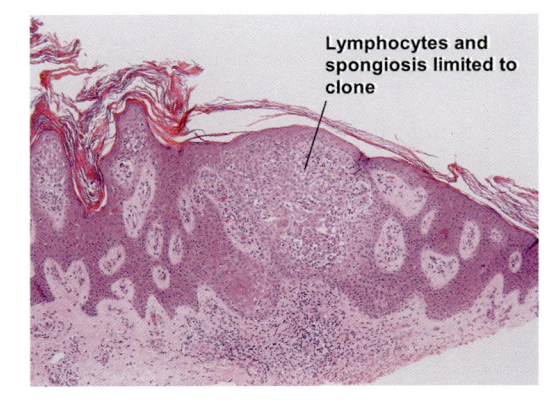

Fig 2-19 Inflamed seborrheic keratosis with lymphocytes and spongiosis

Inflamed seborrheic keratosis is characterized by lymphocytes and spongiosis within the epidermis or the presence of lichenoid interface dermatitis. Some areas of the tumor typically still produce a loose lamellar "shredded-wheat" pattern of keratin, and horn cysts composed of loose lamellar keratin are often present. As in irritated seborrheic keratoses, a zone of loose lamellar keratin may sometimes be seen above a zone of dense eosinophilic keratin. When clonal, the spongiosis and lymphoid infiltrate are typically restricted to the clonal islands.

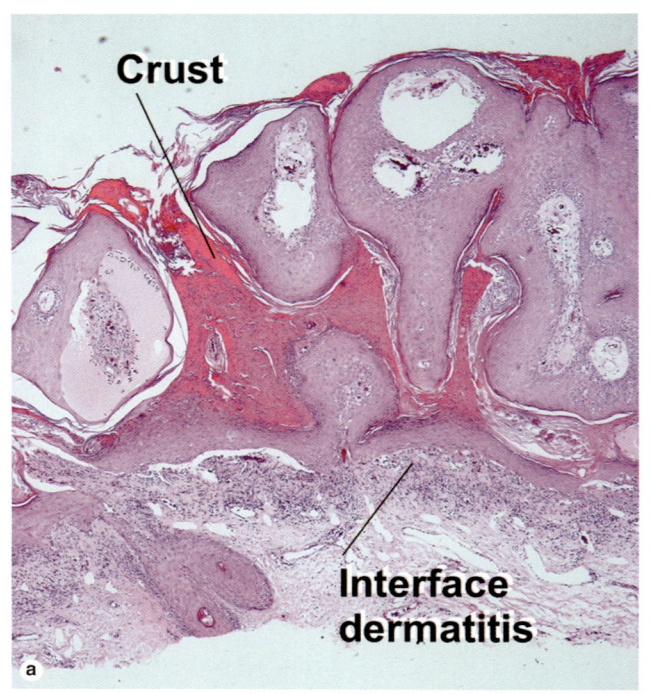

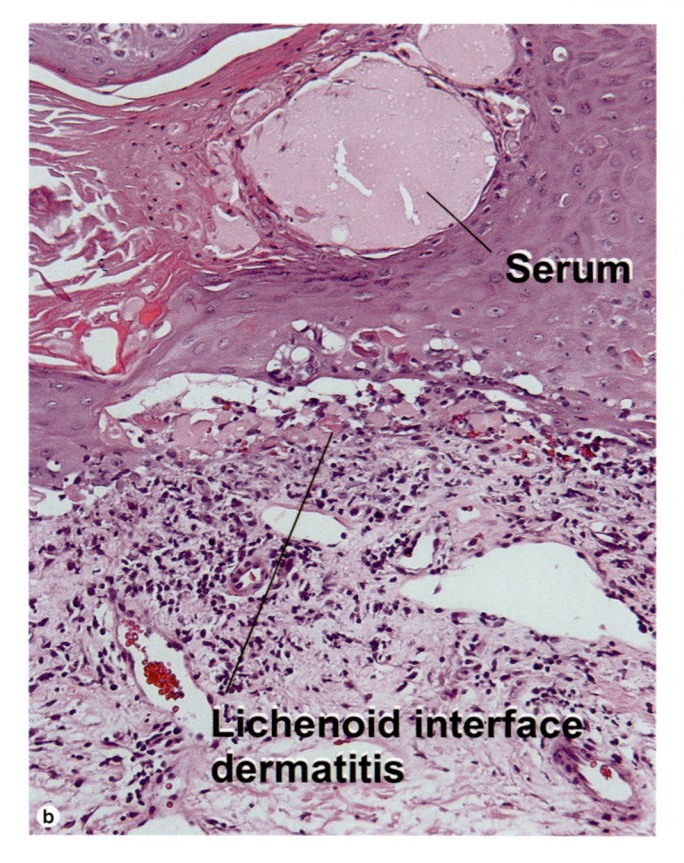

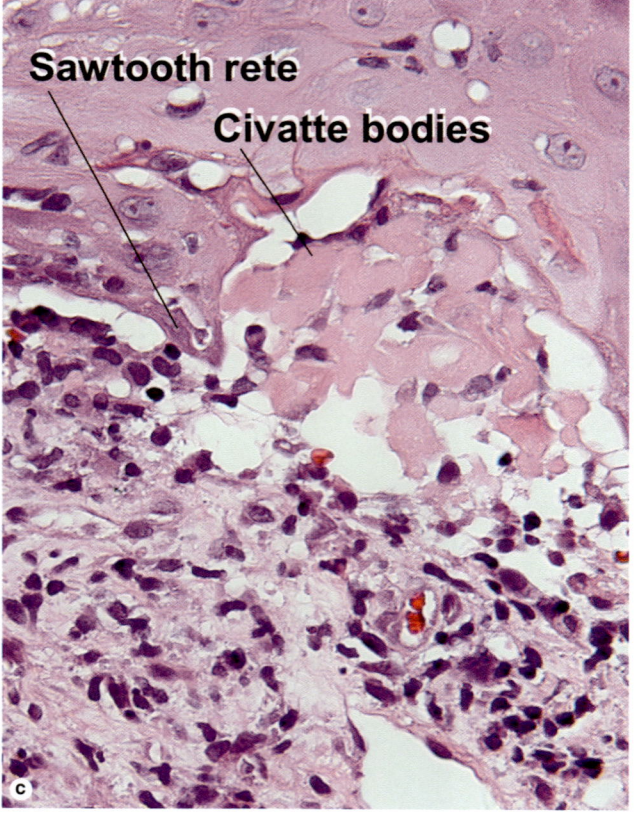

Fig 2-20 Inflamed seborrheic keratosis with lichenoid interface dermatitis

Melanoacanthoma

Key features

- Acanthoma composed of both small keratinocytes and pigmented dendritic melanocytes
- Most pigment is within dendrites
- Overlying stratum corneum is almost always compact eosinophilic and parakeratotic

Cutaneous melanoacanthomas are a type of seborrheic keratosis, composed of both small cuboidal keratinocytes and pigmented dendritic melanocytes. Most melanin pigment is contained within the melanocytic dendrites with little visible pigment within the keratinocytes. Unlike most seborrheic keratoses, horn cysts and loose lamellar horn are typically absent. Instead, the overlying stratum corneum is almost always compact, eosinophilic, and parakeratotic. Cutaneous melanoacanthomas may be clonal. Oral melanoacanthomas are reactive proliferations unrelated to seborrheic keratosis.

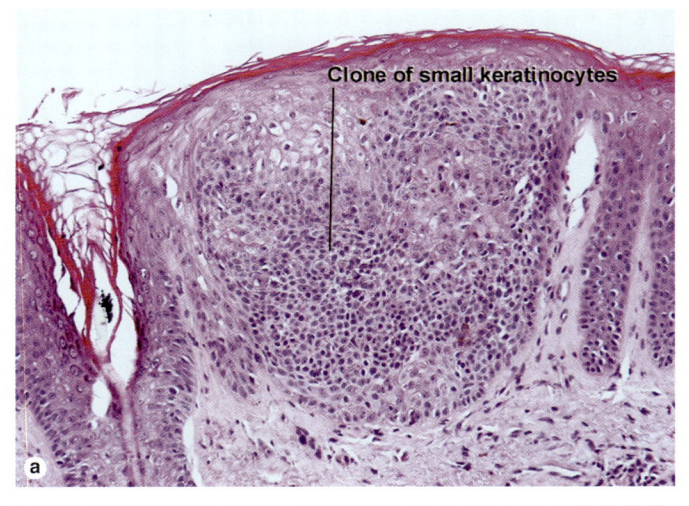

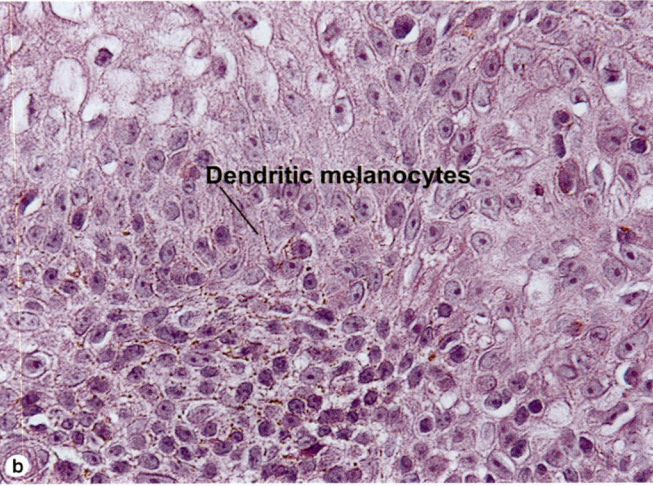

Fig 2-21 Melanoacanthoma

Clear cell acanthoma (pale cell acanthoma)

Key features

- Discrete acanthoma with overlying parakeratosis
- Distinct transition between the normal epidermis and the clearer/paler cells in the stratum spinosum
- Peppered with neutrophils

Clear cell acanthomas are recognizable as a clearly defined acanthotic area of the epidermis with ample clear or pale cytoplasm. A thin overlying parakeratotic scale crust is present, and there is a distinct transition between surrounding normal stratum corneum and the parakeratotic stratum corneum as well as between the normal epidermis and the paler cells comprising the acanthoma. Neutrophils are scattered throughout the lesion. The cells of the acanthoma are deficient in phosphorylase, resulting in an accumulation of glycogen.

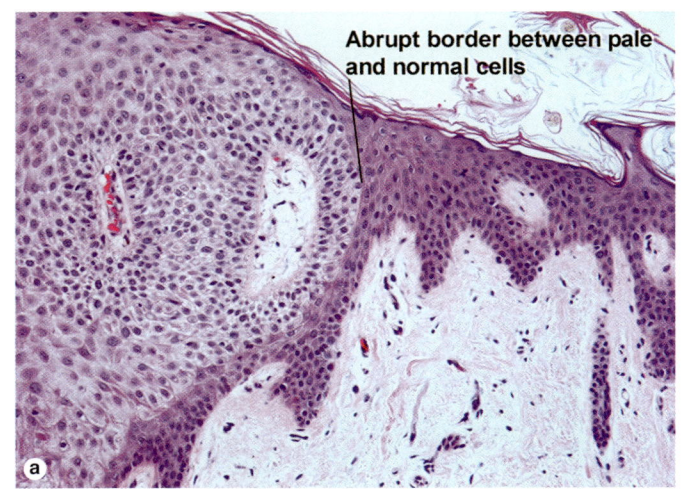

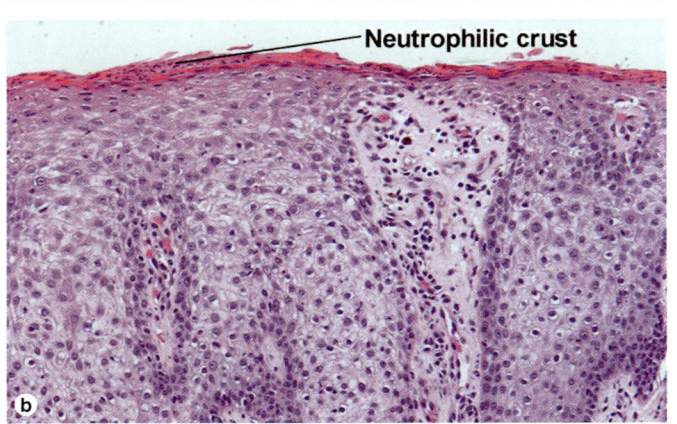

Fig 2-22 Clear cell acanthoma

Large cell acanthoma

Key features

- Discrete acanthoma composed of cells with large nuclei
- Overlying lamellar hyperkeratosis is common
- May be pigmented

Dermatopathology

The rete ridges may be bulbous or there may be a solid plate-like acanthosis. The cells composing the acanthoma have large nuclei, typically twice the size of the nuclei in the surrounding epidermis.

Large cell acanthomas represent a heterogeneous group of lesions. The most common type presents as a slightly hyperkeratotic pigmented patch, resembling a solar lentigo. Other lesions are erythematous. Many appear to represent a histologic variant of solar lentigo, others of Bowen's disease. The cells of some lesions have been shown to be aneuploid, and no histologic features predict which lesions demonstrate aneuploid populations. Because of this, many clinicians prefer to destroy any remaining lesion by means of cryotherapy.

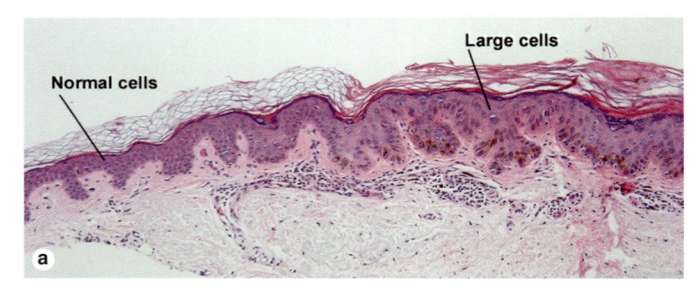

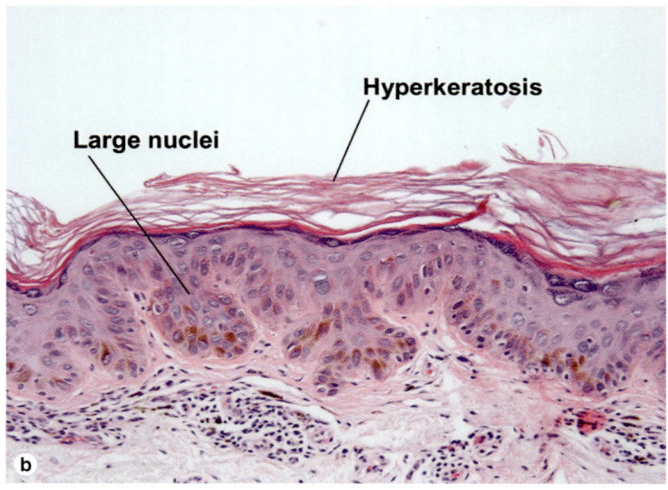

Fig 2-23 Large cell acanthoma

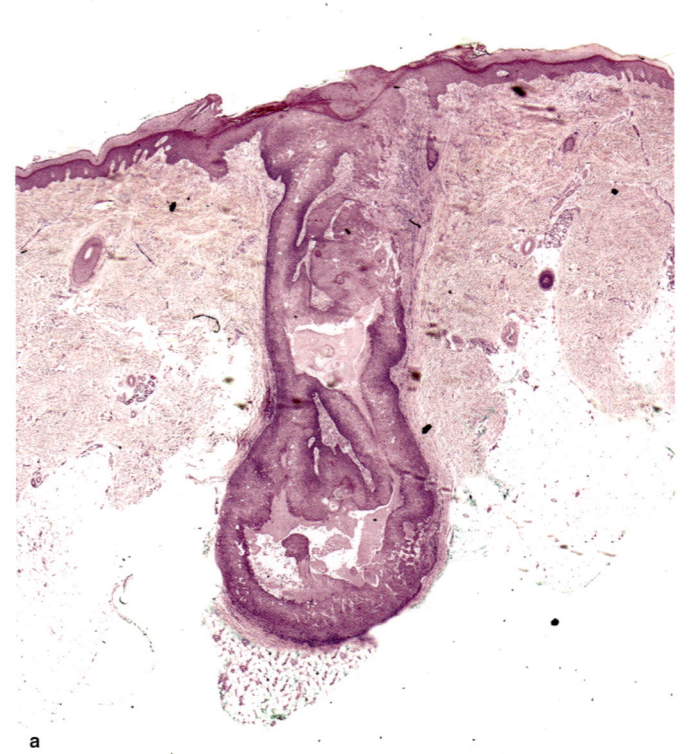

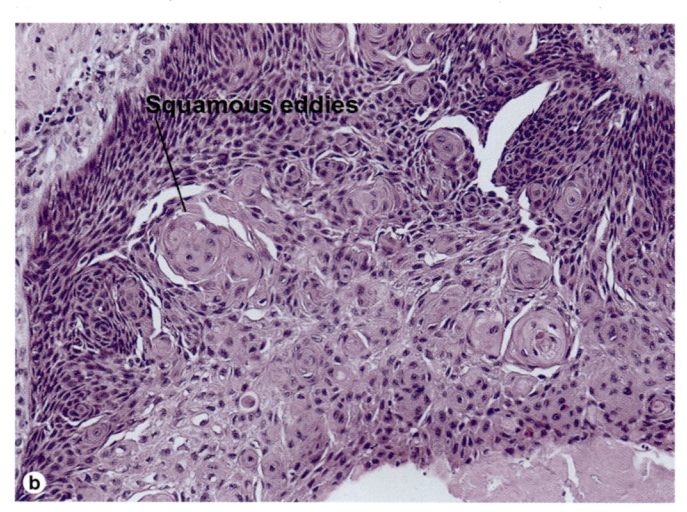

Fig 2-24 Inverted follicular keratosis

Inverted follicular keratosis (IFK)

Key features

- Endophytic lesion resembling an expanded hair follicle
- Squamous eddies

The outline of the epithelial column is smooth, with no evidence of jagged invasive growth.

True inverted follicular keratoses are benign follicular proliferations unrelated to human papillomavirus infection. Multiple lesions may be associated with Cowden's syndrome. Follicular warts may sometimes have squamous eddies and resemble IFK.

Warty dyskeratoma

Key features

- Endophytic growth
- Acantholytic dyskeratosis
- Overlying parakeratotic crust may be present

Two types of dyskeratotic cells are noted. Corps ronds are round dyskeratotic cells that stain pale pink to red, and may have a wide clear halo surrounding the nucleus. Grains are flattened basophilic dyskeratotic cells. Either or both may be present. Some lesions are crateriform; others resemble expanded hair follicles.

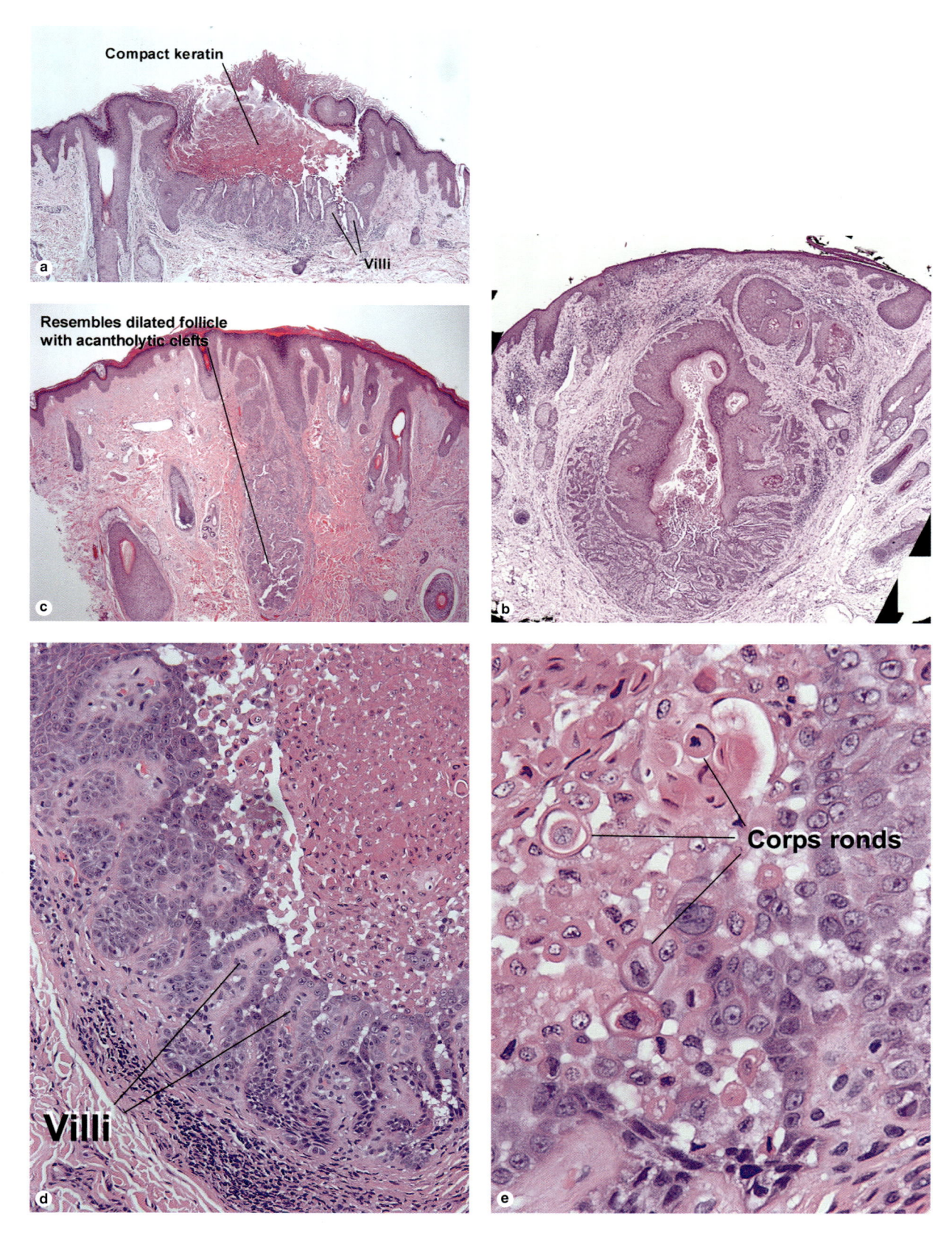

Fig 2-25 Warty dyskeratoma

Acantholytic acanthoma

Key features

- Acanthoma composed of bland keratinocytes
- Acantholysis

The appearance resembles the "dilapidated brick wall" of Hailey–Hailey disease.

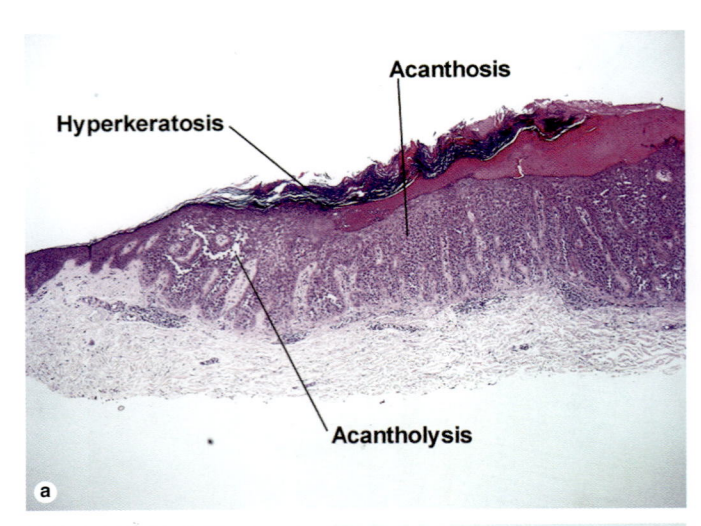

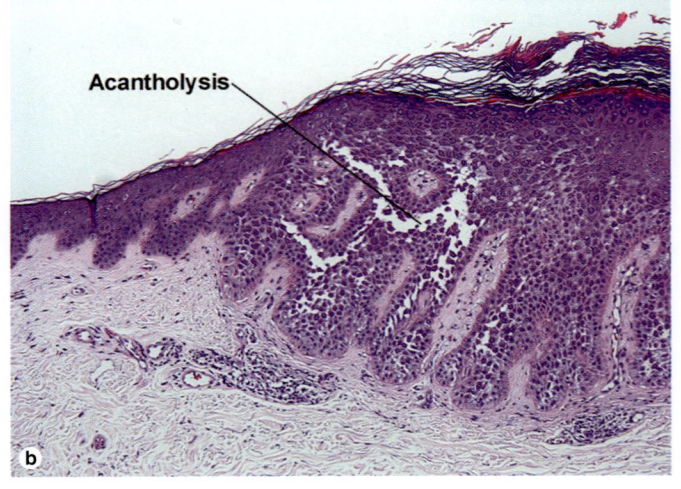

Fig 2-26 Acantholytic acanthoma

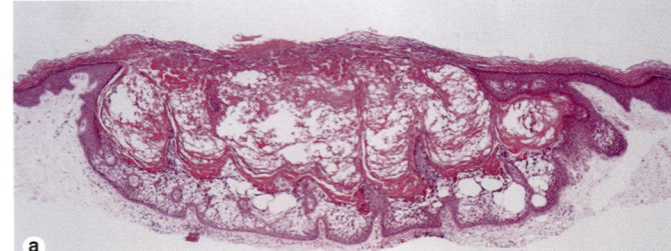

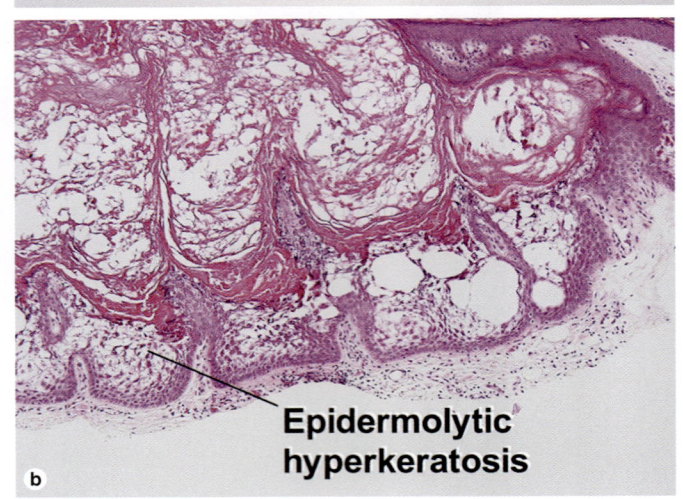

Epidermolytic acanthoma

Key features

- Often crateriform
- Epidermolytic hyperkeratosis

Epidermolytic acanthomas are characterized by epidermolytic hyperkeratosis. The granular layer is thick and contains irregularly shaped keratohyalin granules and cytoplasmic borders are indistinct. Clinically, the lesions are solitary discrete acanthomas resembling seborrheic keratoses.

Fig 2-27 Epidermolytic acanthoma

Epidermal nevi

Key features

- Discrete acanthomas or hyperkeratotic lesions

Epidermal nevi are typically present at or near birth. Linear epidermal nevi follow Blaschko's lines and may represent mosaicism, via post-zygotic somatic mutation, lyonization of X chromosomes, or loss of heterozygosity. Patients with multiple epidermal nevi may have associated eye, central nervous, and musculoskeletal abnormalities.

Common epidermal nevus

Key features

- Resembles seborrheic keratosis

Inflammatory linear verrucous epidermal nevus (ILVEN)

Key features

- Variable acanthosis
- Stratum corneum with alternating orthokeratosis and parakeratosis
- Parakeratotic areas have no granular layer
- Orthokeratotic areas have a granular layer

The name "inflammatory" linear verrucous epidermal nevus relates to the erythematous clinical appearance of the lesions. Orthokeratosis and parakeratosis alternate from right to left.

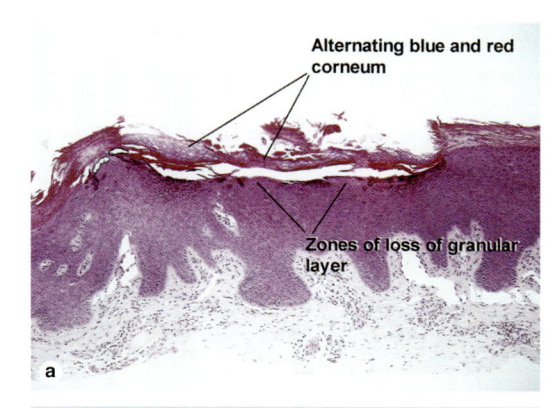

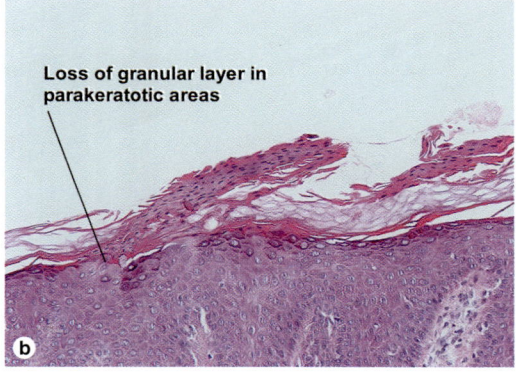

Fig 2-28 ILVEN

Epidermoid cysts often connect to the surface with a visible punctum. This connection may be visible histologically. In a young cyst, a rete ridge pattern may be present. As tension increases within the cyst, the lining is stretched and the rete pattern disappears. Ruptured cysts demonstrate a neutrophilic infiltrate, histiocytes, and foreign-body giant cells. Flat bits of keratin are noted within giant cells.

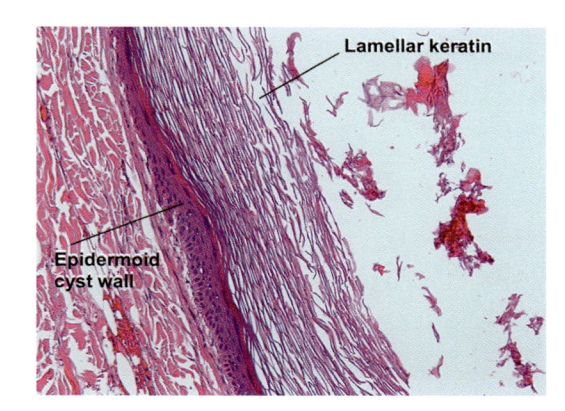

Fig 2-29 Epidermoid cyst

Differential Diagnosis

Blaschkoid epidermolytic hyperkeratosis (EHK)

Key features

- Resembles epidermal nevus clinically
- Epidermolytic hyperkeratosis histologically
- Represents mosaicism for keratin 1 and 10 mutations
- Patient can pass on the mutation and have a child with generalized EHK, known as epidermolytic ichthyosis (bullous congenial ichthyosiform erythroderma)

Widely separated lesions involving different parts of the body suggest that the mutation occurred in the embryo prior to gastrulation. In this case, the affected cell line is more likely to contribute to many organ tissues, including the gonads.

Cysts

Epidermoid cyst (epidermal inclusion cyst, infundibular cyst)

Key features

- Lining resembles the surface epidermis, but with no adnexal structures
- Loose lamellar "onion-skin" keratin within the cyst

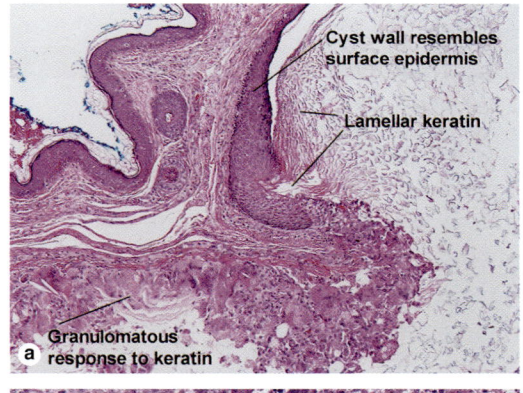

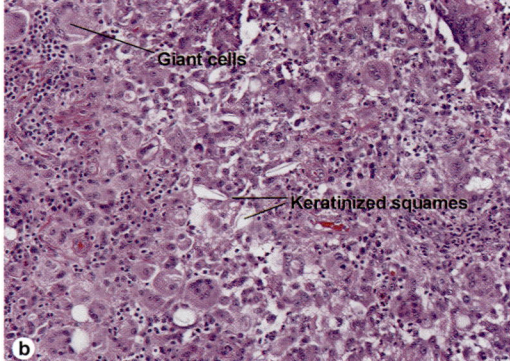

Fig 2-30 Ruptured and inflamed epidermoid cyst

Epidermoid cyst with pilomatrical differentiation

Key features

- Areas of ghost cell keratinization as in a pilomatricoma
- Associated with Gardner's syndrome

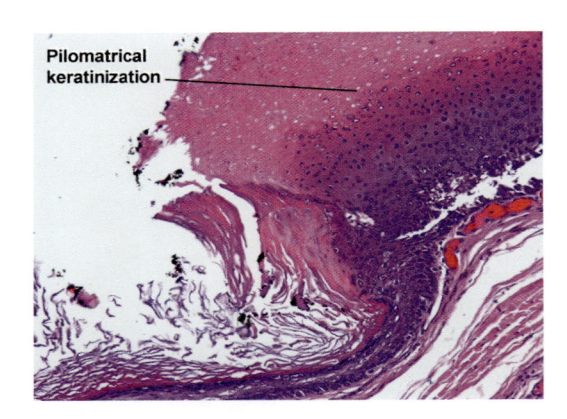

Fig 2-31 Epidermoid cyst with pilomatrical differentiation

Vellus hair cyst

Key features

- Wall resembles that of an epidermoid cyst
- Many small vellus hairs within the cyst
- Frequently arise in an eruptive fashion

Eruptive vellus hair cysts may coexist with steatocystomas, and individual cysts may have features of both. Eruptive vellus hair cysts have been reported in association with renal failure and Lowe syndrome (Fanconi-type renal failure, mental retardation, and eye abnormalities).

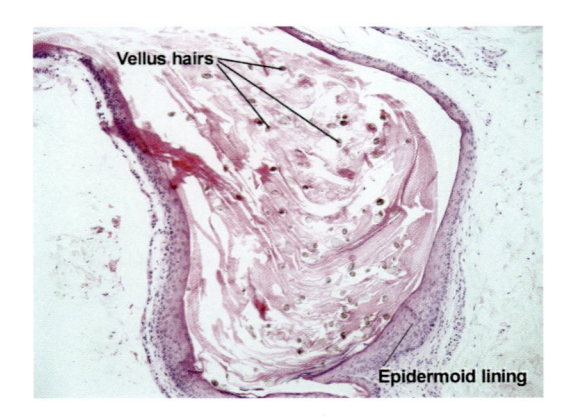

Fig 2-32 Vellus hair cyst

Dermoid cyst

Key features

- Wall commonly resembles that of an epidermoid cyst
- Adnexal structures within cyst wall

Adnexal structures within the cyst wall may include terminal hair follicles, sebaceous glands, eccrine glands, and apocrine glands. Terminal hair shafts are commonly noted within the cyst contents. Lamellar keratin is typically present, although some dermoid cysts demonstrate a bright red "shark-tooth" lining similar to that of a steatocystoma. Dermoid cysts occur in embryonic fusion planes and may be associated with underlying skull defects.

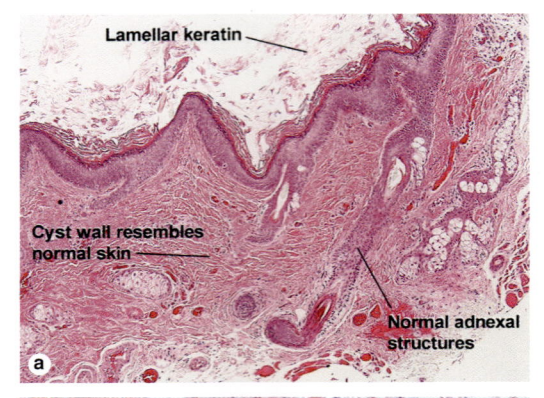

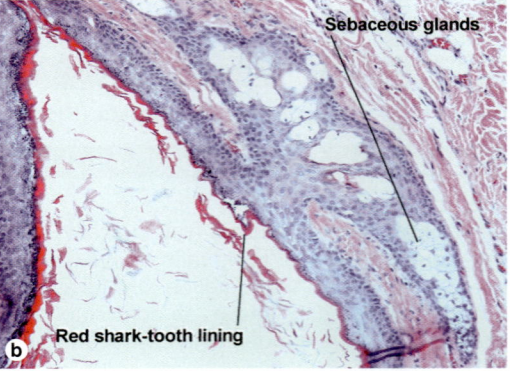

Fig 2-33 Dermoid cyst

Pilar cyst (trichilemmal cyst, isthmus catagen cyst)

Key features

- Abrupt keratinization without a granular layer
- Deeply eosinophilic dense keratin
- Focal calcification of contents common
- Typically on scalp
- Often multiple

Benign tumors and cysts of the epidermis   Chapter 2   51

The abrupt keratinization of pilar cysts resembles that of the outer root sheath (the trichilemma).

As the epithelium proliferates, the wall buckles inward, rolling on itself and producing a trabecular or scroll-like appearance ("rolls and scrolls"). A diagnosis of trichilemmal carcinoma should be suspected in tumors with a location other than scalp, recent rapid growth, size greater than 5 cm, infiltrative growth, significant cytologic atypia, and mitotic activity.

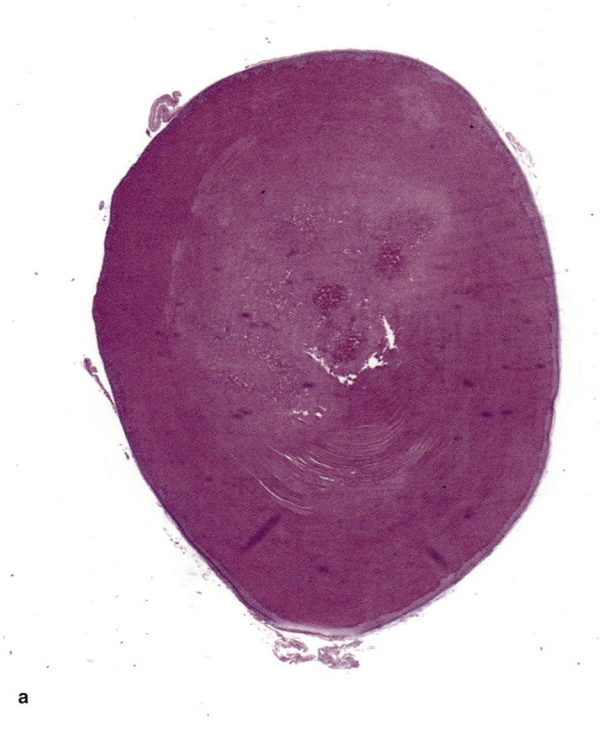

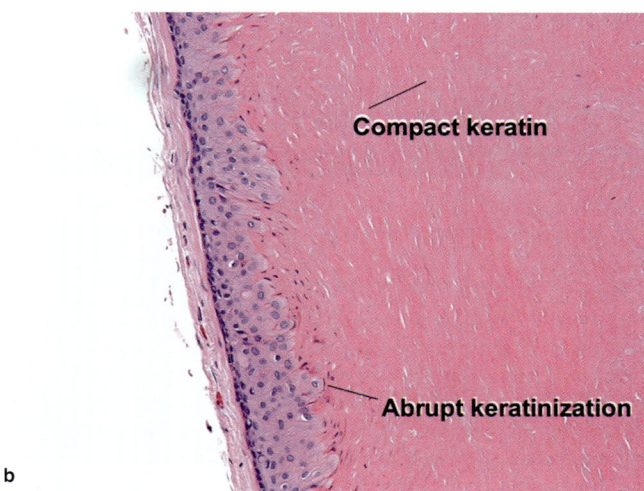

Fig 2-34 Pilar cyst

Proliferating pilar cyst

Key features
- Rolls and scrolls
- May form small new cysts within the confines of the mother cyst
- Trichilemmal keratinization

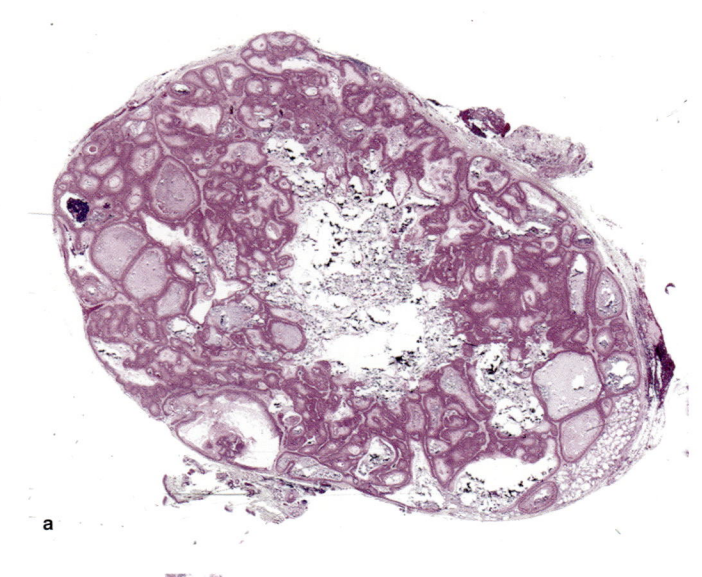

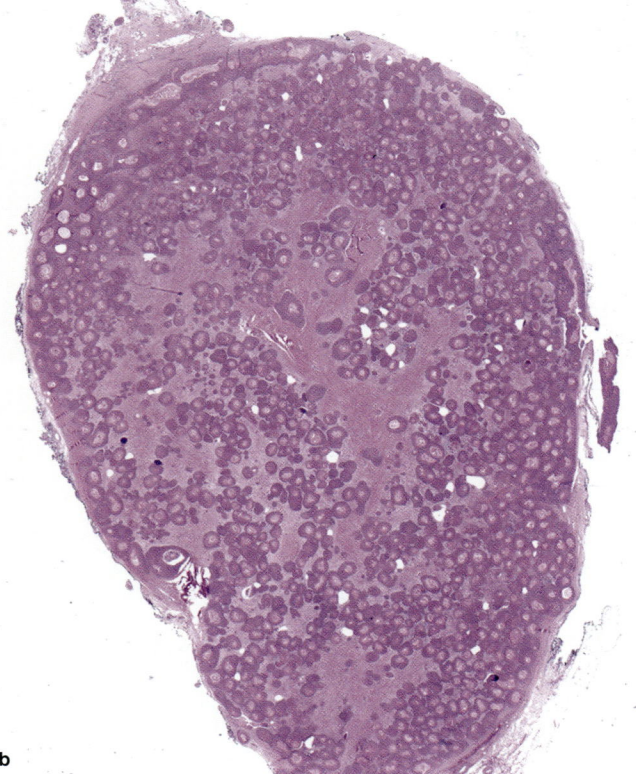

Fig 2-35 Proliferating pilar cyst

Continued

52 Dermatopathology

Fig 2-35, cont'd

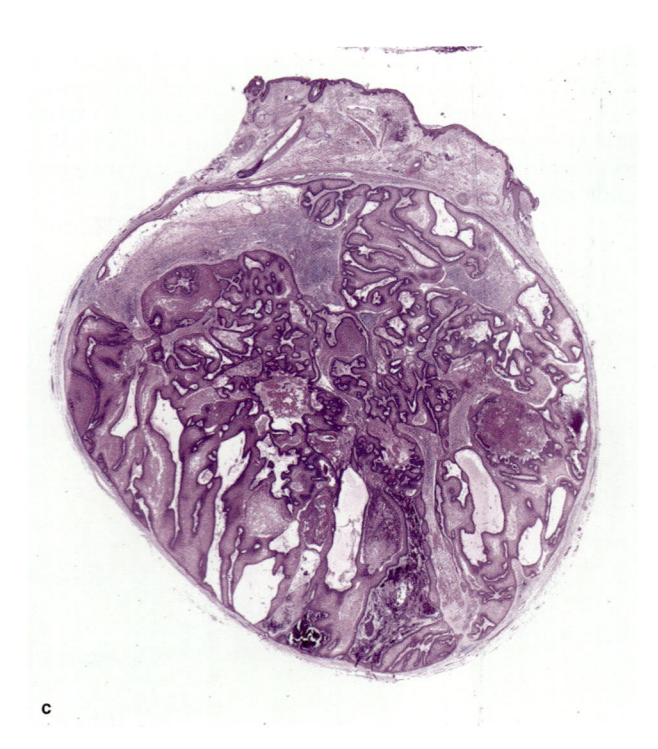

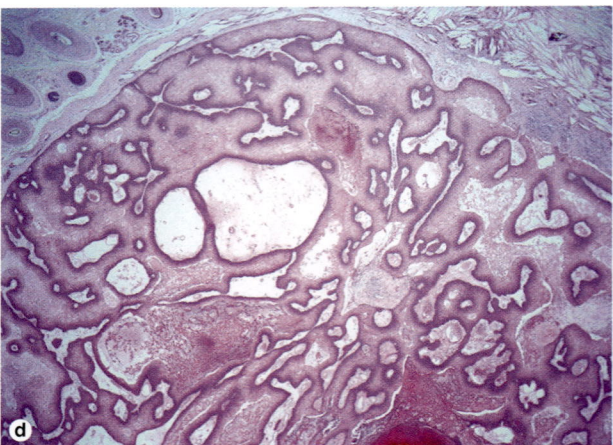

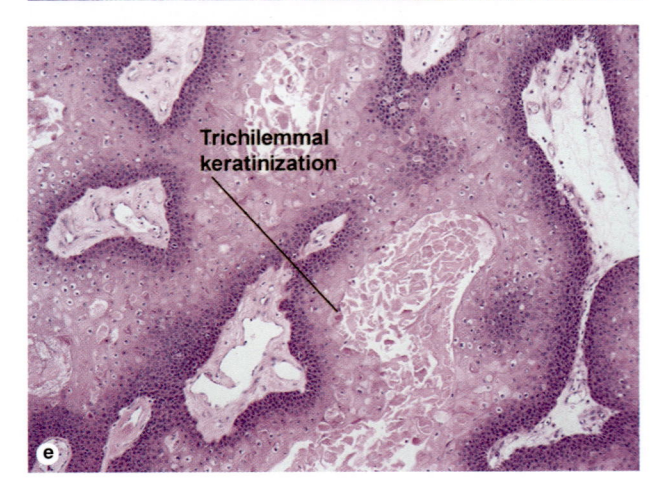

Differential Diagnosis
Pilomatricoma

Key features
- Rolls and scrolls
- Ghost cell keratinization, see page 73

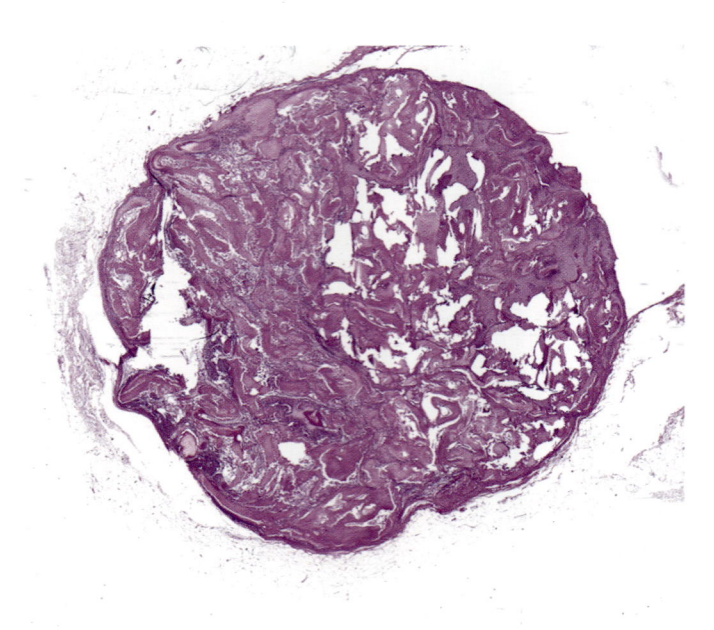

Fig 2-36 Pilomatricoma

Branchial cleft cyst

Key features
- Epidermoid or pseudostratified columnar epithelium
- Lymphoid tissue with germinal centers surrounding the cyst
- Cyst usually appears empty

Branchial cleft cysts are generally found on the lateral part of the neck, anterior to the sternocleidomastoid muscle. They may occur as a result of failure of obliteration of the second branchial cleft in embryonic development. Phylogenetically, the branchial apparatus may be related to gill slits. This analogy is helpful in remembering the typical location on the lateral neck. They are the most common cause of a congenital neck mass, and 2–3% of cases are bilateral.

Although the classic teaching has been that branchial cleft cysts and bronchogenic cysts are embryologically distinct, cases with overlap in distribution and histology occur. In general, branchial cleft cysts are far more likely to occur on the side of the neck, and to demonstrate lymphoid follicles and stratified squamous epithelium. Although smooth muscle may occur, it is rare.

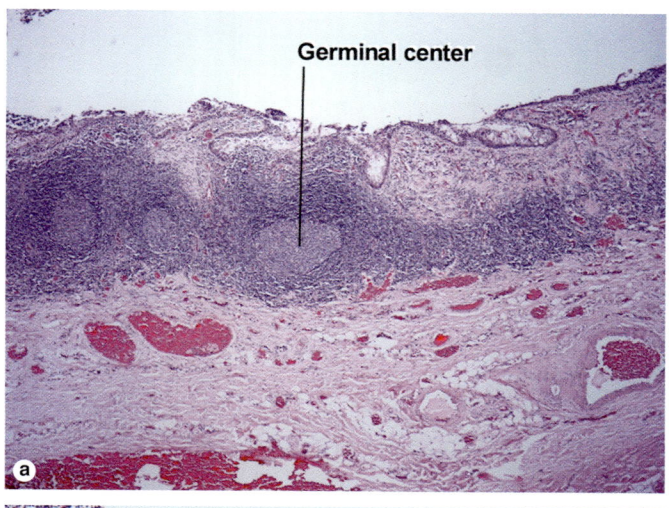

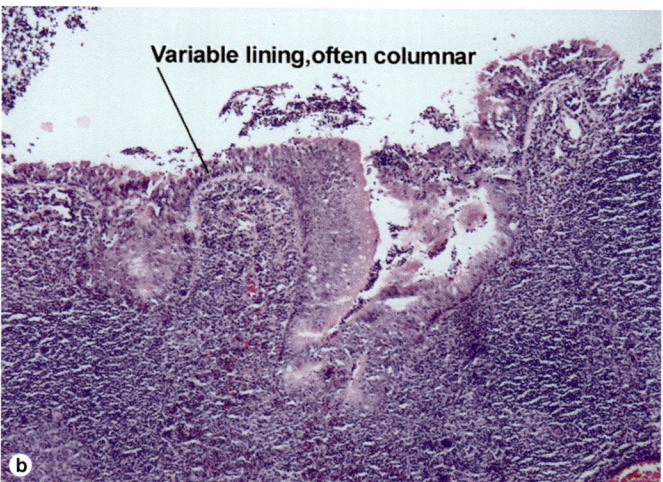

Fig 2-37 Branchial cleft cyst

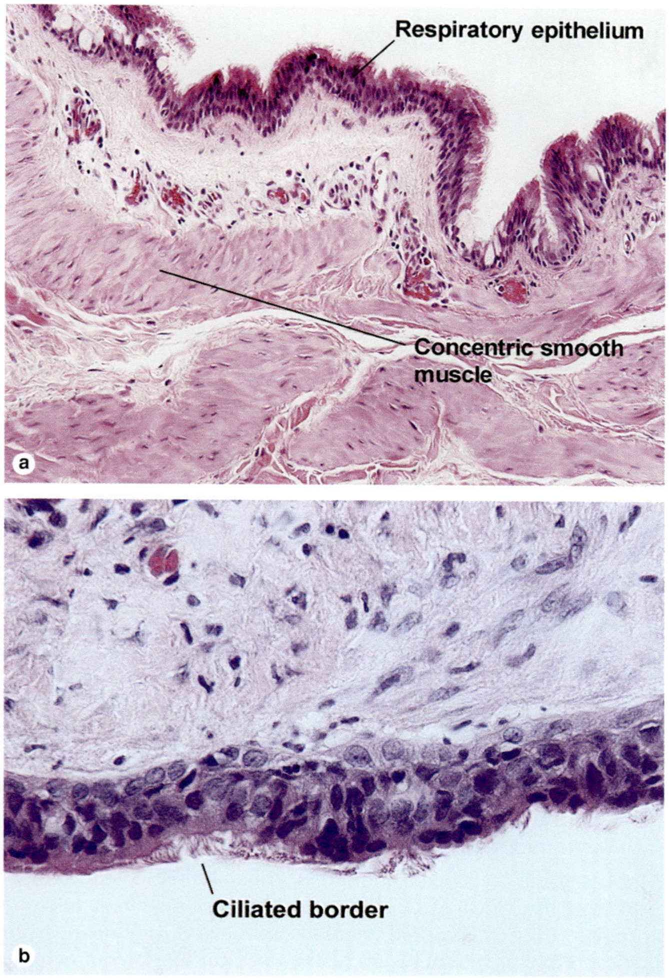

Fig 2-38 Bronchogenic cyst

Bronchogenic cyst

Key features

- Ciliated pseudostratified columnar epithelium
- Goblet cells
- May have circumferential smooth muscle around cyst
- May have cartilage

Bronchogenic cysts are typically midline lesions, located in the suprasternal notch. Bronchogenic cysts are thought to result from remnants of the primitive foregut. Although bronchogenic cysts occur predominantly within the chest, *cutaneous* lesions generally present as neck lesions in children.

As compared with branchial cleft cysts, bronchogenic cysts typically lack lymphoid follicles. They typically demonstrate pseudostratified respiratory-type ciliated epithelium, goblet cells, concentric smooth muscle, and cartilage.

Steatocystoma (simple sebaceous duct cyst)

Key features

- Wavy, eosinophilic "shark's-tooth" cuticle
- Sebaceous glands in cyst wall
- Oily contents, frequently containing vellus hairs

Steatocystomas are commonly inherited, with multiple lesions on the chest. The appearance resembles nodulocystic acne. Solitary lesions are common, and sporadic in occurrence. The cyst lining resembles that of the sebaceous duct. Sebaceous glands are common within the cyst wall, but may not be prominent. Some sections lack visible sebaceous glands, but the cyst can still be identified by the characteristic wavy eosinophilic cuticle.

While dermoid cysts may occasionally demonstrate an identical wavy cuticle, they also commonly demonstrate terminal hair follicles, and may have eccrine or apocrine glands within the cyst wall. Grossly, steatocystomas tend to drain oil and collapse when sectioned, while dermoid cysts tend to remain rigid because they contain keratin.

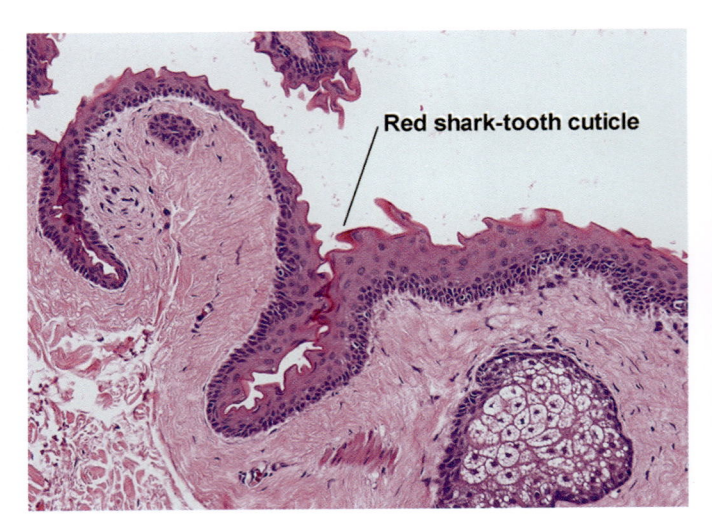

Fig 2-39 Steatocystoma

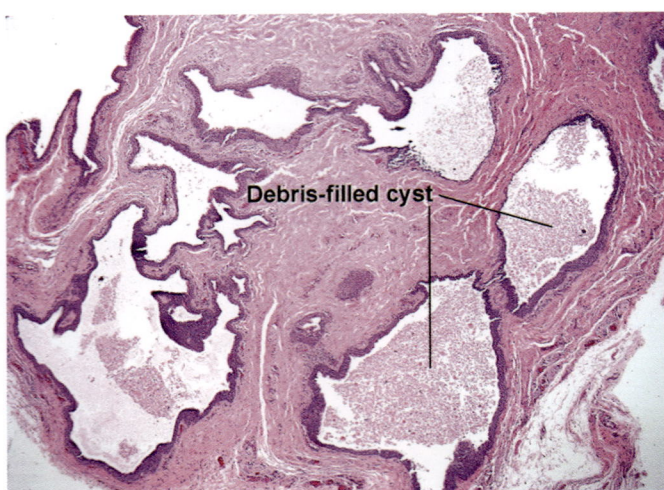

Fig 2-40 Median raphe cyst

Median raphe cyst

Key features

- Midline along anogenital raphe
- Debris-filled cyst
- Lining variable
- Surrounding skin has characteristics of genital skin

Median raphe cysts occur in men in a characteristic ventral location from the meatus to the anus. The cyst may first become apparent after intercourse. Median raphe cysts may result from incomplete embryonic fusion of the urethral folds, from ectopic periurethral glands of Littre, or sequestration of urethral epithelium after closure of the median raphe.

Typically, the cyst is filled with amorphous debris, and the surrounding genital skin is readily identified by the presence of delicate collagen, randomly arranged smooth muscle, many small nerves, and prominent vascularity. Unlike the circumferential smooth muscle of a bronchogenic cyst, the smooth muscle in genital skin has a random, haphazard arrangement throughout the surrounding skin. The cyst wall itself has a highly variable lining. Some areas may appear ciliated, some cuboidal, and some areas may suggest decapitation secretion.

Cutaneous ciliated cyst

Key features

- Similar to median raphe cysts
- Much less likely to occur on genital skin

Although ciliated cysts typically occur on the legs of women, and are thought to relate to Müllerian duct remnants, they are occasionally noted in men. Ciliated cysts are commonly filled with debris, and the appearance of the cyst itself can be indistinguishable from that of a median raphe cyst. Helpful differentiating features are the location, sex of the patient, and characteristics of the surrounding skin. As ciliated cysts commonly occur on the legs, the skin lacks the typical appearance of genital skin.

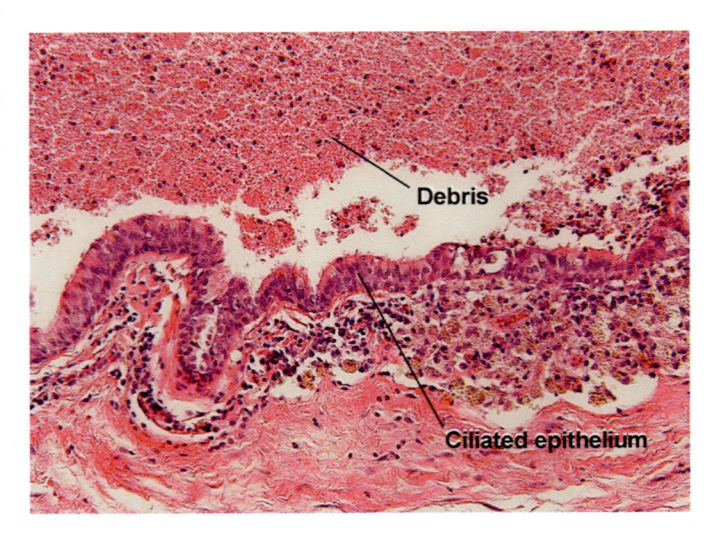

Fig 2-41 Cutaneous ciliated cyst

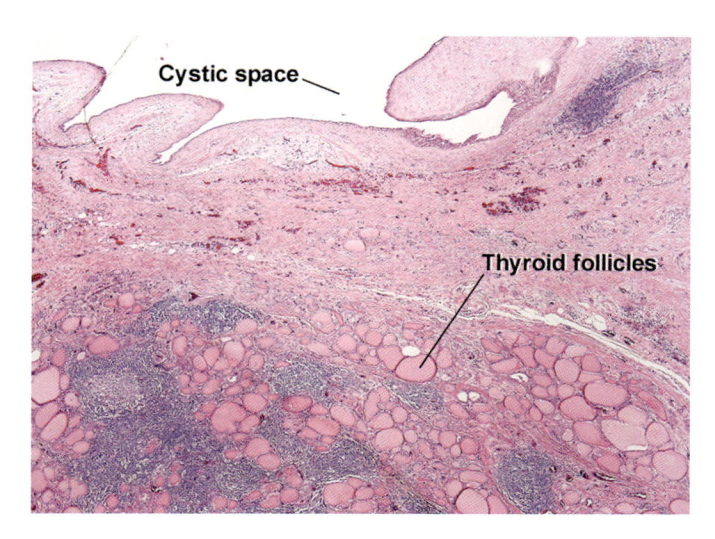

Fig 2-42 Thyroglossal duct cyst

Thyroglossal duct cyst

Key features

- Midline of neck
- Typically lined by respiratory-type epithelium
- May be lined by squamous epithelium
- Surrounding thyroid follicles and lymphoid aggregates may be present

Further reading

Abbas O, Wieland CN, Goldberg LJ. Solitary epidermolytic acanthoma: a clinical and histopathological study. J Eur Acad Dermatol Venereol 2011;25(2):175–180.

Argenyi ZB, Huston BM, Argenyi EE, et al. Large-cell acanthoma of the skin. A study by image analysis cytometry and immunohistochemistry. Am J Dermatopathol 1994;16(2):140–144.

Cho S, Chang SE, Choi JH, et al. Clinical and histologic features of 64 cases of steatocystoma multiplex. J Dermatol 2002;29(3):152–156.

Folpe AL, Reisenauer AK, Mentzel T, et al. Proliferating trichilemmal tumors: clinicopathologic evaluation is a guide to biologic behavior. J Cutan Pathol 2003;30(8):492–498.

Fornatora ML, Reich RF, Haber S, et al. Oral melanoacanthoma: a report of 10 cases, review of the literature, and immunohistochemical analysis for HMB-45 reactivity. Am J Dermatopathol 2003;25(1):12–15.

Jaworsky C, Murphy GF. Cystic tumors of the neck. J Dermatol Surg Oncol 1989;15(1):21–26.

Kaddu S, Dong H, Mayer G, et al. Warty dyskeratoma – "follicular dyskeratoma": analysis of clinicopathologic features of a distinctive follicular adnexal neoplasm. J Am Acad Dermatol 2002;47(3):423–428.

Kim SH, Choi JH, Sung KJ, et al. Acantholytic acanthoma. J Dermatol 2000;27(2):127–128.

Martorell-Calatayud A, Sanmartin-Jimenez O, Traves V, et al. Numerous umbilicated papules on the trunk: multiple warty dyskeratoma. Am J Dermatopathol 2012;34(6):674–675.

Mehregan DR, Hamzavi F, Brown K. Large cell acanthoma. Int J Dermatol 2003;42(1):36–39.

Romaní J, Barnadas MA, Miralles J, et al. Median raphe cyst of the penis with ciliated cells. J Cutan Pathol 1995;22(4):378–381.

Santos LD, Mendelsohn G. Perineal cutaneous ciliated cyst in a male. Pathology 2004;36(4):369–370.

Sharma R, Verma P, Yadav P, et al. Proliferating trichilemmal tumor of scalp: benign or malignant, a dilemma. J Cutan Aesthet Surg 2012;5(3):213–215.

Vidaurri-de la Cruz H, Tamayo-Sánchez L, Durán-McKinster C, et al. Epidermal nevus syndromes: clinical findings in 35 patients. Pediatr Dermatol 2004;21(4):432–439.

Chapter 3

Malignant tumors of the epidermis

Dirk M. Elston

Actinic keratosis

Key features

- Crowding, disorder, and atypia of epidermal keratinocytes
- Arises from the basal layer
- Solar elastosis typically present

Atypical cells commonly surround the follicular infundibulum. In two-dimensional sections, they appear to form a shoulder zone peripheral to the benign follicular epithelium. The overlying stratum corneum may be normal or may have features of a "malignant horn." A malignant horn is a compact eosinophilic stratum corneum with hyperchromatic brick-like parakeratosis. The brightly eosinophilic zones alternate from left to right with pale basophilic lamellar keratin originating from adnexal structures (flag sign). Broad-based buds of atypical keratinocytes are commonly seen extending downward from the epidermis. The budding can become complex, and separation from superficially invasive squamous cell carcinoma may sometimes be difficult.

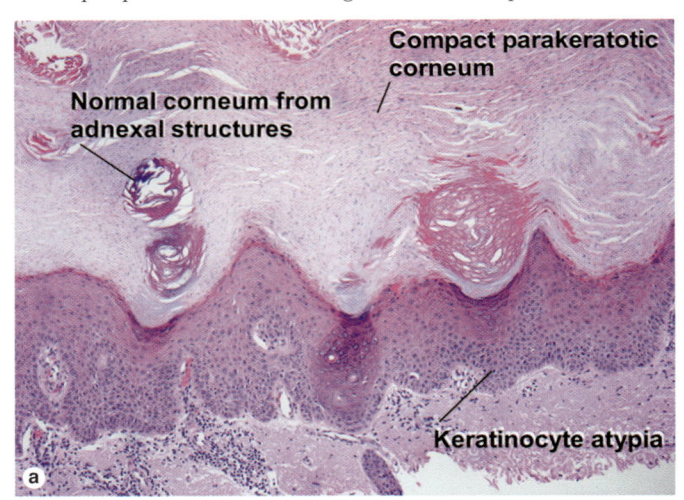

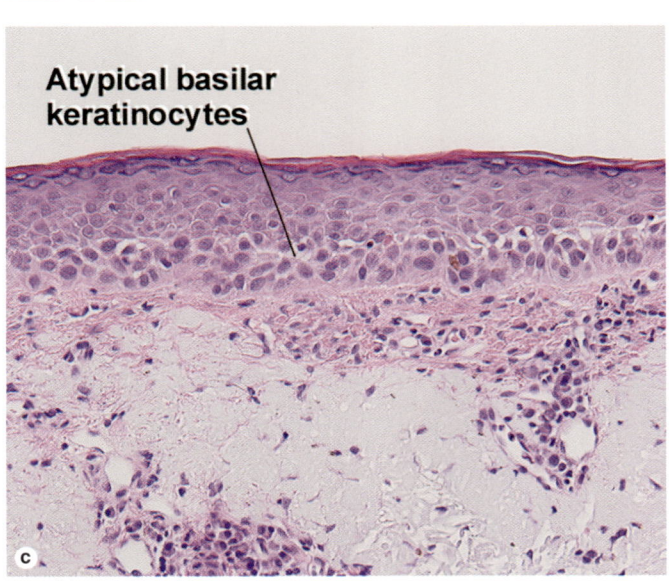

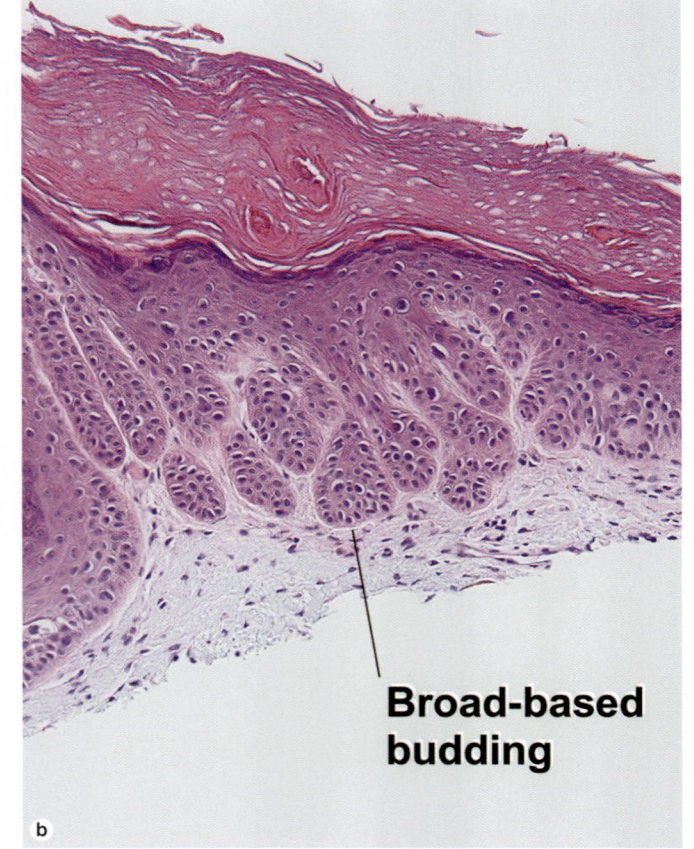

Fig 3-1 Actinic keratosis

Acantholytic actinic keratosis

Key features

- Crowding, disorder, and atypia of epidermal keratinocytes
- Acantholysis in areas of atypia
- Overlying "malignant horn" may be present
- Complex epidermal budding may be present

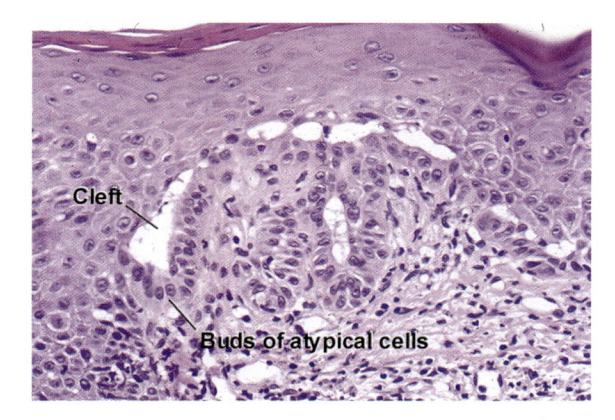

Fig 3-2 Acantholytic actinic keratosis

Lichenoid actinic keratosis

Key features

- Crowding, disorder, and atypia of epidermal keratinocytes
- Areas of lichenoid interface dermatitis
- Overlying "malignant horn" may be present

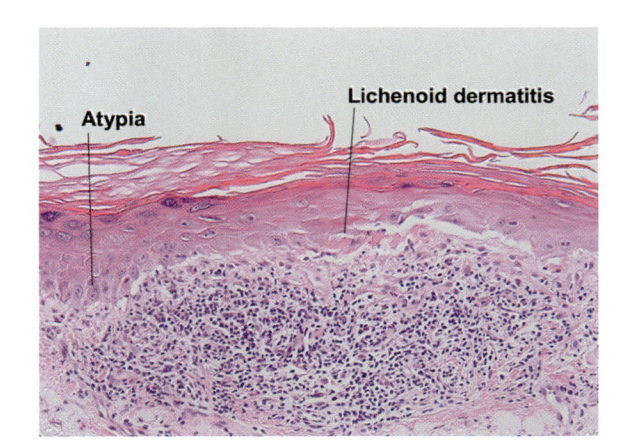

Fig 3-3 Lichenoid actinic keratosis

Hypertrophic actinic keratosis

Key features

- Crowding, disorder, and atypia of epidermal keratinocytes
- Prominent overlying "malignant horn"
- Acanthosis, often with complex epidermal budding

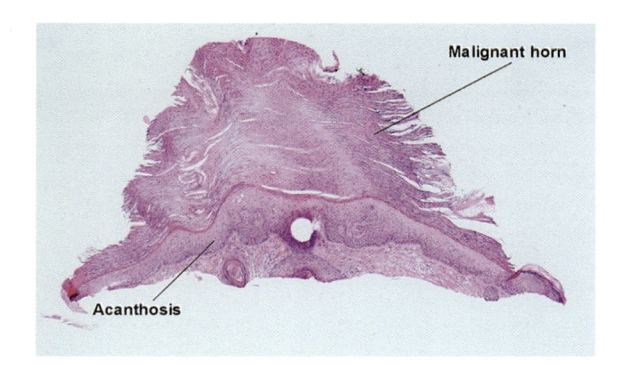

Fig 3-4 Hypertrophic actinic keratosis

Bowenoid actinic keratosis

Key features

- Focal full-thickness atypia

Unlike Bowen's disease, bowenoid actinic keratosis never demonstrates anaplastic nuclei, clonal nesting, buckshot intraepidermal scatter of atypical cells, or full-thickness follicular involvement.

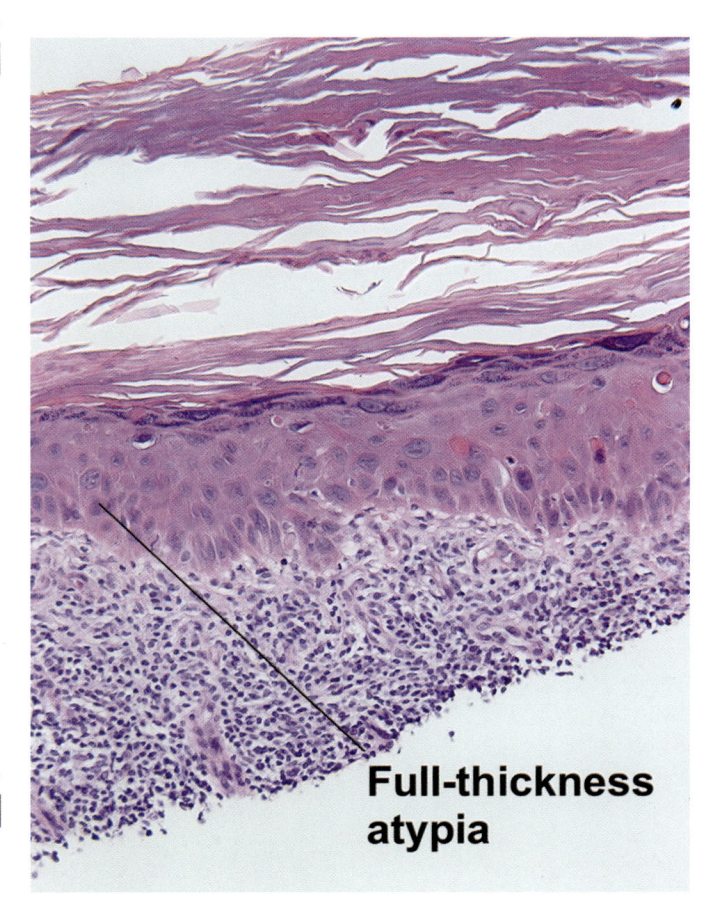

Fig 3-5 Bowenoid actinic keratosis

Bowen's disease

Key features

- Full-thickness atypia with loss of normal maturation (wind-blown pattern)
- Malignant horn typically present
- Atypical cells may occur in an intraepidermal buckshot or nested pattern
- Full-thickness atypia commonly involves follicles

Bowen's disease is a form of squamous cell carcinoma *in situ*. The malignant cells probably originate in the follicular epithelium. As the malignant cells migrate into the epidermis, they create a buckshot or nested pattern. With time, they involve the full-thickness of the epidermis. This is the stage most commonly represented in biopsy specimens. It resembles bowenoid actinic keratosis, except that the cells tend to be more anaplastic with a higher nuclear-to-cytoplasm ratio. Areas with a nested or buckshot pattern may persist. Clear cell change or cells with ample glassy eosinophilic cytoplasm may sometimes be present instead of anaplastic cells. Bowen's disease tends to involve the full-thickness of at least some follicles. Some examples show full-thickness involvement of multiple follicles with relative sparing of the overlying epidermis.

Differential Diagnosis

1. Paget's disease
2. Melanoma
3. Intraepidermal porocarcinoma
4. Sebaceous carcinoma

The malignant keratinocytes of Bowen's disease can keratinize and become part of the stratum corneum. In contrast, the malignant cells of Paget's disease or melanoma often "spit out" into the stratum corneum intact. Bowen's disease contains glycogen and is periodic acid-Schiff (PAS) positive and diastase sensitive. In contrast, Paget's disease contains sialomucin and is PAS positive, diastase resistant. Bowen's disease is negative for carcinoembryonic antigen (CEA) whereas Paget's stains for CEA. Ducts and sebaceous differentiation distinguish porocarcinoma and sebaceous carcinoma.

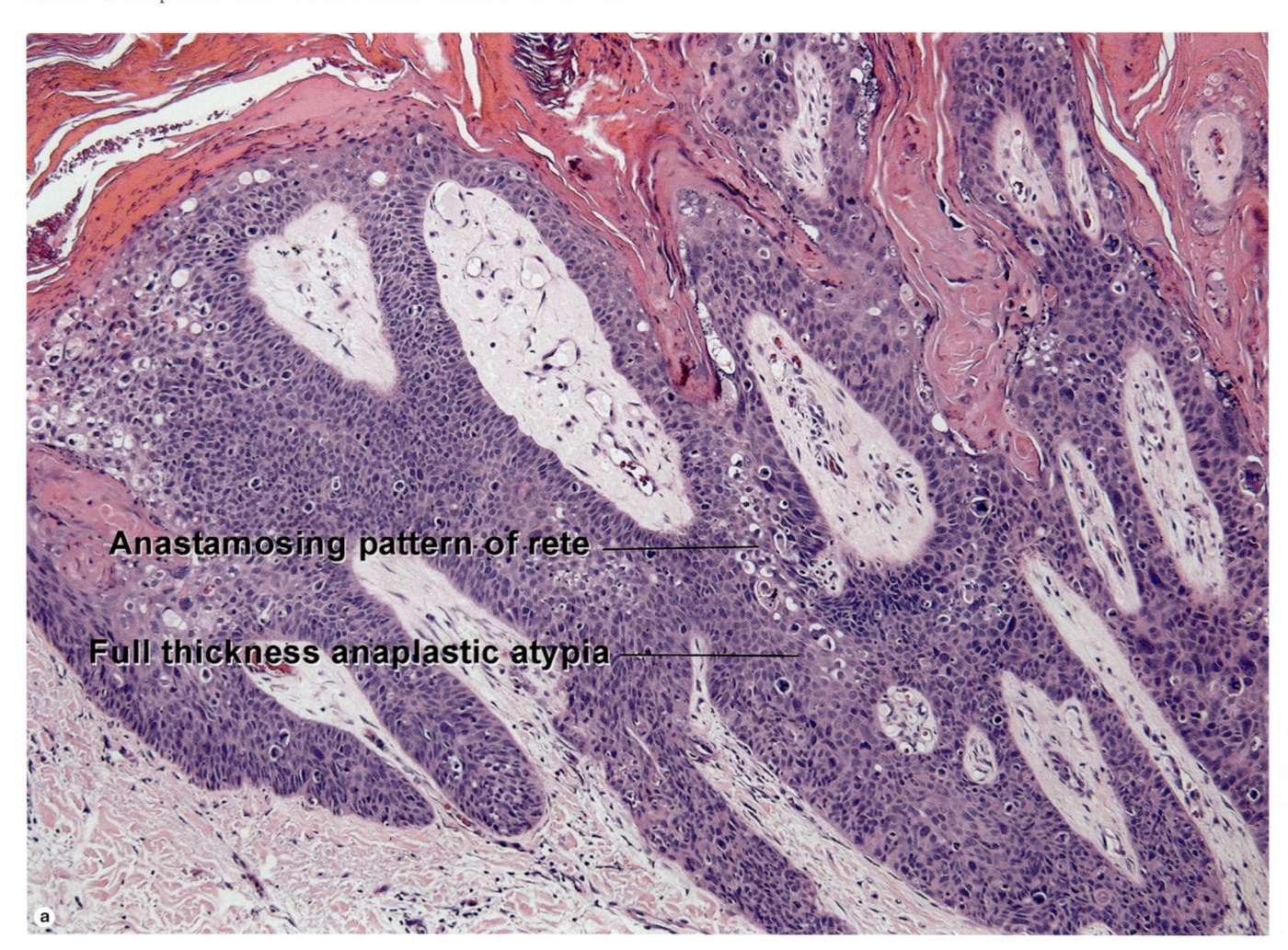

Fig 3-6 Bowen's disease

Malignant tumors of the epidermis

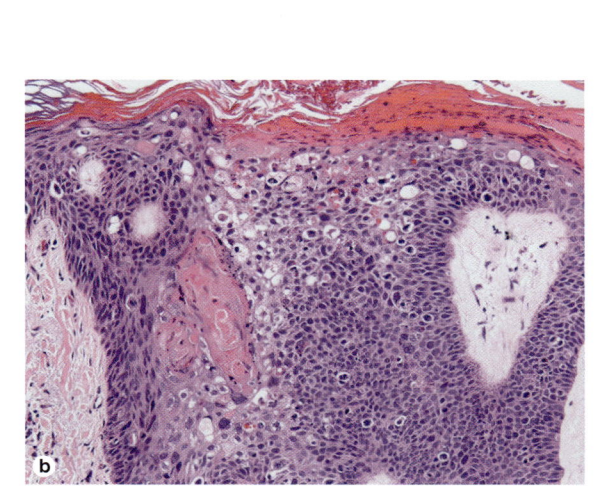

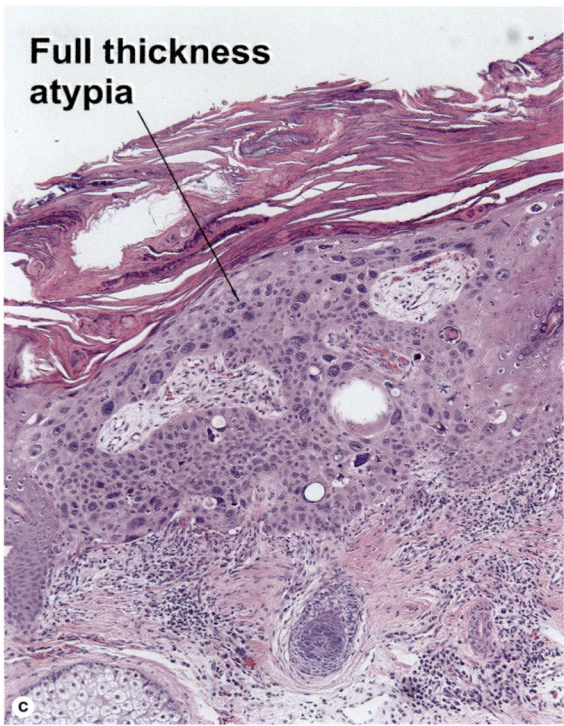

Fig 3-6, cont'd

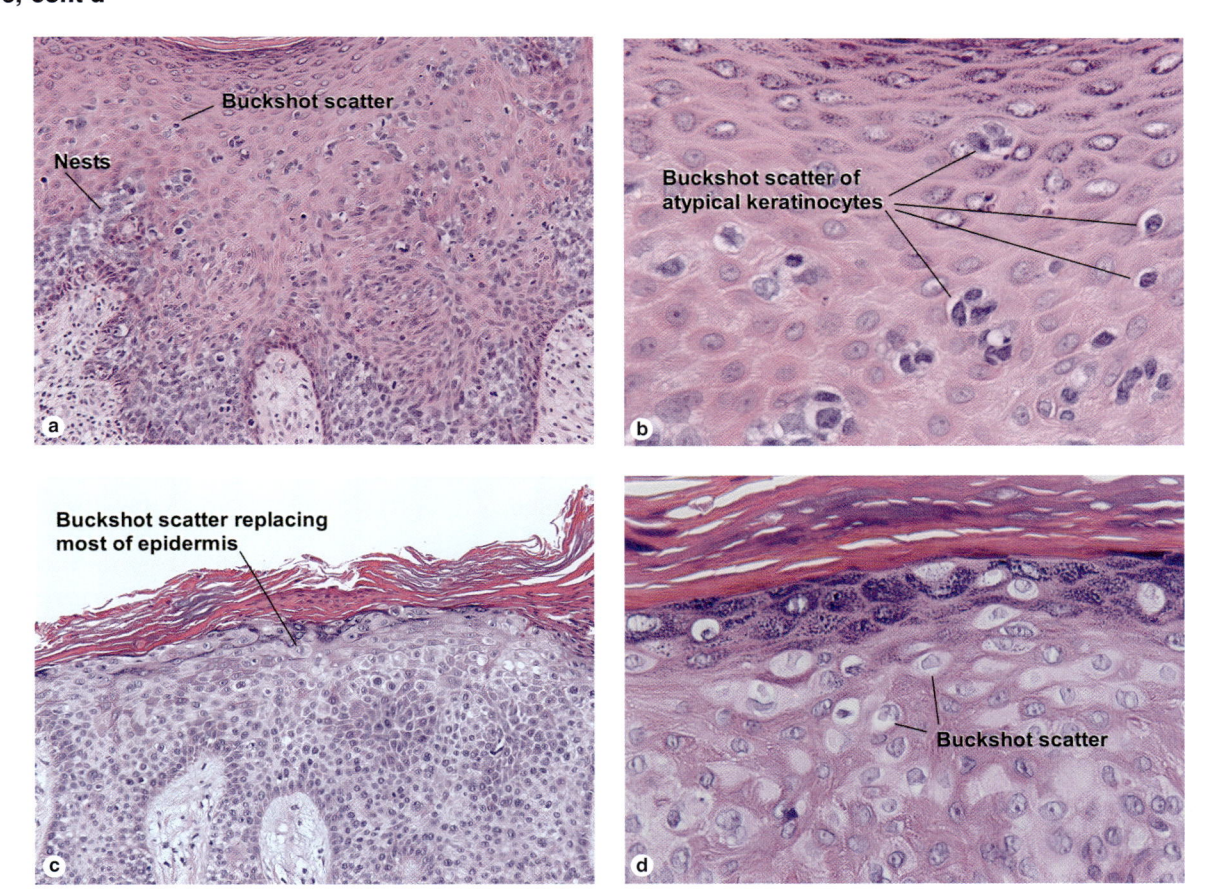

Fig 3-7 Bowen's disease: buckshot scatter of atypical cells

Dermatopathology

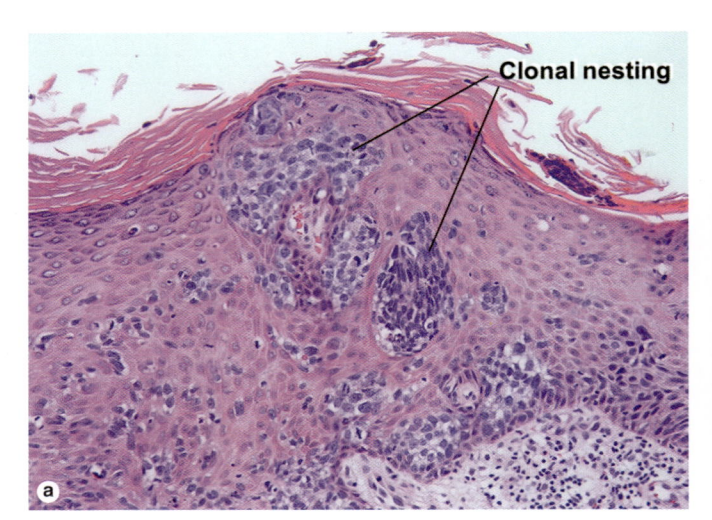

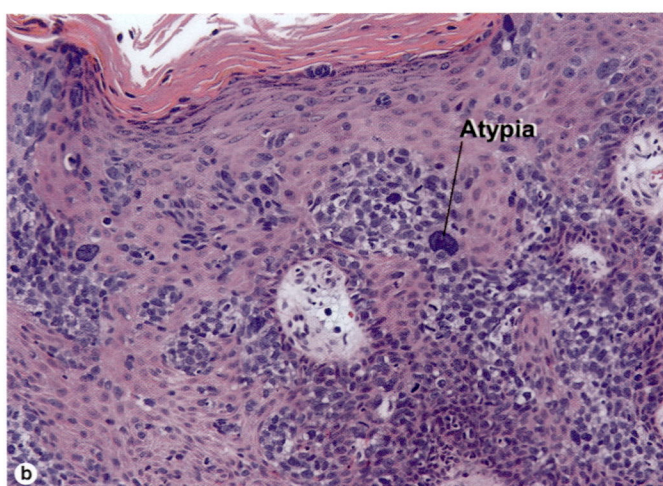

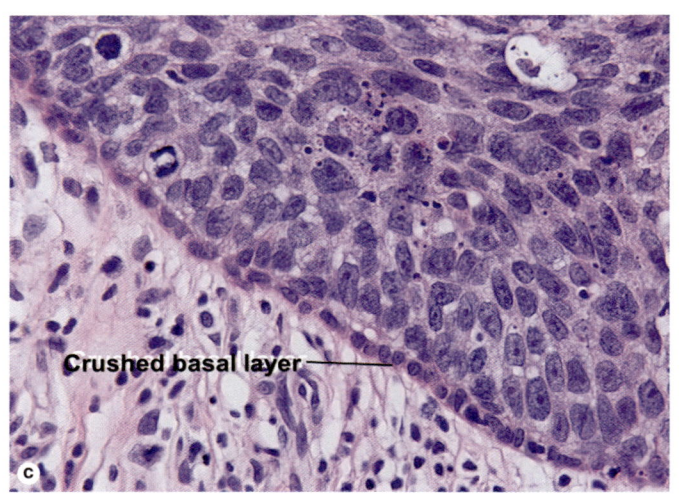

Fig 3-8 Bowen's disease: clonal nesting of atypical cells

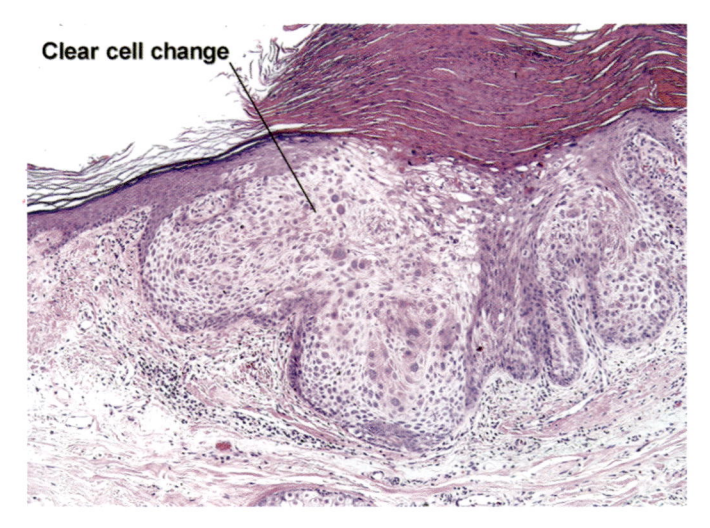

Fig 3-9 Clear cell change in Bowen's disease

Squamous cell carcinoma

Key features

- Atypical keratinocytes invading the dermis
- Acantholysis may be present
- Desmoplasia may be present

Well-differentiated invasive squamous cell carcinoma closely resembles the surface epidermis in staining characteristics, and keratinization is present. Pseudoepitheliomatous hyperplasia is often noted at the periphery of the tumor, and overlying changes of prurigo nodularis may be present in lesions that have been picked. An adequate biopsy is essential to avoid misdiagnosis.

Nodular lymphoid aggregates are an important clue to the presence of desmoplastic squamous carcinoma. Immunostaining can be used to confirm the presence of atypical squamous cells within the stroma.

Moderately differentiated tumors have a higher nuclear/cytoplastic ratio, but still keratinize. Poorly differentiated tumors are spindled or anaplastic. Keratin immunostaining is typically necessary to confirm the diagnosis of a poorly differentiated tumor.

Malignant tumors of the epidermis   Chapter 3   61

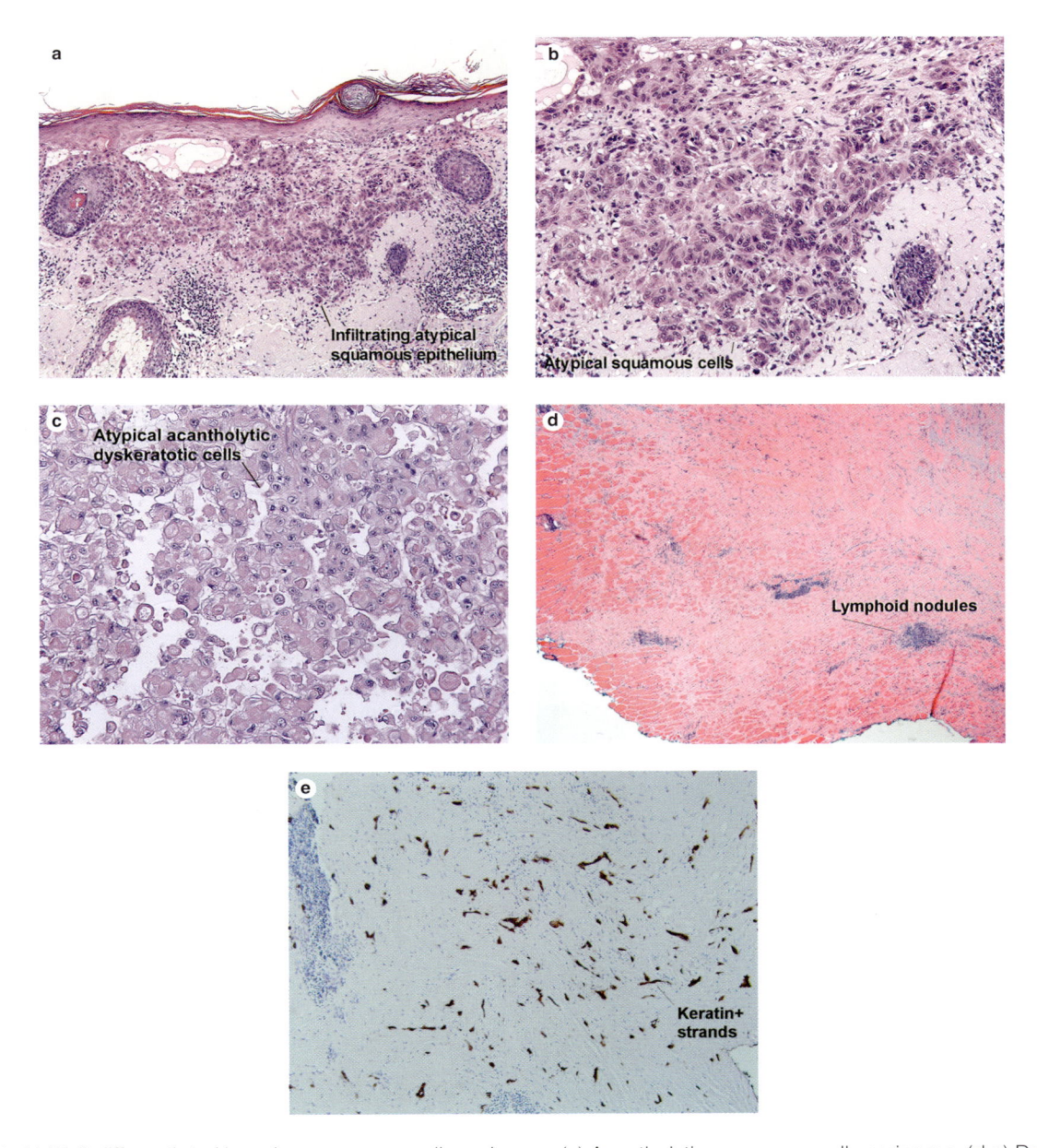

Fig 3-10 (a,b) Well-differentiated invasive squamous cell carcinoma. (c) Acantholytic squamous cell carcinoma. (d,e) Desmoplastic squamous cell carcinoma (H&E and keratin 907 immunostain)

Verrucous carcinoma

Key features

- Well-differentiated glassy squamous epithelium
- Rounded border

Whereas most invasive squamous cell carcinomas have a jagged outline, verrucous carcinomas are composed of well-differentiated glassy eosinophilic keratinocytes and have a blunt, rounded outline. They slowly push into the underlying tissue in a bulldozing fashion.

Dermatopathology

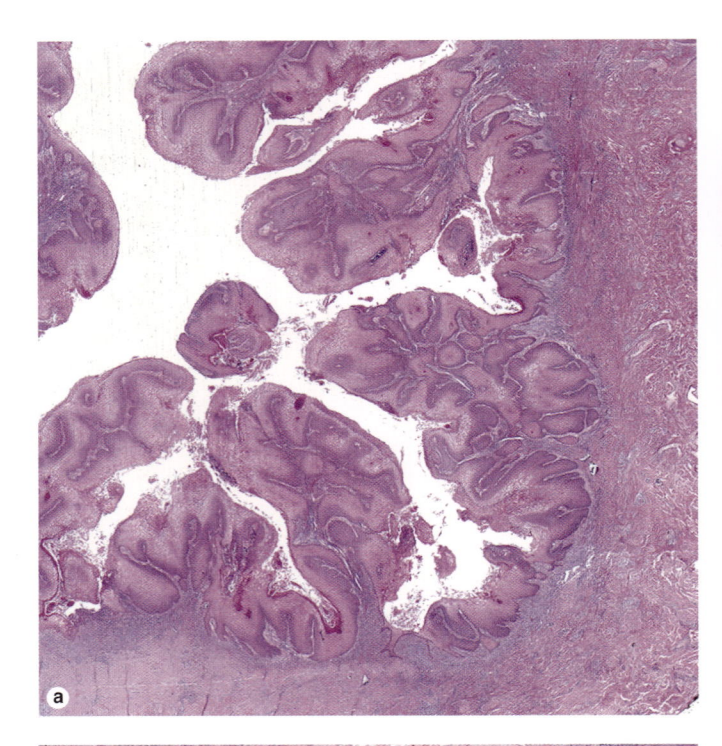

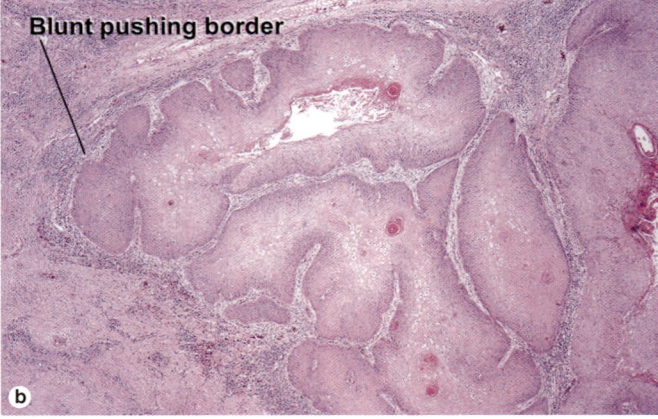

Fig 3-11 Verrucous carcinoma

Spindled squamous cell carcinoma

Key features
- Atypical spindle cells abutting the epidermis

Differential Diagnosis

Spindled squamous cell carcinoma can closely resemble other spindle cell neoplasms. The microscopic differential diagnosis for an atypical spindle cell tumor *SLAM*med up against the epidermis includes:
- *S*quamous cell carcinoma (keratin positive)
- *L*eiomyosarcoma (smooth muscle actin and desmin positive)
- *A*typical fibroxanthoma (diagnosis of exclusion)
- *M*elanoma (S100 positive)

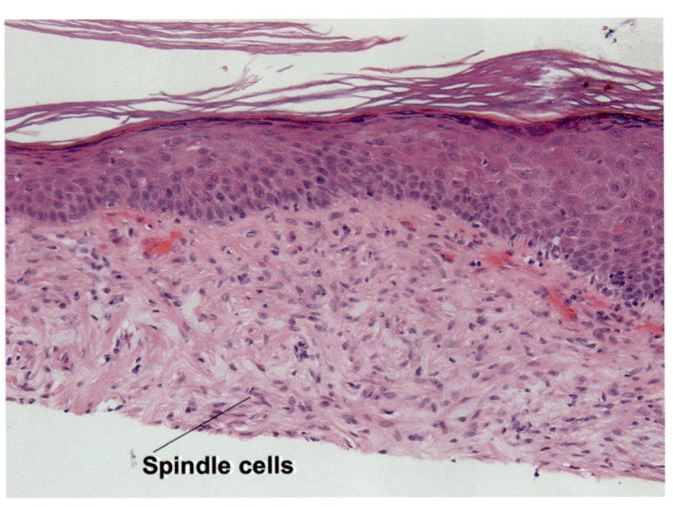

Fig 3-12 Spindled squamous cell carcinoma

Keratoacanthoma

Key features
- Defined by rapid growth and ability to involute spontaneously
- Explosive growth common after biopsy
- Many consider it a form of invasive squamous cell carcinoma capable of regression
- Keratin-filled crater
- Invasive proliferation of glassy red keratinocytes
- Neutrophil microabscesses common
- Eosinophils common in surrounding infiltrate
- Trapping of elastic fibers common at the periphery of the squamous proliferation
- Hypergranulosis and pseudoepitheliomatous hyperplasia prominent in hair follicles towards the center of early lesions
- Acantholysis is *never* present

Keratoacanthomas grow rapidly, then involute. Unfortunately, they can sometimes be difficult to distinguish from well-differentiated invasive squamous cell carcinomas that will never involute. Perineural extension may be seen in both. Explosive growth after a biopsy is consistent with a diagnosis of keratoacanthoma. In contrast, the presence of acantholysis indicates that the lesion will behave like squamous cell carcinoma. Neutrophilic microabscesses, eosinophils, and elastic trapping are common in keratoacanthoma, but rare in squamous cell carcinoma.

Pseudoepitheliomatous hyperplasia and hypergranulosis in follicles occur in the central portion of early keratoacanthomas but only at the periphery of squamous cell carcinomas. The defining feature of a keratoacanthoma is its ability to undergo terminal differentiation, a process whereby the tumor keratinizes itself to death.

Malignant tumors of the epidermis

Table 3-1 Characteristics of keratoacanthoma versus squamous cell carcinoma

Characteristic	Keratoacanthoma	Squamous cell carcinoma
Pseudoepitheliomatous hyperplasia and hypergranulosis	At center of lesion	At periphery of lesion
Cell type	Large light pink glassy cells	Often large, light pink and glassy
Dermal infiltrate	Eosinophils common	Plasma cells common
Gland involvement	Pushes eccrine glands down	Invades eccrine glands
Traps elastic tissue	Commonly	Rarely
Acantholysis	No	Often
Perineural invasion	Yes	Yes
Neutrophilic microabscesses	Common	Rarely
Growth	Explosive	Slow
Terminal differentiation	Yes	No

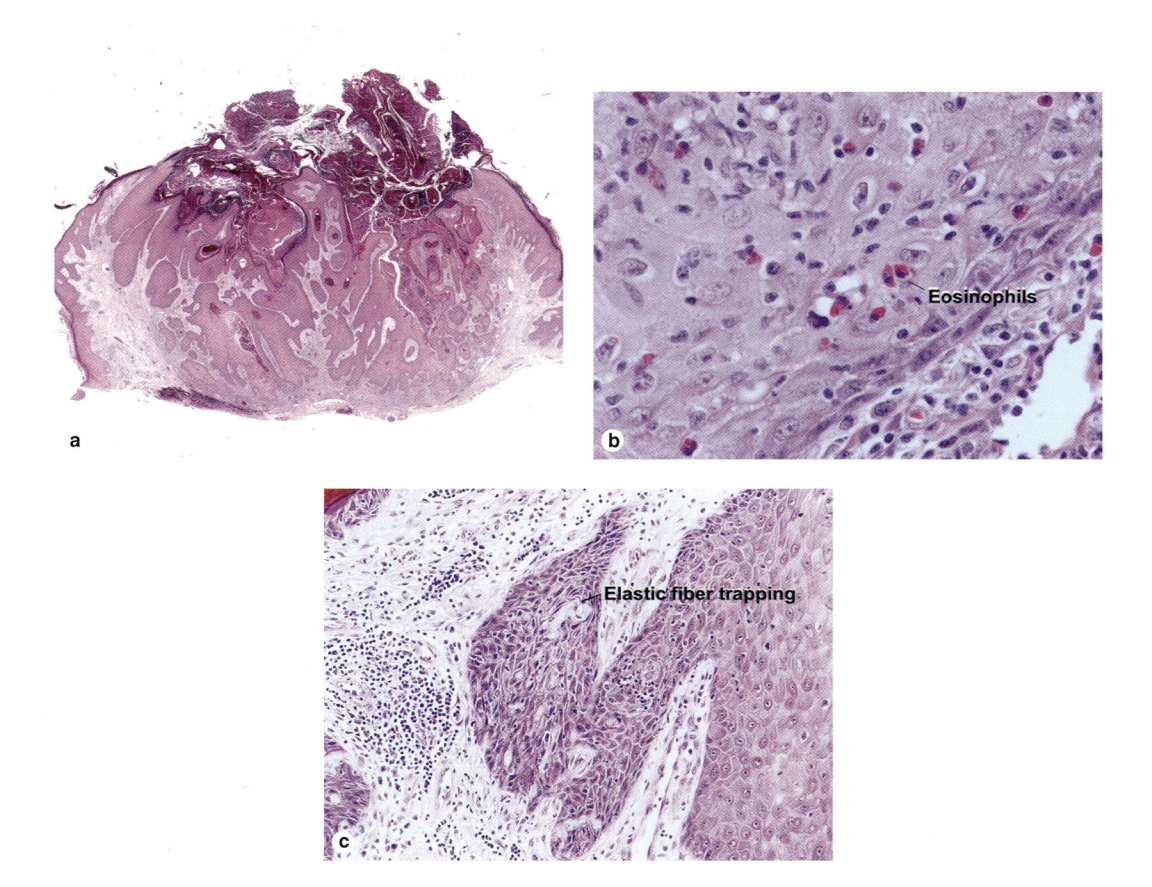

Fig 3-13 Keratoacanthoma

Regressing keratoacanthoma

Key features

- Crater-like outline, often with scalloped outline
- Crater filled with keratin
- Proliferative epithelium has involuted to a thin wall resembling the lining of an epidermoid cyst
- Scar peripheral to regressed epithelium

The most striking feature of a regressing keratoacanthoma is the massive keratin within the crater, out of proportion to the thin epithelium that lines the scalloped crater.

Basal cell carcinoma (BCC)

Key features

- Blue islands
- Peripheral palisading
- High nuclear/cytoplasmic ratio
- Retraction artifact
- Fibromyxoid stroma

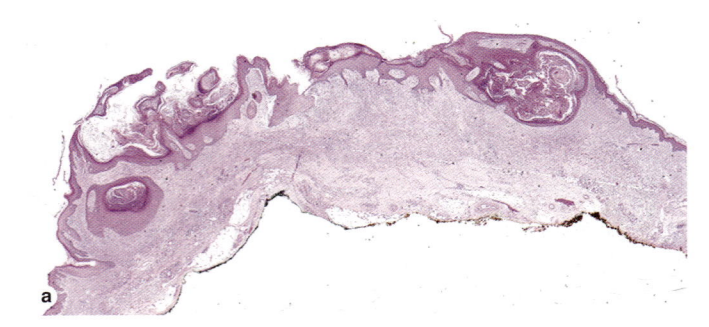

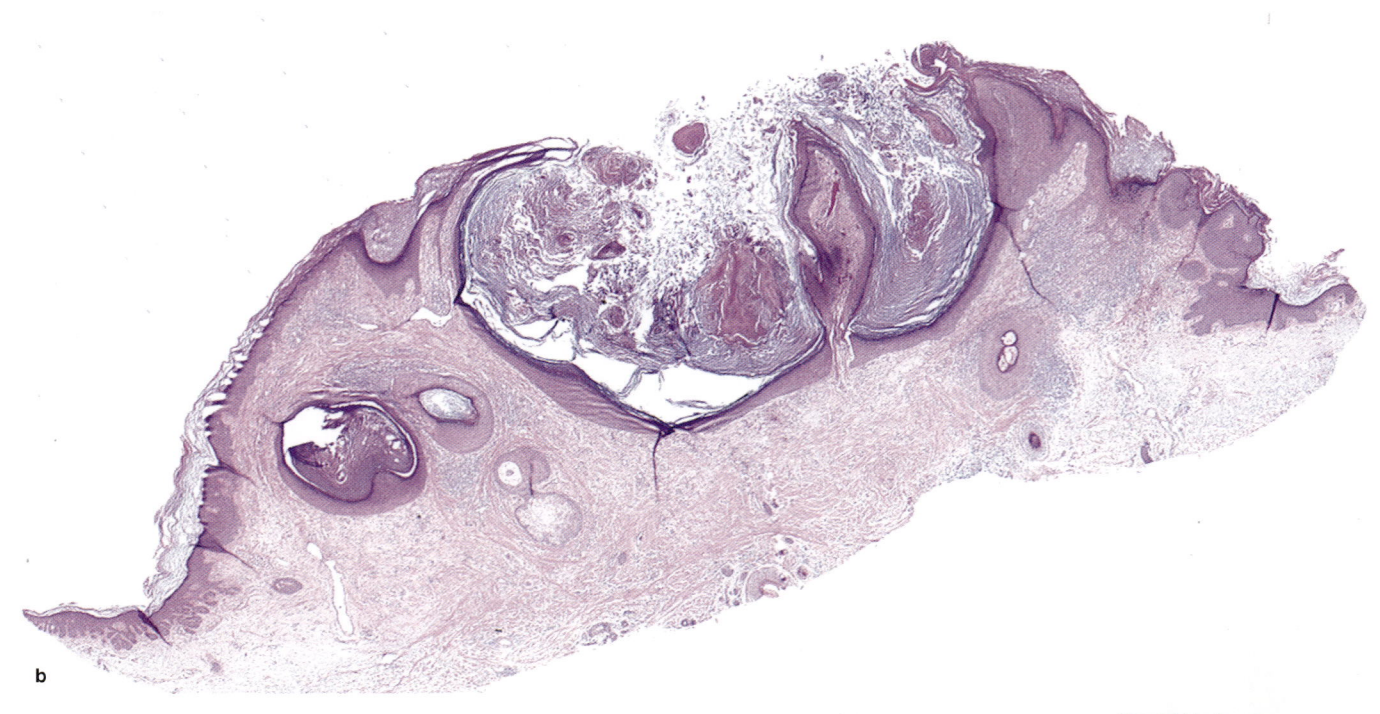

Fig 3-14 Regressing keratoacanthoma

Superficial multifocal BCC

Key features

- Multifocal blue buds
- Distinctive fibromyxoid stroma displaces solar elastosis downward
- Retraction artifact common

Superficial multifocal BCC grows in a pattern resembling garlands draped from the epidermis. In two-dimensional sections, this gives the appearance of multifocal blue buds. Because the buds are spaced far apart, margin evaluation is based largely on the surrounding tumor stroma. The tumor stroma displaces the reticular dermis and solar elastosis downward.

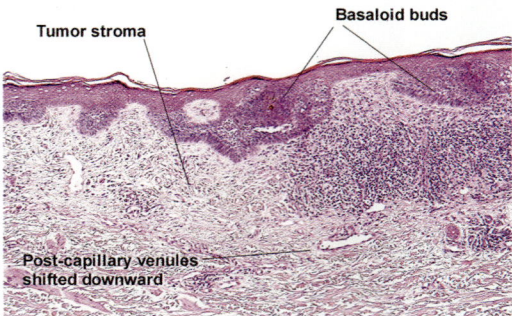

Fig 3-15 Superficial multifocal basal cell carcinoma

Nodular BCC

Key features

- Nodular blue islands
- Peripheral palisading
- Retraction artifact
- Distinctive fibromyxoid stroma

Micronodular BCC is characterized by aggressive worm-like growth into the dermis. In cross-section, the appearance is micronodular. Because of the thick dermal collagen bundles between tumor islands, the tumors are poorly defined clinically, and curettage has a high failure rate.

It should be noted that many ordinary BCCs demonstrate small finger-like projections that appear as small round balls in cross-section. Only tumor stroma separates the islands, with no thick collagen bundles in between. These tumors do not qualify as micronodular BCC.

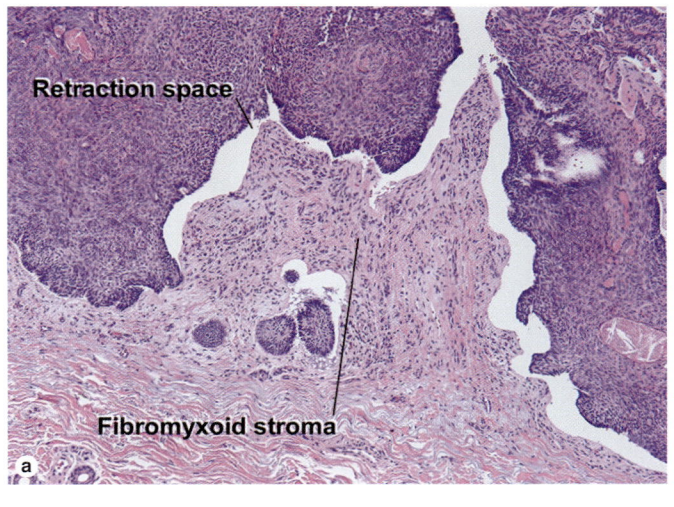

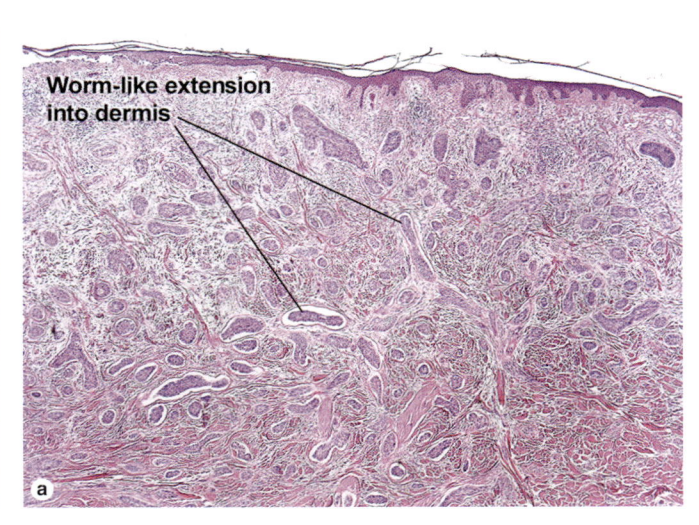

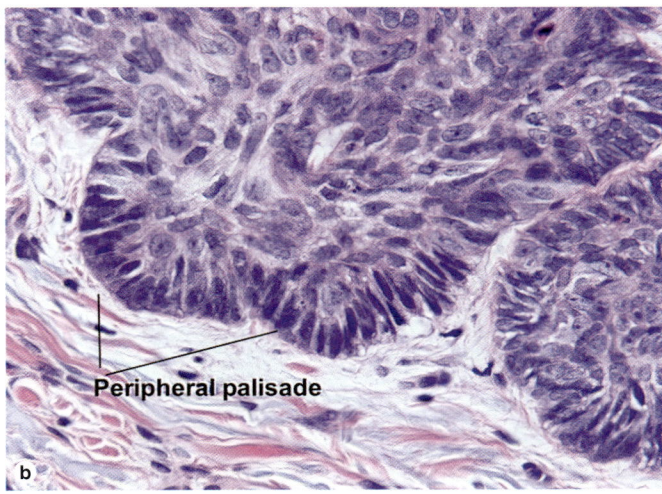

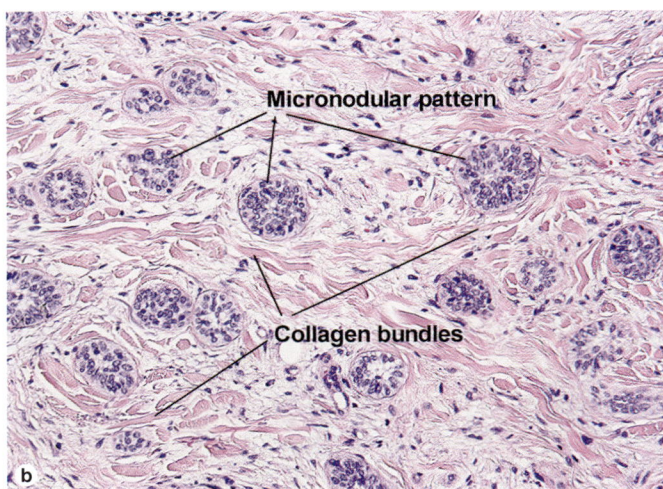

Fig 3-16 Nodular basal cell carcinoma

Fig 3-17 Micronodular basal cell carcinoma

Micronodular BCC

Key features

- Small blue islands
- Peripheral palisading
- Retraction artifact focally
- Distinctive fibromyxoid stroma surrounds individual islands, but normal dermis is present between islands

Morpheaform BCC

> **Key features**
> - Thin infiltrating strands of basaloid cells, usually only two cells thick
> - Sclerotic stroma
> - Tadpole-like islands with small horn cysts may be present focally

Morpheaform BCC presents clinically as scar-like lesions that gradually expand. Perineural extension is common. It is usually deeply infiltrative by the time the diagnosis is made. The pink sclerotic stroma contains little to no mucin, and at first glance may resemble a scar. However, the architecture is not that of a scar. In scars, the collagen has an east/west orientation while blood vessels have a north/south orientation. This is unlike the haphazard structure of the tumor stroma. Occasionally, a superficial biopsy will demonstrate tadpole-like islands with small horn cysts, creating a "paisley-tie" appearance.

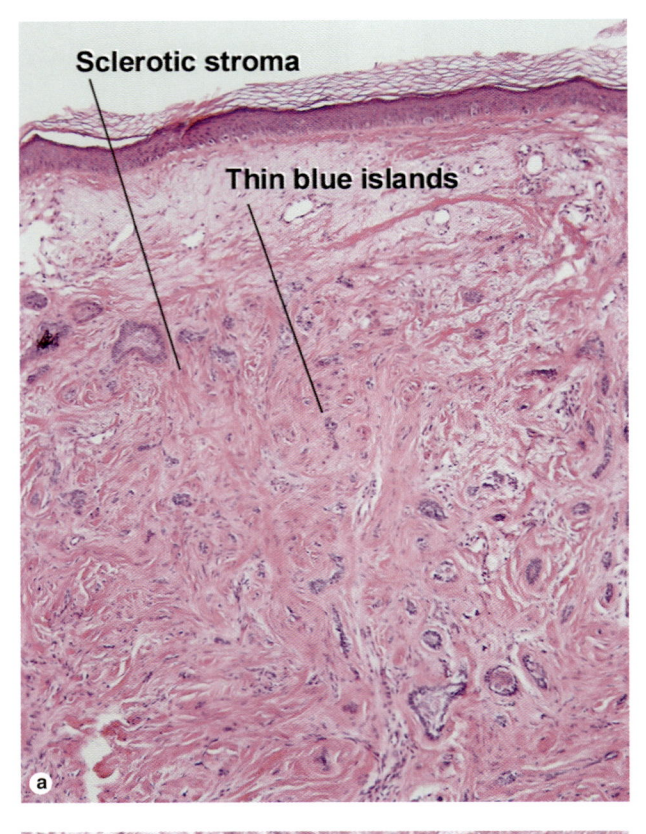

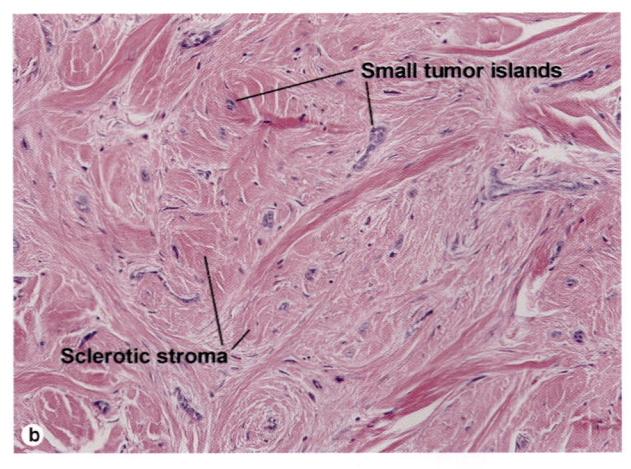

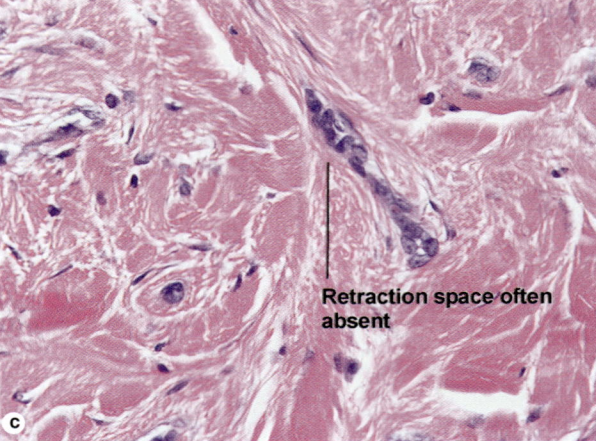

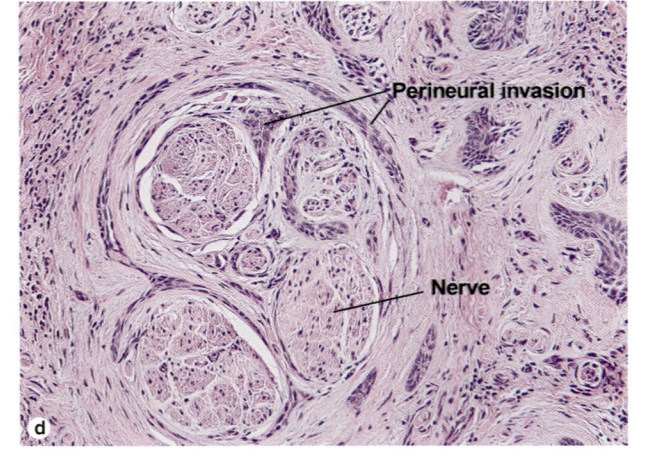

Fig 3-18 Morpheaform basal cell carcinoma

Malignant tumors of the epidermis

Differential Diagnosis

1. Morpheaform BCC (older patient with a scar-like lesion)
2. Microcystic adnexal carcinoma (firm plaque on the upper lip, medial cheek, or chin)
3. Desmoplastic trichoepithelioma (doughnut-like firm lesion with central dell on the cheek of a young female)
4. Syringoma (small papules on the lower lids or widely eruptive papules)
5. Eruptive syringomas (chest and back or penis, often skin type VI)

Infiltrative BCC

Key features

- Spiky growth pattern
- Fibroblast-rich stroma with little mucin
- Areas of squamous differentiation common
- Perineural extension common

At first glance, the fibroblast-rich stroma of an infiltrative BCC can resemble the stroma of a trichoepithelioma. Glance again. Trichoepitheliomas never have spiky islands. If you remember that spiky things are likely to hurt you, it may help you to remember that this feature matches with an aggressive form of BCC. Papillary mesenchymal bodies are absent in infiltrative BCC.

Infundibulocystic BCC

Key features

- Pink strands, blue buds
- Horn cysts
- Fibromyxoid stroma

Infundibulocystic BCC differentiates towards the follicular infundibulum. It is characterized by pink strands of squamous epithelium, blue basaloid buds at the tips of the strands, and horn cysts. It closely resembles basaloid follicular hamartoma. The two entities are best distinguished clinically.

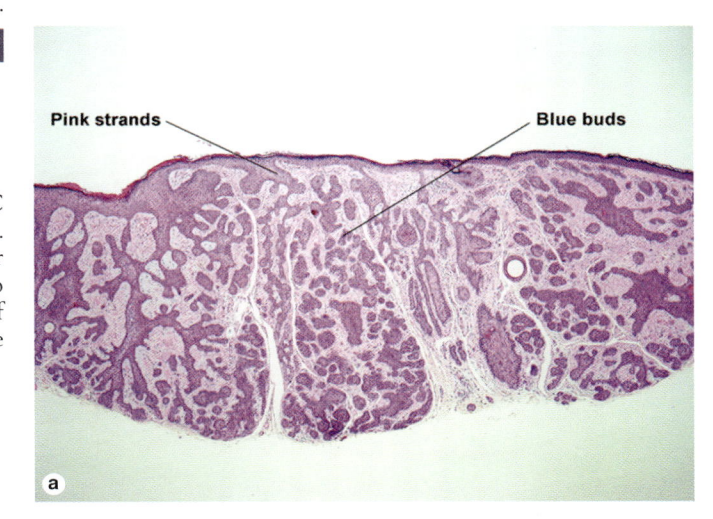

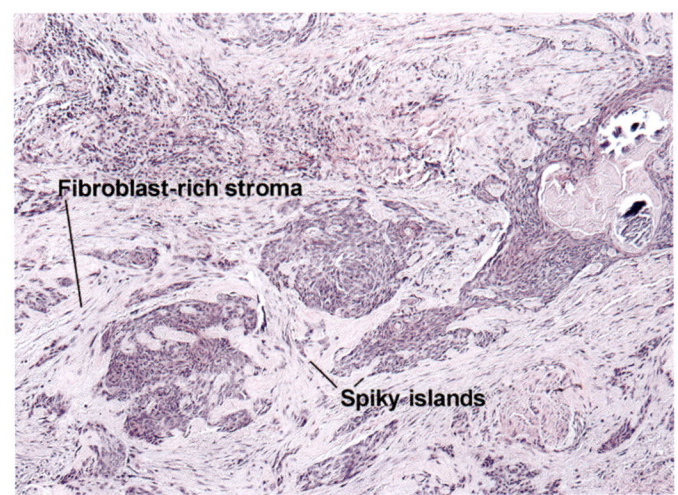

Fig 3-19 Infiltrative basal cell carcinoma

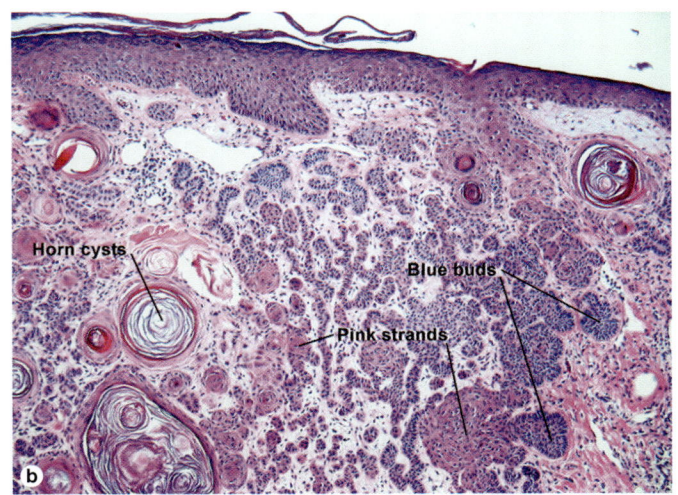

Fig 3-20 Infundibulocystic basal cell carcinoma

Fibroepithelioma of Pinkus

Key features
- Pink strands, blue buds
- Eccrine ducts often visible within strands
- Ample fibromyxoid stroma

Fibroepithelioma of Pinkus is composed of anastomosing pink epithelial strands embedded in a fibromyxoid stroma. Ducts are often visible within the strands. Blue basaloid buds are present at the tips and periphery of strands.

Adenoid BCC

Key features
- Blue islands with adenoid pattern (clear spaces in middle of islands)
- Peripheral palisading
- Fibromyxoid stroma
- Retraction artifact

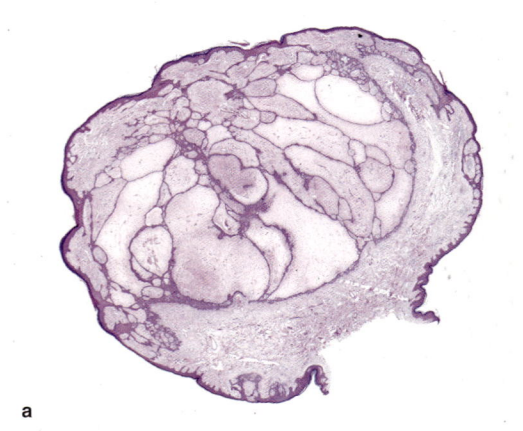

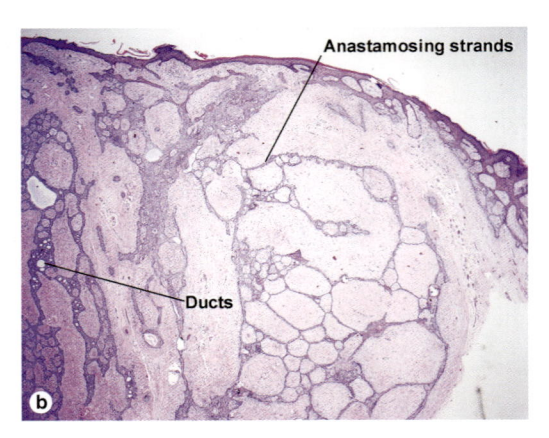

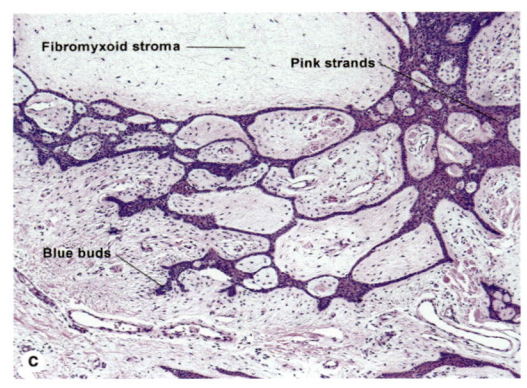

Fig 3-21 Fibroepithelioma of Pinkus

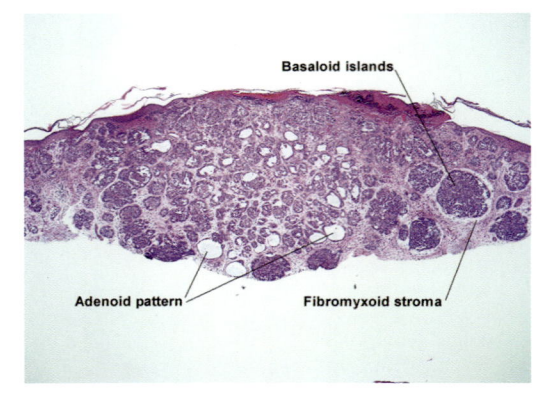

Fig 3-22 Adenoid basal cell carcinoma

Paget's disease

Key features

- Intraepidermal proliferation of large cells with ample amphophilic cytoplasm
- Tumor cells in buckshot distribution or intraepidermal nests
- Atypical cells crush the basal layer
- Atypical cells may "spit out" into the stratum corneum intact
- CK7+
- CEA+
- S100–
- PAS+, diastase resistant (sialomucin)

Paget's disease of the breast represents intraepidermal extension of underlying intraductal carcinoma. Extramammary Paget's disease may represent an extension of an underlying adenocarcinoma, but more commonly arises de novo, probably from pluripotent cells or mammary-like glands along milk lines. Sialomucin stains PAS+, diastase resistant, and with Alcian blue and toluidine blue at high (but not low) pH.

Differential Diagnosis

1. Melanoma (S100+, HMB-45+, never crushes basal layer, cells can spit into stratum corneum)
2. Bowen's disease (keratin+, CEA–, cells rarely spit into stratum corneum intact)
3. Intraepidermal porocarcinoma (related to acrosyringeal keratinocytes, demonstrates focal duct differentiation, may have adjacent benign hidroacanthoma simplex)

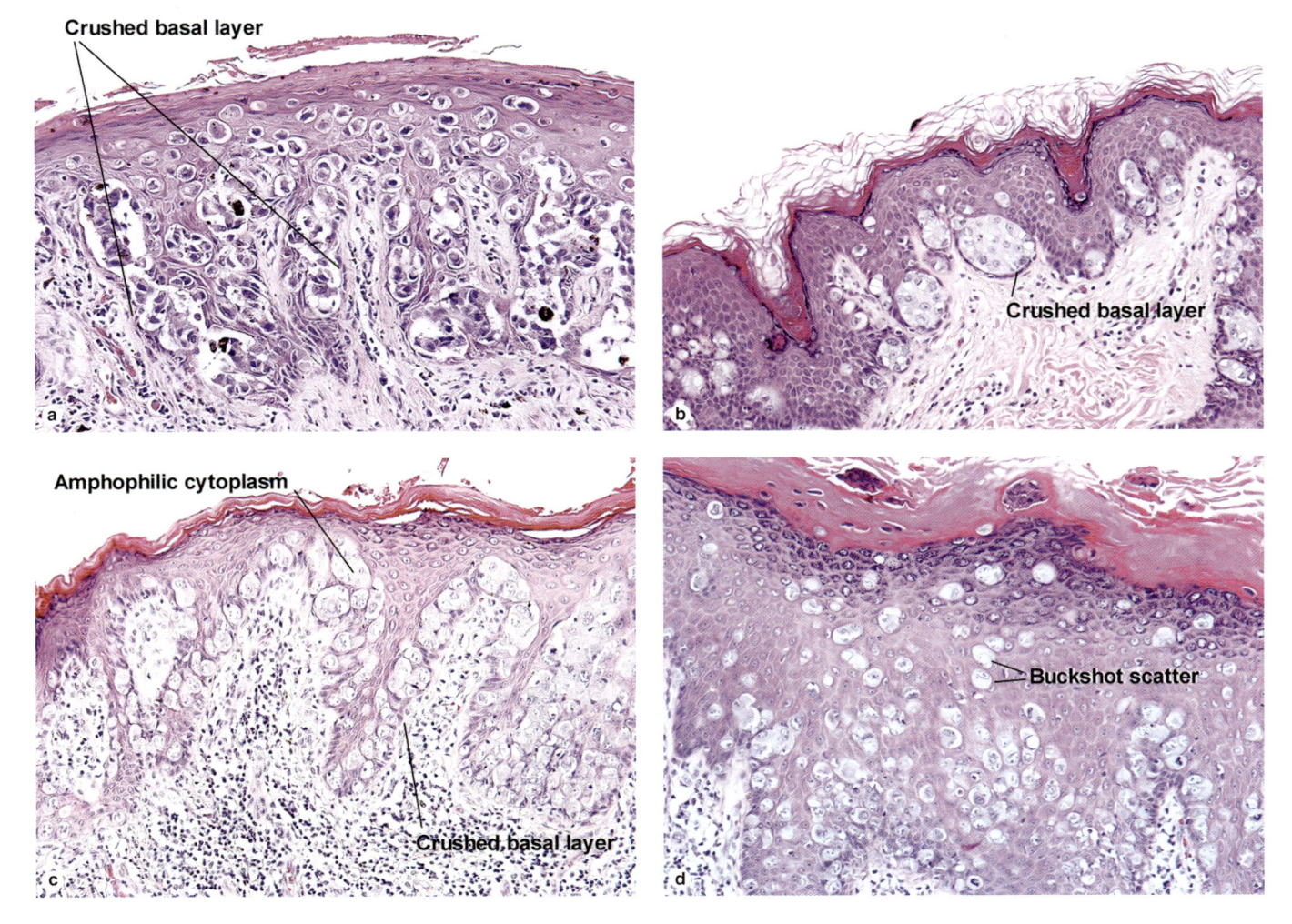

Fig 3-23 Extramammary Paget's disease

Lymphoepithelioma-like carcinoma

Key features
- At scan, mimics a germinal center or lymphoma
- Central keratin-positive atypical epithelial cells
- Surrounding lymphocytes

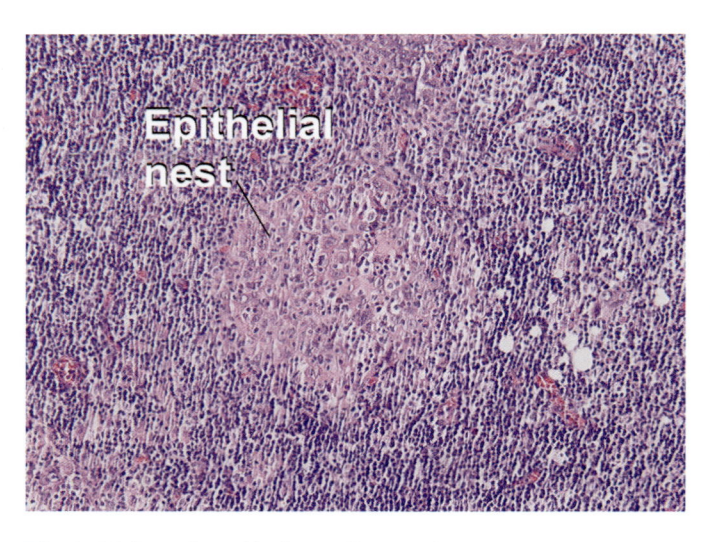

Fig 3-24 Lymphoepithelioma-like carcinoma

Despite the anaplastic character of the cells, the prognosis is generally good. Nasopharyngeal lymphoepithelioma can have a similar appearance, and metastatic disease should be ruled out. Cutaneous lesions are EBV negative, unlike the nasopharyngeal counterpart.

Further reading

Cigna E, Tarallo M, Sorvillo V, et al. Metatypical carcinoma of the head: a review of 312 cases. Eur Rev Med Pharmacol Sci 2012;16(14):1915–1918.

Hernandez-Perez E, Figueroa DE. Warty and clear cell Bowen's disease. Int J Dermatol 2005;44(7):586–587.

Mengjun B, Zheng-Qiang W, Tasleem MM. Extramammary Paget's disease of the perianal region: a review of the literature emphasizing management. Dermatol Surg 2013;39(1 Pt 1):69–75.

Rubin AI, Chen EH, Ratner D. Basal-cell carcinoma. N Engl J Med 2005;353(21):2262–2269.

Rudolph R, Zelac DE. Squamous cell carcinoma of the skin. Plast Reconstr Surg 2004;114(6):82e–94e.

Sah SP, Kelly PJ, McManus DT, et al. Diffuse CK7, CAM5.2 and BerEP4 positivity in pagetoid squamous cell carcinoma in situ (pagetoid Bowen's disease) of the perianal region: a mimic of extramammary Paget's disease. Histopathology 2013;62(3):511–514.

Pilar and sebaceous neoplasms

Dirk M. Elston

Pilar neoplasms

Pilar neoplasms differentiate towards (resemble) various parts of the normal hair follicle. They are named according to what they resemble. Before reading this chapter, review the discussion of hair anatomy in Chapter 1. Blue pilar tumors differentiate towards elements of the inferior segment of the hair follicle. Red pilar tumors differentiate towards the isthmus and infundibulum. Clear cell tumors differentiate towards the glycogenated outer root sheath.

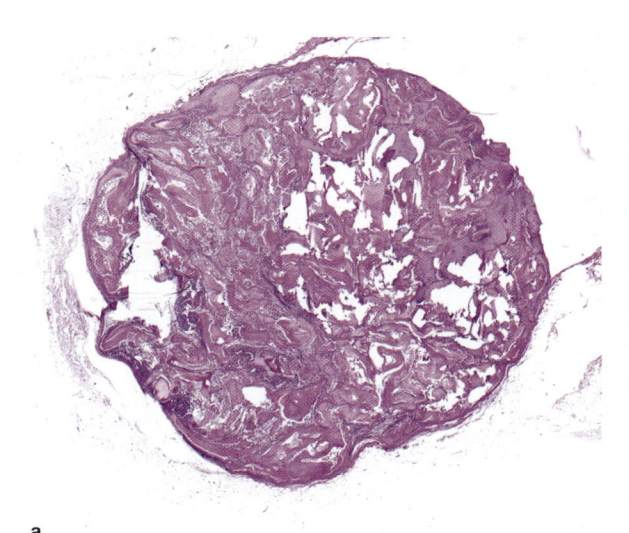

Pilomatricoma (calcifying epithelioma of Malherbe)

Key features

- Low-power architecture is a large ball with internal trabeculae (similar in architecture to a proliferating pilar cyst)
- Basophilic cells that resemble those of the hair matrix keratinize to form shadow cells
- Often calcify
- Giant cell granulomas adjacent to calcifications
- Bone formation common
- Multiple pilomatricomas are associated with myotonic dystrophy

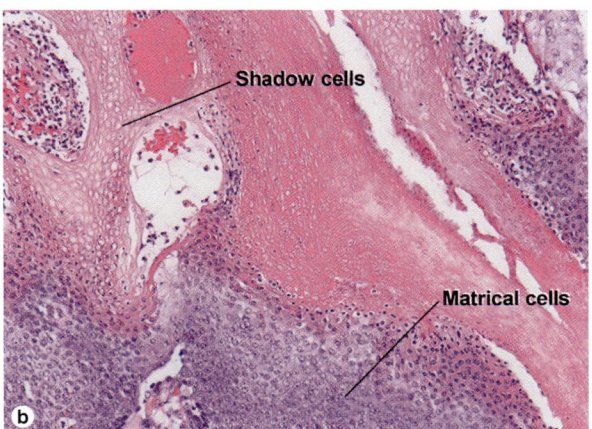

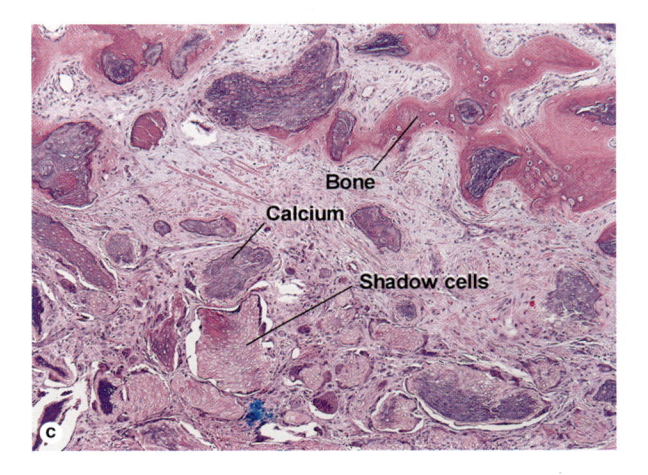

Fig 4-1 Pilomatricoma

Pilomatrical carcinoma

Key features

- Rare
- May arise in long-standing pilomatricomas
- Large
- Infiltrative border
- Atypia, mitoses, necrosis

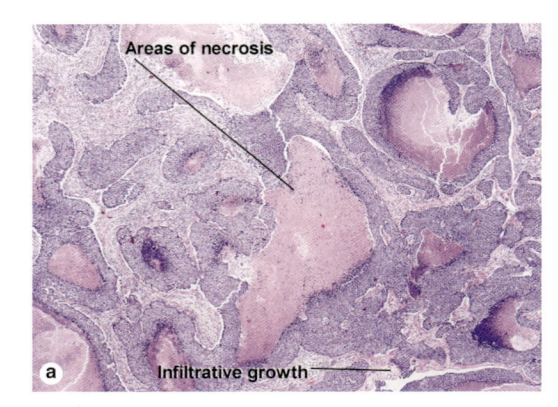

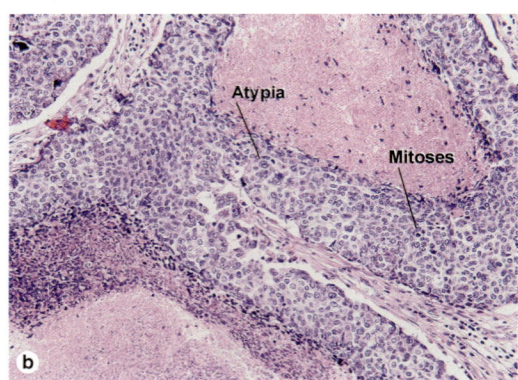

Fig 4-2 Pilomatrical carcinoma

Trichoblastoma

Key features

- Family of blue follicular tumors composed of basaloid cells
- Cells resemble those of basal cell carcinoma
- Stroma resembles the normal fibrous sheath of the hair follicle, with concentric collagen and many fibroblasts
- Papillary mesenchymal bodies may be present in the stroma
- Mucin may be present within tumor islands, but never in the stroma
- No retraction artifact

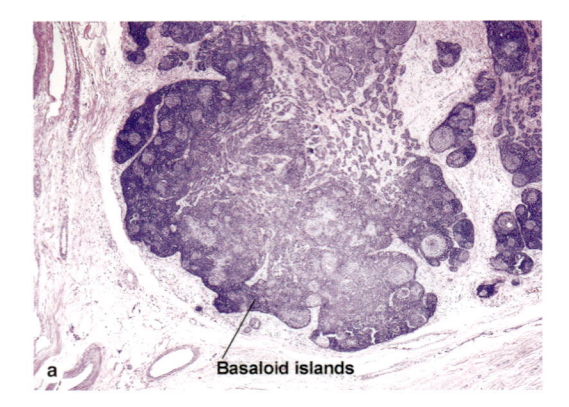

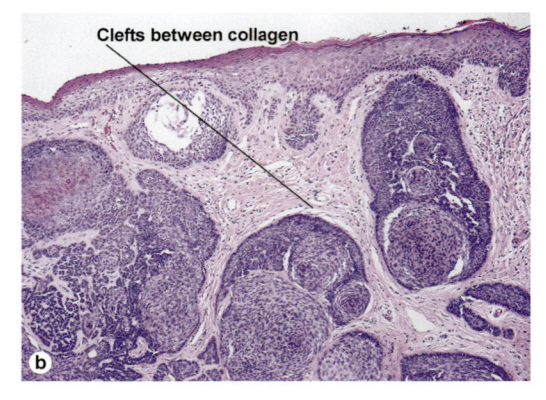

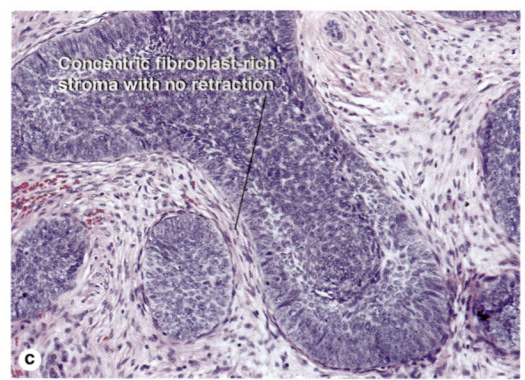

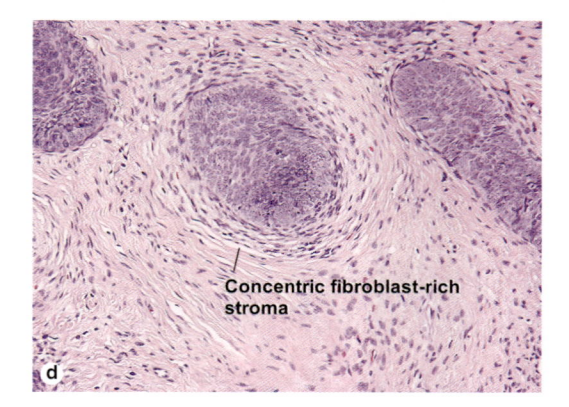

Fig 4-3 Trichoblastoma

Benign trichoblastomas are large basaloid follicular neoplasms. The tumor islands resemble basal cell carcinoma, but the stroma resembles the normal fibrous sheath of the hair follicle. Trichoepitheliomas and lymphadenomas are distinctive forms of benign trichoblastoma. Trichogerminomas are a type of trichoblastoma with differentiation towards the hair germ. Basal cell carcinoma is the most common malignant counterpart of a benign trichoblastoma. Some trichoblastic carcinomas arising in long-standing trichoblastomas have been very aggressive tumors with metastases.

Trichoepithelioma

Key features

- Distinctive type of trichoblastoma
- Blue tumor composed of basaloid cells
- At scan, finger-like projections and cribriform (Swiss-cheese) nodules
- Cells resemble those of basal cell carcinoma
- Stroma resembles the normal fibrous sheath of the hair follicle, with concentric collagen and many fibroblasts (as with any other trichoblastoma)
- Papillary mesenchymal bodies typically prominent
- Mucin may be present within cribriform tumor islands, but never in the stroma
- No retraction artifact

Trichoepitheliomas commonly present as multiple small papules in the nasolabial folds. The multiple type is inherited in an autosomal-dominant fashion. Each papule is composed of basaloid islands in a fibroblast-rich stroma with papillary mesenchymal bodies. Horn cysts and calcification are common. Small clefts may occur between collagen fibers of the tumor stroma, but not between the tumor epithelium and stroma. Papillary mesenchymal bodies are round collections of plump mesenchymal cells resembling those in the follicular papilla.

Table 4-1 Characteristics of trichoepithelioma versus basal cell carcinoma

Characteristic	Trichoepithelioma	Basal cell carcinoma
Basaloid cells	Yes	Yes
Peripheral palisading	Yes	Yes
Finger-like and cribriform	Yes	Sometimes
Stroma	Concentric, fibroblast-rich	Myxoid
Mucin	In tumor islands only, none in stroma	Metachromatic mucin in stroma
Papillary mesenchymal bodies	Common	Rare
Horn cysts	Common	Rare
Calcification	Common	Rare
Clefts	Between collagen fibers within stroma	Between epithelium and stroma
CD34 staining	Strong staining in stroma	+/−
BCL-2 staining	Periphery of islands	Strong, diffuse
CK20+ Merkel cells	Present in tumoral islands	Absent in tumoral islands

PEARLS

- Multiple trichoepitheliomas (epithelioma adenoides cysticum) inherited as autosomal-dominant trait
- Brooke–Spiegler syndrome: multiple trichoepitheliomas and cylindromas
- Rombo syndrome: milia, hypotrichosis, trichoepitheliomas, basal cell carcinoma, atrophoderma, vasodilation with cyanosis

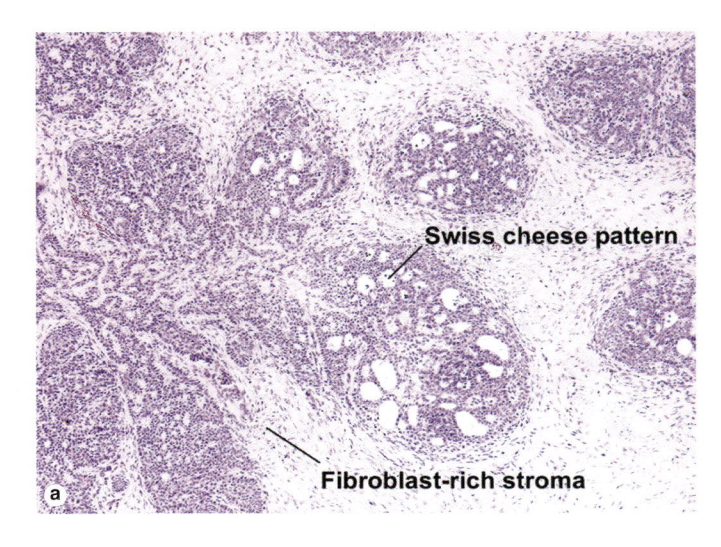

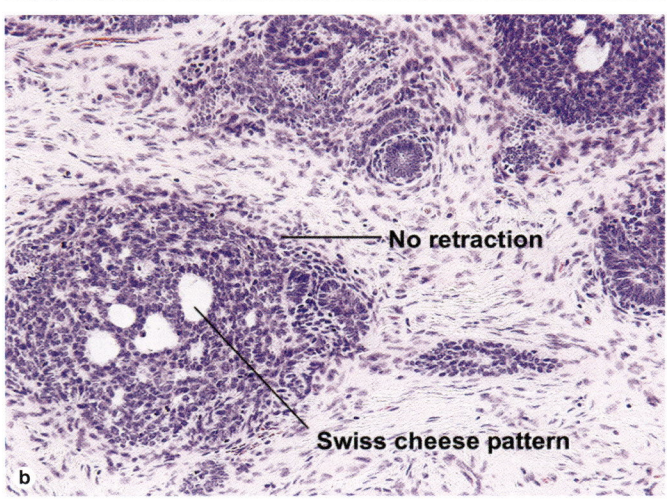

Fig 4-4 Trichoepithelioma

Continued

74 Dermatopathology

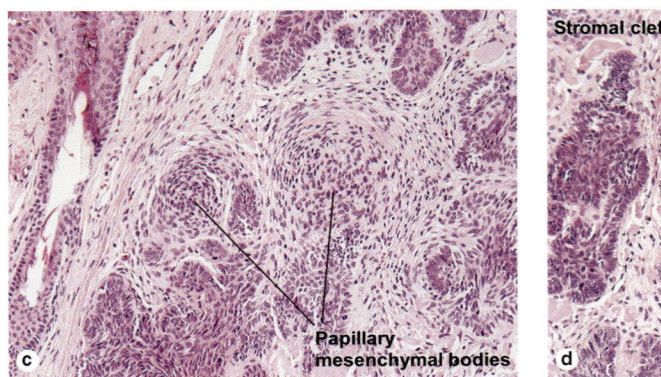

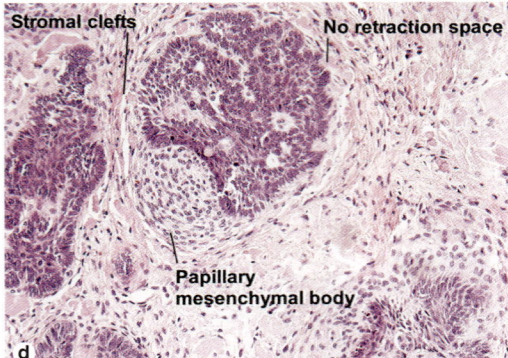

Fig 4-4, cont'd

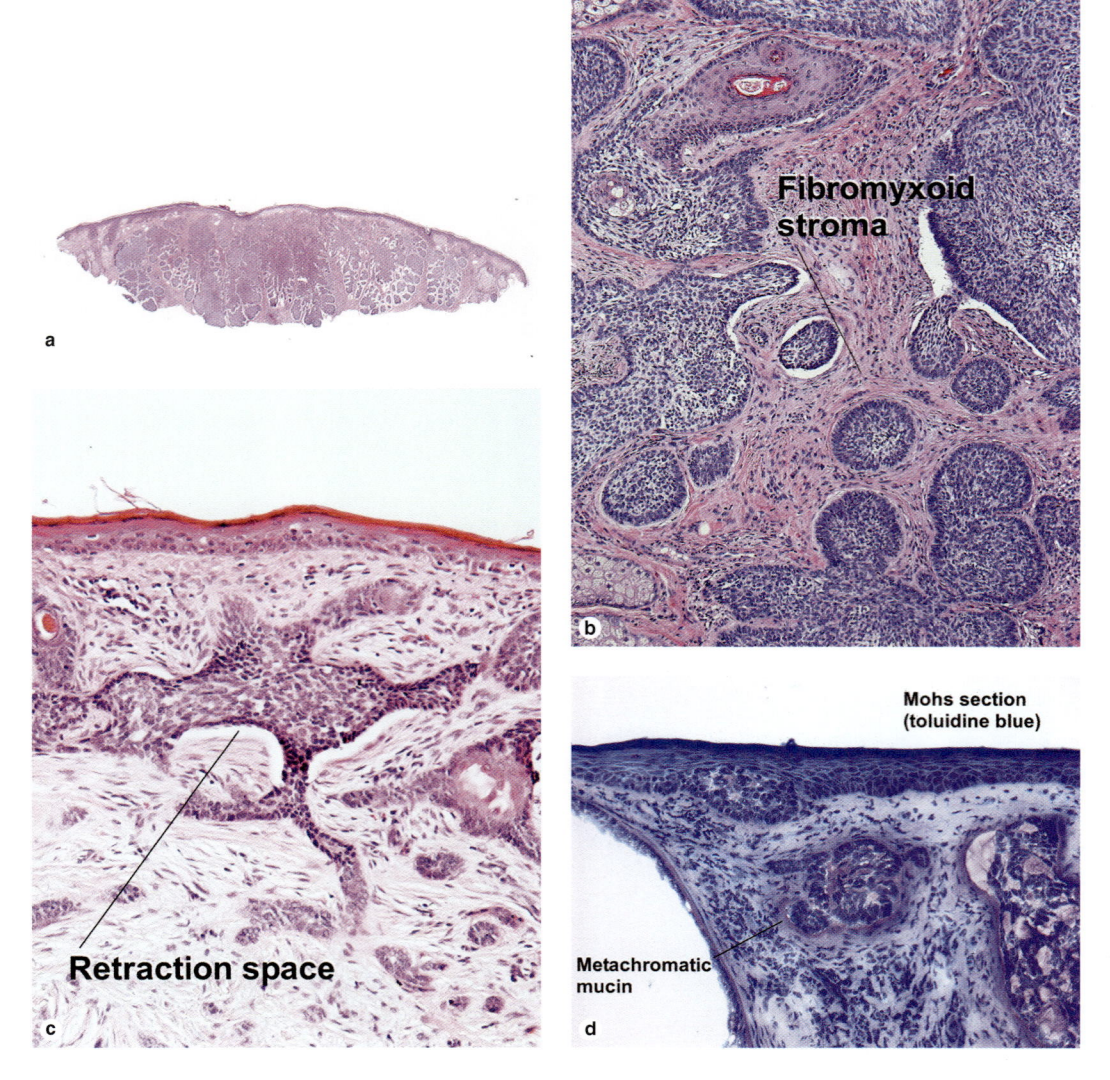

Fig 4-5 Basal cell carcinoma for comparison

Desmoplastic trichoepithelioma

Key features

- Firm doughnut-shaped lesion on a young woman's cheek
- Central dell
- Paisley-tie pattern (tadpole-shaped islands)
- Red desmoplastic stroma
- Calcifications common
- Horn cysts common
- Clefts only within stroma

Table 4-2 Characteristics of desmoplastic trichoepithelioma versus morpheaform basal cell carcinoma

Characteristic	Desmoplastic trichoepithelioma	Morpheaform basal cell carcinoma
Paisley-tie pattern	Yes	Sometimes superficially
Stroma	Red, sclerotic	Red, sclerotic
Horn cysts	Common	Occasional
Calcification	Common	Rare
Clefts	Between collagen fibers within stroma	Between epithelium and stroma
Central dell	Yes	No
Age	Younger	Older
Clinical appearance	Firm doughnut	Scar-like

PEARL

Paisley-tie tumors
- Desmoplastic trichoepithelioma: doughnut-shaped tumor on the cheek of a young female
- Microcystic adnexal carcinoma: firm plaque on the upper lip, medial cheek, or chin
- Morpheaform basal cell carcinoma: scar-like lesion in older patient
- Eruptive syringomas: chest and back or penis, commonly on skin type VI
- Syringomas: small papules on lower lids, very common with Down's syndrome and in Asian females

Table 4-3 Characteristics of desmoplastic trichoepithelioma versus microcystic adnexal carcinoma

Characteristic	Desmoplastic trichoepithelioma	Microcystic adnexal carcinoma
Paisley-tie pattern	Yes	Yes
Stroma	Red, sclerotic	Often red, sclerotic
Horn cysts	Common	Common
Calcification	Common	Rare
Lymphoid aggregates	Rare	Typical
Perineural extension	No	Yes
Clinical appearance	Firm doughnut	Plaque on upper lip, cheek, chin
Central dell	Typical	Absent

Table 4-4 Characteristics of desmoplastic trichoepithelioma versus syringoma

Characteristic	Desmoplastic trichoepithelioma	Syringoma
Paisley-tie pattern	Yes	Yes
Stroma	Red, sclerotic	Red, sclerotic
Horn cysts	Common	May occur
Calcification	Common	Rare
Central dell	Typical	Absent
Shape	Broad	Small and round
Clinical appearance	Firm doughnut	Small papules

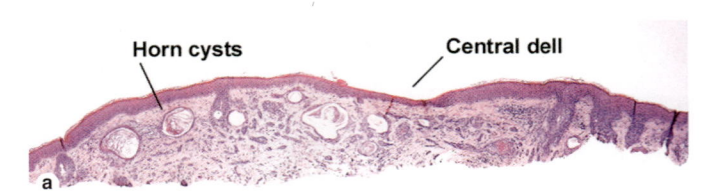

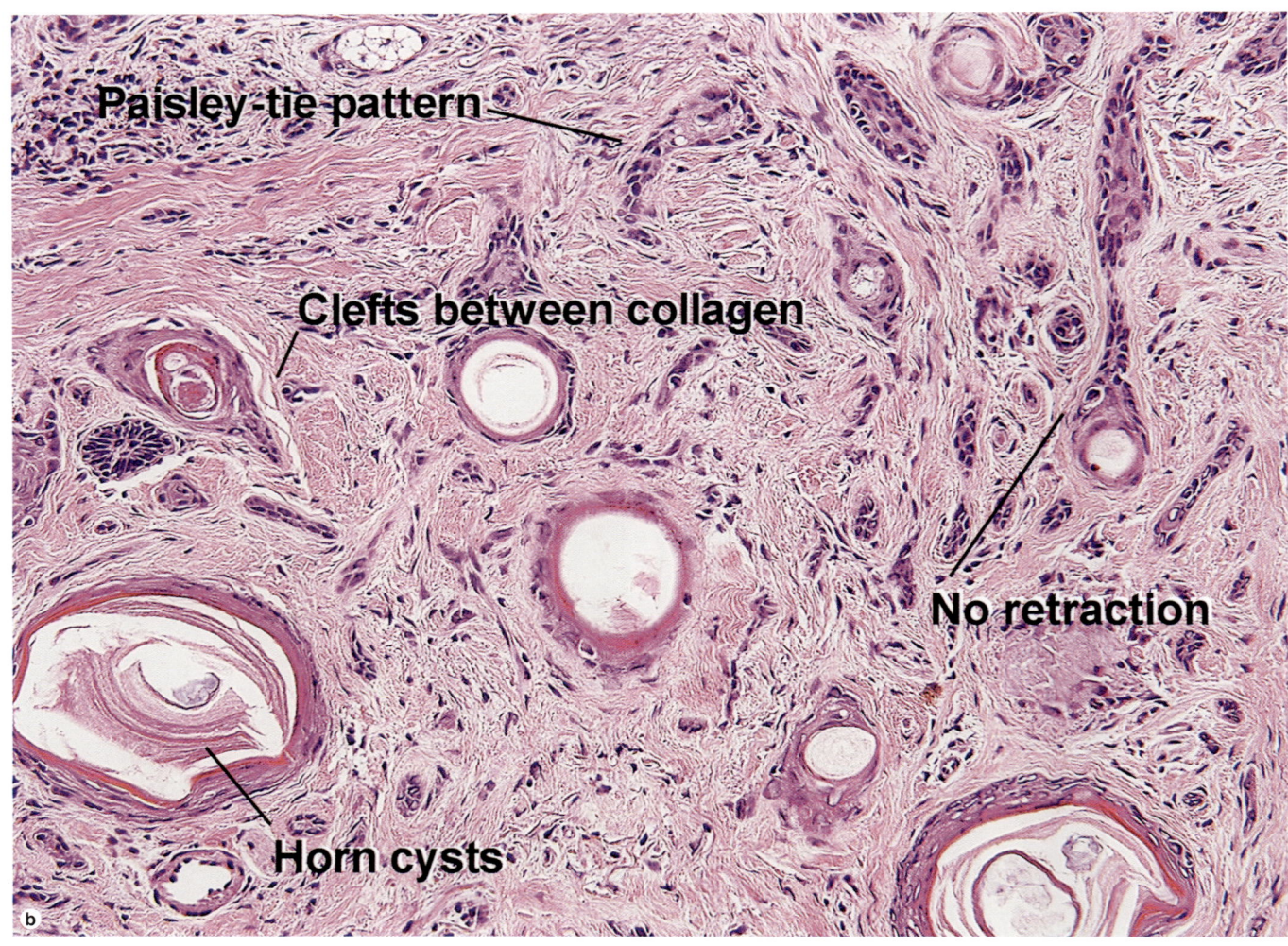

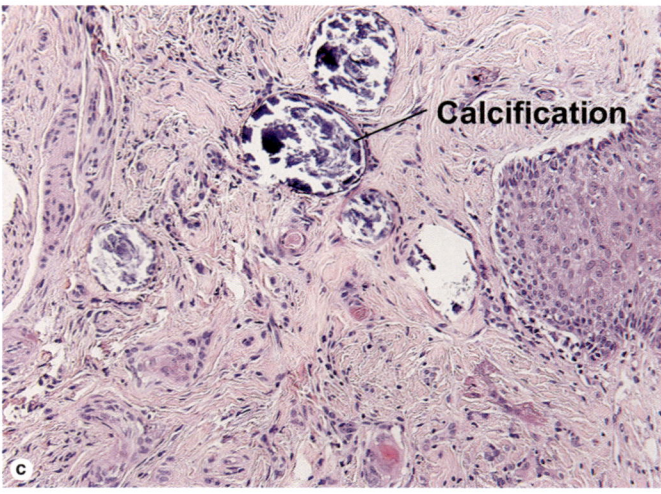

Fig 4-6 Desmoplastic trichoepithelioma

Pilar and sebaceous neoplasms

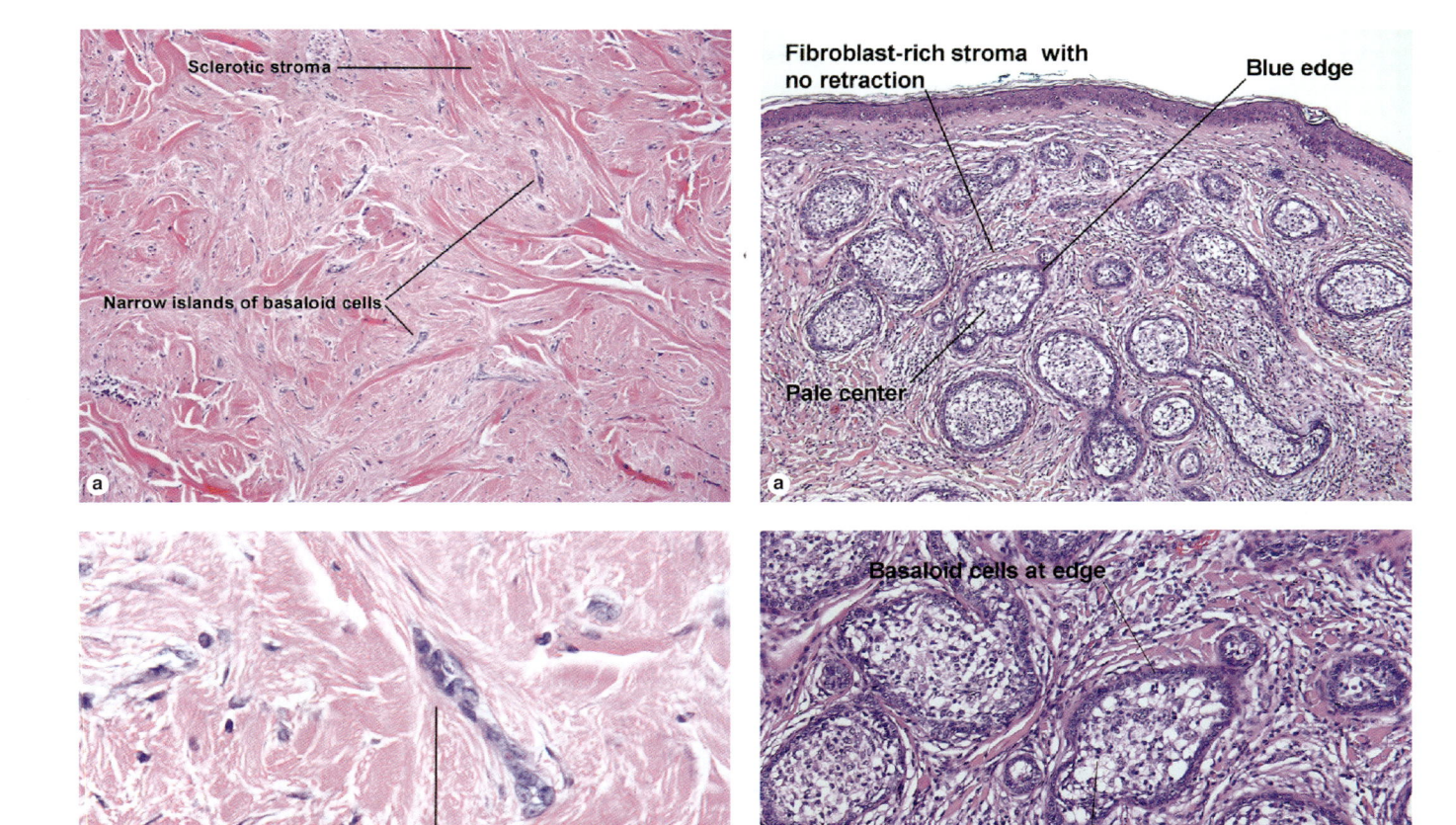

Fig 4-7 Morpheaform basal cell carcinoma for comparison

Lymphadenoma (adamantinoid trichoblastoma)

Key features

- Tumor islands with 1–2 layers of basaloid cells peripherally
- Centers of each island composed of clear cells/inflammatory cells

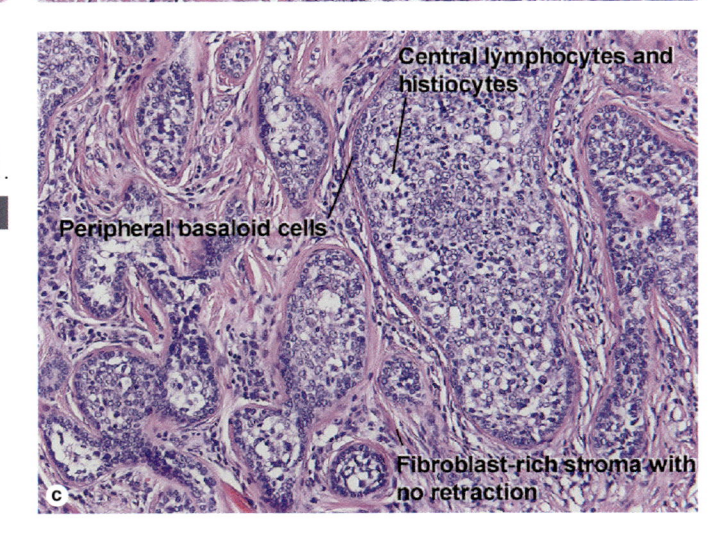

Fig 4-8 Lymphadenoma

Fibrofolliculoma

Key features

- Fibrous pink orb or amphophilic fibromucinous orb
- Epithelial strands radiating outward from central follicle-like structure
- No hair fibers

In fibrofolliculomas, the strands of epithelium are not well enough differentiated to form hair fibers. No bulb, inner or outer root sheath is present. The strands of epithelium may have an anastomosing pattern. *Trichodiscomas* are simply fibrofolliculomas cut in a plane of section that does not reveal the epithelial strands.

PEARL

Birt–Hogg–Dubé syndrome
- Multiple fibrofolliculomas, "trichodiscomas," and "acrochordons" (all three are probably fibrofolliculomas cut at various angles)
- Chromophobe renal carcinoma, renal oncocytoma, spontaneous pneumothorax

Fig 4-9 Fibrofolliculoma

Trichofolliculoma

Key features

- Many small hair follicles emptying into a central large follicular infundibulum (momma and her babies)
- Each small hair follicle has a bulb and root sheath, and produces a hair fiber
- Central infundibulum contains many small hair shafts
- Clinically, there is a tuft of hairs protruding from a central pore

Trichofolliculomas demonstrate miniature follicles converging on a central infundibulum (fingers of *fully formed* follicles forming follicular fibers). Some examples are embedded in an eosinophilic fibrous orb of stroma.

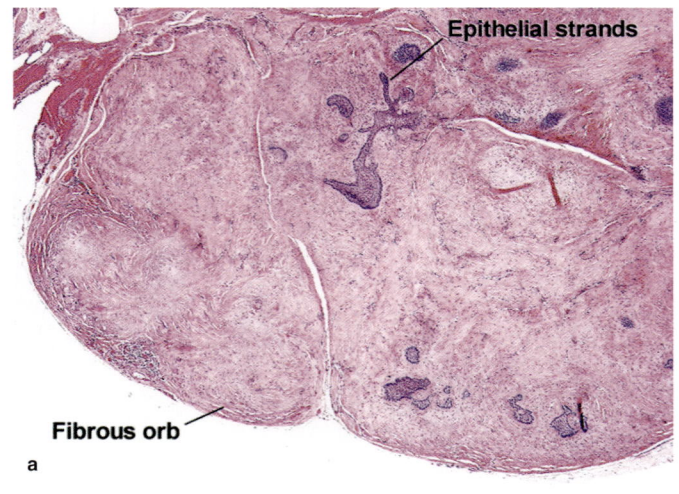

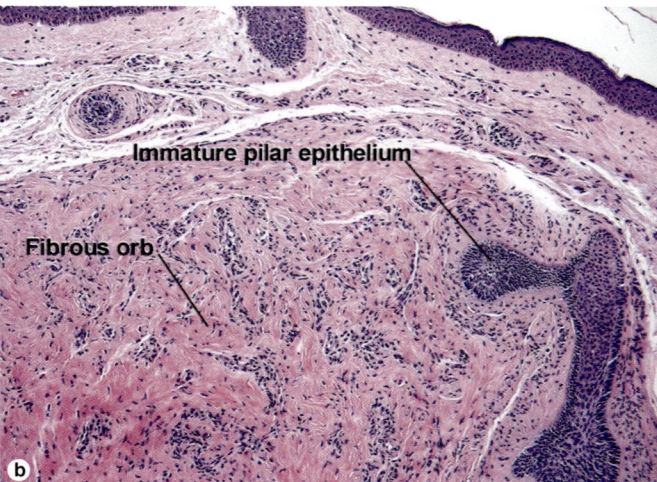

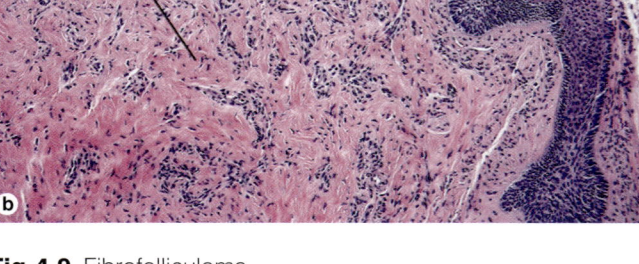

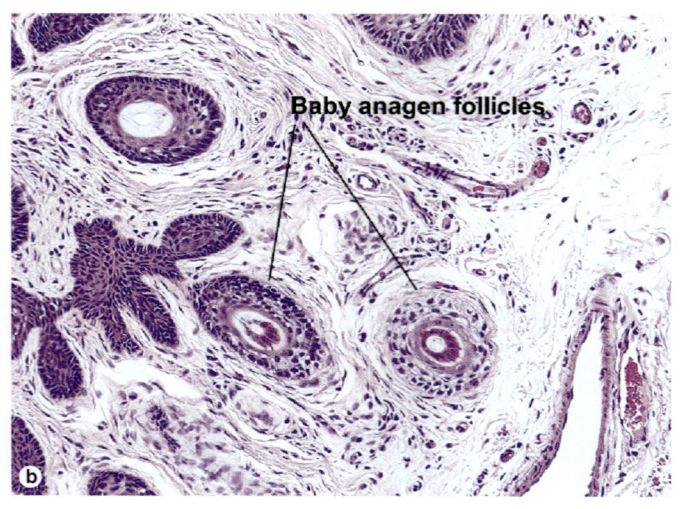

Fig 4-10 Trichofolliculoma

Pilar and sebaceous neoplasms

Trichoadenoma

Key features

- Multiple red doughnuts in the dermis, each resembling a follicular infundibulum
- Often in pairs resembling eyeglasses or toasted oat cereal

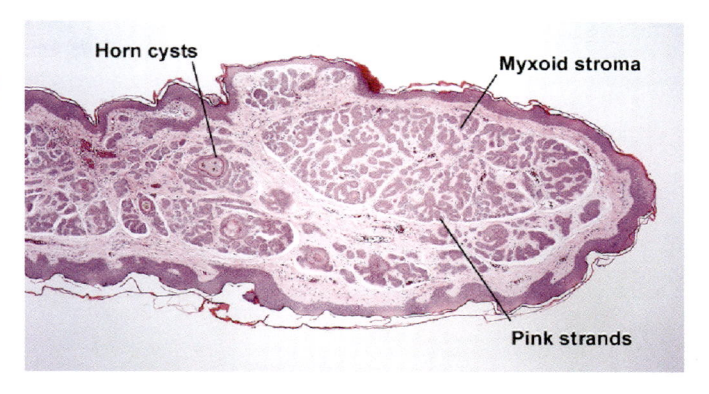

Fig 4-12 Basaloid follicular hamartoma

Differential Diagnosis

Infundibulocystic basal cell carcinoma can appear identical histologically. The two are best distinguished clinically.

Dilated pore of Winer

Key features

- Resembles a dilated follicular infundibulum
- Small radiating red finger-like epithelial projections

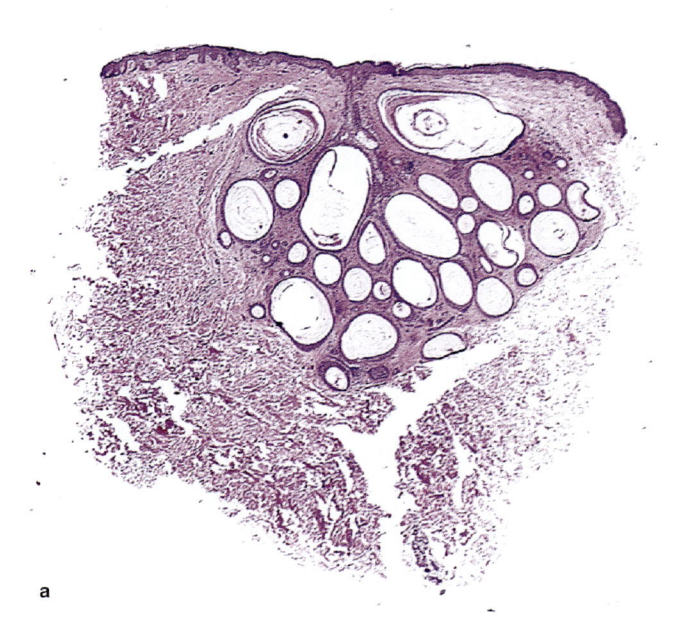

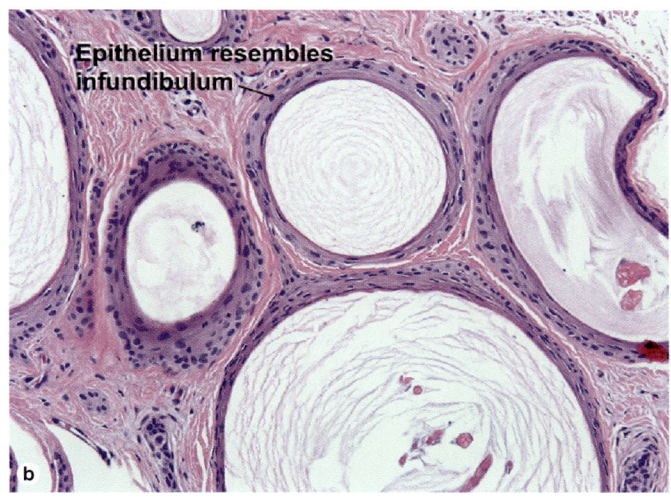

Fig 4-11 Trichoadenoma

Basaloid follicular hamartoma

Key features

- Resembles infundibulocystic basal cell carcinoma histologically
- Often multiple with autosomal-dominant inheritance
- Sometimes segmental Blaschkoid distribution

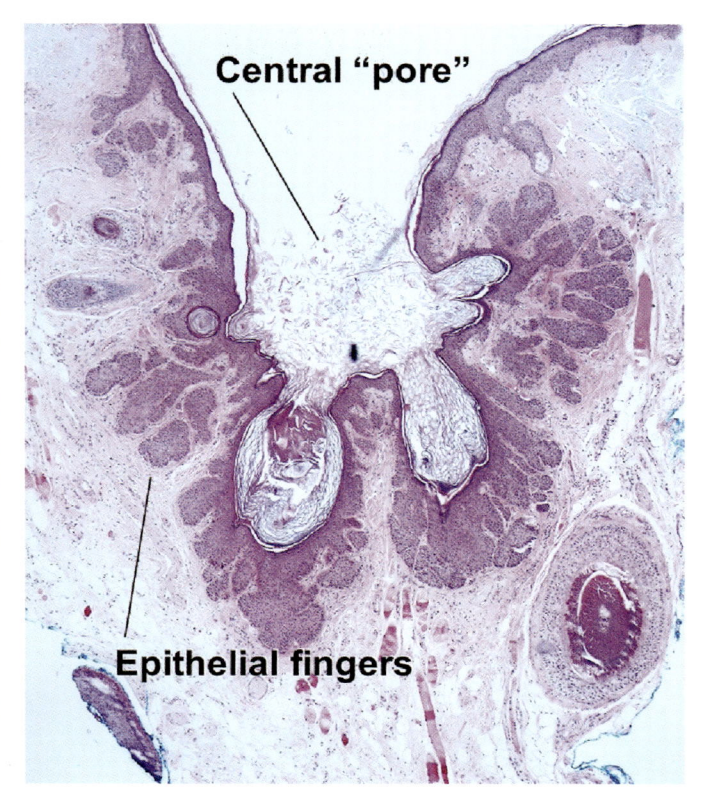

Fig 4-13 Dilated pore of Winer

Pilar sheath acanthoma

Key features

- Similar to dilated pore of Winer, but with thick acanthotic fingers

Pilar sheath acanthoma has been described as a "pore of Winer on steroids".

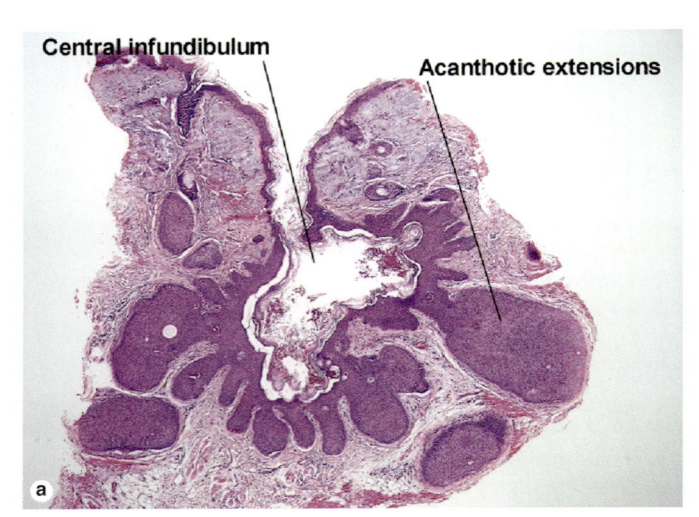

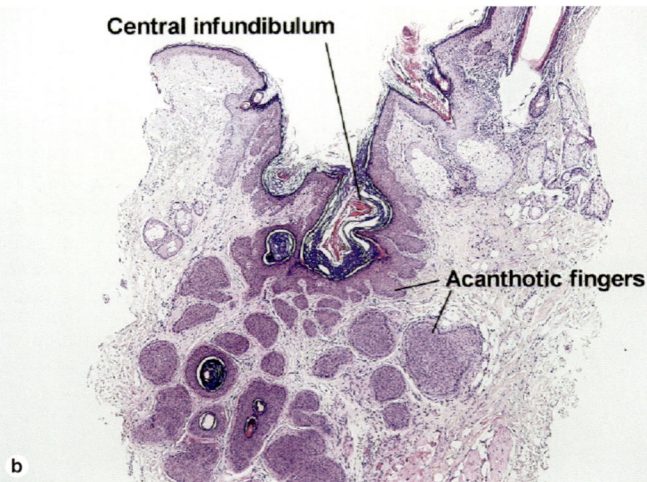

Fig 4-14 Pilar sheath acanthoma

Trichilemmoma

Key features

- Often a warty surface
- Smooth lobules of clear glycogenated cells hanging down from the epidermis
- Peripheral palisading
- Outlined by a thick glassy eosinophilic "vitreous" basement membrane

Trichilemmomas resemble the glycogenated outer root sheath of the hair follicle. When multiple, they may be a marker for Cowden's syndrome.

Differential Diagnosis

Trichilemmomas are composed of lobules of clear glycogenated cells that hang down from the surface epidermis. A clear cell acanthoma is a thickened area of the epidermis. In clear cell acanthoma, a glycogenated pale segment of epidermis is sharply demarcated from the surrounding skin. Neutrophils are noted throughout the lesion and in the overlying crust. There is no thickening of the basement membrane zone.

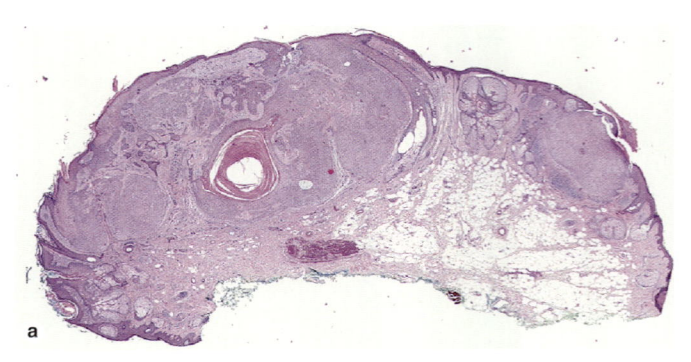

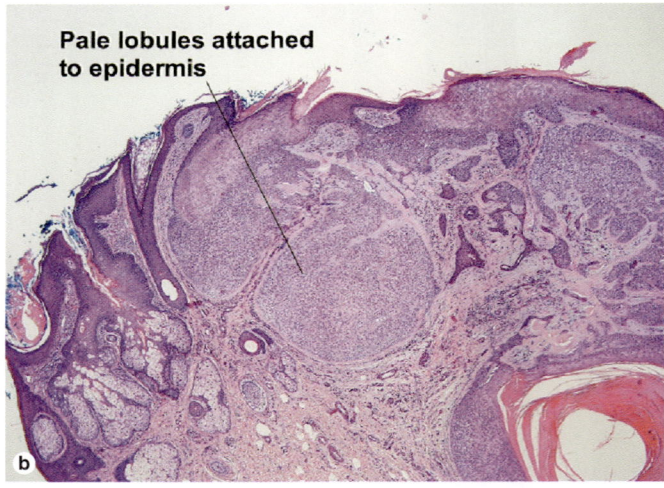

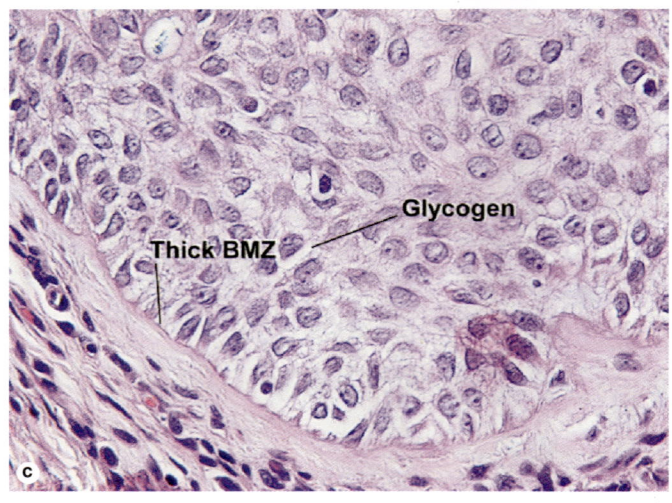

Fig 4-15 Trichilemmoma (BMZ, basement membrane zone)

Desmoplastic trichilemmoma

Key features

- Smooth outline with surrounding glassy basement membrane
- Centrally, broken into jagged islands separated by dense pink stroma

Sebaceous neoplasms

Nevus sebaceus of Jadassohn (organoid nevus)

Postpubertal nevus sebaceus of Jadassohn

Key features

- "Broad, bald, bumpy, and bubbly"
- Present at birth, becomes cerebriform at puberty
- Dilated apocrine glands in underlying dermis

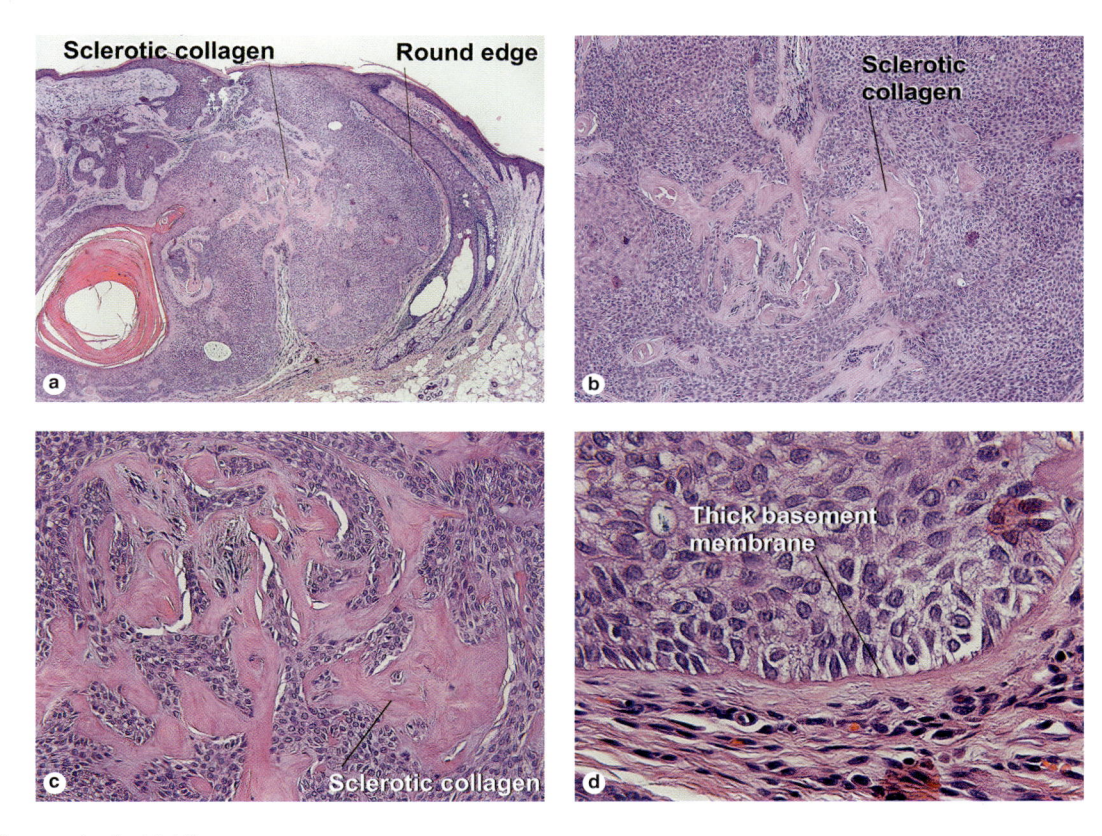

Fig 4-16 Desmoplastic trichilemmoma

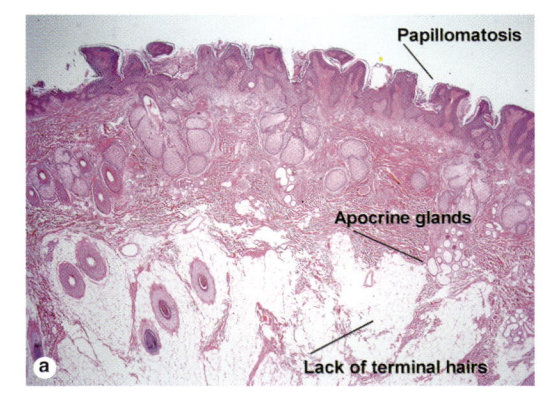

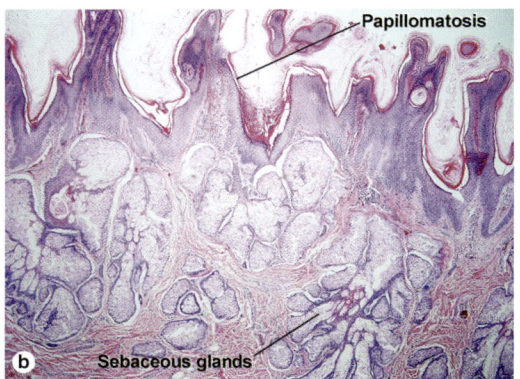

Fig 4-17 Postpubertal nevus sebaceus of Jadassohn

Dermatopathology

- Hyperkeratosis, acanthosis, and papillomatosis common
- Secondary tumors, especially syringocystadenoma papilliferum and small trichoblastomas, are common

Postpubertal cerebriform lesions of nevus sebaceus of Jadassohn appear as *broad*, alopecic (*bald*), acanthotic and papillomatous (*bumpy*) lesions with large sebaceous lobules (*bubbly*) and dilated apocrine glands.

Prepubertal nevus sebaceus of Jadassohn

Key features

- "Broad and bald, but not bumpy or bubbly"
- Present at birth, but will not become cerebriform or develop large sebaceous or apocrine elements until puberty
- Primitive epithelial germs resembling fetal hair germs present

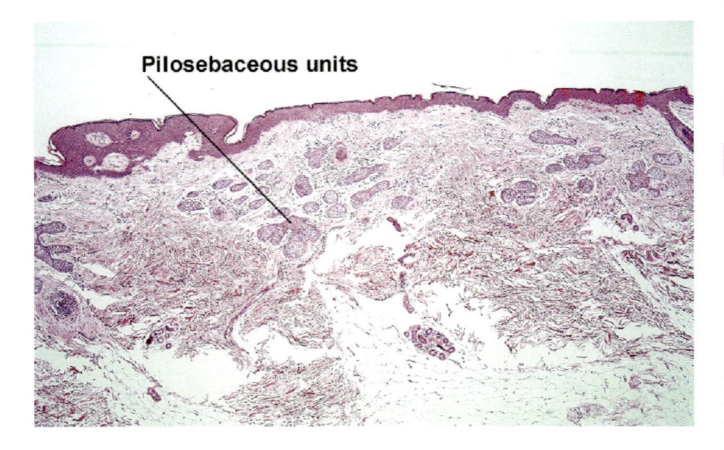

Fig 4-18 Prepubertal nevus sebaceus of Jadassohn

Sebaceous hyperplasia

Key features

- Large cluster of sebaceous glands around a patulous follicular opening
- Normal germinative basaloid layer at periphery of lobule

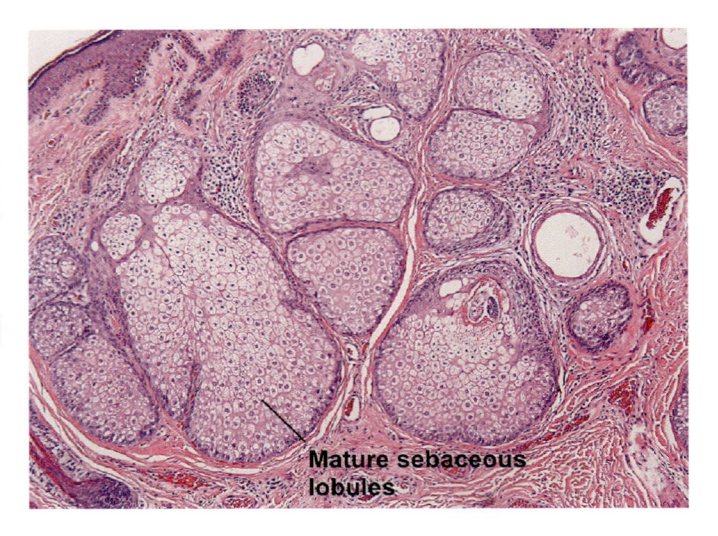

Fig 4-19 Sebaceous hyperplasia

Sebaceoma

Key features

- Usually a single nodule
- Basaloid cells and mature sebocytes in varying proportions
- Some use the term *sebaceous adenoma* for tumors with <50% basaloid cells, and the term *sebaceous epithelioma* for tumors with >50% basaloid cells.

Benign sebaceous neoplasms may be markers for the Muir–Torre syndrome (associated with keratoacanthomas and gut carcinoma). The syndrome is allelic to hereditary non-polyposis colorectal cancer. Gastrointestinal cancers are the most common internal malignancies in the Muir–Torre syndrome (61%), followed by genitourinary tumors (22%). Approximately 15% of female patients with Muir–Torre syndrome develop endometrial cancer. The cancers, although multiple, are usually relatively indolent. Loss of normal nuclear staining for either MSH-2 or MLH-1 suggests microsatellite instability and supports a diagnosis of Muir–Torre syndrome. MSH-6 and PMS staining are less specific in skin. Genetic testing is also available, but is more expensive.

Pilar and sebaceous neoplasms **Chapter 4** 83

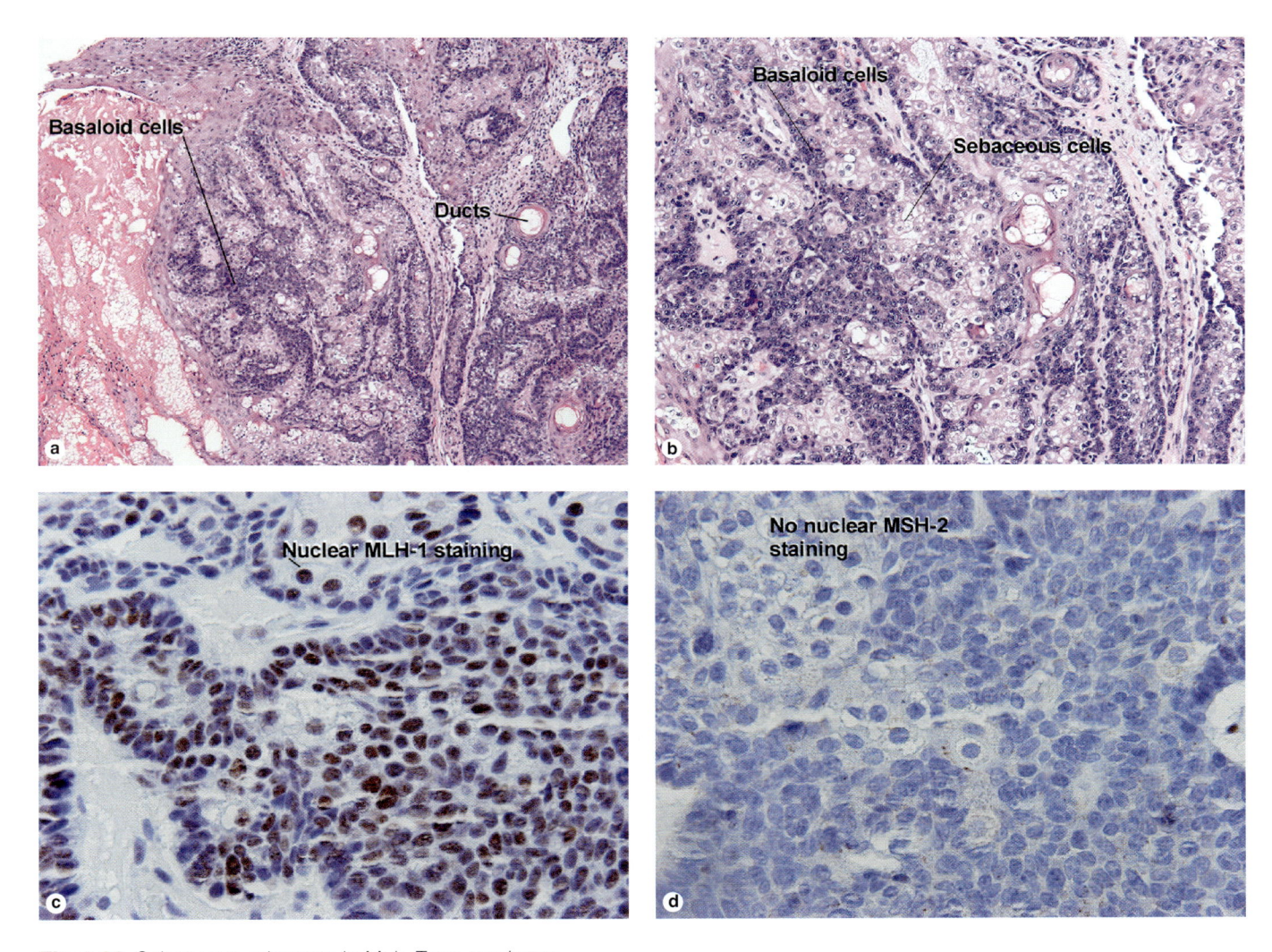

Fig 4-20 Sebaceous adenoma in Muir–Torre syndrome

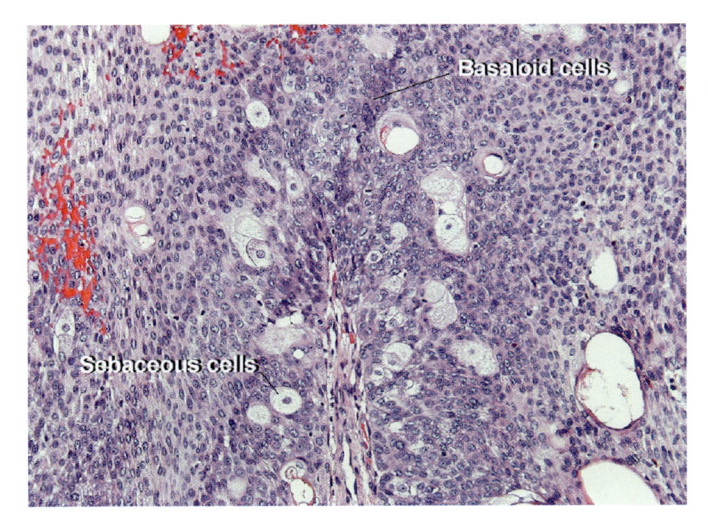

Fig 4-21 Sebaceous epithelioma

Sebaceous carcinoma

Key features

- May be predominantly red or blue at scan
- Atypia and mitoses common
- Infiltrative border may be apparent
- Foamy cells with scalloped nuclei
- Atypical cells may extend into the epidermis or conjunctiva in a nested or buckshot pattern

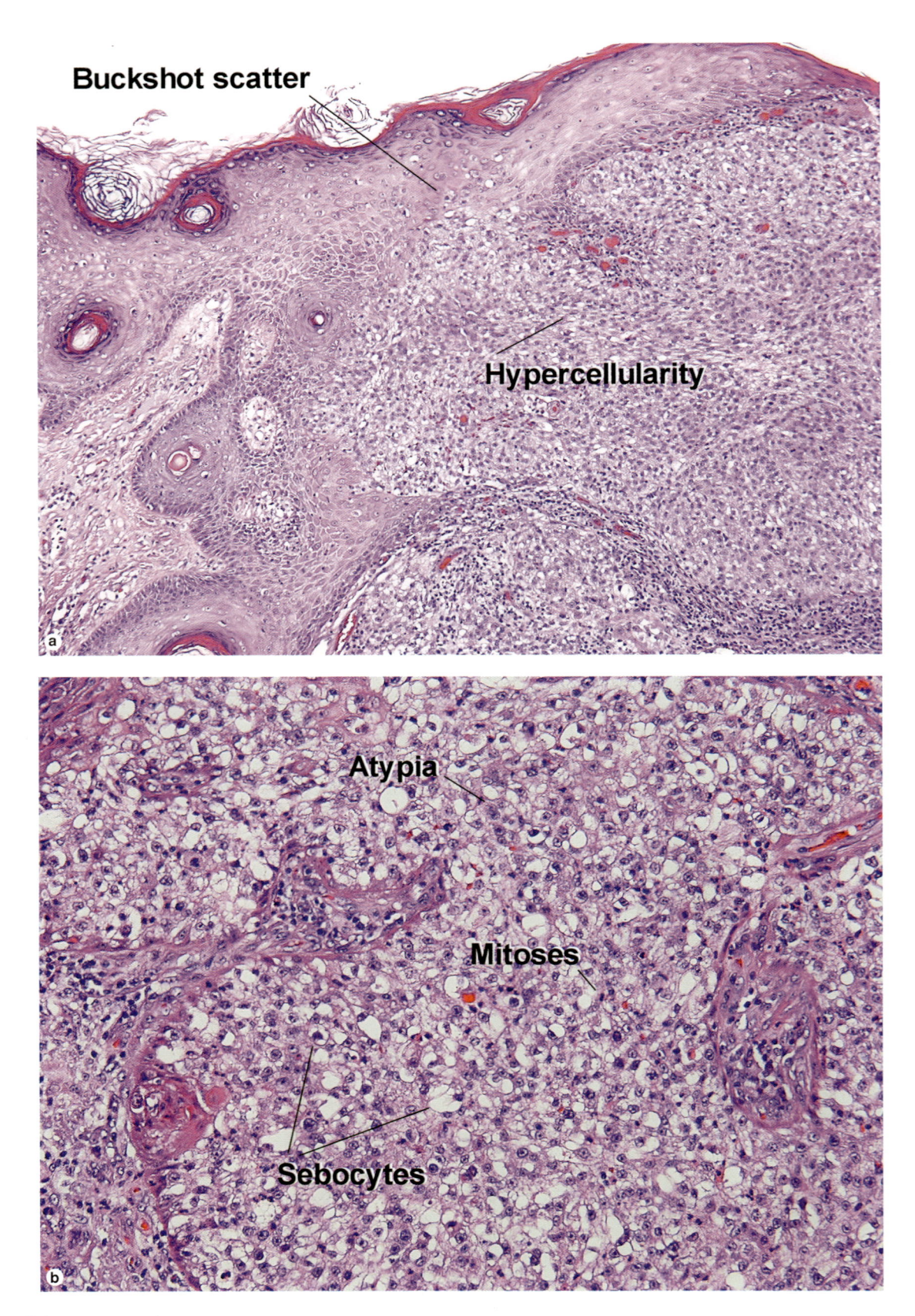

Fig 4-22 Sebaceous carcinoma

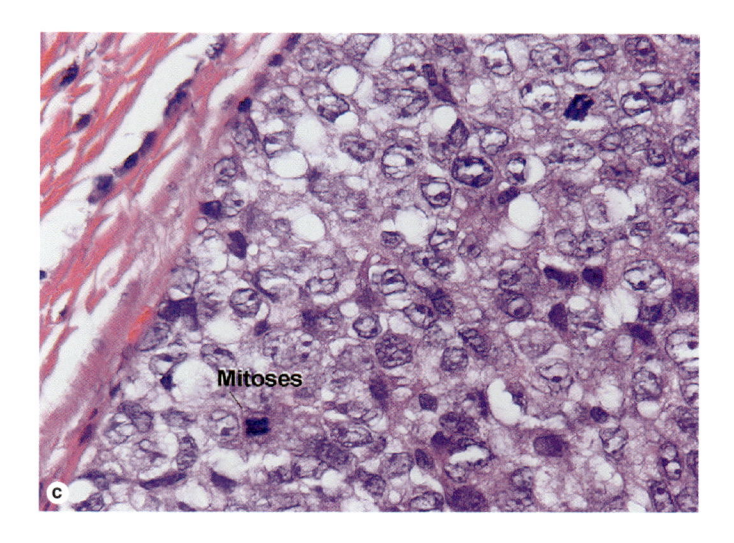

Fig 4-22, cont'd

Further reading

Ansai S, Mitsuhashi Y, Kondo S, et al. Immunohistochemical differentiation of extra-ocular sebaceous carcinoma from other skin cancers. J Dermatol 2004;31(12):998–1008.

Kazakov DV, Kutzner H, Rütten A, et al. Trichogerminoma: a rare cutaneous adnexal tumor with differentiation toward the hair germ epithelium. Dermatology 2002;205(4):405–408.

Pereira PR, Odashiro AN, Rodrigues-Reyes AA, et al. Histopathological review of sebaceous carcinoma of the eyelid. J Cutan Pathol 2005;32(7):496–501.

Ponti G, Longo C. Microsatellite instability and mismatch repair protein expression in sebaceous tumors, keratocanthoma, and basal cell carcinomas with sebaceous differentiation in Muir–Torre syndrome. J Am Acad Dermatol 2013;68(3):509–510.

Sidhu HK, Patel RV, Goldenberg G. Dermatology clinics: what's new in dermatopathology: news in nonmelanocytic neoplasia. Dermatol Clin 2012;30(4):623–641.

Tebcherani AJ, de Andrade HF Jr, Sotto MN. Diagnostic utility of immunohistochemistry in distinguishing trichoepithelioma and basal cell carcinoma: evaluation using tissue microarray samples. Mod Pathol 2012;25(10):1345–1353.

Tse JY, Nguyen AT, Le LP, et al. Microcystic adnexal carcinoma versus desmoplastic trichoepithelioma: a comparative study. Am J Dermatopathol 2013;35(1): 50–55.

Welsch MJ, Krunic A, Medenica MM. Birt–Hogg–Dube Syndrome. Int J Dermatol 2005;44(8):668–673.

Chapter 5

Sweat gland neoplasms

Dirk M. Elston

Blue sweat gland tumors differentiate towards the secretory portion of the sweat gland. Red sweat gland tumors differentiate towards the sweat duct. Sweat duct tumors often demonstrate clear cell change. Most sweat gland tumors can show at least focal decapitation secretion, suggesting they are capable of apocrine differentiation.

Cylindroma (turban tumor)

Key features

- Islands of blue cells with little cytoplasm
- Dark and pale blue nuclei present
- Jigsaw-puzzle pattern
- Islands outlined by a deeply eosinophilic basement membrane
- Deeply eosinophilic hyaline droplets may be noted in islands
- Often inherited and multiple on the scalp

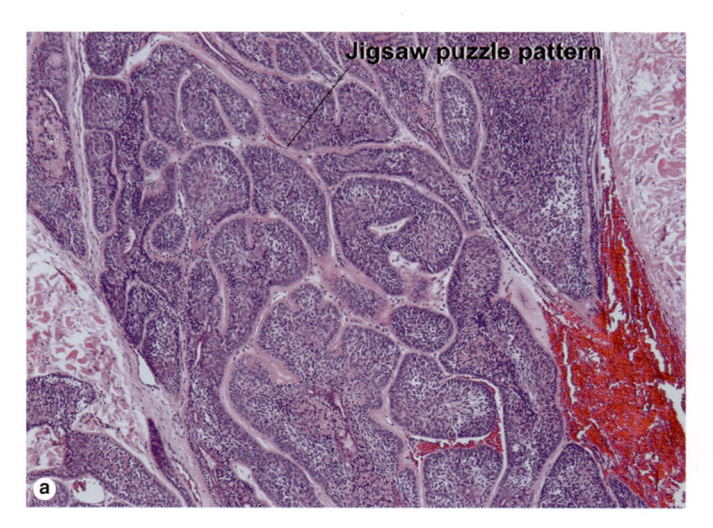

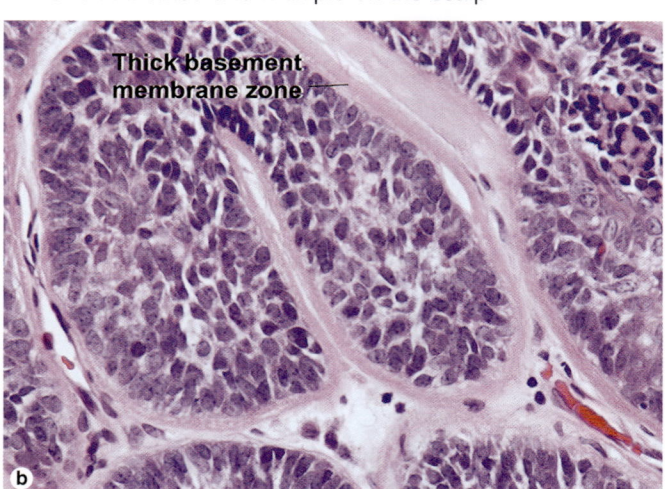

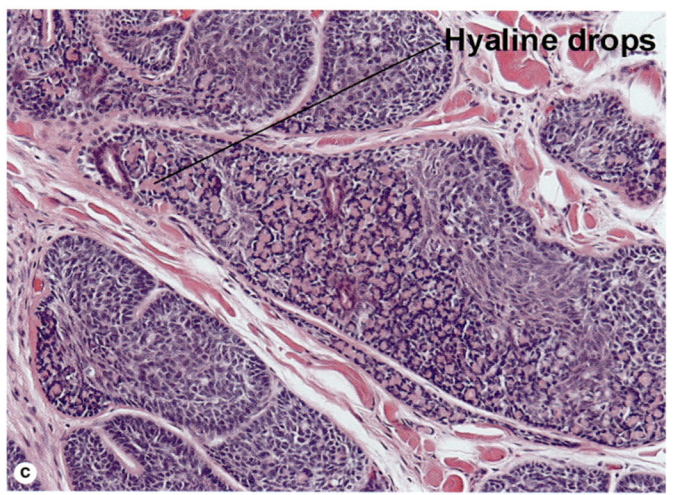

Fig 5-1 Cylindroma

Spiradenoma

Key features

- Larger round islands of blue cells with little cytoplasm
- Dark and pale blue nuclei present
- Islands peppered with black lymphocytes
- Deeply eosinophilic hyaline droplets may be noted in islands
- Usually solitary

Spiradenomas and cylindromas are closely related tumors. Both differentiate towards the secretory portion of the sweat gland. Hybrid tumors occur. Spiradenomas are usually sporadic and solitary, while cylindromas are multiple, inherited, and may occur together with trichoepitheliomas. Spiradenomas are inflamed (lymphocytes) and spontaneously tender.

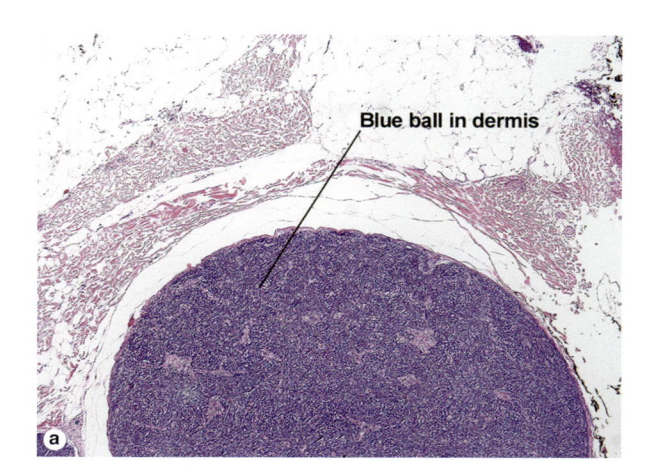

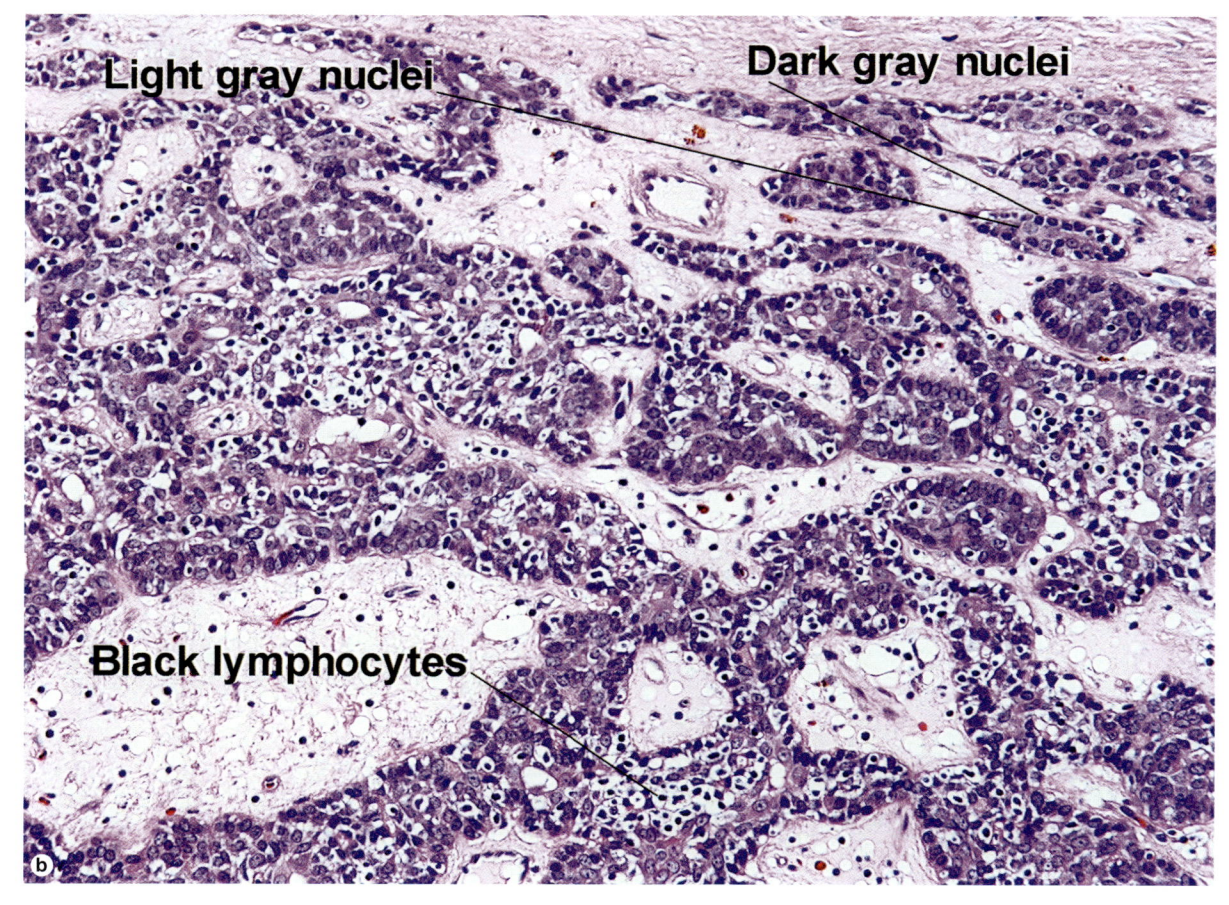

Fig 5-2 Spiradenoma

Dermatopathology

Table 5-1 Characteristics of cylindroma versus spiradenoma

Characteristic	Cylindroma	Spiradenoma
Blue cells with little cytoplasm	Yes	Yes
Dark and pale blue nuclei	Yes	Yes
Peppered with black lymphocytes	No	Yes
Hyaline droplets in nests	Yes	Yes
Jigsaw-puzzle pattern	Yes	No
Deeply eosinophilic basement membrane	Yes	No
Inheritance	Autosomal dominant	Sporadic
Tender	No	Yes

PEARL

Tender tumors: BANGLE
- *B*lue rubber bleb nevus
- *A*ngiolipoma
- *N*euroma, neurilemmoma
- *G*lomus tumor
- *L*eiomyoma
- "*E*ccrine" spiradenoma

These tumors are probably tender because they have:
1. Smooth muscle that can contract to cause pain
2. Compressed nerve
3. Inflammation

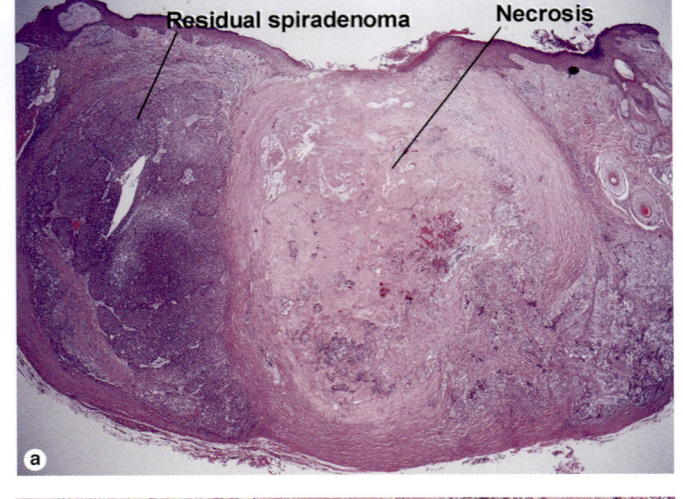

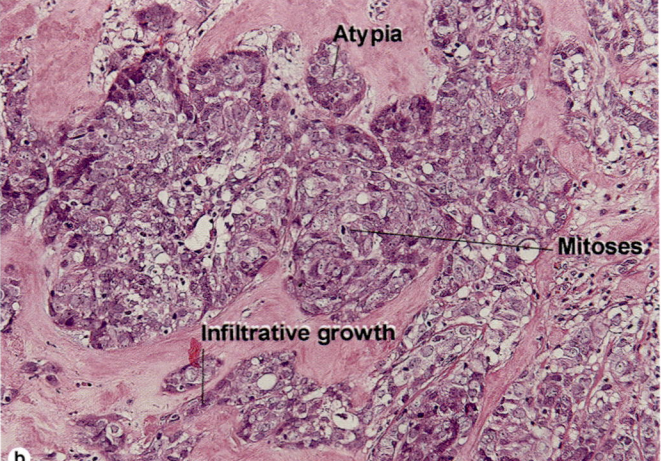

Fig 5-3 Spiradenocarcinoma

Spiradenocarcinoma

Key features
- Rare
- Occurs in long-standing spiradenomas
- Atypia, mitoses, and necrosis

Syringocystadenoma papilliferum

Key features
- Opens to surface
- Blue papillary fronds extending upward into clear spaces: "fjords and fronds"
- Decapitation secretion
- Plasma cells

Syringocystadenoma papilliform (SPAP) differentiates towards the secretory portion of the sweat gland. SPAP opens to the surface, which looks as though one could slide into it. Plasma cells are typically present in the mesenchymal core of each frond. Clinically, they appear as raised warty plaques on the head or neck. One-third of cases occur within nevus sebaceus.

Sweat gland neoplasms   Chapter 5   89

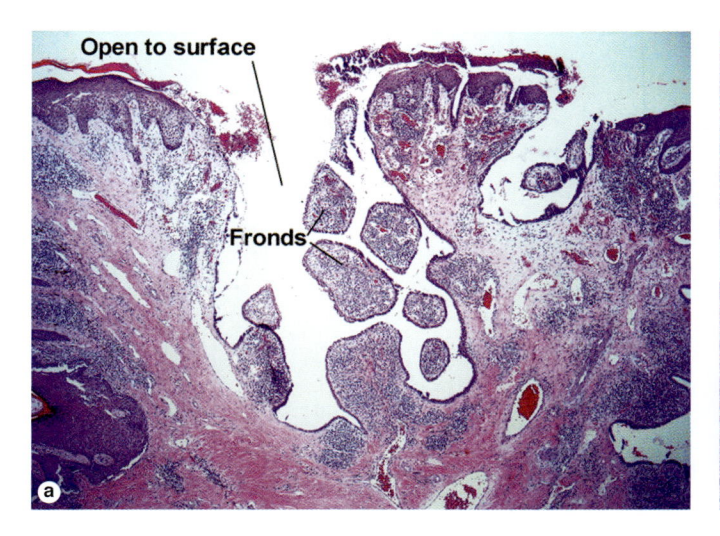

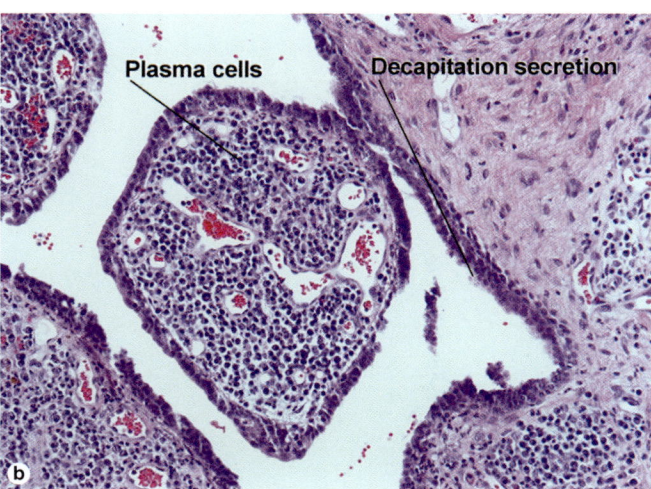

Fig 5-4 Syringocystadenoma papilliferum

Hidradenoma papilliferum

Key features

- Blue dermal nodule with branching cystic spaces
- Papillary fronds
- Decapitation secretion

Hidradenoma papilliferum (HPAP) usually presents clinically as a vulvar dermal nodule, but occasionally presents on a breast, eyelid, or ear. Histologically, HPAP is a maze-like dermal nodule, which looks as though one could *hide* in it. The arborizing pattern of blue fronds demonstrates decapitation secretion. Like SPAP, it differentiates towards the secretory segment.

Papillary digital carcinoma (aggressive digital papillary adenocarcinoma)

Key features

- Blue tumor nodules with cystic change
- Little to no visible cytoplasm
- Papillary fronds
- Atypia, mitoses, and necrosis variable
- Typically involves the hand
- Many patients are young
- Even bland tumors can metastasize

There can be significant histologic similarities to hidradenoma papilliferum. All digital papillary tumors should be considered carcinomas.

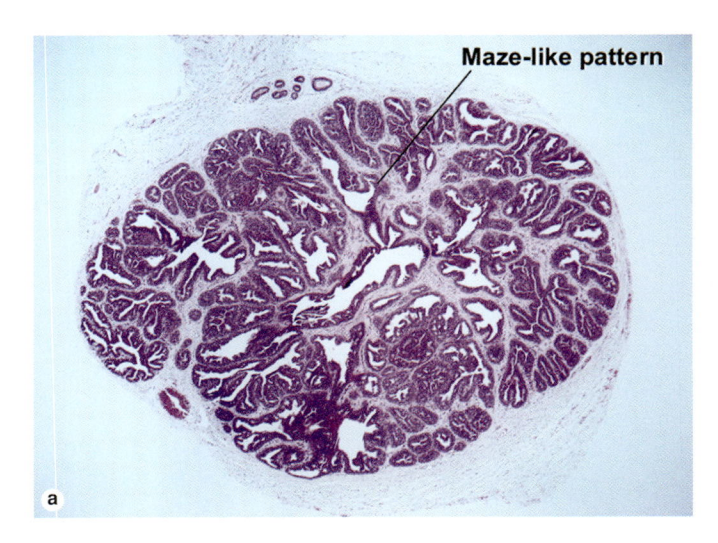

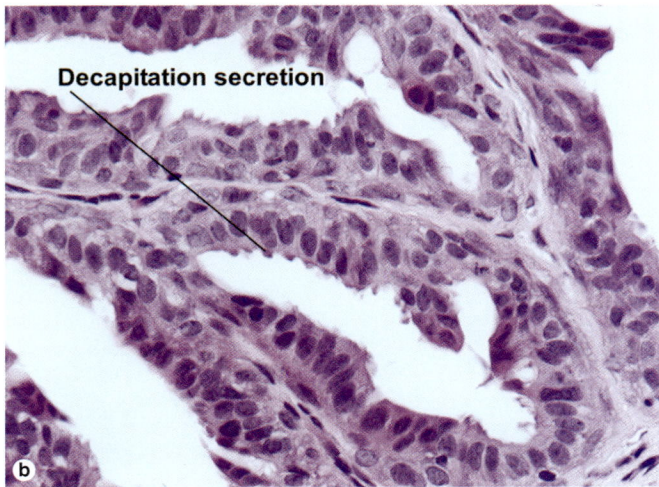

Fig 5-5 Hidradenoma papilliferum

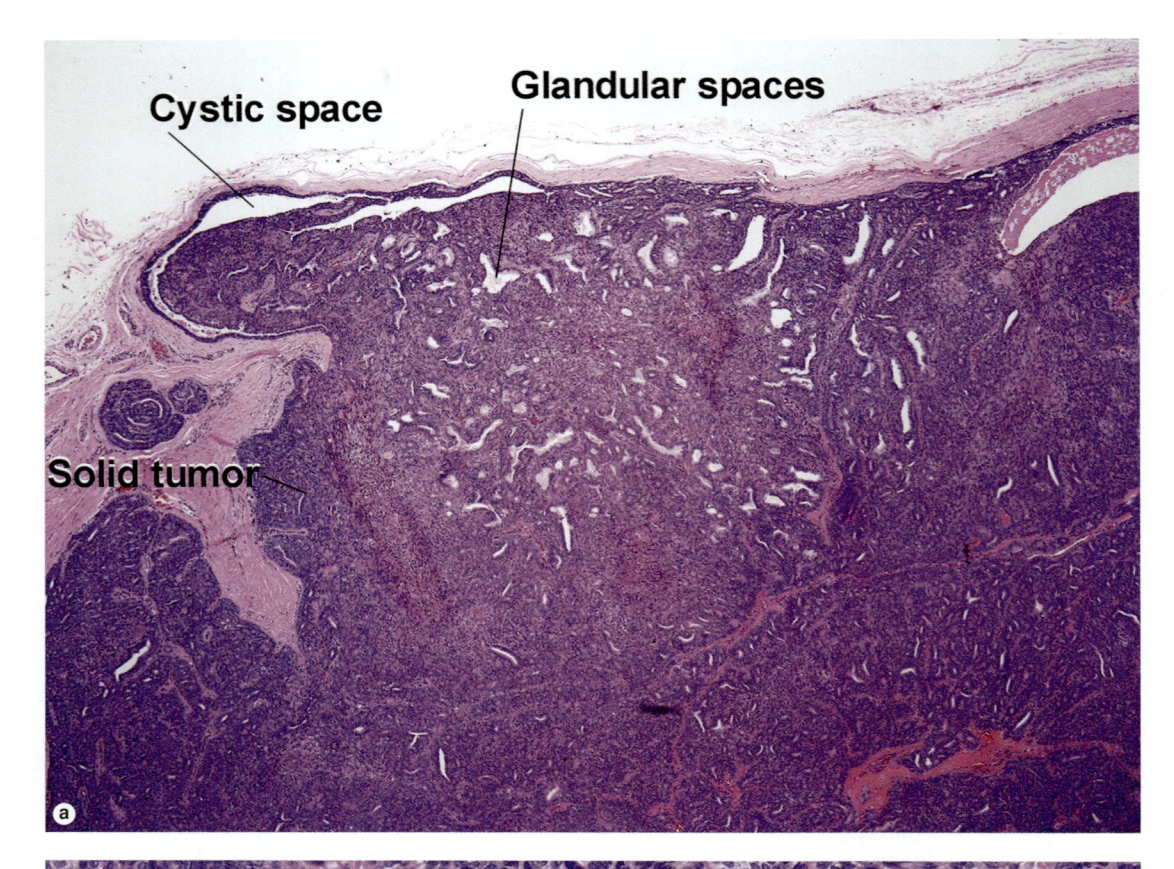

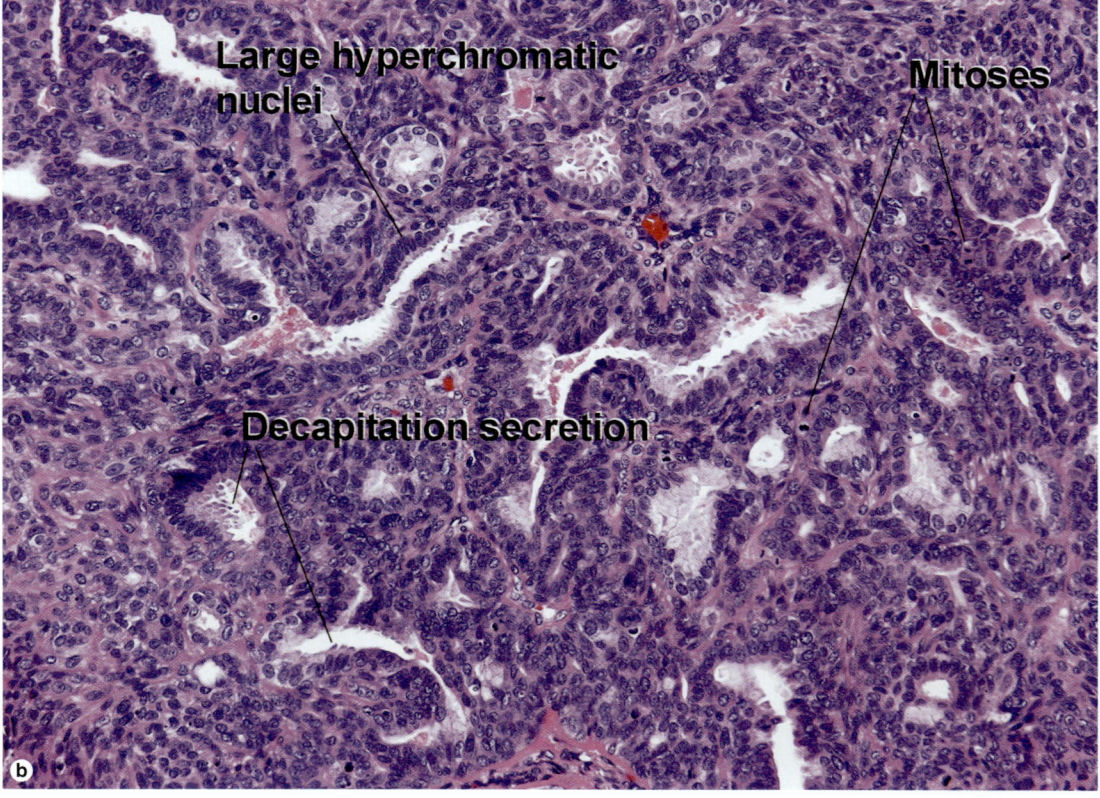

Fig 5-6 Papillary digital carcinoma

Mucinous carcinoma

Key features

- Islands of blue cells surrounded by mucin ("blue islands floating in a sea of snot")
- Primary cutaneous mucinous carcinoma and metastatic mucinous carcinoma look identical

Mucinous carcinoma can be primary in the skin, or can be metastatic from a primary cancer of the breast or gastrointestinal tract. Imaging studies may be required.

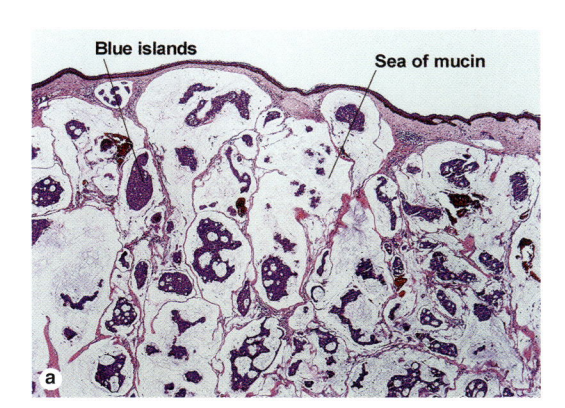

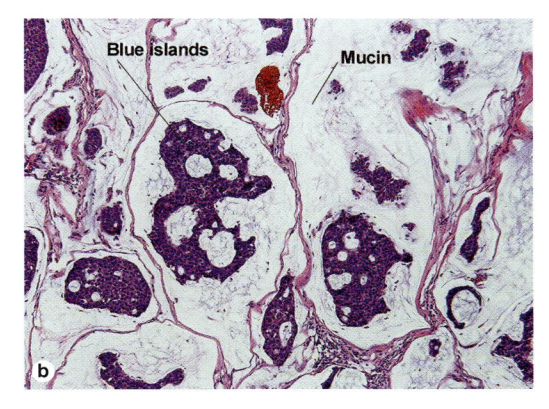

Fig 5-7 Mucinous carcinoma

Syringoma

Key features

- Paisley-tie pattern of tadpole-shaped ducts
- Ample pink cytoplasm
- Dense red sclerotic stroma
- Tumor is small and round

Syrinx refers to a pipe or duct. Syringomas usually appear as small papules on the eyelids. They are especially common in Asian women and in children with Down's syndrome. Eruptive syringomas typically occur on the chest, back, or penis of a dark-skinned patient. Eruptive syringomas appear as small hyperpigmented papules with no tendency to coalesce.

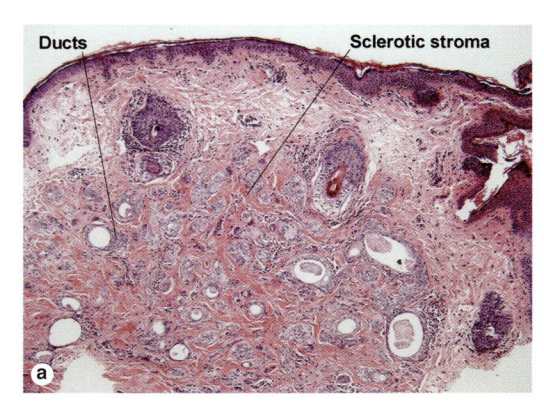

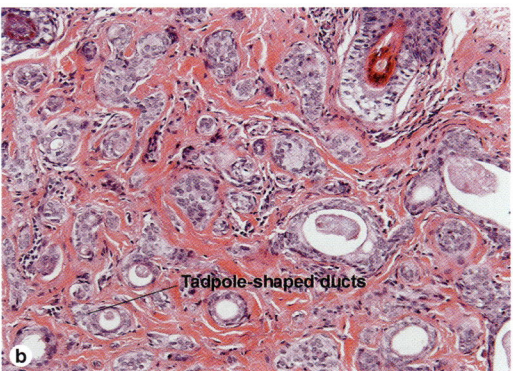

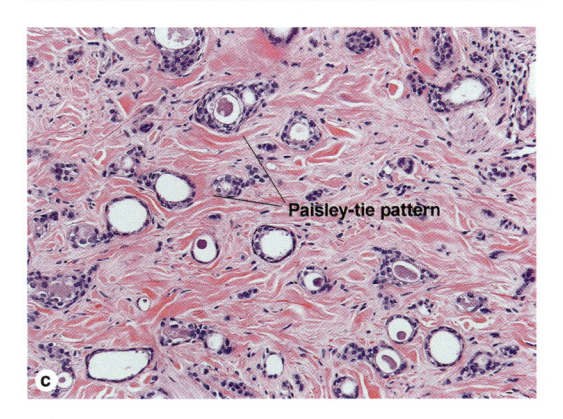

Fig 5-8 Syringoma

Clear cell syringoma

Key features

- Paisley-tie pattern of tadpole-shaped ducts
- Clear cells containing abundant glycogen
- Dense red sclerotic stroma
- Tumor is small and round
- Associated with diabetes mellitus

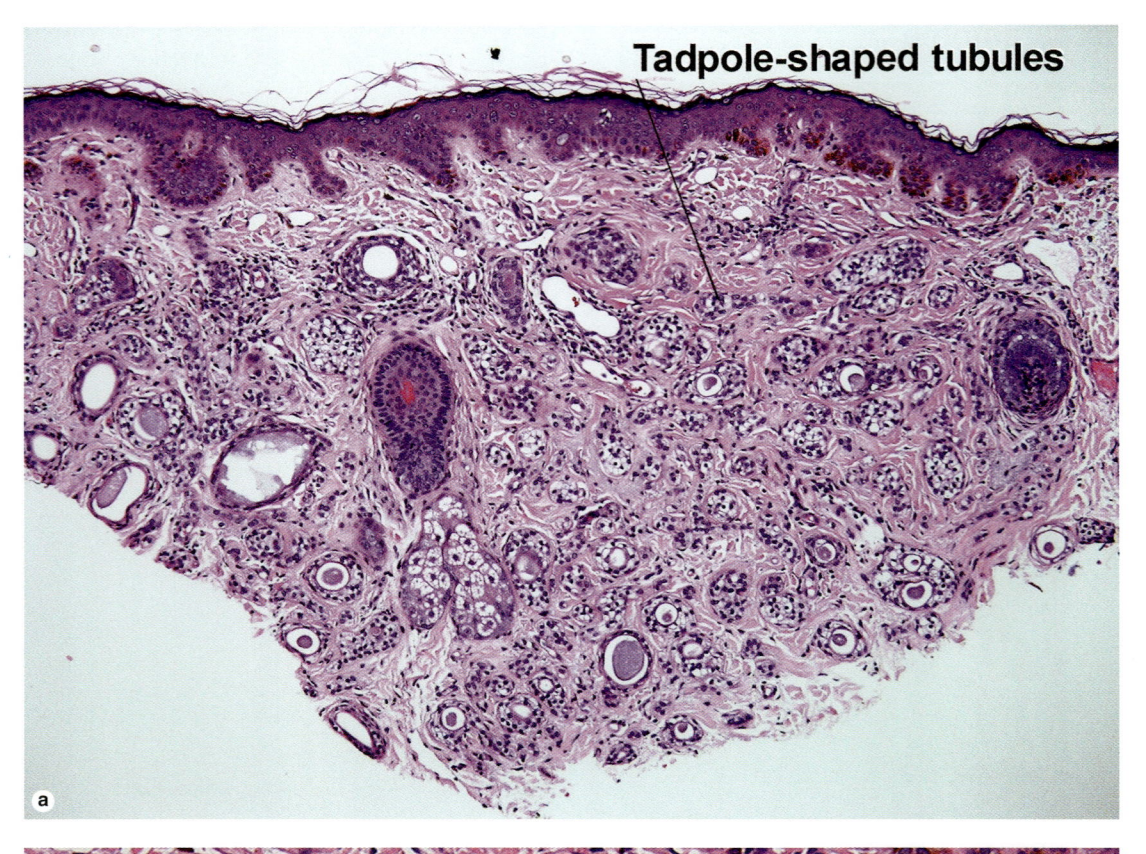

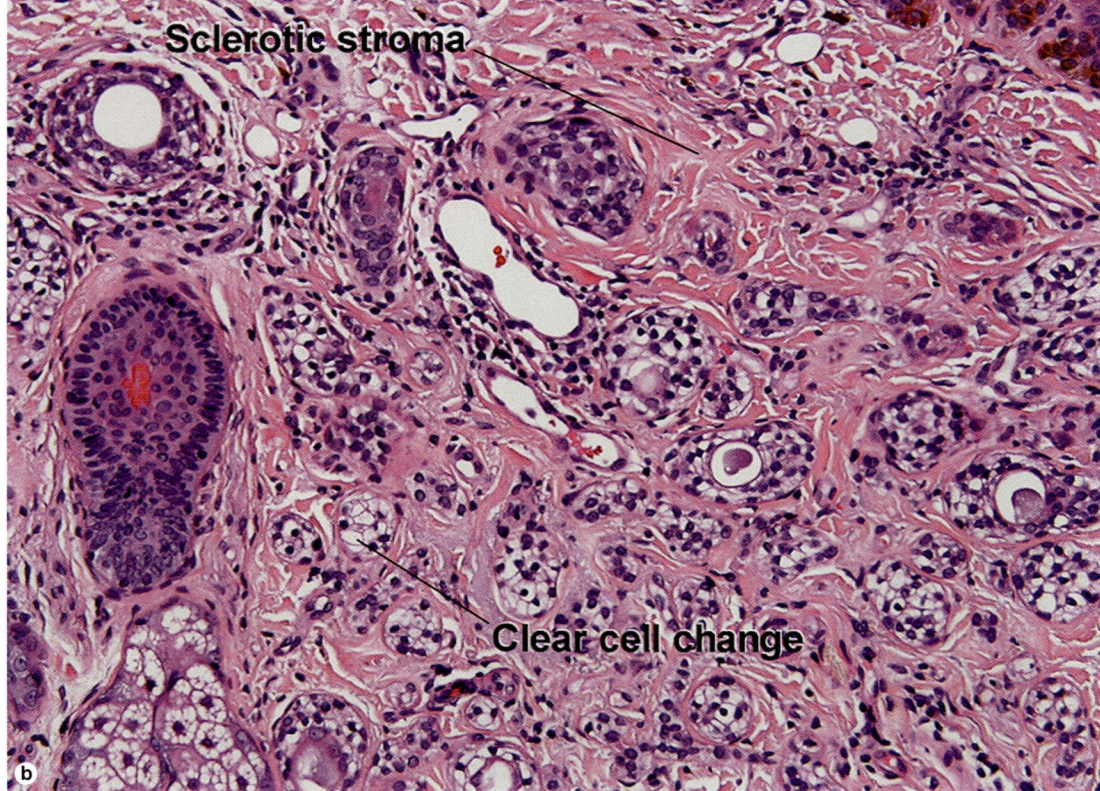

Fig 5-9 Clear cell syringoma

Microcystic adnexal carcinoma

Key features

- Biphasic pattern (sweat duct-like and pilar)
- Paisley-tie tadpole-shaped ducts with ample pink cytoplasm and horn cysts
- Basaloid nests with pilar differentiation common
- Dense pink to red sclerotic stroma
- Deeply invasive
- Lymphoid aggregates
- Perineural extension

Microcystic adnexal carcinoma (MAC) typically presents as a firm plaque on the upper lip, medial cheek, or chin. Histologically, they have a paisley-tie appearance with dense red sclerotic stroma, and must be differentiated from syringoma, morpheaform basal cell carcinoma, and desmoplastic trichoepithelioma.

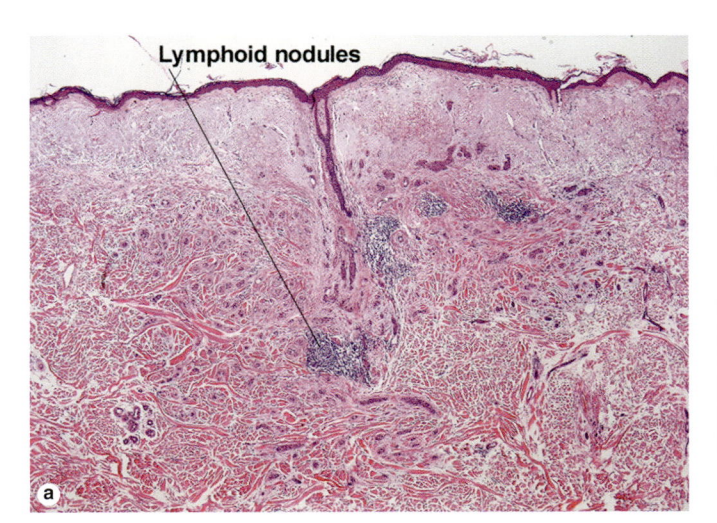

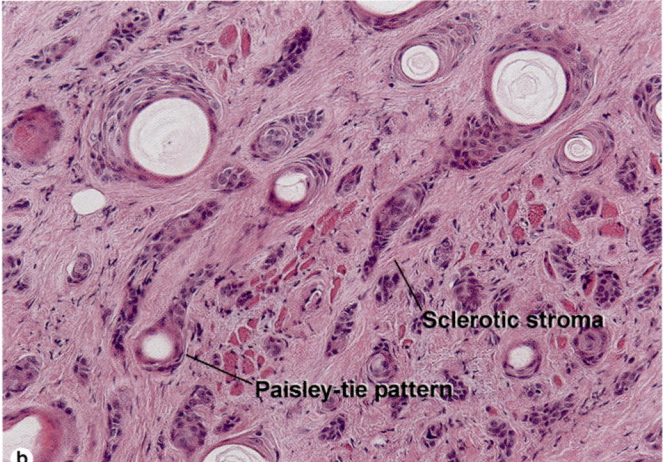

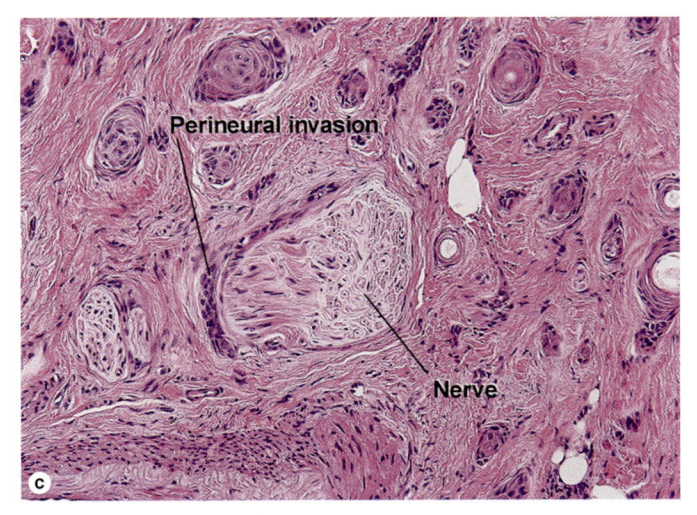

Fig 5-10 Microcystic adnexal carcinoma

Table 5-2 Characteristics of microcystic adnexal carcinoma versus syringoma

Characteristic	Microcystic adnexal carcinoma	Syringoma
Paisley-tie pattern	Yes	Yes
Stroma	Red, sclerotic	Red, sclerotic
Horn cysts	Common	May occur
Size	Large	Small
Shape	Infiltrative	Round
Perineural extension	Yes	No
Basaloid islands	+/−	No
Clinical appearance	Plaque on upper lip, cheek, chin	Small papules on eyelids or eruptive papules

Table 5-4 Characteristics of microcystic adnexal carcinoma versus desmoplastic trichoepithelioma

Characteristic	Microcystic adnexal carcinoma	Desmoplastic trichoepithelioma
Paisley-tie pattern	Yes	Yes
Stroma	Red, sclerotic	Red, sclerotic
Horn cysts	Common	Common
Calcification	Rare	Common
Lymphoid aggregates	Typical	Rare
Perineural extension	Yes	No
Central dell	No	Typical
Clinical appearance	Plaque on upper lip, cheek, chin	Firm doughnut

Table 5-3 Characteristics of microcystic adnexal carcinoma versus morpheaform basal cell carcinoma

Characteristic	Microcystic adnexal carcinoma	Morpheaform basal cell carcinoma
Paisley-tie pattern	Throughout tumor	Sometimes superficially
Stroma	Red, sclerotic	Red, sclerotic
Horn cysts	Common	Occasional
Deeply invasive	Yes	Yes
Perineural invasion	Yes	Yes
Clinical appearance	Plaque on upper lip, cheek, chin	Scar-like

Sclerosing sweat duct carcinoma

Key features
- Monophasic variant of MAC
- No pilar component
- Paisley-tie pattern of tadpole-shaped ducts with ample pink cytoplasm and horn cysts
- Dense pink to red sclerotic stroma
- Deeply invasive
- Lymphoid aggregates
- Perineural extension

Sclerosing sweat duct carcinoma has been described as the "syringoma from hell." Although small fields closely resemble syringoma, the tumor is deeply invasive and demonstrates perineural invasion. The clinical appearance is identical to that of a MAC. Perivascular nodular lymphoid aggregates are common in the tumor stroma.

Sweat gland neoplasms

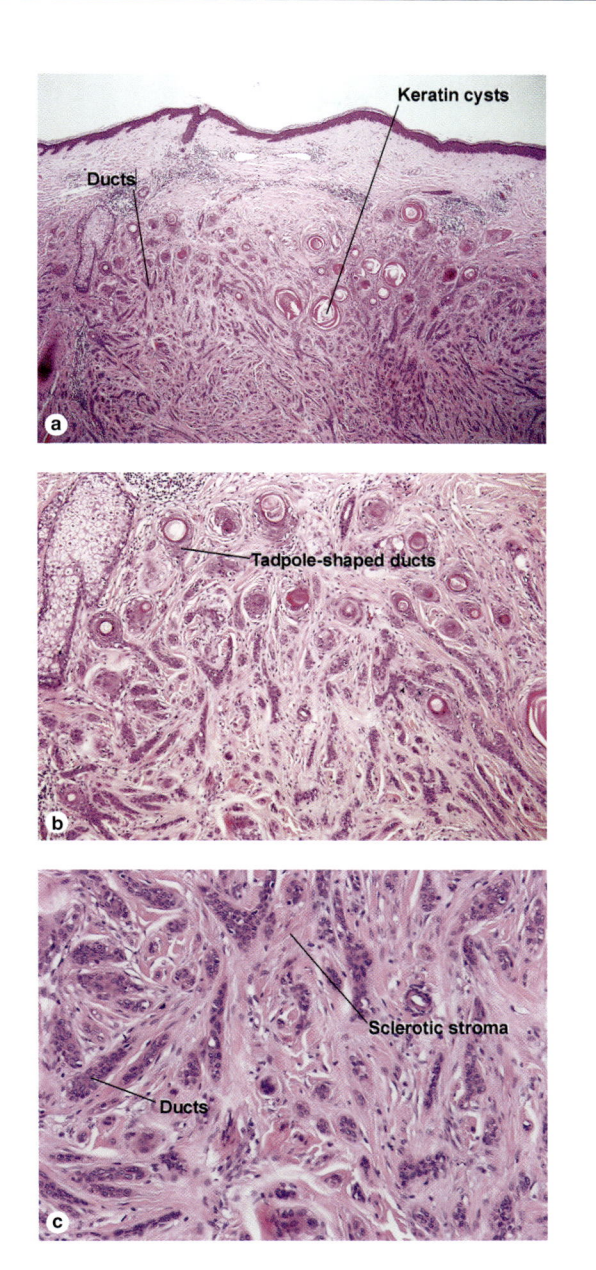

Fig 5-11 Sclerosing sweat duct carcinoma

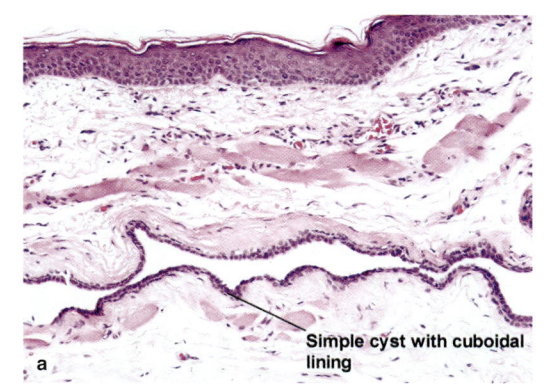

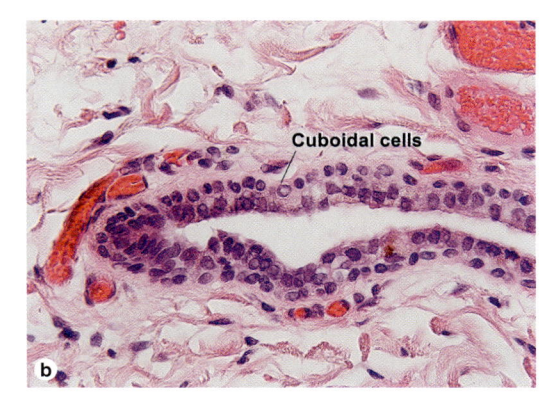

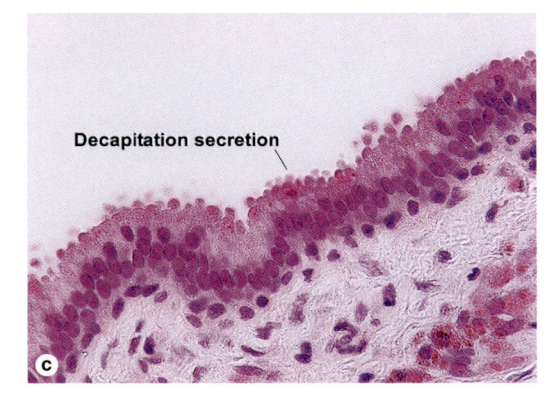

Fig 5-12 Hidrocystoma

Hidrocystoma

Key features
- Simple cyst
- Lined by cuboidal or columnar cells
- Decapitation secretion may be noted

Hidrocystomas typically appear as bluish translucent papules on the cheeks or eyelids.

Mixed tumor (chondroid syringoma)

Key features

- Sweat ducts with ample pink cytoplasm embedded in a mesenchymal stroma
- Secretory elements with blue nuclei and little cytoplasm may be present
- Cartilaginous differentiation common in stroma
- Bone formation may occur

Small tubular type

Key features

- Sweat ducts with ample pink cytoplasm embedded in a mesenchymal stroma
- Cartilaginous differentiation common in stroma
- Small tubules resemble those of a syringoma

Branching alveolar type

Key features

- Sweat ducts embedded in a mesenchymal stroma
- Cartilaginous differentiation common in stroma
- Tubules quite long, with a branching and alveolar pattern
- Decapitation secretion may be seen

While the small tubular type of chondroid syringoma differentiates towards the sweat duct, the branching alveolar type shows differentiation towards both the secretory segment and duct. Mucin within the stroma is sulfated, giving it a deep gray-blue cartilaginous hue.

PEARL

Metachromatic stains for mucin include toluidine blue, methylene blue, and Giemsa (methylene blue plus eosin). Alcian blue and colloidal iron are not metachromatic stains. Chondroitin sulfate stains with Alcian blue and toluidine blue at both high and low pH.

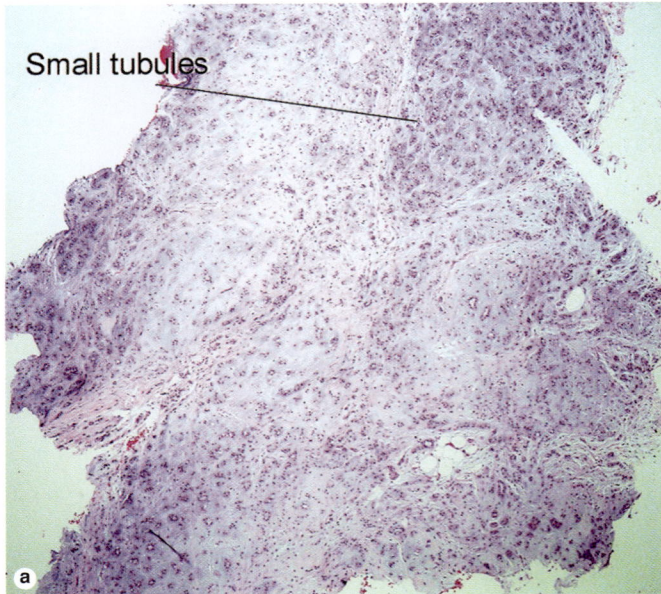

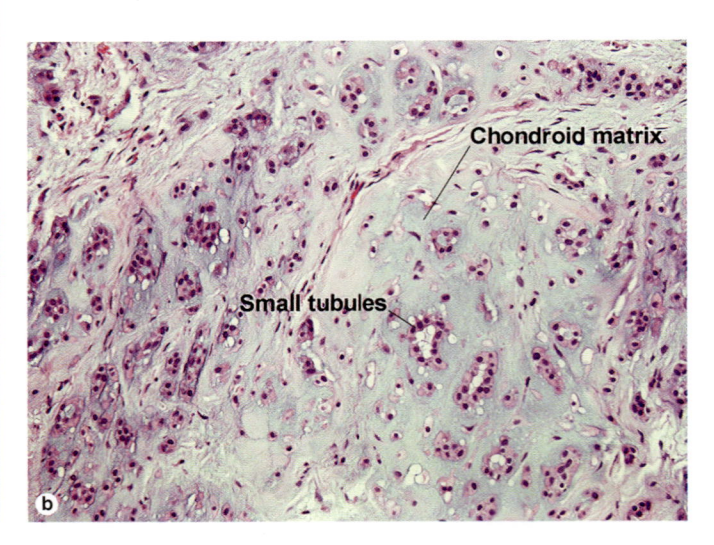

Fig 5-13 Mixed tumor, small tubular type

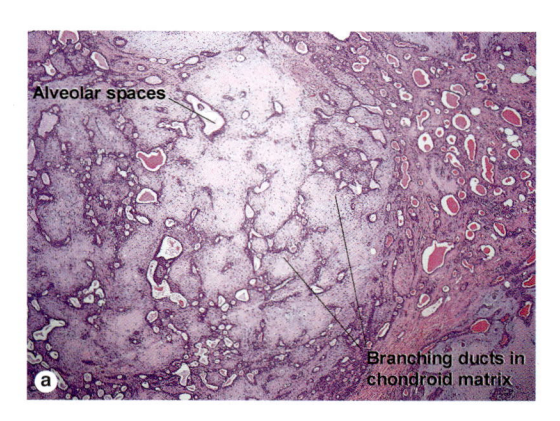

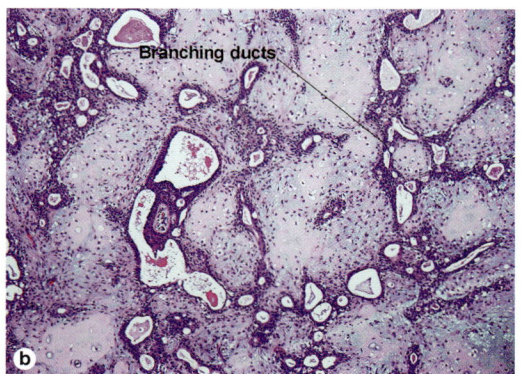

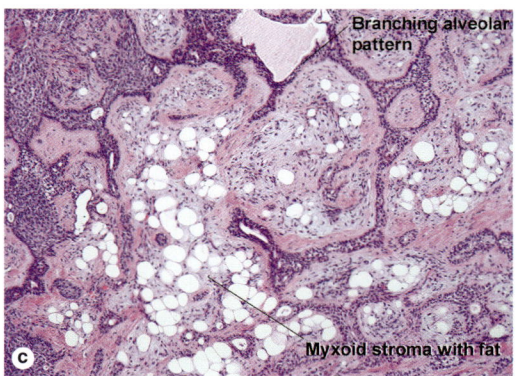

Fig 5-14 Mixed tumor, branching alveolar type

Malignant mixed tumor (malignant chondroid syringoma)

Key features

- Similar to chondroid syringoma, but atypia, mitoses, and sometimes necrosis are noted

Acrospiromas

Key features

- Differentiate towards the acrosyringium (the intraepidermal portion of the sweat duct)
- Cuboidal cells with ample pink cytoplasm
- Tendency towards clear cell degeneration
- Cuticle-lined ducts
- Pink sweat may be seen within ducts

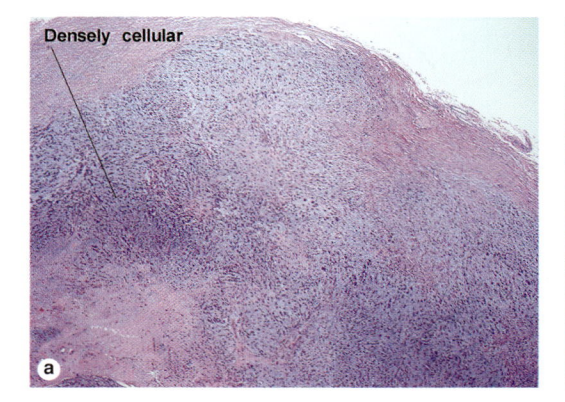

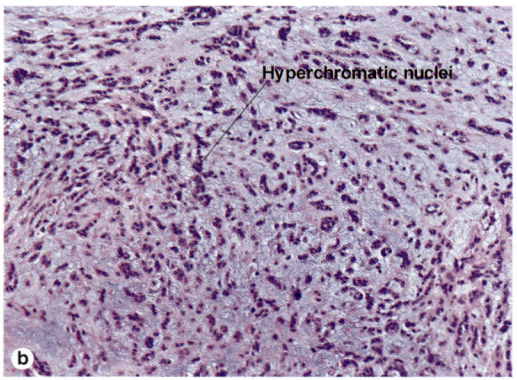

Fig 5-15 Malignant mixed tumor

Dermatopathology

Acrospiromas comprise a large family of sweat gland tumors that includes poromas, hidradenomas, dermal duct tumors, and hidroacanthoma simplex. They are all composed of cells that resemble those of the acrosyringium. They all demonstrate duct differentiation within tumor islands. Hybrid forms are common.

Poroma

Key features
- Cuboidal cells with ample pink cytoplasm
- Cuticle-lined ducts
- Connects with the epidermis
- Commonly found on the foot

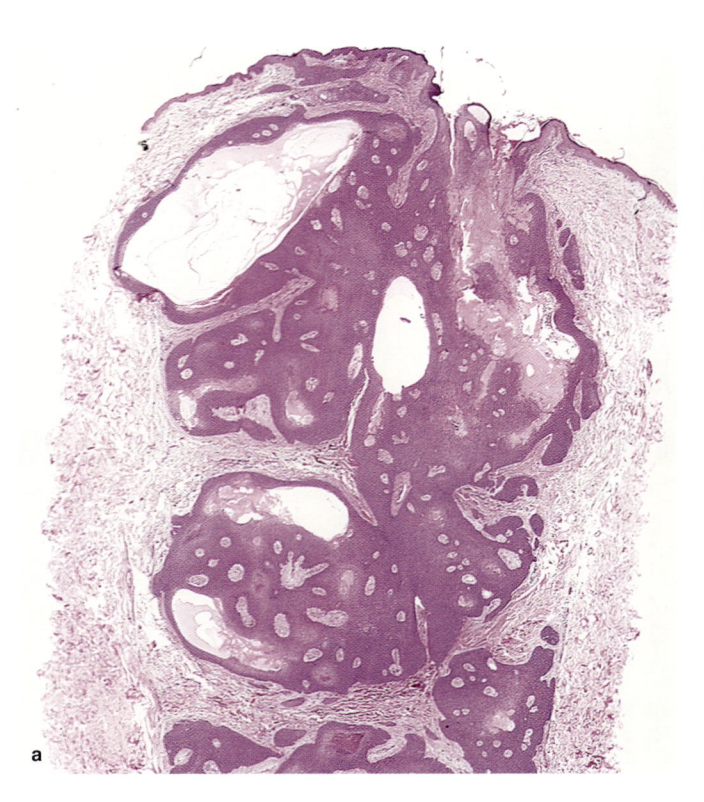

Fig 5-16 Hybrid acrospiroma

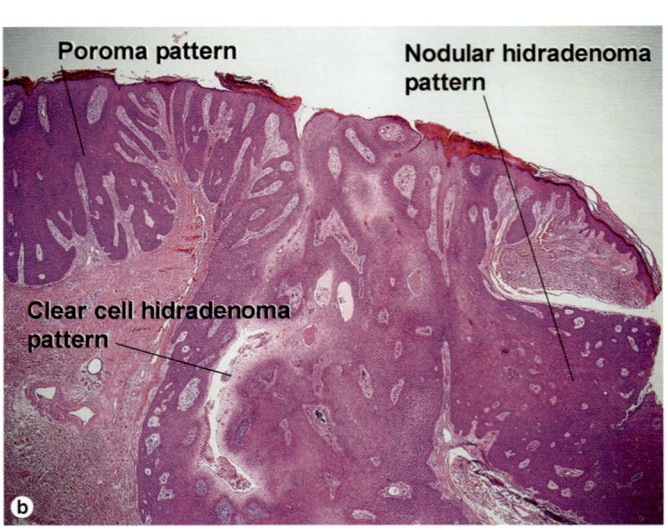

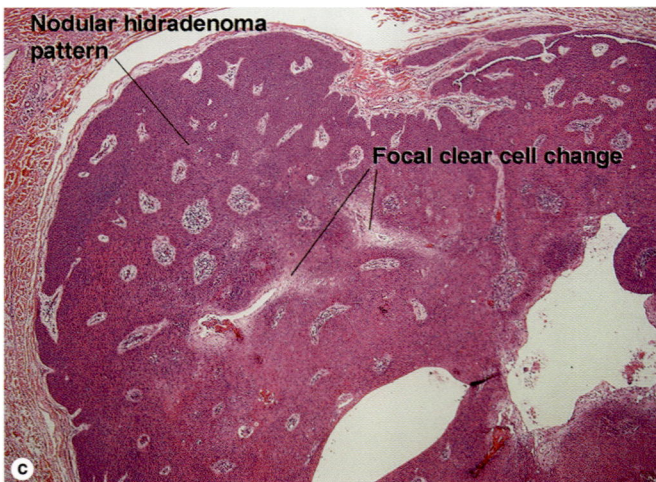

Sweat gland neoplasms

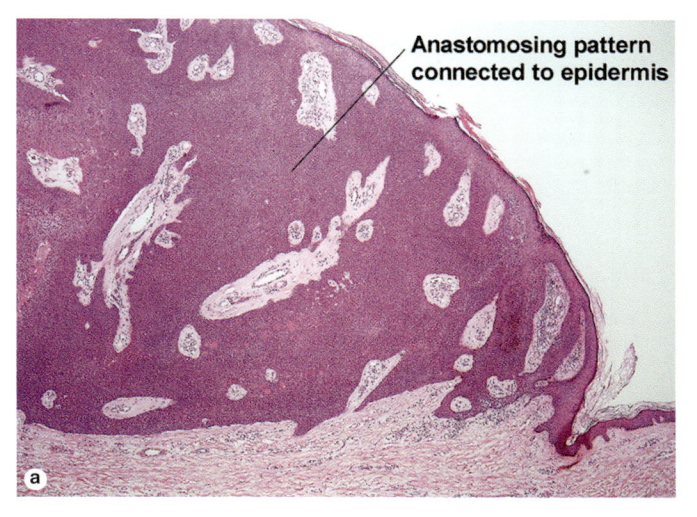

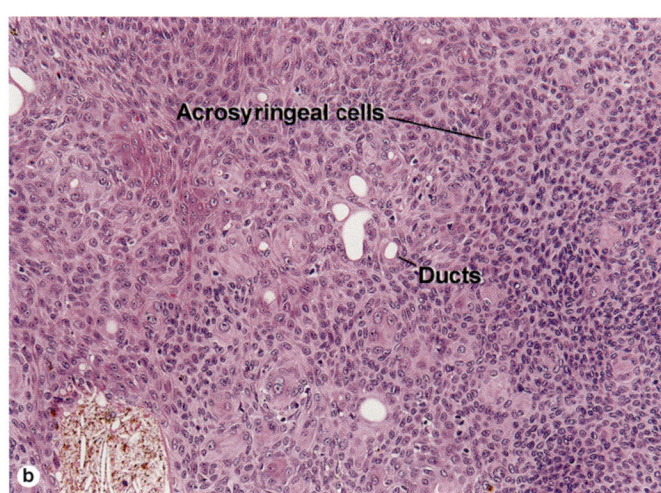

Fig 5-17 Poroma

Hidroacanthoma simplex

Key features

- Intraepidermal nests
- Cuboidal cells with ample pink cytoplasm
- Cuticle-lined ducts

Differential Diagnosis

Resembles clonal seborrheic keratosis, but contains ducts.

Fig 5-18 Hidroacanthoma simplex

Dermal duct tumor

Key features

- Cuboidal cells with ample pink cytoplasm
- Cuticle-lined ducts
- Small dermal nodules

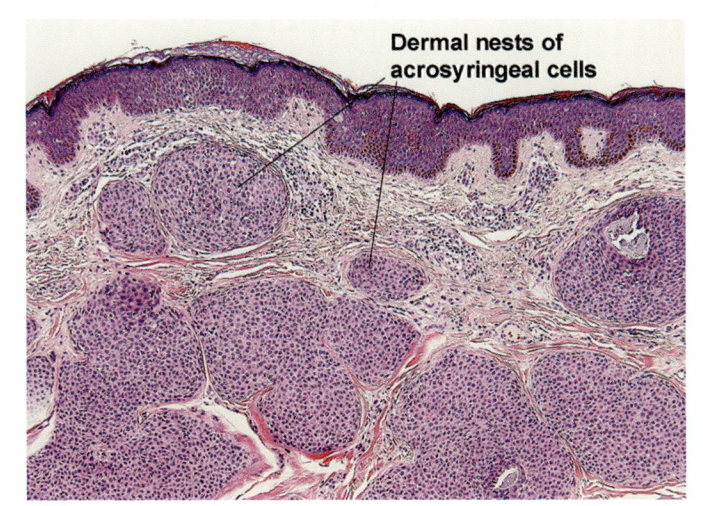

Fig 5-19 Dermal duct tumor

100 Dermatopathology

Nodular hidradenoma

Key features

- Cuboidal cells with ample pink cytoplasm
- Cuticle-lined ducts
- Large dermal nodule
- Bright red zones of basement membrane zone reduplication commonly surround vessels

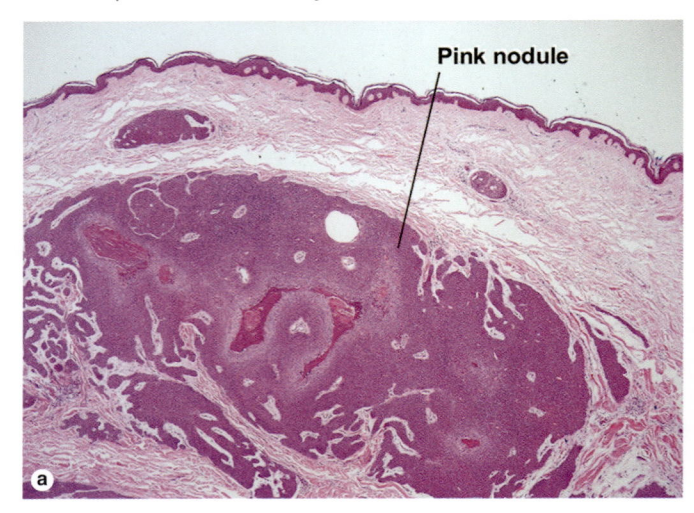

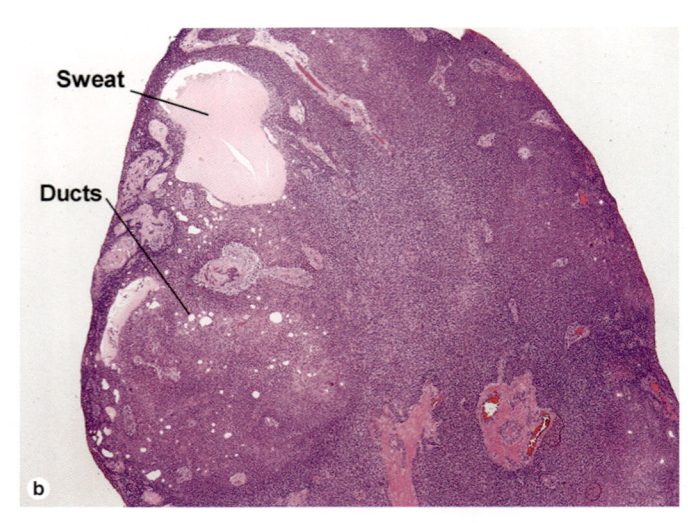

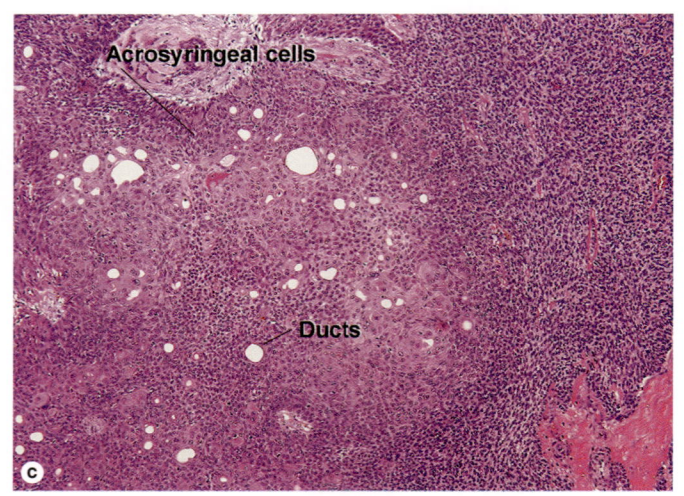

Fig 5-20 Nodular hidradenoma

Clear cell hidradenoma

Key features

- Cuboidal cells with ample pink cytoplasm
- Cuticle-lined ducts
- Large dermal nodule
- Clear cell degeneration
- Cystic degeneration common
- Bright red zones of basement membrane zone reduplication commonly surround vessels

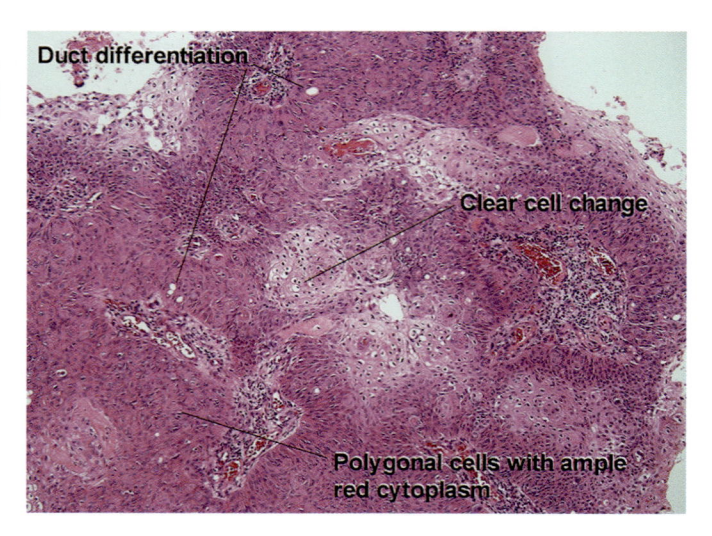

Fig 5-21 Clear cell hidradenoma

Sweat gland neoplasms   Chapter 5   101

Malignant acrospiroma (porocarcinoma, malignant poroma)

Key features

- Invasive growth pattern
- Atypia, mitoses, and necrosis variable
- Some bland-appearing tumors metastasize

Syringofibroadenoma of Mascaro

Key features

- Most cases reactive; only a few are truly neoplastic
- Parallel or anastomosing ducts
- Fibromyxoid stroma

Most examples of syringofibroadenoma represent a reactive proliferation of eccrine ducts, and would be better termed "reactive syringofibroadenomatosis." Some cases have been associated with hidrotic ectodermal dysplasia and Schopf syndrome.

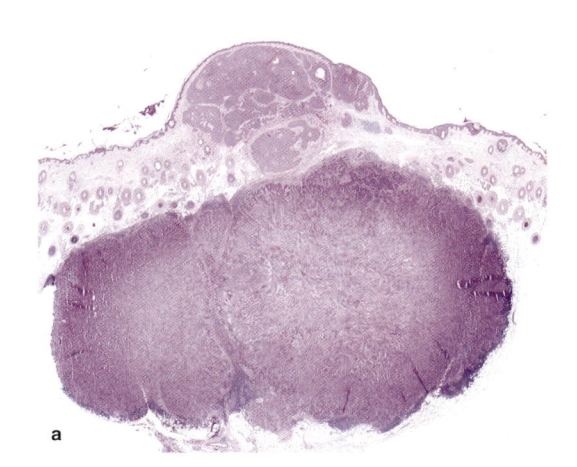

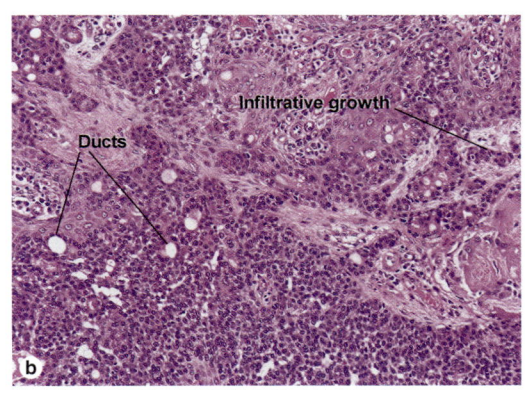

Fig 5-22 Malignant acrospiroma

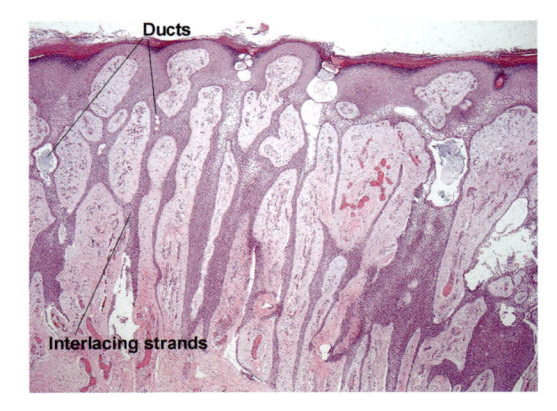

Fig 5-23 Reactive syringofibroadenomatosis

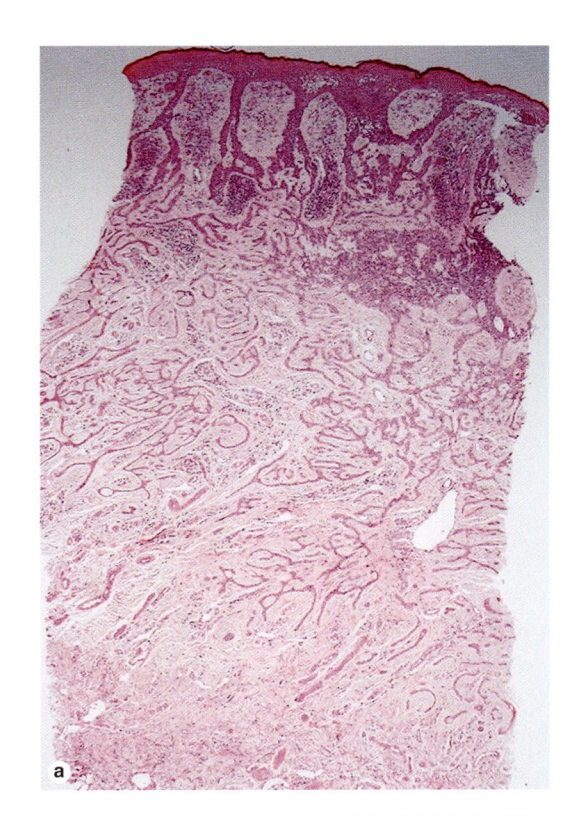

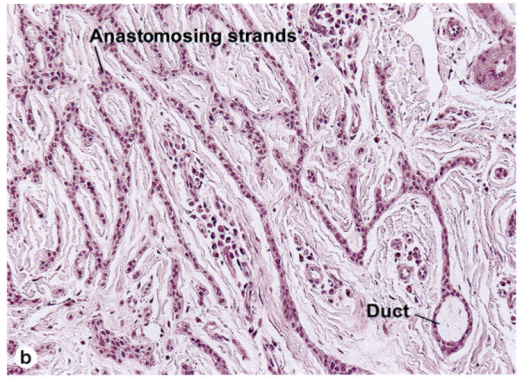

Fig 5-24 Syringofibroadenoma of Mascaro, neoplastic type

Papillary "eccrine" adenoma (tubular apocrine adenoma)

Key features

- No true distinction between papillary eccrine adenoma and tubular apocrine adenoma
- Differentiation towards both secretory segment and duct
- Dilated duct-like spaces
- Blue papillary projections into spaces variable

The variant called papillary "eccrine" adenoma is often found on the dorsal hand or foot of a black child. The tubular variant has a more varied presentation and may occur in the axilla, breast, cheek, or within a nevus sebaceus of Jadassohn.

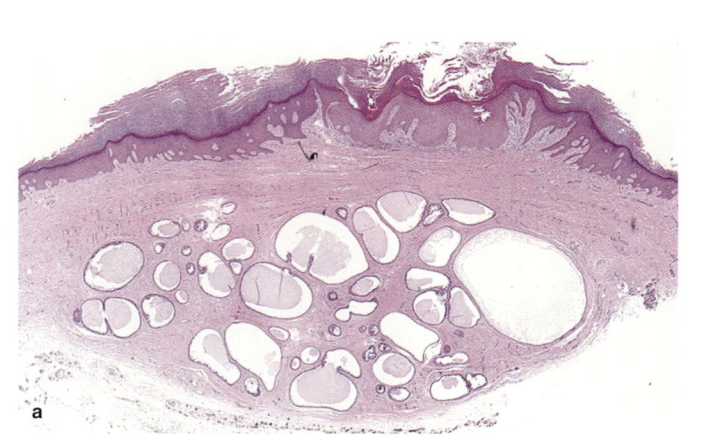

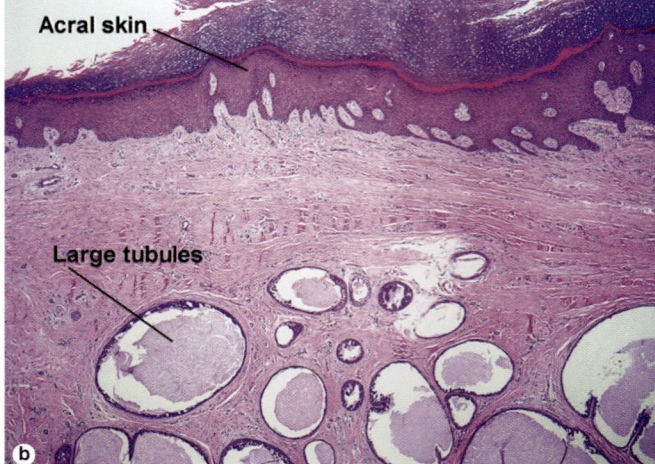

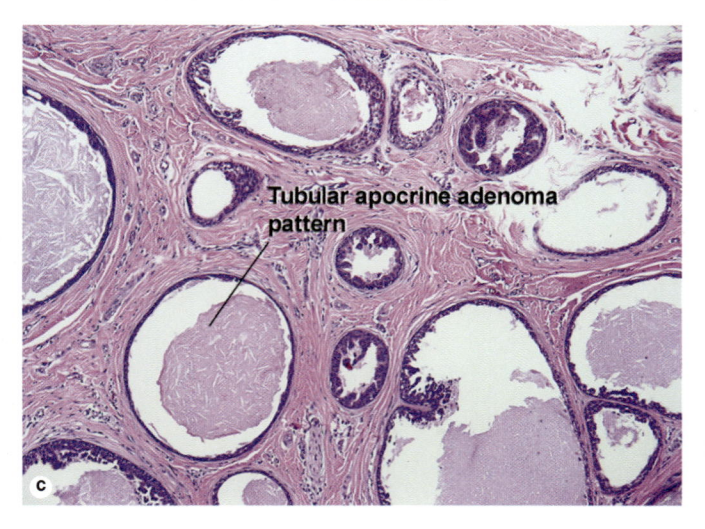

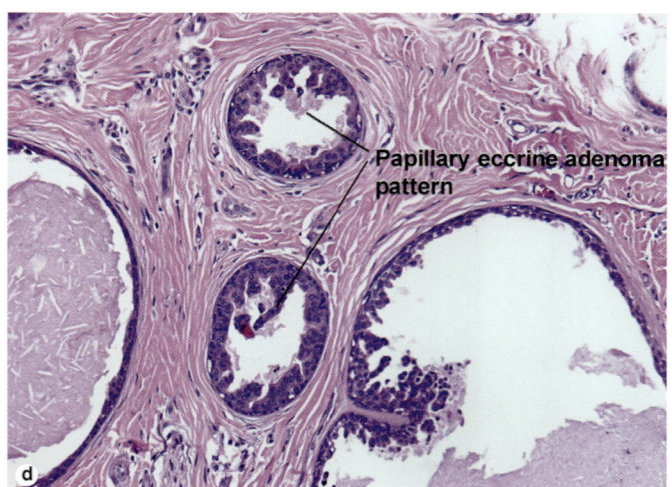

Fig 5-25 Papillary "eccrine" adenoma

Adenoid cystic carcinoma

Key features

- Sieve-like (cribriform) appearance in some areas
- Tubular appearance in other areas
- Atypia and mitoses variable

Adenoid cystic carcinoma typically occurs in the vulva, breast, and salivary glands. Mucin is present in the cribriform areas, so the tumor has been likened to a pink sponge containing pale blue ink.

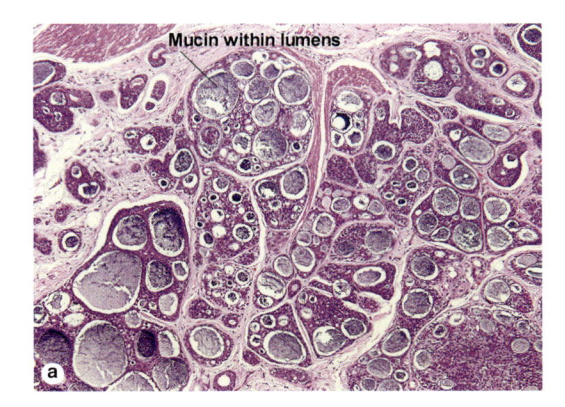

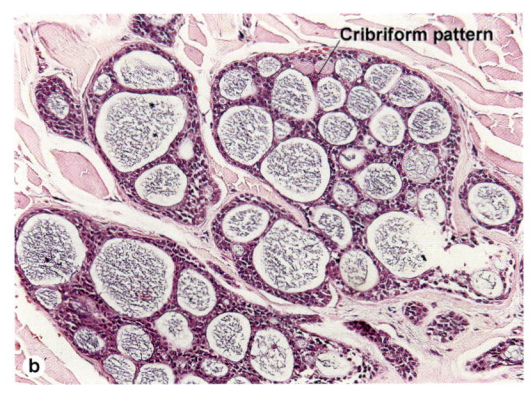

Fig 5-26 Adenoid cystic carcinoma

Differential Diagnosis

Trichoepithelioma is a blue tumor with a cribriform pattern. Adenoid cystic carcinoma is a red tumor with a cribriform pattern.

Eccrine angiomatous hamartoma

Key features

- Often present as tender, dusky nodules in children
- Mature sweat glands and vessels

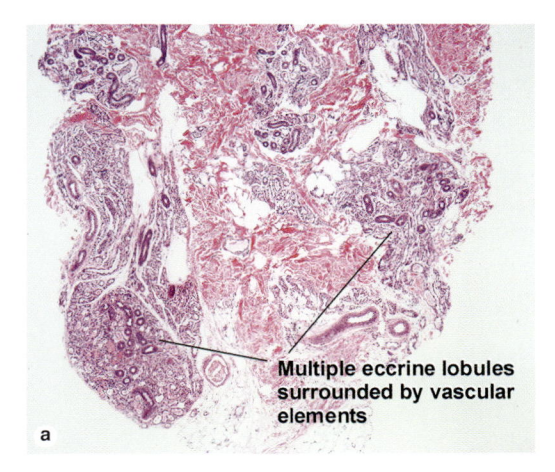

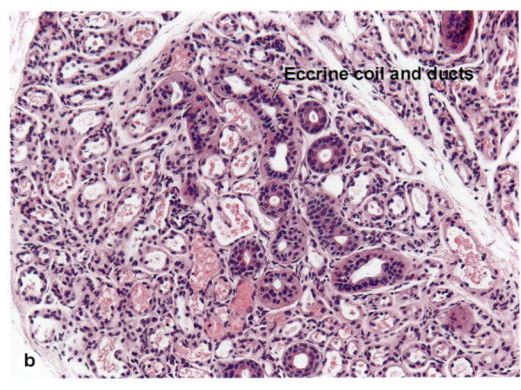

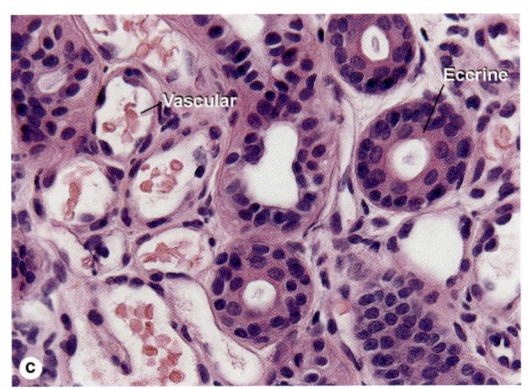

Fig 5-27 Eccrine angiomatous hamartoma

Further reading

Duke WH, Sherrod TT, Lupton GP. Aggressive digital papillary adenocarcinoma (aggressive digital papillary adenoma and adenocarcinoma revisited). Am J Surg Pathol 2000;24(6):775–784.

Fischer S, Breuninger H, Metzler G, et al. Microcystic adnexal carcinoma: an often misdiagnosed, locally aggressive growing skin tumor. J Craniofac Surg 2005;16(1):53–58.

Halachmi S, Lapidoth M. Approach to the rare eccrine tumors. Dermatol Surg 2011;37(8):1194–1195.

Ishiko A, Shimizu H, Inamoto N, et al. Is tubular apocrine adenoma a distinct clinical entity? Am J Dermatopathol 1993;15(5):482–487.

Komine M, Hattori N, Tamaki K. Eccrine syringofibroadenoma (Mascaro): an immunohistochemical study. Am J Dermatopathol 2000;22(2):171–175.

Lago EH, Piñeiro-Maceira J, Ramos-e-Silva M, et al. Primary adenoid cystic carcinoma of the skin. Cutis 2011;87(5):237–239.

Matin RN, Gibbon K, Rizvi H, et al. Cutaneous mucinous carcinoma arising in extramammary Paget disease of the perineum. Am J Dermatopathol 2011;33(7):705–709.

Melanocytic neoplasms

Dirk M. Elston

Solar lentigo

Key features

- Thin rete with bulbous tips "dipped in chocolate"

Differential Diagnosis

Reticulated seborrheic keratosis looks similar to a lentigo but with anastomosis of rete and horn cysts.

Melanotic macule

Key features

- Common on the lips and genitalia
- Rete are broad and squared-off with pigment at basal layer

Melanotic macules are typically light brown and evenly pigmented, but those in the genitalia may sometimes have strikingly irregular pigment. The histologic changes are the same, regardless of location and clinical appearance.

Benign melanocytic nevus

Key features

- Sharply defined
- Well nested at the dermal–epidermal junction
- Matures[a]
- Disperses at the base of the lesion[a]
- No deep mitoses[a]
- No deep pigment in melanocytic nests[a]

[a]*These features are only if there is a dermal component.*

Benign nevi are bilaterally symmetrical from right to left, but they are asymmetrical from top to bottom. In contrast, melanoma metastases are radially symmetrical in all directions, like a cannonball.

A biopsy of a nevus demonstrates a discrete well-nested melanocytic proliferation in the upper portion of the lesion. Melanocytes disperse into individual units in the deeper portions of the lesion. Maturation refers to melanocytes becoming progressively smaller and spindled in the deeper portions of the lesion. Melanin should not be present in deep melanocytic nests,

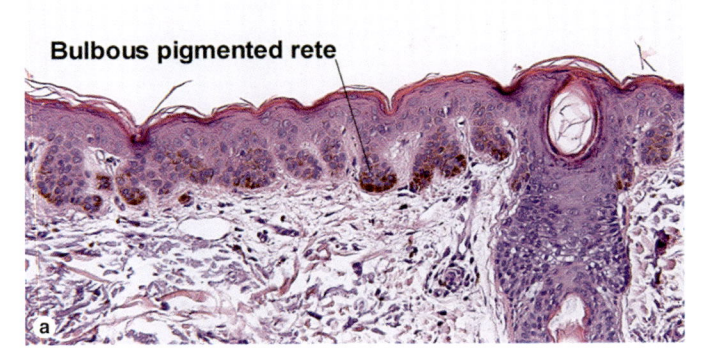

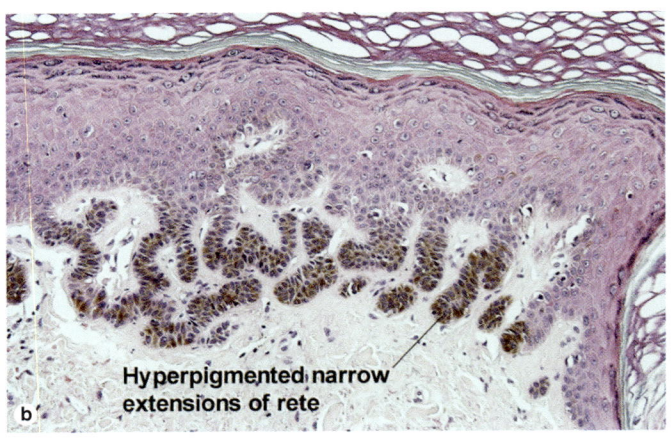

Fig 6-1 Solar lentigo

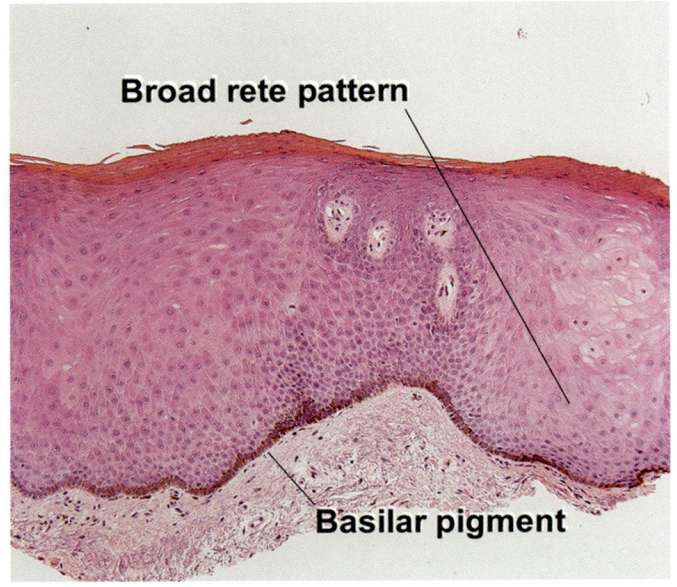

Fig 6-2 Melanotic macule

106 Dermatopathology

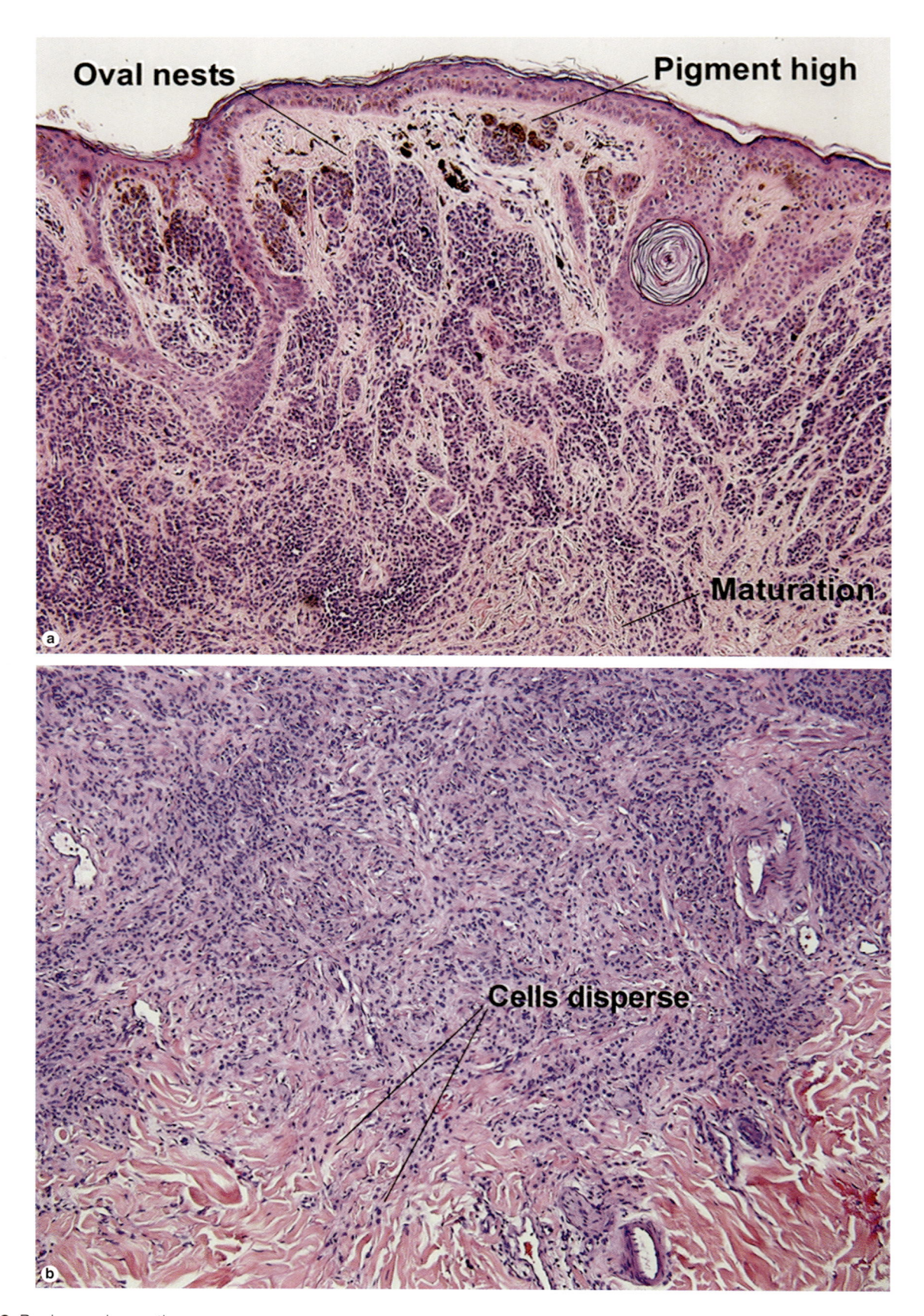

Fig 6-3 Benign melanocytic nevus

Melanocytic neoplasms · Chapter 6

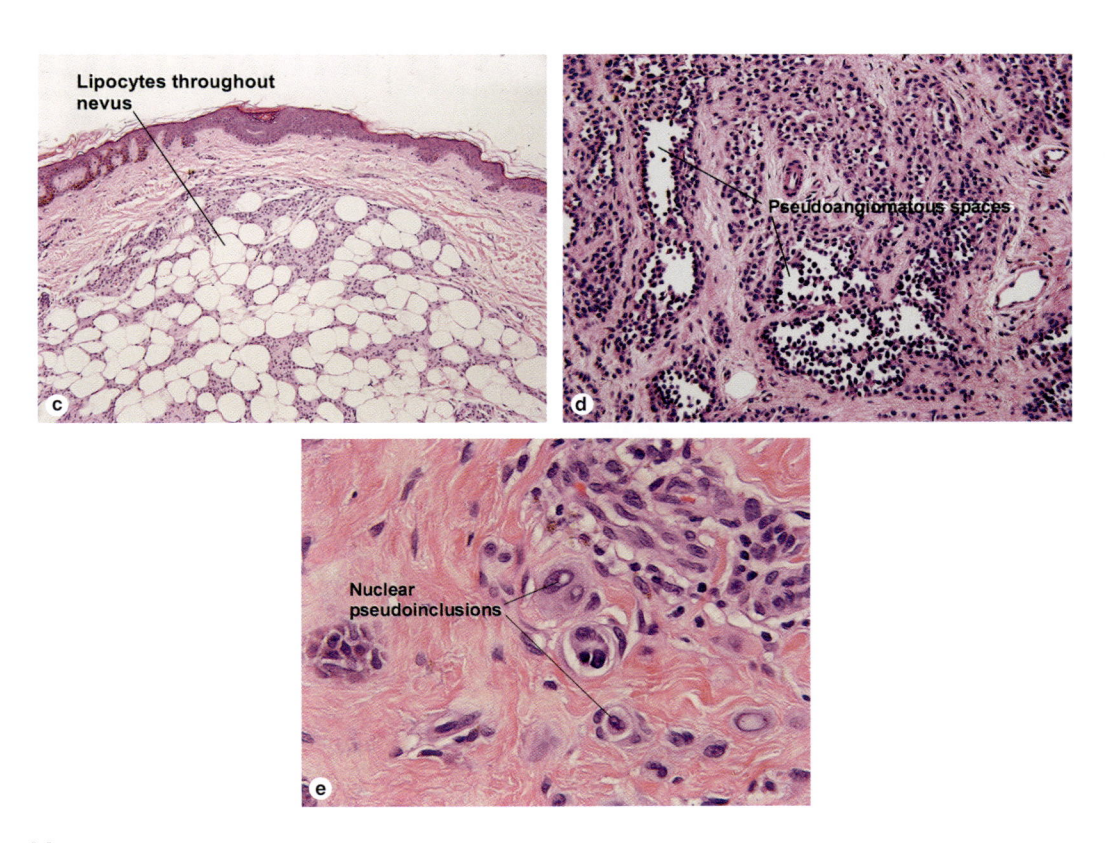

Fig 6-3, cont'd

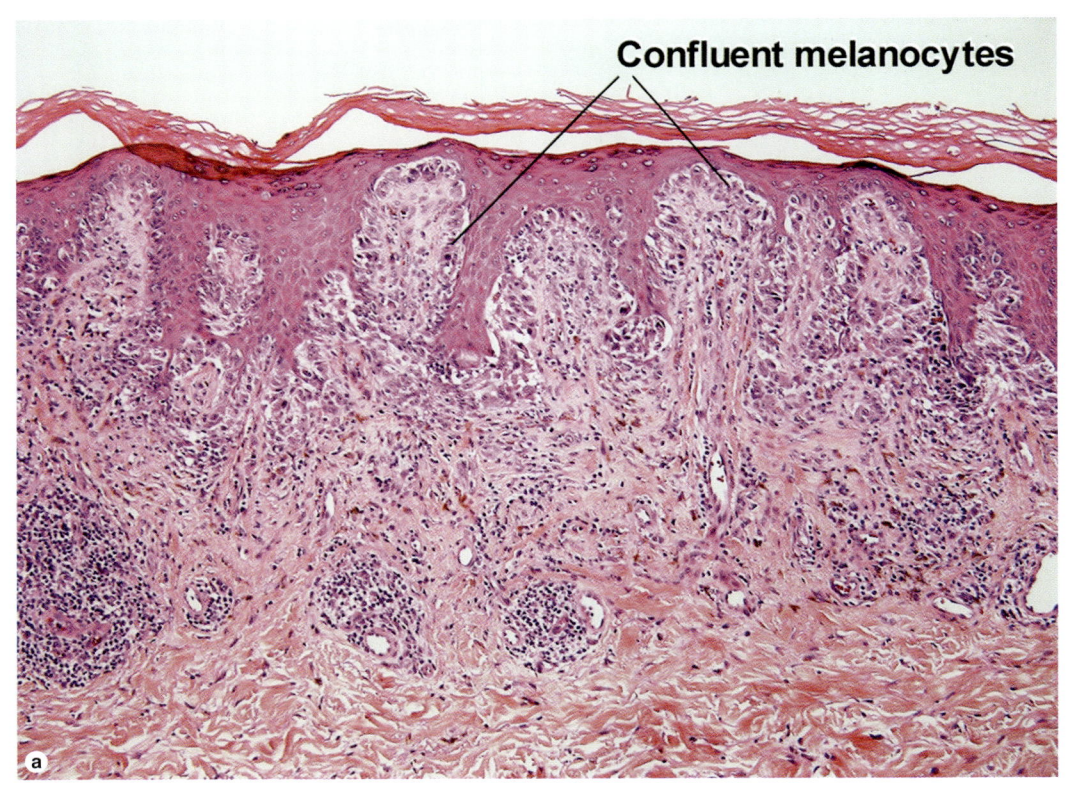

Fig 6-4 Malignant melanoma for comparison: Confluent melanocytes involving the arches between rete

108 Dermatopathology

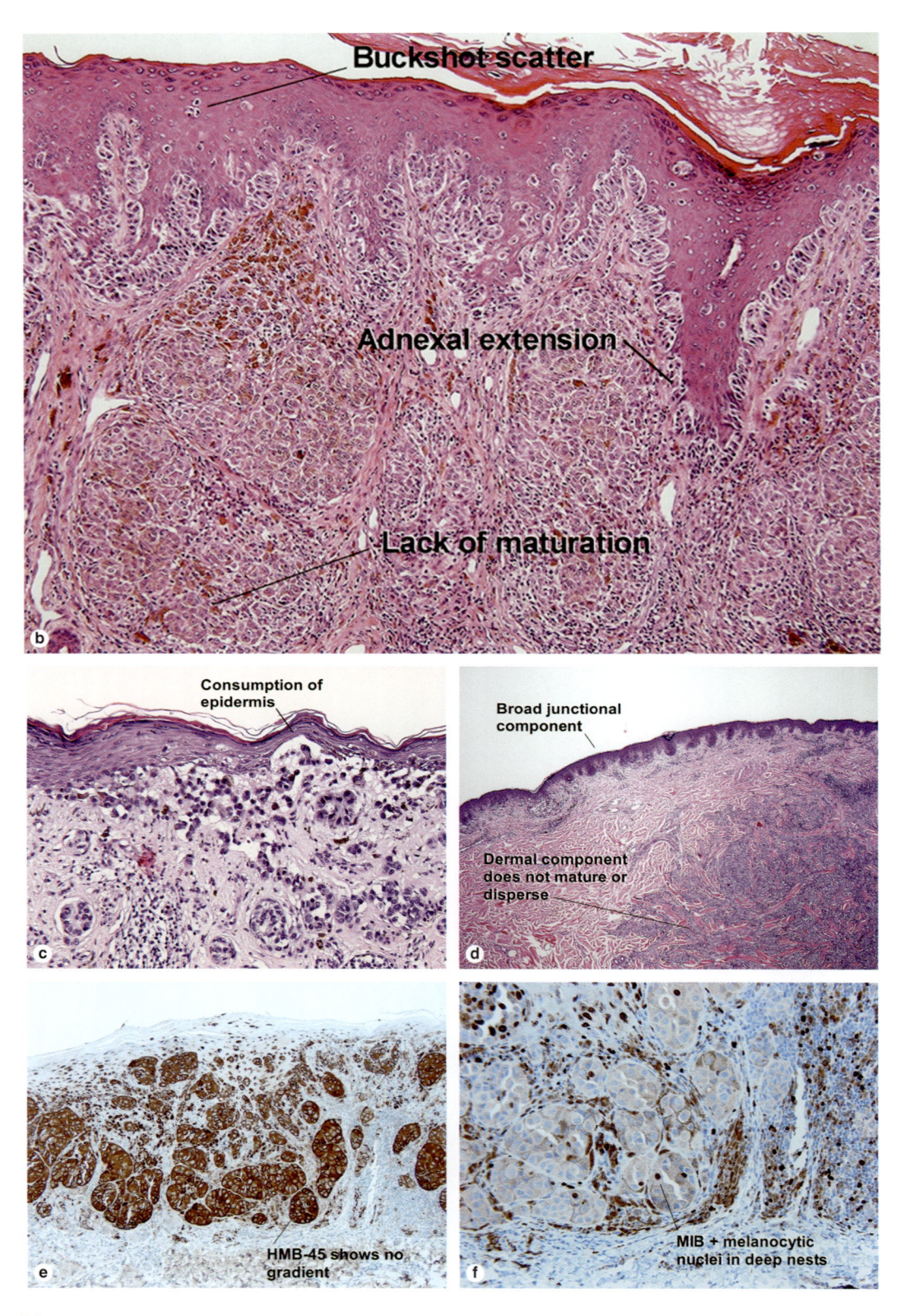

Fig 6-4, cont'd

although melanophages may be present. In cases with questionable maturation, top-heavy HMB-45 immunostaining (loss of staining in the deep component) is a surrogate marker of maturation. Deep mitoses are absent. In unusual lesions, MIB-1 immunostaining is sometimes performed. MIB-1 is expressed in all active phases of the cell cycle – G1, M, G2 and S phase (but not resting G0) – and is not a mitotic marker. There should be no staining of deep melanocytic nuclei.

> **PEARLS**
>
> 1. Broad junctional lesions on heavily sun-damaged skin are usually melanoma, regardless of how bland they appear.
> 2. Small well-nested lesions are almost always benign.
> 3. Horn cysts can occur in the epidermis overlying melanocytic lesions. Horn cysts visible with dermoscopy are *not* diagnostic of seborrheic keratosis.

Table 6.1 gives general rules, and is a good starting point for the evaluation of pigmented lesions. There are exceptions to the rules. For example, blue nevi show no evidence of maturation or dispersion. They are commonly deeply pigmented to the base of the lesion. They are readily recognized by their wedge-like or bulbous outline and characteristic cytologic features.

Balloon cell nevus

> **Key features**
>
> - Balloon cells
> - Sharply defined
> - Well nested at the dermal–epidermal junction
> - Matures
> - Disperses at the base of the lesion
> - No deep mitoses
> - No deep pigment in melanocytic nests

Balloon change is a degenerative feature. Ultrastructurally, it is characterized by swelling of cellular organelles.

Table 6-1 Characteristics of nevus versus melanoma

Characteristic	Nevus	Melanoma
Lateral circumscription	Sharp	Variable
Bilateral (right to left) symmetry	Yes	Commonly asymmetrical
Top to bottom symmetry	No	Variable
Size	Small	Usually quite broad
Dermal–epidermal junction	Well nested	Non-nested melanocytes usually outnumber nests in areas
Shape of junctional nests	Round to oval	Often elongated and bizarre
Location of junctional nests	Tips and sides of rete	Tops of dermal papillae often involved as well
Spacing of junctional nests	Regular	Usually irregular
Buckshot scatter in epidermis	Absent except in the center of Spitz nevi, pigmented spindle cell nevi, acral nevi, traumatized nevi, and sunburned nevi	Variable (present in superficial spreading malignant melanoma, usually not prominent in lentigo maligna and acral lentiginous malignant melanoma)
Maturation	Cells become smaller and more neuroid from top to bottom	Typically fails to mature
Dispersion	Disperses to single units at base of lesion	Generally remains nested at base
Junctional vs dermal nests	Dermal nests smaller than junctional nests; from top to bottom, nests become smaller, melanocytes disperse	Dermal nests often larger than junctional nests
Deep mitoses	Rare	Variable
Deep pigment	No	Variable
HMB-45	Top-heavy	Commonly stains strongly to base
MIB-1	No deep nuclei positive	Deep nuclei commonly positive
S100A6	Spitz nevi usually stain diffusely	Usually patchy

110 Dermatopathology

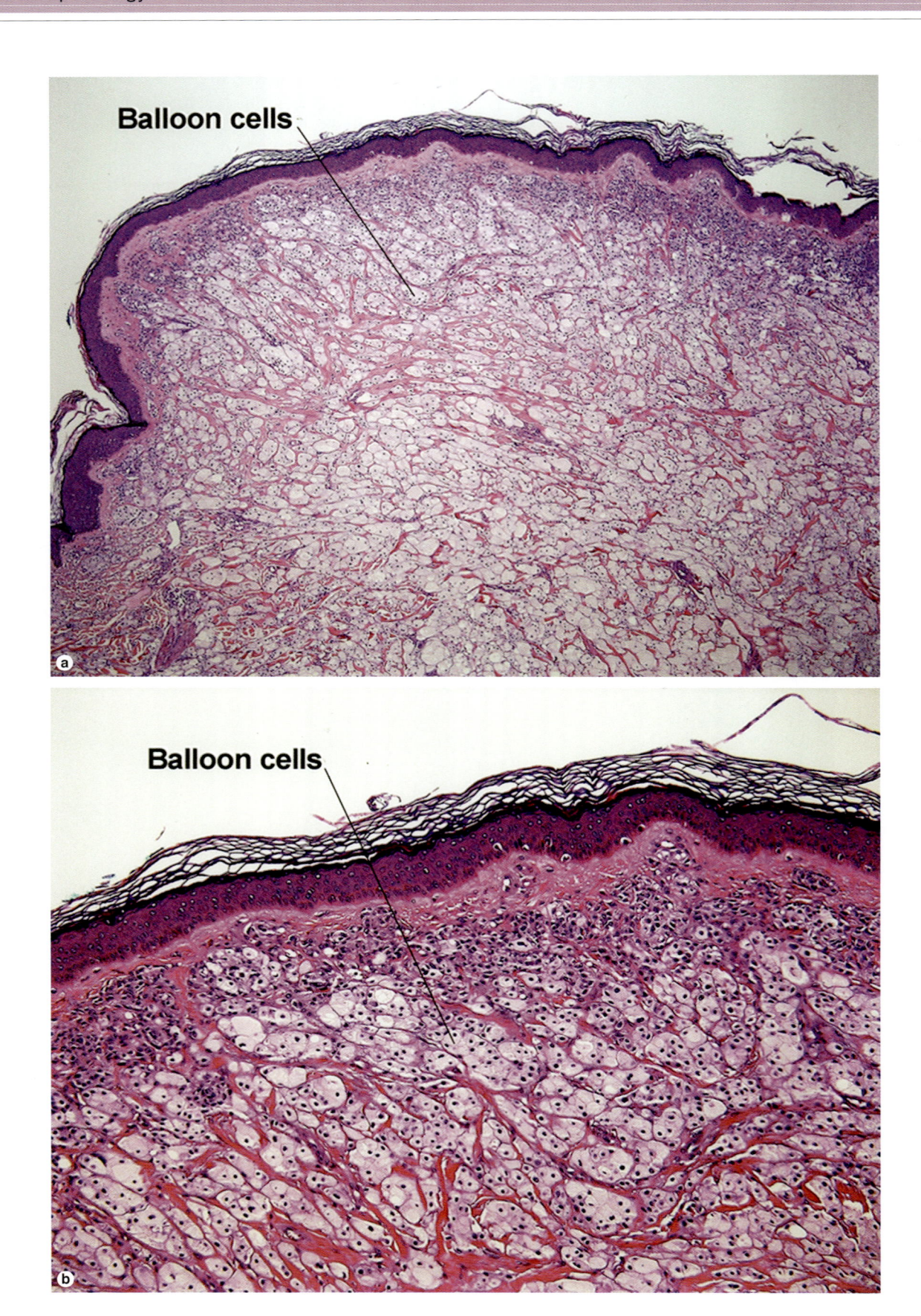

Fig 6-5 Balloon cell nevus

"Neural" nevus

Key features

- S-shaped spindle cells similar to those of a neurofibroma
- Nevic corpuscles resembling Meissner corpuscles
- Sharply defined
- Disperses at the base of the lesion
- No deep mitoses
- No deep pigment

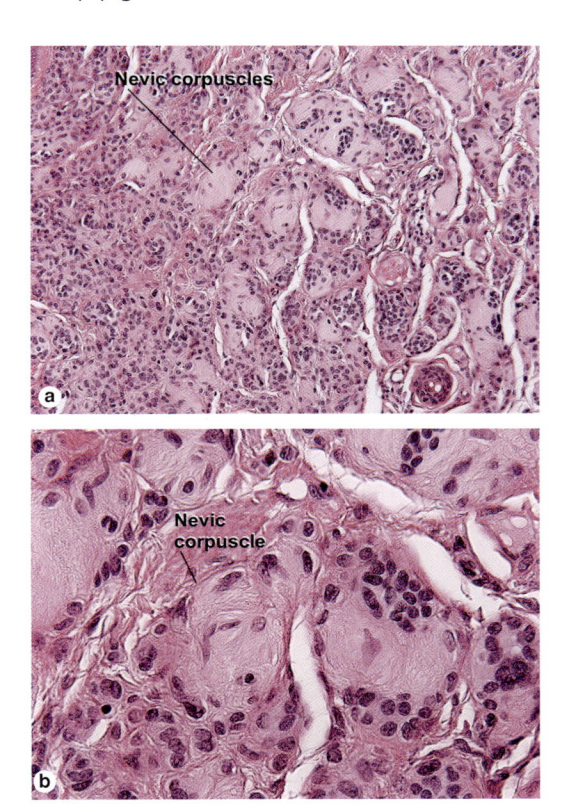

Fig 6-6 Neural nevus

Congenital nevus

Key features

- Broad
- Bland cytologically
- Matures
- Cells disperse at base
- Often within or aggregated about follicles, vessel walls, and nerves
- Patchy perivascular pattern
- Single-file interstitial pattern

A typical congenital nevus demonstrates a well-defined melanocytic proliferation with bland nuclei. The lesion is symmetrical from right to left, with a patchy perivascular, periadnexal, and interstitial pattern. Cells mature and disperse in the deeper portions of the lesion.

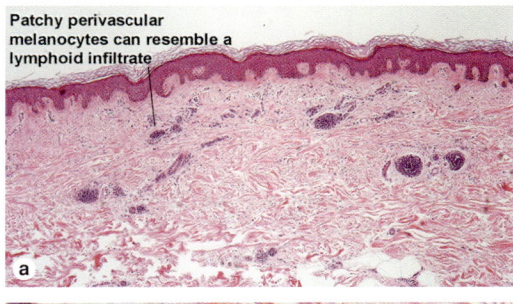

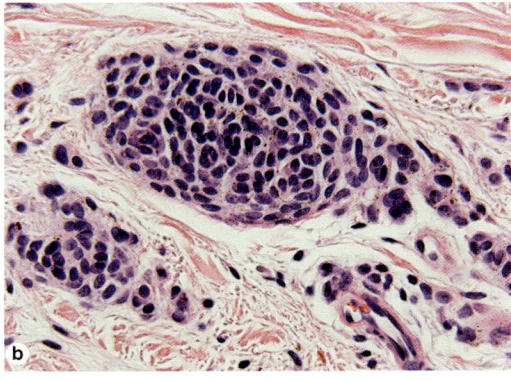

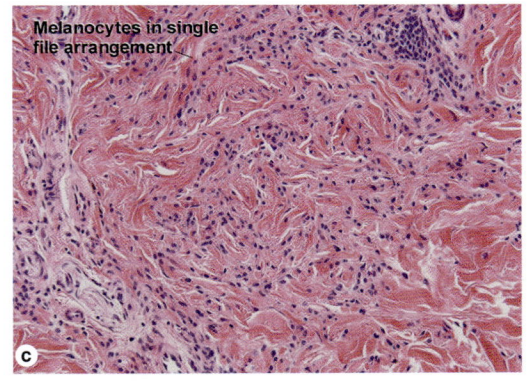

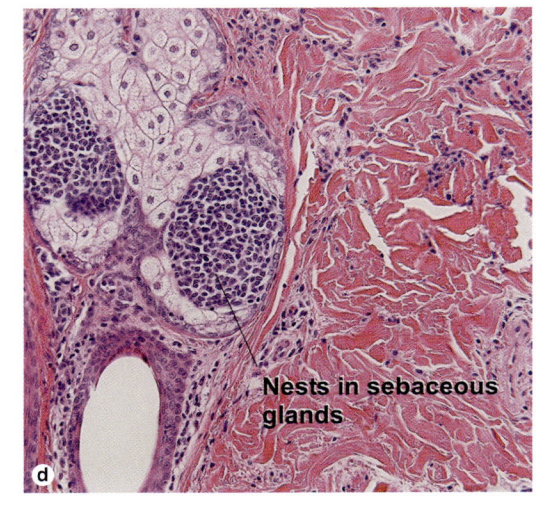

Fig 6-7 Congenital nevus

Spitz nevus

Key features

- Hyperkeratosis, hypergranulosis, pseudoepitheliomatous hyperplasia (PEH)[a]
- Well nested at the dermal–epidermal junction[a]
- Nests vertically oriented along rete ("raining-down pattern," "bananas on the tree")[a]
- Melanocytes within the nests share the vertical orientation[a]
- Clefts around nests[a]
- Kamino bodies[a]
- Large spindle and epithelioid cells
- Nuclei as large as or larger than keratinocyte nuclei
- Nuclei vesicular with prominent nucleoli
- Two-tone cytoplasm
- Sharply defined laterally
- Line symmetry from left to right
- Matures from top to bottom
- Disperses at the base of the lesion
- No deep mitoses
- No deep pigment in nests
- Buckshot scatter OK in center of lesion[a]

[a]*These features are only present if there is a junctional component.*

Benign spindle and epithelioid cell (Spitz) nevi occur in adults, but most commonly present as pink papules on the face or scalp of a child. Unfortunately, melanomas can demonstrate large spindle and epithelioid cells, hyperkeratosis, hypergranulosis, and pseudoepitheliomatous hyperplasia. These features are especially common among melanomas in the pediatric age group. Critical distinguishing features include sharp lateral circumscription, maturation, and dispersion, all of which should be present in benign Spitz nevi.

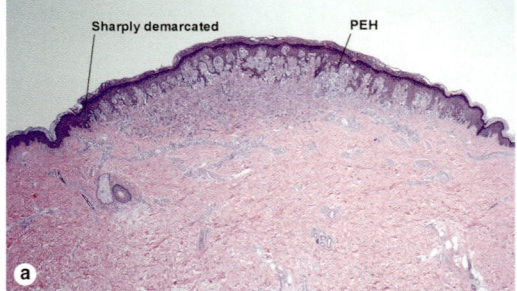

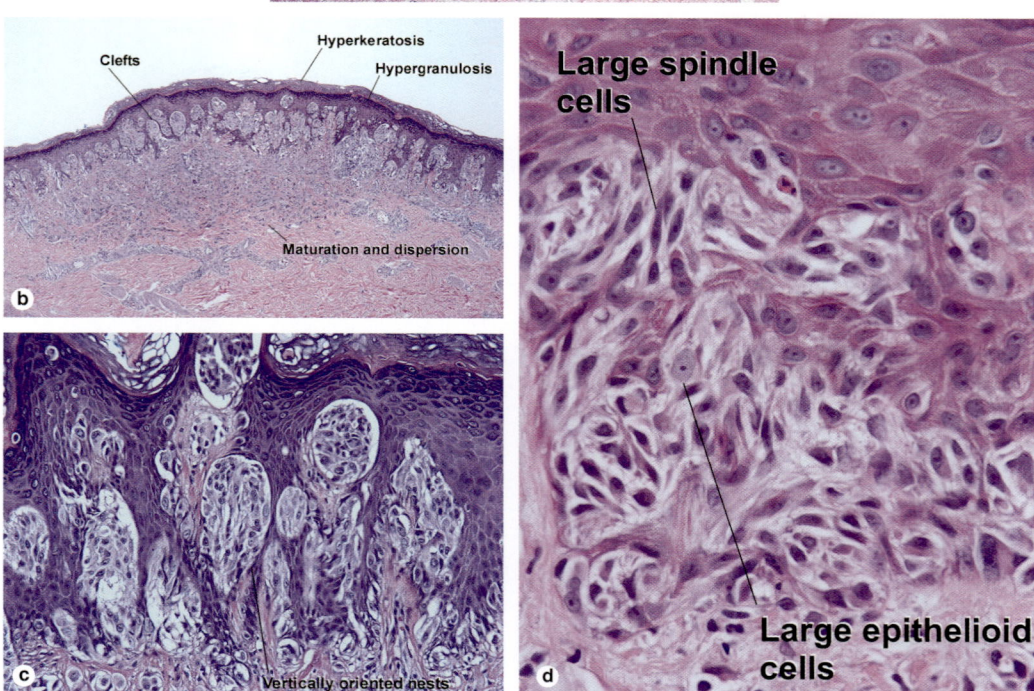

Fig 6-8 Spitz nevus (PEH, pseudoepitheliomatous hyperplasia)

Melanocytic neoplasms   Chapter 6   113

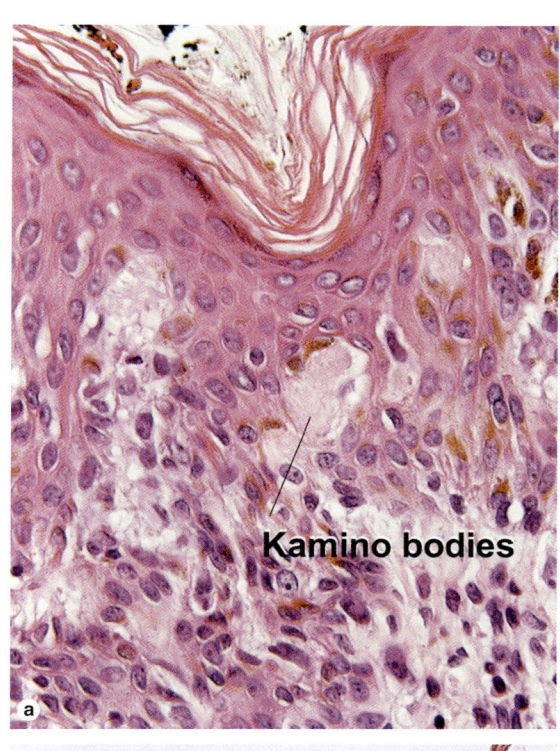

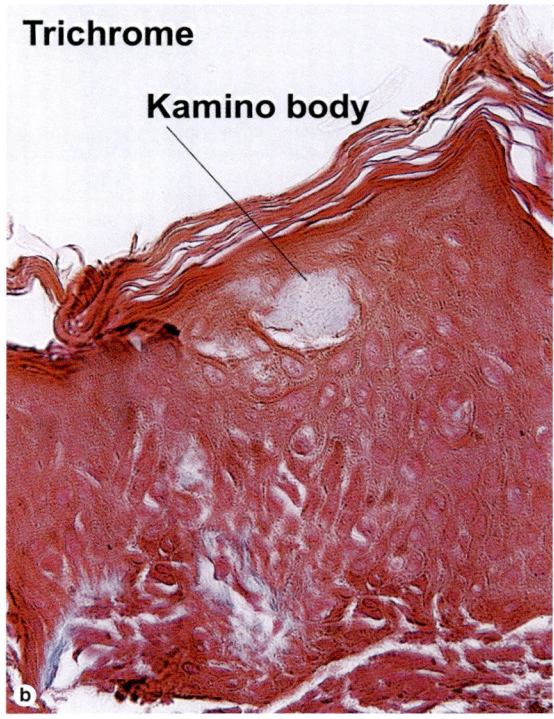

Fig 6-9 Kamino body (trichrome stain)

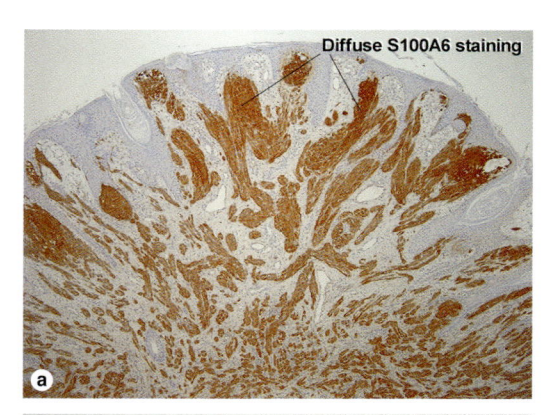

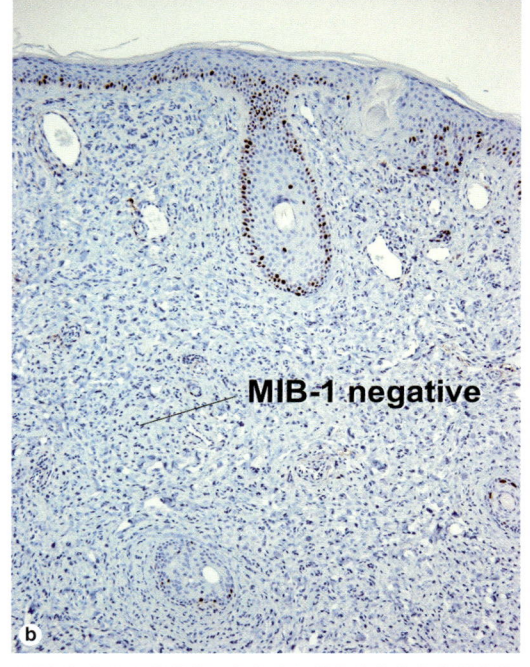

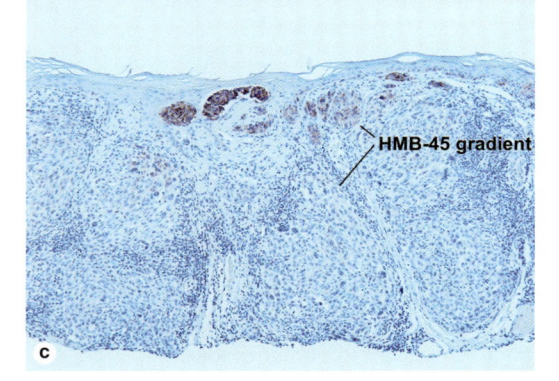

Fig 6-10 Immunostaining pattern of Spitz nevus

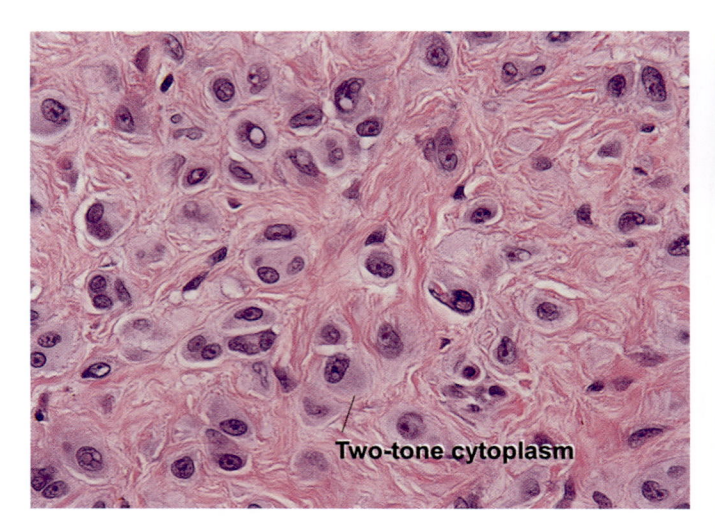

Fig 6-11 Intradermal Spitz nevus (Two-tone cytoplasm)

Deep mitoses should be absent. Kamino bodies are dull pink areas of trapped basement membrane material within the epidermis. They stain blue to green with a trichrome stain and mark with immunostains for type IV collagen.

In lesions with any atypical feature, immunostaining is commonly performed. HMB-45 immunostaining should be top-heavy, and the lesion should stain diffusely for S100A6. MIB-1 staining should be absent in melanocyte nuclei at the base of the lesion.

Comparative genomic hybridization and chromosome deletion analysis by fluorescent *in situ* hybridization are promising techniques. The majority of Spitz nevi have a normal chromosome complement. Some large Spitz nevi have an 11p gain.

Pigmented spindle cell nevus of Reed

Key features

- Hyperkeratosis, hypergranulosis, pseudoepitheliomatous hyperplasia
- Well nested at the dermal–epidermal junction
- Clefts around nests variable
- Kamino bodies variable
- Small spindle cells
- Sharply defined
- Line symmetry from left to right
- Matures from top to bottom if compound
- Disperses at the base of the lesion if compound
- No deep mitoses
- No deep pigment in nests
- Buckshot scatter OK in center of lesion

Benign pigmented spindle cell nevus is considered by many to be a variant of Spitz nevus. They typically present as deeply pigmented macular lesions on the thighs or lower legs of young women. The spindled melanocytes are smaller than those in a Spitz nevus. Epithelioid cells are rare.

Table 6-2 Characteristics of Spitz nevus versus pigmented spindle cell nevus of Reed

Characteristic	Spitz nevus	Pigmented spindle cell nevus of Reed
Age	Children	Young women
Color	Usually pink	Usually dark brown
Location	Head	Legs
Hyperkeratosis, hypergranulosis, and pseudoepitheliomatous hyperplasia	Yes	Yes
Cytology	Large spindle and epithelioid cells	Small spindle cells
Kamino bodies	Common	Variable
Buckshot scatter in epidermis	Normal in center lesion	Normal in center lesion
S100A6	Strongly +	Weak and patchy

"Special site" nevus

Key features

- Occur in the anogenital region, axillae, umbilicus, breast, scalp, ears
- One pattern resembles a dysplastic nevus
- Second pattern characterized by large junctional nests that appear poorly cohesive (white space surrounding each melanocyte)

Acral nevus

Key features

- On volar skin, nests are commonly elongated and follow dermatoglyphs
- Buckshot scatter OK in center of lesion
- Sharply defined
- Well nested at the dermal–epidermal junction
- Matures
- Disperses at the base of the lesion
- No deep mitoses
- No deep pigment in melanocytic nests

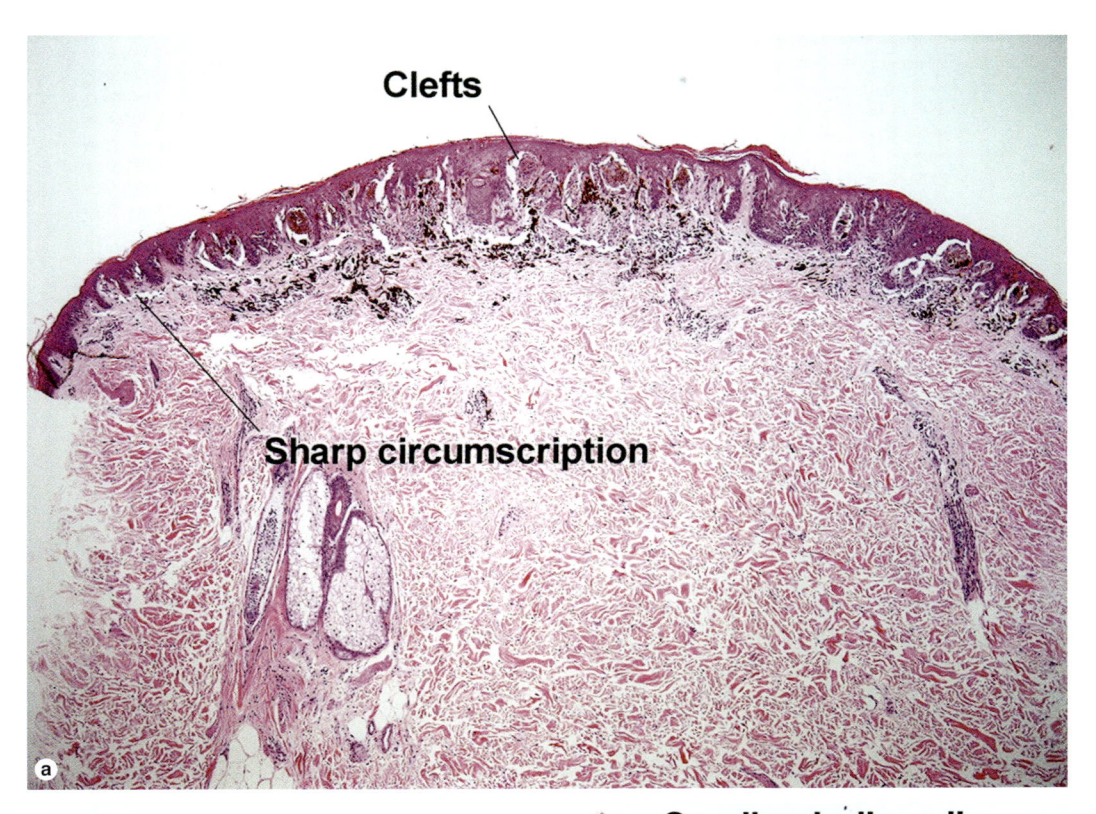

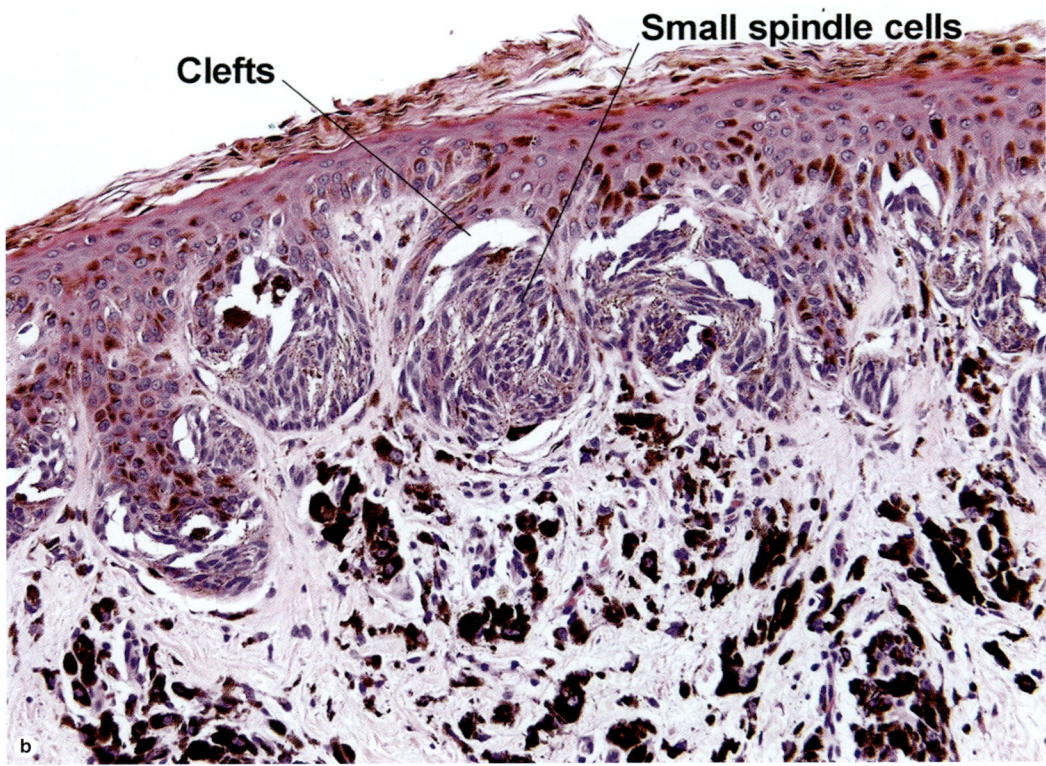

Fig 6-12 Pigmented spindle cell nevus

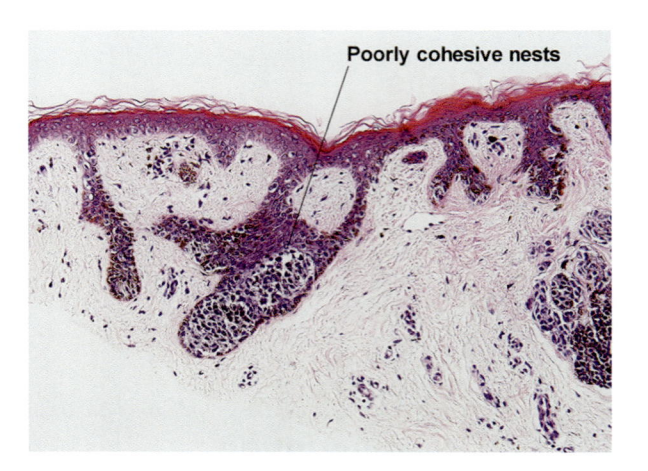

Fig 6-13 Genital nevus

Within the central portion of an acral nevus, melanocytes are commonly noted above the dermal–epidermal junction. As long as it is confined to the center of the lesion, "buckshot scatter" by itself is not a worrisome feature in an acral nevus.

If volar nevi are bisected perpendicular to the dermatoglyphs, the nests will appear round. The rete pattern will be regular. If they are inappropriately sectioned parallel to the dermatoglyphs, the nests will appear long and confluent. The rete pattern may appear effaced in such sections. Oblique sections will give the appearance of irregular nesting and Swiss-cheese rete. It is important to communicate carefully with the lab when submitting a specimen from acral skin. Some clinicians prefer to bisect the specimen themselves, perpendicular to the dermatoglyphs.

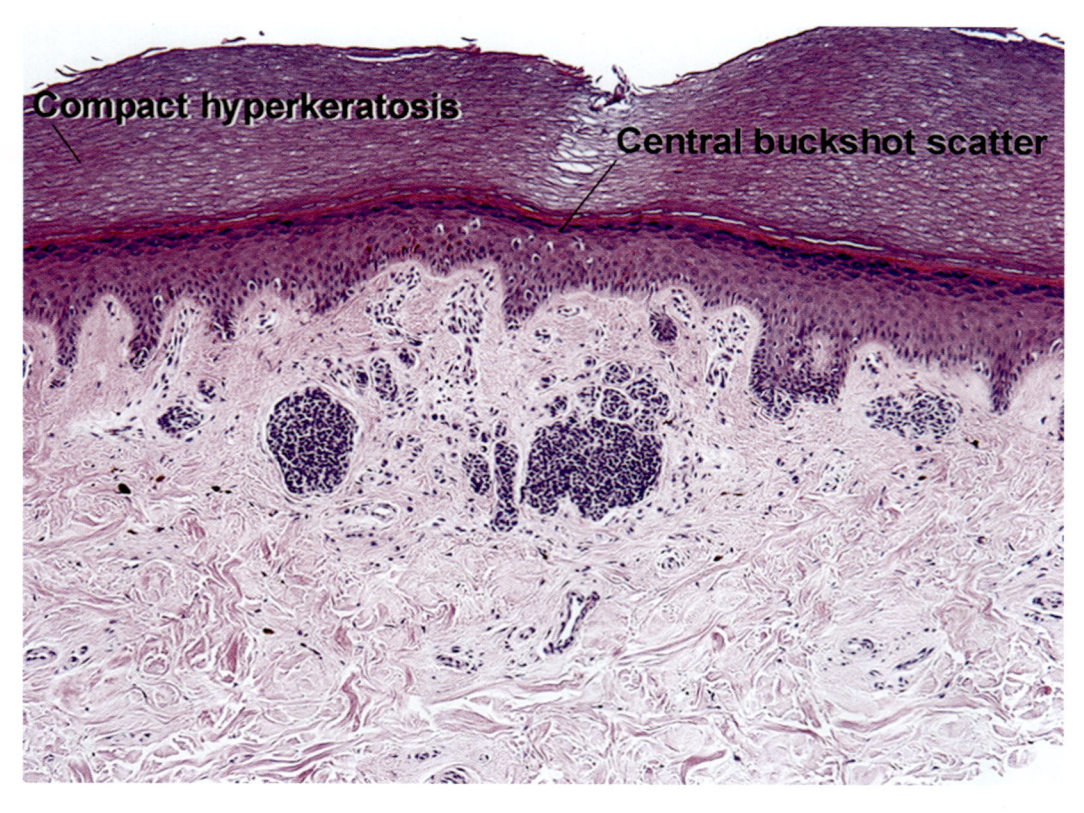

Fig 6-14 Acral nevus

"Ancient" nevus

Key features

- Large, hyperchromatic nuclei
- No confluent growth
- No expansile growth pattern
- No mitoses
- Sharply defined
- Well nested at the dermal–epidermal junction
- Matures
- Disperses at the base of the lesion
- No deep pigment in nests

The term "ancient" atypia has been applied to atypical nuclei in benign lesions. Mitoses, confluent growth or an expansile growth pattern (nodule) should never be present.

Halo nevus

Key features

- Band-like lymphoid infiltrate through the lesion
- Sharply defined
- Well nested at the dermal–epidermal junction
- Matures
- Disperses at the base of the lesion
- No deep mitoses
- No deep pigment in nests (melanophages may be present)

PEARL

The pattern of the lymphoid infiltrate of a halo nevus resembles a cocktail party, with lymphocytes and melanocytes mingling together. In contrast, the pattern of the lymphoid infiltrate of a melanoma resembles a wall of riot police trying to hold back an angry mob (band of lymphocytes at the periphery of melanocytic nests).

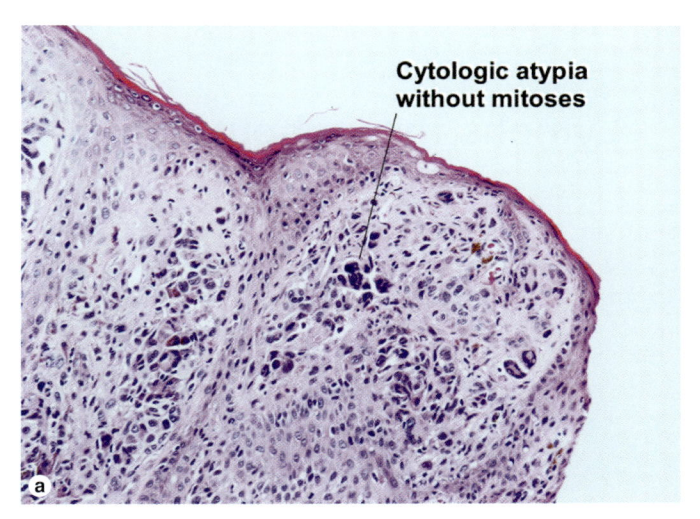

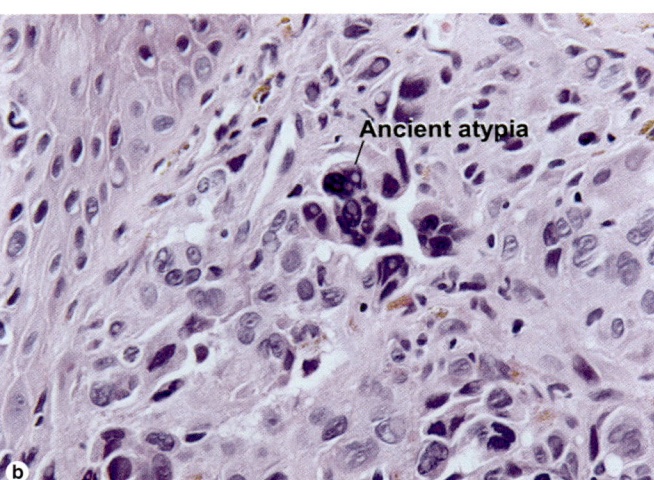

Fig 6-15 Ancient nevus

118   Dermatopathology

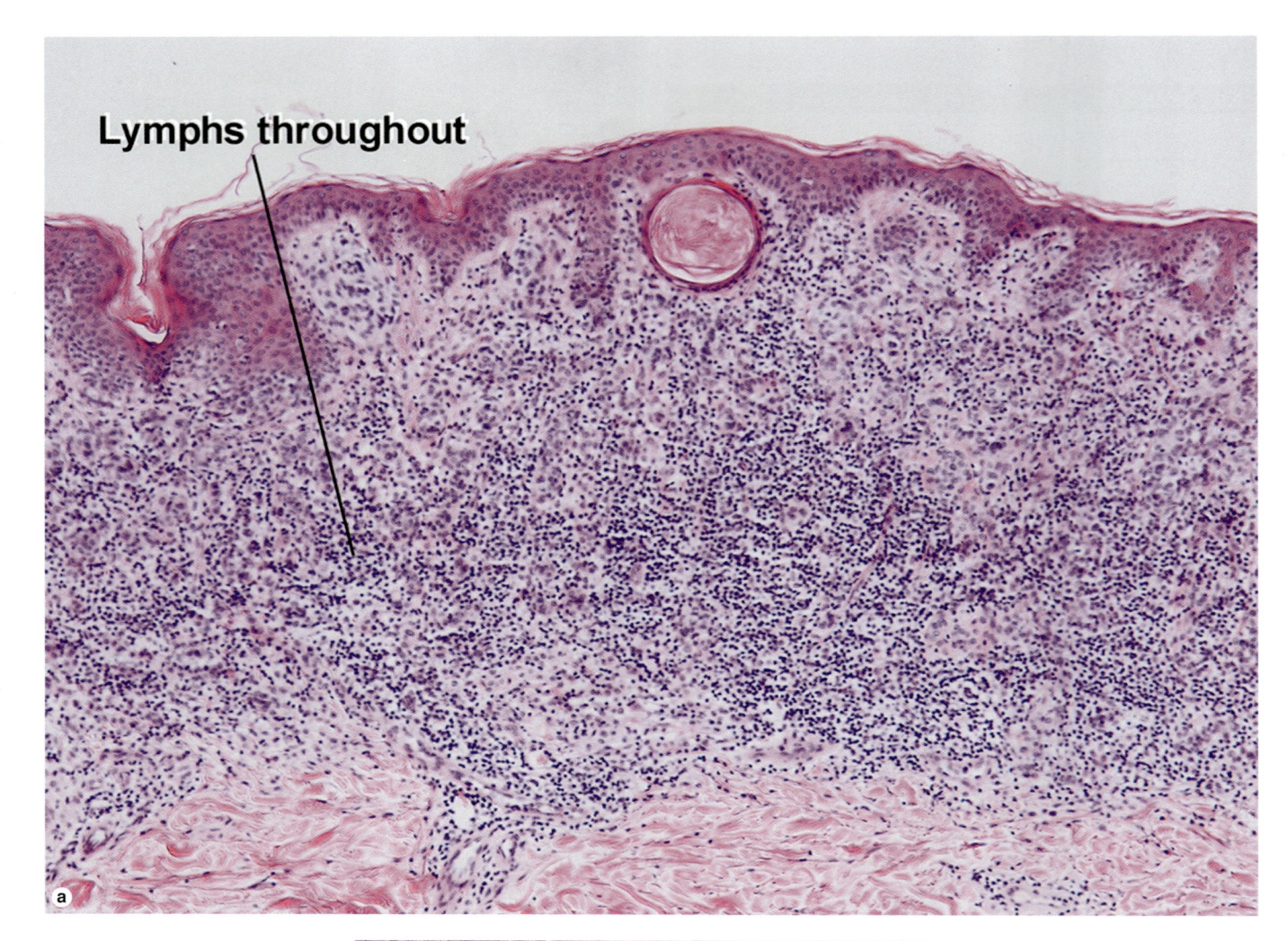

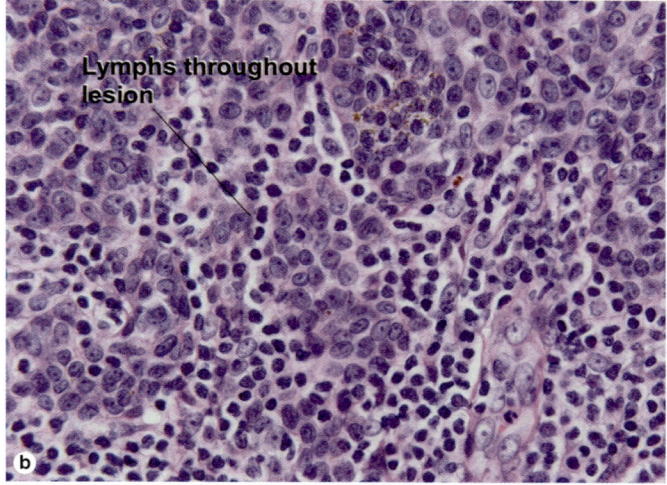

Fig 6-16 Halo nevus

Melanocytic neoplasms — Chapter 6 — 119

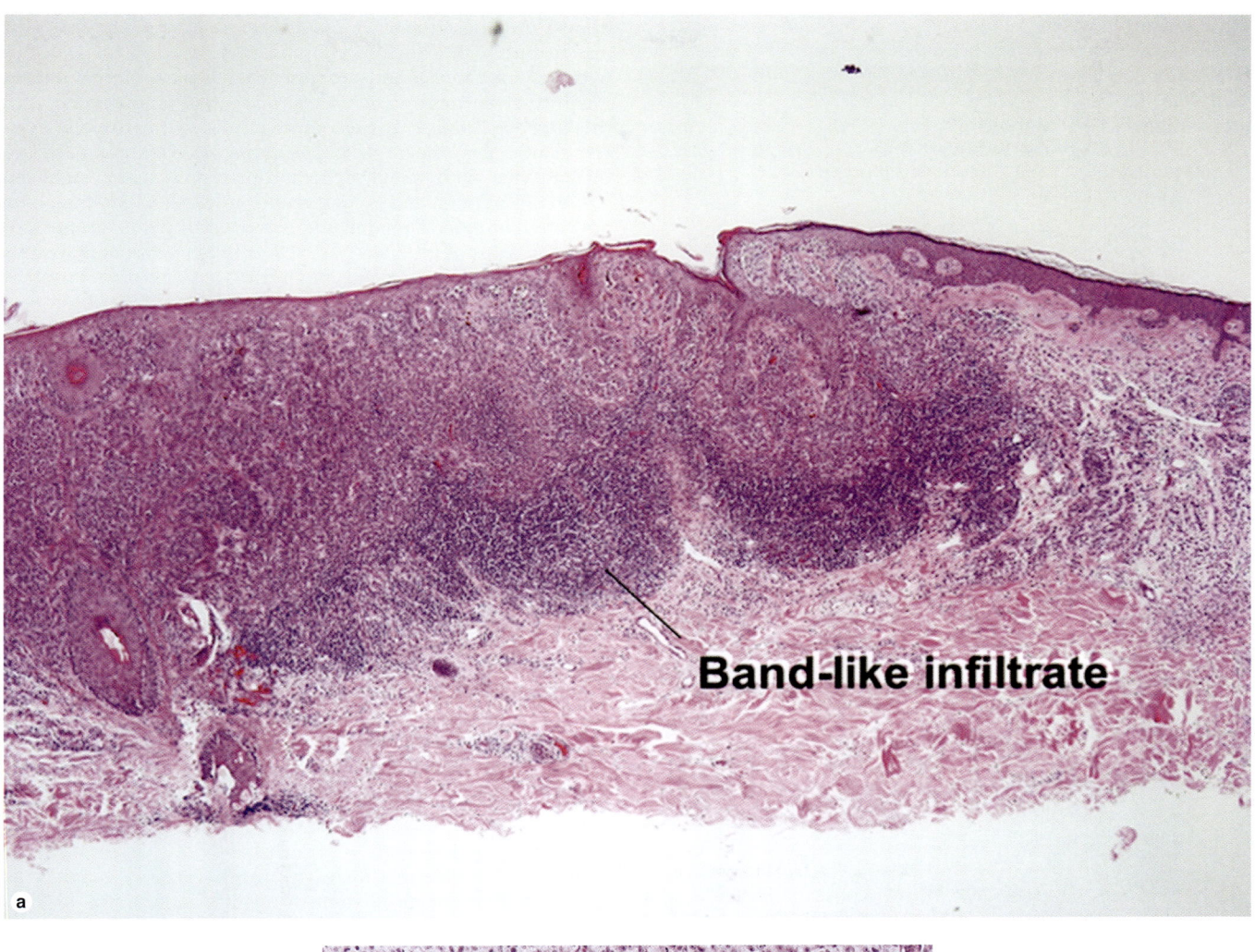

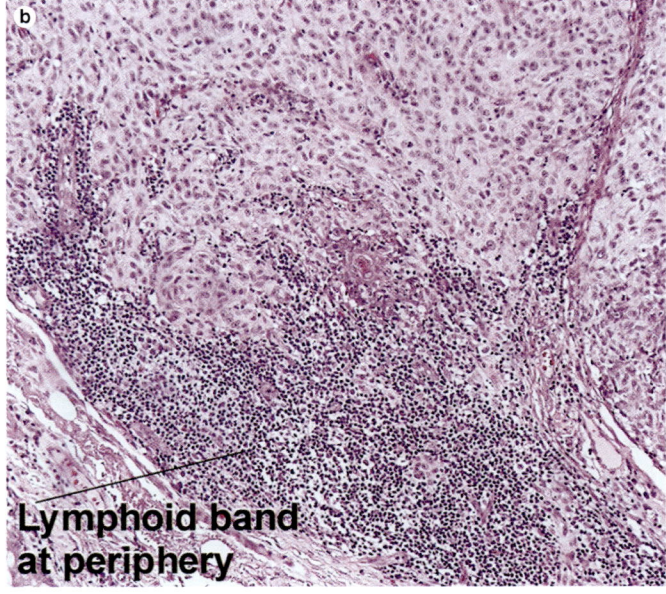

Fig 6-17 Melanoma for comparison

Blue nevus

> **Key features**
> - Wedge or bulbous outline
> - Pigment typically extends to base
> - Melanocytes do not mature or disperse
> - No deep mitoses
> - No necrosis
> - Typically have a distinctive sclerotic red stroma
> - Distinctive cytology

Variants of blue nevus are defined by the cytologic characteristics of the melanocytes. *Common blue nevi* are often seen on the dorsal hands and feet, face, and scalp. They are composed of dendritic melanocytes. *Cellular blue nevi* are commonly seen on the buttocks. They are composed of fusiform melanocytes with vesicular nuclei and prominent nucleoli. A closely related lesion referred to as an *epithelioid blue nevus* is associated with the Carney complex. It lacks the sclerotic stroma usually associated with blue nevi. *Deep penetrating nevi* are composed of melanocytes with small hyperchromatic nuclei, a smudged chromatin pattern, and inconspicuous nucleoli. Combined blue nevi are common. They include lesions with mixed features of different types of blue nevi, as well as lesions with components of blue and ordinary nevus. Dendritic "equine-type" melanomas are quite rare; they can be differentiated from blue nevi by the presence of nuclear atypia and the lack of sclerotic stroma.

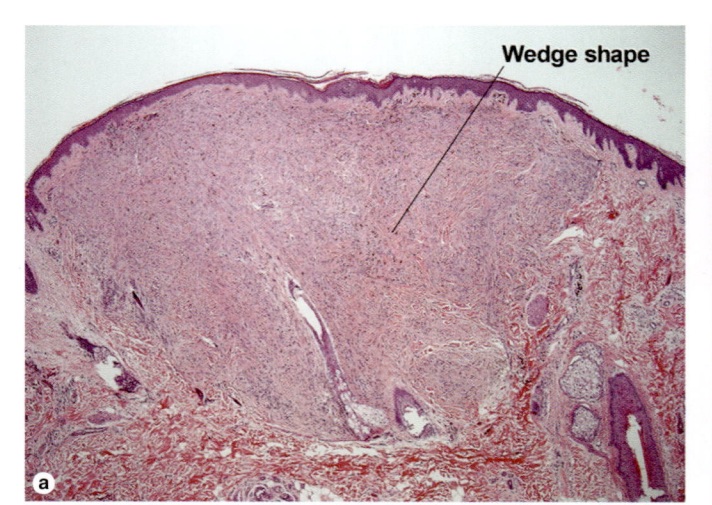

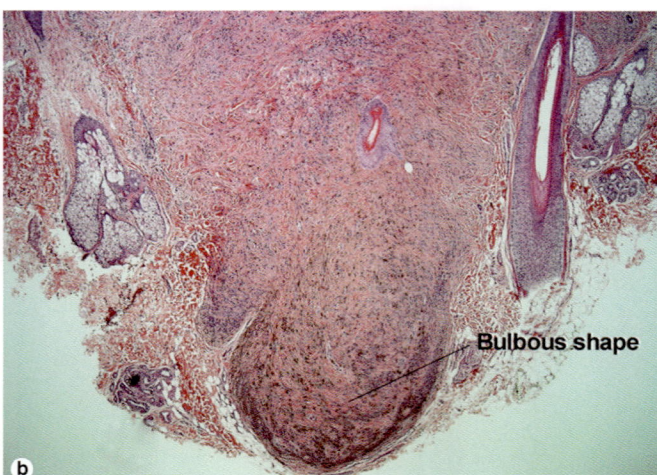

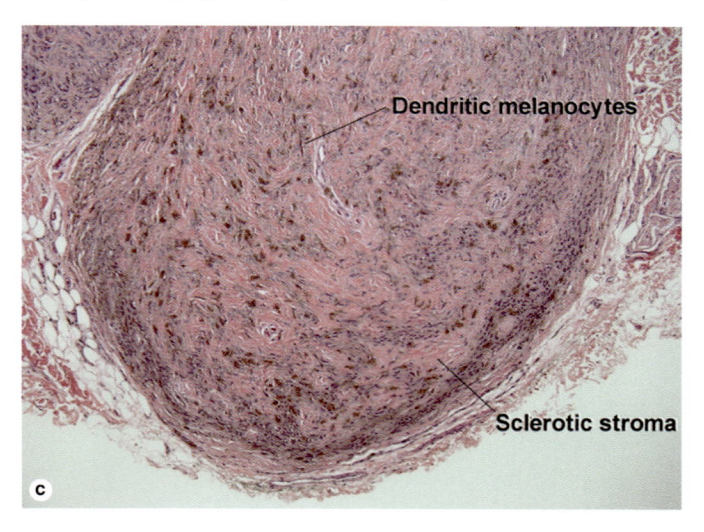

Fig 6-18 Common blue nevus

Melanocytic neoplasms   Chapter 6

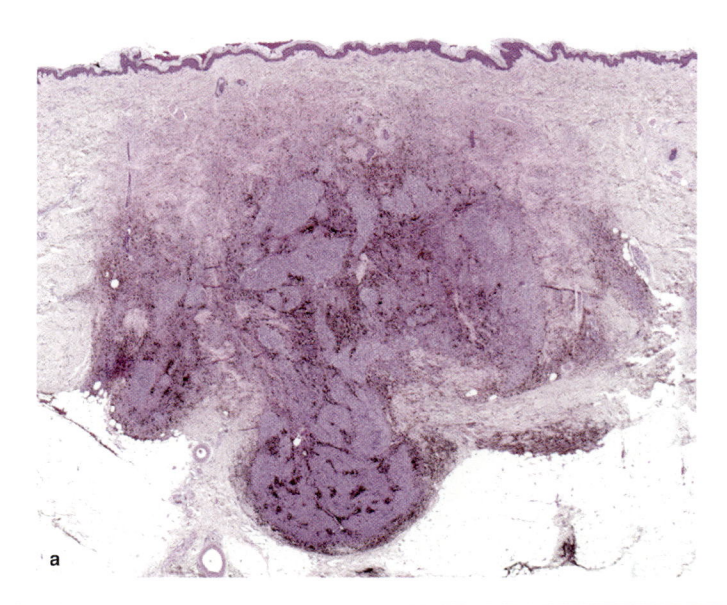

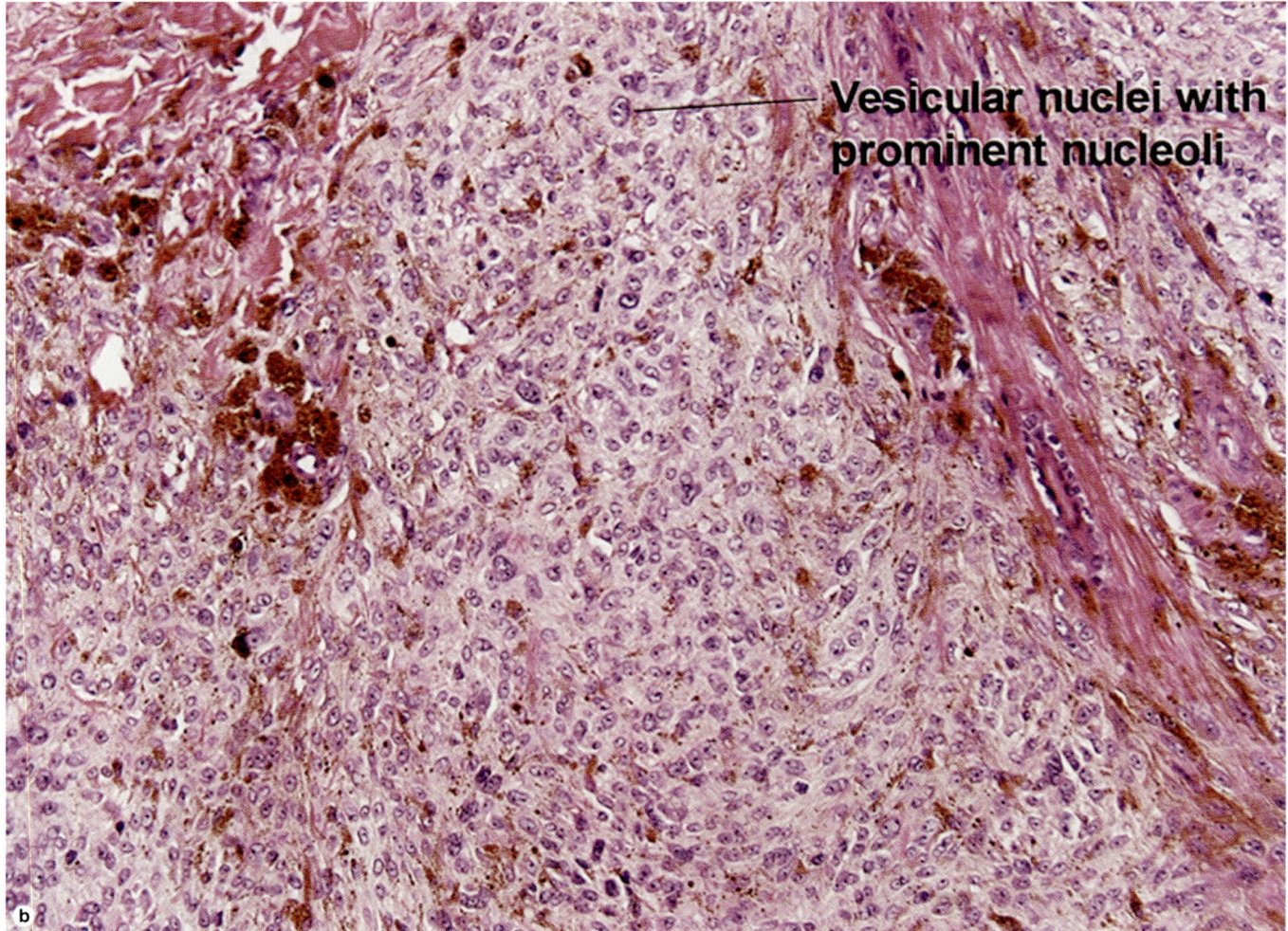

Fig 6-19 Cellular blue nevus

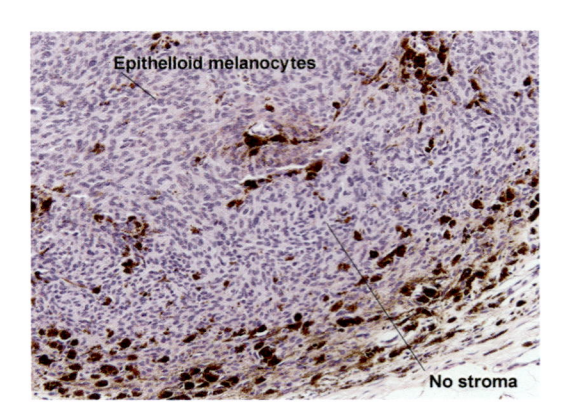

Fig 6-20 Epithelioid blue nevus

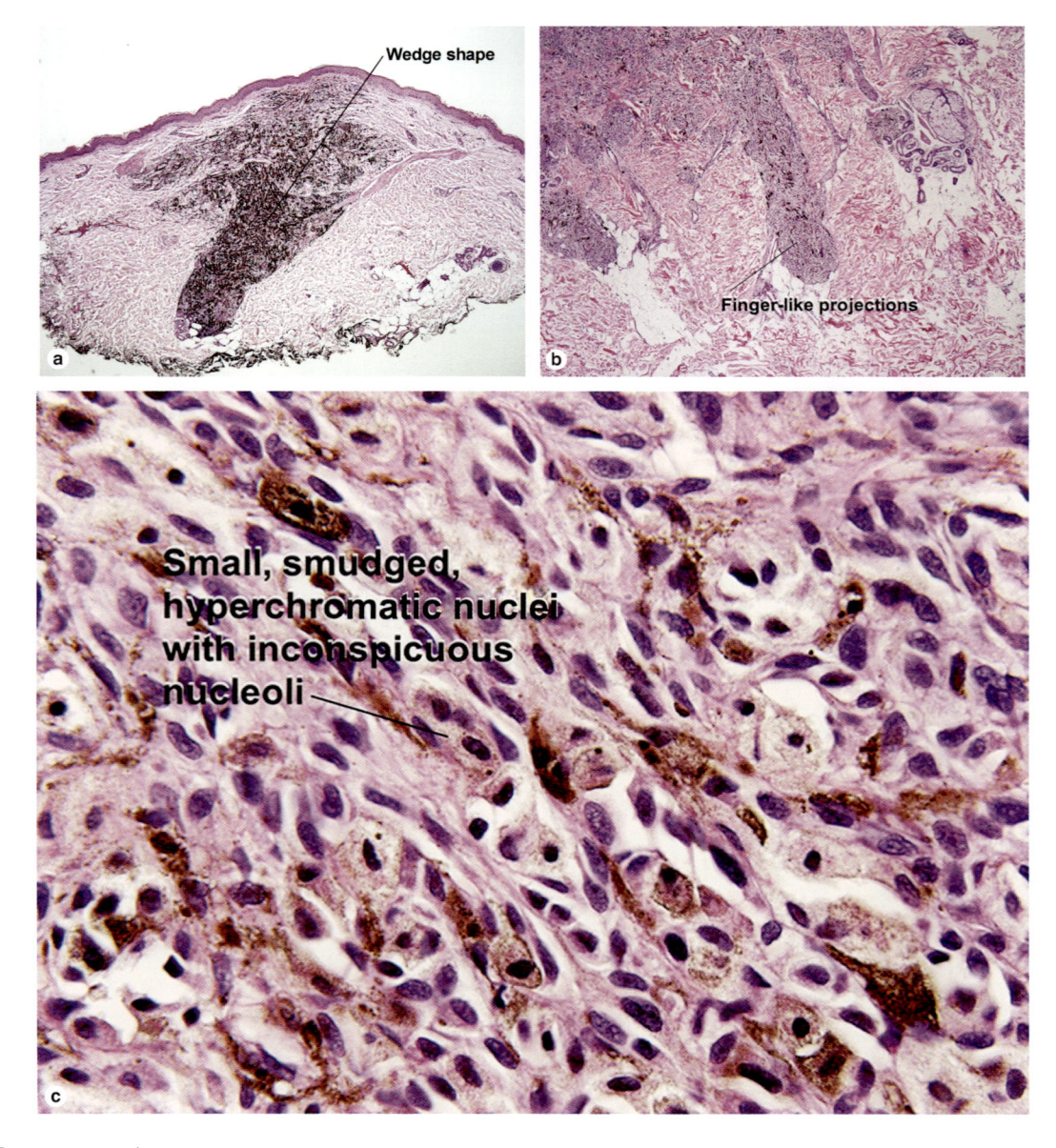

Fig 6-21 Deep penetrating nevus

Combined nevus

Key features

- Two or more populations of nevus cells

Combined nevi most commonly demonstrate a banal (ordinary) nevus component as well as a blue nevus component, but any variant of nevus can be represented within a combined nevus.

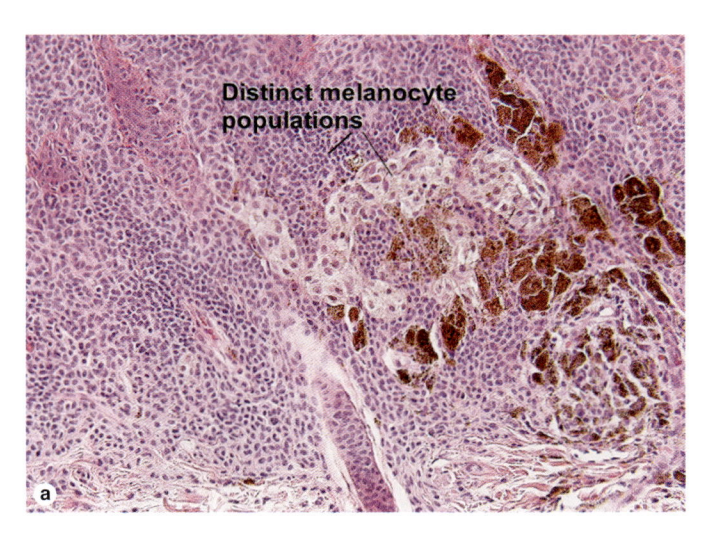

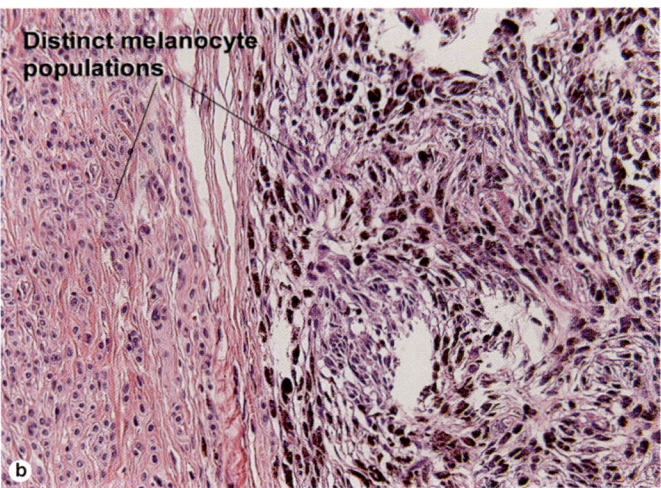

Fig 6-22 Combined nevus

Dysplastic nevus

Key features

- Commonly large, oval, and multiple
- Irregular pigment common
- Fading border or fried-egg appearance clinically (central papule, surrounding macule)
- Fading macular border corresponds to the "shoulder" region
- Junctional component extends at least 3 retia beyond the intradermal component
- Club-shaped hyperplasia of the rete
- Horizontally oriented nests with bridging of adjacent rete
- Nests are at tips and sides of rete
- Concentric papillary dermal fibrosis
- Large oval melanocytes, especially in shoulder region
- Well nested at the dermal–epidermal junction
- Matures
- Disperses at the base of the lesion
- No deep mitoses
- No deep pigment in nests

Dysplastic nevi occur in patients with the B-K mole/melanoma syndrome (dysplastic nevus syndrome) as well as sporadically. Any growing mole will have some features in common with a dysplastic nevus. "Special site" nevi can be indistinguishable from dysplastic nevi. Some refer to these as "atypical" nevi.

Grading dysplastic nevi

- Low-grade: atypia restricted to shoulder region
- Moderate: atypia in both shoulder region and central portion, some irregularity and confluence of nests
- High-grade: high-grade cytologic atypia in areas, not entirely well nested at junction, irregular nests, may be marginal in distinction from malignant melanoma *in situ*

Some have questioned the significance of grading of dysplastic nevi. Others prefer to divide them into high-grade and low-grade lesions.

Management

The management of dysplastic nevi is controversial. Most of the atypical cells are found in the shoulder region at the lateral edges of the specimen. The shoulder extends up to 2 mm beyond the clinically apparent edge of the specimen. A broad saucerization that includes a 0.5–2 mm margin of normal-appearing skin will provide the pathologist with the entire lesion, including the entire shoulder region.

In the author's opinion, high-grade lesions are best managed like malignant melanoma *in situ*. The risk of melanoma arising in a lesion with low-grade or moderate atypia is low. A greater risk is that a recurrent nevus within the scar will be misdiagnosed as melanoma. This can lead to overly aggressive management. For a low-grade dysplastic nevus that involves a margin, I will often include a comment:

The patient can be reassured that the lesion appears benign histologically. When they recur, lesions such as these commonly appear atypical clinically and histologically. This creates a potential for diagnostic confusion. In the case of recurrence, it is best if the patient is evaluated by a clinician who is familiar with the preceding lesion. Prompt removal of any recurrent lesion will minimize the potential for future diagnostic confusion.

124 Dermatopathology

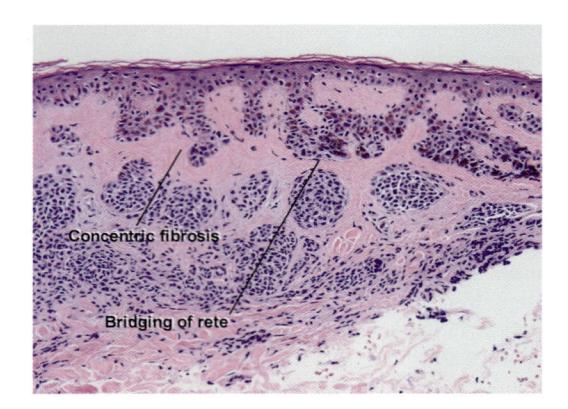

Fig 6-23 Dysplastic nevus

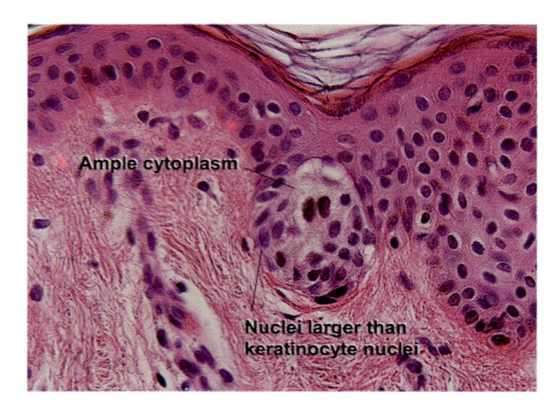

Fig 6-24 Atypia in the shoulder region of a dysplastic nevus

Junctional lentiginous nevus

Key features

- Club-shaped epidermal hyperplasia
- Round to oval melanocytic nests at the dermal–epidermal junction
- Nests restricted to the tips and sides of rete

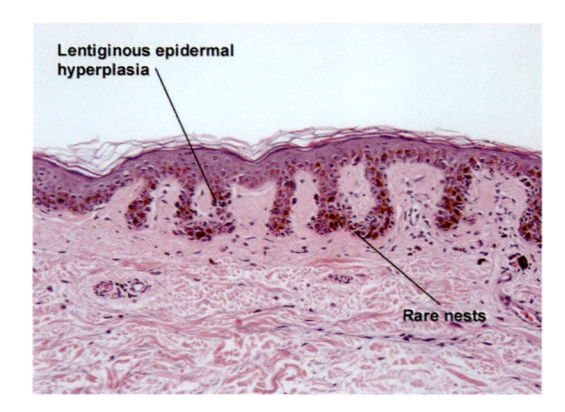

Fig 6-25 Junctional lentiginous nevus

Recurrent nevus (persistent nevus, pseudomelanoma)

Key features

- Confluent, poorly nested, or irregularly nested junctional melanocytic proliferation
- Underlying scar
- Melanocytic proliferation confined to the area overlying the scar
- May see residual bland nevus under scar

Recurrent nevi may simulate melanoma. History is critical, and review of the prior biopsy material may be necessary.

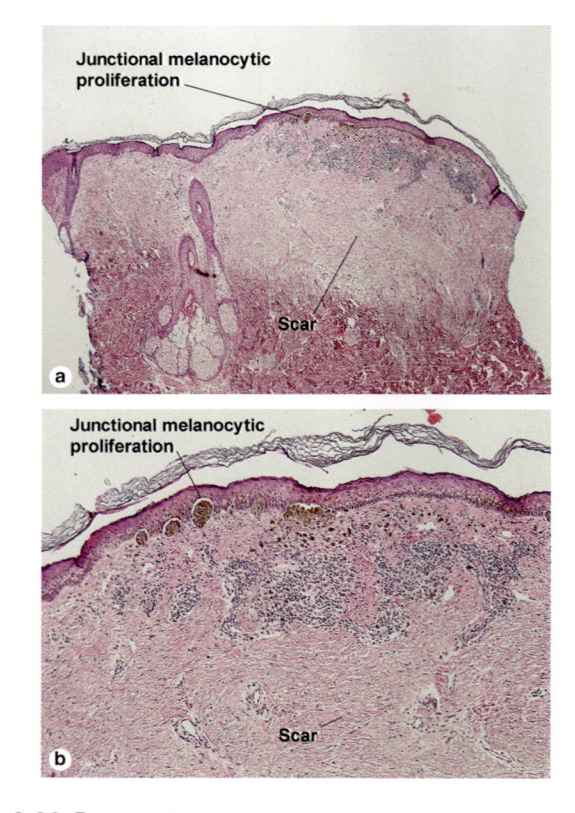

Fig 6-26 Recurrent nevus

Nevus of Ota/nevus of Ito

Key features

- Dendritic melanocytes scattered between collagen bundles in the upper third of the dermis
- Melanocytes oriented east to west
- No sclerotic stroma

A biopsy will demonstrate a subtle band of dendritic melanocytes in the upper dermis. There is no associated sclerotic stroma. Clinically, they present as deep blue patches on the face (Ota) or shoulder (Ito).

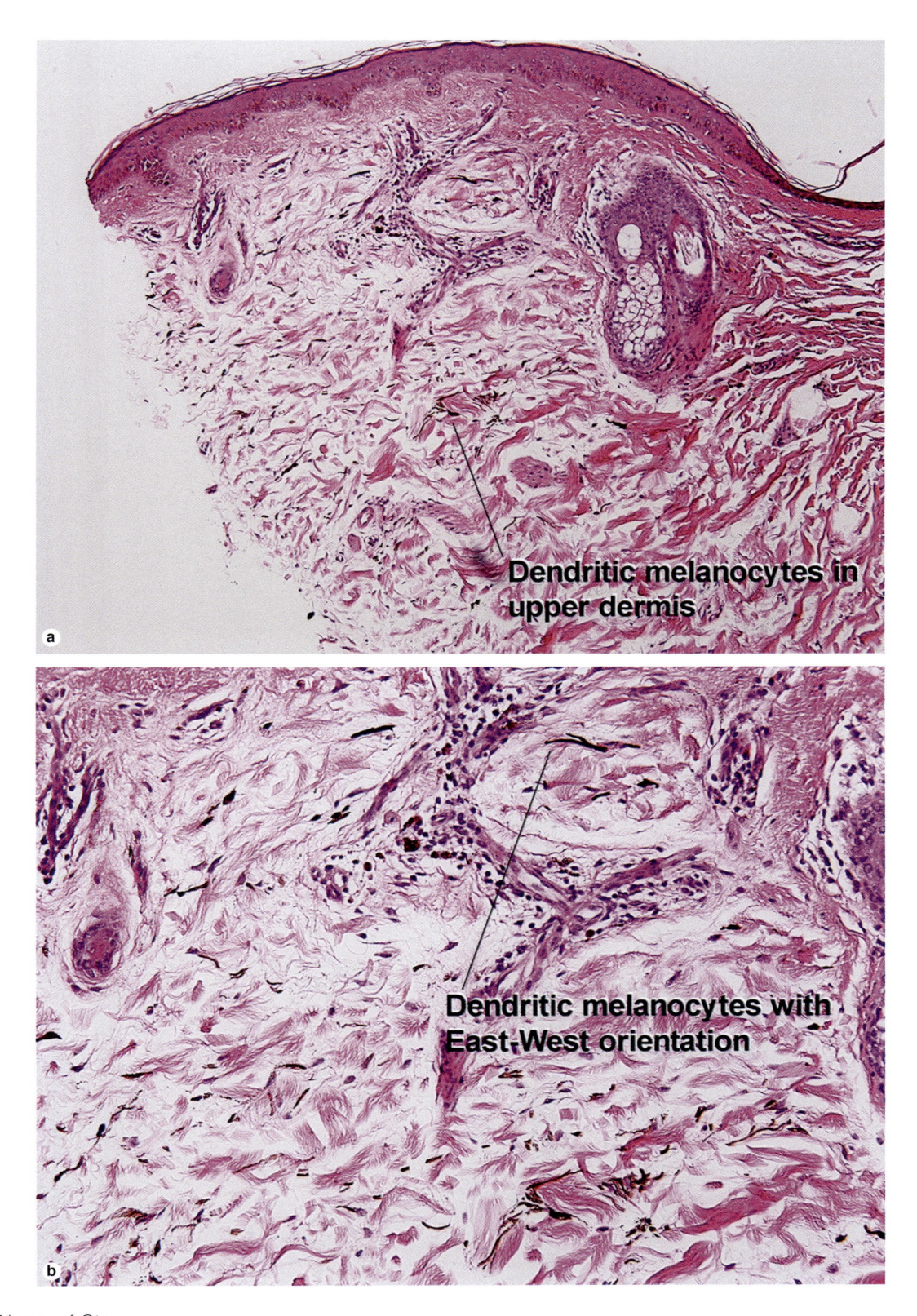

Fig 6-27 Nevus of Ota

126 Dermatopathology

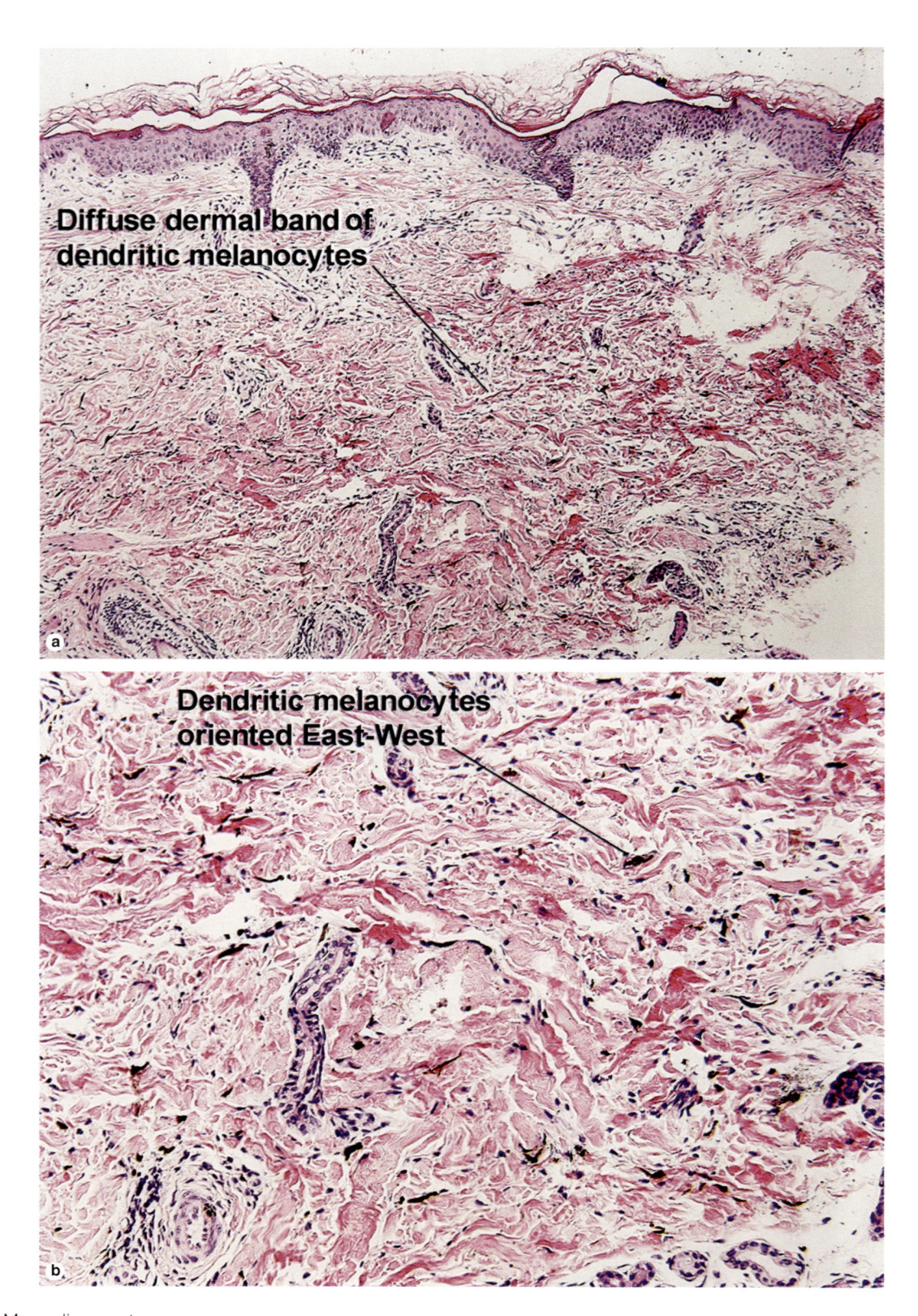

Fig 6-28 Mongolian spot

Melanocytic neoplasms | Chapter 6 | 127

Table 6-3 Distinguishing features of melanomas

Type of melanoma	Distinguishing features
Superficial spreading melanoma	Radial growth phase characterized by buckshot scatter in epidermis
Nodular melanoma	Lacks radial growth phase
Lentigo maligna	Malignant melanoma *in situ*
	Poorly nested and confluent melanocytes at the dermal–epidermal junction
	Adnexal extension
	Heavily sun-damaged skin
Lentigo maligna melanoma	Lentigo maligna with vertical growth phase
Acral lentiginous melanoma	Poorly nested and confluent melanocytes at the dermal–epidermal junction
Desmoplastic melanoma	Commonly arises in subtle *in situ* lesions of a lentiginous type
	Desmoplastic stroma
	Spindle cells with variable atypia
	Nodular lymphoid aggregates
Mucosal melanoma	Oral, genital, or conjunctival mucosa
	Often has a lentiginous growth pattern

Mongolian spot

Key features

- Dendritic melanocytes scattered between collagen bundles in the lower half of the dermis
- Melanocytes oriented east to west
- No sclerotic stroma

PEARLS

1. In the *in situ* portion of lentiginous types of melanoma, the atypical melanocytes proliferate predominantly at the dermal–epidermal junction, with little to no buckshot scatter.
2. The vertical growth phase is an expansile dermal nodule. It typically invades the reticular dermis (into the zone of bundled collagen or solar elastosis) or appears as a dermal nest larger than the largest junctional nest. Mitoses or necrosis may be noted in the nodule. The vertical growth phase may have different cytologic features from the radial growth phase. Metastases typically resemble the vertical growth phase cytologically.
3. Measure the depth of invasion from the granular layer, the base of an ulcer, or the inner root sheath (if invading outward from a follicle).
4. Clark's levels:
   I. Confined to the epidermis (*in situ* melanoma)
   II. Into the papillary dermis
   III. To the papillary dermis–reticular dermis interface
   IV. Into the reticular dermis
   V. Into the subcutaneous fat.

Superficial spreading malignant melanoma

Key features

- Broad lesion
- Buckshot scatter of atypical melanocytes within the epidermis
- Non-nested melanocytes outnumber nests in areas
- Nests vary in size and shape (often elongated, bizarre, or confluent)
- Nests not evenly spaced
- Nests not confined to tips and sides of rete
- Typically not symmetrical (right to left)
- Typically fails to mature from top to bottom
- Typically fails to disperse at base
- Dermal nests often larger than junctional nests
- Deep pigment may be present within melanocytic nests
- Lymphoid infiltrate frequent at base, walling off lesion ("riot police")
- Plasma cells common in infiltrate
- Deep mitoses may be present
- Cytologic atypia
- Melanocytes often have ample amphophilic cytoplasm
- HMB-45 staining typically strong to base
- S100A6 staining typically patchy
- MIB-1 staining of deep melanocyte nuclei common

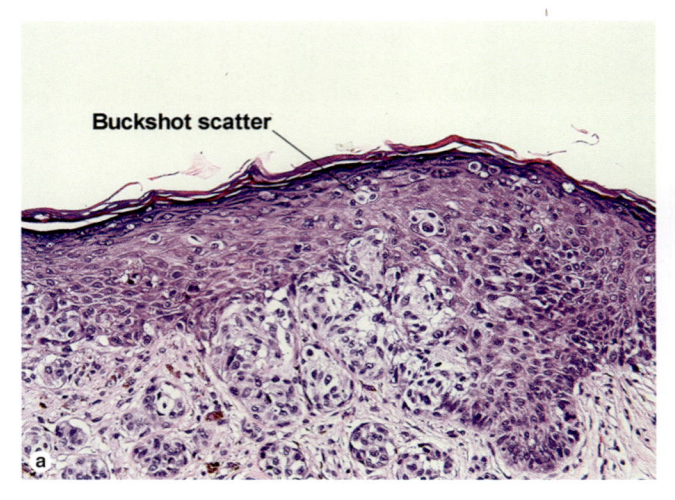

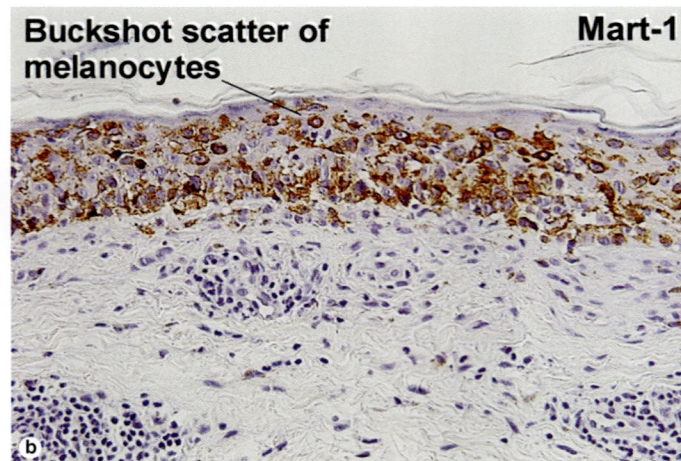

Fig 6-29 Superficial spreading melanoma

Lentigo maligna

Key features

- Broad lesion on sun-damaged skin
- Rete ridge pattern commonly effaced
- Predominantly junctional growth of atypical melanocytes
- Multinucleated giant cells may be seen at dermal–epidermal junction (DEJ)
- Non-nested melanocytes usually outnumber nests in areas
- Nests vary in size and shape (often elongated, bizarre, or confluent)
- Nests not evenly spaced
- Extends down adnexal structures
- Nests not confined to tips and sides of rete
- Often lacks sharp lateral circumscription
- Often not symmetrical (right to left)
- Cytologic atypia

Lentigo maligna typically exhibits asymmetrical growth. As the atypical melanocytes are only one cell thick at the dermal–epidermal junction, the lateral borders are poorly defined clinically. The lesion often extends far beyond the clinically apparent margin.

PEARLS

1. Small biopsies are likely to result in misdiagnosis. Skip areas are common. Lichenoid regression can mimic a lichenoid actinic keratosis or benign lichenoid keratosis. Benign pigmented lesions (pigmented actinic keratosis and solar lentigo) occur in collision with lentigo maligna in about half of all cases. Small biopsies may sample only the benign lesion. The false-negative rate of a small biopsy is up to 80%. The best biopsy technique for a large macular facial lesion may be a broad thin shave, or multiple small shave biopsies, to sample every color within the lesion.
2. Although effacement of the rete is typical, lentiginous epidermal hyperplasia may occur, and lentigo maligna may closely resemble a junctional lentiginous nevus or junctional dysplastic nevus. A broad junctional lesion on sun-damaged skin is probably melanoma *in situ*.

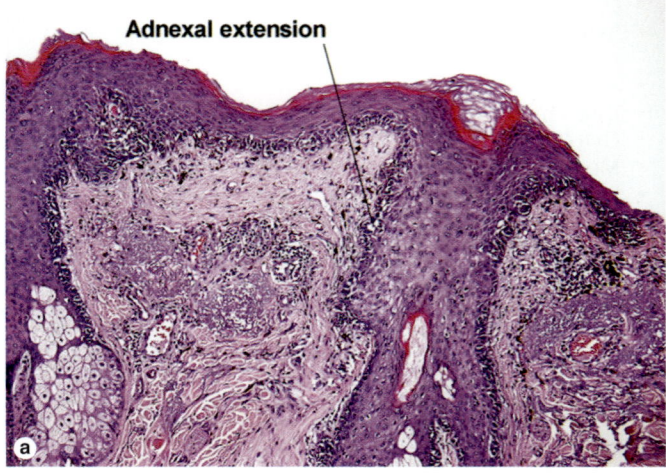

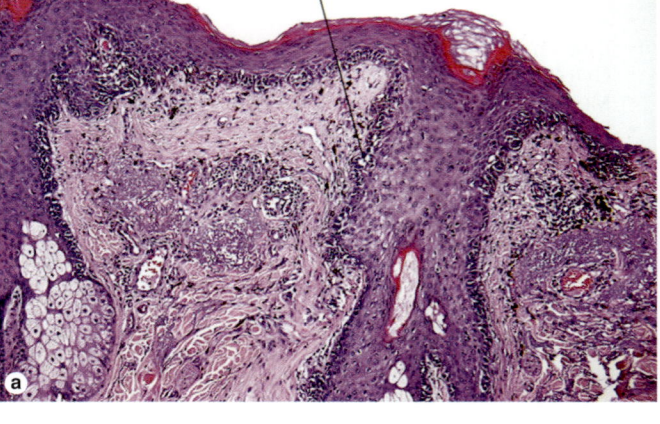

Fig 6-30 Lentigo maligna (DEJ, dermal–epidermal junction)

Lentigo maligna melanoma

Key features

- Lentigo maligna with a vertical growth phase
- Vertical growth phase may be epithelioid, spindled, or desmoplastic

Spindle cell melanoma

Key features

- Spindled cytology
- Most reliable immunostain are S100 and SOX10

Desmoplastic melanoma

Key features

- Dense desmoplastic stroma
- Nodular lymphoid aggregates
- May see a subtle overlying lentigo maligna
- S100 and SOX10 are generally reliable, but other immunostains like HMB-45 are unreliable in desmoplastic melanoma
- Atypia of spindle cells is variable
- Perineural extension common

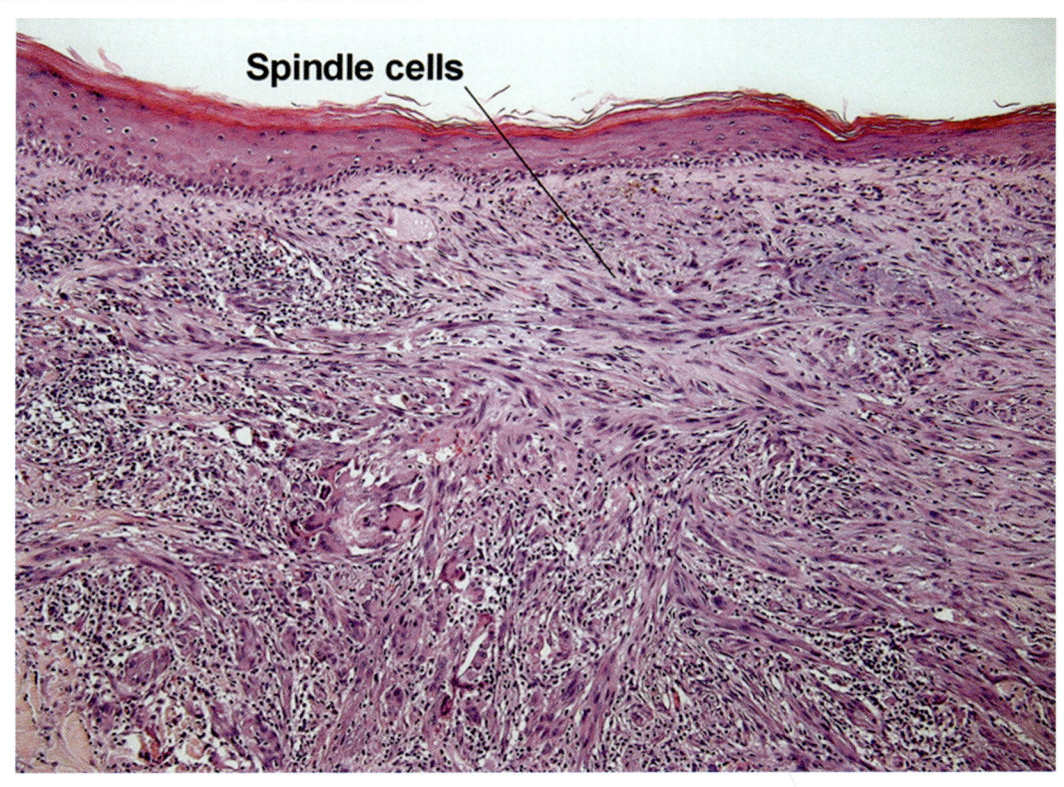

Fig 6-31 Spindle cell melanoma

Differential Diagnosis

Spindled melanomas can closely resemble other spindle cell neoplasms. The microscopic differential diagnosis for an atypical spindle cell tumor *slam*med up against the epidermis includes:

- *S*quamous cell carcinoma (keratin-positive)
- *L*eiomyosarcoma (smooth muscle actin-positive, desmin-positive)
- *A*typical fibroxanthoma (diagnosis of exclusion)
- *M*elanoma (S100-positive)

Nodular melanoma

Key features

- No apparent radial growth phase
- May be symmetrical in all directions
- Typically fails to mature from top to bottom
- Typically fails to disperse at base
- Deep pigment may be present in melanocytic nests
- Lymphoid infiltrate frequent at base, walling off lesion ("riot police")
- Plasma cells commonly present in infiltrate
- Deep mitoses may be present
- Cytologic atypia
- Necrosis
- HMB-45 staining typically strong to base
- S100A6 staining typically patchy
- MIB-1 staining of deep melanocyte nuclei common

130 Dermatopathology

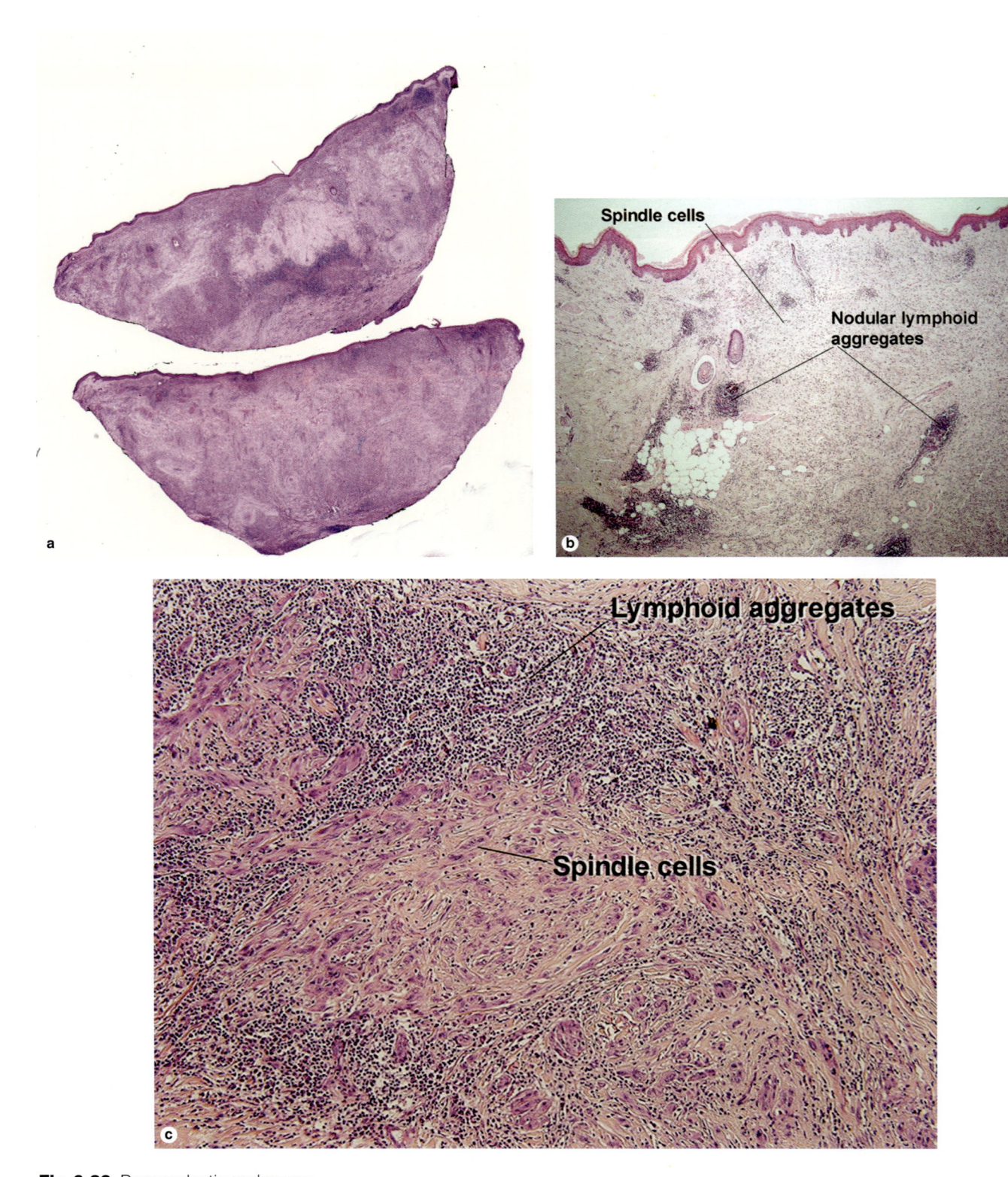

Fig 6-32 Desmoplastic melanoma

Melanocytic neoplasms Chapter 6

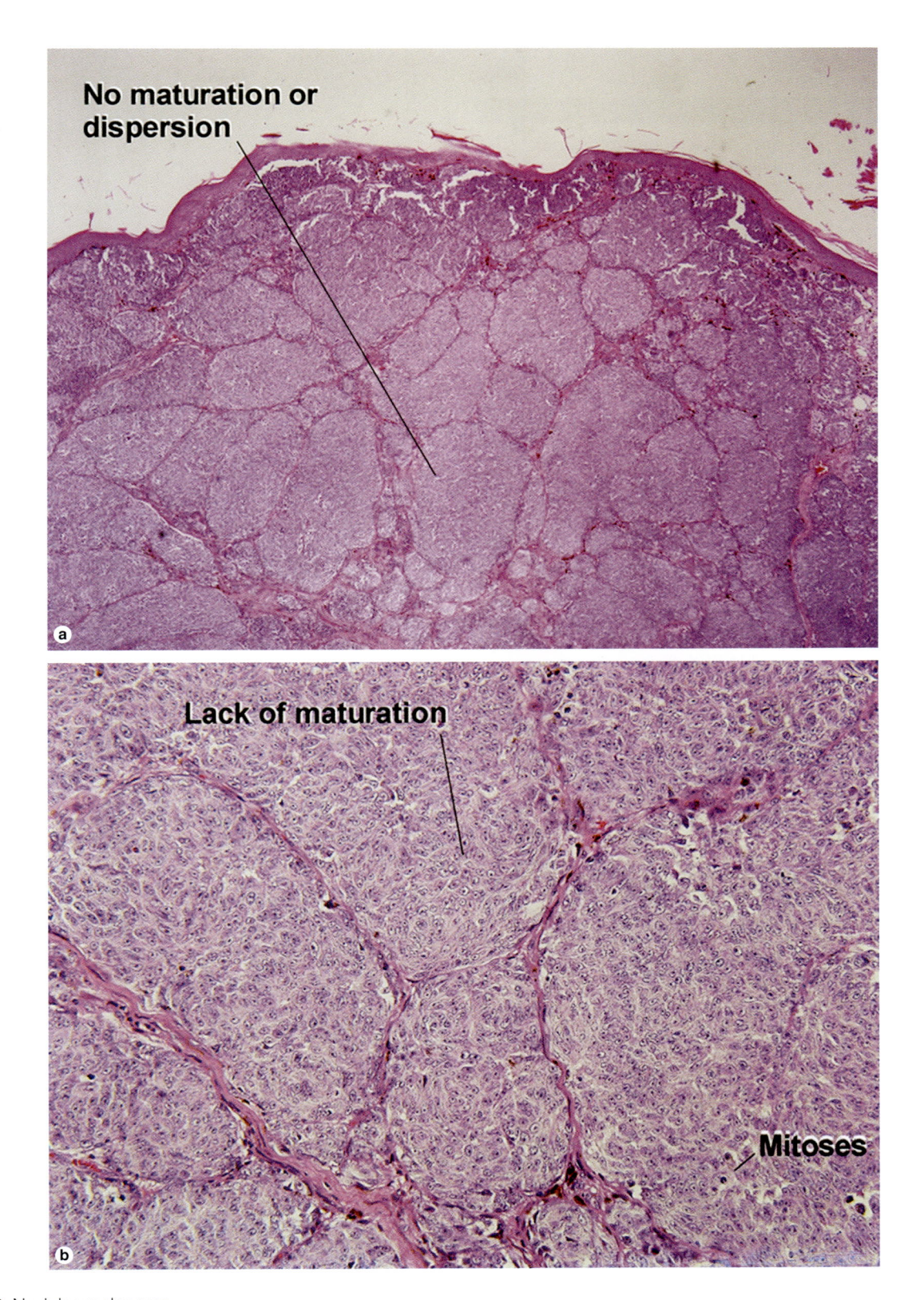

Fig 6-33 Nodular melanoma

Regressing melanoma

Key features

- Lichenoid regression may occur in lentigo maligna
- Regression in other melanomas is probably secondary to genomic instability rather than inflammatory response
- May appear as zones of fibrosis and melanophages
- Adverse prognostic indicator
- "Tumoral melanosis" may be regressed melanoma

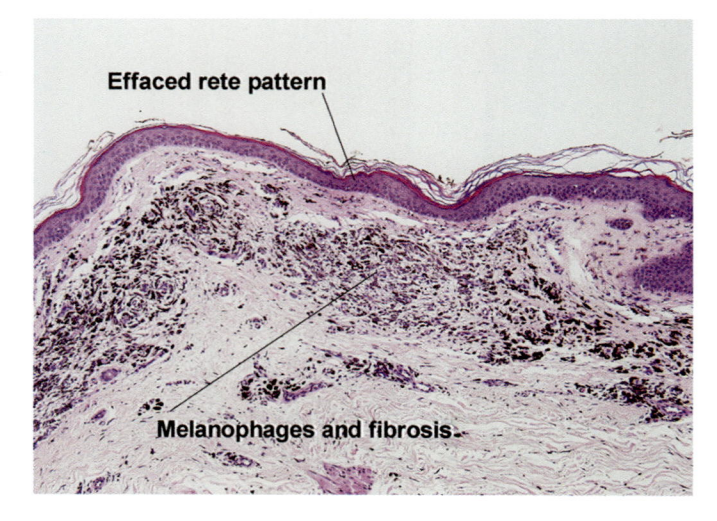

Fig 6-34 Regressing melanoma

Metastatic melanoma

Key features

- May be a radially symmetrical "cannonball"
- May be epidermotropic and nevoid
- Atypical cells may be noted in lymphatic vessels
- Cytologic atypia may be marked
- Mitoses common
- Necrosis common
- MIB-1 positivity common
- HMB-45 positive to base, or may be patchy or negative

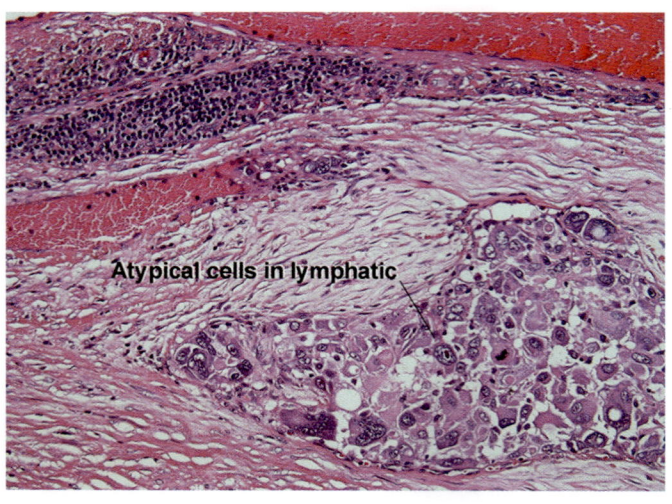

Fig 6-35 Metastatic melanoma

Epidermotropic nevoid metastases typically fail to mature or disperse well at the base. This helps to distinguish them from nevi. In lymph nodes, metastatic melanoma is typically subcapsular in location. Nodal nevi occur, but are typically located within the capsule and are composed of bland nuclei.

Clear cell sarcoma

Key features

- Soft-tissue tumor
- Clear cytoplasm
- Nuclear atypia
- S100-positive

Clear cell sarcoma is regarded by some as a form of primary soft-tissue clear cell melanoma. The tumor is also defined by a characteristic chromosome translocation t(12;22)(q13;q12).

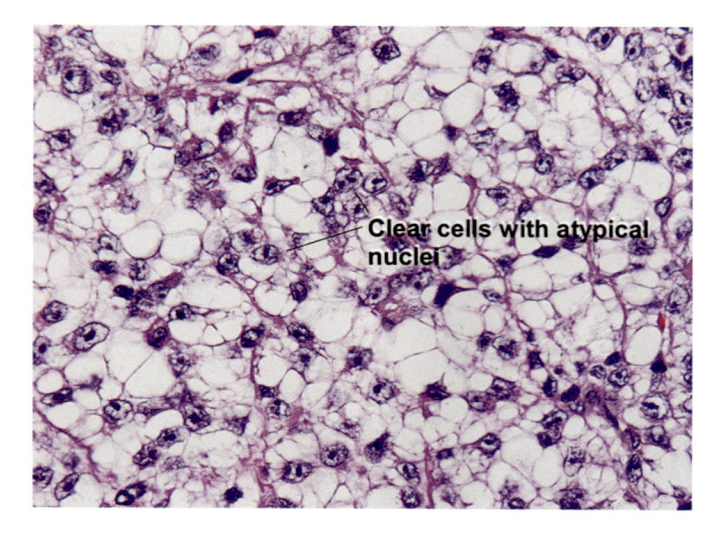

Fig 6-36 Clear cell sarcoma

Further reading

Bauer J, Bastian BC. Distinguishing melanocytic nevi from melanoma by DNA copy number changes: comparative genomic hybridization as a research and diagnostic tool. Dermatol Ther 2006;19(1):40–49.

Boyd AS, Rapini RP. Acral melanocytic neoplasms: a histologic analysis of 158 lesions. J Am Acad Dermatol 1994;31(5 Pt 1):740–745.

Cerroni L. A new perspective for spitz tumors? Am J Dermatopathol 2005;27(4):366–367.

Cesinaro AM. Clinico-pathological impact of fibroplasia in melanocytic nevi: a critical revision of 209 cases. APMIS 2012;120(8):658–665.

Dalton SR, Gardner TL, Libow LF, et al. Contiguous lesions in lentigo maligna. J Am Acad Dermatol 2005;52(5):859–862.

Farrahi F, Egbert BM, Swetter SM. Histologic similarities between lentigo maligna and dysplastic nevus: importance of clinicopathologic distinction. J Cutan Pathol 2005;32(6):405–412.

Ferrara G, Argenziano G, Soyer HP, et al. The spectrum of Spitz nevi: a clinicopathologic study of 83 cases. Arch Dermatol 2005;141(11):1381–1387.

Griewank KG, Ugurel S, Schadendorf D, et al. New developments in biomarkers for melanoma. Curr Opin Oncol 2013;25(2):145–151.

Kapur P, Selim MA, Roy LC, et al. Spitz nevi and atypical Spitz nevi/tumors: a histologic and immunohistochemical analysis. Mod Pathol 2005;18(2):197–204.

King R, Page RN, Googe PB, et al. Lentiginous melanoma: a histologic pattern of melanoma to be distinguished from lentiginous nevus. Mod Pathol 2005;18(10):1397–1401.

Moore DA, Pringle JH, Saldanha GS. Prognostic tissue markers in melanoma. Histopathology 2012;60(5):679–689.

Nambiar S, Mirmohammadsadegh A, Hengge UR. Cutaneous melanoma: fishing with chips. Curr Mol Med 2008;8(3):235–243.

Ribé A, McNutt NS. S100A6 protein expression is different in Spitz nevi and melanomas. Mod Pathol 2003;16(5):505–511.

Strungs I. Common and uncommon variants of melanocytic naevi. Pathology 2004;36(5):396–403.

Tannous ZS, Mihm MC Jr, Sober AJ, et al. Congenital melanocytic nevi: clinical and histopathologic features, risk of melanoma, and clinical management. J Am Acad Dermatol 2005;52(2):197–203.

Urso C. A new perspective for spitz tumors? Am J Dermatopathol 2005;27(4):364–366.

Xu X, Elder DE. A practical approach to selected problematic melanocytic lesions. Am J Clin Pathol 2004;121.

7 Interface dermatitis

Dirk M. Elston

Lichenoid interface dermatitis

Key features
- Basal layer is destroyed
- Civatte bodies
- Sawtooth rete pattern

Causes of lichenoid interface dermatitis
- Lichen planus
- Benign lichenoid keratosis (BLK, lichen planus-like keratosis)
- Lichenoid drug eruption
- Lichenoid graft-versus-host disease (GvHD)
- Hypertrophic lupus erythematosus
- Lichenoid regression of a melanocytic lesion (usually lentigo maligna)

The biopsy in each of these conditions demonstrates a sawtooth rete ridge pattern with destruction of the basal layer, a band-like lymphoid infiltrate, and presence of Civatte bodies. Compact hyperkeratosis and beaded hypergranulosis are typically present. The cells of the stratum spinosum are enlarged and more eosinophilic than the normal epidermis. Vacuoles may be present in the lowest cells of stratum spinosum, but the basal layer is gone. An underlying band-like lymphoid infiltrate is common.

If neither parakeratosis nor eosinophils are noted, the changes are consistent with lichen planus. Lichenoid interface dermatitis with neither eosinophils nor parakeratosis may also be seen in BLK (lichen planus-like keratosis), lichenoid drug eruption, lichenoid GvHD, hypertrophic lupus erythematosus, and lichenoid regression of lentigo maligna. Clinical correlation is essential. Direct immunofluorescence (DIF) will distinguish hypertrophic lupus erythematosus (continuous granular band of immunoglobulins and complement plus cytoid bodies) from lichen planus (shaggy fibrin, cytoid bodies).

When parakeratosis is present, lichen planus is very unlikely. The differential diagnosis still includes BLK, lichenoid drug eruption, lichenoid GvHD, and lichenoid regression of a melanocytic lesion. Hypertrophic lupus erythematosus rarely demonstrates parakeratosis.

The presence of eosinophils strongly favors a diagnosis of lichenoid drug eruption. The presence of eosinophils weighs strongly against a diagnosis of lichen planus. They are rarely seen in hypertrophic lupus erythematosus, BLK, lichenoid GvHD, or lichenoid regression of a melanocytic lesion.

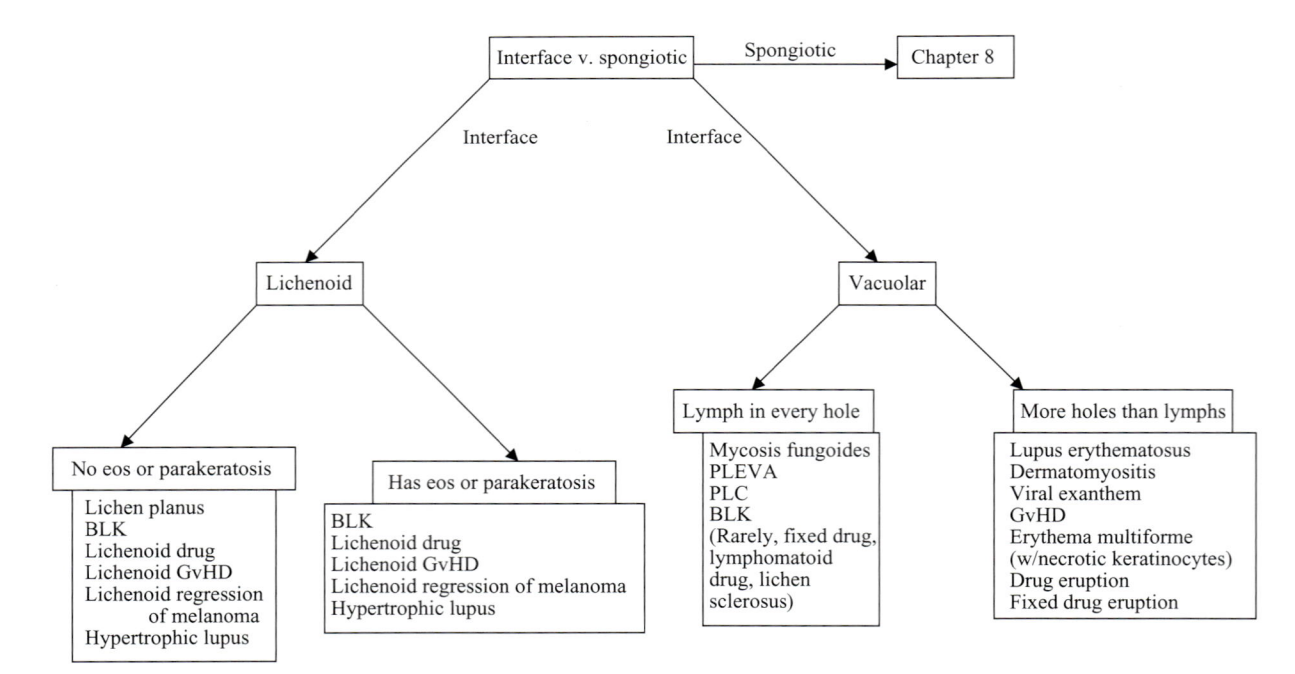

Fig 7-1 Interface versus spongiotic dermatitis (eos, eosinophils; PLEVA, Pityriasis lichenoides chronica; PLC, pleomorphic lobular carcinoma)

Interface dermatitis | Chapter 7 | 135

PEARL

An analogy that those with teenagers may appreciate:
- Lichen planus is like a strict parent: "You will not hang around with eosinophils or parakeratosis"
- Lichenoid drug eruption and the remaining lichenoid processes are more permissive: "You don't have to have eosinophils or parakeratosis, but if you want to, it's OK"

Late-phase (burnt-out) lichenoid dermatitis

Key features

- Effacement of the rete pattern
- Melanin pigment incontinence (melanoderma)
- Civatte bodies

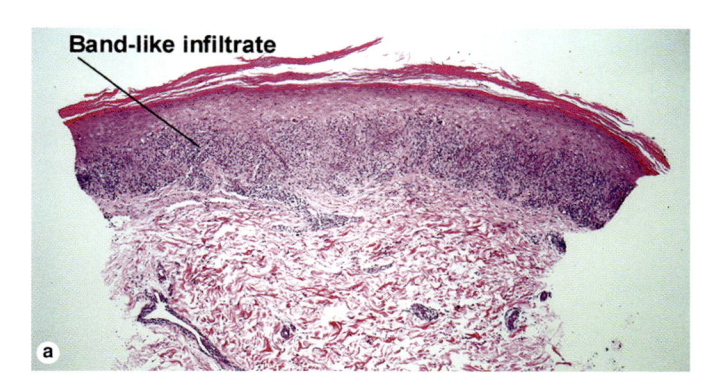

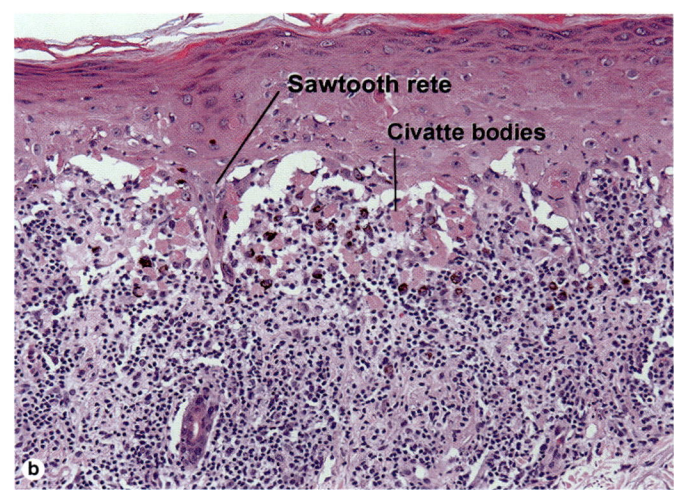

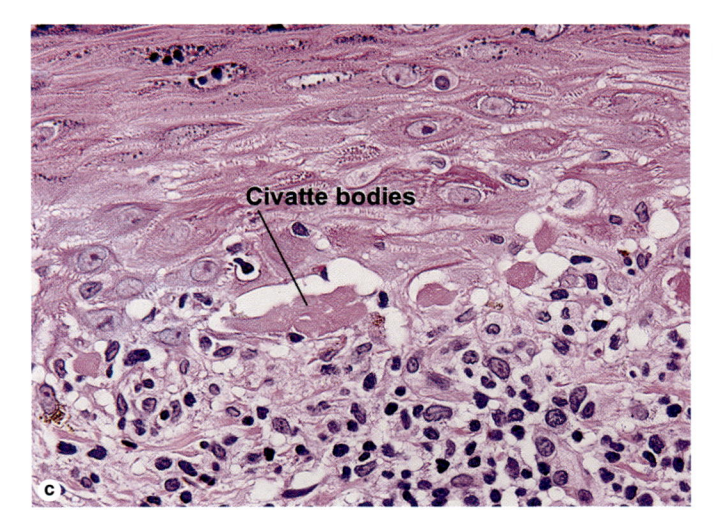

Fig 7-2 Lichenoid interface dermatitis

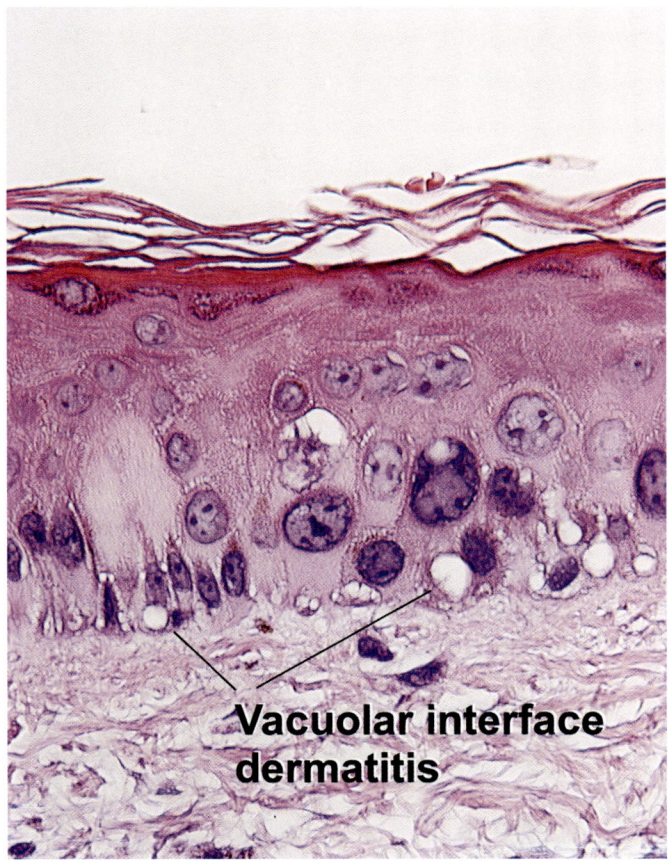

Fig 7-3 Vacuolar interface dermatitis for comparison

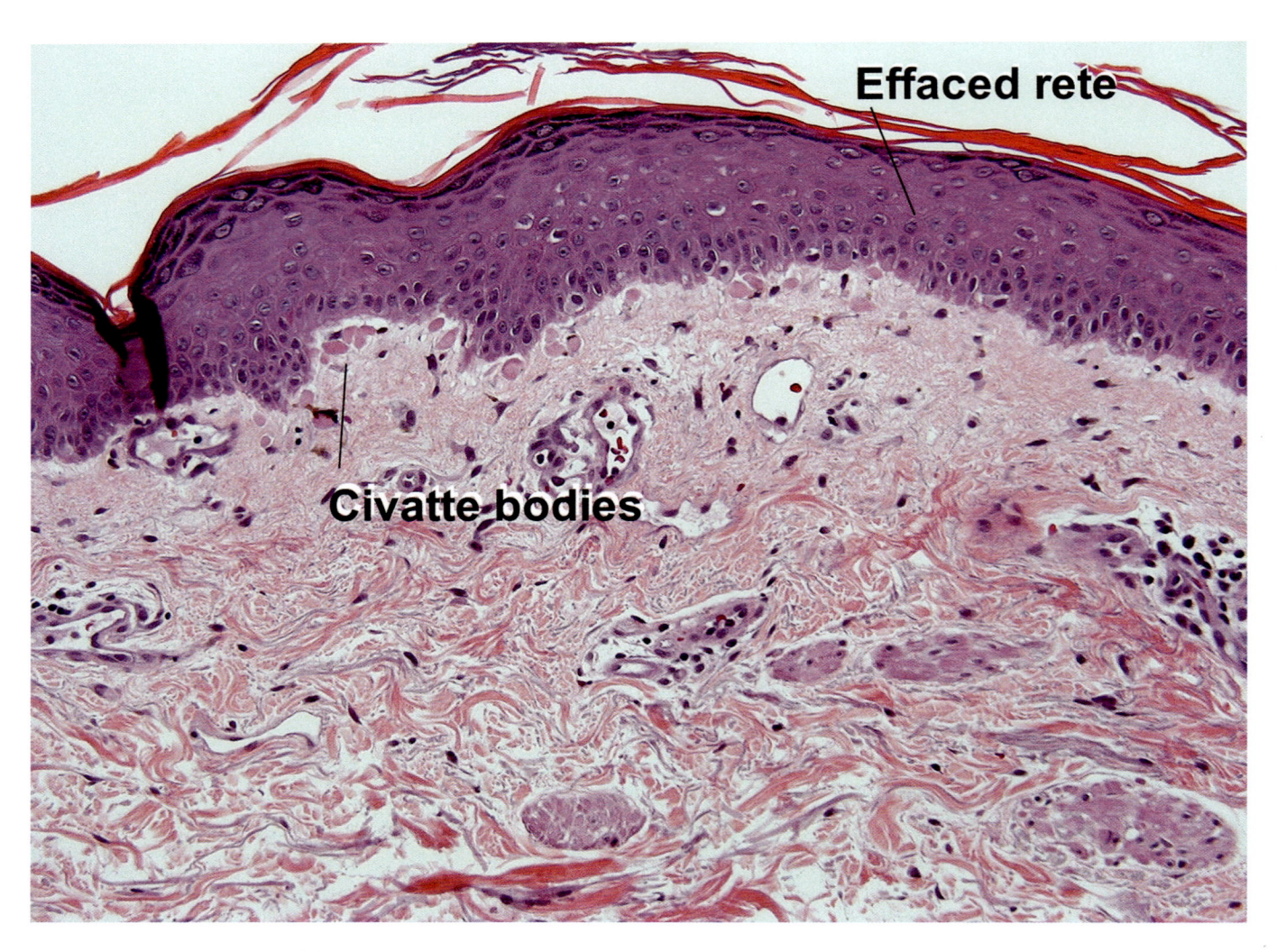

Fig 7-4 Late-stage lichenoid dermatitis

Lichen planus

Key features
- Lichenoid interface dermatitis
- No parakeratosis or eosinophils
- Sawtooth rete ridges

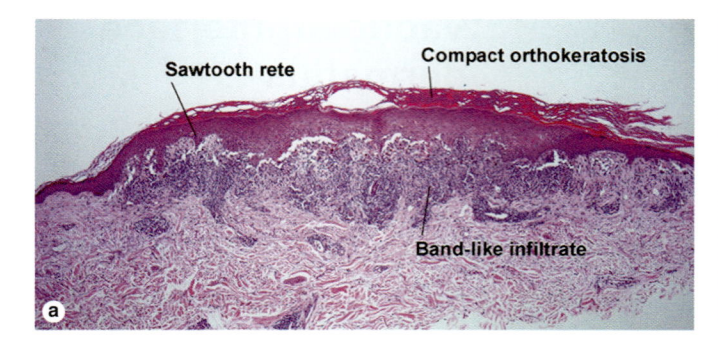

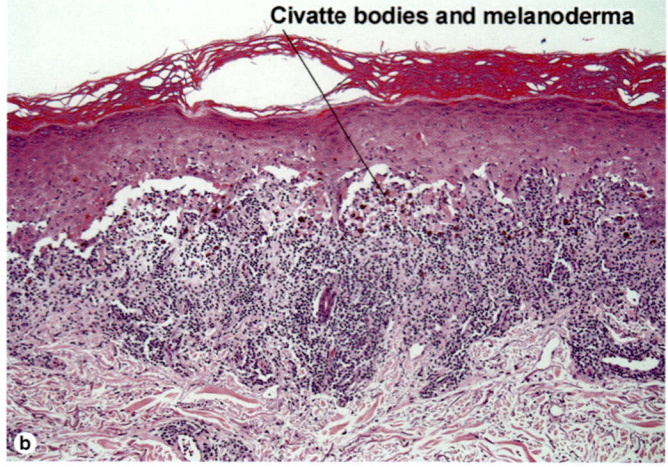

Fig 7-5 Lichen planus

Interface dermatitis   Chapter 7   137

Lichenoid drug eruption

Key features

- Lichenoid interface dermatitis
- Typically has eosinophils
- Often has parakeratosis

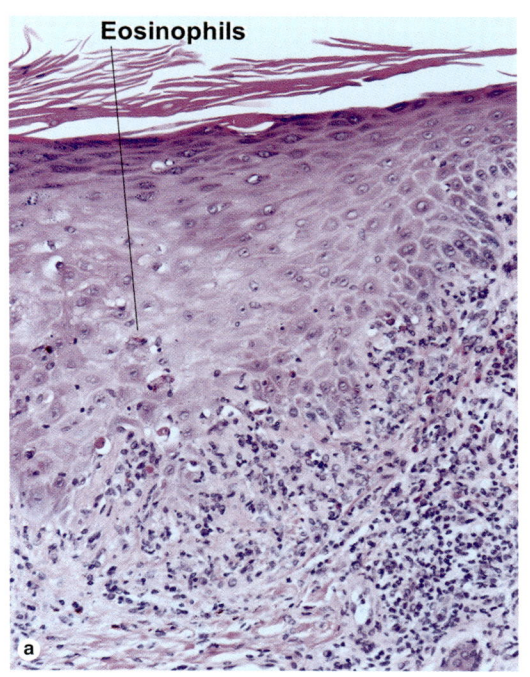

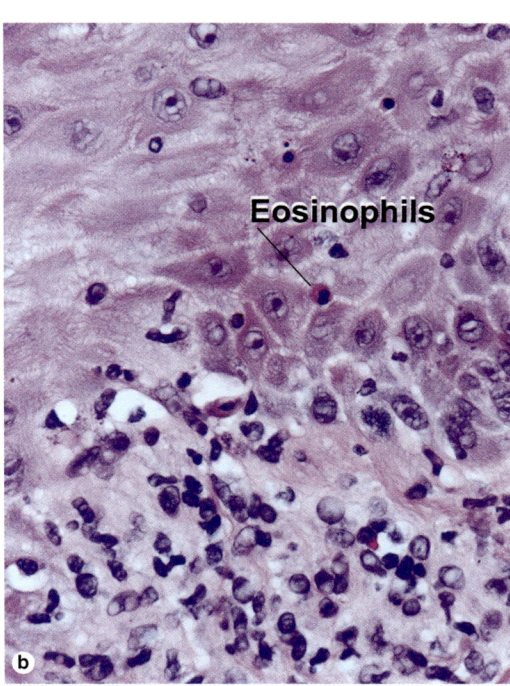

Fig 7-6 Lichenoid drug eruption

Benign lichenoid keratosis

Key features

- Lichenoid interface dermatitis
- May have parakeratosis
- Rarely has eosinophils
- Solar lentigo commonly present at the margin

BLK usually presents as a solitary pearly pink macule on the trunk or an extremity. The biopsy is usually performed to rule out basal cell carcinoma. Most lesions represent lichenoid regression of benign solar lentigines. The earliest stage of evolution may show vacuolar interface dermatitis with a lymphocyte in every vacuole.

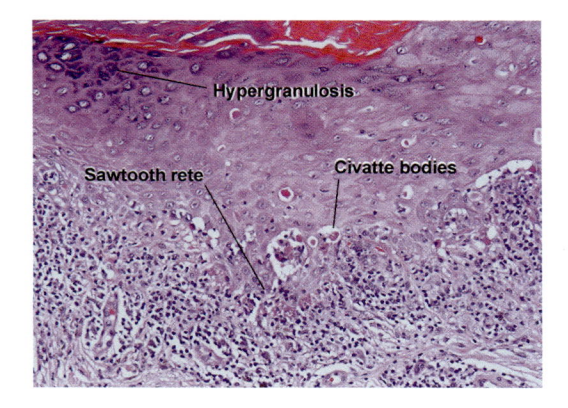

Fig 7-7 Benign lichenoid keratosis

Lichenoid graft-versus-host disease

Key features

- Lichenoid interface dermatitis
- May have parakeratosis
- Rarely has eosinophils

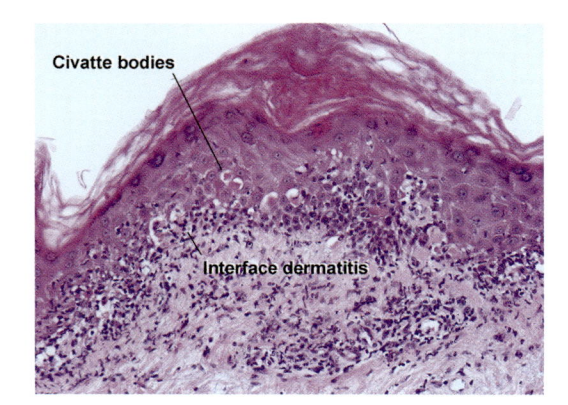

Fig 7-8 Lichenoid GvHD

Hypertrophic lupus erythematosus

Key features

- Lichenoid interface dermatitis
- Rarely has parakeratosis
- Rarely has eosinophils
- DIF: continuous granular band of immunoglobulin (Ig) G/A/M and C3 (full house) at the basement membrane zone (BMZ)
- Superficial and deep infiltrate
- Follicular plugging
- Many CD123+ plasmacytoid dendritic cells adjacent to epithelium (helps differentiate from squamous cell carcinoma in situ)

Hypertrophic lupus erythematosus is lichenoid histologically. It is distinguished from lichen planus by the DIF pattern, occasional presence of basement membrane zone thickening or dermal mucin, and by clinical history and serologic findings. This is the form of chronic cutaneous lupus erythematosus that is most likely to give rise to invasive squamous cell carcinoma.

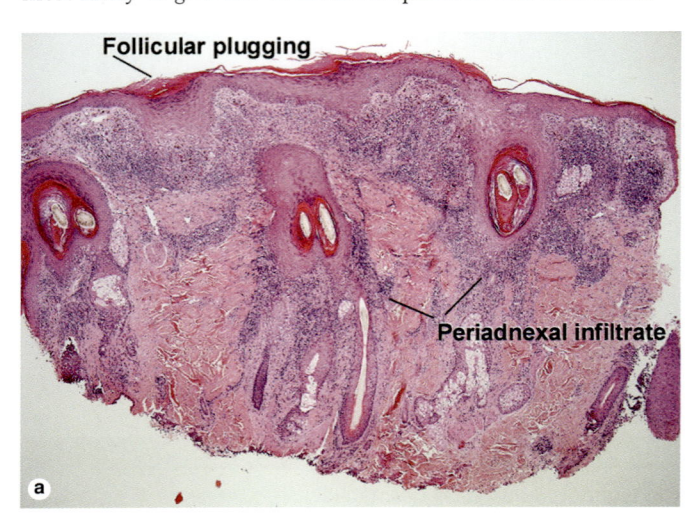

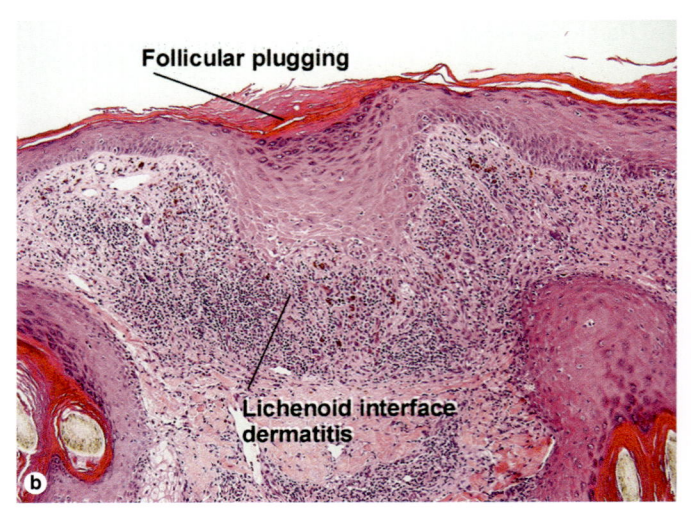

Fig 7-9 Hypertrophic lupus erythematosus

Lichenoid regression of lentigo maligna

Key features

- Lichenoid interface dermatitis
- Heavily sun-damaged skin
- Adjacent rete pattern may be effaced
- May have parakeratosis
- Rarely has eosinophils

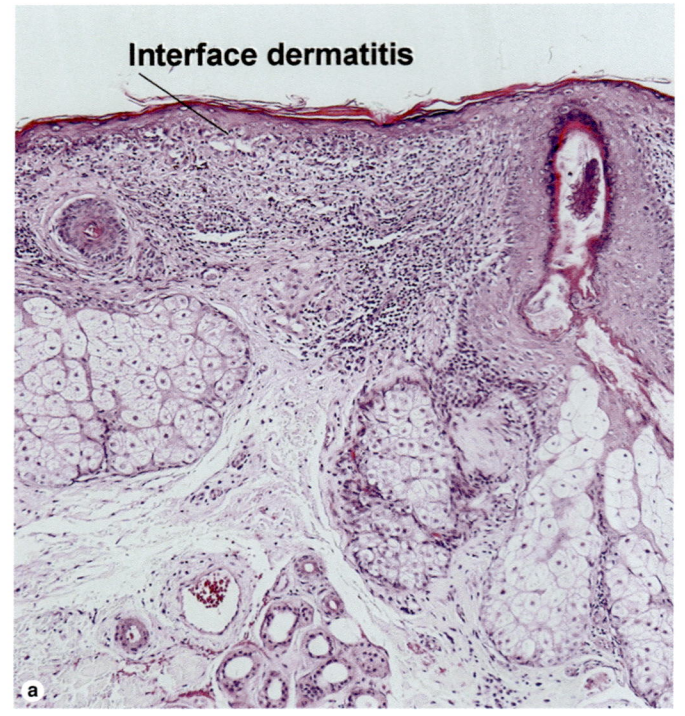

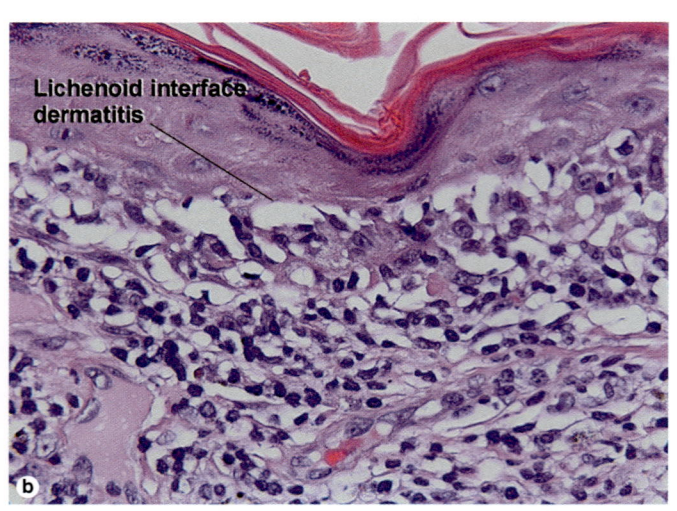

Fig 7-10 Lichenoid regression within a lentigo maligna

Porokeratosis

Key features

- Cornoid lamella (column of parakeratosis at 45° angle, dyskeratotic cells below)
- Zone between cornoid lamellae may appear lichenoid or psoriasiform

Vacuolar interface dermatitis

Key features

- Basal layer intact
- Vacuoles within basal layer
- Rounded rete pattern

Vacuolar interface dermatitis with a lymphocyte in nearly every vacuole

Vacuolar interface dermatitis with a lymphocyte in nearly every vacuole is characteristic of mycosis fungoides (MF), pityriasis lichenoides, and the early evolving stage of a BLK. Rarely, a similar pattern may be seen in fixed drug eruption, lymphomatoid drug eruption, or lichen sclerosus.

Mycosis fungoides

Key features

- Vacuolar interface dermatitis
- A lymphocyte in nearly every vacuole ("a lymph in every hole")
- Lymphocytes hyperchromatic and surrounded by white space (lump of coal on a pillow)
- Lymphocytes tend to line up along the dermal–epidermal junction (DEJ)
- Lymphocytes tend to form small aggregates
- Epidermal lymphocytes larger, darker, and more angulated than lymphocytes in dermis
- Little spongiosis in adjacent epidermis
- Papillary dermal fibrosis
- Bare underbelly sign
- Pautrier microabscess

The biopsy demonstrates epidermotropism of large atypical lymphocytes with little accompanying spongiosis. These lymphocytes show some tendency to form small aggregates and to line up along the dermal–epidermal junction. Papillary dermal fibrosis is prominent. The bare underbelly sign refers to the tendency for the superficial perivascular lymphoid infiltrate to predominate above the vessel, with few lymphocytes below the vessel. It has been likened to a vacuum cleaner sucking the lymphocytes towards the surface. Immunostaining and gene rearrangement studies can be helpful. Selective loss of CD7 expression in the atypical intraepidermal lymphocytes is a common finding. As the disease progresses from patch, to plaque, to tumor stage, atypical cells appear in the dermal infiltrate, and epidermotropism is lost.

Differential Diagnosis

The pattern of vacuolar interface dermatitis with a lymphocyte in every vacuole may also be seen in pityriasis lichenoides and the early stage of a BLK. The pattern of large dark nuclei with surrounding vacuoles at the dermal–epidermal junction may also be seen in lentigo maligna and lymphomatoid drug eruption.

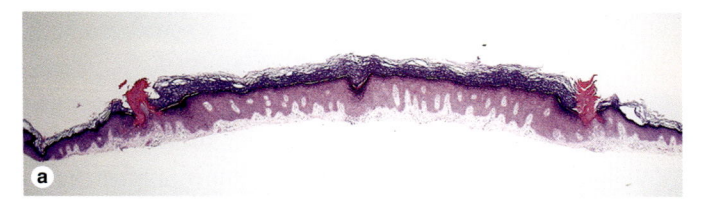

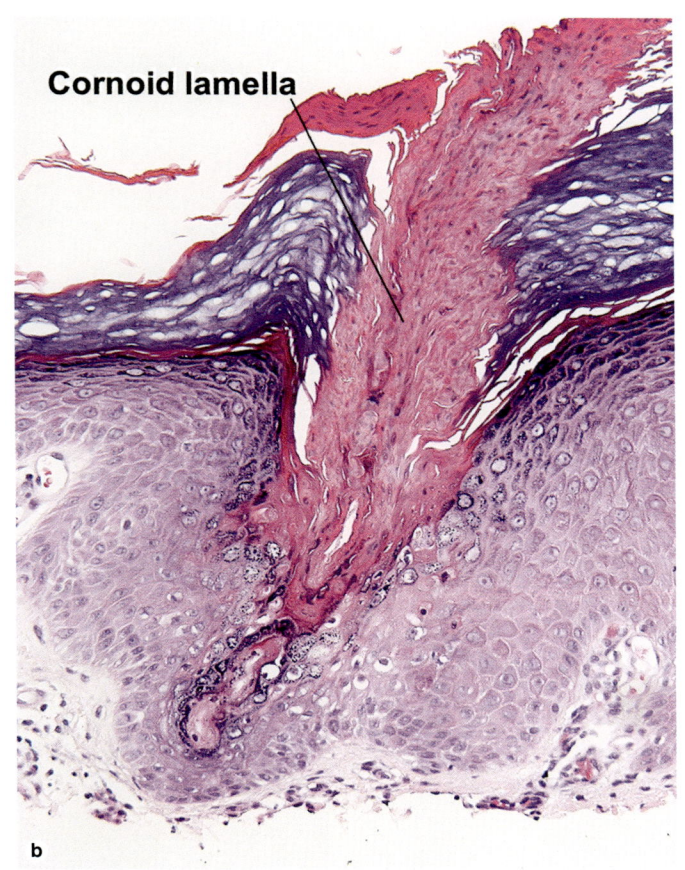

Fig 7-11 Porokeratosis

140 Dermatopathology

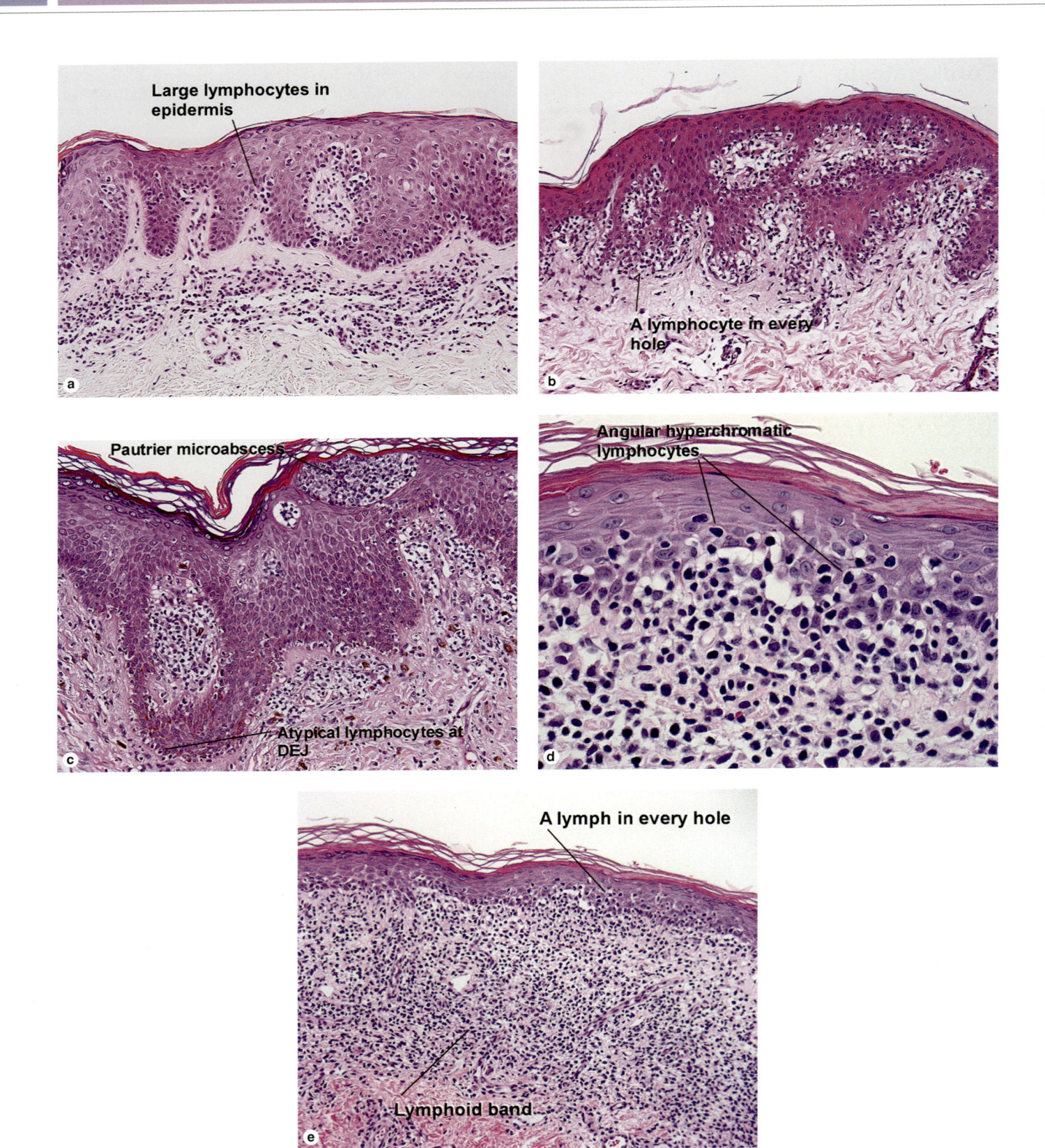

Fig 7-12 Mycosis fungoides

Pityriasis lichenoides et varioliformis acuta (PLEVA)

Key features

- Vacuolar interface dermatitis
- A lymphocyte in nearly every vacuole
- Compact stratum corneum ± ulceration or crust
- No papillary dermal fibrosis
- Erythrocyte extravasation
- Transepidermal elimination of erythrocytes
- Neutrophil margination within dermal vessels

The biopsy demonstrates vacuolar interface dermatitis with a lymphocyte in every vacuole. Keratinocyte necrosis, central ulceration, and crusting may be noted. Erythrocyte extravasation with transepidermal elimination of erythrocytes is common. The infiltrate is purely lymphoid, with a superficial and deep perivascular pattern. Prominent intravascular margination of neutrophils is typical. The infiltrate in PLEVA is characterized by CD8-positive cytotoxic T cells. A clone can often be detected by gene rearrangement studies.

Pityriasis lichenoides chronica

Key features

- Vacuolar interface dermatitis
- A lymphocyte in nearly every vacuole
- Transepidermal elimination of erythrocytes variable

Early stage of benign lichenoid keratosis

Key features

- Vacuolar interface dermatitis
- A lymphocyte in nearly every vacuole

Vacuolar interface dermatitis with vacuoles or cell death out of proportion to lymphocytes

Lupus erythematosus

Key features

- Interface change usually vacuolar, but may be lichenoid (as in hypertrophic lupus erythematosus)
- Compact hyperkeratosis
- Follicular hyperkeratosis
- Basement membrane zone thickening
- Melanin pigment incontinence (melanoderma) underlying the dermal–epidermal junction
- Vertical columns of lymphocytes within fibrous tract remnants
- Perivascular lymphoid aggregates
- Lymphoid aggregates within the eccrine coil
- Dermal mucin between collagen bundles
- Underlying lupus panniculitis may be present
- DIF: continuous granular band of IgG/A/M and C3 (full house) at the basement membrane zone

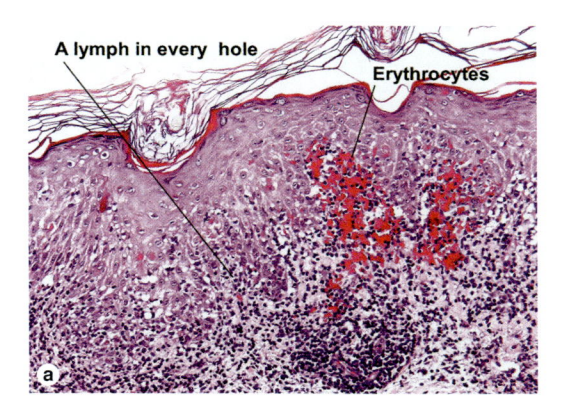

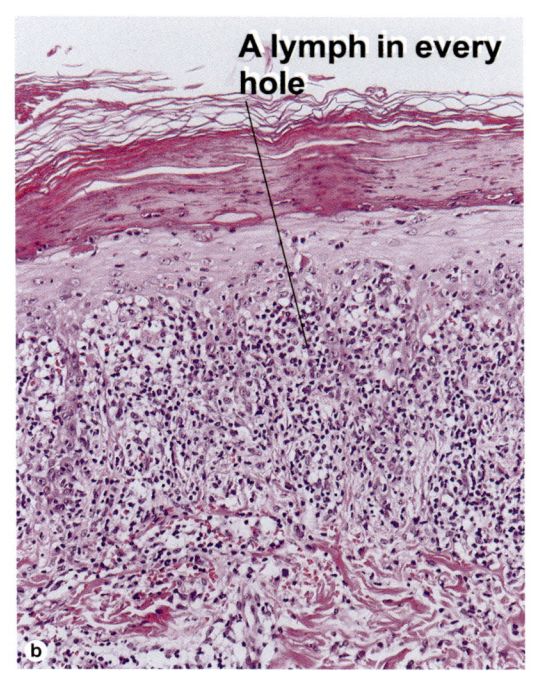

Fig 7-13 Pityriasis lichenoides et varioliformis acuta (PLEVA)

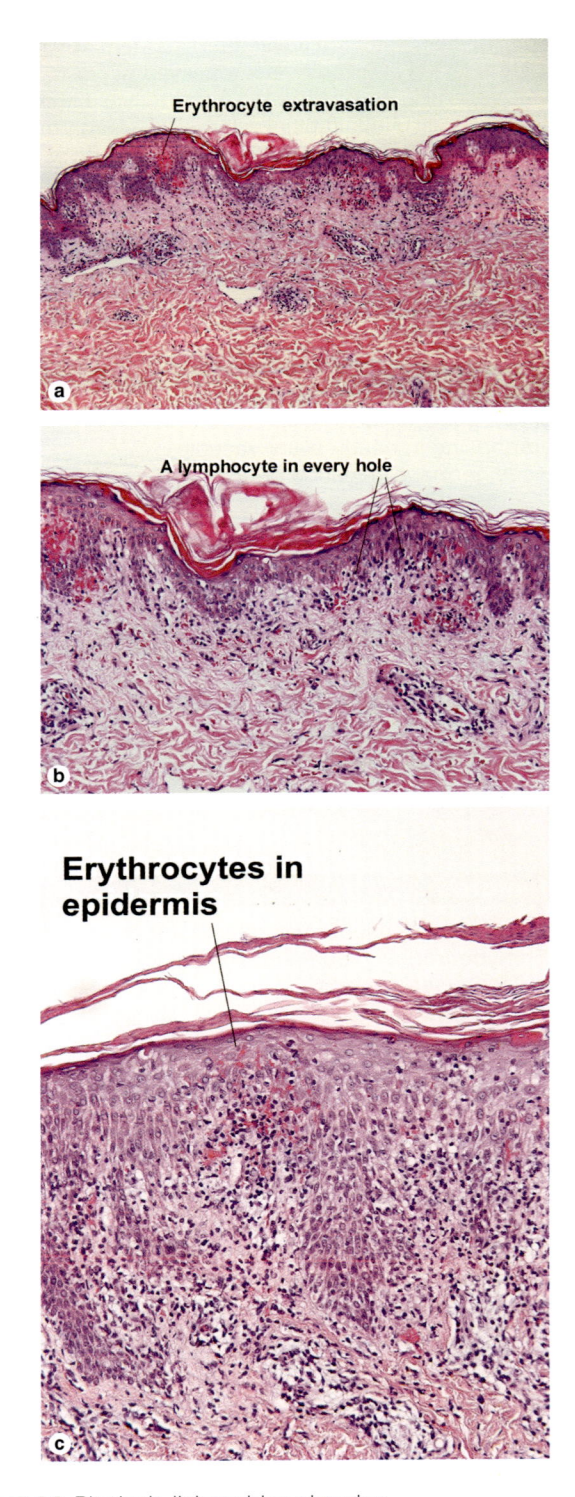

Fig 7-14 Pityriasis lichenoides chronica

The features of discoid lupus erythematosus appear in a time-dependent fashion. Biopsies of acute lupus erythematosus show only vacuolar interface dermatitis. DIF will usually be negative at this stage. Subacute lesions of lupus erythematosus show vacuolar interface dermatitis, hyperkeratosis, and follicular plugging, as well as a variable dermal infiltrate. DIF is positive in about one-third of cases. Well-established discoid lesions (of at least 3 months' duration) typically demonstrate strong DIF. Histologically, established discoid lupus erythematosus lesions are characterized by hyperkeratosis, follicular plugging, vacuolar interface dermatitis, basement membrane zone thickening, a patchy superficial and deep perivascular and periadnexal lymphoid infiltrate, and interstitial mucin. Underlying lupus panniculitis may be present.

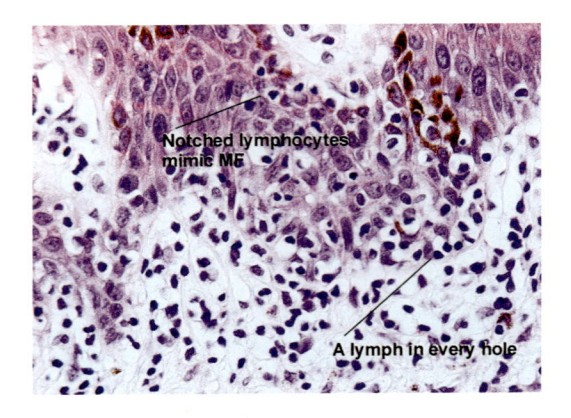

Fig 7-15 Early benign lichenoid keratosis (BLK)

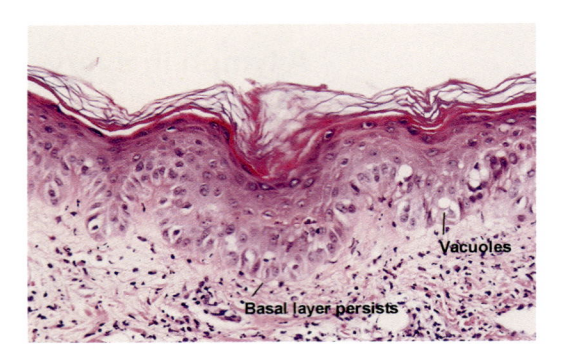

Fig 7-16 Acute lupus erythematosus

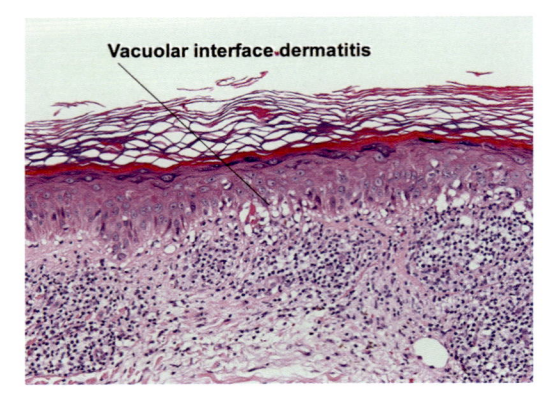

Fig 7-17 Subacute lupus erythematosus

Interface dermatitis — Chapter 7 — 143

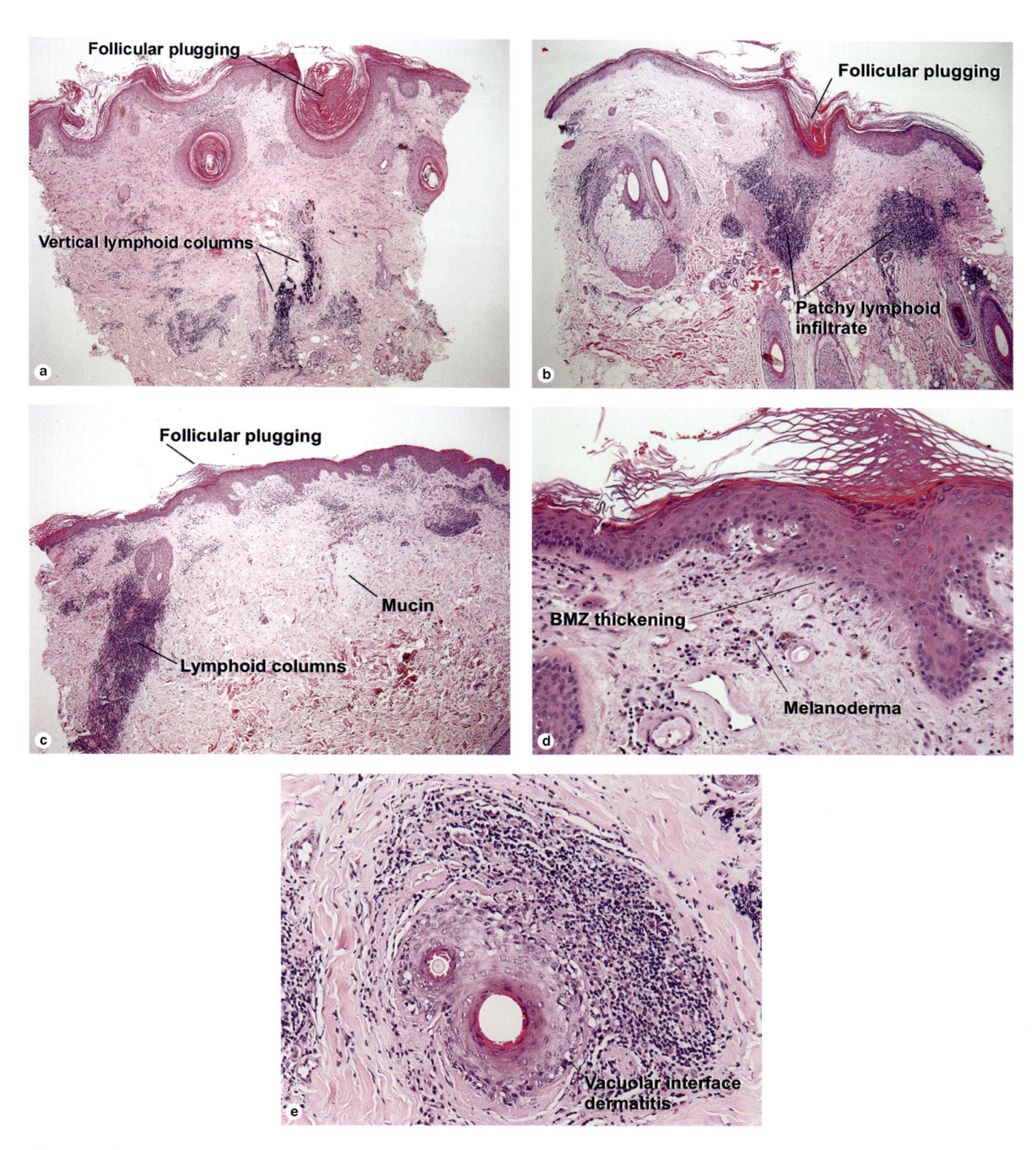

Fig 7-18 Chronic discoid lupus erythematosus (BMZ, basement membrane zone)

Dermatopathology

Differential Diagnosis

1. Dermatomyositis may look identical to lupus erythematosus, although the former usually demonstrates epidermal atrophy.
2. Tumid lupus lacks interface changes.
3. Lichen striatus lacks dermal mucin.
4. Differential diagnosis of nodular lymphoid infiltrate – the seven *L*s:
   Lupus
   Light (polymorphous light eruption): papillary dermal edema usually prominent
   Lymphoma
   Lymphocytoma cutis
   Lichen striatus (eccrine coil involved like lupus)
   Lymphocytic eruption of Jessner–Kanof
   Lues (vacuolar interface dermatitis typically paired with elongation of rete, interstitial busy dermis, endothelial swelling, lymphocytes with ample cytoplasm or plasma cells
5. Viral exanthem (may have erythrocyte extravasation; lacks hyperkeratosis, papillary dermal fibrosis)
6. Drug eruption (may be mix of inflammatory patterns, lacks hyperkeratosis, papillary dermal fibrosis)
7. Phototoxic eruption (lacks hyperkeratosis, papillary dermal fibrosis)

Polymorphous light eruption

Key features

- Plaque variant has papillary dermal edema and dense perivascular lymphoid infiltrate
- Papulovesicular variant is spongiotic

Lichen striatus

Key features

- Blaschkoid interface dermatitis
- Lymphoid aggregates perivascular and in eccrine coil

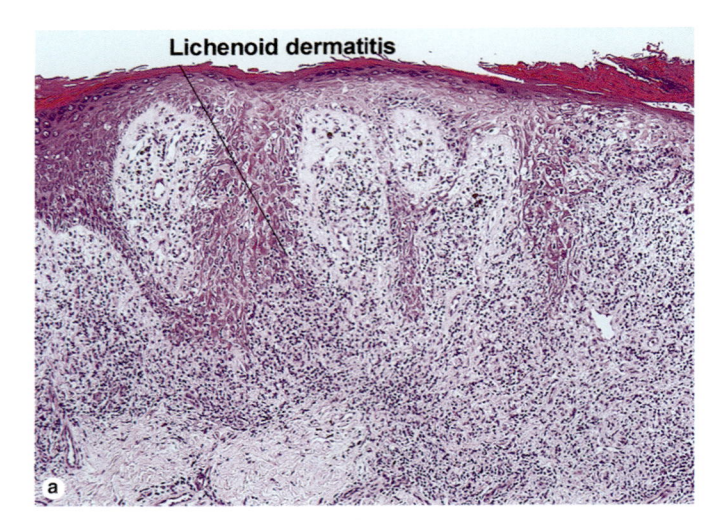

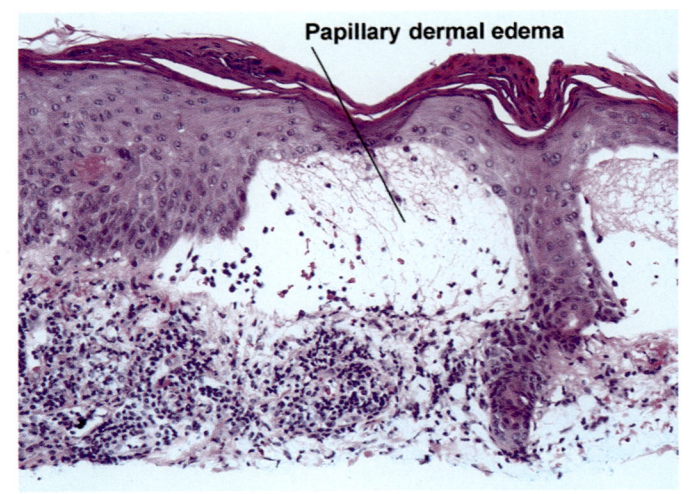

Fig 7-19 Polymorphous light eruption

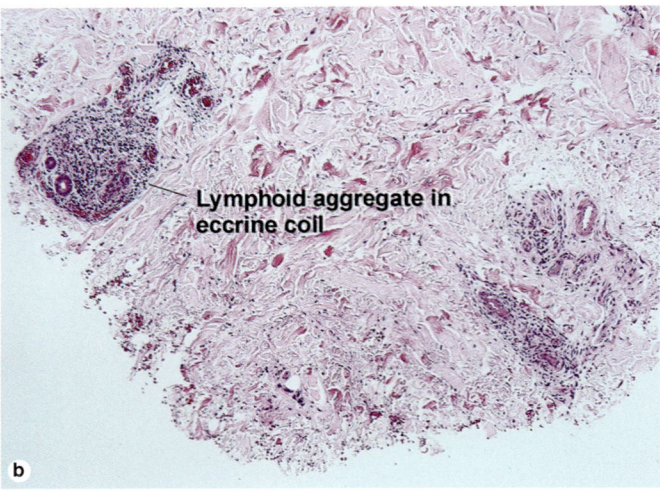

Fig 7-20 Lichen striatus

Dermatomyositis

Key features
- Similar to lupus erythematosus
- Typically demonstrates epidermal atrophy

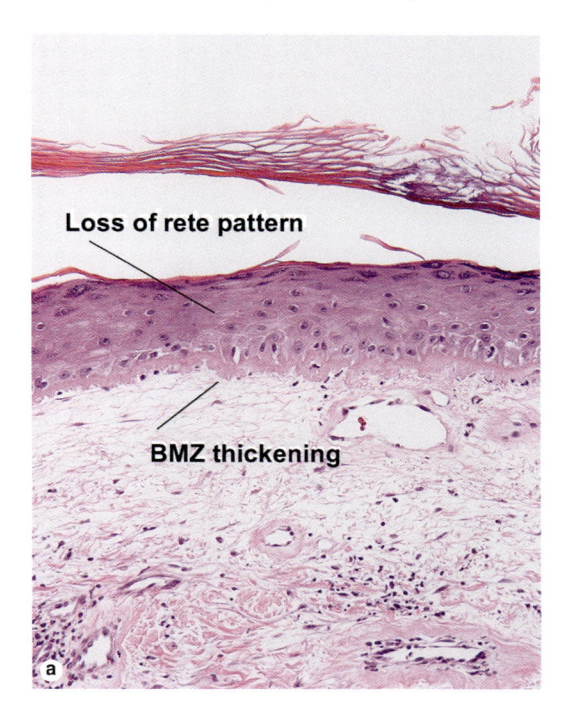

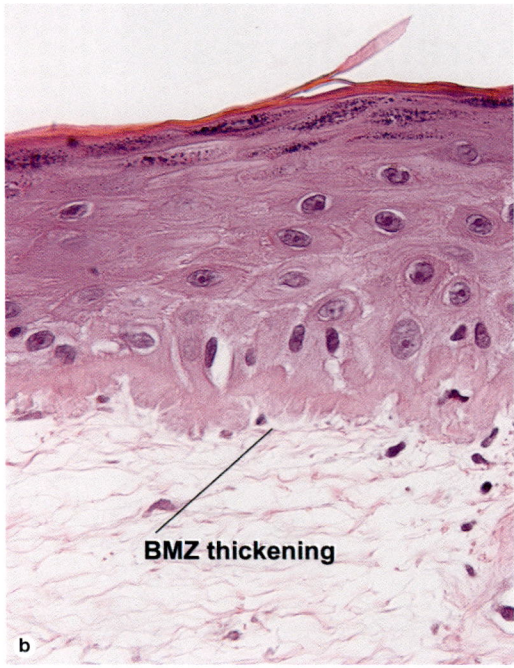

Fig 7-21 Dermatomyositis

Syphilis

Key features

Vacuolar interface dermatitis together often with slender acanthosis
- Vacuolar interface dermatitis together with an interstitial pattern (busy dermis)
- Interface-predominant pattern may have an atrophic epidermis
- Neutrophils in the stratum corneum
- Plasma cells present in about two-thirds of cases
- Endothelial swelling obliterates the lumen of small vessels
- Perivascular lymphocytes and histiocytes with visible cytoplasm

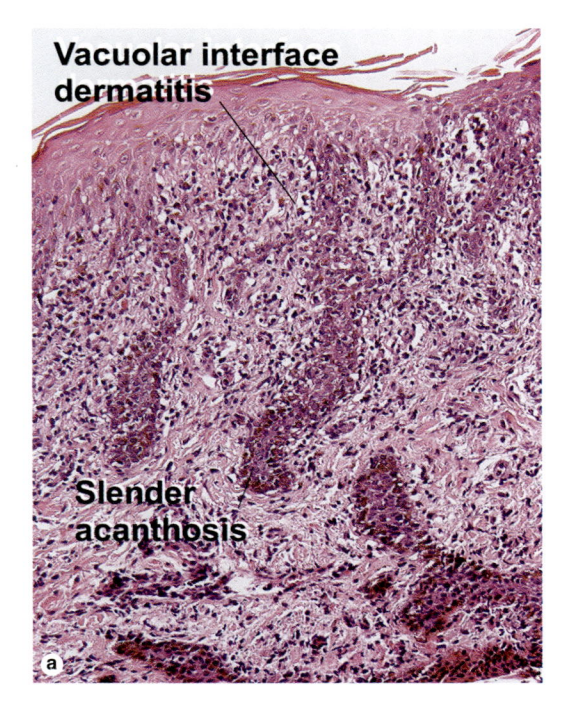

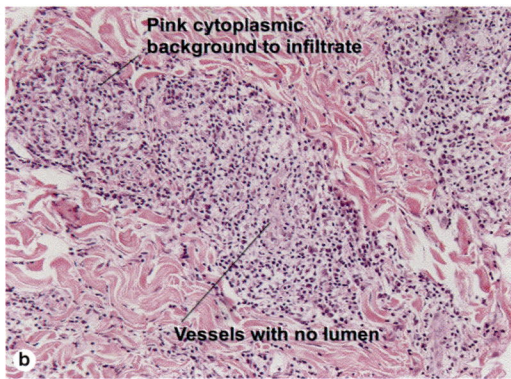

Fig 7-22 Lues (syphilis)

Dermatopathology

Erythema multiforme

Key features

- Acute (normal) basket-weave stratum corneum
- Individual necrotic keratinocytes
- May progress to confluent epidermal necrosis
- Cell death out of proportion to lymphocytes
- In late stage, bulla and re-epithelialization occur

The typical picture of erythema multiforme includes a normal stratum corneum with "death and squalor" in the underlying epidermis. In the acute stage, the infiltrate is purely lymphoid.

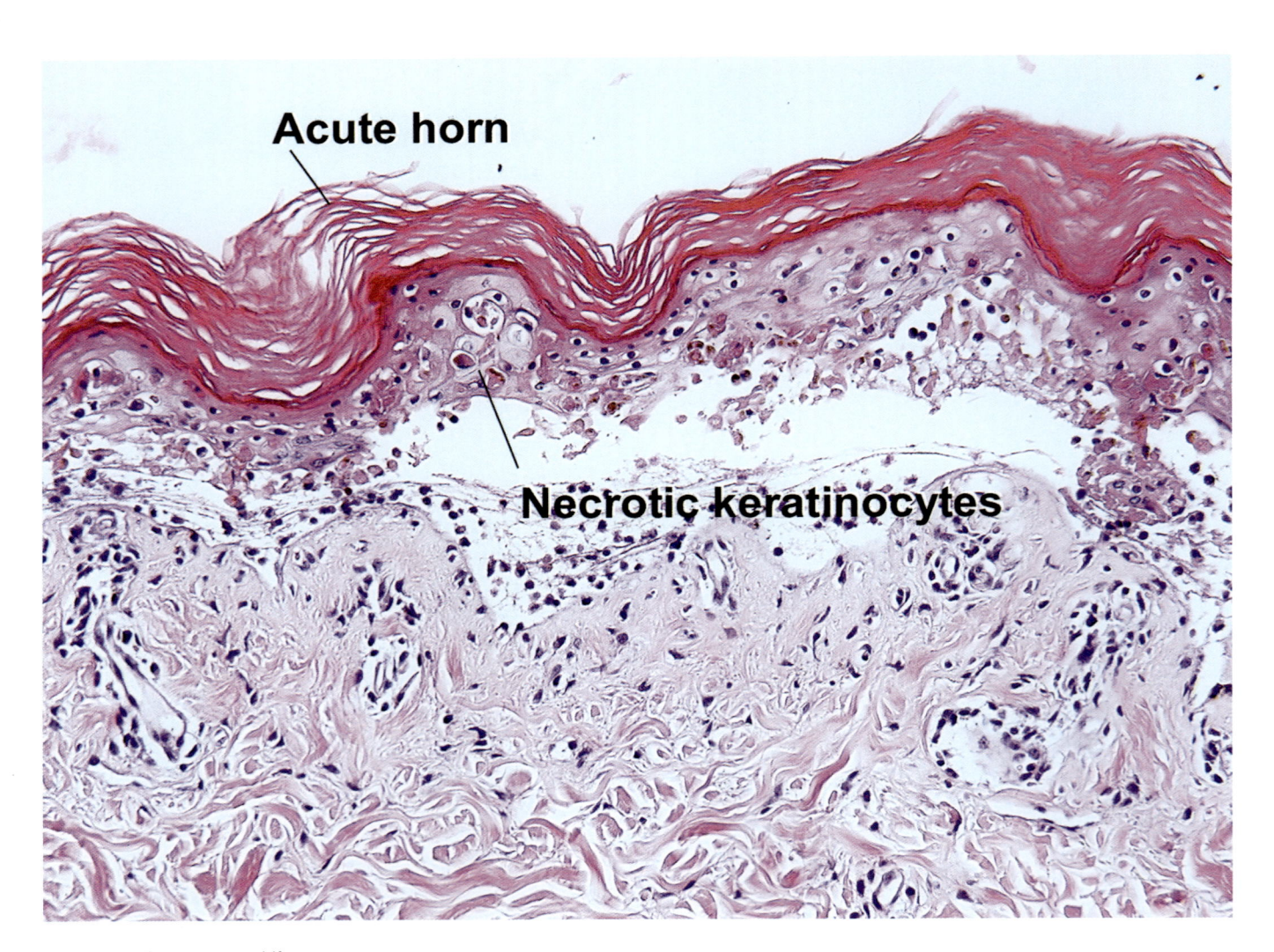

Fig 7-23 Erythema multiforme

Toxic epidermal necrolysis

Key features

- Looks like erythema multiforme

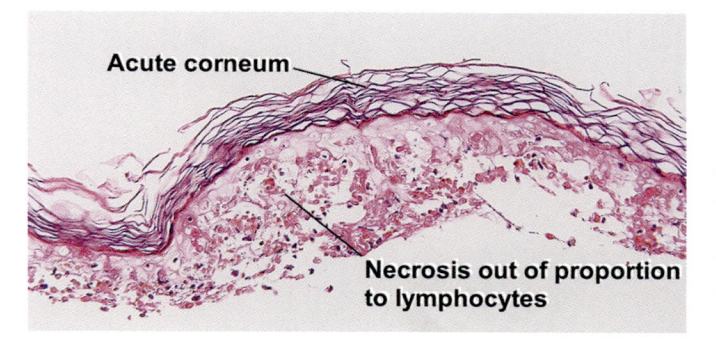

Fig 7-24 Toxic epidermal necrolysis

Paraneoplastic pemphigus

Key features

- Acantholysis may or may not be present
- May be lichenoid
- May look like erythema multiforme (see Chapter 9)

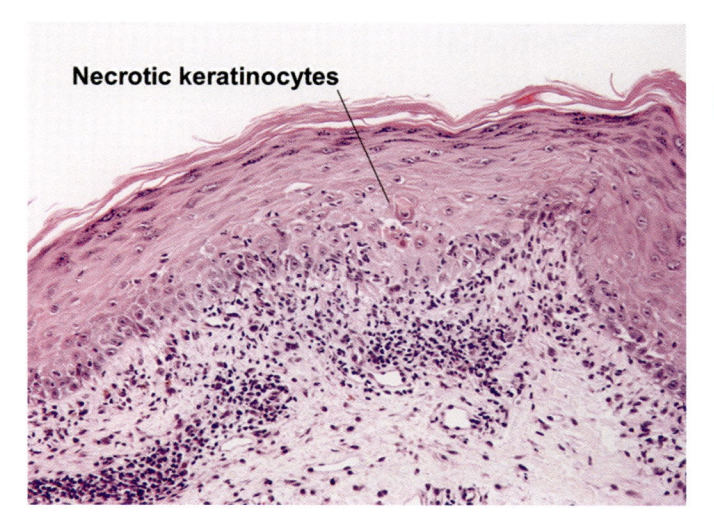

Fig 7-25 Paraneoplastic pemphigus

Fixed drug eruption

Key features

- Vacuolar interface dermatitis
- Proportion of lymphocytes and vacuoles variable
- Polymorphous infiltrate (typically with eosinophils)
- Acute (normal) stratum corneum
- Chronic dermal changes:
  - *Papillary dermal fibrosis*
  - *Melanin pigment incontinence in perivascular location*

The most important diagnostic feature is the mismatch between the normal stratum corneum and chronic changes in the superficial dermis. Fixed drug eruption is episodic. The biopsy is likely to occur during an acute inflammatory phase, but dermal changes from past episodes are present. The result is a normal stratum corneum, consistent with an acute process. In contrast, there is papillary dermal fibrosis, consistent with a chronic process. Pigment has had time to be carried to a perivascular location. The polymorphous infiltrate typically includes eosinophils and may include neutrophils.

PEARL

The normal stratum corneum whispers, "Look at me, I'm an acute process." The papillary dermal fibrosis and pigment around vessels respond, "Liar! There are chronic changes in the dermis."

Graft-versus-host disease

Key features

- Subacute (fairly compact) stratum corneum
- Vacuolar interface dermatitis
- Necrotic keratinocytes
- Epithelial atypia and disorder

Dermatopathology

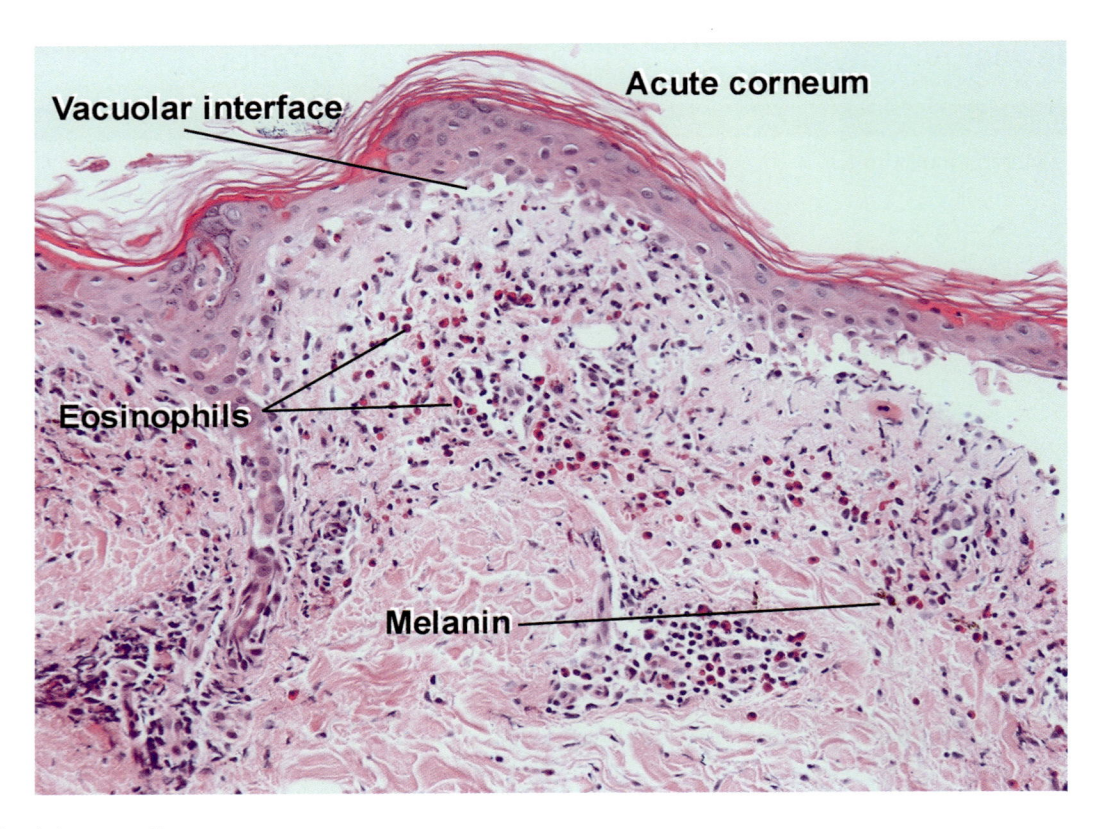

Fig 7-26　Fixed drug eruption

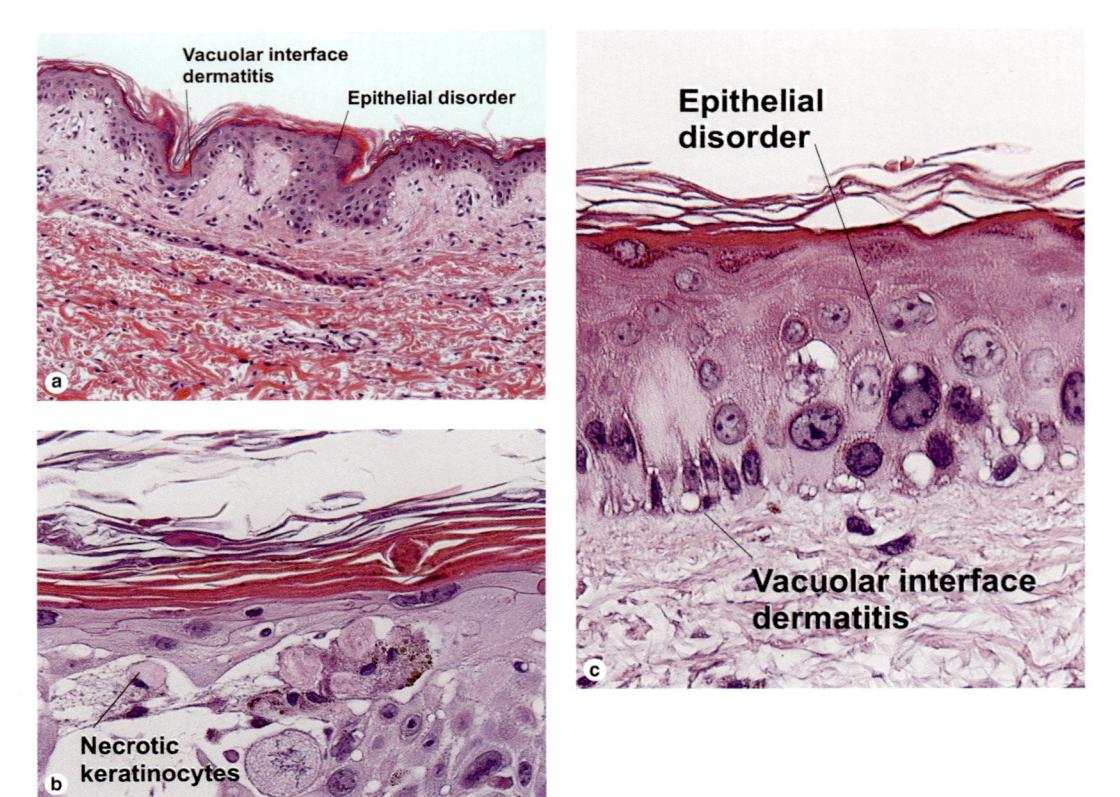

Fig 7-27　Graft-versus-host disease (GvHD)

Further reading

Acikalin A, Bagir E, Tuncer I, et al. Contribution of T-cell receptor gamma gene rearrangement by polymerase chain reaction and immunohistochemistry to the histological diagnosis of early mycosis fungoides. Saudi Med J 2013;34(1):19–23.

Brönnimann M, Yawalkar N. Histopathology of drug-induced exanthems: is there a role in diagnosis of drug allergy? Curr Opin Allergy Clin Immunol 2005;5(4):317–321.

Dalton SR, Chandler WM, Abuzeid M, et al. Eosinophils in mycosis fungoides: an uncommon finding in the patch and plaque stages. Am J Dermatopathol 2012;34(6):586–591.

Dalton SR, Fillman EP, Altman CE, et al. Atypical junctional melanocytic proliferations in benign lichenoid keratosis. Hum Pathol 2003;34(7):706–709.

Demartini CS, Dalton MS, Ferringer T, et al. Melan-A/MART-1 positive "pseudonests" in lichenoid inflammatory lesions: an uncommon phenomenon. Am J Dermatopathol 2005;27(4):370–371.

Kaley J, Pellowski DM, Cheung WL, et al. The spectrum of histopathologic findings in cutaneous eruptions associated with influenza A (H1N1) infection. J Cutan Pathol 2013;40(2):226–229.

Massone C, Kodama K, Kerl H, et al. Histopathologic features of early (patch) lesions of mycosis fungoides: a morphologic study on 745 biopsy specimens from 427 patients. Am J Surg Pathol 2005;29(4):550–560.

Morgan MB, Stevens GL, Switlyk S. Benign lichenoid keratosis: a clinical and pathologic reappraisal of 1040 cases. Am J Dermatopathol 2005;27(5):387–392.

Smith SB, Libow LF, Elston DM, et al. Gloves and socks syndrome: early and late histopathologic features. J Am Acad Dermatol 2002;47(5):749–754.

Yawalkar N, Pichler WJ. Immunohistology of drug-induced exanthema: clues to pathogenesis. Curr Opin Allergy Clin Immunol 2001;1(4):299–303.

Zhang Y, Wang Y, Yu R, et al. Molecular markers of early-stage mycosis fungoides. J Invest Dermatol 2012;132(6):1698–1706.

Chapter 8

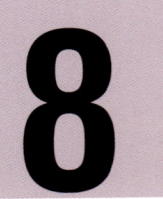

Psoriasiform and spongiotic dermatitis

Dirk M. Elston

Psoriasis

Key features

- Neutrophils above parakeratosis in stratum corneum
- Little to no serum in stratum corneum
- Alternating neutrophils and parakeratosis in the stratum corneum (sandwich sign)
- Neutrophilic spongiform pustules
- Little spongiosis in adjacent epidermis
- Tortuous blood vessels in dermal papillae

The appearance of psoriasis depends on the stage of the lesion and type of lesion. Early guttate lesions demonstrate no acanthosis. Established plaques demonstrate a characteristic pattern of regular acanthosis. Pustular psoriasis may never demonstrate acanthosis. Acral and intertriginous lesions of psoriasis commonly demonstrate a background of spongiosis, but spongiosis is distinctly absent from the surrounding epidermis in most other locations. *Reiter's disease* and *geographic tongue* histologically look like psoriasis.

PEARL

Collections of neutrophils within the stratum corneum:
- Psoriasis, tinea, impetigo, *Candida*, seborrheic dermatitis, syphilis (PTICSS)

Plaque psoriasis

Key features

- Regular bulbous club-shaped acanthosis
- Thin superpapillary plates
- Alternating neutrophils and parakeratosis in the stratum corneum (sandwich sign)
- Little to no serum in stratum corneum
- Neutrophilic spongiform pustules
- Little spongiosis in adjacent epidermis

Pustular psoriasis

Key features

- Collections of neutrophils within stratum corneum
- Subcorneal pustules
- Spongiform pustules

PEARL

Subcorneal pustules: *Candida*, acropustulosis of infancy, transient neonatal pustular melanosis, Sneddon–Wilkinson (and IgA pemphigus), impetigo, pustular psoriasis, *Staphylococcus* scalded-skin syndrome (CAT SIPS, or an anagram of SIPS)

Guttate psoriasis

Key features

- Neutrophils above parakeratosis

The key histologic feature of guttate psoriasis is a focus of neutrophils on top of parakeratosis (half of the sandwich sign, jelly up). The neutrophilic focus may be small and only visible in step sections. The focus often has a hump-like configuration or resembles a child's drawing of a seagull.

Psoriasiform and spongiotic dermatitis

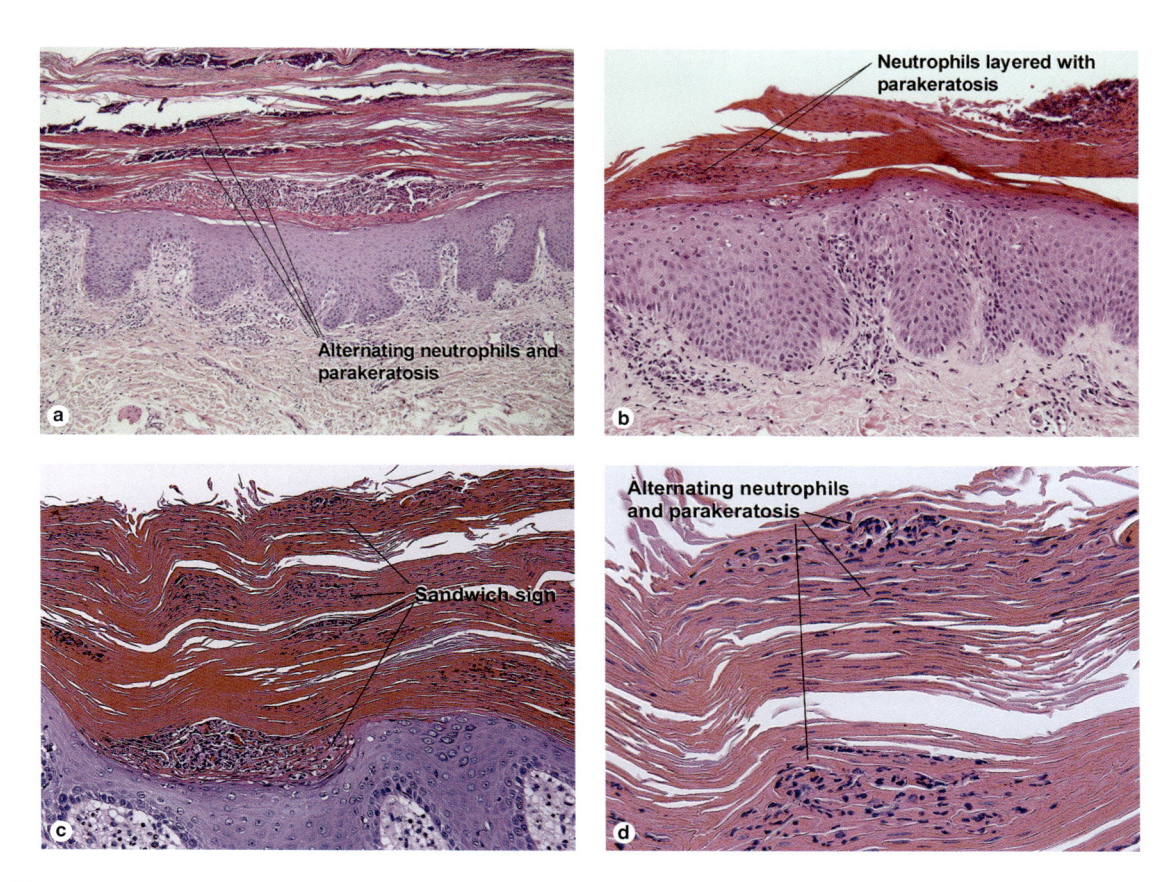

Fig 8-1 Plaque psoriasis

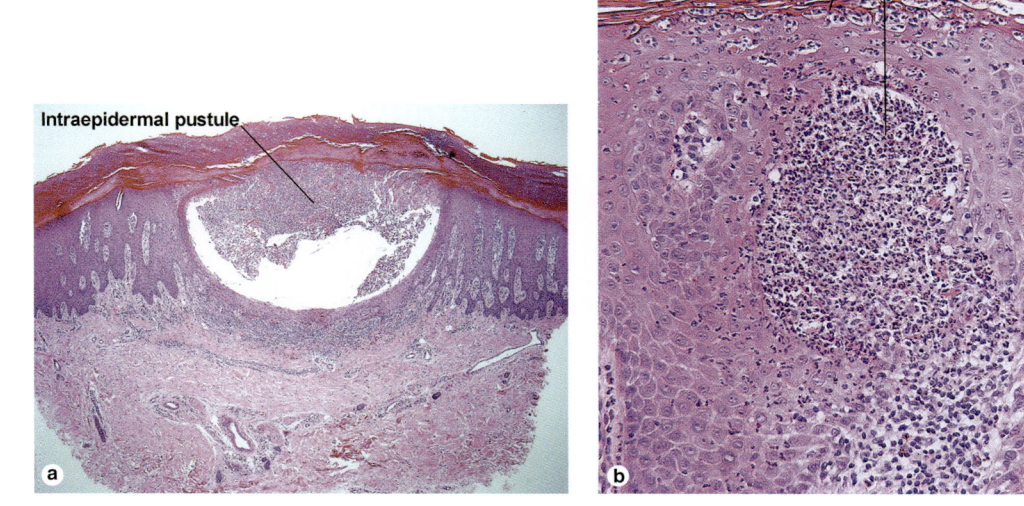

Fig 8-2 Pustular psoriasis

Dermatopathology

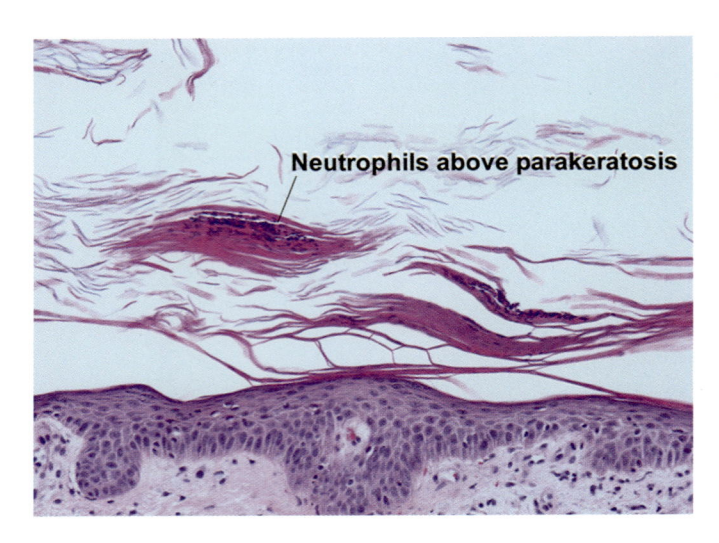

Fig 8-3 Guttate psoriasis (Neutrophils above parakeratosis)

Inflammatory linear verrucous epidermal nevus (ILVEN)

Key features

- Alternating ortho- and parakeratosis from left to right
- Areas of orthokeratosis have a prominent granular layer
- Areas of parakeratosis lack an underlying granular layer (see Chapter 2)

Mycosis fungoides

Key features

- Epidermal collections of lymphocytes
- Lymphocytes hyperchromatic and surrounded by white space (lump of coal on a pillow)
- Epidermal lymphocytes larger, darker, and more angulated than lymphocytes in dermis
- Little spongiosis in adjacent epidermis
- Papillary dermal fibrosis
- In areas, lymphocytes may also line up along the dermal epidermal junction
- Bare underbelly sign (see Chapters 7 and 24)

Syphilis

Key features

- Vacuolar interface dermatitis together with elongated psoriasiform acanthosis
- Vacuolar interface dermatitis together with interstitial dermal infiltrate (busy dermis)
- Neutrophils in the stratum corneum
- Plasma cells present in about two-thirds of cases
- Endothelial swelling obliterates the lumen of small vessels
- Perivascular lymphocytes and histiocytes with visible cytoplasm (see Chapters 7 and 17)

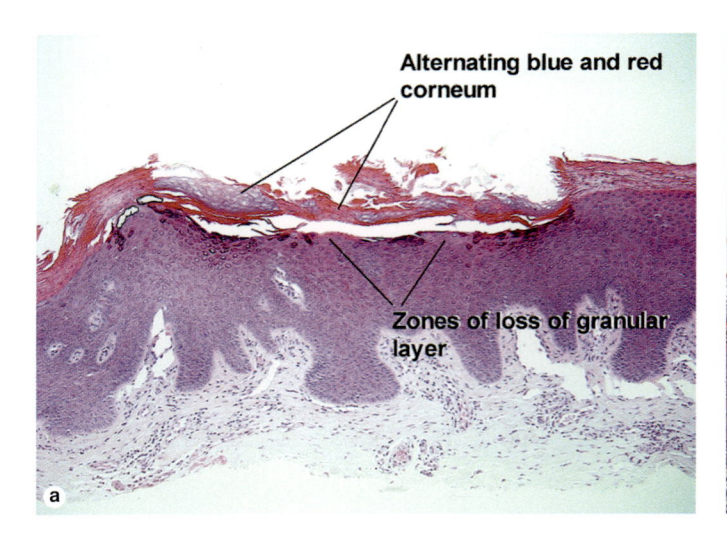

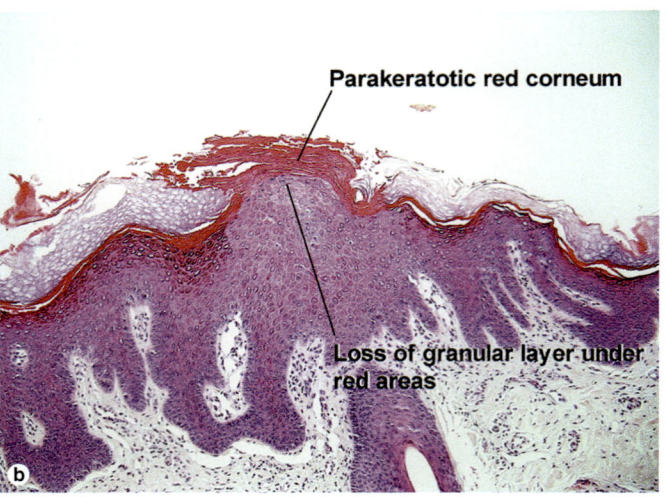

Fig 8-4 Inflammatory linear verrucous epidermal nevus (ILVEN)

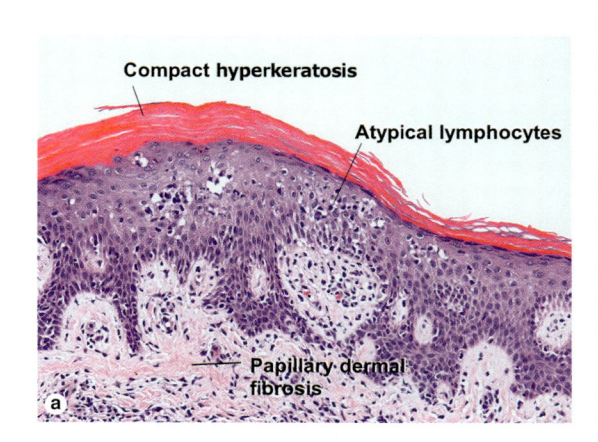

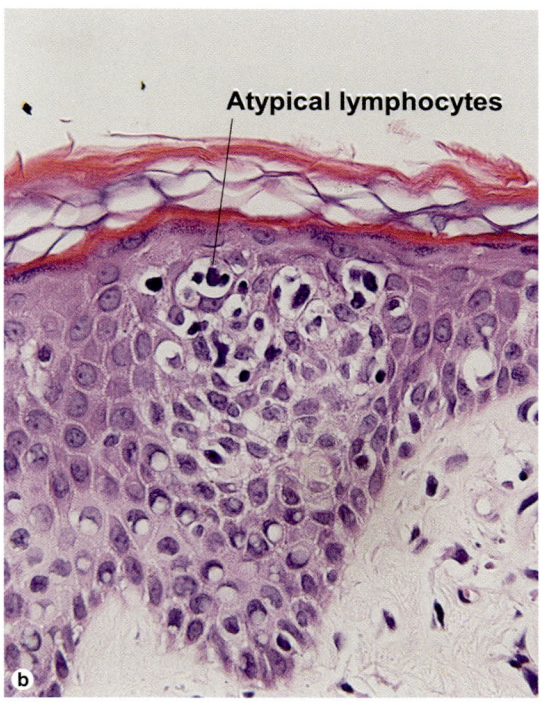

Psoriasiform and spongiotic dermatitis   Chapter 8   153

Fig 8-5 Psoriasiform mycosis fungoides

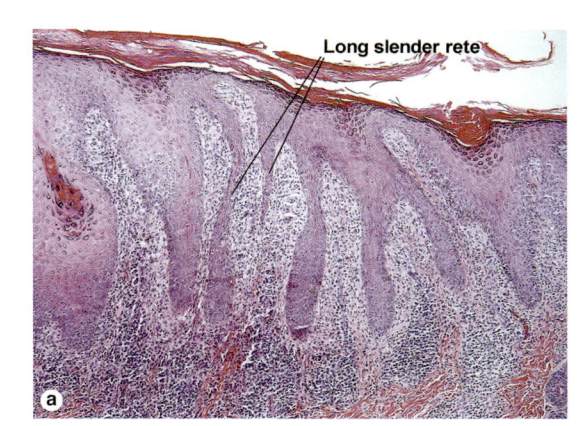

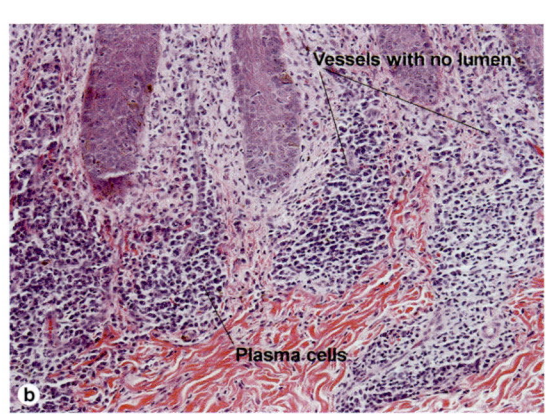

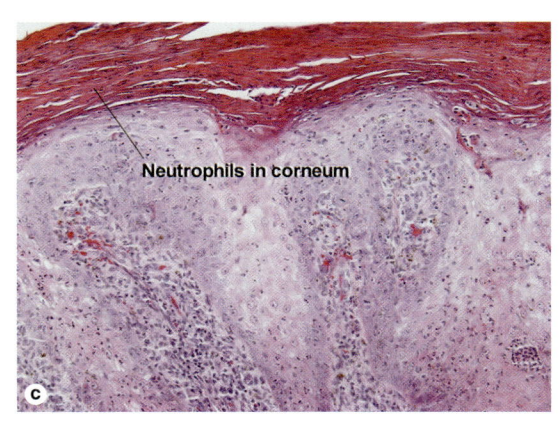

Fig 8-6 Syphilis

PEARL

Plasma cells are commonly associated with:

Diagnoses:
- Kaposi's sarcoma
- Syphilis
- Leishmaniasis
- Rhinoscleroma
- Melanoma
- Squamous cell carcinoma

Body locations that recruit plasma cells:
- Face
- Mucosa
- Back of neck
- Axillae
- Breasts
- Anogenital area
- Shins

Nutritional-deficiency dermatitis

Key features
- Pallor and ballooning of upper epidermis

Causes include glucagonoma (necrolytic migratory erythema), pellagra, and acrodermatitis enteropathica. Although pallor and ballooning of the upper epidermis are characteristic, many biopsies demonstrate only non-specific dermatitis with diffuse parakeratosis.

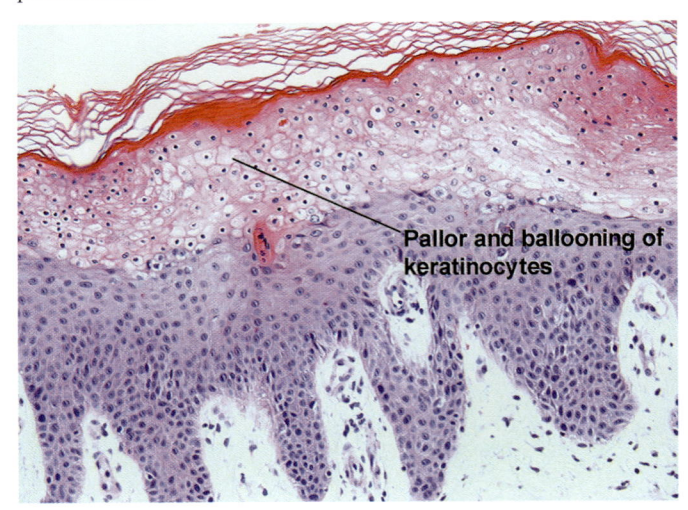

Fig 8-7 Necrolytic migratory erythema

Granular parakeratosis

Key features
- Compact hyperkeratosis with parakeratosis
- Granules in stratum corneum
- Granular layer preserved

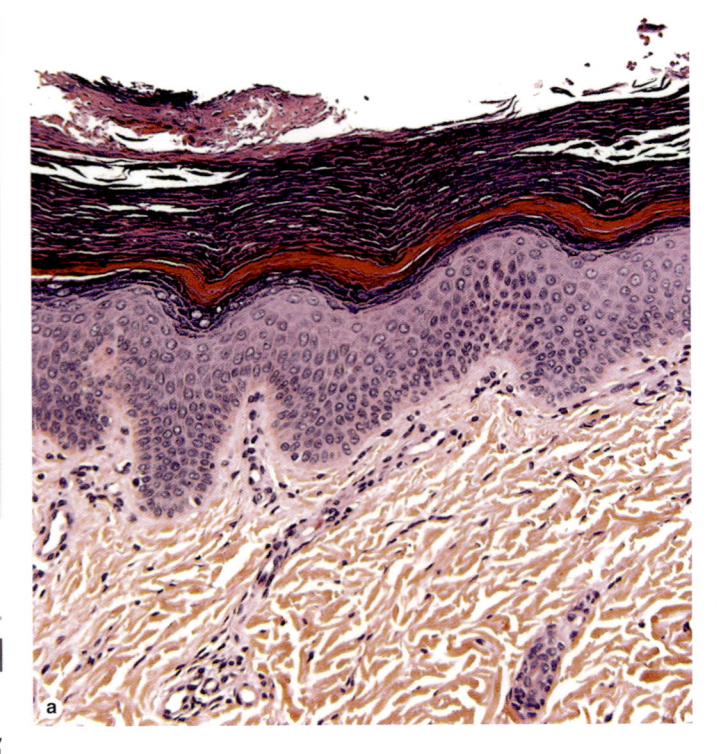

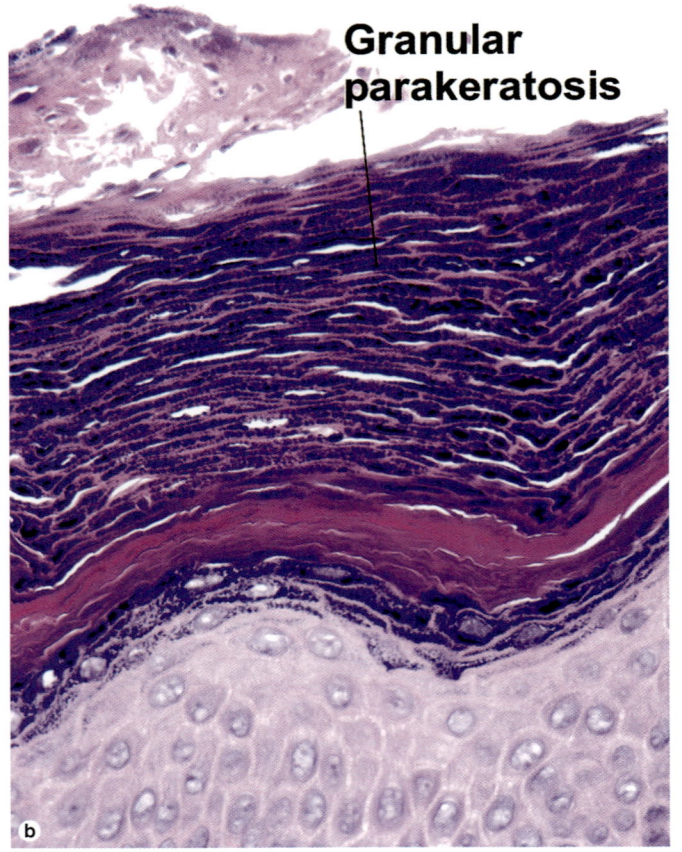

Fig 8-8 Granular parakeratosis

Porokeratosis

Key features

- Cornoid lamella (column of parakeratosis at 45° angle, dyskeratotic cells below)
- Zone between cornoid lamellae may appear lichenoid or psoriasiform (see Chapter 7)

Acute spongiotic dermatitis

Key features

- Spongiosis (intercellular edema)
- Exocytosis of lymphocytes

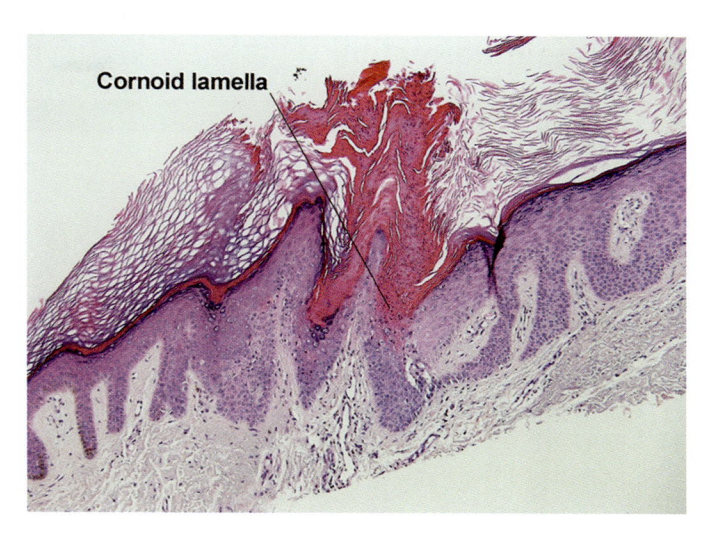

Fig 8-9 Porokeratosis

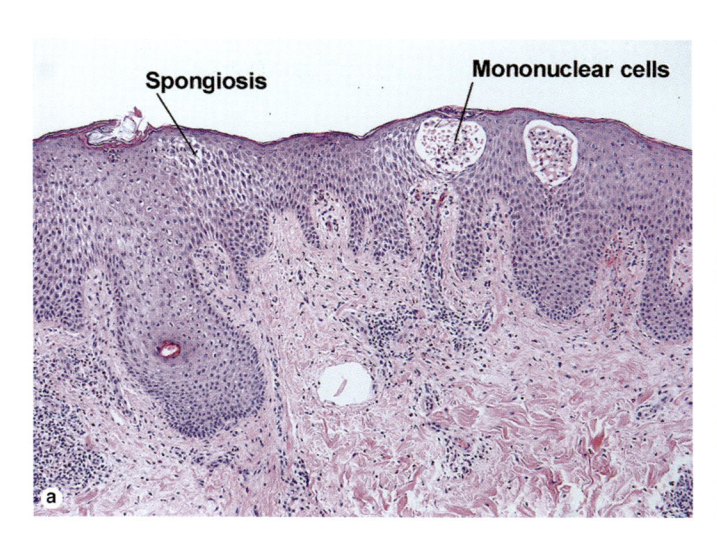

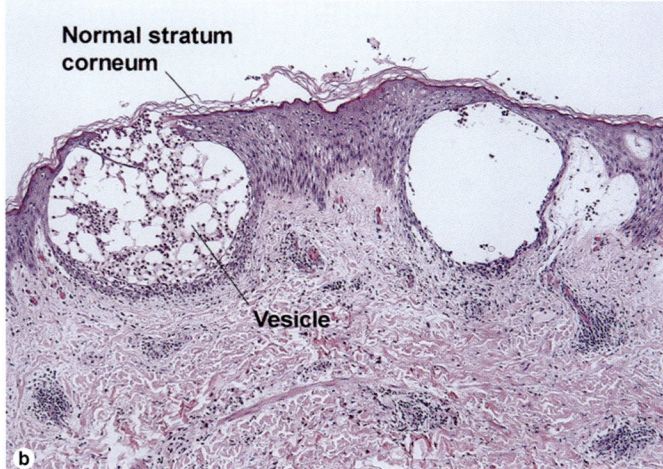

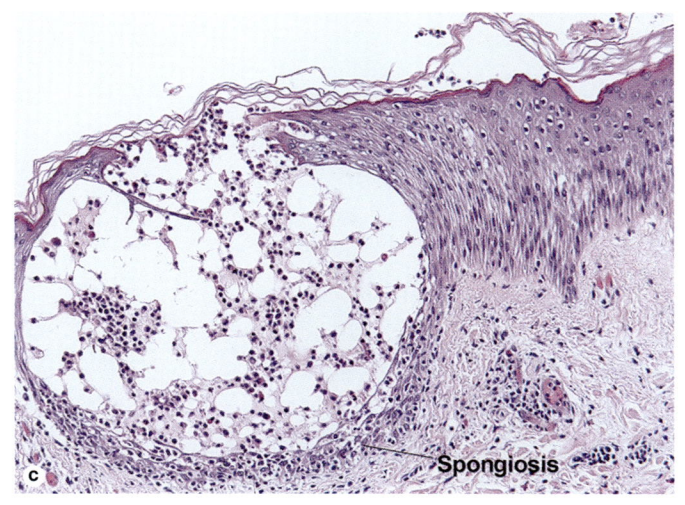

Fig 8-10 Acute spongiotic dermatitis

Seborrheic dermatitis

Key features

- Psoriasiform spongiotic dermatitis
- Neutrophilic scale/crust at edges of follicular ostium

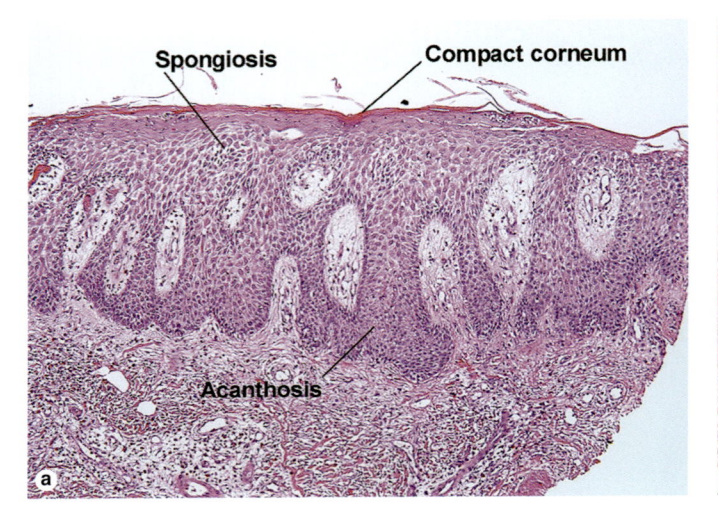

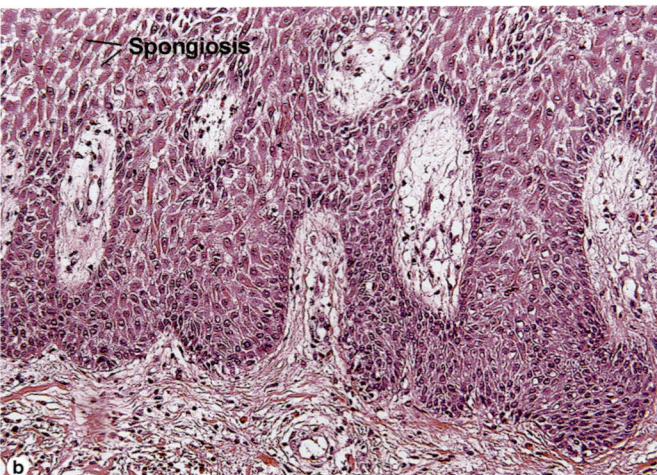

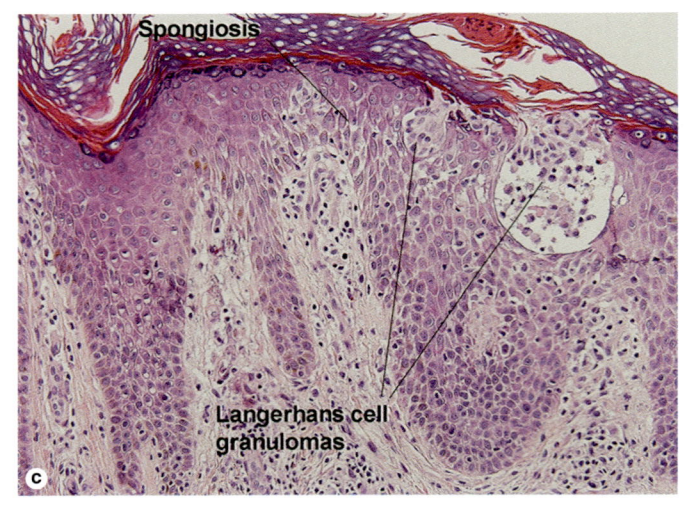

Subacute spongiotic dermatitis

Key features

- Parakeratosis
- Acanthosis
- Spongiosis (intercellular edema)
- Exocytosis of lymphocytes

Common causes of spongiotic dermatitis
- Allergic contact dermatitis
- Dyshidrotic dermatitis
- Nummular dermatitis
- Stasis dermatitis
- Id reaction
- Pityriasis rosea
- Spongiotic pigmenting purpura
- Tinea

Fig 8-11 Subacute spongiotic dermatitis

Chronic dermatitis (lichen simplex chronicus)

Key features

- Compact stratum corneum
- Stratum lucidum as in volar skin, but follicles are present (hairy palm appearance)
- Irregular acanthosis
- Papillary dermal fibrosis

The histologic findings of chronic dermatitis are those of lichen simplex chronicus. Excoriation commonly produces focal superficial epidermal necrosis. Papillary dermal fibrosis is commonly accompanied by capillary proliferation (angiofibroplasia). Vertical streaking of papillary dermal collagen is common.

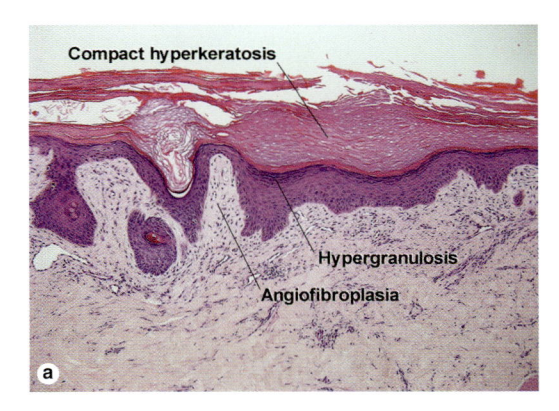

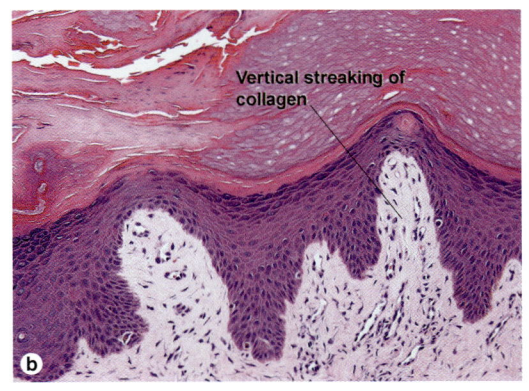

Fig 8-12 Lichen simplex chronicus

Pityriasis rosea

Key features

- Subacute spongiotic dermatitis
- Erythrocyte extravasation
- Transepidermal elimination of erythrocytes

The herald patch of pityriasis rosea is broad and fairly uniform in appearance. The subsequent lesions demonstrate a migrating spongiotic focus, followed by a trailing scale. The focus and scale form a roughly 45° angle.

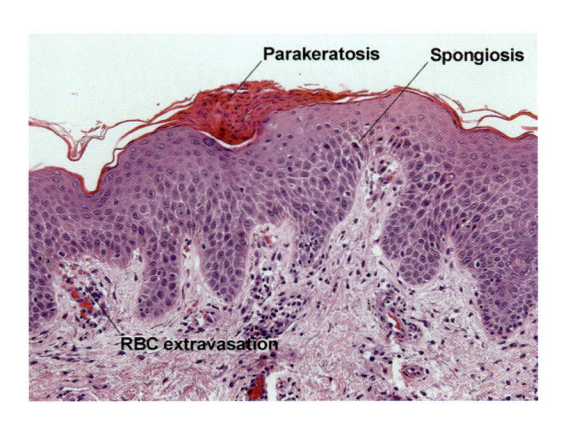

Fig 8-13 Pityriasis rosea (RBC, red blood cell)

Spongiotic pigmented purpuric eruption (PPE)

Key features

- Spongiosis
- Inflammation purely lymphoid
- Surrounds capillaries (centered above the level of the post-capillary venule)
- Erythrocyte extravasation
- Hemosiderin deposits over time

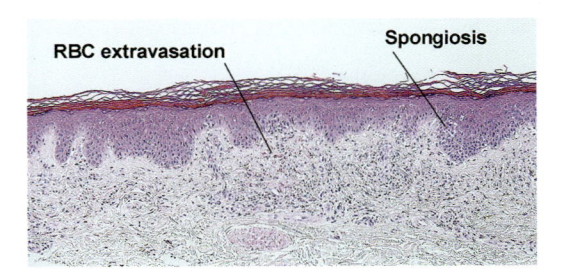

Fig 8-14 Pigmented purpuric eruption (RBC, red blood cell)

Stasis dermatitis

Key features

- Subacute spongiotic dermatitis
- Cannonball-like angioplasia in the superficial dermis
- Hemosiderin

PEARL

Hemosiderin is refractile, whereas melanin is not.

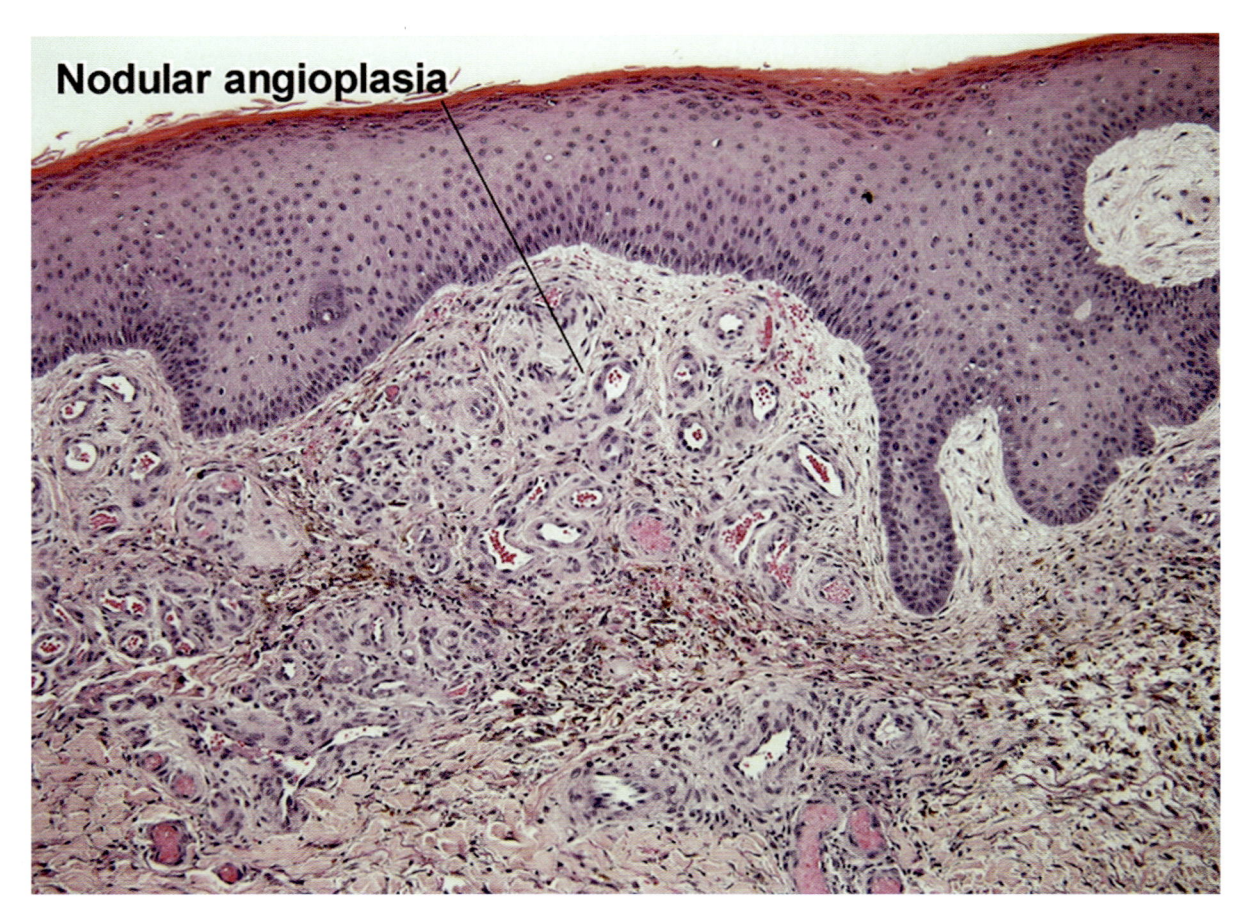

Fig 8-15 Stasis dermatitis

Spongiotic dermatitis with intraepidermal eosinophils

Key features
- Spongiosis
- Eosinophils within the epidermis ("eosinophilic spongiosis")

PEARL
Causes include *herpes gestationis*, arthropod bite, allergic contact dermatitis, pemphigus, pemphigoid, incontinentia pigmenti, erythema toxicum (spongiosis adjacent to a follicle) (HAAPPIE).

Zoon's balanitis

Key features
- Spongiosis
- Flattened, diamond-shaped keratinocytes
- Dermal plasma cells

Zoon's balanitis (balanitis circumscripta plasmacellularis) demonstrates subacute spongiotic mucositis with an underlying dense plasmacytic infiltrate and flattened keratinocytes with intercellular edema.

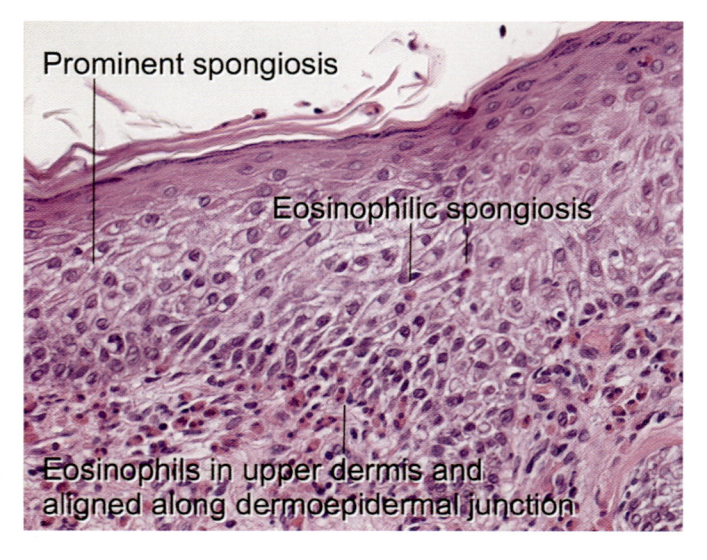

Fig 8-16 Pemphigoid

Psoriasiform and spongiotic dermatitis — Chapter 8 — 159

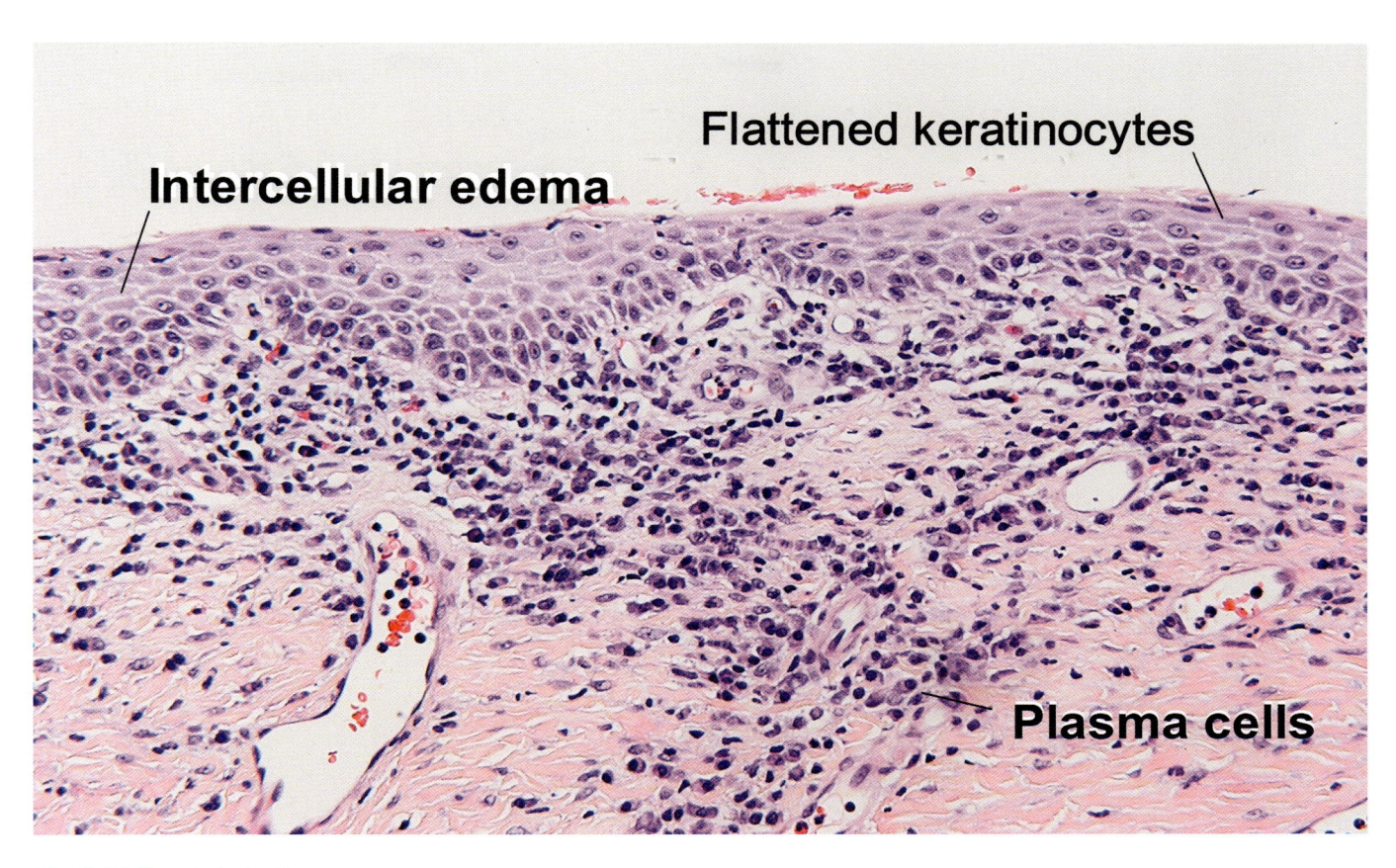

Fig 8-17 Zoon's balanitis

Pityriasis rubra pilaris

Key features

- Acanthosis with thick superpapillary plates
- Parakeratosis adjacent to follicles
- Vertical and horizontal alternating (checkerboard) ortho- and parakeratosis
- Occasional spongiosis
- Occasional acantholysis in follicles or eccrine ducts

Dermatopathology

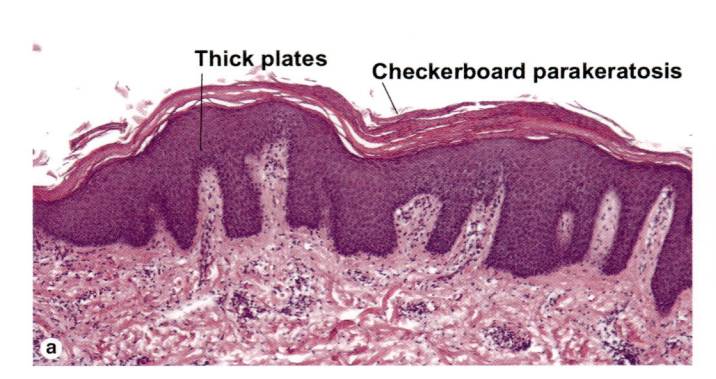

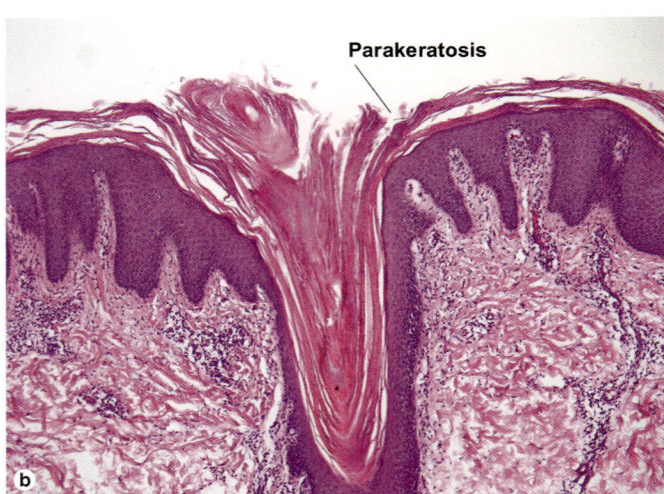

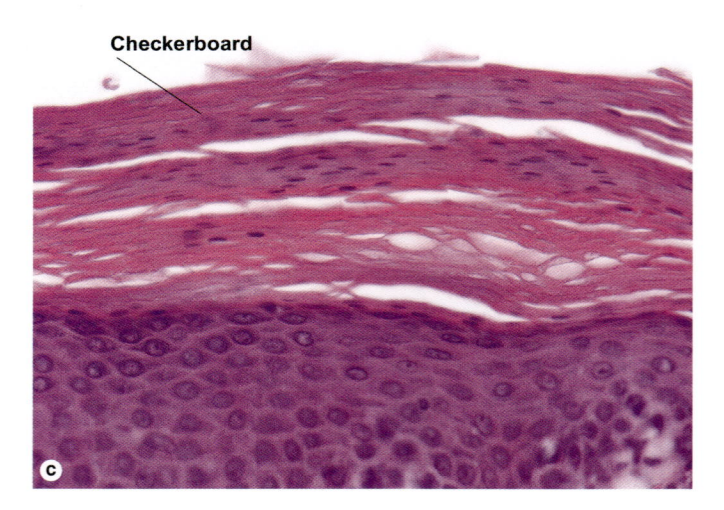

Fig 8-18 Pityriasis rubra pilaris

Further reading

Behrhof W, Springer E, Bräuninger W, et al. PCR testing for Treponema pallidum in paraffin-embedded skin biopsy specimens: test design and impact on the diagnosis of syphilis. J Clin Pathol 2008;61(3):390–395.

Chen CY, Chi KH, George RW, et al. Diagnosis of gastric syphilis by direct immunofluorescence staining and real-time PCR testing. J Clin Microbiol 2006;44(9):3452–3456.

Hugel H. Histological diagnosis of inflammatory skin diseases. Use of a simple algorithm and modern diagnostic methods. Pathologe 2002;23(1):20–37.

Meymandi S, Silver SG, Crawford RI. Intraepidermal neutrophils – a clue to dermatophytosis? J Cutan Pathol 2003;30(4):253–255.

Pujol RM, Wang CY, el-Azhary RA, et al. Necrolytic migratory erythema: clinicopathologic study of 13 cases. Int J Dermatol 2004;43(1):12–18.

Blistering diseases

Whitney A. High

Chapter 9

Subcorneal vesiculobullous disorders

Pemphigus foliaceus

Key features

- Subcorneal split
- Acantholysis (loss of attachments between keratinocytes)
- Dyskeratosis may occur within the granular layer
- Direct immunofluorescence demonstrates "net-like" deposition of immunoglobulin (Ig) G and C3 between keratinocytes in upper epidermis

Pemphigus foliaceus is a subcorneal vesiculobullous disorder caused by autoantibodies directed at an intercellular keratinocyte adhesion protein, desmoglein 1 (160 kD). The disease usually presents with superficial crusted erosions upon the face and upper trunk. The superficial nature of the blisters makes them fragile and most patients lack intact bullae.

The presence of a subcorneal blister, with acantholytic cells and scattered eosinophils, is highly suggestive of pemphigus foliaceus. Direct immunofluorescence (DIF) is diagnostic and demonstrates intercellular IgG and C3 deposition, primarily confined to the upper half of the epidermis. The split occurs in the granular layer, as in staphylococcal scalded-skin syndrome. Pemphigus foliaceus may demonstrate neutrophils within the vesicle, making distinction from bullous impetigo difficult. A tissue Gram stain may be helpful, but the presence of an impetiginized crust does not rule out pemphigus foliaceus.

Pemphigus erythematosus blends the immunohistologic findings of pemphigus foliaceus with lupus erythematosus. Patients often have a positive serum antinuclear antibody. Immunofluorescence yields both an intercellular deposition of immunoreactants and a "lupus band" of immunoreactants along the basement membrane zone.

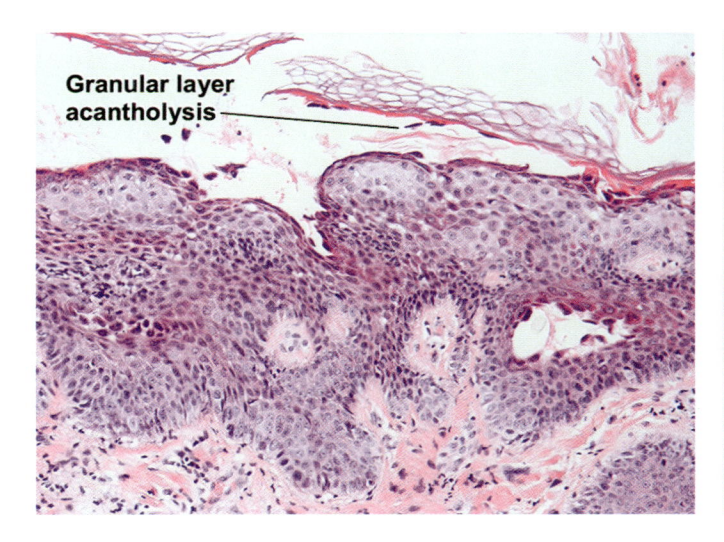

Fig 9-1 Pemphigus foliaceus

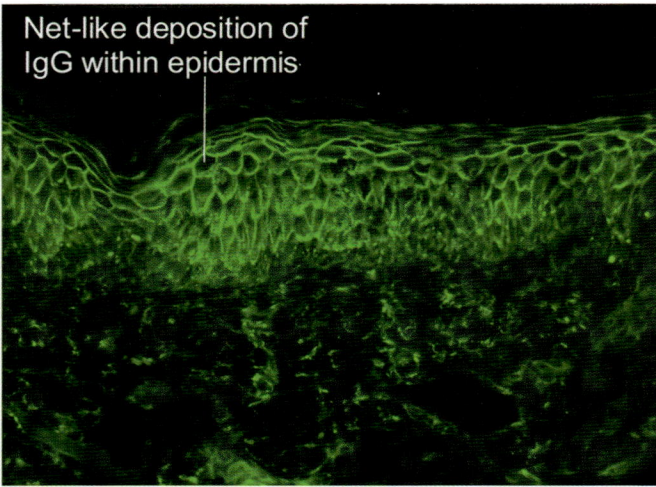

Fig 9-2 Direct immunofluorescence of "net-like" staining in the upper epidermis of pemphigus foliaceus

Subcorneal pustular dermatosis (Sneddon–Wilkinson disease)

Key features

- Subcorneal pustule
- Pustule "sits" upon the epidermis without depressing it
- Superficial mixed perivascular infiltrate with occasional neutrophils
- Dyskeratosis is uncommon
- Immunofluorescence is negative (distinguishing it from IgA pemphigus)

Cases of subcorneal pustular dermatosis with intercellular deposition of IgA have been reclassified as IgA pemphigus. Subcorneal pustular dermatosis may represent a subclass of pustular psoriasis, although mitotic figures within the underlying epidermis, common to psoriasis, are not identified in subcorneal pustular dermatosis. The classic patient is an older woman with annular or polycyclic lesions of the trunk or groin with pustules at the periphery.

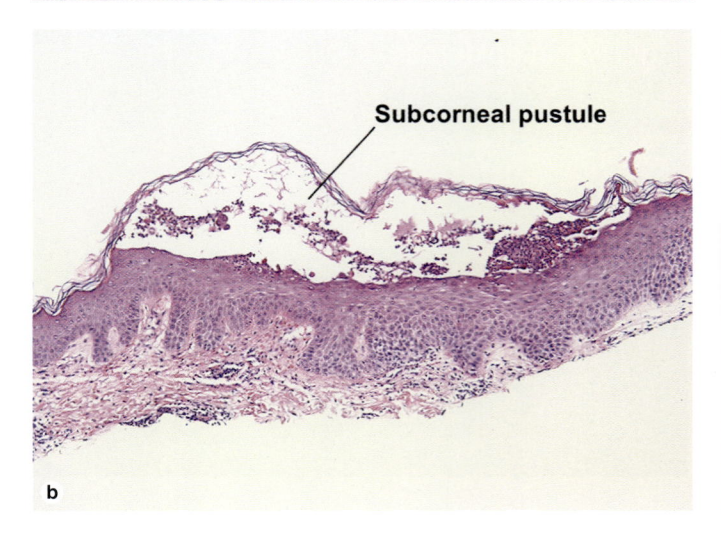

Fig 9-3 (a) Subcorneal pustular dermatosis. (b) "Subcorneal pustular dermatosis" type of IgA pemphigus

Acute generalized exanthematous pustulosis

Key features

- Subcorneal or superficial epidermal pustules
- Mild spongiosis in the surrounding epidermis
- Superficial mixed infiltrate in an edematous papillary dermis
- Occasional eosinophils within the dermal infiltrate
- Immunofluorescence is negative

Acute generalized exanthematous pustulosis is an uncommon reaction to exogenous medications. Beta-lactam antibiotics are most often implicated, but a myriad of drug associations have been described. The presence of eosinophils in the inflammatory infiltrate helps distinguish the condition from pustular psoriasis. Early pustules may be noted in association with hair follicles or sweat ducts.

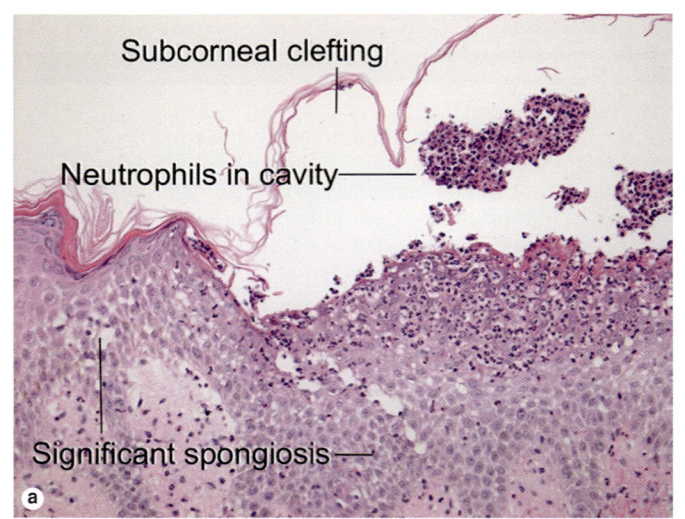

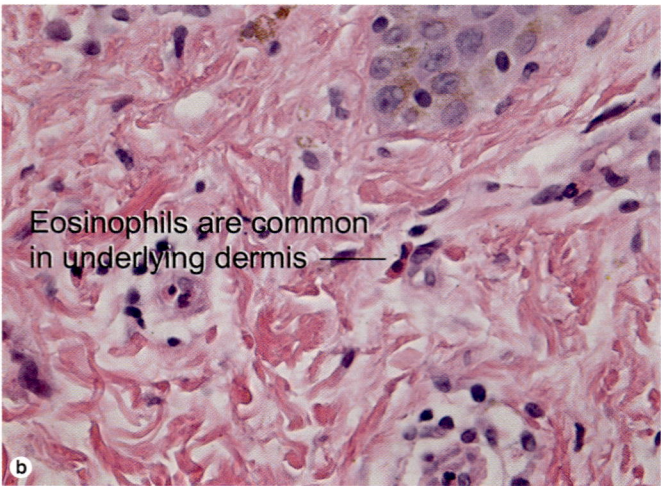

Fig 9-4 Acute generalized exanthematous pustulosis

Intraepidermal vesiculobullous disorders

Pemphigus vulgaris

Key features

- Split immediately above basal layer leaves a "tombstone row" of basal keratinocytes
- Tracking of separation down hair follicles ("follicular extension")
- Eosinophils may occur in spongiotic foci or within the blister cavity
- Superficial lymphocytic inflammatory infiltrate in dermis
- Eosinophils may be seen within the dermal infiltrate
- Direct immunofluorescence demonstrates "net-like" deposition of IgG and C3 between keratinocytes in lower epidermis

Pemphigus vulgaris is an intraepidermal vesiculobullous disorder caused by autoantibodies directed at an intercellular keratinocyte adhesion protein, desmoglein 3 (130 kD). The disease presents with erosions of the skin and mucosa. Often the disease begins in the posterior oropharynx weeks before cutaneous lesions are noted. Most patients lack intact bullae. Erythematous skin shears away easily when lateral pressure is applied (Nikolsky sign).

Clefting above the basal layer, with acantholysis of the remaining basilar keratinocytes, leads to a visual impression likened to "rows of tombstones" sitting upon the dermal papillae.

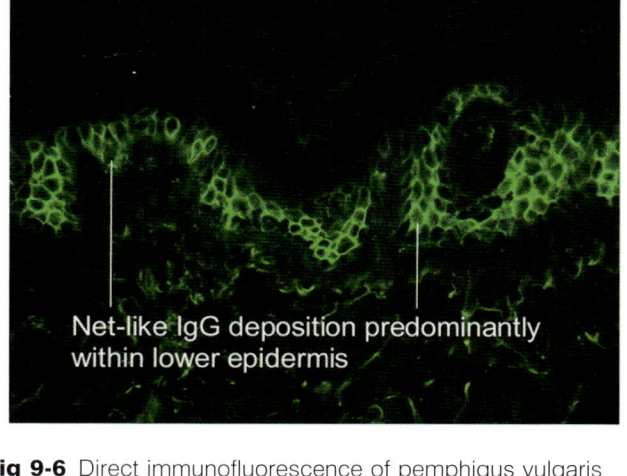

Fig 9-6 Direct immunofluorescence of pemphigus vulgaris

Tracking of the blistering process down adnexal structures is often demonstrated. Direct immunofluorescence is diagnostic and demonstrates intercellular IgG and C3 deposition, primarily confined to the lower half of the epidermis.

Pemphigus vegetans is a related disorder which demonstrates vegetative cutaneous lesions with epidermal hyperplasia and lesser vesiculation. Suprabasilar crypts containing eosinophils may be identified within the acanthotic epidermis in many cases of pemphigus vegetans.

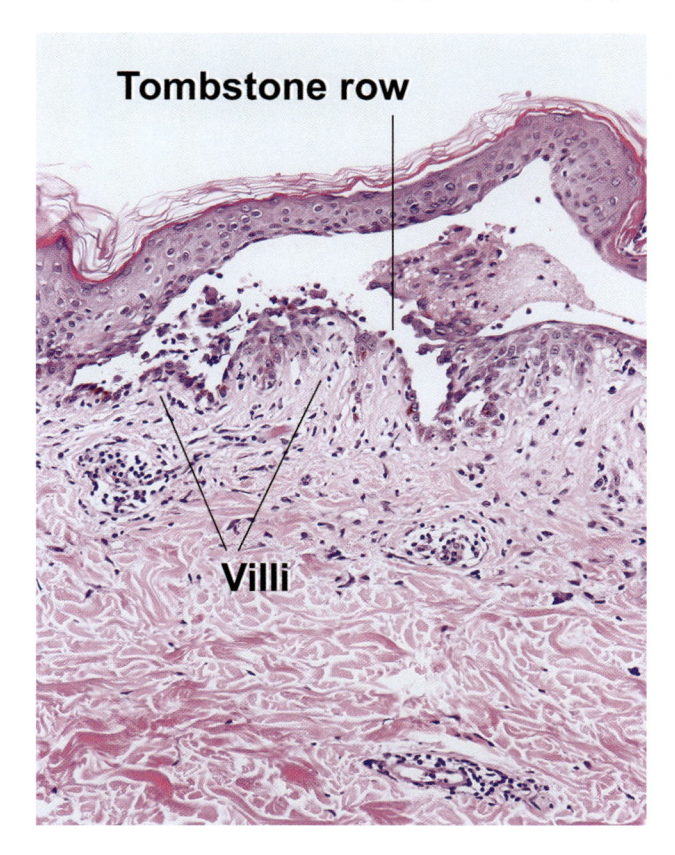

Fig 9-5 Pemphigus vulgaris

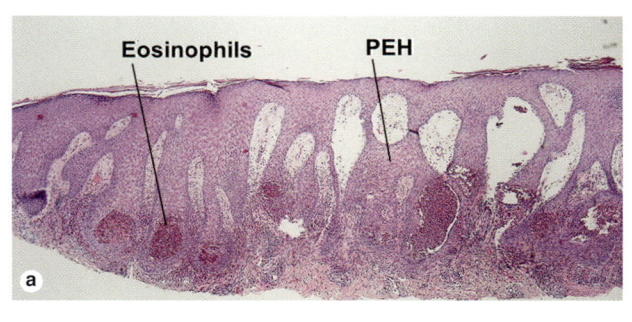

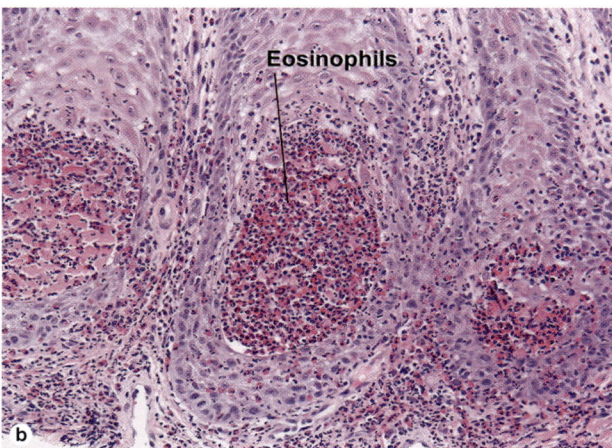

Fig 9-7 Pemphigus vegetans–pseudoepitheliomatous hyperplasia (PEH) and eosinophils

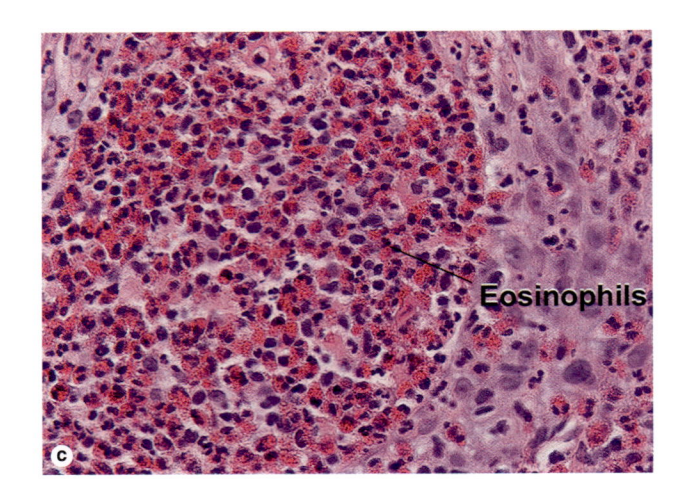

Fig 9-7, cont'd

Familial benign chronic pemphigus (Hailey–Hailey disease)

Key features

- An inherited disorder with defective cell–cell adhesion
- Not antibody-mediated
- Acantholysis at all levels of the epidermis resembles a "dilapidated brick wall"
- Acanthosis
- Red dyskeratotic rim surrounds nucleus
- Immunofluorescence is negative

Hailey–Hailey disease is an autosomal-dominant, inherited disease caused by mutations in the *ATP2C1* gene. This gene encodes for a portion of a calcium pump essential for proper keratinocyte differentiation and adhesion. Skin of the intertriginous areas is most prominently affected and yields a clinical appearance likened to "wet tissue paper." Acantholysis at all levels of the epidermis yields the histologic appearance of a "dilapidated brick wall." While the disease itself is not immunologically mediated, superinfection of macerated skin by bacteria or yeast may engender an underlying inflammatory infiltrate within the superficial dermis.

Differential Diagnosis

The Hailey–Hailey variant of Grover's disease has similar histologic findings; however, in contrast to the broad lesions of benign familial pemphigus, there is less extensive and focal involvement in Grover's disease.

The negative direct immunofluorescence, dyskeratosis and follicular sparing in Hailey–Hailey disease allows distinction from pemphigus vulgaris. The acanthosis of benign familial pemphigus is a feature not typically identified in other blistering disorders.

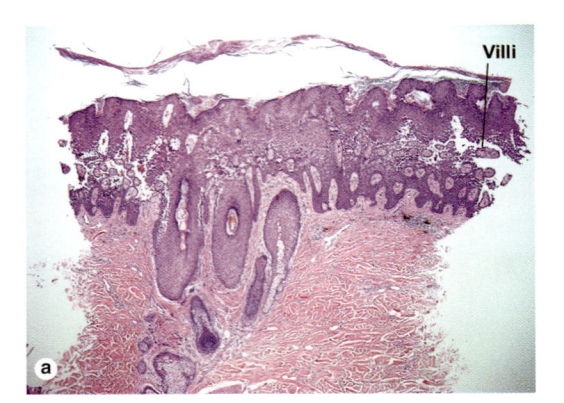

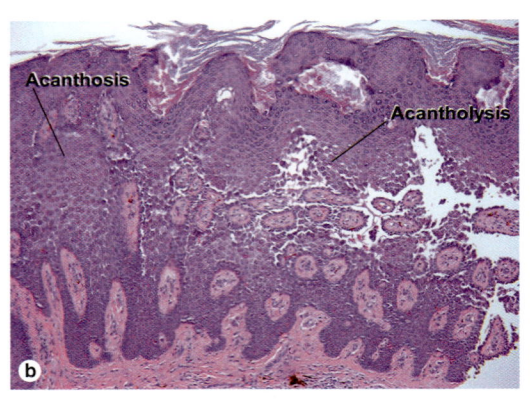

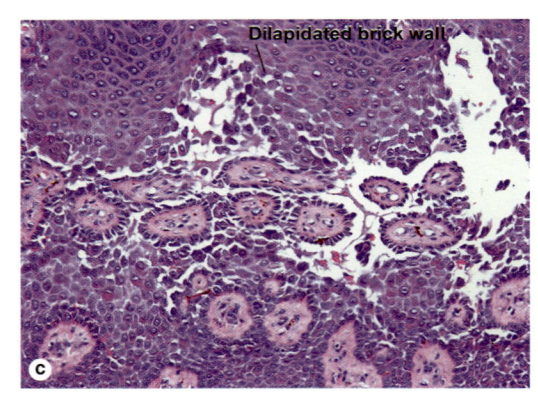

Fig 9-8 Hailey–Hailey disease

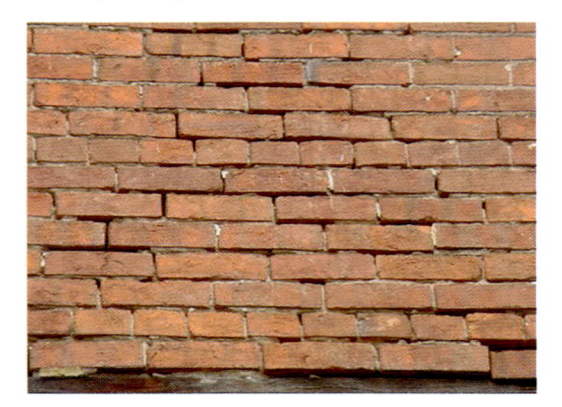

Fig 9-9 Dilapidated brick wall for comparison

Keratosis follicularis (Darier's disease)

Key features

- Acantholytic dyskeratosis
- Acantholysis accentuated in the lower epidermis yielding suprabasilar clefting
- More dyskeratosis than Hailey–Hailey disease
- Less acantholysis than Hailey–Hailey disease
- Grains (basophilic keratinocytes with elongated nuclei in or near the granular layer)
- Corps ronds (dyskeratotic keratinocytes with a round nucleus surrounded by a blue rim or clear halo)
- Hyperkeratosis and parakeratosis in the overlying stratum corneum
- Immunofluorescence is negative

PEARL

- Dyskeratotic keratinocytes in Hailey–Hailey disease have a red rim around the nucleus, while those in Darier's disease usually have blue or clear rim.

The acantholysis results in suprabasal clefts (lacunae) that contain projections of papillary dermis covered by a single layer of basal cells (villi). There are two types of dyskeratotic cells. The granular layer and horny layer contain corps ronds, round dyskeratotic cells with pyknotic nuclei, a clear perinuclear halo, and pale to bright eosinophilic cytoplasm. Grains are seen in the granular layer as flattened basophilic dyskeratotic cells.

Darier's disease is an autosomal-dominant disorder with greasy, yellow-brown crusted and hyperkeratotic lesions in the seborrheic areas. Other cutaneous findings include cobblestone papules of the mucosa, palmoplantar pits, verrucous lesions on the dorsal hands and feet (acrokeratosis verruciformis of Hopf) and red and white longitudinal nail streaks with distal "V" nicking. Similar to Hailey–Hailey disease, the gene responsible, *ATP2A2*, encodes a calcium pump.

Differential Diagnosis

The differential diagnosis of acantholytic dyskeratosis includes the Darier's type of Grover's disease where the degree of dyskeratosis is less extensive and more localized. The acantholysis and dyskeratosis of warty dyskeratoma are isolated to a solitary, cup-shaped, follicular configuration. Acantholytic dyskeratosis unrelated to Darier's disease may occur in the genital region.

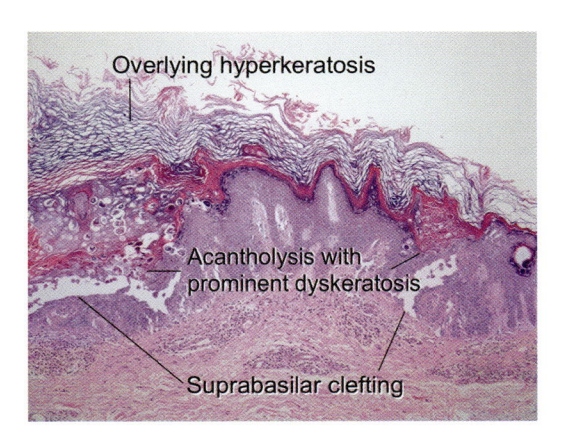

Fig 9-10 Darier's disease

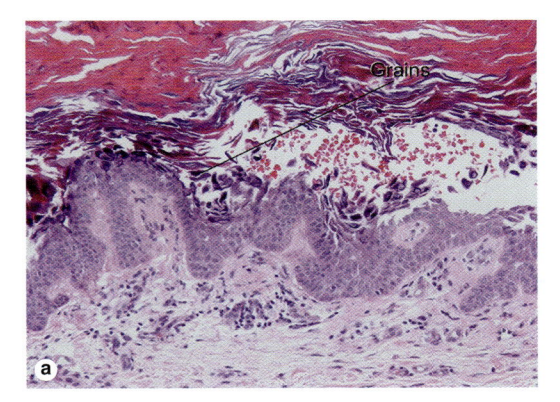

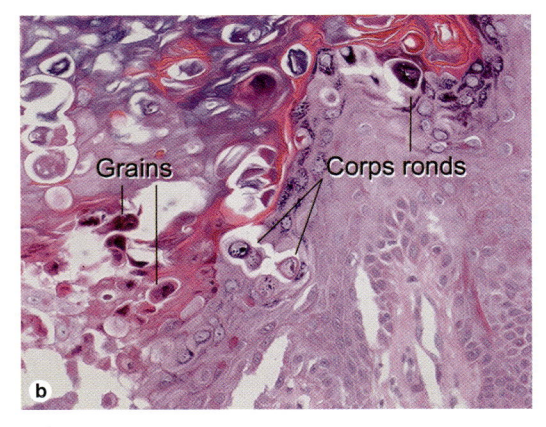

Fig 9-11 Darier's disease, corps ronds and grains

Transient acantholytic dermatosis (Grover's disease)

Key features

- Darier's pattern with acantholysis and dyskeratosis
- Hailey–Hailey-like full-thickness acantholysis
- Pemphigus pattern with partial-thickness acantholysis
- Spongiotic pattern with rare acantholytic cells

More than one of these patterns may be found in the same specimen. The clinical presentation, the mixture of histologic patterns, and the focal nature of the lesions help distinguish the disease from the histologic mimics. Eosinophils, if present, aid in differentiation from Darier's disease. Direct immunofluorescence is typically negative, in contrast to pemphigus.

Grover's disease is an acquired, pruritic disorder most commonly affecting older men on the trunk. Typically there is a sudden onset of discrete, crusted papules. Despite the name, the eruption may or may not be transient. Heat, fever, and sweating precipitate this disorder. Despite the histologic similarity to some genodermatoses, Grover's disease is not an inherited disorder.

Paraneoplastic pemphigus

Key features

- Variable intraepidermal acantholysis
- Dermal infiltrate of lymphocytes which is often heavy and band-like ("lichenoid")
- Interface reaction with necrotic keratinocytes and vacuolar change
- Subepidermal clefting is possible, though less common
- Focal epidermal spongiosis is possible
- Direct immunofluorescence demonstrates "net-like" epidermal deposition of IgG and C3 (similar to pemphigus) and linear deposition at the dermoepidermal junction
- Indirect immunofluorescence on rat bladder epithelium is used for screening purposes

Paraneoplastic pemphigus demonstrates a wide variety of histologic patterns. The most common form represents a hybrid of classic pemphigus (intraepidermal acantholysis) and erythema multiforme (lichenoid lymphocytic infiltrate with interface reaction and necrotic keratinocytes). In one single study, 27% of cases had only suprabasilar acantholysis alone.

Multiple autoantibodies have been detected in paraneoplastic pemphigus, including those directed at: desmoglein 1 (160 kD), desmoglein 3 (130 kD), desmoplakin I (250 kD), bullous pemphigoid antigen 1 (230 kD), envoplakin (210 kD), periplakin (190 kD), and an unnamed 170-kD antigen. Paraneoplastic pemphigus is more severe and recalcitrant to treatment than is pemphigus vulgaris. The disease often remits with cancer remission, and recurs with cancer recurrence.

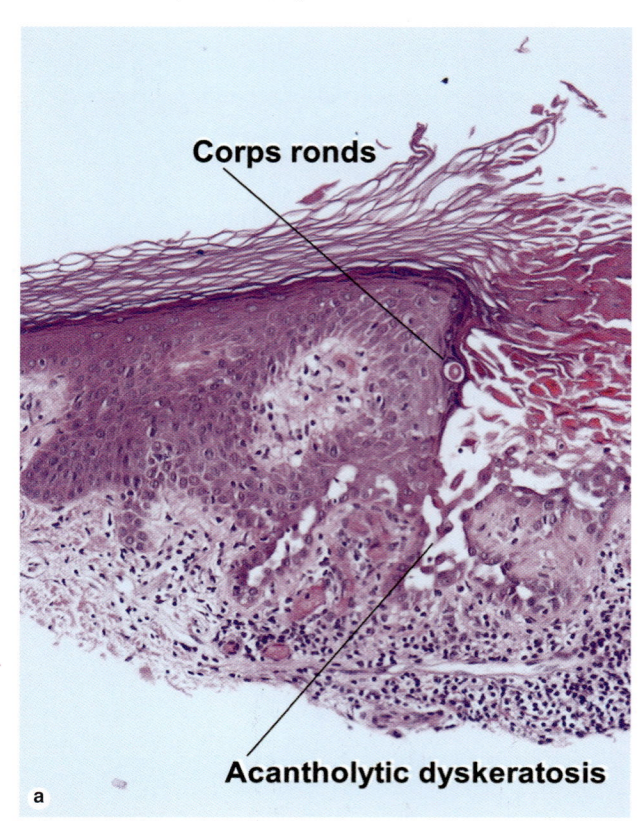

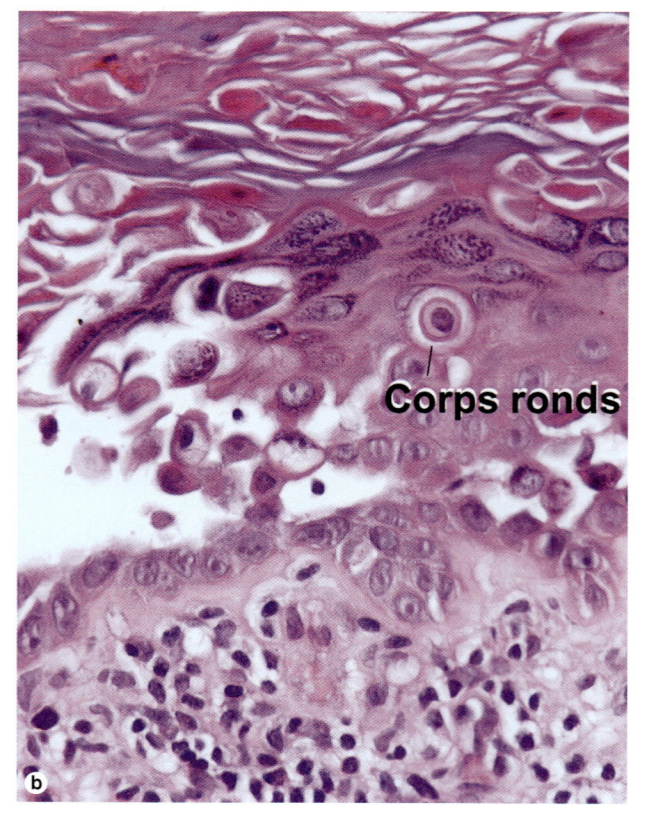

Fig 9-12 Darier-type Grover's disease

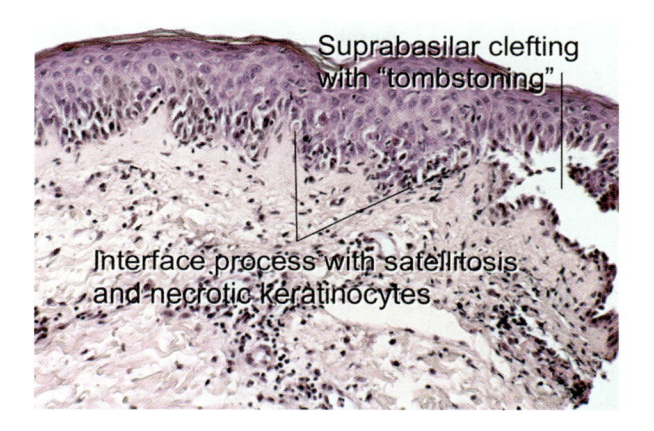

Fig 9-13 Paraneoplastic pemphigus with intraepidermal acantholysis and interface dermatitis

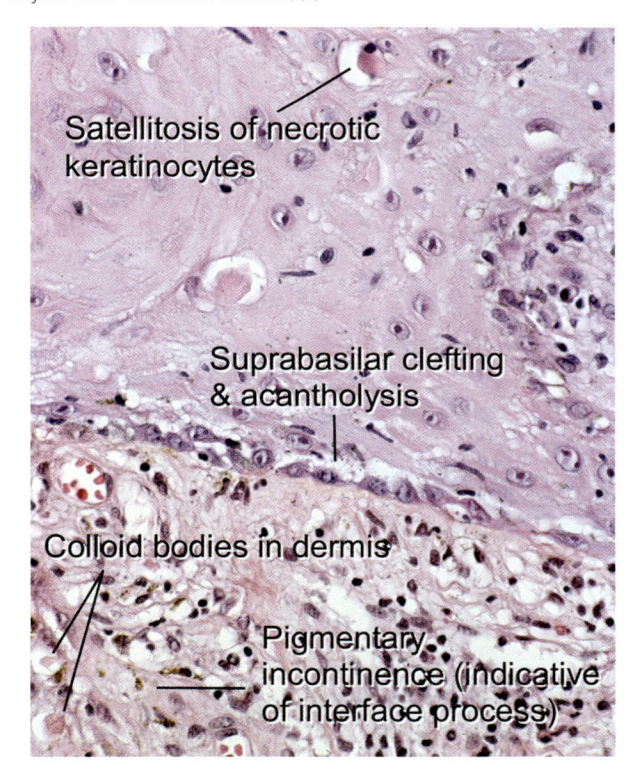

Fig 9-14 Paraneoplastic pemphigus

Subepidermal vesiculobullous disorders: pauci-inflammatory subepidermal conditions

Porphyria cutanea tarda

Key features

- Subepidermal vesiculation
- Acral skin with compact orthokeratosis
- Solar elastosis (due to patient age and characteristic acral location)
- Minimal inflammatory infiltrate
- Protuberance of rigid dermal papillae into blister cavity ("festooning")
- Entrapped amphophilic basement membrane within the overlying epidermis ("caterpillar bodies")
- Perivascular hyaline material deposited in superficial dermis
- Periodic acid-Schiff staining may accentuate the perivascular deposition of hyaline material
- Direct immunofluorescence demonstrates IgM and C3 in vessels (adsorbed by the hyaline material like a sponge)

Porphyria cutanea tarda is the most common form of porphyria in the USA. It is commonly associated with hepatitis C, alcohol ingestion, and iron overload. Inherited types result from reduced activity of uroporphyrinogen decarboxylase, an enzyme involved in heme synthesis. Blisters, erosions, and milia occur on the hands and other photo-exposed locations.

Pseudoporphyria results in *essentially identical* clinical and histopathologic changes, but is instead due to an exogenous medication. Naproxen sodium causes the majority of cases. No disturbance of porphyrin synthesis has been detected in pseudoporphyria. Pseudoporphyria may occur in young patients, and solar elastosis may not be demonstrated. Limited evidence suggests that occasional eosinophils may be more common in pseudoporphyria and festooning of the papillary dermis may not be as prominent.

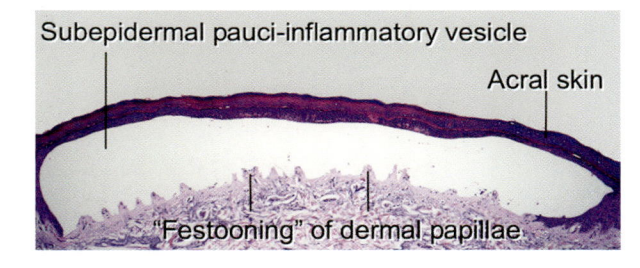

Fig 9-15 Porphyria cutanea tarda (PCT)

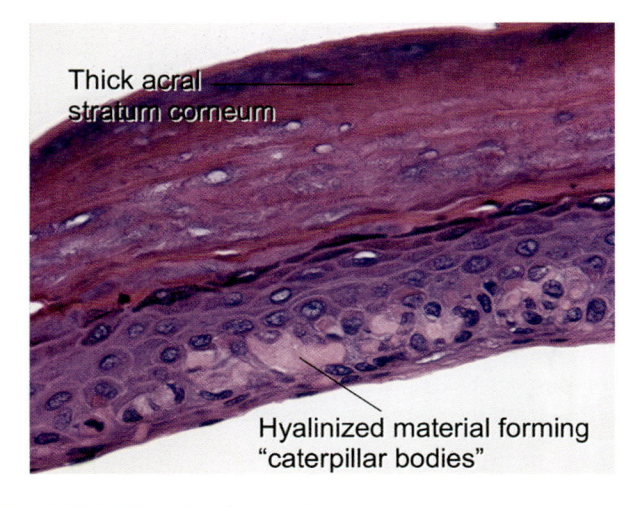

Fig 9-16 PCT: caterpillar bodies

Dermatopathology

Epidermolysis bullosa acquisita

Key features

- Subepidermal vesiculation
- Fibrin deposition in the floor of the blister cavity
- Some cases may show neutrophils within the papillary dermis, while other cases are histologically indistinguishable from bullous pemphigoid
- Dermal fibrosis (scar) may be present in the dermis
- Milia formation may be seen in late lesions
- Direct immunofluorescence of adjacent skin demonstrates linear deposition of IgG and C3 at the dermoepidermal junction in a u-serrated pattern; IgA has been demonstrated in a significant number of cases

Epidermolysis bullosa acquisita (EBA) is caused by an antibody to type VII collagen, a major component of the anchoring fibrils. It is thought that deposition of immune complexes leads to the neutrophilic inflammation present in some specimens.

The histology may overlap with bullous pemphigoid, and indirect immunofluorescence on salt-split skin is sometimes used to distinguish the conditions when the typical u-serrated pattern of EBA is not apparent on DIF. In bullous pemphigoid, the immunoreactants are deposited within the basement membrane zone and highlight the roof of salt-split skin. Conversely, in epidermolysis bullosa, the immunoreactants mark the floor of salt-split skin.

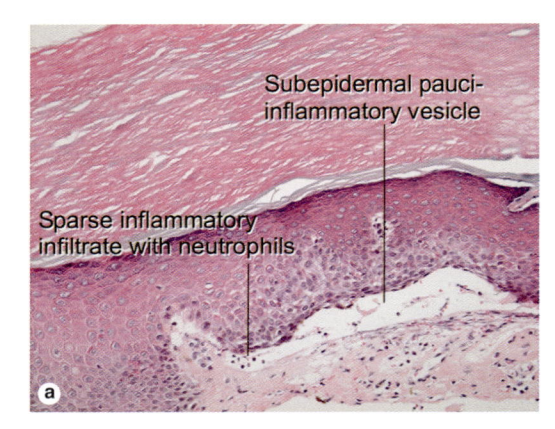

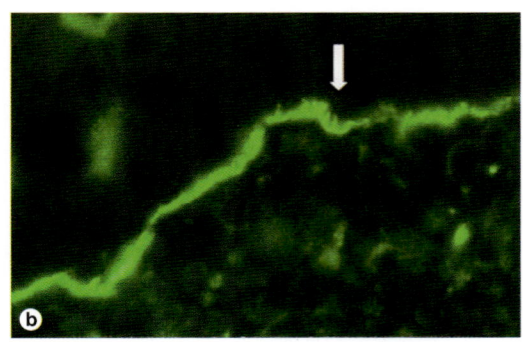

Fig 9-17 (a) Epidermolysis bullosa acquisita. (b) Epidermolysis bullosa acquisita, DIF showing characteristic u-serrated pattern (arrow).

Toxic epidermal necrolysis/Stevens–Johnson syndrome

Key features

- Subepidermal vesiculation/sloughing with confluent necrosis of the epidermis
- Minimal inflammatory infiltrate
- Some cases may show a sparse superficial perivascular inflammatory infiltrate
- Overlap between toxic epidermal necrolysis and Stevens–Johnson syndrome exists
- Immunofluorescence is negative

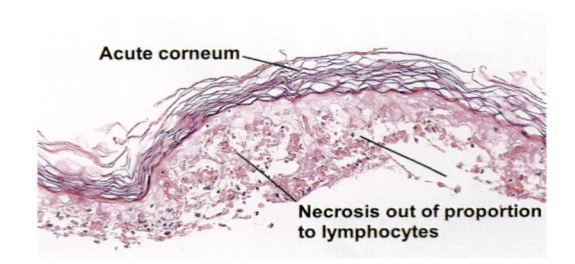

Fig 9-18 Toxic epidermal necrolysis

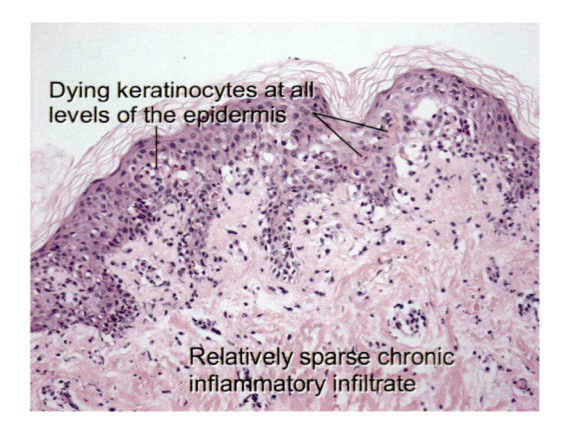

Fig 9-19 Stevens–Johnson syndrome

Inflammatory subepidermal conditions

Bullous pemphigoid

Key features

- Subepidermal bulla
- Eosinophils typically present within blister cavity
- In some patients, neutrophils predominate in the blister cavity
- Early lesions may demonstrate exocytosis of eosinophils within a mildly spongiotic epidermis ("eosinophilic spongiosis")
- Urticarial lesions may demonstrate eosinophils "lined up" along the dermal–epidermal junction

- Direct immunofluorescence of adjacent skin demonstrates linear deposition of C3 and IgG along the dermoepidermal junction in an n-serrated pattern
- Indirect immunofluorescence on salt-split skin demonstrates immunoreactants in the roof of the blister (compared with same test in epidermolysis bullosa acquisita, which marks the floor)

Bullous pemphigoid usually occurs in older patients, although children are occasionally affected. The disease is associated with autoantibodies to bullous pemphigoid antigen I (230 kD) and/or bullous pemphigoid antigen II (180 kD). The latter antigen is most clearly linked to pathogenesis. The subepidermal vesiculation results in firm and tense blisters. Intensely pruritic urticarial plaques, without clinically apparent vesiculation, may predate frankly bullous lesions ("urticarial pemphigoid"). Mucosal involvement is sometimes present, but, unlike pemphigus, it is rarely the first site of involvement.

Pemphigoid gestationis (also known as herpes gestationis) is a related vesiculobullous condition occurring in gravid women; it has essentially identical histopathologic and immunohistologic findings.

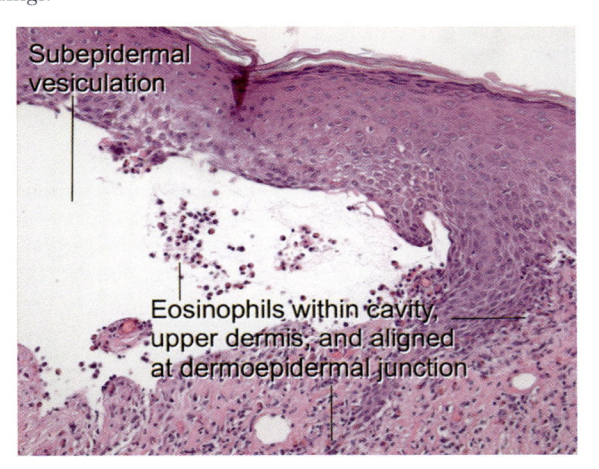

Cicatricial pemphigoid

Key features

- Subepidermal vesiculation
- Variable degree of inflammation in the dermis
- Neutrophilic microabscesses in the dermis may be identified in new lesions
- Cicatricial pemphigoid usually demonstrates fewer eosinophils than bullous pemphigoid
- Direct immunofluorescence of adjacent skin demonstrates linear deposition of IgG and C3 along the dermoepidermal junction in 80% of cases (also seen along appendageal structures)

Cicatricial pemphigoid refers to a heterogeneous group of scarring, subepidermal blistering disorders caused by a variety of autoantibodies. Tense bullae that heal with scarring are a common theme. Most subtypes involve oral or ocular mucosa. Recurring lesions may demonstrate extensive dermal scarring. Paraneoplastic variants have been described in the literature.

Fig 9-20 Bullous pemphigoid

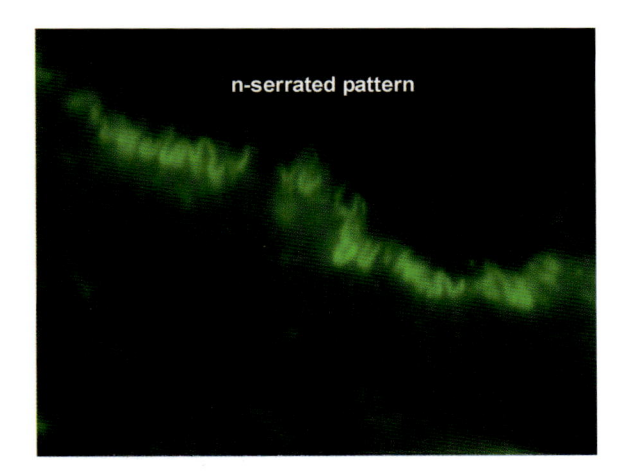

Fig 9-22 Direct immunofluorescence of bullous pemphigoid showing linear deposition of IgG at the dermal–epidermal junction

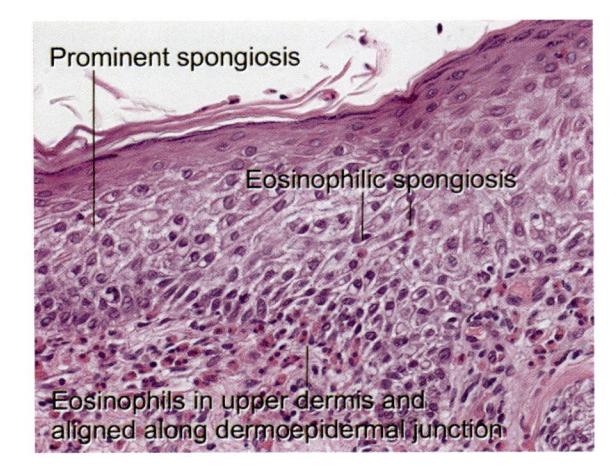

Fig 9-21 Urticarial pemphigoid

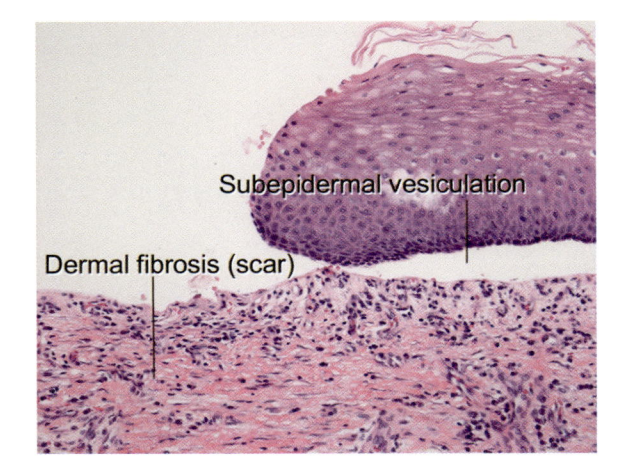

Fig 9-23 Cicatricial pemphigoid

Dermatitis herpetiformis

Key features

- Subepidermal vesiculation
- Neutrophilic abscesses in tips of dermal papillae
- Slight fibrin deposition in the tips of dermal papillae at points of vesiculation
- DIF demonstrates granular deposition of IgA within dermal papillae ± along dermal–epidermal junction. Granules have a vertical "picket fence" appearance.

Dermatitis herpetiformis is an intensely pruritic vesiculobullous disorder. Lesions are common upon the elbows, knees, buttocks, and scalp. Recent research indicates that epidermal transglutaminase-3 is the autoantigen in dermatitis herpetiformis. The disease is highly correlated with celiac sprue. Essentially, all patients have some level of gastrointestinal pathology, even if it is subclinical. Strict gluten-free diets prevent clinical manifestations of disease activity.

The granular deposition of IgA distinguishes dermatitis herpetiformis from linear IgA bullous dermatosis. Deposition is most marked in perilesional skin, with the densest deposits within dermal papillae. A vertical "picket fence" granule pattern may be apparent. Other immunoglobulins may be present in dermatitis herpetiformis; IgM is identified concurrently in up to 30% of cases.

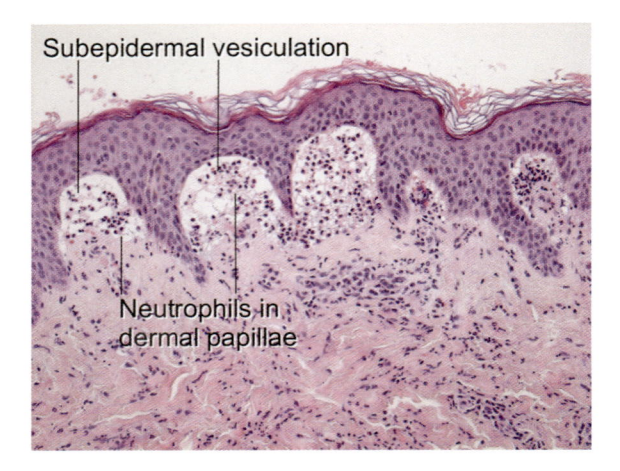

PEARL

The differential diagnosis for neutrophils within dermal papillae or subepidermal collections of neutrophils:
Plaid
- Bullous **p**emphigoid
- **L**upus (bullous)
- EB**A**
- Linear **i**mmunoglobulin A
- **D**ermatitis herpetiformis

Linear IgA bullous dermatosis

Key features

- Subepidermal vesiculation
- Neutrophils are the predominant inflammatory cell
- Some cases may demonstrate scattered eosinophils and a mild perivascular lymphocytic inflammatory infiltrate
- Direct immunofluorescence of adjacent skin demonstrates linear deposition of IgA along the dermoepidermal junction (the only immunoreactant present in 80% of cases)

Linear IgA is a heterogeneous subepidermal vesiculobullous disorder. In children, the disease is referred to as chronic bullous dermatosis of childhood. Both disorders are caused by autoantibodies targeting proteins (97–120 kD) that form as degradation products of bullous pemphigoid antigen II. Classically, the disease results in grouped annular lesions of tense bullae which have been likened to a "string of pearls." Drug-induced cases have been described with vancomycin.

By light microscopy, linear IgA bullous dermatosis overlaps significantly with dermatitis herpetiformis. It may be difficult to separate the two conditions without direct immunofluorescence examination.

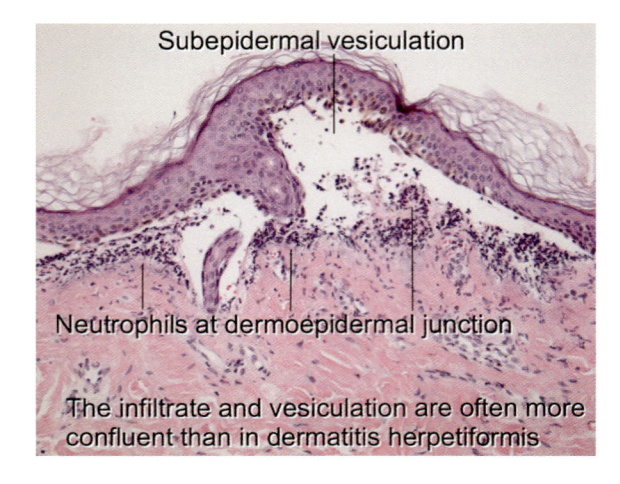

Fig 9-24 Dermatitis herpetiformis

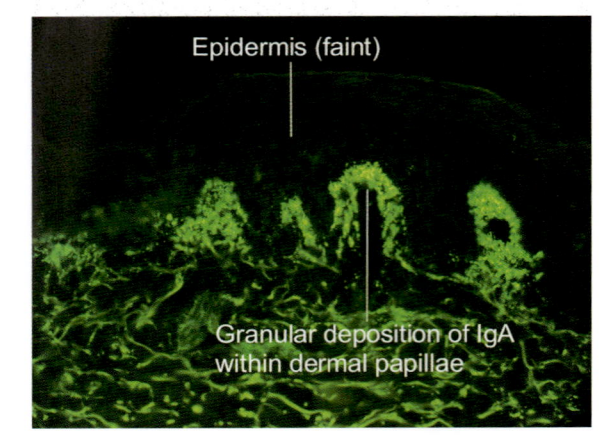

Fig 9-25 Direct immunofluorescence of dermatitis herpetiformis showing granular deposition of IgA in the dermal papillae

Fig 9-26 Linear IgA bullous dermatosis

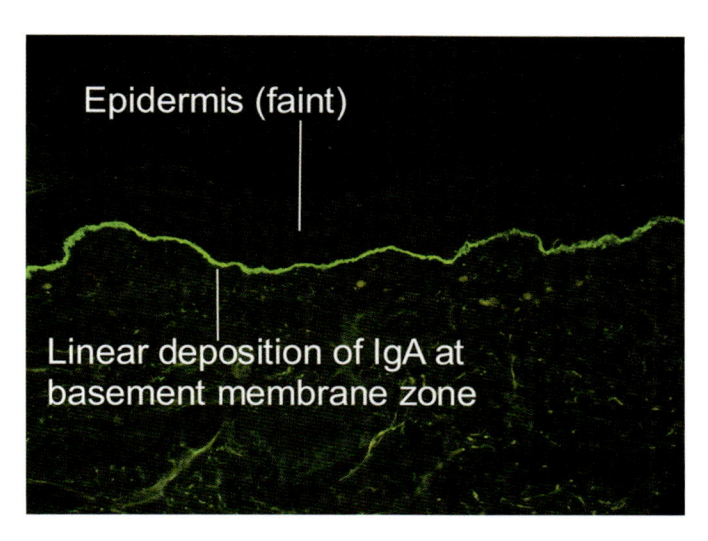

Fig 9-27 Direct immunofluorescence showing linear deposition of IgA along dermoepidermal junction

Bullous lupus erythematosus

Key features

- Subepidermal bulla with neutrophils
- Immunoreactants on floor of salt-split skin
- Other features of lupus may be present

Friction blister

Key features

- Mid-epidermal necrosis
- Serum may be present

Further reading

Chhabra S, Minz RW, Saikia B. Immunofluorescence in dermatology. Indian J Dermatol Venereol Leprol 2012;78(6):677–691.

Connor BL, Marks R, Jones EW. Dermatitis herpetiformis: histologic discriminants. Trans St Johns Hosp Dermatol Soc 1972;58:191–198.

Fung MA, Murphy MJ, Hoss DM, et al. The sensitivity and specificity of "caterpillar bodies" in the differential diagnosis of subepidermal blistering disorders. Am J Dermatopathol 2003;25:287–290.

Horn TD, Anhalt GJ. Histologic features of paraneoplastic pemphigus. Arch Dermatol 1992;128:1091–1095.

Jeong SJ, Lee CW. Bullous pemphigoid: persistent lesions of eczematous/urticarial erythemas. Cutis 1995;56:225–226.

Letko E, Papaliodis DN, Papaliodis GN, et al. Stevens–Johnson syndrome and toxic epidermal necrolysis: a review of the literature. Ann Allergy Asthma Immunol 2005;94:419–436.

Liu AY, Valenzuela R, Helm TN, et al. Indirect immunofluorescence on rat bladder transitional epithelium: a test with high specificity for paraneoplastic pemphigus. J Am Acad Dermatol 1993;28:696–699.

Nishioka K, Hashimoto K, Katayama I, et al. Eosinophilic spongiosis in bullous pemphigoid. Arch Dermatol 1984;120:1166–1168.

Quirk CJ, Heenan PJ. Grover's disease: 34 years on. Australas J Dermatol 2004;45:83–86.

Sardy M, Karpati S, Merkl B, et al. Epidermal transglutaminase (TGase 3) is the autoantigen of dermatitis herpetiformis. J Exp Med 2002;195:747–757.

Schmidt E, Zillikens D. Pemphigoid diseases. Lancet 2013;381(9863):320–332.

Tsuruta D, Dainichi T, Hamada T, et al. Molecular diagnosis of autoimmune blistering diseases. Methods Mol Biol 2013;961:17–32.

Yeh SW, Ahmed B, Sami N, et al. Blistering disorders: diagnosis and treatment. Dermatol Ther 2003;16:214–223.

Chapter 10

Granulomatous and histiocytic diseases

Tammie Ferringer

Granulomas are discrete collections of histiocytes with or without multinucleate giant cells. Histiocytes are bone marrow-derived or mesenchymal. In granulomas, their cytoplasmic membranes touch with no intervening connective tissue. Infectious etiologies, especially fungal and mycobacterial, should be excluded with special stains in any granulomatous process without obvious etiology. Examination under polarized light is required to exclude birefringent foreign material.

Granulomas can be categorized into: sarcoidal, tuberculoid, palisading, and suppurative. Sarcoidal granulomas, composed of epithelioid histiocytes, are "naked" granulomas with a paucity of surrounding infiltrate. Tuberculoid granulomas are associated with a peripheral mononuclear infiltrate and may show central caseous necrosis. Palisading granulomas surround devitalized collagen (necrobiosis), mucin, or foreign material. Suppurative granulomas have a central collection of neutrophils (stellate abscess).

Granuloma annulare

Key features

Interstitial pattern
- Patchy interstitial histiocytes, lymphocytes, and mucin give the appearance of a "busy dermis" at low power

Palisading pattern
- Histiocytes surround altered dermal collagen and mucin

Granuloma annulare typically involves the upper- to mid-reticular dermis. The mucin in palisading lesions is usually apparent with routine staining as faint feathery blue material; however, colloidal iron or other mucin stains can be used for confirmation. Sparse multinucleate histiocytes are typically identified and eosinophils occur in approximately half of cases. Rarely, perforation of the process through the epidermis (transepidermal elimination) occurs.

The subcutaneous tissue can be involved. Subcutaneous or deep granuloma annulare typically consists of histiocytes palisading around fibrin rather than mucin. It may be indistinguishable from rheumatoid nodule, resulting in its designation as pseudorheumatoid nodule. This subtype of granuloma annulare typically occurs on the lower legs, hands, head, and buttock in young individuals without rheumatoid disease.

The microscopic differential diagnosis of granuloma annulare and other palisading granulomas includes epithelioid sarcoma. Clues to this malignant neoplasm include necrosis and mild cytologic atypia. Epithelioid sarcoma demonstrates a biphasic pattern with transition between epithelioid and spindle cells. Cells stain for both keratin and vimentin.

Table 10.1 shows distinctions between granuloma annulare and necrobiosis lipoidica.

Table 10-1 Features of granuloma annulare and necrobiosis lipoidica

Feature	Granuloma annulare	Necrobiosis lipoidica
Distribution	Focal and patchy	Diffuse and full-thickness
Granuloma	Palisaded or interstitial	Horizontal tiers (layers)
Mucin	Yes	No
Shape of punch biopsy	Tapered	Rectangular
Plasma cells	Rare	Common
Cholesterol clefts	No	Occasional

Granulomatous and histiocytic diseases — Chapter 10

Differential Diagnosis

The microscopic differential for a "busy dermis" includes:
- Blue nevus
- Dermatofibroma
- Dermal Spitz nevus
- Metastatic breast carcinoma
- Kaposi's sarcoma (patch stage)
- Granuloma annulare
- Scleromyxedema
- Neurofibroma

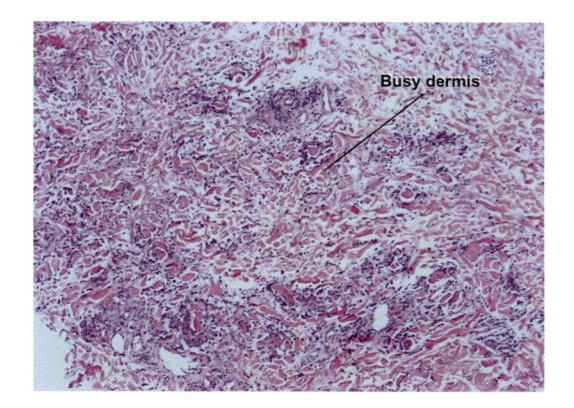

Fig 10-1 Interstitial granuloma annulare

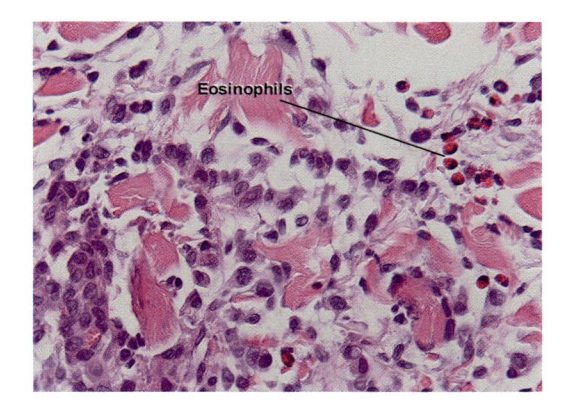

Fig 10-2 Interstitial granuloma annulare

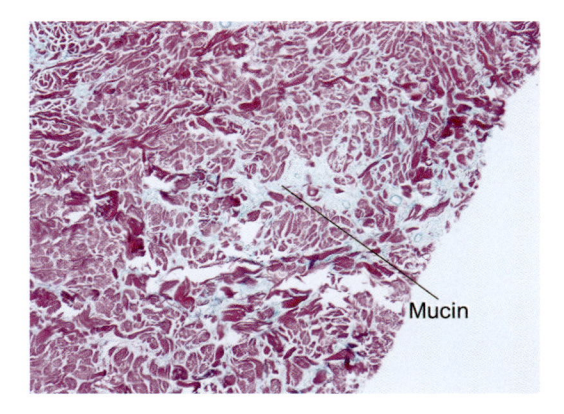

Fig 10-3 Interstitial granuloma annulare (colloidal iron)

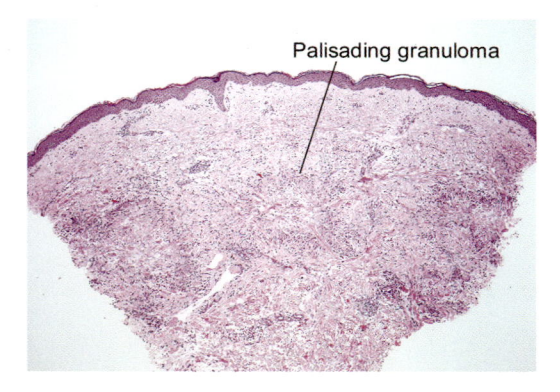

Fig 10-4 Palisading granuloma annulare

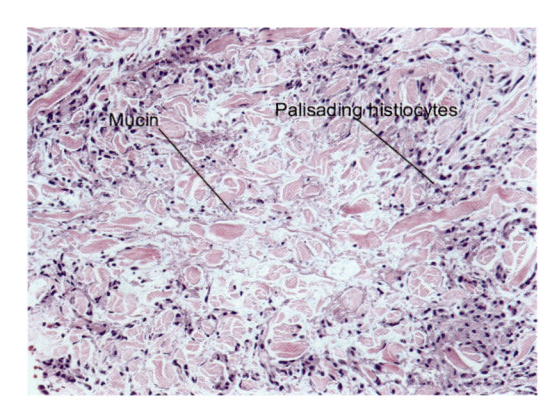

Fig 10-5 Palisading granuloma annulare

Actinic granuloma

Key features
- Solar elastosis
- Similar palisade to granuloma annulare but no mucin
- Elastic fibers are engulfed by palisading giant cells and histocytes (elastolysis)
- Central loss of elastic tissue

These lesions occur on areas of chronic sun damage such as the face, neck, hands, and arms. They have a raised border and atrophic finely wrinkled center. The granulomas consume actinically damaged elastic tissue. Other names have included Miescher's facial granuloma, atypical necrobiosis lipoidica of the face and scalp, and annular elastolytic giant cell granuloma. Some consider it to be a variant of granuloma annulare on sun-damaged skin. The central loss of elastic tissue, absence of mucin, and conspicuous multinucleated histiocytes are the primary basis for distinguishing these lesions.

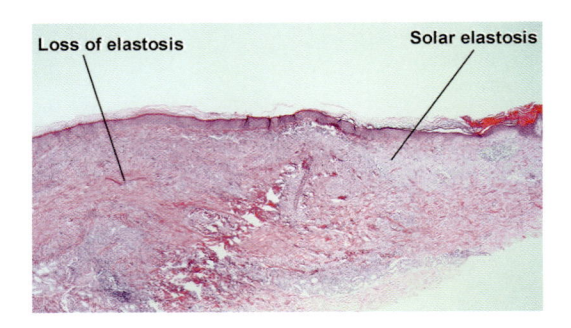

Fig 10-6 Actinic granuloma

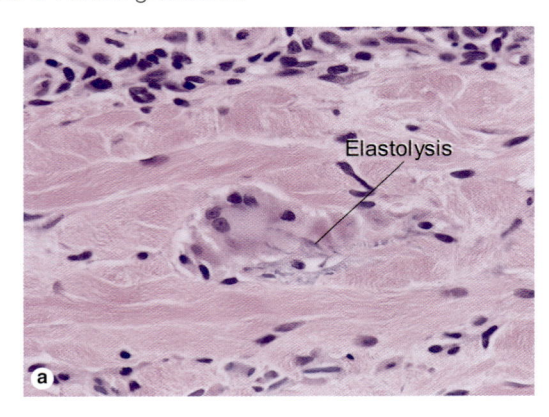

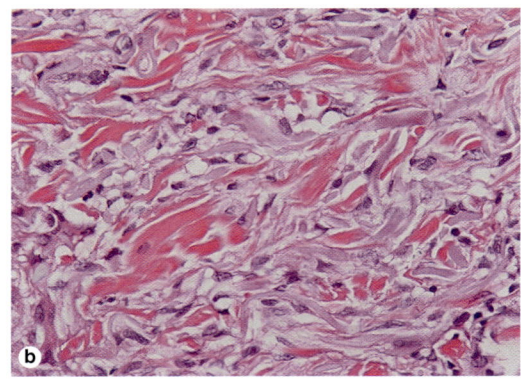

Fig 10-7 Actinic granuloma

Necrobiosis lipoidica

Key features

- Horizontal acellular, pale, degenerated collagen between layers of granuloma
- Top-to-bottom and side-to-side involvement
- Plasma cells common in the deep dermis
- No mucin
- Rectangular punch due to sclerosis
- May see cholesterol clefts or lymphoid nodules
- Very early lesions can resemble interstitial granuloma annulare

A large proportion of patients with necrobiosis lipoidica have diabetes, thus the original name necrobiosis lipoidica diabeticorum. However, fewer than 1% of patients with diabetes have necrobiosis lipoidica. The pretibial area is the most common site but other areas of the lower extremities, arms, hands, and trunk can rarely be involved.

Necrobiosis lipoidica is considered a palisading granulomatous dermatitis. The palisade is horizontally arranged in tiers like the layers of lasagna. The full thickness of the dermis and often the subcutis is involved.

The term "necrobiosis" refers to alteration of dermal connective tissue with loss of definition, pale staining, and absence of nuclei.

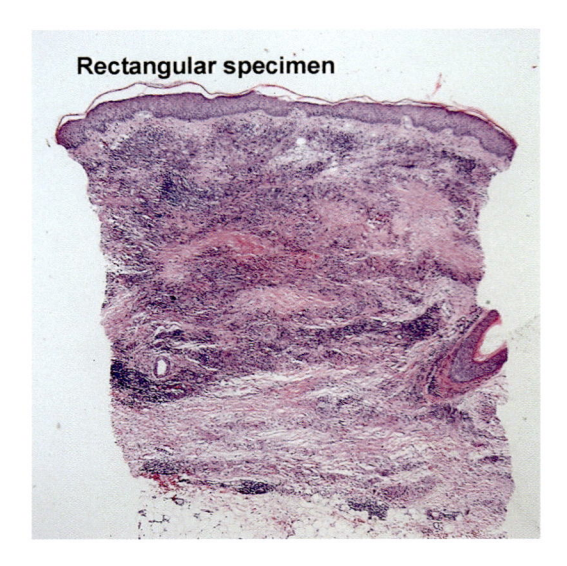

Fig 10-8 Necrobiosis lipoidica

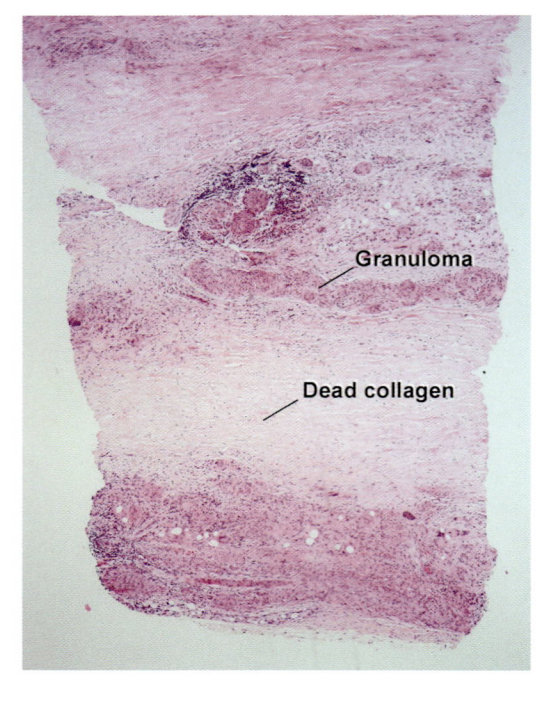

Fig 10-9 Necrobiosis lipoidica (medium-power)

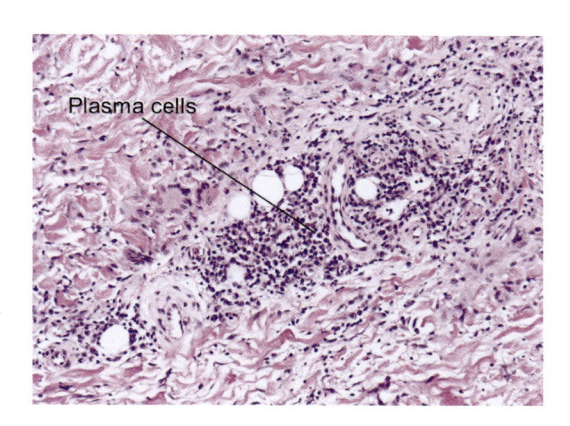

Granulomatous and histiocytic diseases Chapter 10 175

Fig 10-10 Necrobiosis lipoidica

Rheumatoid nodule

Key features

- Large palisading granuloma surrounding deeply staining eosinophilic fibrin
- Deep dermis and subcutis
- No mucin

The histology mimics subcutaneous granuloma annulare and rheumatic fever nodules. Rarely similar nodules occur in systemic lupus erythematosus.

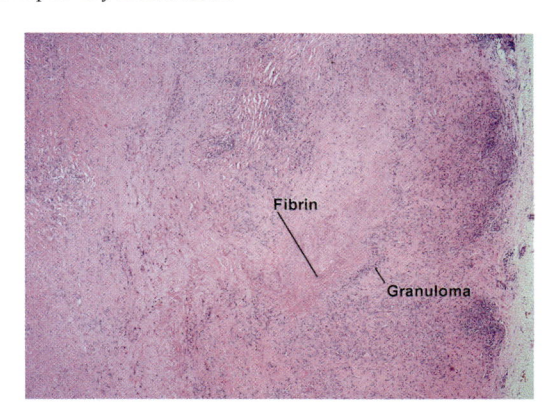

Fig 10-11 Rheumatoid nodule

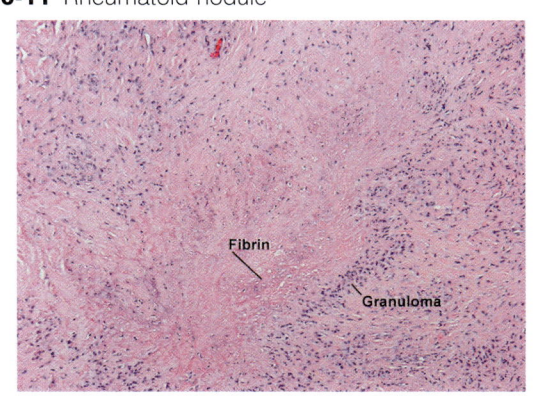

Fig 10-12 Rheumatoid nodule

Lupus miliaris disseminatus faciei (LMDF: acne agminata)

Key features

- Small pea-like palisaded granuloma with central caseous necrosis

Despite its histologic resemblance to miliary tuberculosis, LMDF is a variant of rosacea. LMDF can be distinguished from miliary tuberculosis by the absence of acid-fast bacilli.

Caseation has a dull, pale pink amorphous appearance, unlike the deeply staining fibrin of a rheumatoid nodule.

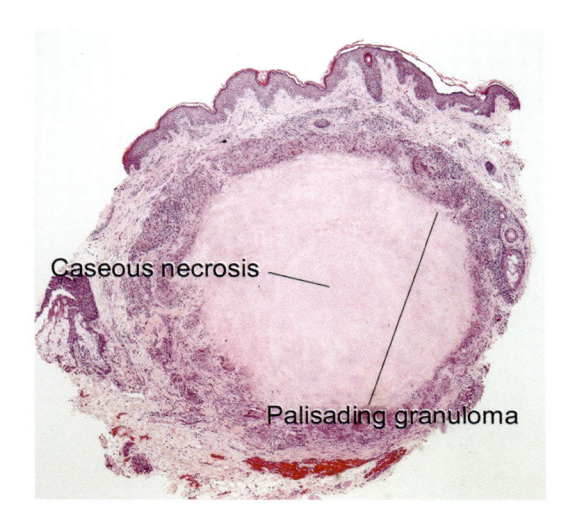

Fig 10-13 Lupus miliaris disseminatus faciei (LMDF)

Sarcoidosis

Key features

- Epithelioid histiocytes forming discrete "naked" granulomas with minimal lymphocytic infiltrate
- No necrosis

Cutaneous lesions are present in up to one-quarter of patients with systemic sarcoidosis, but cutaneous lesions can occur in the absence of systemic disease in one-quarter of patients.

Asteroid bodies and Schaumann bodies can be found in sarcoidosis but are not specific and have been observed in other granulomas such as tuberculosis, leprosy, and berylliosis. An eosinophilic star-burst inclusion within a giant cell is an asteroid body. Schaumann bodies are cytoplasmic, laminated calcifications.

Sarcoidosis is a diagnosis of exclusion requiring clinicopathologic correlation. Infectious etiologies, including acid-fast bacilli and fungi, should be sought with special stains. The granulomas should be polarized to rule out foreign body. However, the presence of small crystalline refractile silica material does not exclude the possibility of sarcoidosis. In fact, silica granulomas may be the earliest manifestation of sarcoidosis ("scar sarcoid").

Differential Diagnosis

The microscopic differential for "naked" granulomas includes:

- Sarcoidosis
- Cutaneous Crohn's disease: perioral or perianal lesions with bowel symptoms
- Cheilitis granulomatosa (Melkersson–Rosenthal syndrome): on the lip
- Tuberculoid leprosy: granulomas follow nerves and acid-fast bacilli may be present
- Silica granuloma/scar sarcoid: polarizable material
- Granulomatous rosacea: adjacent to follicles
- Zirconium and beryllium granulomas: require high index of suspicion and spectrographic analysis

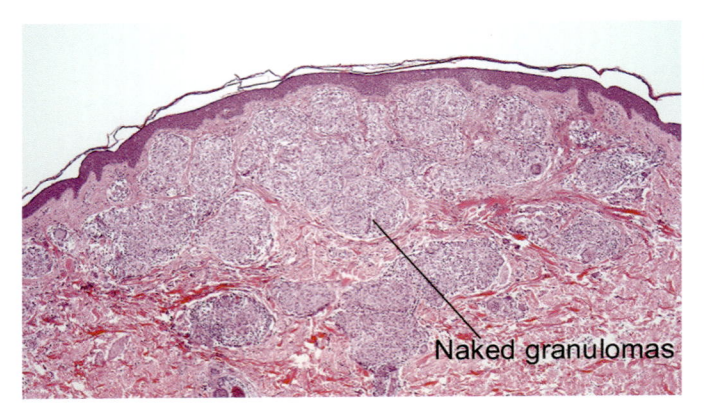

Fig 10-14 Sarcoidosis

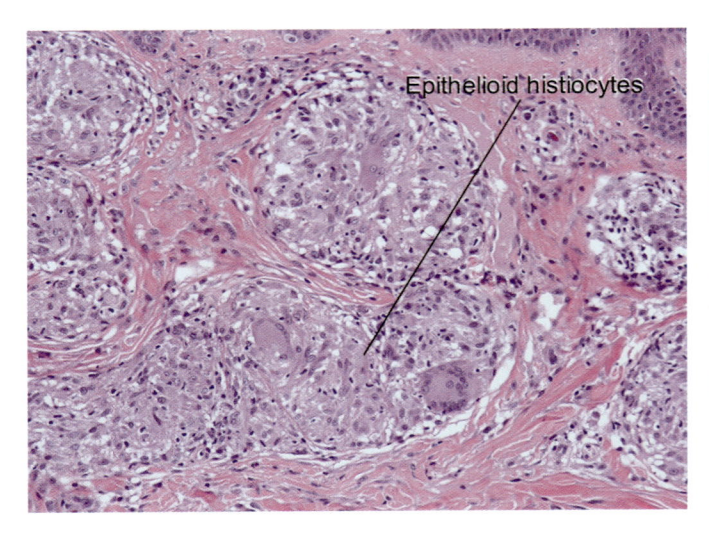

Fig 10-15 Sarcoidosis

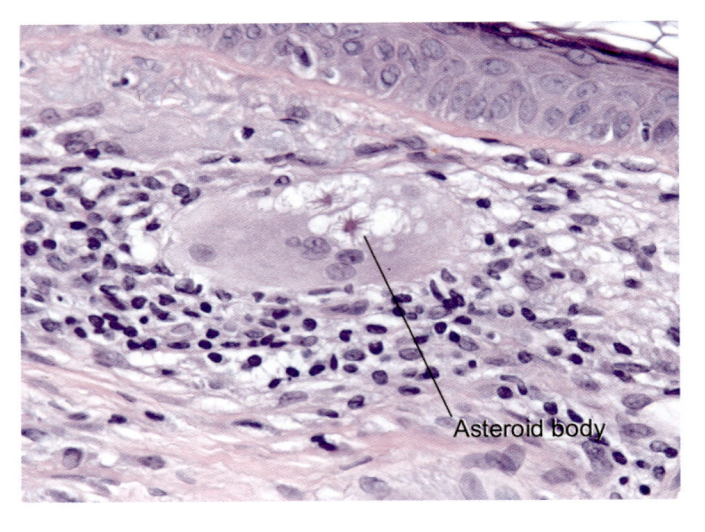

Fig 10-16 Asteroid body

Necrobiotic xanthogranuloma

Key features

- X-shaped red zones of necrosis within granulomatous nodule (X-shaped necrosis in N**X**G)
- Lipidized histiocytes and multinucleate wreath giant cells, including Touton giant cells
- Dermis and subcutis involved
- Neutrophilic debris within necrotic areas
- Cholesterol clefts
- Plasma cells and lymphoid follicles

If the layered appearance of necrobiosis lipoidica is likened to strips of bacon, then the appearance of necrobiotic xanthogranuloma resembles "pepper bacon" or "dirty cholesterol-laden bacon," with karyorrhectic debris making up the "pepper" or "dirt." The differentiation from necrobiosis lipoidica can be made clinically by the periorbital predominance and associated

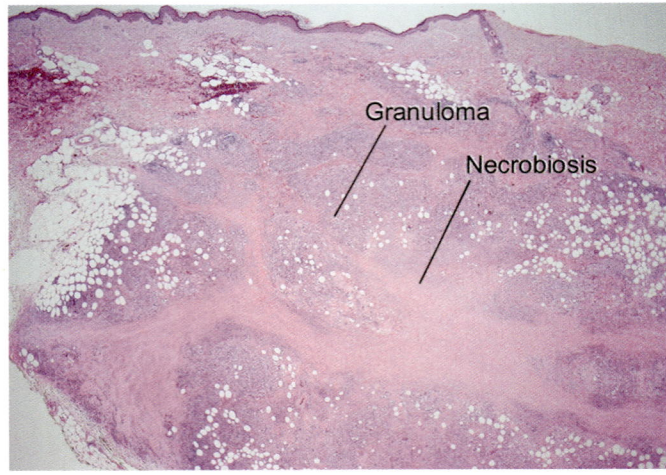

Fig 10-17 Necrobiotic xanthogranuloma

Granulomatous and histiocytic diseases

immunoglobulin (Ig) G (usually kappa) paraproteinemia in necrobiotic xanthogranuloma. Necrobiotic xanthogranuloma is more cellular, has a greater proportion of foamy histiocytes, and contains more giant cells than necrobiosis lipoidica.

Touton giant cells have a ring of nuclei and a peripheral rim of foamy cytoplasm. Touton giant cells are also common in juvenile xanthogranuloma, dermatofibroma, and necrobiotic xanthogranuloma.

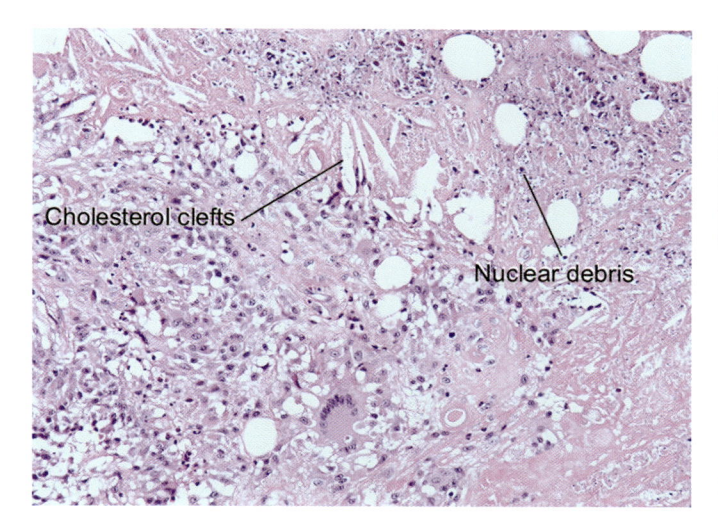

Fig 10-18 Necrobiotic xanthogranuloma

Xanthogranuloma

Key features

- Early: sea of histiocytes in the papillary and reticular dermis
- Later: wreath giant cells appear
- Late: lipidized histiocytes and Touton giant cells
- Secondarily inflamed with lymphocytes and eosinophils

Xanthogranulomas can be seen at any age but are most common in children, giving rise to the name juvenile xanthogranulomas.

Early xanthogranulomas are clinically red and consist of numerous histiocytes with abundant cytoplasm, giving the impression of a sea of lavender histologically. Over time, the histiocytes become lipidized and the lesion clinically becomes yellow-orange. At this point, Touton giant cells, with a wreath of nuclei surrounded by foamy cytoplasm, are identified. Regressing lesions show a proliferation of fibroblasts and fibrosis. In contrast to those in dermatofibromas, the Touton giant cells in xanthogranulomas never contain hemosiderin.

In children with multiple xanthogranulomas, an eye exam should be considered as ocular involvement can result in glaucoma or anterior-chamber hemorrhage. Visceral xanthogranulomas with pericarditis have been reported. An association between xanthogranuloma, neurofibromatosis I, and juvenile chronic myelogenous leukemia has been identified.

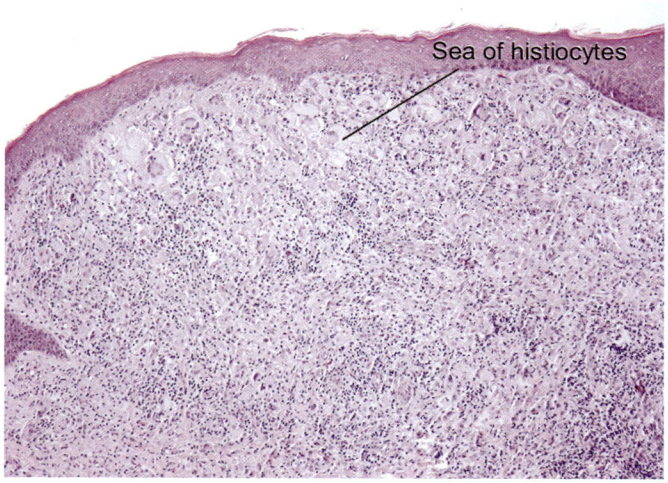

Fig 10-19 Xanthogranuloma

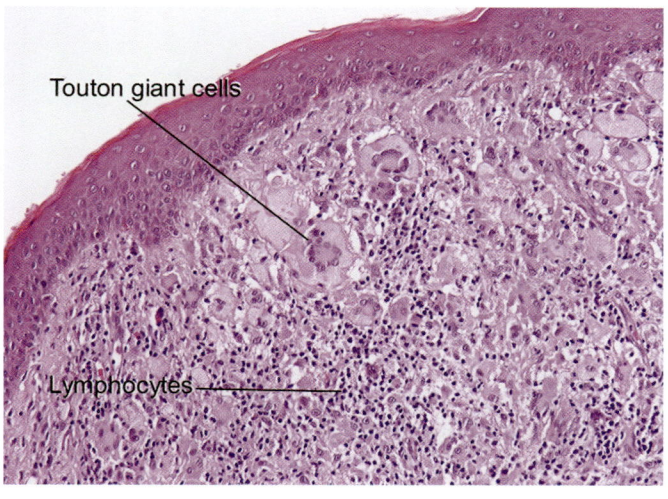

Fig 10-20 Xanthogranuloma

Reticulohistiocytic granuloma (solitary reticulohistiocytoma)

Key features

- Sea of histiocytes in dermis
- Each histiocyte often sits in a punched-out lacuna
- Cytoplasm of histiocyte is two-toned with darker and lighter areas
- Cytoplasm is dusty rose or ground glass
- Binucleate and multinucleate cells occur

Dermatopathology

Multinucleate cells typically have irregularly arranged vesicular nuclei containing prominent nucleoli. There are admixed lymphocytes and lesser numbers of eosinophils and neutrophils. Older lesions are less inflammatory and reveal cells with artifactual halos around them due to retraction.

Lesions can be solitary or multiple. When multiple they may be associated with systemic findings. Multicentric reticulohistiocytosis consists of multiple lesions with deforming arthritis, coral beading around the nail folds, and an associated internal malignancy in 10% of cases.

Differential Diagnosis

Xanthogranulomas have more foamy cells, including Touton giant cells, and are much less likely to have cells with ground-glass cytoplasm.

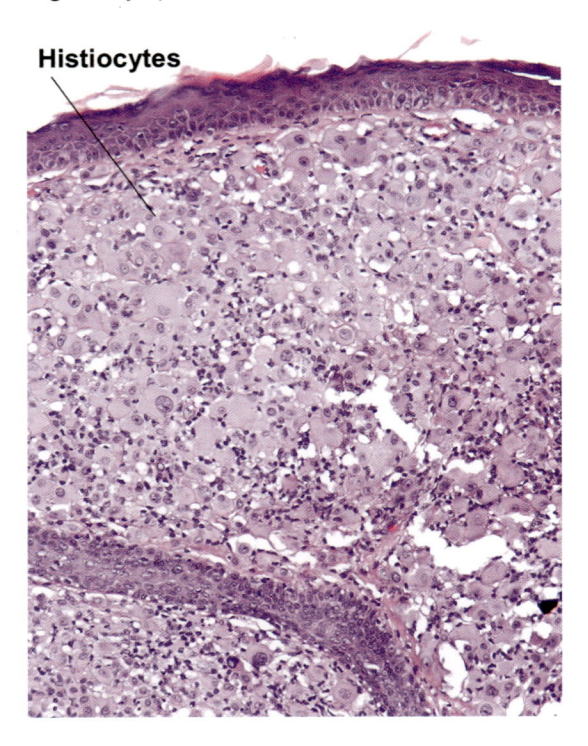

Fig 10-21 Reticulohistiocytic granuloma

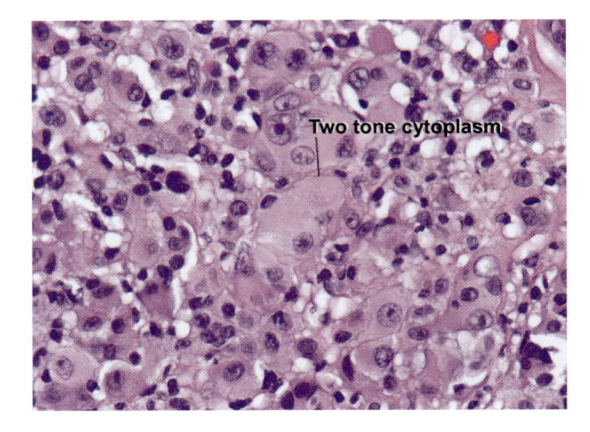

Fig 10-22 Reticulohistiocytic granuloma

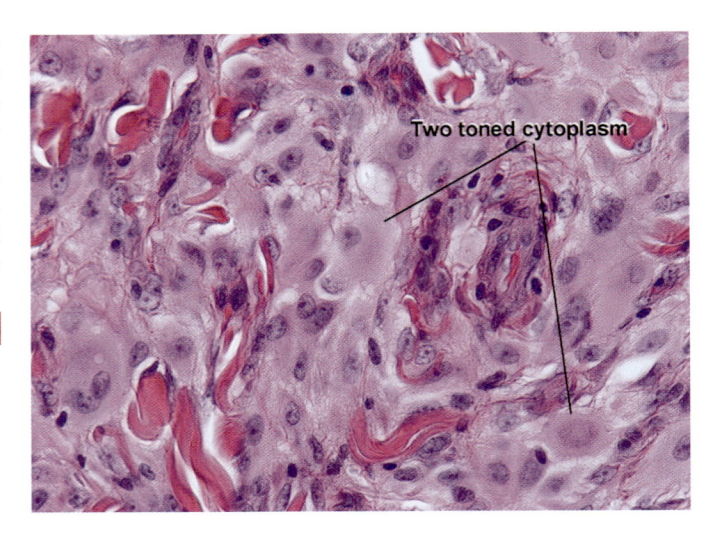

Fig 10-23 Reticulohistiocytic granuloma

Rosai–Dorfman disease (sinus histiocytosis with massive lymphadenopathy)

Key features

- Fibrotic nodules
- Sheets of lymphocytes and histiocytes
- Emperipolesis (intact cells, especially lymphocytes and plasma cells, passing through histiocytes)
- S100-positive, CD1a-negative, CD68+

Rosai–Dorfman disease typically occurs in the first two decades of life as painless cervical adenopathy and fever. There is extranodal involvement in one-third of cases. Skin lesions are found in approximately 10% with a predilection for the eyelids and the malar area. Occasionally, the skin is the only site of involvement. Emperipolesis is a phenomenon where lymphocytes and plasma cells pass through histiocytes, but are not found within phagolysosomes.

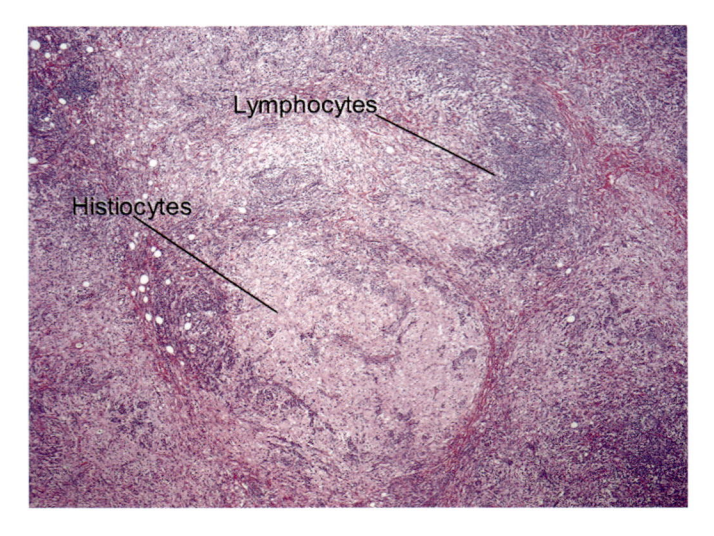

Fig 10-24 Rosai–Dorfman disease

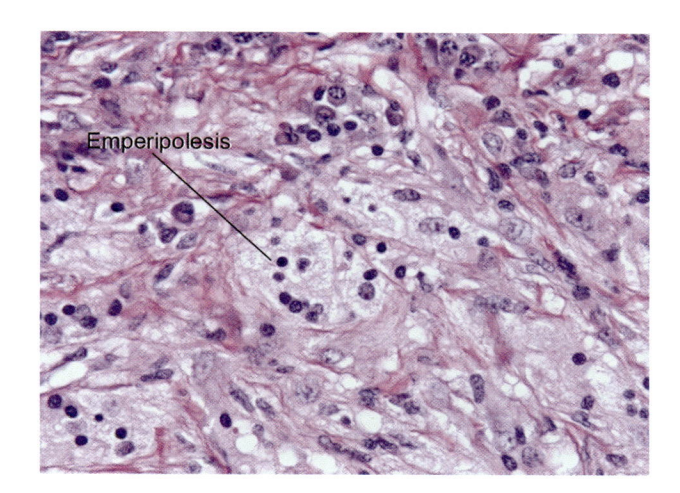

Granulomatous and histiocytic diseases

Fig 10-25 Rosai–Dorfman disease emperipolesis

Langerhans cell histiocytosis (histiocytosis X)

Key features

- Polymorphous infiltrate with prominent edema and hemorrhage
- Reniform (kidney bean-shaped) nuclei
- Folliculotropism common in acute type
- S100-positive, CD1a-positive, peanut agglutinin-positive, langerin positive

The infiltrate can be a perivascular, band-like, or periappendageal pattern. Variable eosinophils, lymphocytes, and sparse neutrophils accompany the characteristic large cells with lobulated, notched, or grooved nuclei that resemble kidney beans. Due to the edema, these cells appear to be "floating in the sea." Acute Langerhans cell histiocytosis is described in further detail in Chapter 15.

In the past, Langerhans cell histiocytosis was subclassified into Letterer–Siwe disease, Hand–Schüller–Christian disease, or eosinophilic granuloma, based on the clinical findings. Eosinophilic granuloma is typically localized to one site, such as bone or skin, whereas the other two affect several organ systems. Hand–Schüller–Christian disease is typically associated with the triad of diabetes insipidus, exophthalmos, and lytic bone lesions. Letterer–Siwe disease is more disseminated and involves multiple organs. As many patients do not clearly fit into these categories, the prognosis is currently based on the patient's age, number of organs involved, and the degree of organ dysfunction. Children are most commonly affected but adult cases have been observed. The scalp, ears, and intertriginous areas are preferred cutaneous sites.

Similar to Langerhans cells of normal skin, Birbeck granules, with the appearance of a tennis racket, are pathognomonic ultrastructural markers.

Congenital self-healing "reticulohistiocytosis" is a form of Langerhans cell histiocytosis that generally presents with one or several cutaneous nodules, at or shortly after birth, and resolves spontaneously.

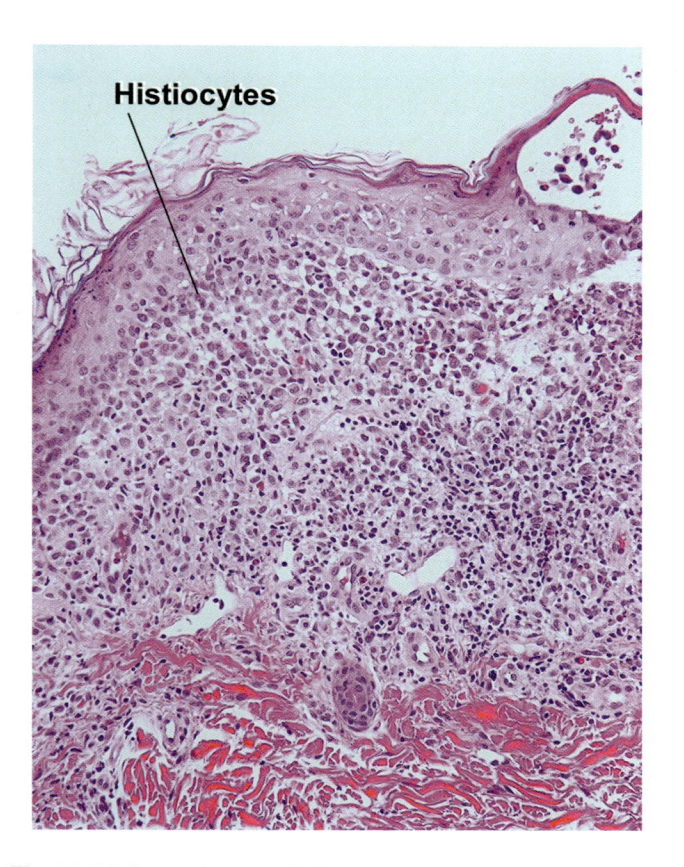

Fig 10-26 Langerhans cell histiocytosis

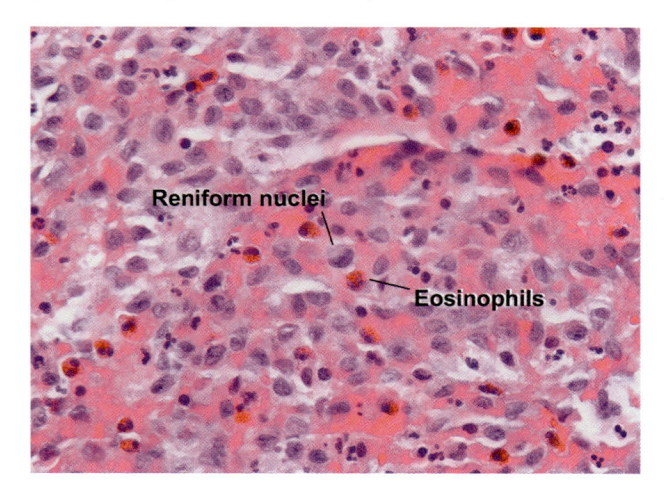

Fig 10-27 Langerhans cell histiocytosis

Xanthomas

Xanthomas represent the accumulation of lipid in histiocytes, known as foam cells or xanthoma cells. Xanthomas can be subdivided by clinical morphology, anatomic location, and mode of development into: tuberous, tendinous, eruptive, planar, and verruciform. Many are associated with inherited or acquired disorders of lipoprotein metabolism but normolipemic planar xanthoma is related to plasma cell dyscrasia.

Planar xanthomas are further subdivided on the basis of their location into xanthelasma, intertriginous xanthomas, xanthoma striatum palmaris, and diffuse (generalized) plane xanthomas.

Intertriginous xanthomas are pathognomonic of homozygous familial hypercholesterolemia. Xanthoma striatum palmaris is characteristic of familial dysbetalipoproteinemia (type III) and, as the name describes, are identified in the palmar creases. The great majority of patients with diffuse plane xanthomas are normolipemic, and there is an association with IgG paraproteinemia and progression to myeloma.

Xanthelasma

Key features

- Thin skin, many vellus follicles, and striated muscle suggest the eyelid location
- Foam cells form a band in the superficial or mid dermis

Xanthelasma are the most common form of xanthoma and are characterized by periorbital yellowish plaques. Lipid levels are normal in around half of patients.

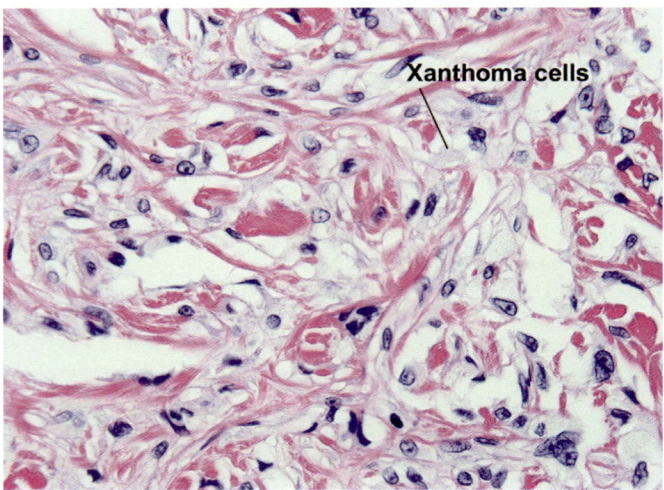

Tuberous xanthoma

Key features

- Fibrotic nodule with variable and occasionally sparse foam cells
- Cholesterol clefts may be found

Tuberous xanthomas are typically seen on the elbows, knees, and buttock, in cases with an increase in chylomicron and very-low-density lipoprotein remnants. These lesions are most characteristic of familial dysbetalipoproteinemia (type II), but can also be seen in homozygous and heterozygous hypercholesterolemia, hepatic cholestasis, cerebrotendinous xanthoma, and ß-sitosterolemia.

Tendinous xanthomas are histologically similar to tuberous xanthomas, except they occur in ligaments, fasciae, and tendons, especially the tendons of the hands and feet and the Achilles tendon. These lesions are most common with severe familial hypercholesterolemia.

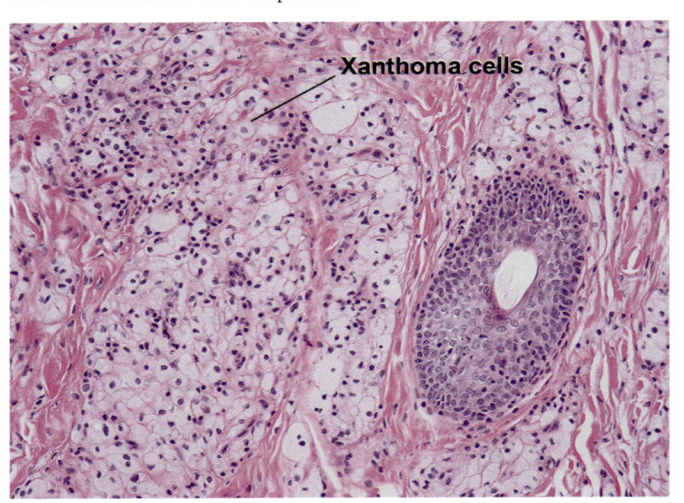

Fig 10-28 Xanthelasma

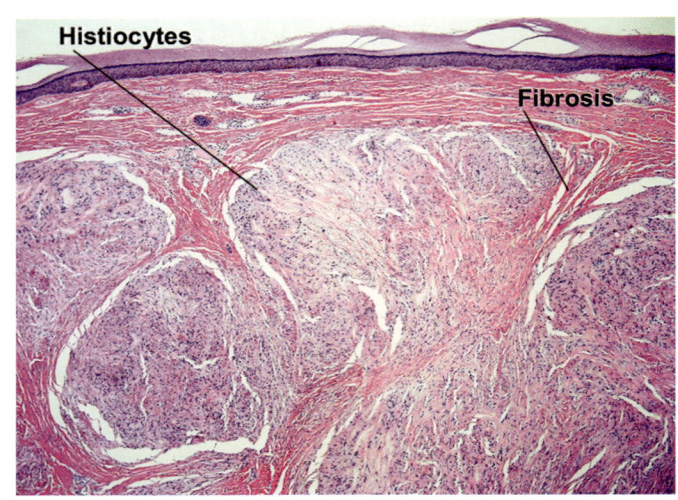

Fig 10-30 Tuberous xanthoma

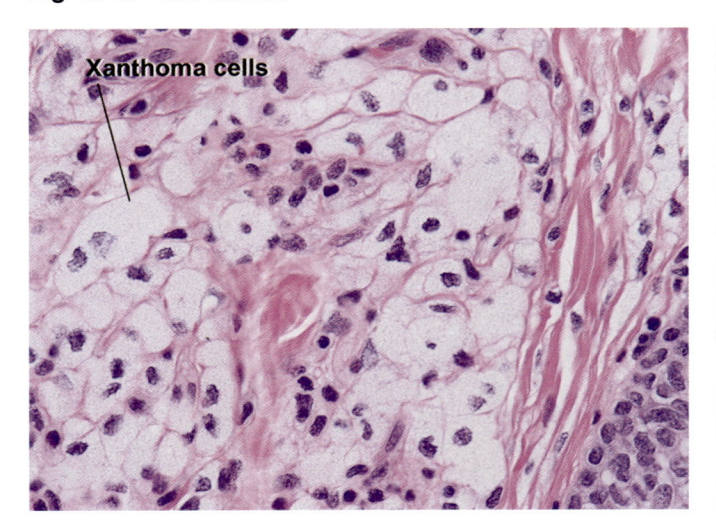

Fig 10-29 Xanthelasma

Fig 10-31 Tuberous xanthoma

Granulomatous and histiocytic diseases — Chapter 10

Eruptive xanthoma

Key features

- Foam cells and extracellular lipid
- Scattered lymphocytes and neutrophils, especially in early lesions

The lipid deposition in the dermis is so rapid in eruptive lesions that the phagocytic capacity of the histiocytes is overwhelmed, resulting in free or extracellular lipid.

Eruptive lesions are most common on the buttock and thigh as crops of yellow papules with a red halo. These lesions are associated with an increase in serum chylomicrons, as in uncontrolled diabetes, hypothyroidism, following alcohol ingestion, and use of exogenous estrogens or retinoids. Genetic associations include lipoprotein lipase deficiency type I, type IV, and type V (less commonly type III) for eruptive xanthoma.

Differential Diagnosis

Histologically, eruptive xanthomas may be confused with granuloma annulare at scan. However, on close inspection, there is intracellular and extracellular lipid in the xanthoma rather than extracellular mucin of granuloma annulare. Gout may also be considered in the differential diagnosis but the material deposited in gout is feathery and there are no foam cells.

Verruciform xanthoma

Key features

- Papillomatosis
- Foam cells in the dermal papillae
- Orange-hued parakeratosis forms V-shapes pointing downward towards xanthoma cells

Verruciform xanthomas are not associated with increased serum lipids and may be due to degeneration of or damage to cells in the overlying epidermis. Oral lesions are common, although genital sites, extragenital skin, and nail beds may be involved.

Differential Diagnosis

The low-power appearance is that of verruca. Close inspection reveals the foamy histiocytes.

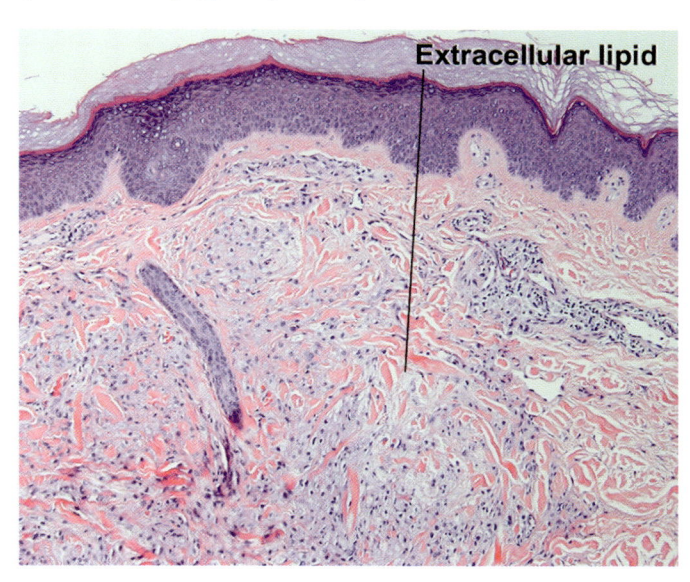

Fig 10-32 Eruptive xanthoma

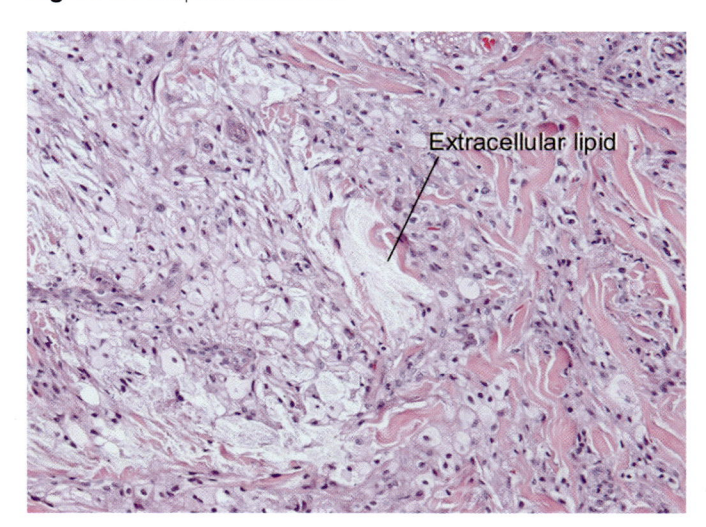

Fig 10-33 Eruptive xanthoma

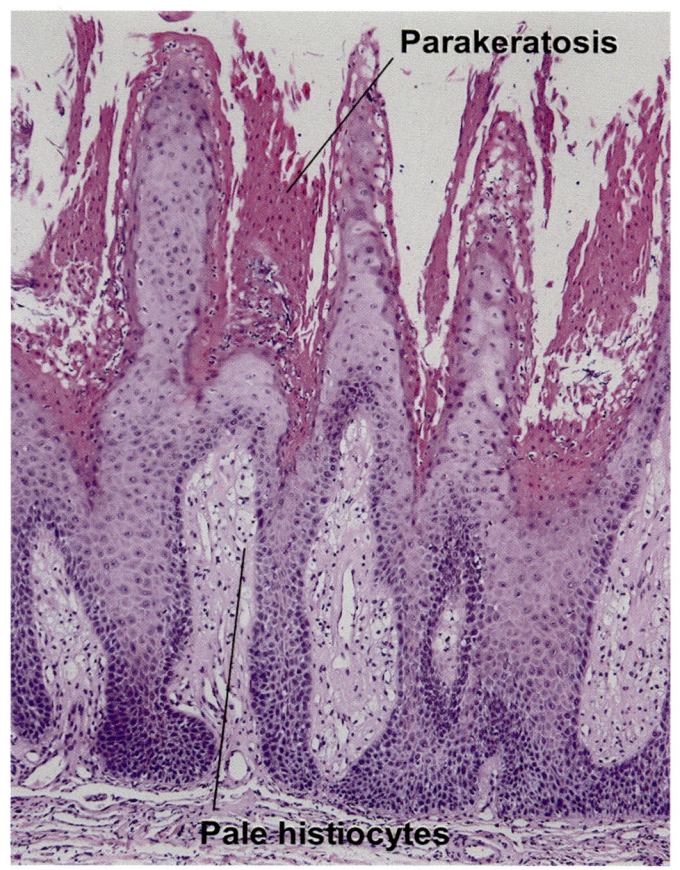

Fig 10-34 Verruciform xanthoma

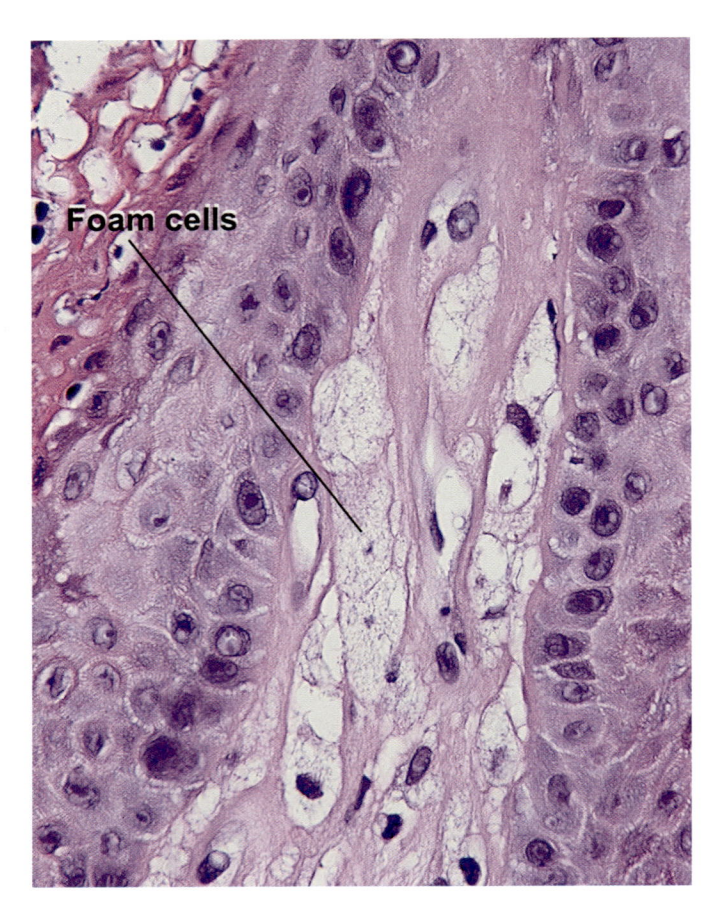

Fig 10-35 Verruciform xanthoma

Further reading

Beatty EC Jr. Rheumatic-like nodules occurring in nonrheumatic children. AMA Arch Pathol 1959;68(2):154–159.

de Oliveira FL, de Barros Silveira LK, Machado Ade M, et al. Hybrid clinical and histopathological pattern in annular lesions: an overlap between annular elastolytic giant cell granuloma and granuloma annulare? Case Rep Dermatol Med 2012:102915.

Eisen RN, Buckley PJ, Rosai J. Immunophenotypic characterization of sinus histiocytosis with massive lymphadenopathy (Rosai–Dorfman disease). Semin Diagn Pathol 1990;7(1):74–82.

el Darouti M, Zaher H. Lupus miliaris disseminatus faciei – pathologic study of early, fully developed, and late lesions. Int J Dermatol 1993;32(7):508–511.

Finan MC, Winkelmann RK. Necrobiotic xanthogranuloma with paraproteinemia. A review of 22 cases. Medicine (Baltimore) 1986;65(6):376–388.

Hanke CW, Bailin PL, Roenigk HH Jr. Annular elastolytic giant cell granuloma. A clinicopathologic study of five cases and a review of similar entities. J Am Acad Dermatol 1979;1(5):413–421.

Hanno R, Needelman A, Eiferman RA, et al. Cutaneous sarcoidal granulomas and the development of systemic sarcoidosis. Arch Dermatol 1981;117(4):203–207.

Helm KF, Lookingbill DP, Marks JG Jr. A clinical and pathologic study of histiocytosis X in adults. J Am Acad Dermatol 1993;29(2 Pt 1):166–170.

Mehregan AH, Altman J. Miescher's granuloma of the face. A variant of the necrobiosis lipoidica–granuloma annulare spectrum. Arch Dermatol 1973;107(1):62–64.

Mohsin SK, Lee MW, Amin MB, et al. Cutaneous verruciform xanthoma: a report of five cases investigating the etiology and nature of xanthomatous cells. Am J Surg Pathol 1998;22(4):479–487.

O'Brien JP. Actinic granuloma. An annular connective tissue disorder affecting sun- and heat-damaged (elastotic) skin. Arch Dermatol 1975;111(4):460–466.

Silverman RA, Rabinowitz AD. Eosinophils in the cellular infiltrate of granuloma annulare. J Cutan Pathol 1985;12(1):13–17.

Walsh NM, Hanly JG, Tremaine R, et al. Cutaneous sarcoidosis and foreign bodies. Am J Dermatopathol 1993;15(3):203–207.

Inflammatory vascular diseases

Dirk M. Elston

Leukocytoclastic vasculitis (LCV)

Key features

- Perivascular infiltrate with neutrophils
- Karyorrhexis (nuclear dust, leukocytoclasis)
- Expansion of the vessel wall
- Fibrin deposition within the vessel wall
- Erythrocyte extravasation

Clinical lesions of leukocytoclastic vasculitis are purpuric, and often palpable. Vasculitis involving arterioles commonly produces livedo reticularis or stellate infarcts.

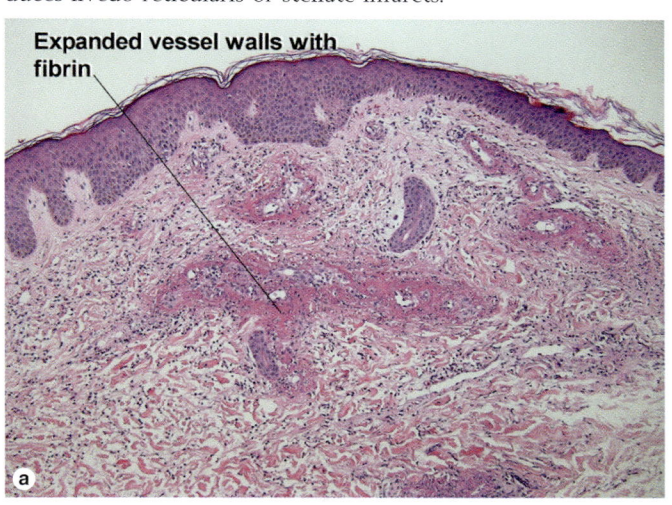

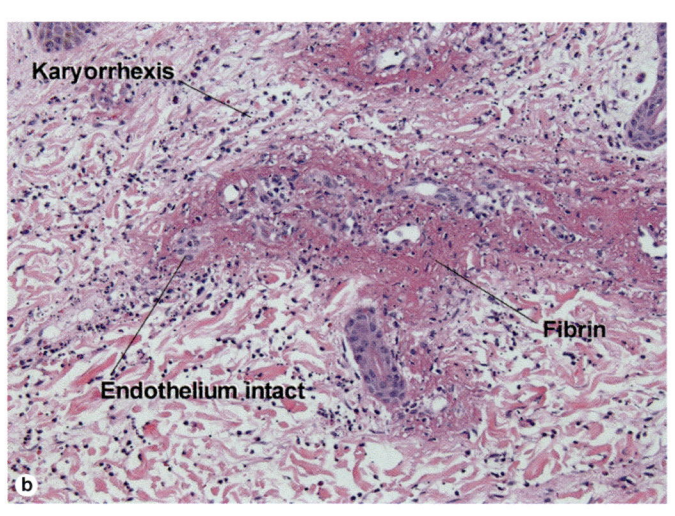

Fig 11-1 Leukocytoclastic vasculitis

Classification of vasculitis

Vasculitis is classified by the type of inflammatory infiltrate, type of vessel involved, the presence or absence of endothelial necrosis, associated systemic findings, immunofluorescent patterns, and serologic findings. American College of Rheumatology (ACR) classification criteria are mostly clinical, with little emphasis on histologic findings. The Chapel Hill criteria include histologic features, especially vessel size. As many entities demonstrate involvement of vessels of various sizes, any classification will have limitations.

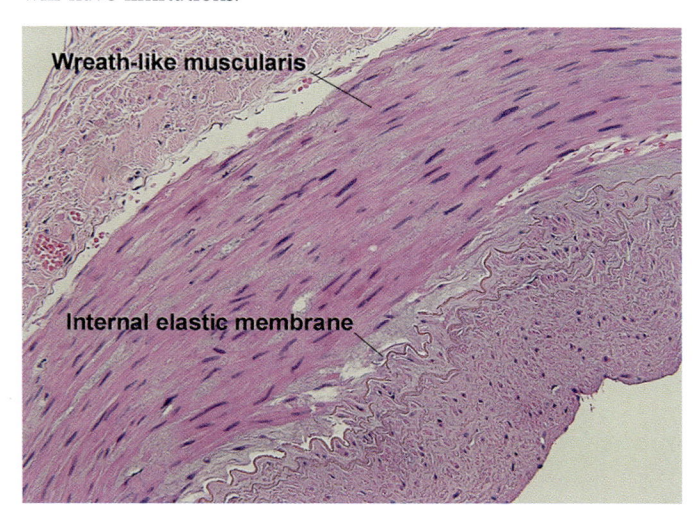

Fig 11-2 Characteristic features of an artery

Large vessel vasculitis

When a large vessel is involved by vasculitis, it is critical to determine whether the involved vessel is an artery or a vein. Arteries are characteristically round, with a wreath-like muscularis and an internal elastic membrane. Veins are characteristically oval, with a bundled muscularis. They may have visible valves, and lack an internal elastic membrane. So-called "arterialization" of veins occurs when they are subjected to elevated hydrostatic pressure. This phenomenon is occasionally noted in cutaneous vessels, but is best demonstrated in coronary artery bypass grafts. The grafted vein develops a prominent internal elastic membrane, but retains the bundled muscularis characteristic of a vein.

Giant cell arteritis (temporal arteritis)

Key features

- Muscular artery with wreath-like muscularis and prominent internal elastic membrane

Dermatopathology

- Subendothelial granulomatous inflammation
- With progression, becomes transmural inflammation
- Incidental atherosclerotic changes (calcification, subintimal plaques) often present in the vessel

Temporal arteritis often involves the vessel in a focal, beaded fashion, so an adequate length of temporal artery (ideally 2 cm) should be submitted for examination.

Chapel Hill criteria
Granulomatous arteritis involving the major branches of the aorta, with a predilection for the extracranial branches of the carotid artery. The temporal artery is frequently involved. Patients are usually >50 years of age. Frequently associated with polymyalgia rheumatica.

American College of Rheumatology criteria
Age >50; new headache; abnormal temporal artery clinically; elevated sedimentation rate; positive temporal artery biopsy (three criteria give >93% sensitivity, >91% specificity).

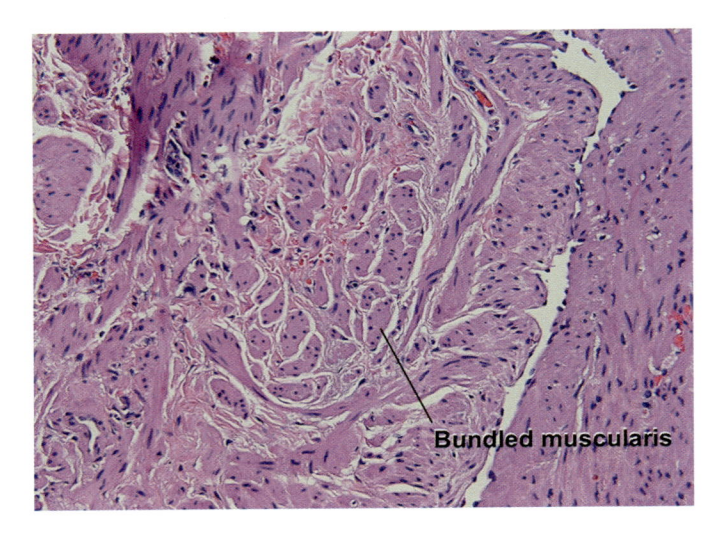

Fig 11-3 Characteristic features of a vein

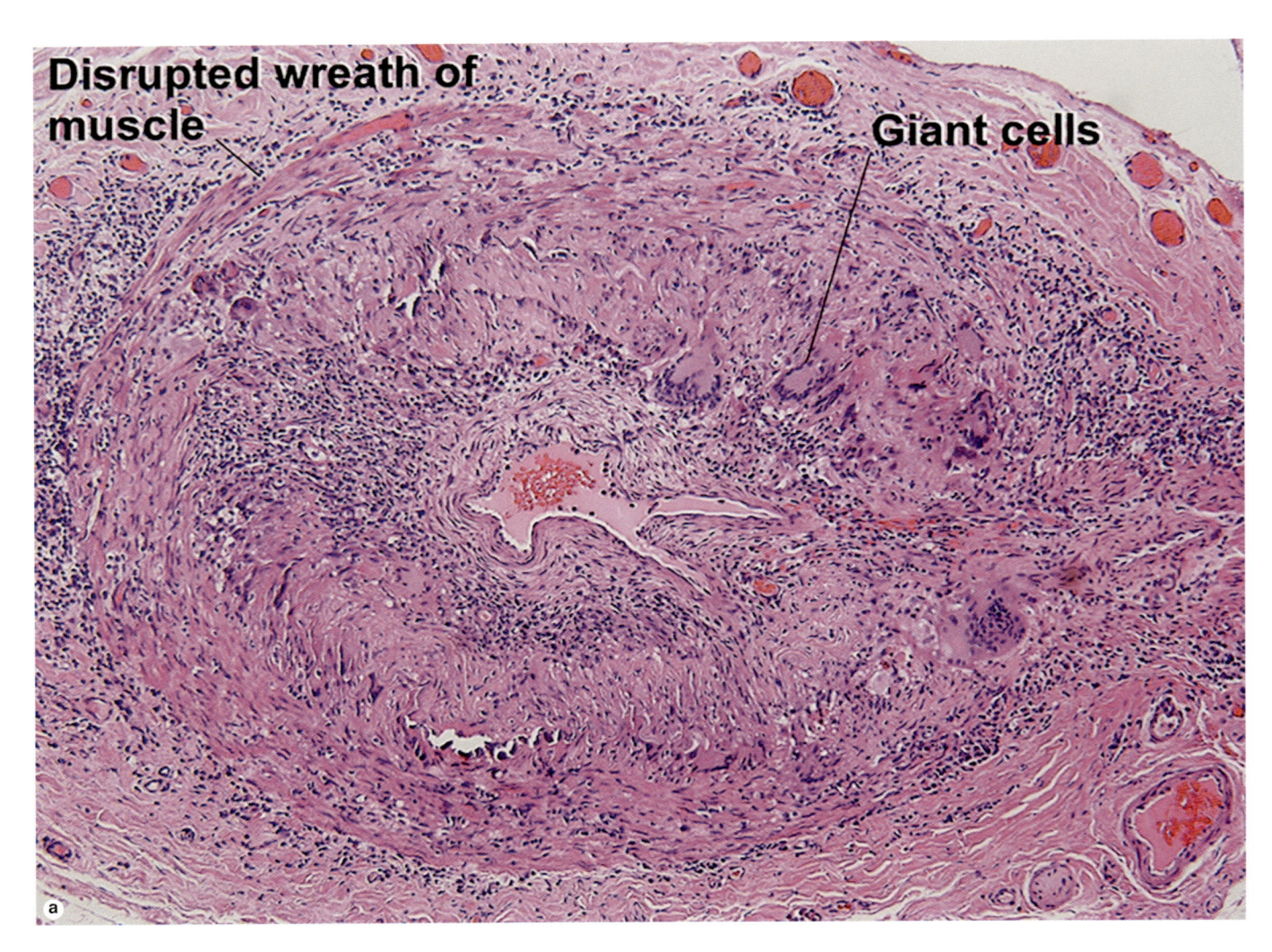

Fig 11-4 Temporal arteritis

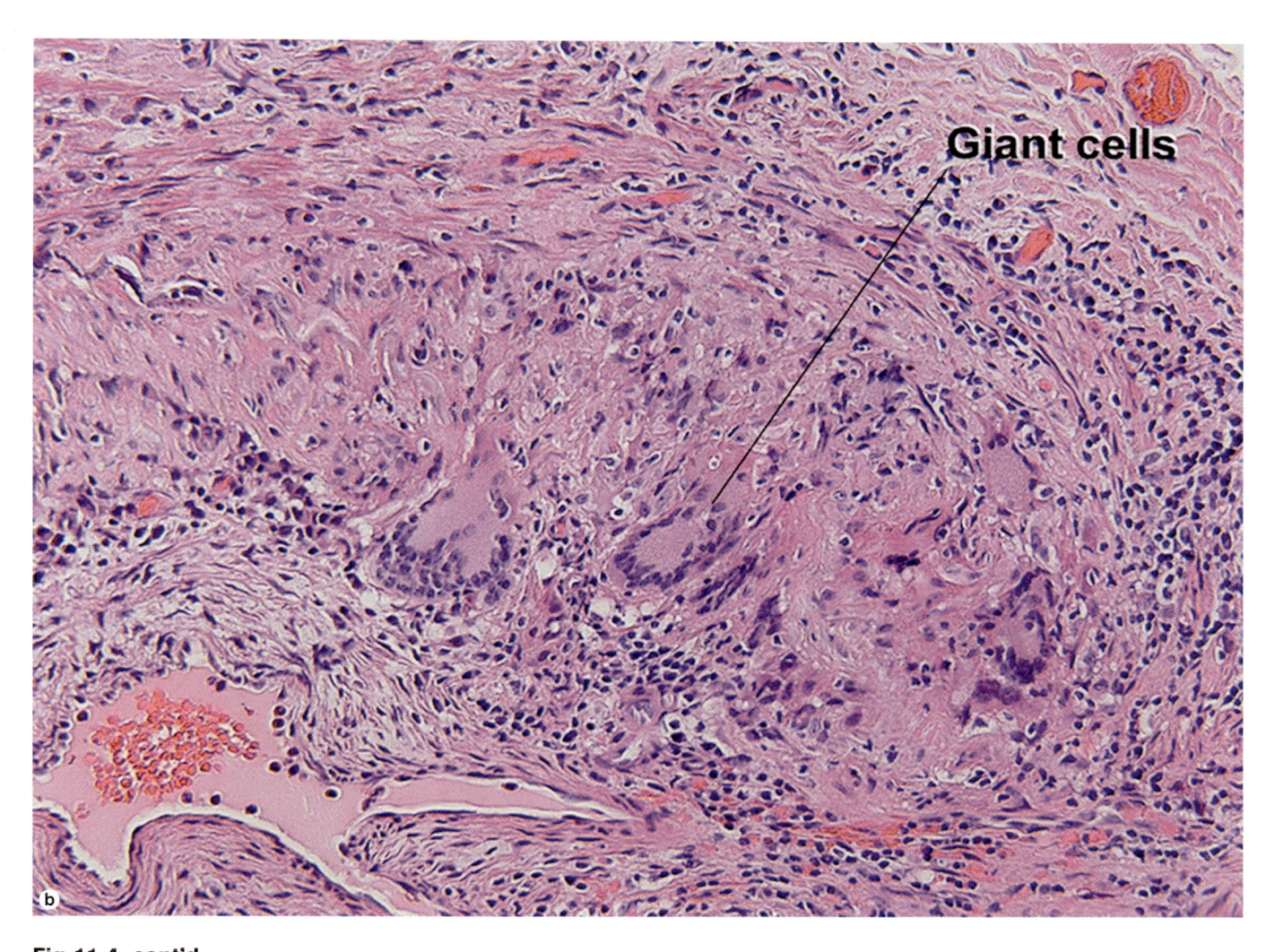

Inflammatory vascular diseases **Chapter 11** 185

Fig 11-4, cont'd
Takayasu arteritis

Key features

- Granulomatous vasculitis involving large muscular arteries

Chapel Hill criteria
Granulomatous arteritis involving the aorta and its major branches. Usually <50 years of age.

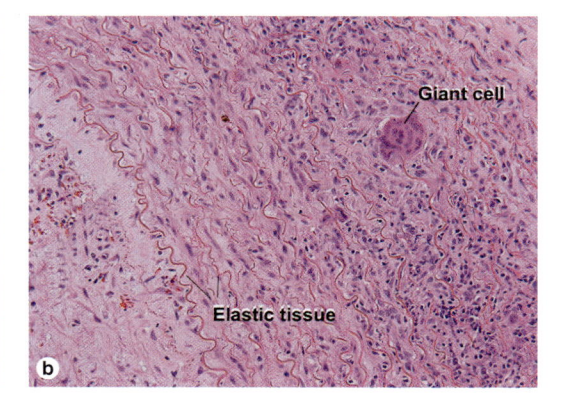

Fig 11-5 Takayasu arteritis

Continued

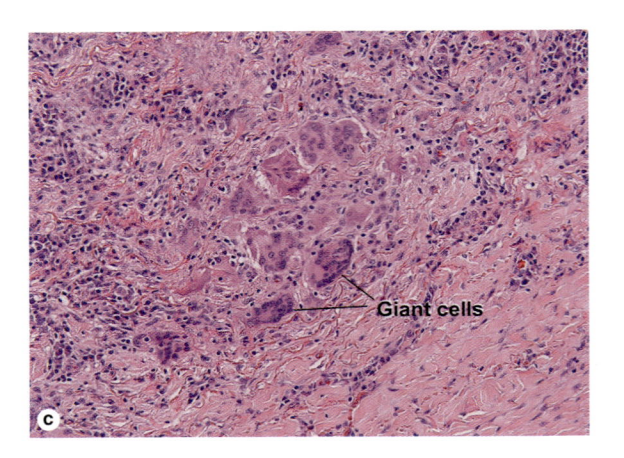

Fig 11-5, cont'd

American College of Rheumatology criteria
Age <40; claudication; decreased pulses; >10 mmHg difference in pressure between arms; bruits; abnormal arteriogram (three criteria give >90% sensitivity, >97% specificity).

Polyarteritis nodosa

> **Key features**
> - Large artery involved, typically in the deep dermis or subcutaneous tissue
> - Often involves branch points of vessels
> - Acute phase is neutrophilic with karyorrhexis
> - Chronic phase may demonstrate a granulomatous component
> - Fat necrosis is common

Polyarteritis nodosa commonly presents with livedo reticularis and subcutaneous erythematous or hyperpigmented nodules. The biopsy typically demonstrates neutrophilic vasculitis involving an artery within the subcutaneous fat. Surrounding lobular necrosis is present.

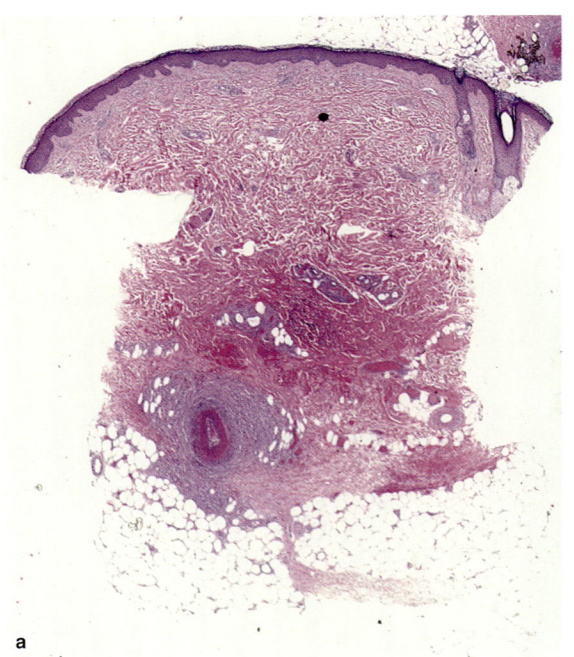

Chapel Hill criteria
Necrotizing inflammation involving medium or small arteries without glomerulonephritis or vasculitis in arterioles, capillaries or venules.

American College of Rheumatology criteria
Weight loss >4 kg; livedo reticularis; testicular pain or tenderness; myalgia/myopathy, or muscle tenderness; neuropathy; hypertension (diastolic >90); renal impairment; hepatitis B infection; abnormal arteriogram; biopsy of an artery with neutrophilic inflammation (three criteria give >82% sensitivity, >86% specificity).

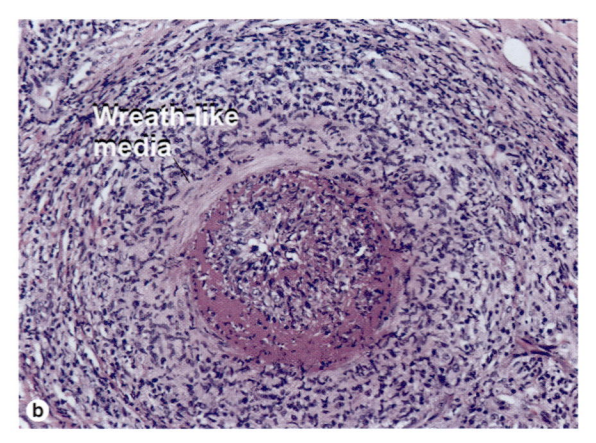

Fig 11-6 Polyarteritis nodosa

Inflammatory vascular diseases — Chapter 11

Thrombophlebitis

Key features

- Vasculitis involving an oval vessel with bundled muscularis
- Vessel lacks an internal elastic membrane and may contain valves
- Thrombus present within vessel

Thromboangiitis obliterans (Buerger's disease)

Key features

- Endarteritis
- Prominent neutrophilic inflammation involving the thrombus

Buerger's disease is a rare disease typically seen in male smokers. It is characterized by a combination of acute inflammation and thrombosis of large distal extremity vessels.

American College of Rheumatology criteria

Age >50; history of smoking; distal peripheral vascular obstructive disease (below knee or elbow); and three additional criteria, such as thrombophlebitis saltans/migrans; involvement of upper extremity; characteristic angiography.

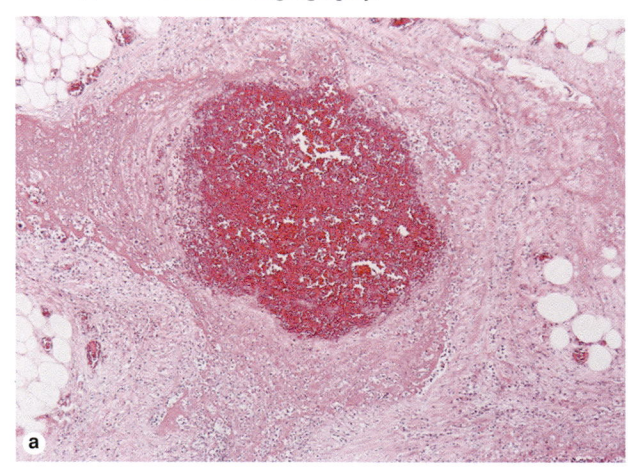

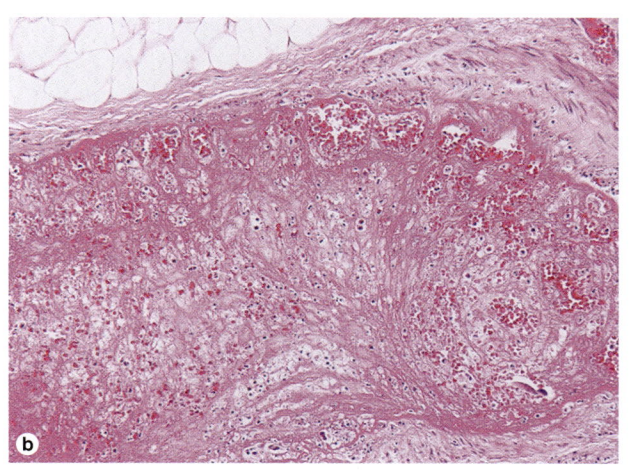

Fig 11-7 Buerger's disease

Medium vessel vasculitis

Key features

- Involves a mix of vessel sizes (post-capillary venules *plus* larger deeper vessels)
- Endothelial necrosis is common
- Often ANCA (anti-neutrophil cytoplasmic antibody)-associated
- The most common causes include:
  - *Wegener's granulomatosis (commonly c-ANCA/anti-proteinase 3)*
  - *Churg–Strauss syndrome (commonly p-ANCA/anti-myeloperoxidase)*
  - *Microscopic polyangiitis (commonly p-ANCA/anti-myeloperoxidase)*
  - *Septic vasculitis*
  - *Rheumatoid vasculitis*
- This group of five disorders is sometimes referred to as the "big 5" because the vessels include those bigger than the post-capillary venule and the patients are often in bigger trouble.

These diseases are characterized by leukocytoclastic vasculitis involving vessels larger than the post-capillary venule. The endothelium is frequently necrotic. The biopsy demonstrates a superficial and deep perivascular infiltrate with neutrophils, karyorrhexis, expansion of the vessel wall, fibrin deposition within the vessel wall, and erythrocyte extravasation.

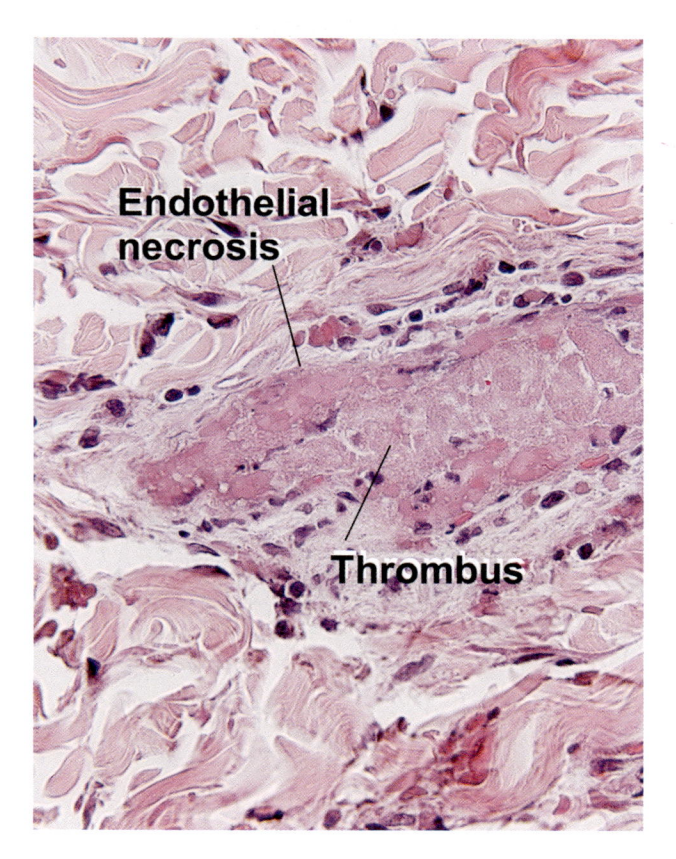

Fig 11-8 "Big 5" pattern of vasculitis

Wegener's granulomatosis

Key features

- Leukocytoclastic vasculitis involving a mix of vessel sizes (post-capillary venule plus larger deeper vessels)
- Endothelial necrosis is common
- May involve skin, upper respiratory tract, kidneys
- LCV evolves into stellate abscess (palisaded granuloma with central neutrophils)
- Giant cells present in the granuloma

Wegener's granulomatosis commonly involves the upper airway. The skin of the nose may become necrotic. Skin lesions may occur in other locations, especially the extremities. The histologic pattern is that of a "big 5" vasculitic disorder. Individual vasculitic foci may evolve into stellate abscesses (palisaded granulomas with a central stellate collection of neutrophils). Multinucleate giant cells are present in the granulomas. Granulomatous vasculitis may be present in medium-sized vessels.

Chapel Hill criteria
Granulomatous inflammation of the respiratory tract; necrotizing vasculitis of small to medium vessels; necrotizing glomerulonephritis common.

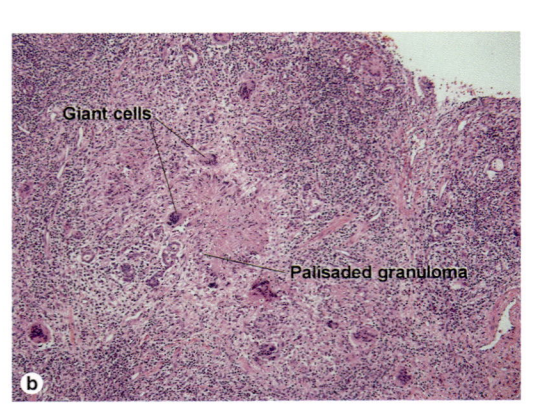

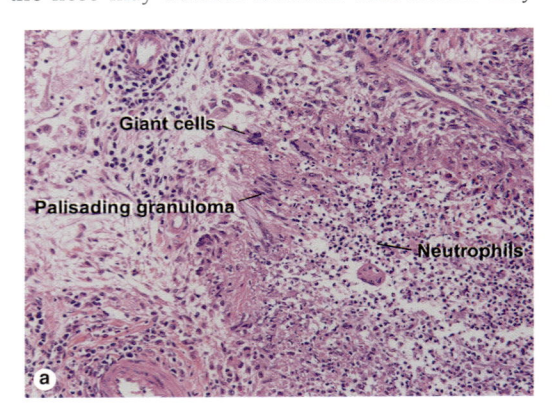

Fig 11-9 Wegener's granulomatosis, palisading granuloma with stellate abscess

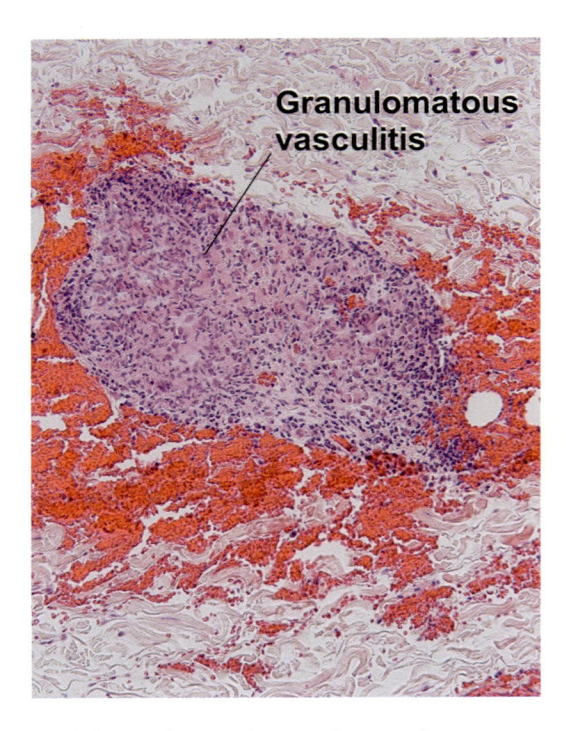

American College of Rheumatology criteria
Nasal or oral inflammation; chest X-ray with nodules; infiltrate or cavities; microscopic hematuria or red cell casts; granulomatous inflammation on biopsy (two criteria give >88% sensitivity, >92% specificity).

Differential Diagnosis

Palisaded granulomatous dermatitis with stellate abscess formation may be seen in Wegener's granulomatosis (giant cells peripherally, neutrophils centrally), Churg–Strauss syndrome (epithelioid cells peripherally, eosinophils centrally), atypical mycobacterial infection, sporotrichosis, nocardiosis, cat scratch disease, lymphogranuloma venereum, and tularemia.

Churg–Strauss syndrome

Key features

- Leukocytoclastic vasculitis involving a mix of vessel sizes (post-capillary venule plus larger deeper vessels)
- Endothelial necrosis is common
- Asthma common
- May involve skin and kidneys
- LCV may produce stellate abscesses (palisaded granuloma with central eosinophils)
- Granuloma composed of epithelioid cells without giant cells

Fig 11-10 Wegener's granulomatosis, granulomatous vasculitis

The Churg–Strauss syndrome is a vasculitic disorder that commonly presents with a prodrome of asthma. Some cases have been induced by leukotriene inhibitors.

Inflammatory vascular diseases

The histologic pattern is that of a "big 5" vasculitic disorder. Palisaded granulomas with central stellate abscesses are commonly seen. Unlike those of Wegener's granulomatosis, these rarely contain multinucleated giant cells and the central abscess is composed of eosinophils rather than neutrophils. Flame figures (eosinophil granules adherent to collagen fibers) similar to those of Well's syndrome may be present.

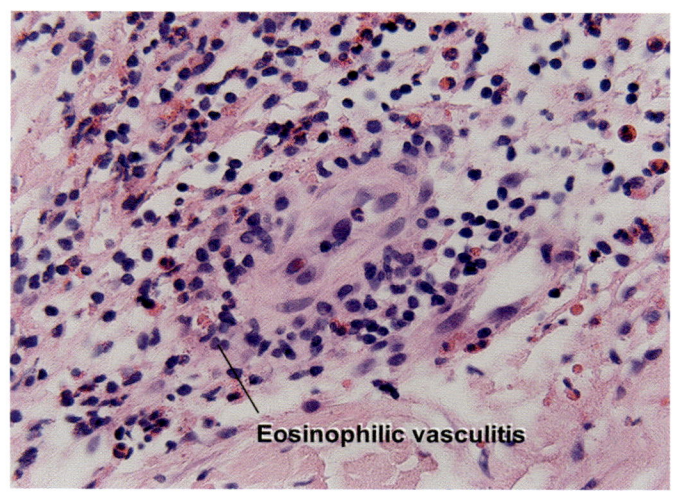

Fig 11-11 Churg–Strauss syndrome, vasculitis with eosinophils

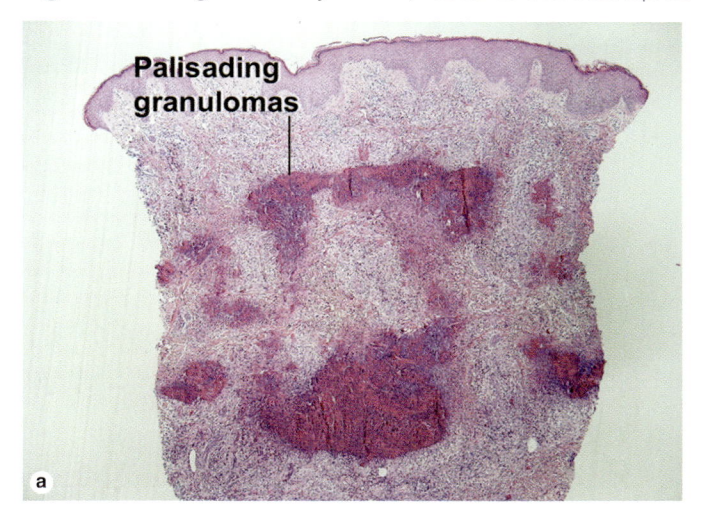

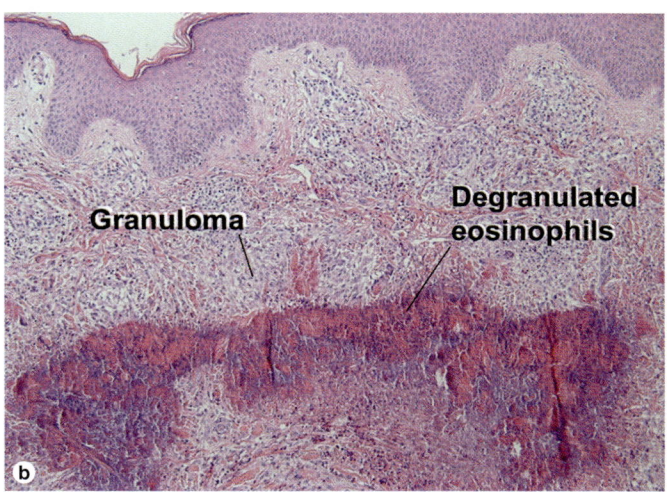

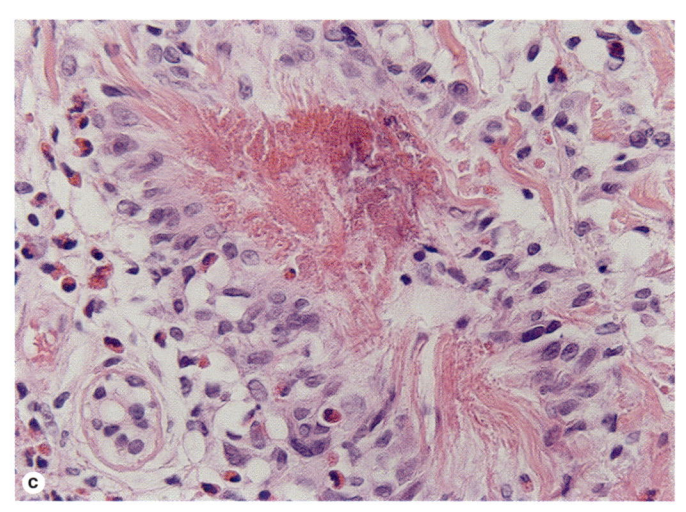

Fig 11-12 Churg–Strauss syndrome, palisading granuloma with stellate abscess

Chapel Hill criteria
Eosinophil-rich and granulomatous inflammation involving respiratory tract; necrotizing vasculitis of small to medium vessels; associated asthma and peripheral eosinophilia.

American College of Rheumatology criteria
Asthma; eosinophilia (>10%); neuropathy; pulmonary infiltrates; paranasal sinus involvement; extravascular eosinophils in tissue (four criteria give >85% sensitivity, >99% specificity).

Microscopic polyangiitis

> **Key features**
> - Leukocytoclastic vasculitis involving a mix of vessel sizes (post-capillary venules plus larger deeper vessels)
> - Endothelial necrosis is common

The histologic pattern is that of a "big 5" vasculitic disorder. Endothelial necrosis is a prominent feature. The histologic pattern, ANCA positivity and systemic involvement define the syndrome.

Chapel Hill criteria
Necrotizing vasculitis, few or no immune deposits, small to medium vessels involved, necrotizing arteriolitis may be present, necrotizing glomerulonephritis and pulmonary capillaritis common.

Rheumatoid vasculitis

> **Key features**
> - Leukocytoclastic vasculitis involving a mix of vessel sizes (post-capillary venules plus larger deeper vessels)
> - Endothelial necrosis is common

The histologic pattern resembles that of the other "big 5" vasculitides. The vasculitis is associated with a rheumatoid factor and rheumatoid arthritis. Unlike most other connective tissue disease-associated vasculitis, rheumatoid vasculitis commonly ulcerates and scars.

Septic vasculitis

> **Key features**
> - Vasculitis involves a mix of vessel sizes (post-capillary venules plus larger deeper vessels)
> - Endothelial necrosis is common
> - "Dirty" necrosis with ample neutrophilic debris

Septic vasculitis is typically associated with dirty necrosis of arterioles. Because of the arteriolar involvement, livedo reticularis and stellate infarcts are commonly seen clinically.

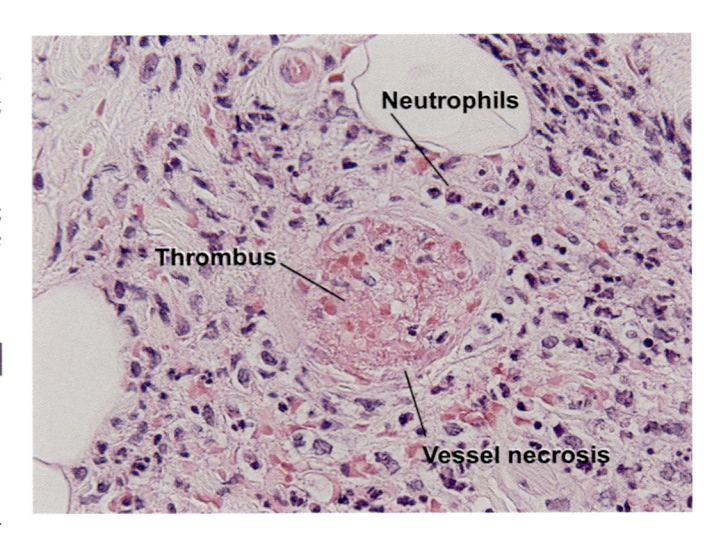

Fig 11-13 Septic vasculitis

Small vessel leukocytoclastic vasculitis

> **Key features**
> - Involves principally post-capillary venules
> - Endothelial necrosis is rare
> - Rarely ANCA-associated
> - The most common causes include:
>   - *Drug-induced*
>   - *Most connective tissue diseases (other than rheumatoid vasculitis)*
>   - *Mixed cryoglobulin disease*
>   - *Serum sickness*
>   - *Henoch–Schönlein purpura*
> - This group of five disorders is sometimes referred to as the "little 5" because only the post-capillary venule is involved.

The biopsy demonstrates a superficial perivascular infiltrate with neutrophils, karyorrhexis, expansion of the vessel wall, fibrin deposition within the vessel wall, and erythrocyte extravasation. The vasculitis involves primarily the post-capillary venules, although an occasional perforating vessel may be involved. These perforating vessels connect the subpapillary and deep plexus, and are vertically oriented. Endothelial necrosis is exceedingly rare. Direct immunofluorescence may be helpful, especially in the case of Henoch–Schönlein purpura. A urinalysis should routinely be performed to look for signs of active renal involvement.

Inflammatory vascular diseases — Chapter 11

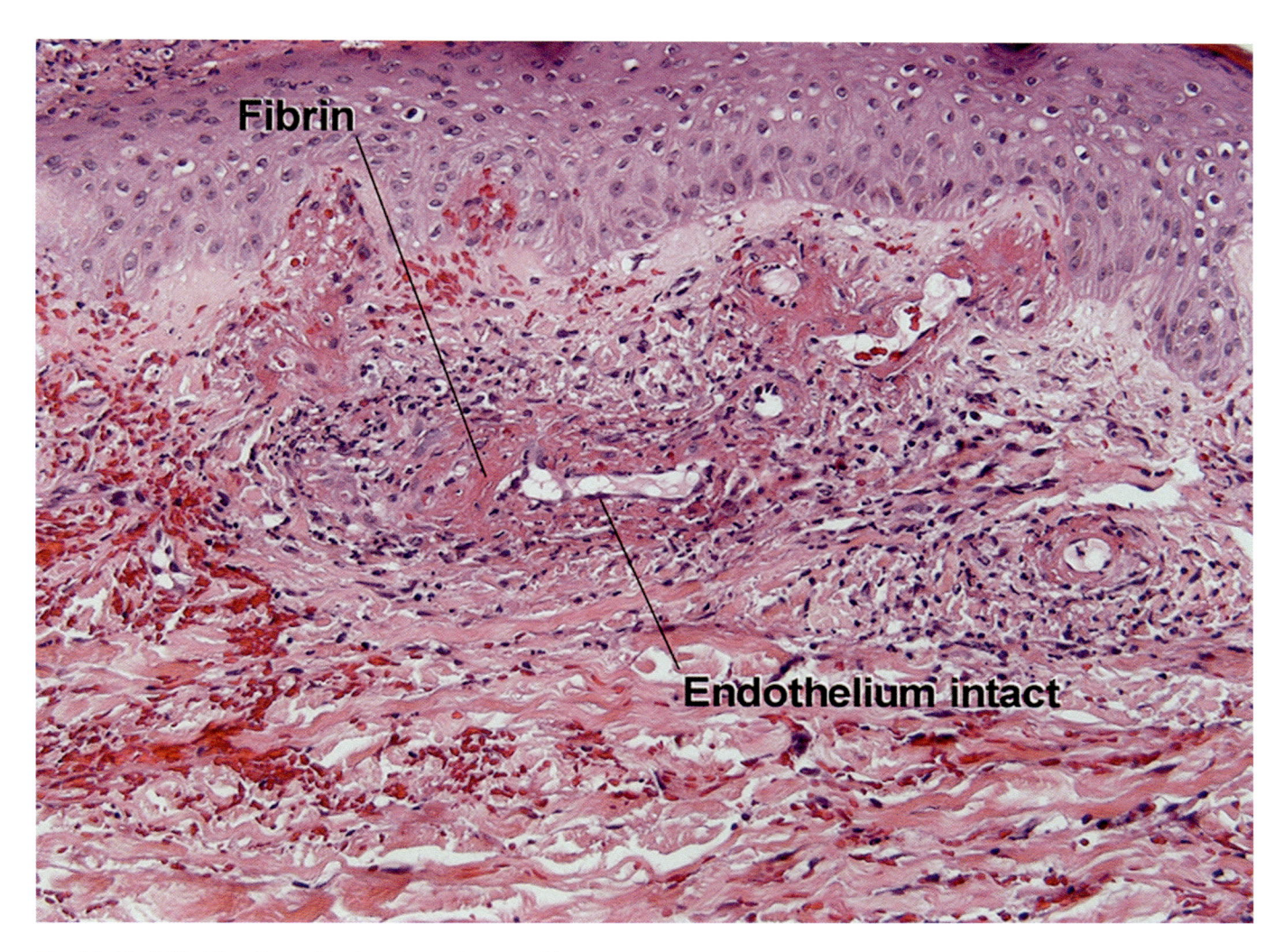

Fig 11-14 "Little 5" pattern of leukocytoclastic vasculitis

Henoch–Schönlein purpura

Key features

- "Little 5" pattern of LCV
- IgA in vessels on direct immunofluorescence (DIF)
- Typically children
- Extensor involvement with large mottled patches of purpura
- Bone, joint gut and renal involvement

Henoch–Schönlein purpura is the most common IgA vasculitis. The clinical features and DIF pattern are distinctive, but the H&E findings are like that of the other "little 5" disorders.

Chapel Hill criteria
Vasculitis with IgA dominant deposits; small to medium vessels; involves skin, gut and glomeruli; associated with arthralgia or arthritis.

American College of Rheumatology criteria
Palpable purpura; age <20; bowel pain; vessel wall neutrophils on biopsy (two criteria give 87% sensitivity, 88% specificity).

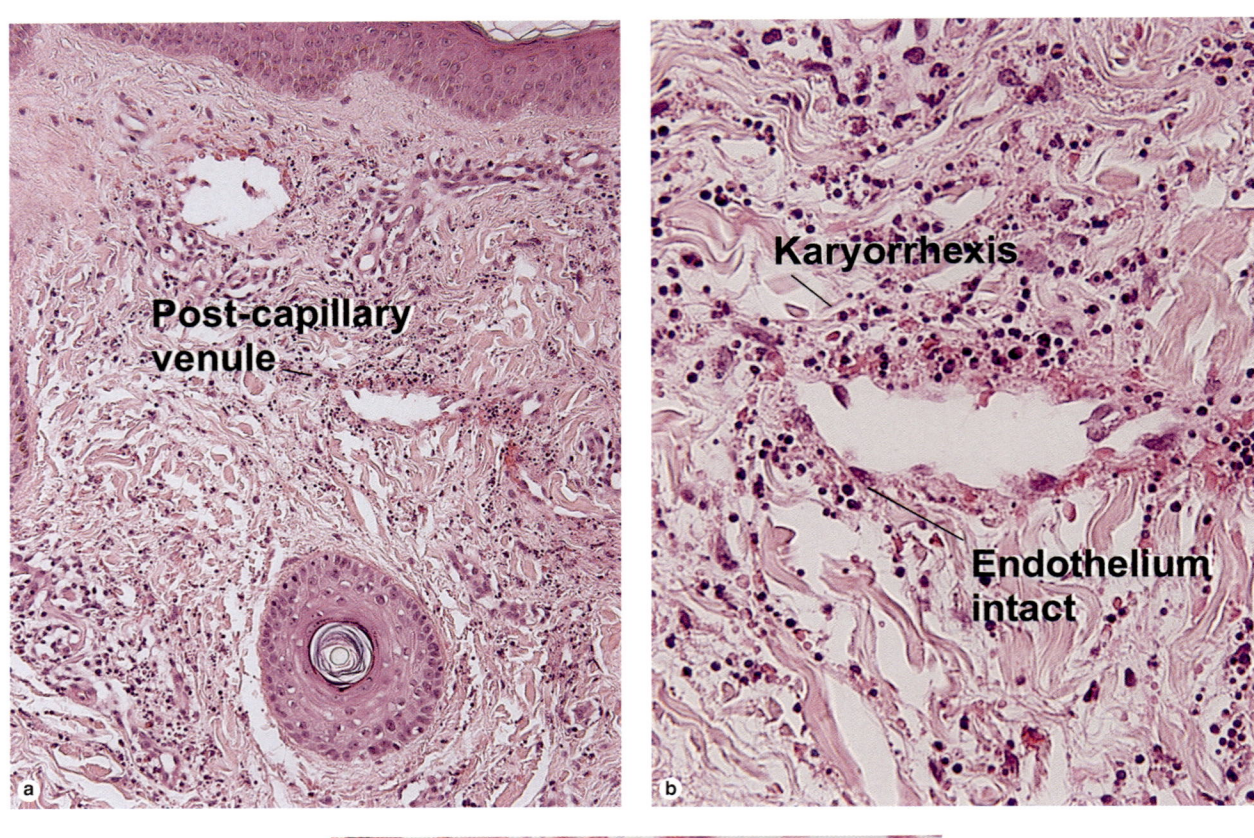

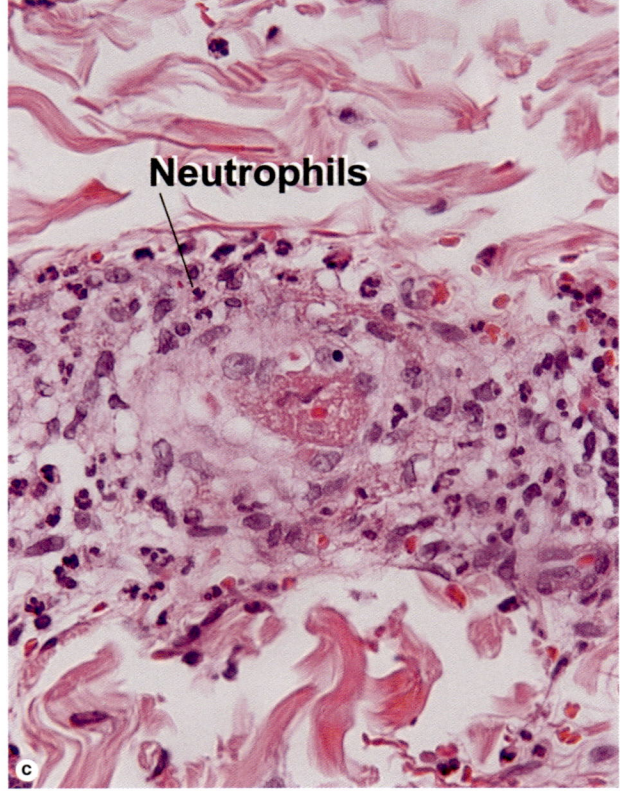

Fig 11-15 Henoch–Schönlein purpura, "Little 5" pattern of leukocytoclastic vasculitis

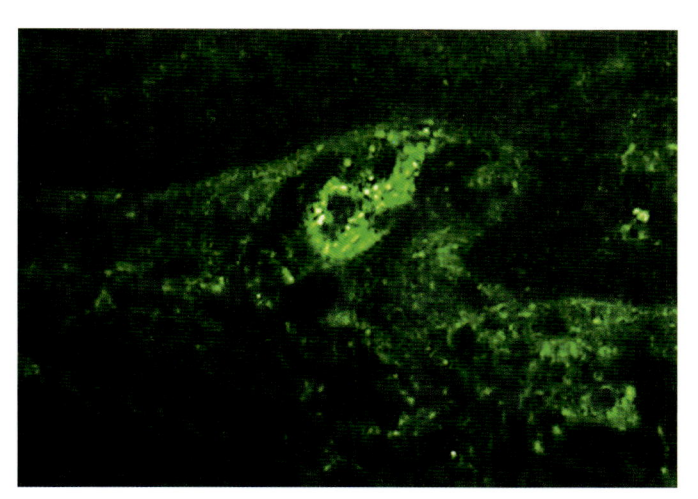

Fig 11-16 Henoch–Schönlein purpura, IgA deposition in vessels (DIF)

Mixed cryoglobulin disease

Key features

- "Little 5" pattern of LCV
- Cryoglobulins present

Mixed cryoglobulin disease is often associated with chronic infection, especially with hepatitis C. The H&E findings are like that of the other "little 5" disorders.

Chapel Hill criteria

Vasculitis of small to medium vessels; cryoglobulin deposits; skin and glomeruli often involved.

Drug-induced and idiopathic leukocytoclastic vasculitis (idiopathic leukocytoclastic angiitis)

Key features

- "Little 5" pattern of LCV

We use the term idiopathic leukocytoclastic vasculitis here, for cases with no known cause. The ACR criteria lump drug-induced vasculitis into this category. The histologic features of both fall into the "little 5" pattern.

Chapel Hill criteria

Isolated leukocytoclastic angiitis without systemic vasculitis or glomerulonephritis.

American College of Rheumatology criteria

Age >16; implicated drug; palpable purpura; cutaneous eruption; positive biopsy (three criteria give 71% sensitivity, >83% specificity).

Unique forms of vasculitis

Granuloma faciale

Key features

- Typically facial skin (sebaceous follicles, *Demodex* mites)
- Grenz zone
- LCV with eosinophils
- Onion-skin fibrosis in chronic cases
- "Granuloma" in the name ONLY – not on the slide

Granuloma faciale presents clinically as reddish brown macules or plaques with patulous follicular openings. Histologically, it is a chronic leukocytoclastic vasculitis with eosinophils. Over time, onion-skin fibrosis develops around vessels. A grenz (border) zone commonly separates the infiltrate from the adjacent follicular epithelium. Despite the name, there are no granulomas in the tissue.

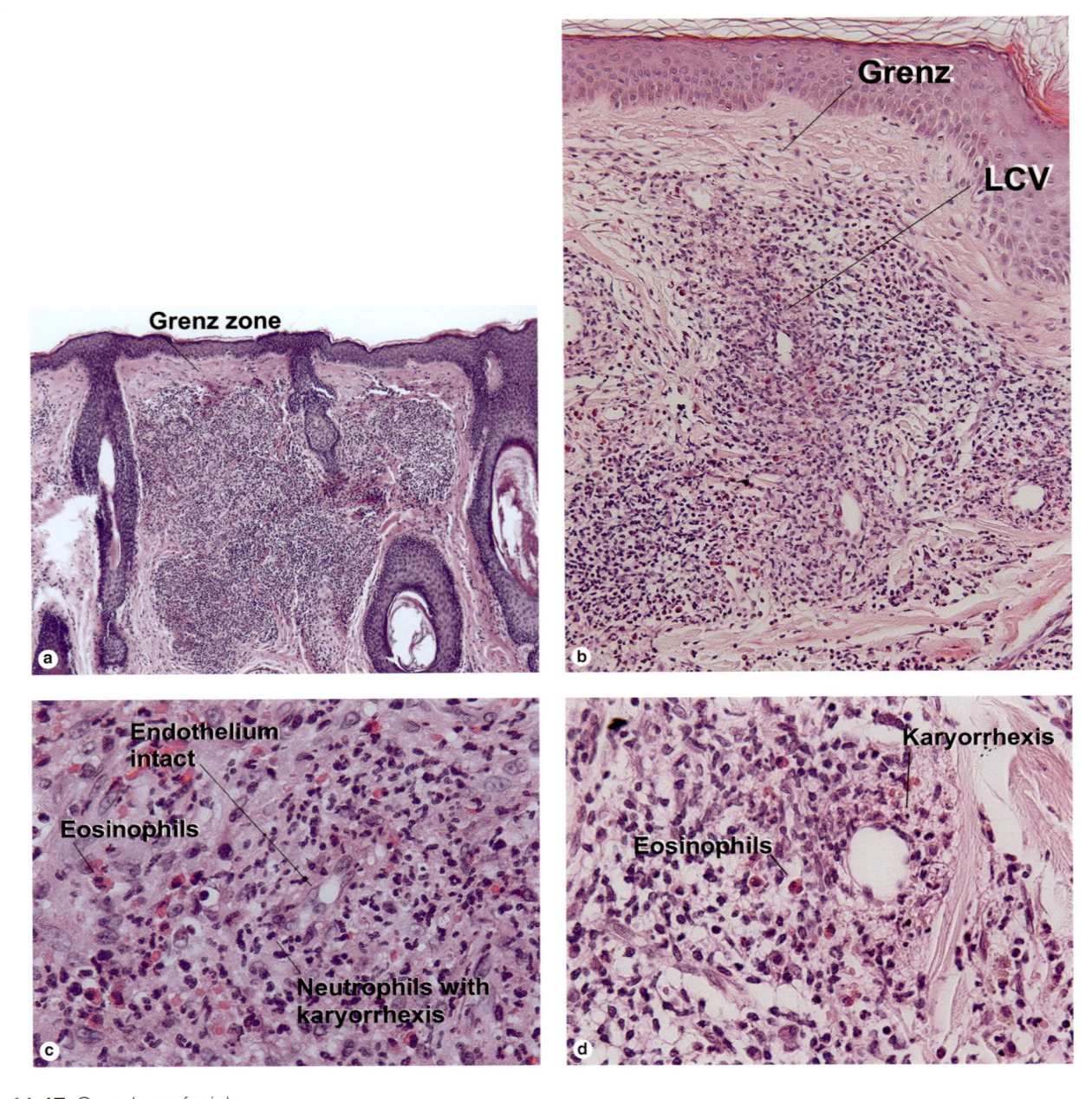

Fig 11-17 Granuloma faciale

> **PEARL**
>
> Question: Where is the granuloma in granuloma faciale?
> Answer: In the name. (Not in the skin.)

Erythema elevatum diutinum

Key features

- Not facial skin
- LCV ± eosinophils
- Onion-skin fibrosis

Erythema elevatum diutinum (EED) presents with red to orange plaques on extensor surfaces. Like granuloma faciale, EED represents a chronic fibrosing form of leukocytoclastic vasculitis. It is distinguished histologically by a non-facial location and greater fibrosis. EED has been associated with chronic streptococcal infection, HIV infection, and IgA gammopathy. The histologic changes are similar to those of granuloma faciale, but the surrounding skin has features of acral skin. Extracellular cholesterol clefts deposit in some chronic cases as a result of years of erythrocyte extravasation.

Inflammatory vascular diseases

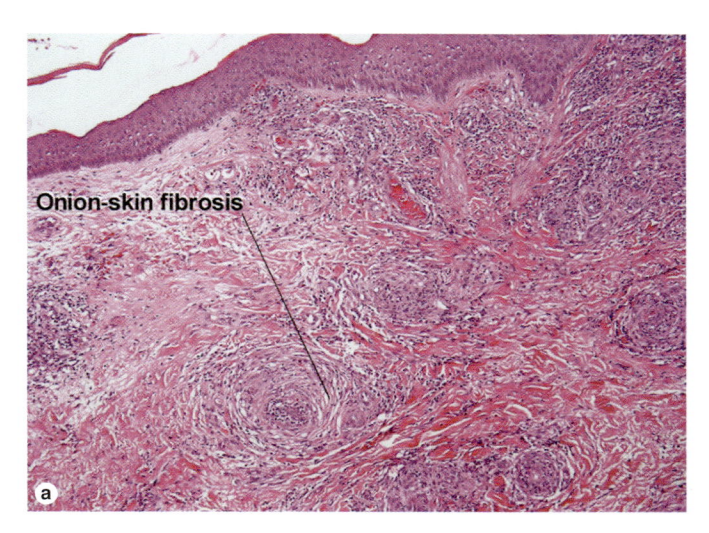

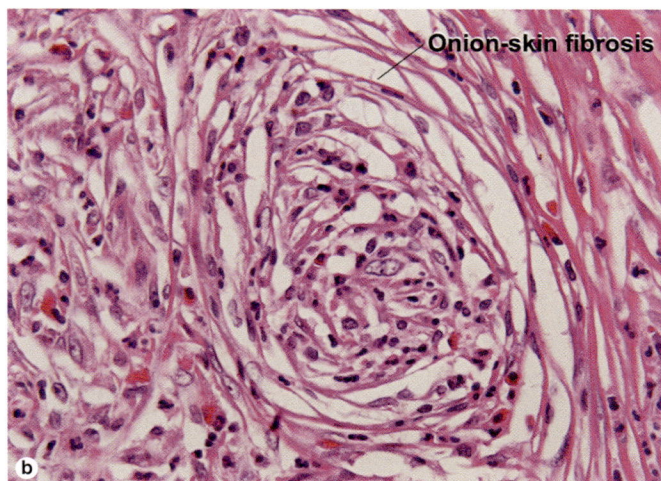

Fig 11-18 Erythema elevatum diutinum

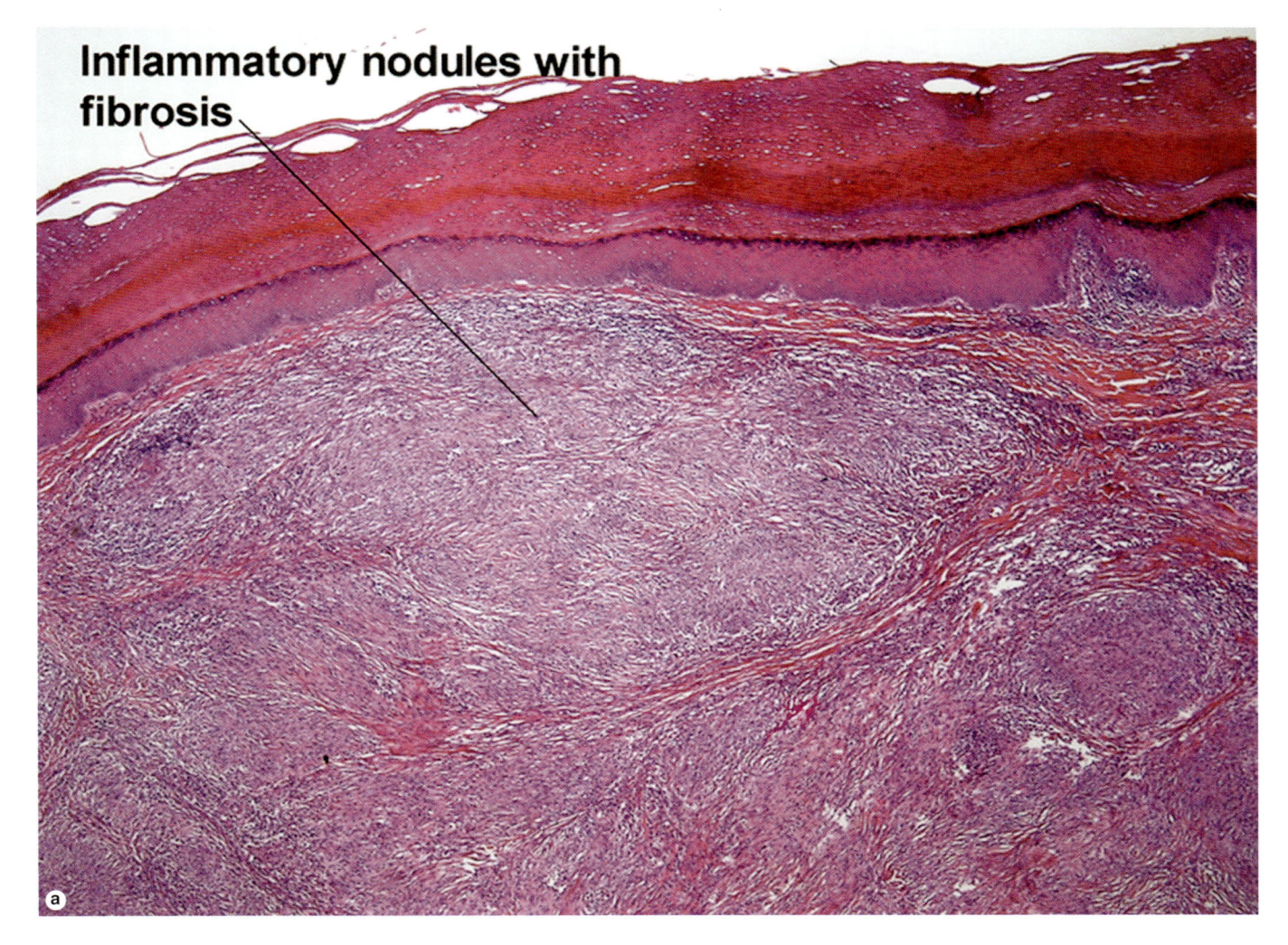

Fig 11-19 Erythema elevatum diutinum with extensive fibrosis

Continued

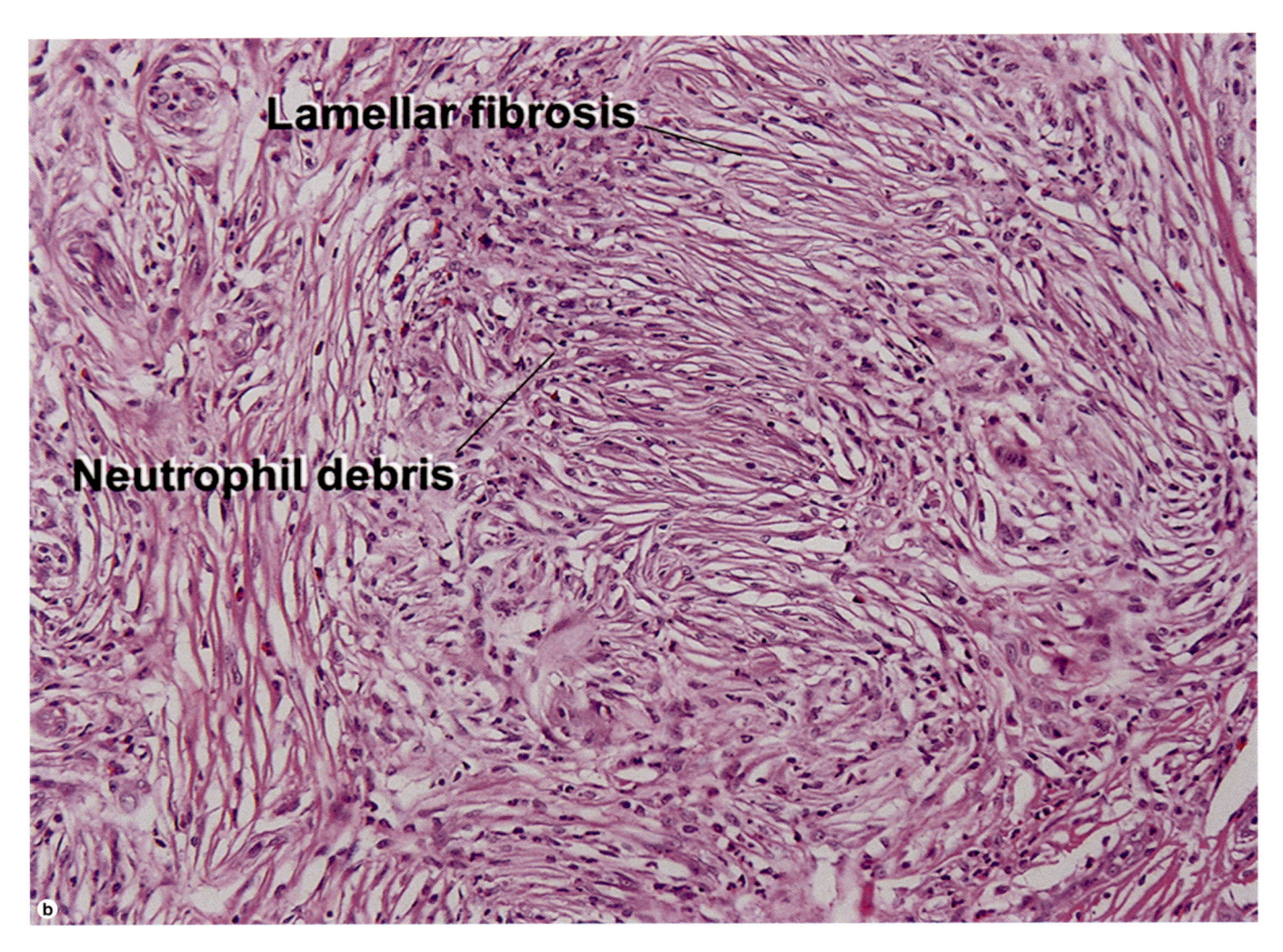

Fig 11-19, cont'd

Kawasaki disease

> **Key features**
>
> - Diagnosis is made clinically
> - Coronary arteritis presents histologically

Chapel Hill criteria
Involves large, medium and small arteries, with associated mucocutaneous lymph node syndrome; coronary arteries often involved; usually affects children.

Incidental vasculitis

> **Key features**
>
> - Not associated with immune complex disease
> - Occurs in ulcers and adjacent to suppurative folliculitis
> - May mimic "big 5" or "little 5" pattern

Leukocytoclastic vasculitis is frequently seen as an incidental finding in the base of a chronic ulcer or adjacent to a focus of suppurative folliculitis. Focal incidental leukocytoclastic vasculitis also occurs in Sweet's syndrome, bowel bypass syndrome, pyoderma gangrenosum, and neutrophilic dermatosis of the dorsal hands.

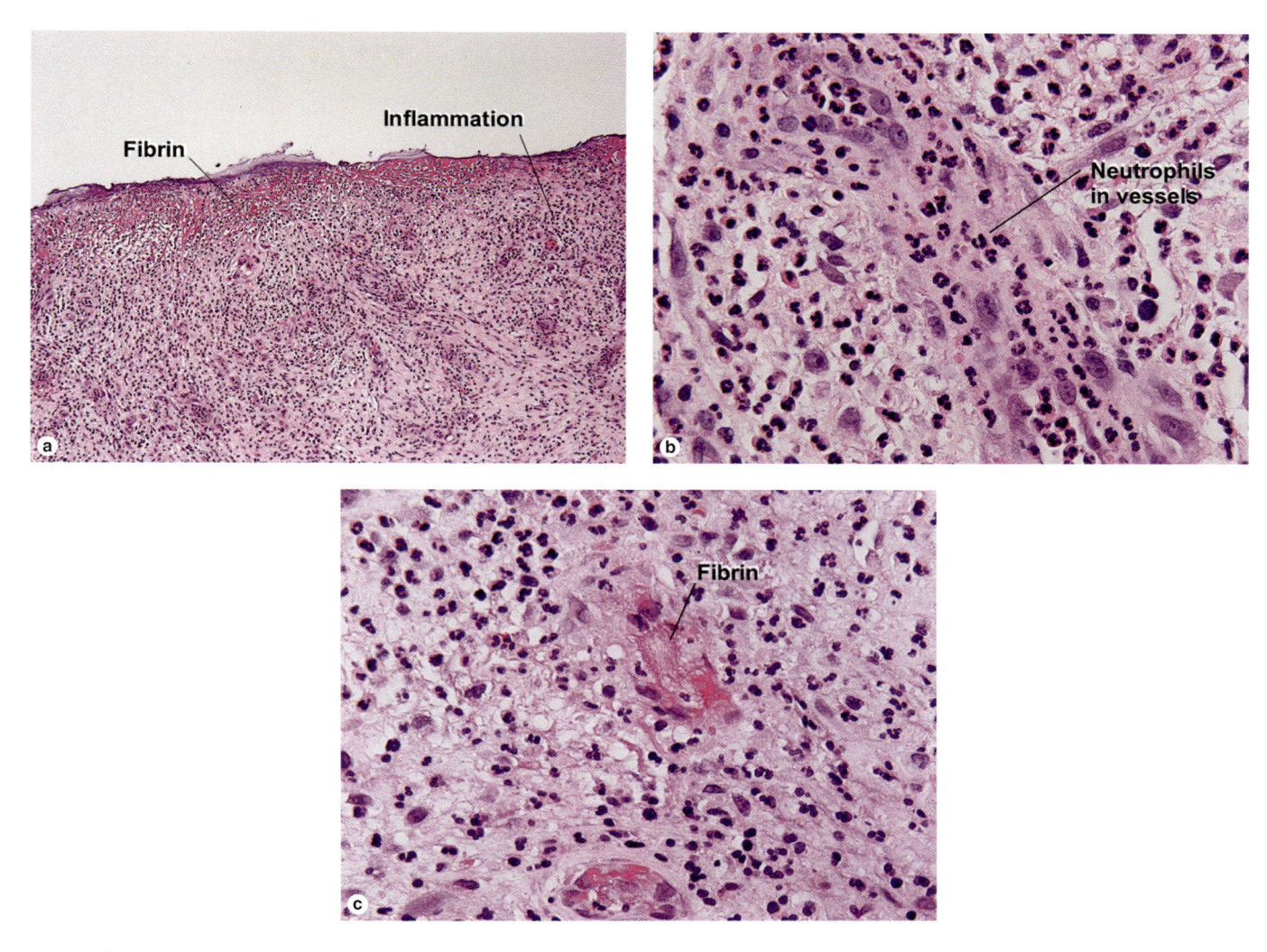

Fig 11-20 Incidental leukocytoclastic vasculitis in the base of a chronic ulcer

Neutrophilic dermatoses

Sweet's syndrome (acute febrile neutrophilic dermatosis)

Key features

- Marked papillary dermal edema
- Nodular and diffuse infiltrate of neutrophils with karyorrhexis
- Focal LCV is common

Sweet's syndrome is a distinct syndrome characterized by bouts of red, hot, tender erythematous plaques, fever and peripheral leukocytosis. Most cases follow bouts of upper respiratory infection in predisposed individuals. About 10% of patients have an associated myeloproliferative disorder. The most striking histologic features of Sweet's syndrome are the nodular and diffuse infiltrates of neutrophils, karyorrhexis, and marked papillary dermal edema. In the presence of these findings, and a characteristic clinical presentation, the presence of focal leukocytoclastic vasculitis does not alter the diagnosis of Sweet's syndrome.

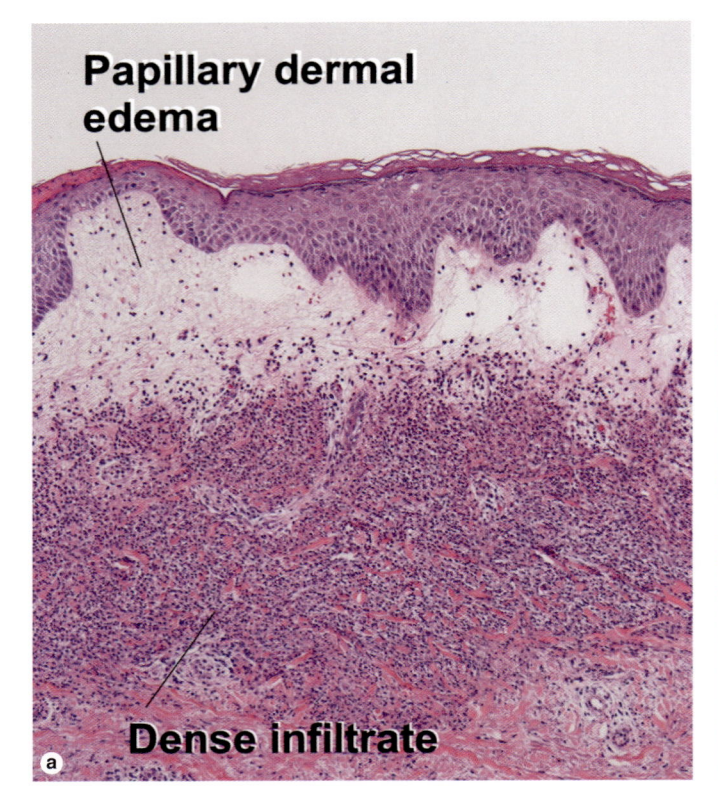

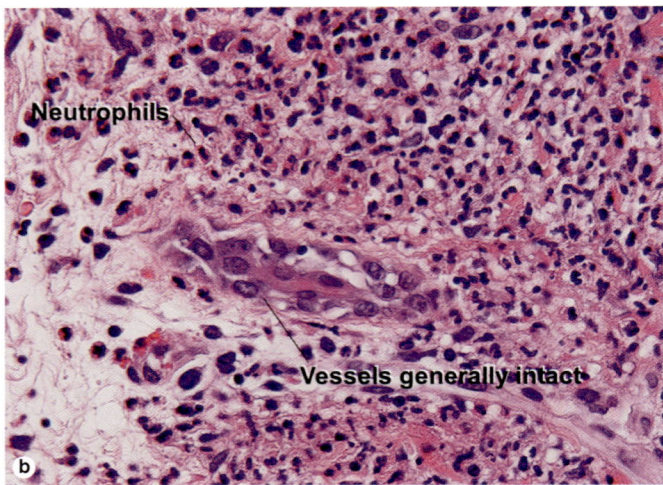

Fig 11-21 Sweet's syndrome

Other neutrophilic dermatoses

> **Key features**
> - Look like Sweet's syndrome
> - Marked papillary dermal edema
> - Nodular and diffuse infiltrate of neutrophils with karyorrhexis
> - Focal LCV is common

Neutrophilic dermatosis of the dorsal hands, pyoderma gangrenosum, bowel-bypass syndrome, and the autoinflammatory syndromes such as familial Mediterranean Fever and Muckle–Wells syndrome have a similar appearance to the lesions of Sweet's syndrome. Ulcerative lesions typically demonstrate more prominent foci of leukocytoclastic vasculitis. *Erythema marginatum* is a superficial gyrate erythema characterized by a superficial perivascular neutrophilic infiltrate. The papillary dermal edema is less prominent.

Urticaria

> **Key features**
>
> **Early lesions of urticaria**
> - Superficial dermal vessels filled with neutrophils
>
> **Late lesions of urticaria**
> - Perivascular and interstitial polymorphous infiltrate
> - Superficial dermal vessels often still contain neutrophils within the lumen
> - Diapedesis of neutrophils through the vessel wall into the surrounding dermis
> - Distinct absence of karyorrhexis
> - No fibrin in vessel walls
> - No expansion of vessel walls
> - Interstitial neutrophils, eosinophils and mononuclear cells

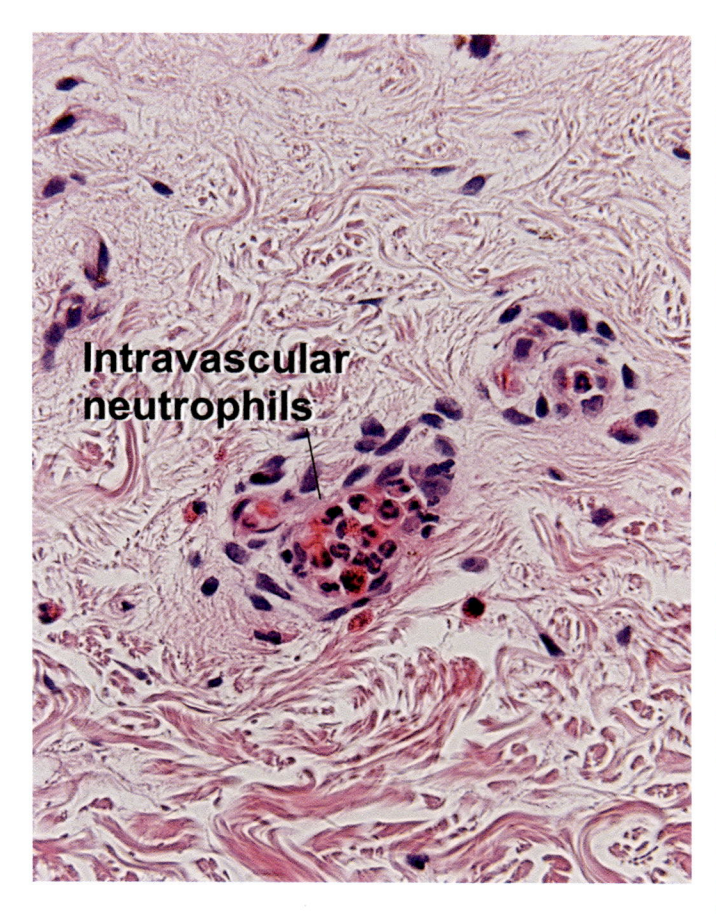

Inflammatory vascular diseases Chapter 11   199

Fig 11-22 Acute stage of a wheal

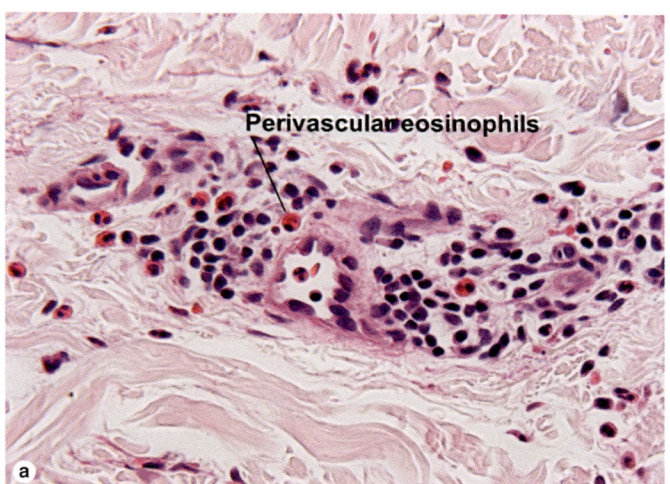

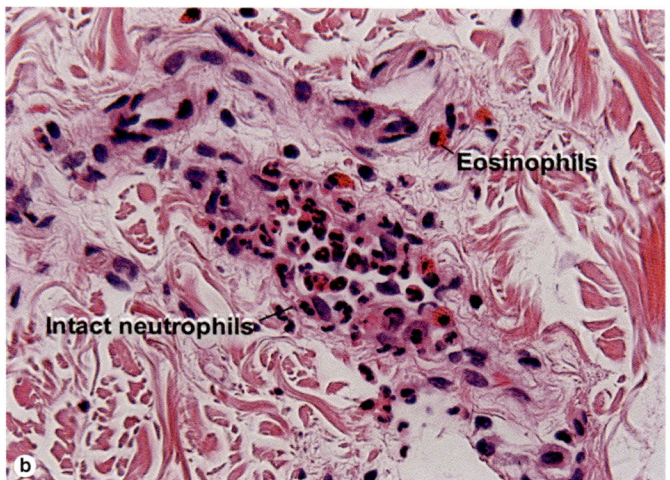

Fig 11-23 Chronic stage of an urticarial wheal

The edema of an urticarial wheal is not visible histologically. Instead, the only significant finding in acute lesions of urticaria is intravascular margination of neutrophils. With time, the neutrophils travel through the vessel wall into the surrounding dermis and are joined by eosinophils and mononuclear cells. In contrast to leukocytoclastic vasculitis, karyorrhexis is absent, the vessels walls are not expanded, and no fibrin is seen in the vessel walls. Erythrocyte extravasation is uncommon.

Wells' syndrome (eosinophilic cellulitis)

Key features

- Flame figures (eosinophil degranulation onto collagen)

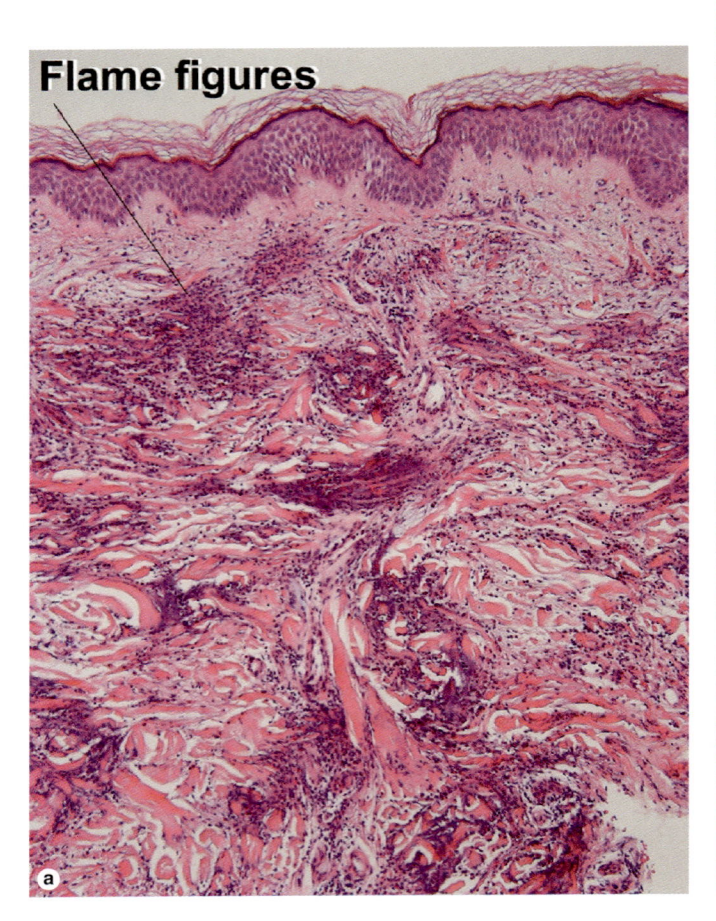

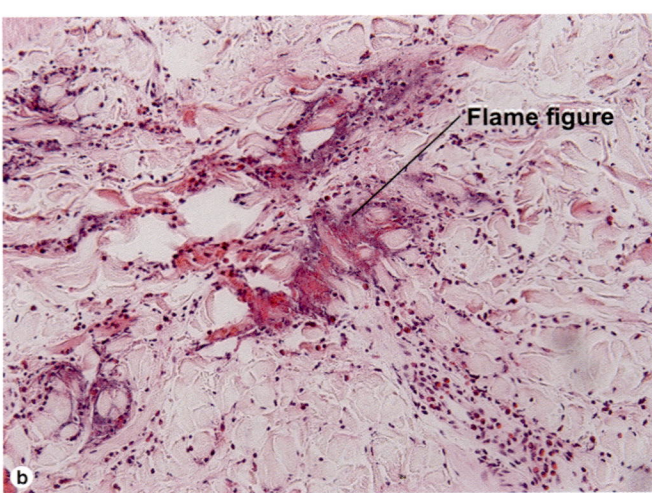

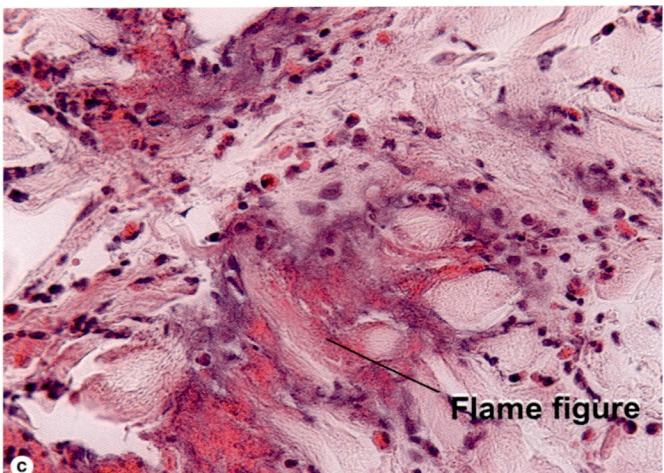

Fig 11-24 Wells' syndrome

Wells' syndrome is characterized by recurrent erythematous plaques that demonstrate flame figures histologically. Some cases may represent a distinct entity, while most represent exaggerated arthropod reactions.

Perivascular lymphoid infiltrates

Pigmenting purpuric eruption

> **Key features**
> - Inflammation purely lymphoid
> - Surrounds capillaries (centered above the level of the post-capillary venule)
> - Erythrocyte extravasation
> - Hemosiderin deposits over time

All types of pigmenting purpura represent forms of chronic lymphocytic capillaritis. Clinical variants include thumbprint hemosiderosis with cayenne pepper spots (Schamberg's disease); annular telangiectatic purpura (Majocchi's purpura); lichenoid

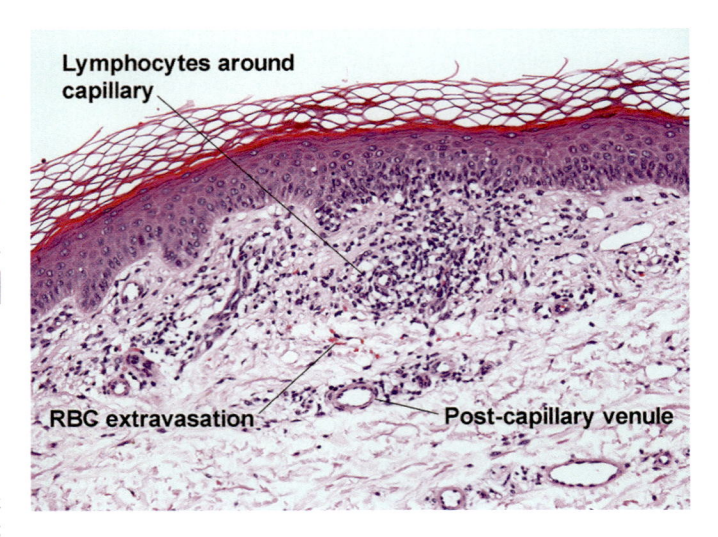

Fig 11-25 Pigmenting purpuric eruption

purpura (Gougerot–Blum purpura); and eczematous purpura (pigmenting purpura of Doucas and Kapetanakis). In all forms, an iron stain (Perl's, Prussian blue, ferricyanide, Gomori iron) can be used to demonstrate hemosiderin.

Gyrate erythemas

Key features
- Dense "coat-sleeve" perivascular lymphoid infiltrate
- Vessels are intact

Superficial gyrate erythemas include erythema marginatum (discussed under the neutrophilic disorders) and *erythema annulare centrifugum*. Erythema annulare centrifugum is characterized clinically by an expanding erythematous ring with a characteristic trailing scale. Histologically, the erythematous ring corresponds to a focus of superficial perivascular coat-sleeve lymphoid infiltrate. Trailing behind this is a small spongiotic focus, and trailing behind that is a small focus of parakeratosis. The infiltrate, spongiotic and parakeratotic foci line up at about a 45° angle. Deep gyrate erythemas lack epidermal changes, and are characterized by a dense superficial and deep coat-sleeve perivascular lymphoid infiltrate.

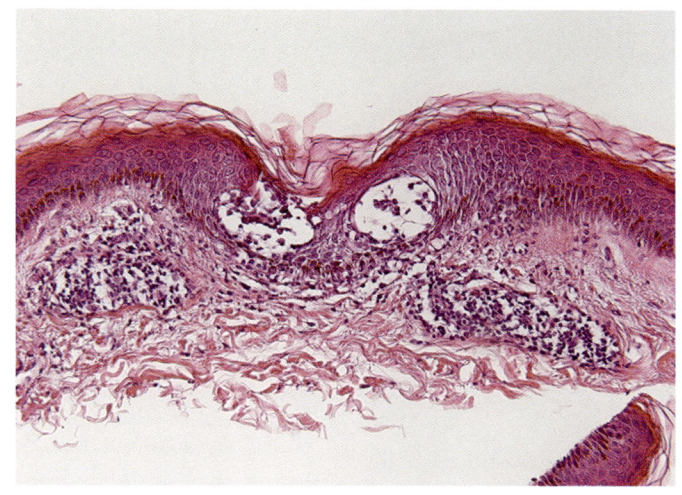

Fig 11-26 Erythema annulare centrifugum

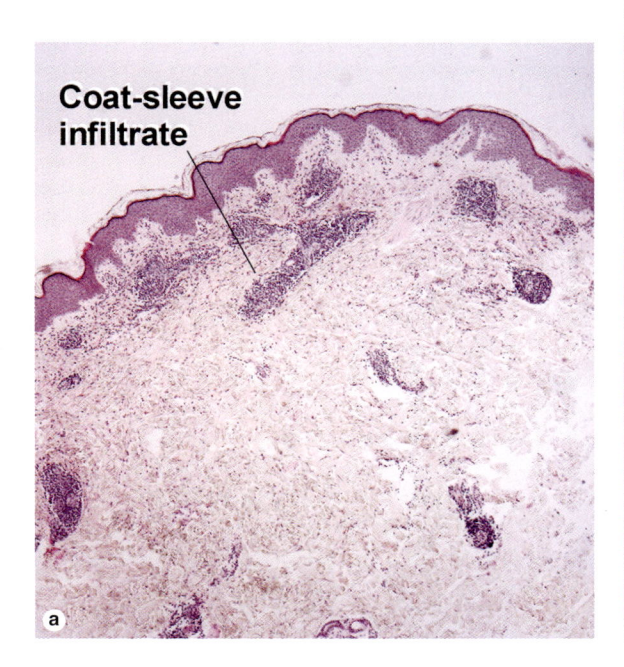

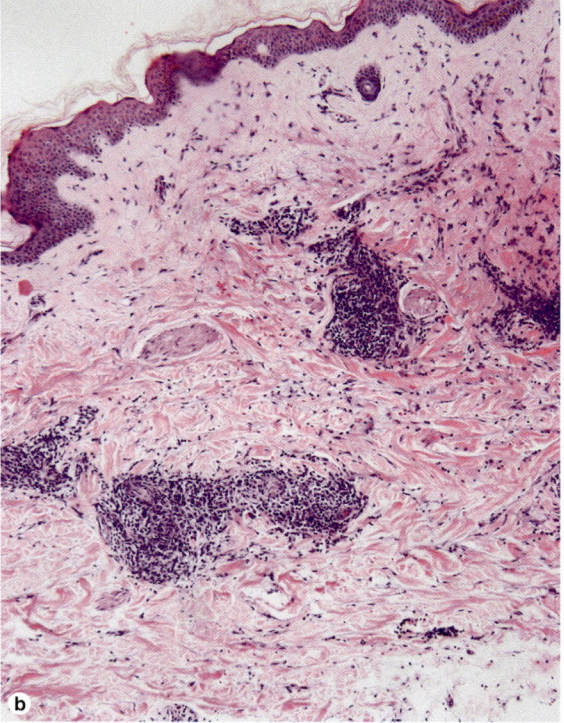

Fig 11-27 Deep gyrate erythema

Tumid lupus erythematosus

Key features
- Perivascular lymphoid inflammation
- Lymphocytes in eccrine coil
- Dermal mucin

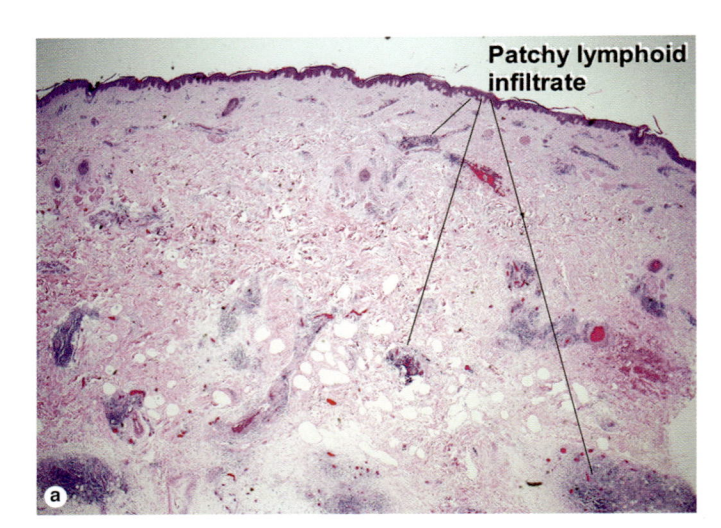

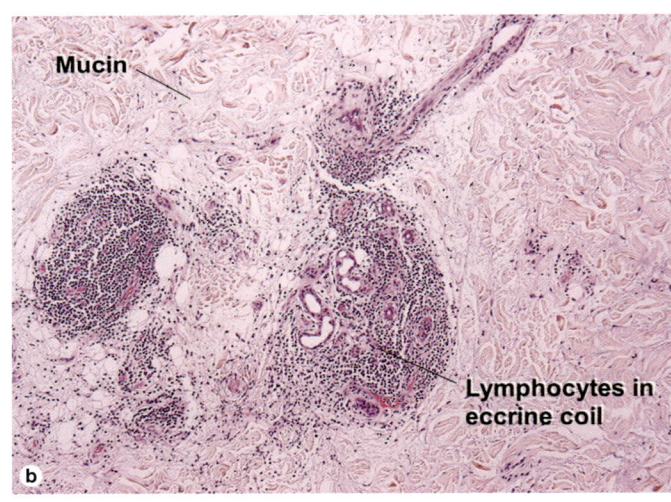

Fig 11-28 Tumid lupus erythematosus

Polymorphous light eruption

Key features
- Perivascular lymphoid inflammation
- Papillary dermal edema
- ± spongiosis

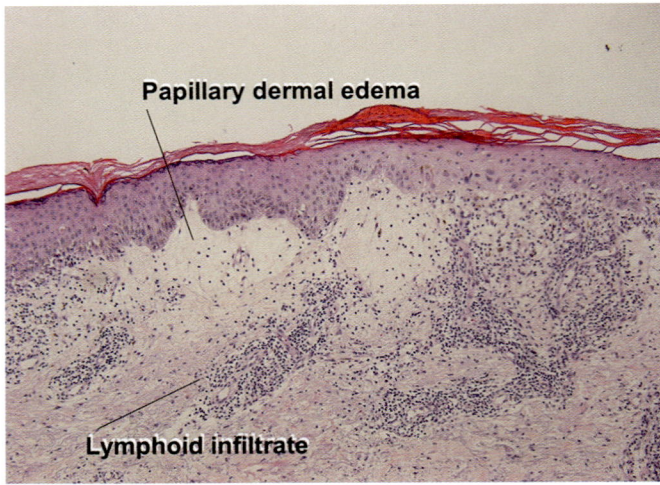

Fig 11-29 Polymorphous light eruption

Morbilliform drug eruptions

Key features
- Evidence of an acute process (basket-weave corneum, papillary dermal edema, dilated superficial vessels, neutrophils in vessels, red cell extravasation)
- Mild vacuolar interface commonly present

Features that suggest a drug eruption include presence of a polymorphous infiltrate, as well as combinations of findings not corresponding to any well-defined disease.

Features that weigh against a diagnosis of a morbilliform drug eruption include signs of chronicity (acanthosis, hyperkeratosis, papillary dermal fibrosis, macrophages in dermis).

Lymphoid vasculitis

Key features
- Perivascular lymphoid infiltrate with damage to the vessel wall

True lymphoid vasculitis may be seen in Degos disease, insect bites, rickettsial disease, pityriasis lichenoides, and perniosis.

Degos disease (malignant atrophic papulosis)

Key features
- Red papules that develop ivory white atrophic centers
- Bowel perforation and stroke
- Wedge-shaped superficial and deep perivascular lymphoid infiltrate with vascular damage
- Over time, central epidermal depression and atrophy, avascular necrosis of dermal structures, and marked dermal mucinosis

Degos disease is a distinct clinical picture that may be a manifestation of lupus erythematosus.

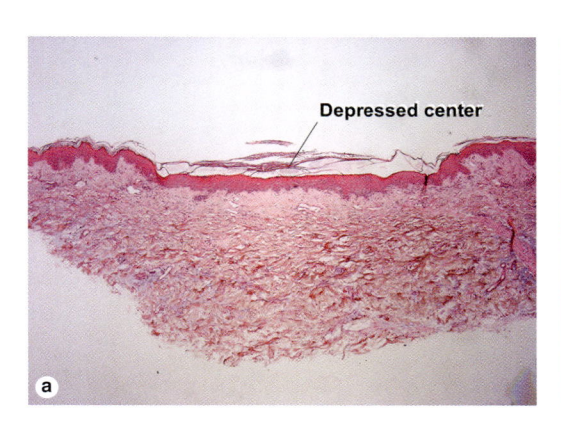

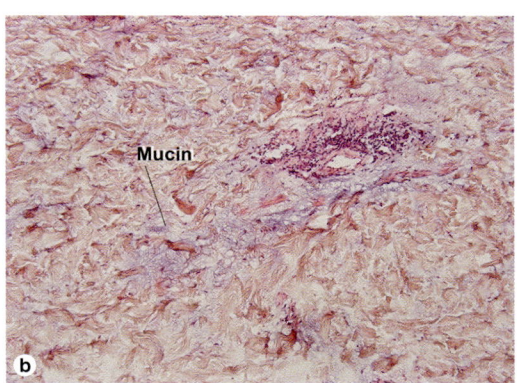

Fig 11-30 Degos disease

Insect bite

Key features

- Dense wedge-shaped perivascular lymphoid infiltrate
- Eosinophils
- Variable vascular damage
- Variable atypical lymphocytes
- Focal leukocytoclastic vasculitis may be present
- Papillary dermal edema may be prominent

Perniosis

Key features

- Superficial and deep perivascular lymphoid infiltrate
- Fluffy edema and expansion of vessel walls without fibrin
- Acral skin

The so-called "fluffy edema" of perniosis is often more prominent in deeper dermal vessels. The vessel wall is expanded, and white space surrounds lymphocyte nuclei within the vessel wall.

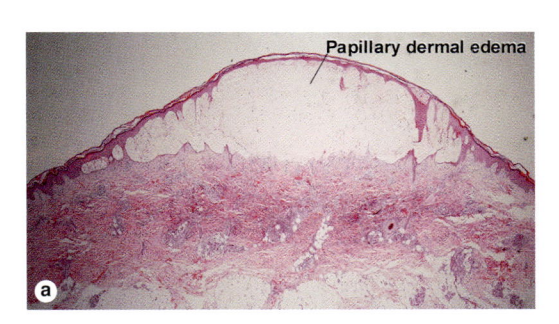

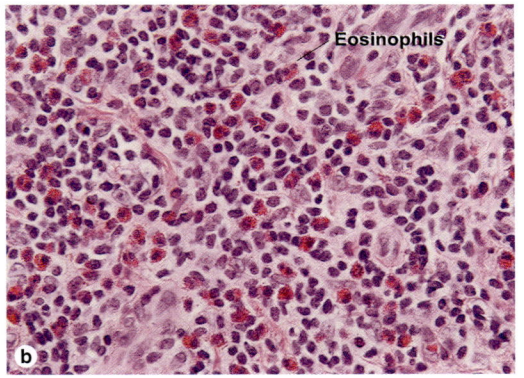

Fig 11-31 Insect bite

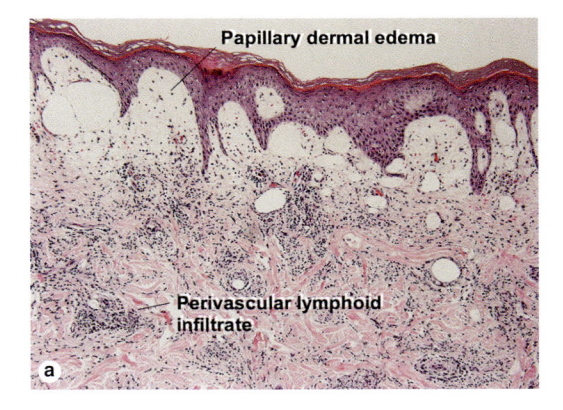

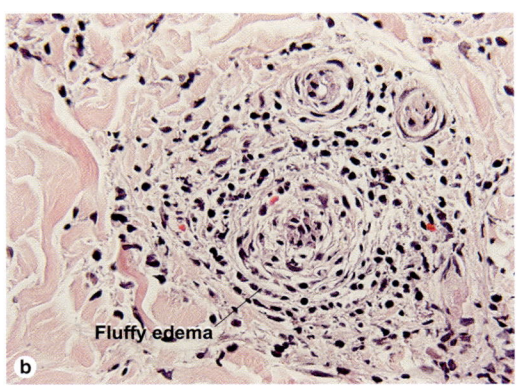

Fig 11-32 Perniosis

Occlusive vascular diseases

Type I cryoglobulinemia

Key features
- Vessels occluded by pink jelly-like substance
- Erythrocyte extravasation

Type I, monoclonal, cryoglobulinemia is a manifestation of plasma cell dyscrasia. The intravascular deposits have an appearance resembling dark pink to red jelly.

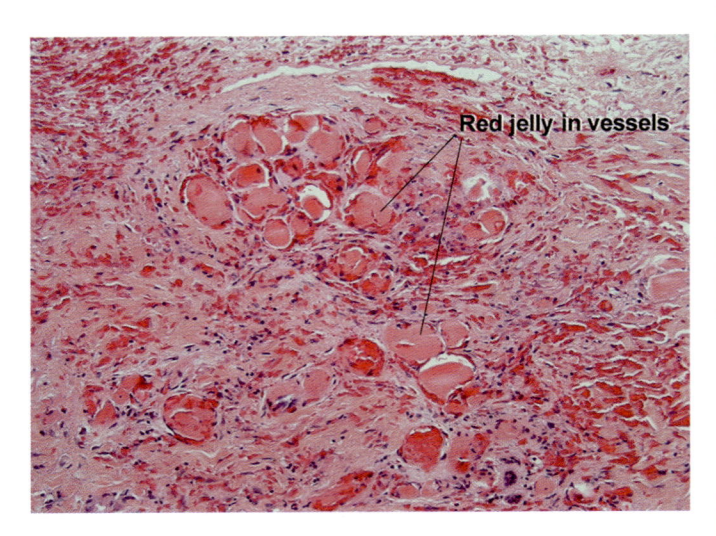

Fig 11-33 Type I cryoglobulinemia

Cholesterol embolization

Key features
- Arteriole containing cholesterol clefts

Cholesterol embolization typically occurs after catheterization or anticoagulation. Spontaneous embolization may also occur. The patient presents with livedo reticularis, dark mottled toes and worsening renal function.

Livedoid vasculopathy

Key features
- Hyalinized vessel walls
- Thrombi
- Cannon-ball tufting of vessels often present in superficial dermis (stasis change)

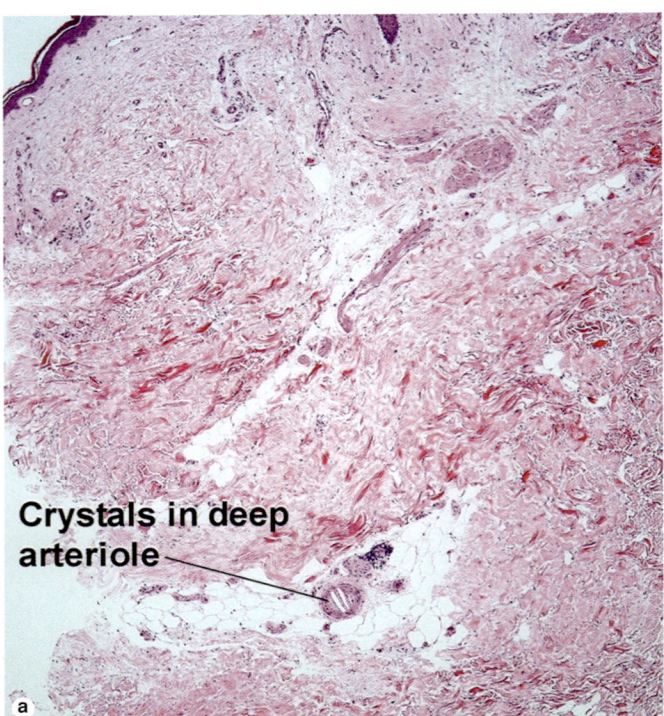

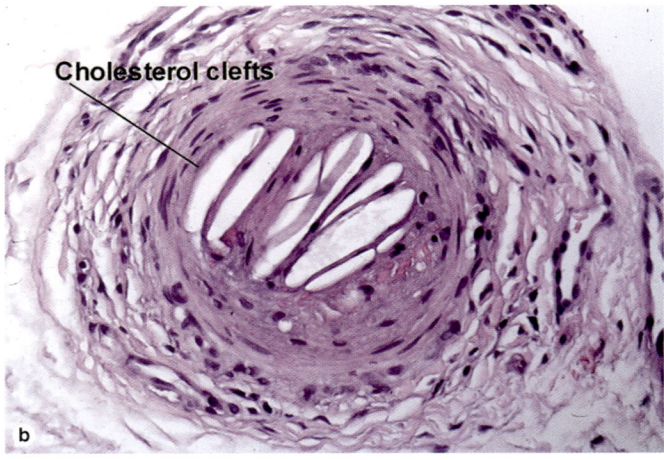

Fig 11-34 Cholesterol embolization

Stasis change

Key features
- Cannon-ball tufting of vessels often present in superficial dermis (stasis change)
- Erythrocyte extravasation
- Dermal hemosiderin
- Small thrombi may be present

Inflammatory vascular diseases

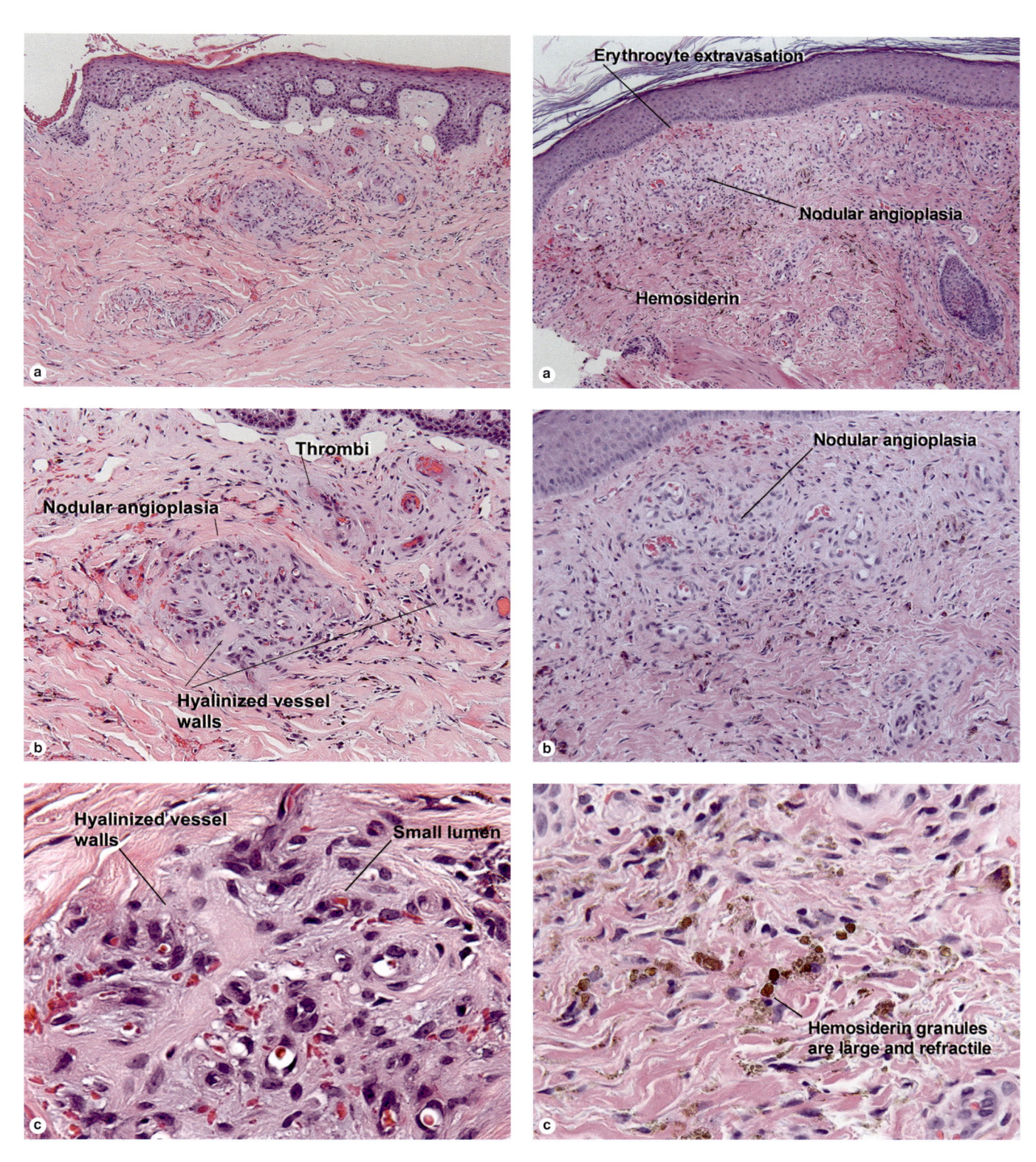

Fig 11-35 Livedoid vasculopathy

Fig 11-36 Stasis change

Coagulopathy

Key features
- Thrombi in vessels

Purpura fulminans, antiphospholipid syndrome, and inherited deficiencies or mutations affecting protein C, protein S, antithrombin III, factor V Leyden, and prothrombin all result in vascular thrombi with variable purpura and necrosis. Levamisole-induced necrosis may have both thrombi and vasculitis.

Non-inflammatory purpura

Scurvy

Key features
- Follicular hyperkeratosis
- Corkscrew hairs
- Perifollicular hemorrhage

Solar ("senile") purpura (Bateman's or actinic purpura)

Key features
- Solar elastosis
- Erythrocyte extravasation

Other non-inflammatory purpura

Key features
- Erythrocyte extravasation

Ecchymoses and thrombocytopenic purpura present with erythrocyte extravasation in the absence of inflammation.

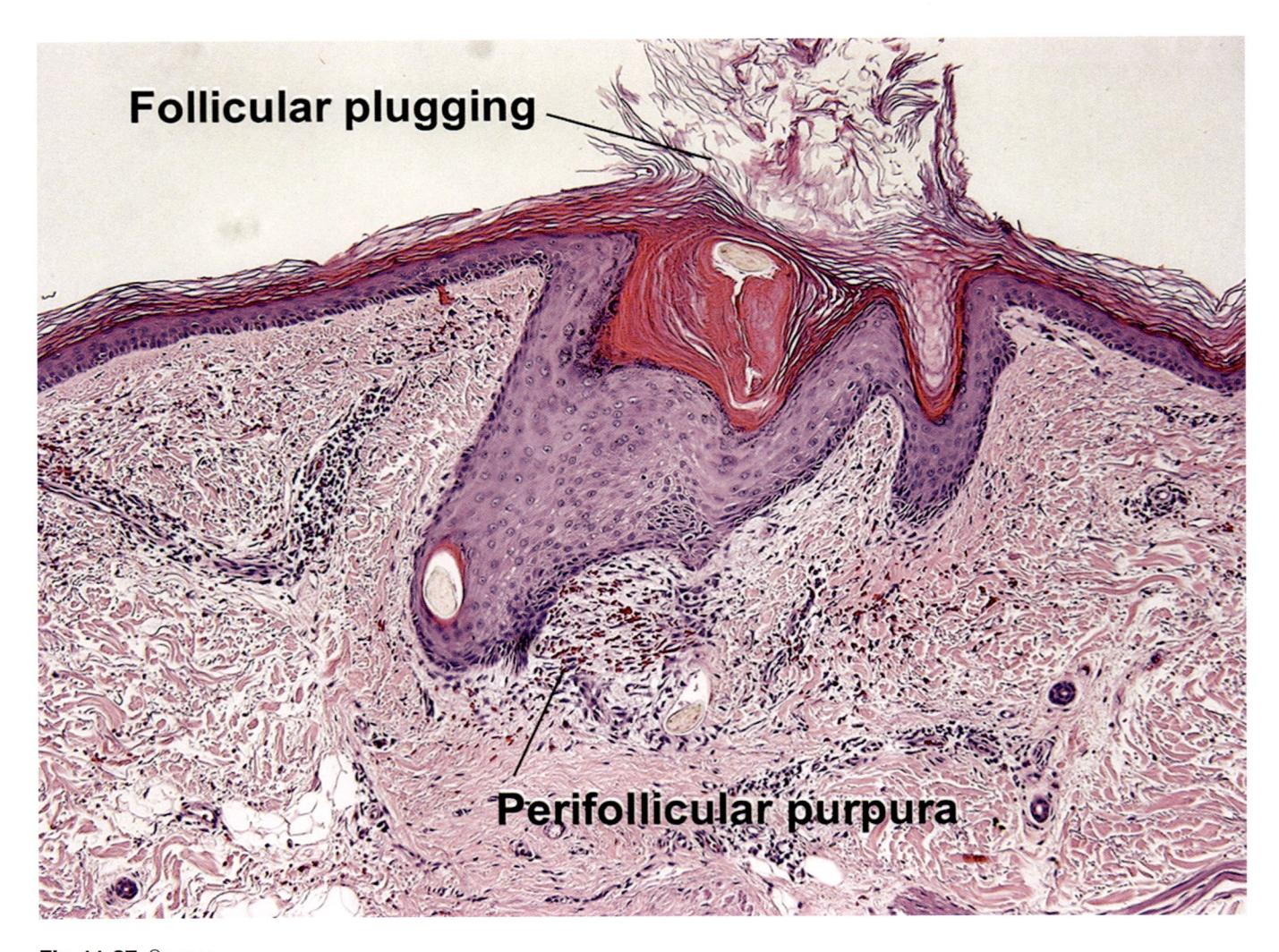

Fig 11-37 Scurvy

Further reading

Bertoli AM, Alarcón GS. Classification of the vasculitides: are they clinically useful? Curr Rheumatol Rep 2005;7(4):265–269.

Carlson JA, Ng BT, Chen KR. Cutaneous vasculitis update: diagnostic criteria, classification, epidemiology, etiology, pathogenesis, evaluation and prognosis. Am J Dermatopathol 2005;27(6):504–528.

Knütter I, Hiemann R, Brumma T, et al. Automated interpretation of ANCA patterns – a new approach in the serology of ANCA-associated vasculitis. Arthritis Res Ther 2012;14(6):R271.

Lionaki S, Blyth ER, Hogan SL, et al. Classification of antineutrophil cytoplasmic autoantibody vasculitides: the role of antineutrophil cytoplasmic autoantibody specificity for myeloperoxidase or proteinase 3 in disease recognition and prognosis. Arthritis Rheum 2012;64(10):3452–3462.

Ozen S. Problems in classifying vasculitis in children. Pediatr Nephrol 2005;20(9):1214–1218.

Pagnoux C, Guillevin L. Cardiac involvement in small and medium-sized vessel vasculitides. Lupus 2005;14(9): 718–722.

Saleh A, Stone JH. Classification and diagnostic criteria in systemic vasculitis. Best Pract Res Clin Rheumatol 2005;19(2):209–221.

Watts RA, Scott DG. ANCA vasculitis: to lump or split? Why we should study MPA and GPA separately. Rheumatology (Oxford) 2012;51(12):2115–2117.

Chapter 12

Genodermatoses

Tammie Ferringer

A summary table of the 'Key histologic features of genodermatoses' can be found in the on-line content for this book.

Pseudoxanthoma elasticum

Key features

- Curled and frayed, calcified elastic fibers in the reticular dermis (pink or blue squiggles)
- Elastic tissue (Verhoeff–Van Gieson) and calcium (Von Kossa) stains highlight the distorted elastic fibers

Pseudoxanthoma elasticum is an autosomal-recessive and, less commonly, autosomal-dominant disorder due to a mutation in the *ABCC6* transporter gene. It results in calcification of the elastic fibers of the skin, eyes, and artery walls. The skin changes become apparent around the second decade and simulate "plucked chicken skin" in the flexural areas. Biopsy of a scar may reveal the elastic tissue abnormalities in a patient with no cutaneous lesions. Eye changes include angioid streaks and retinal hemorrhage that may cause blindness. The vascular changes may lead to hypertension, stroke, myocardial infarction, mitral valve prolapse, and gastrointestinal hemorrhage.

Similar histologic findings can also be seen after topical exposure to calcium salts. Periumbilical perforating pseudoxanthoma elasticum (perforating calcific elastosis) affects multiparous black women but is limited to an isolated area. Patients on long-term penicillamine for Wilson's disease may develop altered elastic fibers with overlapping features of pseudoxanthoma elasticum and elastosis perforans serpiginosa. The penicillamine-induced, altered elastic fibers have small lateral buds arranged perpendicularly to the primary elastic fiber resembling the twigs on a bramble bush.

Differential Diagnosis

Angioid streaks, due to rupture in Bruch's membrane, are associated with other disorders. The mnemonic "PEPSI LiTe" is helpful in remembering the associated diseases:

- *P*enicillamine
- *E*hlers–Danlos syndrome
- *P*seudoxanthoma elasticum/Paget's disease of bone
- *S*ickle cell anemia
- *I*ncreased phosphate
- *L*ead poisoning
- *T*halassemia

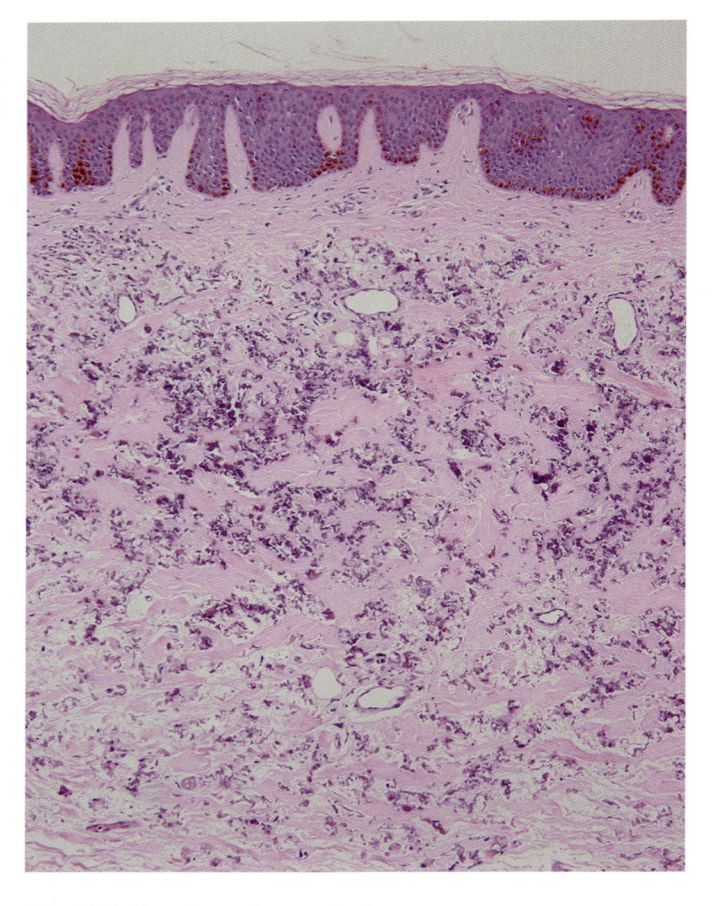

Fig 12-1 Pseudoxanthoma elasticum

Ichthyosis vulgaris

Key features

- Compact orthohyperkeratosis with paradoxically diminished or absent granular layer

In most other conditions, hyperorthokeratosis is associated with a prominent granular layer and parakeratosis is associated with a diminished or absent granular layer. Ichthyosis vulgaris (in which there is little to no granular layer despite hyperkeratosis) and axillary granular parakeratosis (in which there is a granular layer despite the presence of parakeratosis) are exceptions to this rule.

Ichthyosis vulgaris is an autosomal-dominant disorder with retention of the stratum corneum (rather than hyperproliferation) resulting in hyperkeratosis. There is a deficiency in profilaggrin resulting in inadequate keratohyaline granule synthesis. There are fine brown to transparent scales that spare the flexures. Accentuation of the palmoplantar creases, keratosis pilaris, and coexisting atopic dermatitis may be present.

Acquired ichthyosis in association with malignancy, especially Hodgkin's lymphoma, may clinically and histologically mimic ichthyosis vulgaris. Acquired ichthyosis may also occur with niacin therapy.

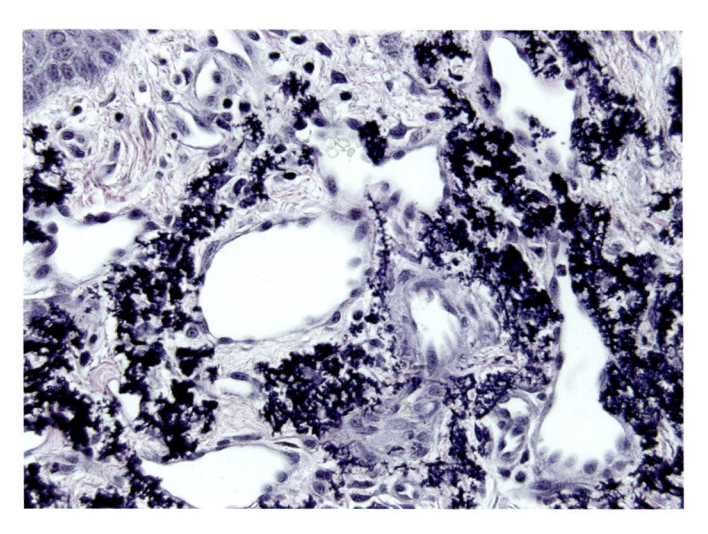

Fig 12-2 'Bramble bush' elastic fibers induced by penicillamine

Incontinentia pigmenti (Bloch–Sulzberger syndrome)

Key features

Vesicular stage
- Eosinophilic spongiosis (spongiosis resulting in intraepidermal vesicles with prominent exocytosis of eosinophils)
- Occasional dyskeratotic cells may be present

Verrucous stage
- Hyperkeratosis and papillomatosis with few eosinophils and little spongiosis
- Prominent dyskeratosis in whorls and clusters

Pigmented stage
- Pigment incontinence
- Hypopigmented lesions reveal normal to decreased melanocytes with or without dermal fibrosis

This X-linked dominant disorder is typically lethal in males. A mutation in the *NEMO* gene leads to defective nuclear factor kappa-B (NF-κB) activation. There is evolution through overlapping stages. At birth or soon after, there are linear vesicular lesions that evolve into verrucous lesions weeks to months later. At 3–6 months of age there are streaks and whorls of hyperpigmentation that do not correlate with the areas of prior vesicles. The pattern has been likened to marble cake. Hypopigmentation may replace the hyperpigmentation decades later. Other cutaneous findings include alopecia and nail dystrophy. Ocular, dental (peg teeth), skeletal, and neurologic abnormalities may be present.

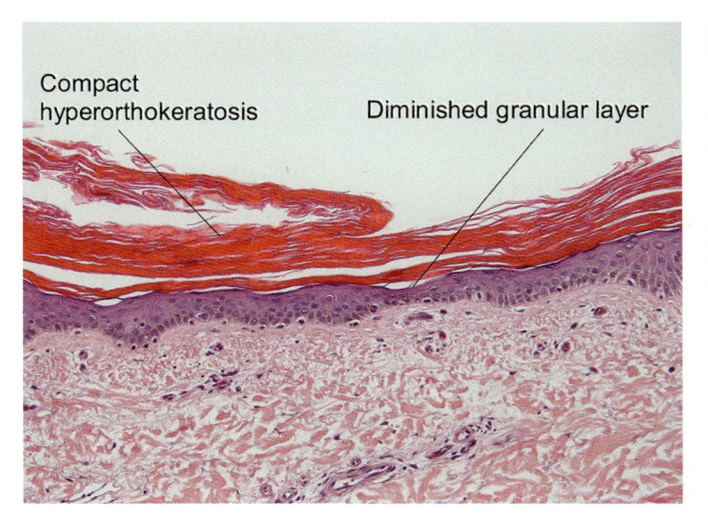

Fig 12-3 Ichthyosis vulgaris

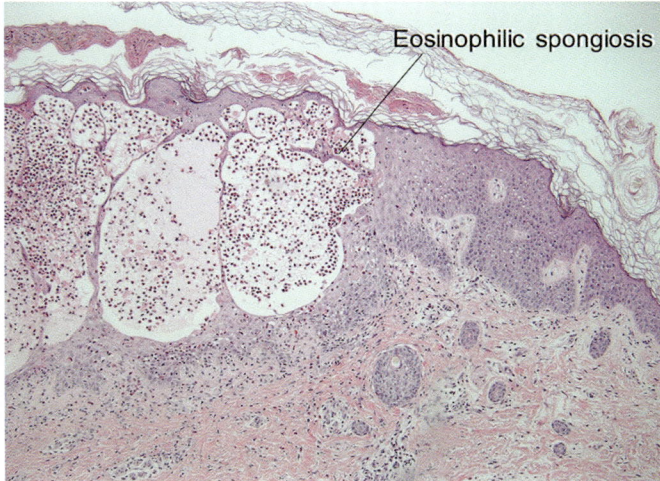

Fig 12-4 Incontinentia pigmenti, vesicular stage

- Subepidermal bullae, basal layer hyperpigmentation, and scattered eosinophils may be present
- Subtle increase in perivascular spindle-shaped hyperchromatic mast cells in telangiectasia macularis eruptiva perstans (TMEP)

Mastocytosis comprises a spectrum of diseases. A solitary mastocytoma may occur in childhood with a tendency to spontaneous involution. Urticaria pigmentosa is a sporadic rather than inherited disorder, characterized by multiple tan macules, papules, or nodules. There is a congenital or early-onset form that is rarely associated with systemic disease and typically clears by puberty. In contrast, adult-onset urticaria pigmentosa persists and can be associated with systemic involvement, especially bone marrow. The majority of lesions urticate with stroking (Darier's sign). Mutations in *c-kit* have been found in sporadic adult cases and in children with extensive or persistent disease but not in typical pediatric urticaria pigmentosa. TMEP is a rare adult form of mastocytosis with erythema, telangiectasia, and faint tan macules on the trunk and extremities, rarely with a Darier's sign.

In macular and TMEP lesions, the mast cells are limited to a superficial perivascular infiltrate. The mast cells may have small round nuclei with ample cytoplasm and resemble fried eggs or they may be spindle-shaped and simulate large hyperchromatic fibroblasts. The presence of more than five perivascular mast cells around each vessel is suggestive of mastocytosis. Special stains are recommended for identification. Mast cells can be identified with Leder stain (ASD-chloroacetate esterase) or via metachromatic staining of granules with toluidine blue and Giemsa methods. Immunohistochemistry for CD117 (the c-kit encoded tyrosine kinase receptor) and mast cell tryptase also identifies mast cells. Lesions degranulated by stroking (Darier's sign) may show no intracellular granules with Giemsa staining. A Leder stain is preferred in this setting.

Multiple or solitary nodular lesions reveal closely packed, uniformly spaced, round to cuboidal mast cells that fill the papillary dermis and may extend into the reticular dermis and subcutaneous tissue. These mast cells may be visibly granular and

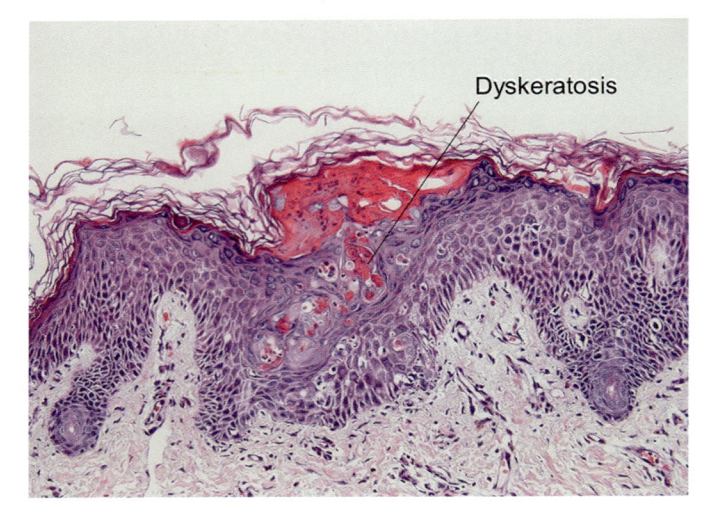

Fig 12-5 Incontinentia pigmenti, verrucous stage

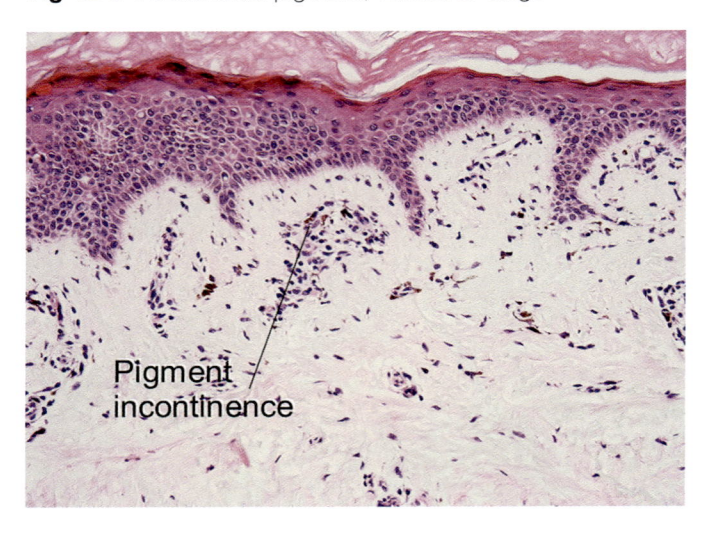

Fig 12-6 Incontinentia pigmenti, pigmented stage

Differential Diagnosis

The microscopic differential for spongiosis with eosinophils ("eosinophilic spongiosis") can be remembered by the mnemonic "HAAPPIE." The dyskeratotic cells help distinguish incontinentia pigmenti from the other conditions.

- *H*erpes gestationis
- *A*rthropod bite/*A*llergic contact dermatitis
- *P*emphigus
- *P*emphigoid
- *I*ncontinentia pigmenti
- *E*rythema toxicum neonatorum

Mastocytosis

Key features

- Uniformly spaced "fried-egg" mast cells fill the papillary dermis and extend into the reticular dermis in nodular lesions

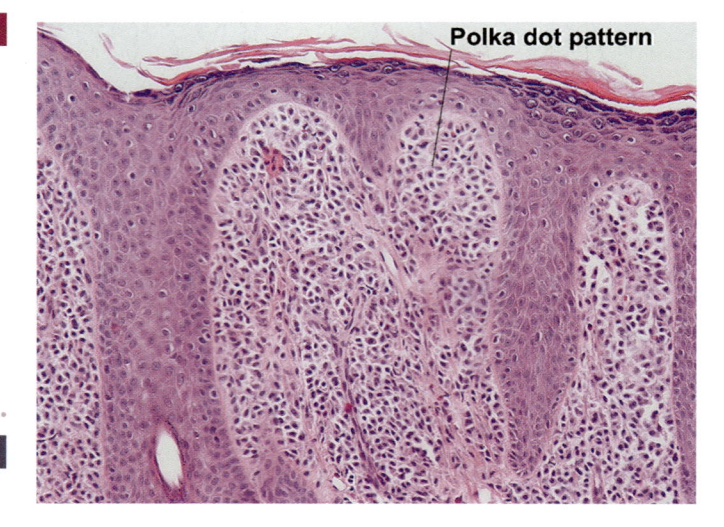

Fig 12-7 Mastocytoma

Genodermatoses 211

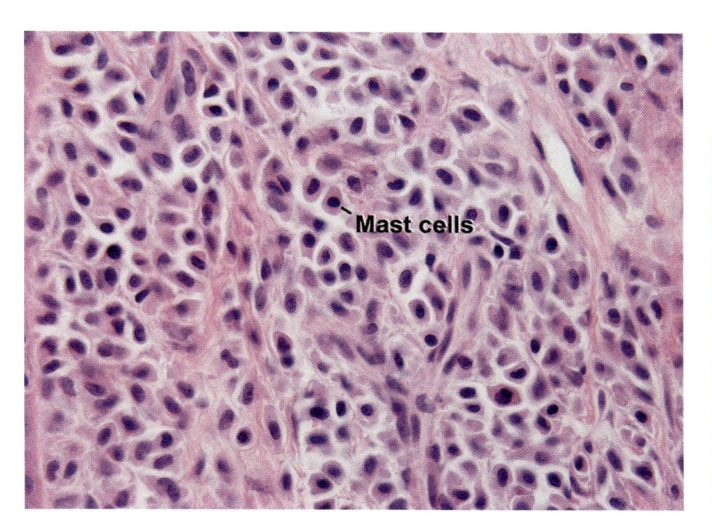

Fig 12-8 Mastocytoma

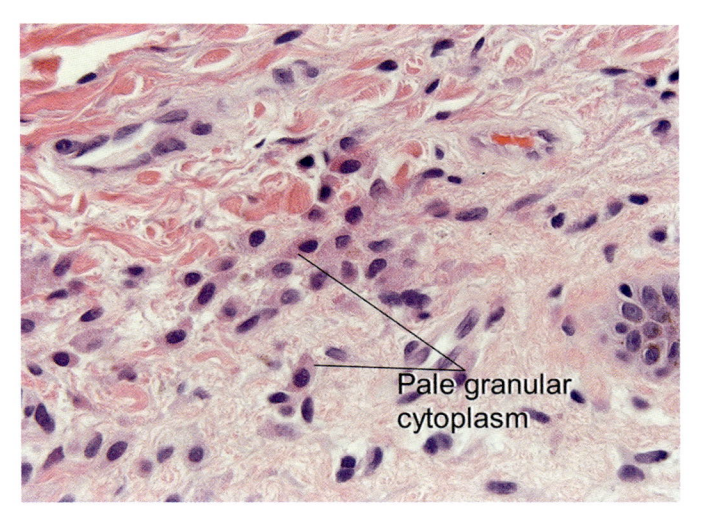

Fig 12-9 Mast cells

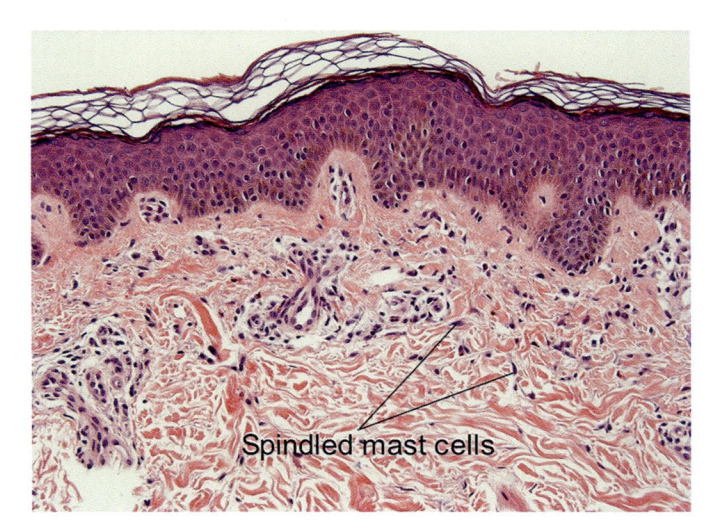

Fig 12-10 Telangiectasia macularis eruptiva perstans

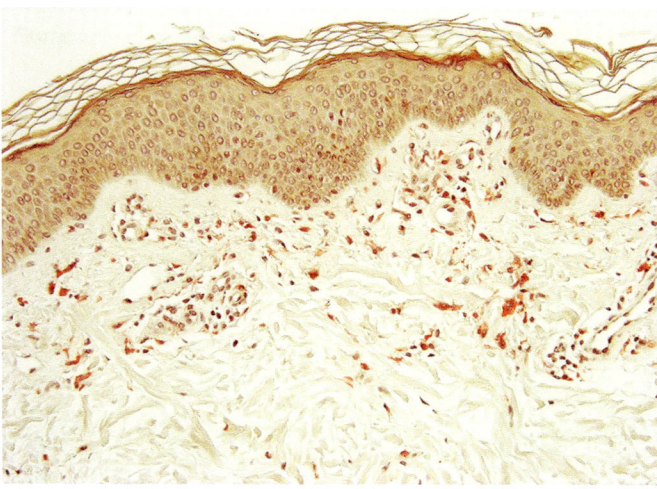

Fig 12-11 Telangiectasia macularis eruptive perstans (Leder stain)

may have a "fried-egg" appearance with a central nucleus and eosinophilic to pale gray cytoplasm. A scattering of eosinophils is usually present and basal hyperpigmentation may be identified. These lesions can be distinguished from Langerhans cell histiocytosis by the absence of epidermal involvement, absence of folliculotropism, absence of reniform nuclei, and with special stains. The cuboidal cells may resemble nevus cells but mast cell lesions lack junctional and dermal nesting and lack the nuclear pseudoinclusions typical of melanocytes.

Epidermolytic ichthyosis (bullous congenital ichthyosiform erythroderma)

Key features

- Compact hyperorthokeratosis
- Granular and vacuolar degeneration of the upper layers of the epidermis
- Red and blue clumped keratohyaline granules and vacuoles – granular layer "chewed up"

Epidermolytic hyperkeratosis is a histologic pattern that can be seen in several clinical settings, including palmoplantar keratoderma, solitary epidermolytic acanthoma, and epidermolytic ichthyosis. Not uncommonly, epidermolytic hyperkeratosis is an incidental finding in biopsies of another lesion such as a dysplastic nevus.

Epidermolytic ichthyosis is an autosomal-dominant condition characterized by widespread blistering and erythema at birth that evolve into generalized furrowed hyperkeratosis with accentuation in the flexures. There is a wide morphologic spectrum. Mutations in keratin genes (*K1* and *K10*) have been identified. This generalized disorder has been reported in the offspring of patients with linear epidermal nevi that histologically reveal epidermolytic hyperkeratosis, suggesting that these "epidermal nevi" represent mosaicism for the trait.

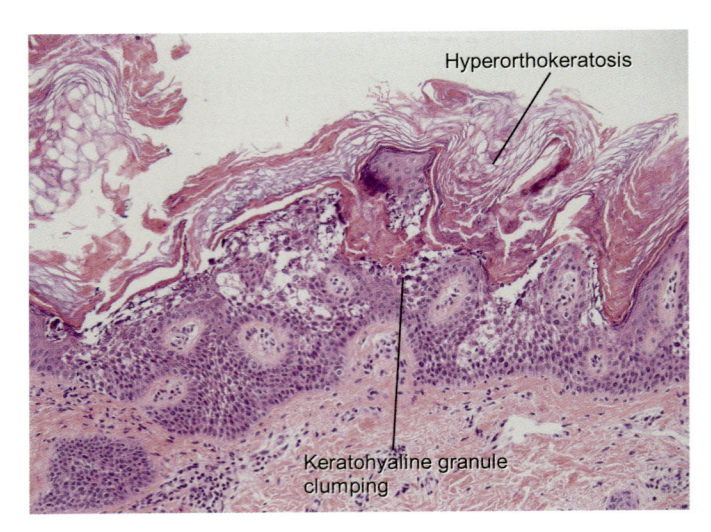

Fig 12-12 Epidermolytic hyperkeratosis

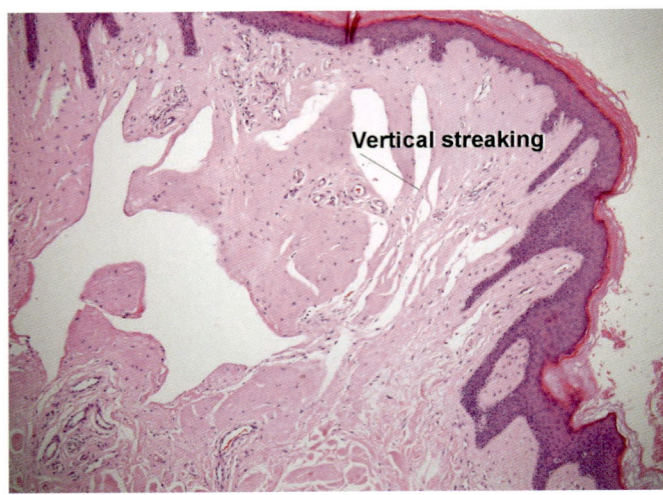

Fig 12-13 Lipoid proteinosis

Lipoid proteinosis

Key features

- Hyperkeratosis
- Extensive deposits of perpendicular hyaline material in the papillary dermis
- Concentric deposits around hair follicles, and eccrine glands

Differential Diagnosis

The deposits are more prominent and extend deeper than in porphyria. The vertical orientation is not seen in porphyria.

Further reading

Bolognia JL, Braverman I. Pseudoxanthoma-elasticum-like skin changes induced by penicillamine. Dermatology 1992;184(1):12–18.

Davis MD, Dinneen AM, Landa N, et al. Grover's disease: clinicopathologic review of 72 cases. Mayo Clin Proc 1999;74(3):229–234.

Eng AM, Bryant J. Clinical pathologic observations in pseudoxanthoma elasticum. Int J Dermatol 1975;14(8):586–605.

Lebwohl M, Phelps RG, Yannuzzi L, et al. Diagnosis of pseudoxanthoma elasticum by scar biopsy in patients without characteristic skin lesions. N Engl J Med 1987;317(6):347–350.

Meyrick Thomas RH, Kirby JD. Elastosis perforans serpiginosa and pseudoxanthoma elasticum-like skin change due to D-penicillamine. Clin Exp Dermatol 1985;10(4):386–391.

Shukla SA, Veerappan R, Whittimore JS, et al. Mast cell ultrastructure and staining in tissue. Methods Mol Biol 2006;315:63–76.

Sybert VP, Dale BA, Holbrook KA. Ichthyosis vulgaris: identification of a defect in synthesis of filaggrin correlated with an absence of keratohyaline granules. J Invest Dermatol 1985;84(3):191–194.

Chapter 13

Alterations in collagen and elastin

Tammie Ferringer

Lichen sclerosus (et atrophicus)

Key features

- Red (compact stratum corneum)
- White (papillary dermal pallor)
- Blue (lymphoid band beneath zone of pallor)
- Synonymous with balanitis xerotica obliterans on the glans penis

Lichen sclerosus may involve skin or mucosa. Follicular plugging is common, and the plugs may resemble comedones clinically. The epidermis is commonly atrophic and the rete pattern is commonly effaced; however, scratching may produce pseudoepitheliomatous hyperplasia, especially in vulvar lesions. Squamous cell carcinoma rarely develops in long-standing genital lesions of lichen sclerosus and must be distinguished from pseudoepitheliomatous hyperplasia. Papillary dermal edema may produce a subepidermal bulla. Vacuolar interface dermatitis and pigment incontinence are common. Epidermotropic lymphocytes may be hyperchromatic and may mimic mycosis fungoides (Table 13.1). The differential diagnosis also includes radiation dermatitis and morphea.

Chronic radiation dermatitis

Key features

- Papillary dermal pallor without vacuolar change or lymphoid band
- Large stellate radiation fibroblasts
- Radiation elastosis
- Loss of adnexa
- Dilated ectatic vessels superficially

There is typically hyperkeratosis and epidermal atrophy with effaced rete that may alternate with hyperplasia. Stellate cells with large nuclei are usually present (radiation fibroblasts). The eccrine glands are atrophic and the pilosebaceous structures are absent; however, the arrector pili muscle may survive. The dermal collagen is hyalinized. Radiation elastosis may resemble solar elastosis but extends into follicular fibrous tracts. The superficial blood vessels are dilated, whereas the deeper vessels have thick walls.

The severity of radiation damage varies with the total dose, its fractionation, and the depth of penetration. Acute radiodermatitis occurs within weeks of irradiation and presents as erythema and edema followed by hyperpigmentation. Although typically diagnosed clinically, there is vacuolization and sparse degenerated keratinocytes similar to a phototoxic eruption. Chronic changes arise months to years after the initial exposure. There is atrophy, fragility, telangiectasias, altered pigmentation, and alopecia. Non-melanoma skin cancers can develop years later and may behave in an aggressive manner with increased risk of metastasis, especially in squamous cell carcinoma.

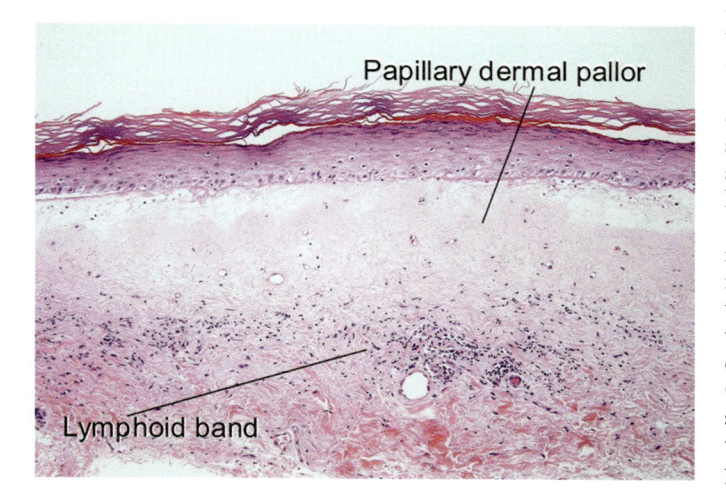

Fig 13-1 Lichen sclerosus

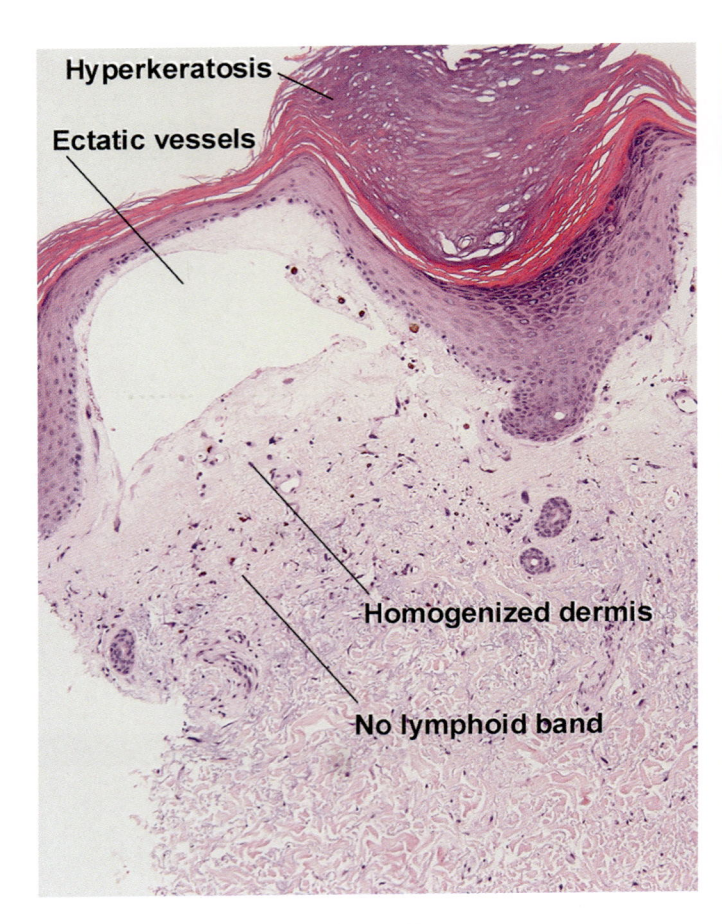

Fig 13-2 Chronic radiation dermatitis

Table 13-1 Features of lichen sclerosus and chronic radiation dermatitis

Feature	Lichen sclerosus	Chronic radiation dermatitis
Compact red stratum corneum	Yes	Yes
Superficial dermal pallor	Yes	Yes
Epidermal atrophy	Variable	Variable
Follicular plugging	Common	Rare
Vacuolar interface dermatitis	Yes	No
Lymphoid band	Yes	No
Pigment incontinence	Common	Usually absent
Superficial dermal vessels	Normal to slight dilatation	Widely ectatic
Radiation elastosis	No	Yes
Adnexal structures	Present	Absent
Large stellate fibroblasts	No	Yes
Deep dermis	Normal	Sclerotic
Shape of punch biopsy	Tapered	Square

- Loss of adventitial fat resulting in "trapped" eccrine glands
- Sparse deep lymphoplasmacytic infiltrate
- Reduced number of CD34+ cells in the dermis
- Superficial dermal pallor may be present, but the vacuolar interface dermatitis and lymphoid band of lichen sclerosus are lacking

Scleroderma encompasses a group of diseases. Localized cutaneous disease may present as morphea or linear scleroderma (including *en coup de sabre*). In addition to cutaneous lesions, Raynaud's phenomenon and variable organ involvement characterize diffuse systemic scleroderma and limited systemic scleroderma (CREST). Although the histologic features are similar, morphea is usually more inflammatory and lacks the intimal thickening and luminal obliteration of vessels seen in systemic scleroderma.

There is controversy concerning the relationship of lichen sclerosus and morphea. Some regard lichen sclerosus as a superficial expression of morphea, explaining the lichen sclerosus-like changes in the papillary dermis overlying some lesions of morphea. However, lesions of morphea with superficial pallor never demonstrate a superficial lymphoid band, vacuolar interface dermatitis, or follicular plugging. Deep dermal sclerosis is always present.

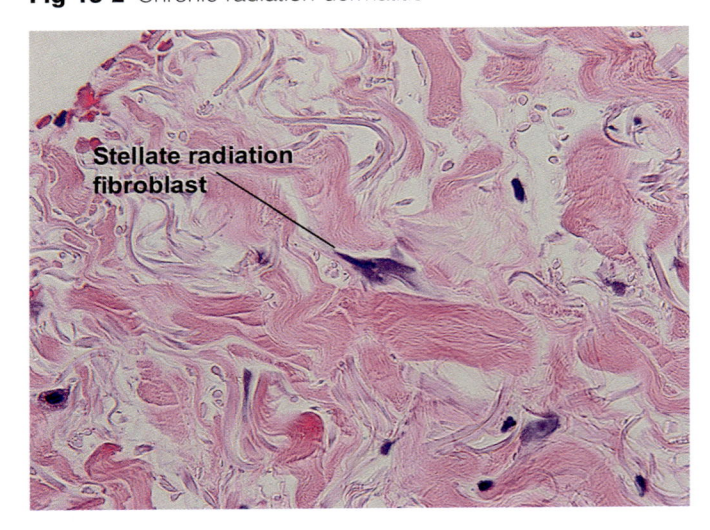

Fig 13-3 Chronic radiation dermatitis

Morphea/scleroderma

Key features

- Rectangular punch
- Thick, closely packed, hyalinized collagen bundles in the lower dermis

The sclerotic process in linear scleroderma and deep morphea (morphea profunda) extends into the subcutaneous fat and possibly fascia and bone. Unlike chronic radiation dermatitis, radiation elastosis is absent and radiation fibroblasts are not identified. Elastic fibers in morphea are often brightly eosinophilic.

Other disorders with dermal sclerosis include sclerodermoid graft-versus-host (GvHD) disease, porphyria cutanea tarda, vinyl chloride exposure, and reactions to bleomycin. There are conflicting data regarding the relationship with *Borrelia burgdorferi* infection and morphea and lichen sclerosus. A relationship has been found in some studies in Europe; however other studies, especially those in North America, have resulted in negative findings.

Differential Diagnosis

Typical punch biopsies exhibit a tapered or cone-shaped outline. However, a thickened or sclerotic dermis can result in a square or rectangular biopsy. This can be seen in:
- Morphea/scleroderma
- Chronic GvHD
- Chronic radiodermatitis
- Scar
- Normal skin of the back
- Connective tissue nevi
- Scleroderma

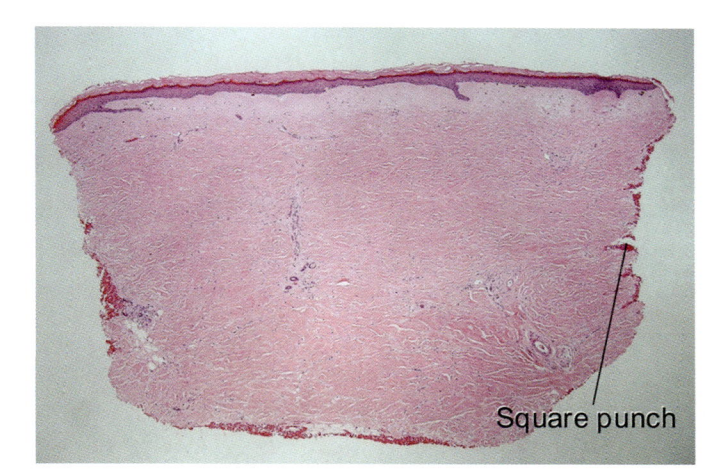

Fig 13-4 Morphea

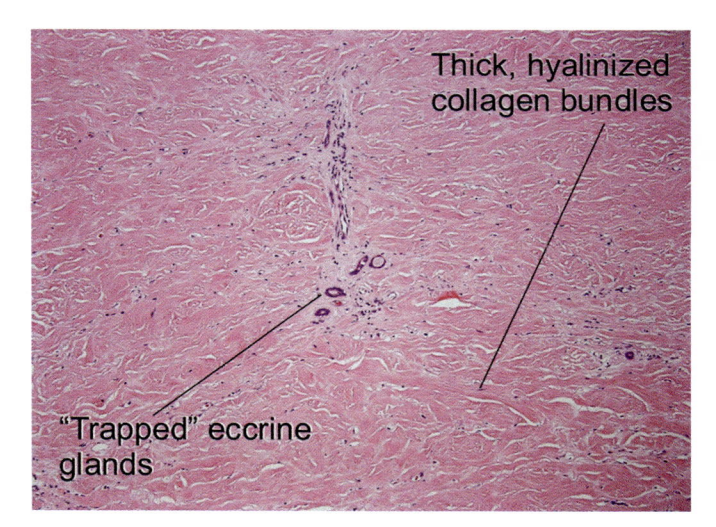

Fig 13-5 Morphea

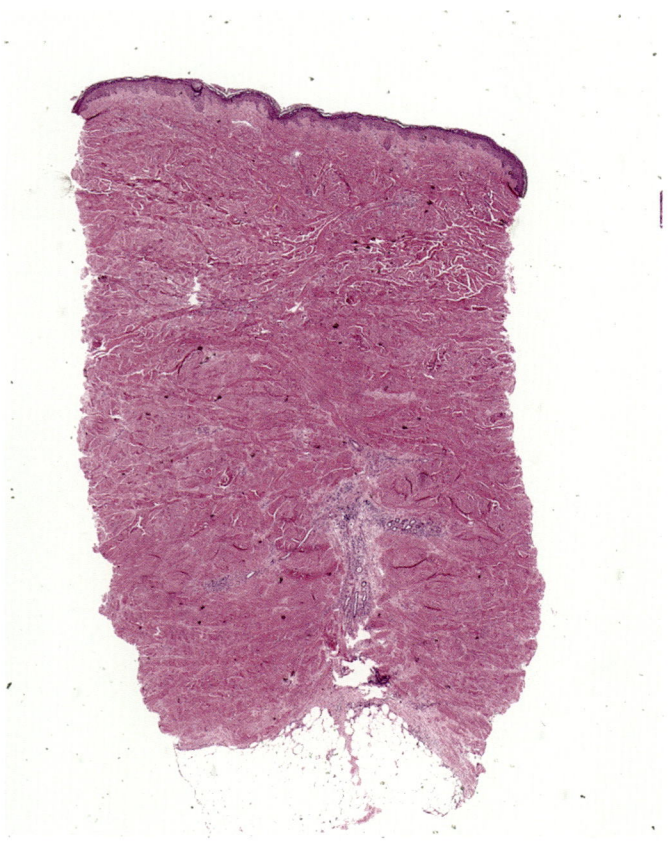

Fig 13-6 Morphea

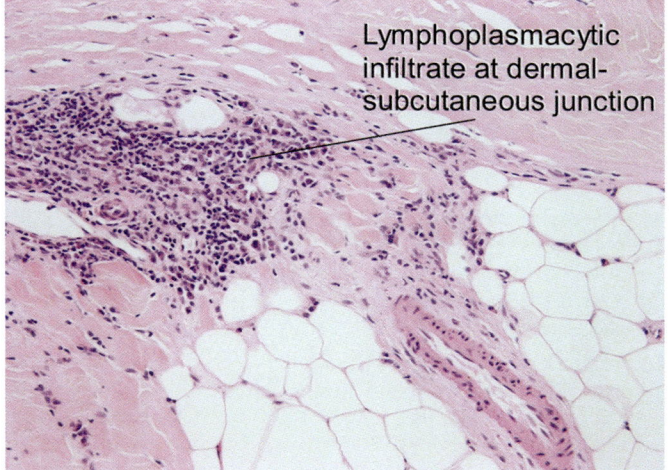

Fig 13-7 Morphea

216 Dermatopathology

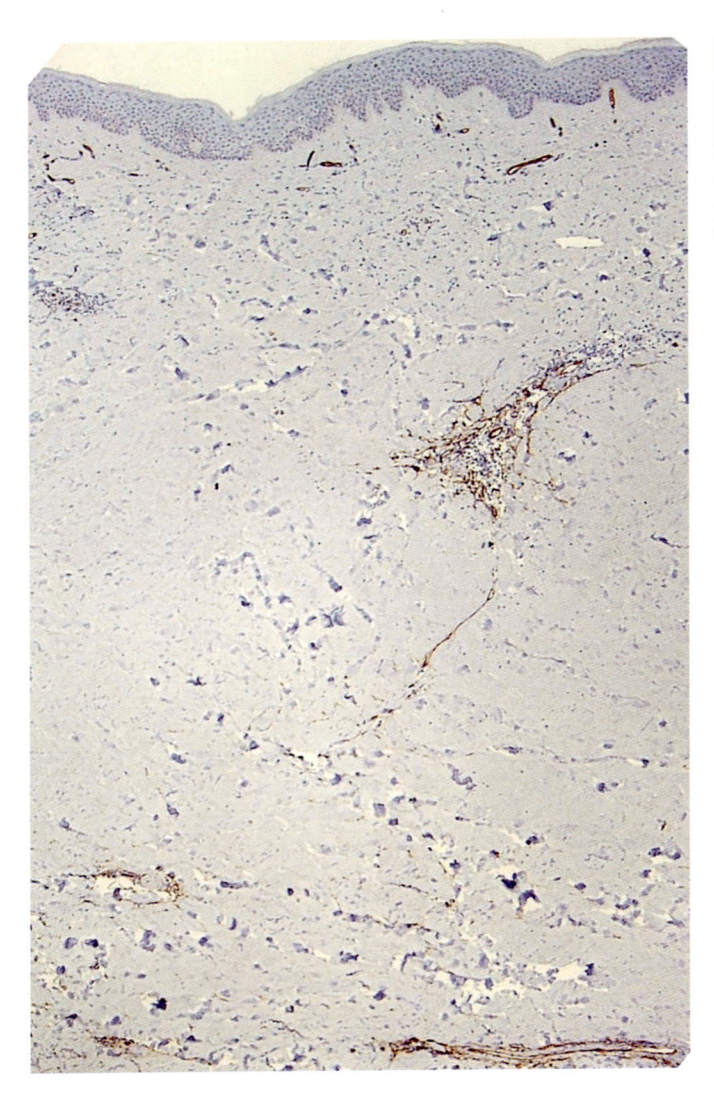

Fig 13-8 Morphea, CD34 revealing loss of interstitial reactivity

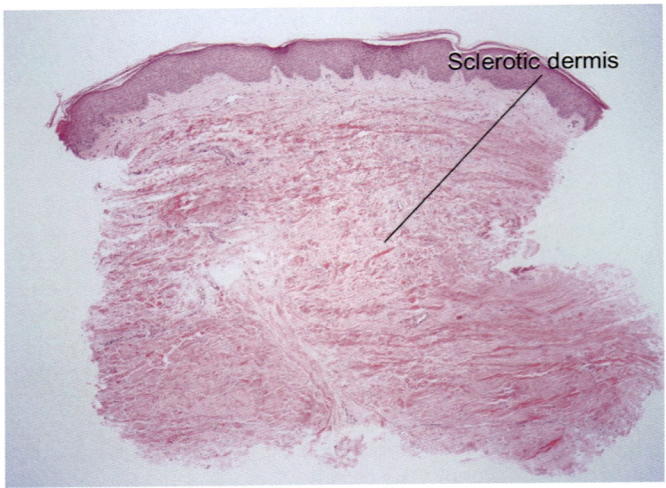

Fig 13-9 Sclerodermoid graft-versus-host disease

Eosinophilic fasciitis (Shulman's syndrome)

Key features

- Thick eosinophilic fascia due to fibrosis and hyalinization of collagen
- Variable infiltrate of lymphocytes, plasma cells, and occasional eosinophils

Eosinophilic fasciitis is a scleroderma-like disorder of the fascia that can be distinguished by the sudden onset of painful edema and progressive induration, typically involving an extremity or extremities following strenuous exercise. The condition is named for its association with peripheral eosinophilia. Eosinophils may be found in the tissue but are not required, and are typically absent. The fibrosis and hyalinization involve the fascia and deep subcutaneous septa. In many cases, the overlying adipose tissue shows no significant changes. A deep incisional biopsy to include fascia is required for diagnosis.

Sclerodermoid graft-versus-host disease

Key features

- Minimal basal vacuolization
- Dermis is thickened and sclerotic
- Adnexal structures are destroyed

Dermal sclerosis begins in the papillary dermis and may extend into the subcutaneous tissue. In the chronic phase of GvHD, an early lichenoid stage and a later sclerotic stage can be distinguished. Each stage can occur without the other. Unlike radiation dermatitis, vascular ectasia and radiation fibroblasts are not identified. Clinically, the skin often has a corrugated appearance.

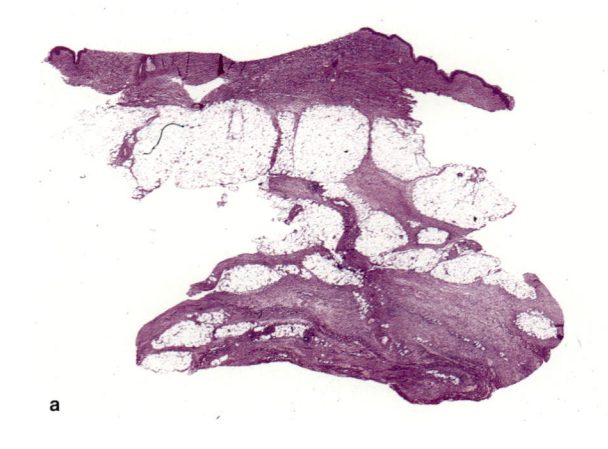

Fig 13-10 Eosinophilic fasciitis

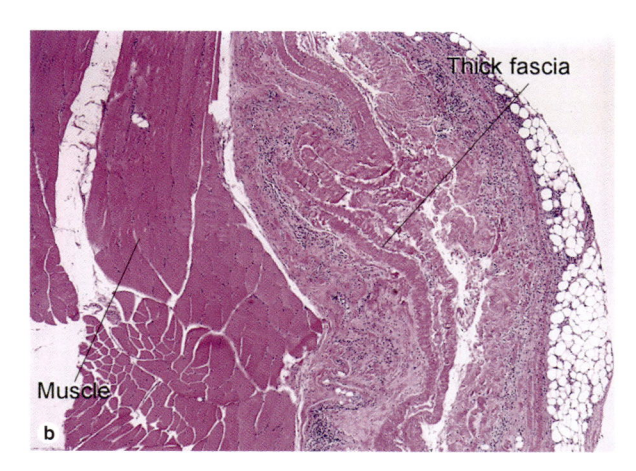

Fig 13-10, cont'd

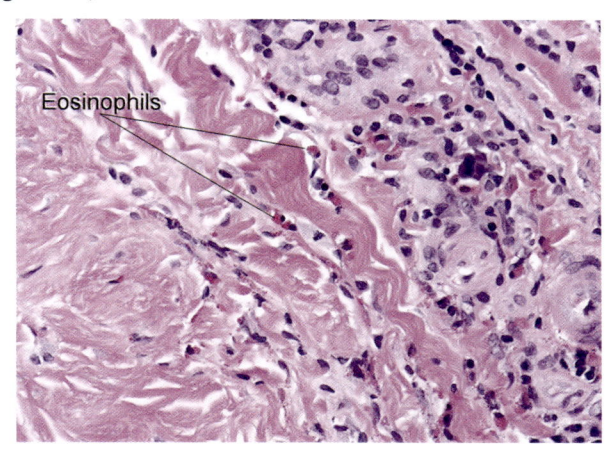

Fig 13-11 Eosinophilic fasciitis

Scleroderma with fascial involvement may appear similar histologically, but can be distinguished clinically. Similar changes are described in eosinophilia-myalgia syndrome secondary to L-tryptophan ingestion, although there is greater dermal involvement in eosinophilia-myalgia syndrome and the late stage is characterized by dermal mucinosis.

Elastosis perforans serpiginosa

Key features

- Tortuous channel through an acanthotic epidermis with extrusion of altered elastic fibers
- Large bulky red elastic fibers

The papules of elastosis perforans serpiginosa coalesce in an arcuate or serpiginous pattern, most commonly on the neck, face, or upper extremity. Elastic tissue stains reveal increased abnormal, thickened elastic fibers in the dermis in the vicinity of the channel.

Patients on long-term penicillamine for Wilson's disease may develop altered elastic fibers with overlapping features of pseudoxanthoma elasticum and elastosis perforans serpiginosa. The penicillamine-induced, altered elastic fibers have small lateral buds arranged perpendicularly to the primary elastic fiber, resembling the twigs on a bramble bush.

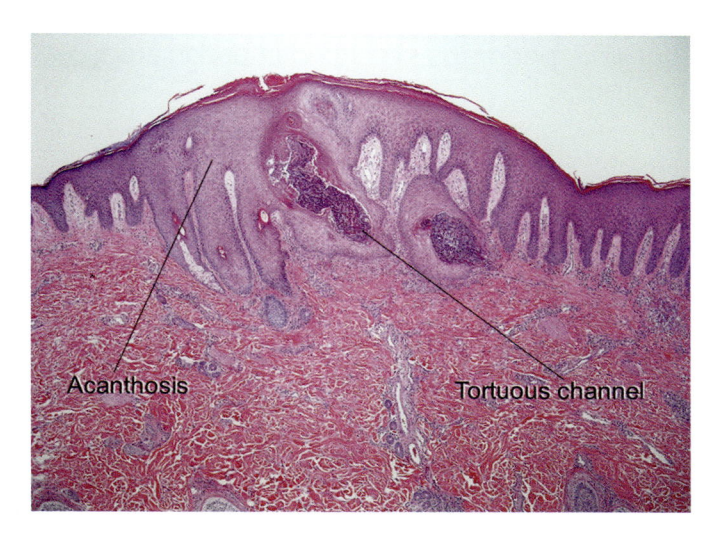

Fig 13-12 Elastosis perforans serpiginosa

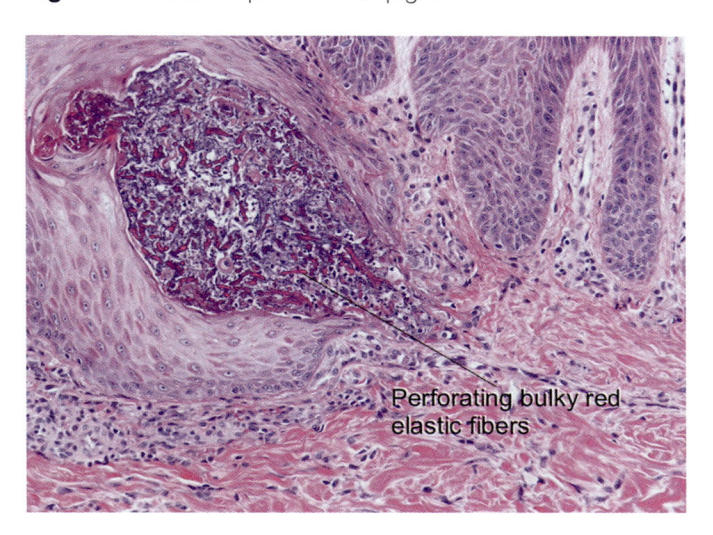

Fig 13-13 Elastosis perforans serpiginosa

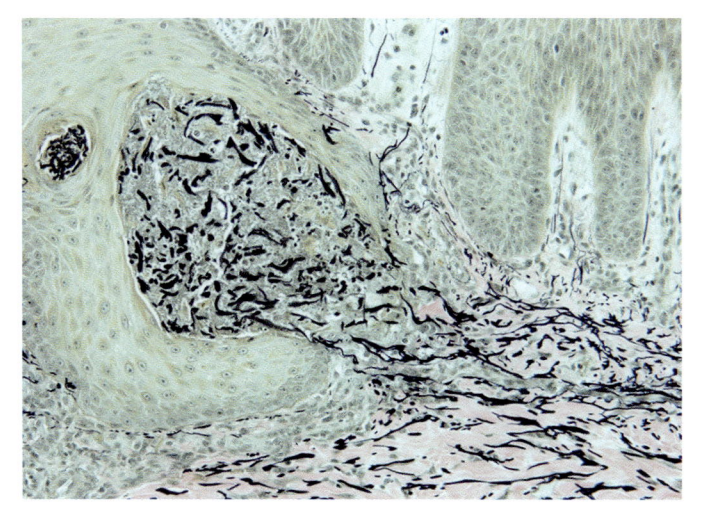

Fig 13-14 Elastosis perforans serpiginosa (elastic tissue stain)

Elastosis perforans serpiginosa-associated disorders

The mnemonic "RAP MOPED" is helpful in remembering the associated diseases.
- *R*othmund–Thompson syndrome
- *A*crogeria
- *P*enicillamine
- *M*arfan's syndrome
- *O*steogenesis imperfecta
- *P*seudoxanthoma elasticum
- *E*hlers–Danlos syndrome
- *D*own's syndrome

Reactive perforating collagenosis

Key features
- Broad channel
- Vertical extrusion of degenerated basophilic collagen bundles
- Masson trichrome stain distinguishes the extruded collagen from elastic tissue

The primary lesion is a small papule with a hyperkeratotic central umbilication. Classic, true reactive perforating collagenosis is an inherited genodermatosis, most often in an autosomal-dominant pattern. These lesions occur in children and are precipitated by minor trauma.

An adult, acquired form has been described in association with diabetes and chronic renal failure. This form, known as acquired perforating dermatosis or perforating disorder of renal disease, encompasses features of Kyrle's disease and perforating folliculitis.

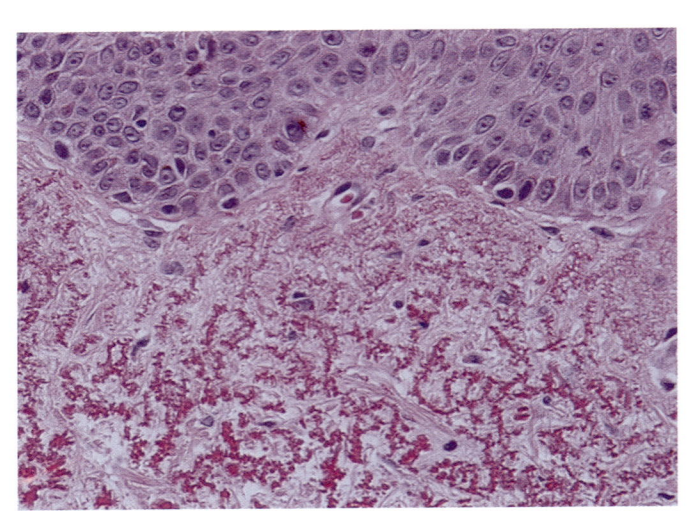

Fig 13-15 Penicillamine-induced altered elastic fibers

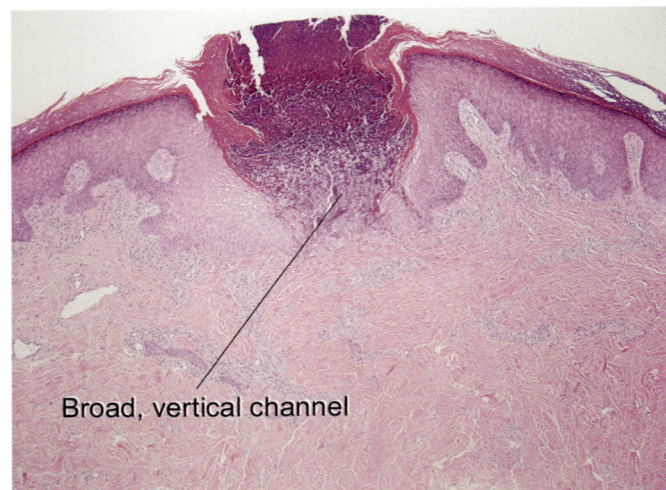

Fig 13-17 Reactive perforating collagenosis

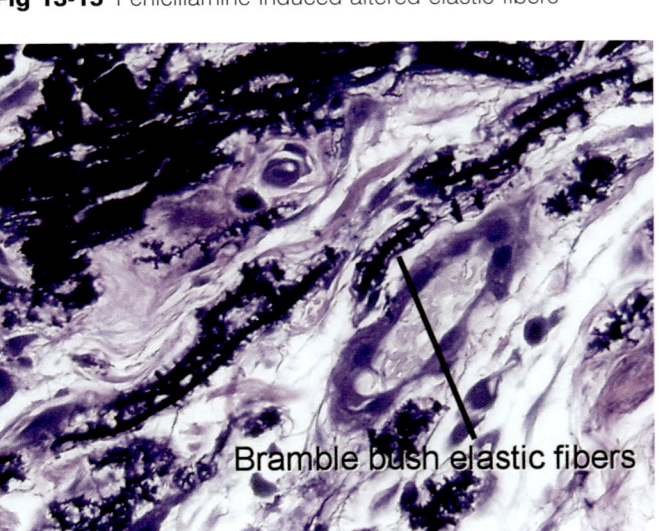

Fig 13-16 Penicillamine-induced altered elastic fibers (Verhoeff–van Gieson)

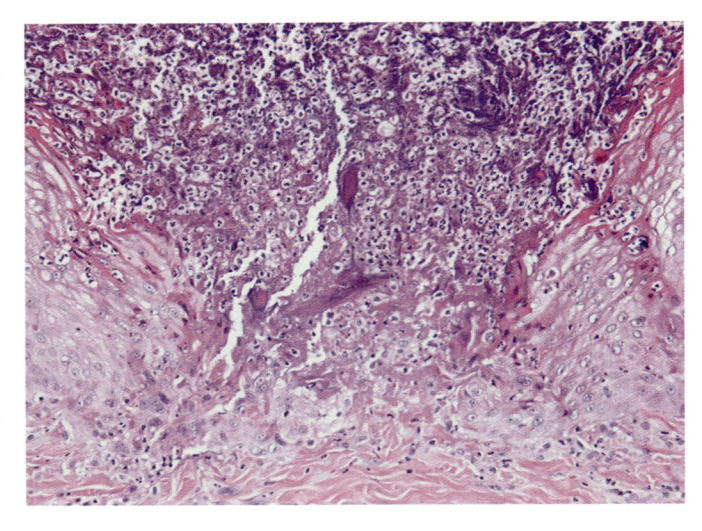

Fig 13-18 Reactive perforating collagenosis

Scar and keloid

Scar

Key features

- Fibroblasts with east–west orientation
- Blood vessels with north–south orientation
- Loss of elastic tissue (see Chapter 20)
- Epidermis is often effaced

Hypertrophic scar

Key features

- Nodules or whorls of thickened collagen and fibroblasts

Keloid

Key features

- Background of hypertrophic scar
- Broad, hyalinized, eosinophilic "bubble gum" collagen fibers

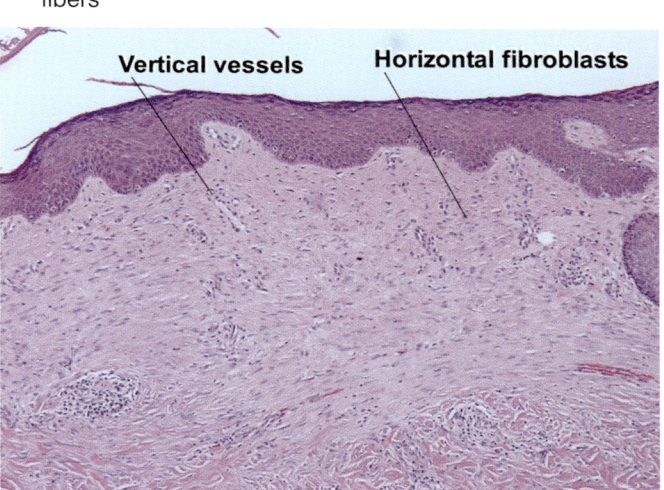

Fig 13-19 Scar

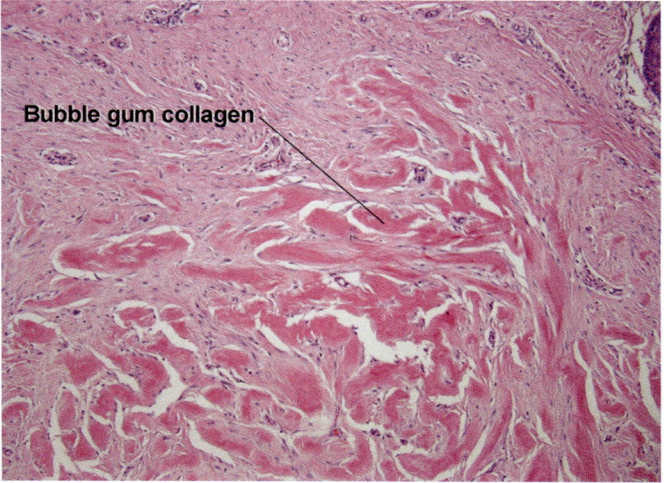

Fig 13-20 Scar

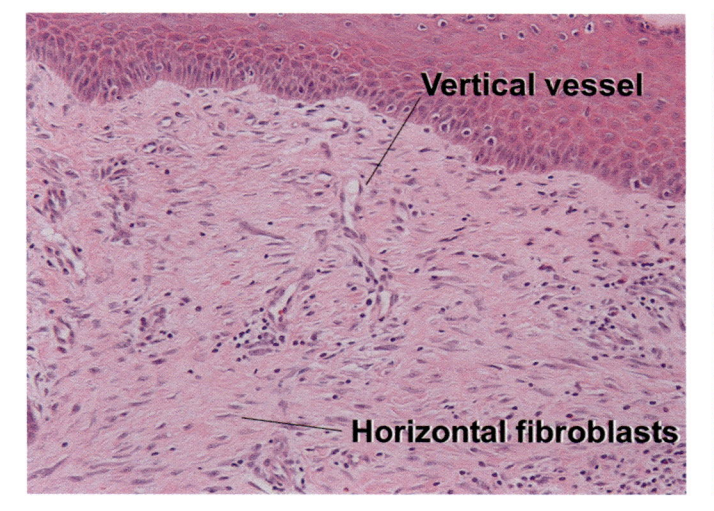

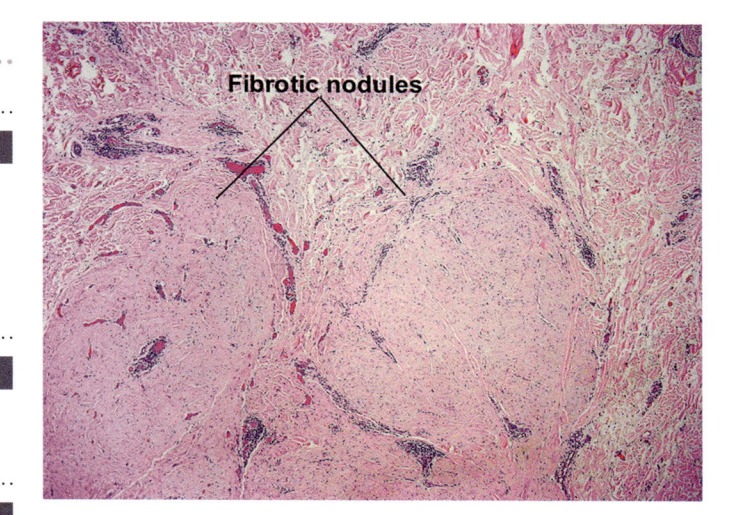

Fig 13-21 Hypertrophic scar

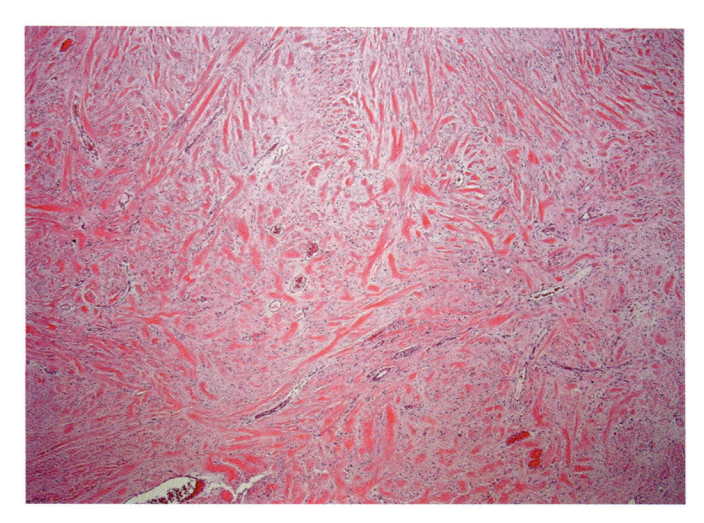

Fig 13-22 Keloid

Fig 13-23 Keloid

Keloids clinically differ from hypertrophic scars by extending beyond the confines of the original wound. Elastic fibers and adnexal structures are diminished or absent in both scars and keloids. Recent surgical scars may also contain signs of Monsel's solution, gelfoam, or aluminum chloride.

Acne keloidalis nuchae

Key features
- Hypertrophic scar (not keloid)
- Suppurative folliculitis with hair shafts free in the dermis
- Plasma cell infiltrate

The plasma cell infiltrate is related to the predominance on the posterior neck. Plasma cells are typically a component of the inflammatory infiltrate on the face, occipital scalp/posterior neck, axillae, breast, genital area, and shins. Hair shafts free in the dermis are surrounded by microabscesses and/or giant cells.

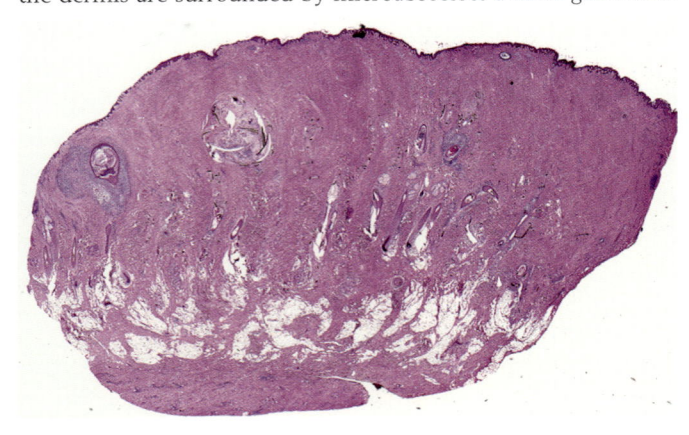

Fig 13-24 Acne keloidalis nuchae

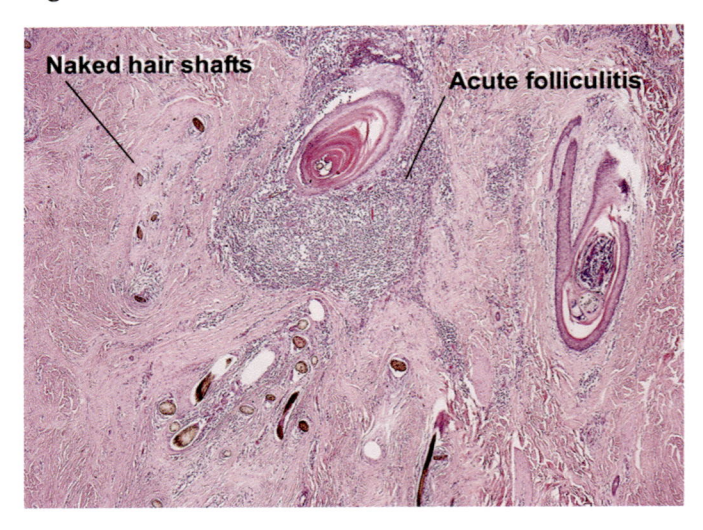

Fig 13-25 Acne keloidalis nuchae

PEARL
There is no mycosis in mycosis fungoides, no granuloma in granuloma faciale, and no keloid in acne keloidalis.

Favre–Racouchot syndrome (nodular elastosis with cysts and comedones)

Key features
- Dilated, keratin-filled follicles
- Small cysts
- Solar elastosis

This solar degeneration condition presents with yellowish plaques lateral to the eyes that are studded with cysts and multiple open comedones. Smoking may act in conjunction with the solar damage to create this syndrome. Solar elastosis is a bluish, amorphous material that is primarily sun-damaged elastic and/or collagen fibers.

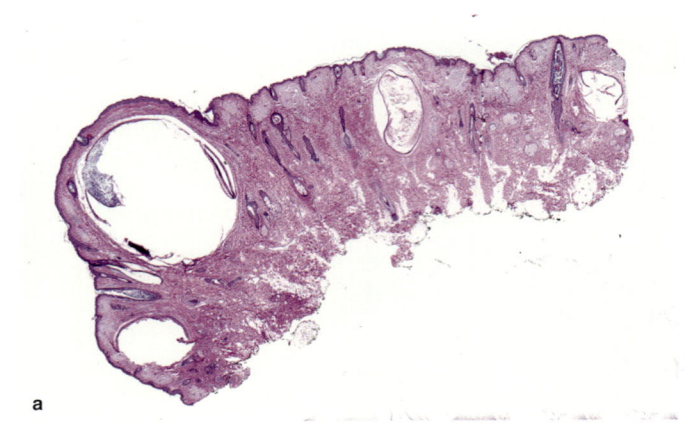

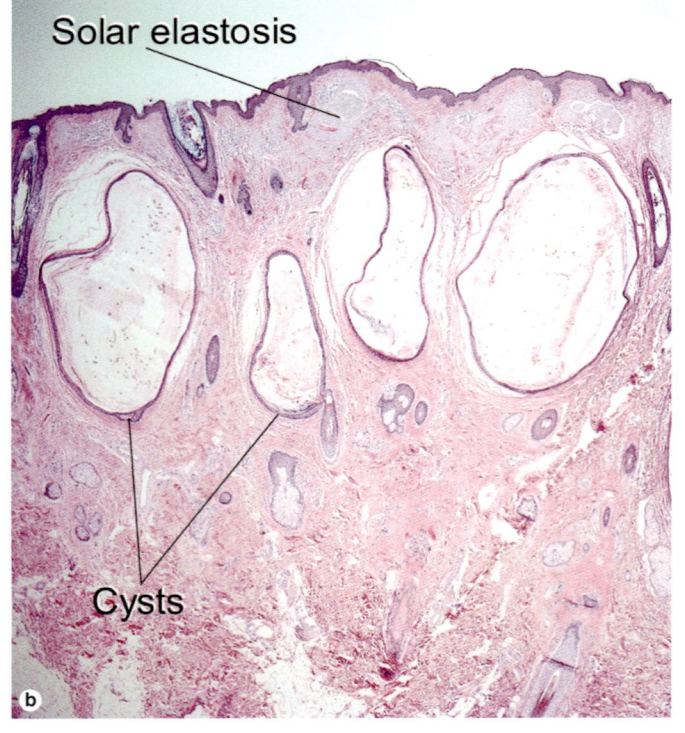

Fig 13-26 Favre–Racouchot syndrome

Chondrodermatitis nodularis helicis

Key features

- Ulcer or erosion with adjacent acanthosis overlying a zone of fibrin
- Fibrin is flanked on either side by granulation tissue

Depending on the depth of the biopsy, cartilage may be present but is not required for diagnosis. Collagen degeneration occurs from a combination of pressure, poor vascularity, and solar damage (see Chapter 15).

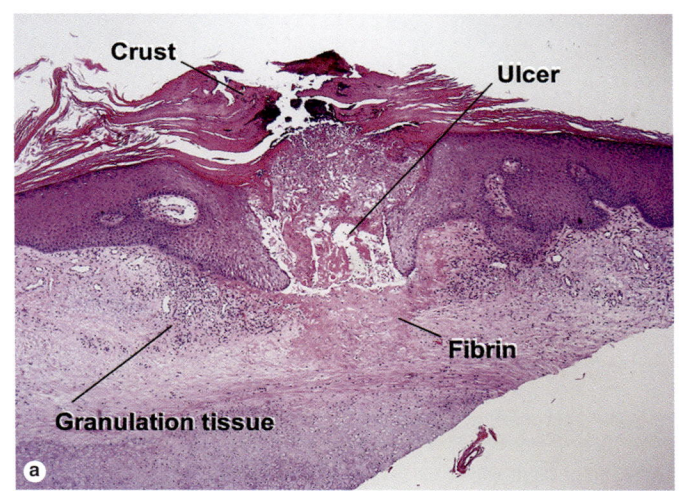

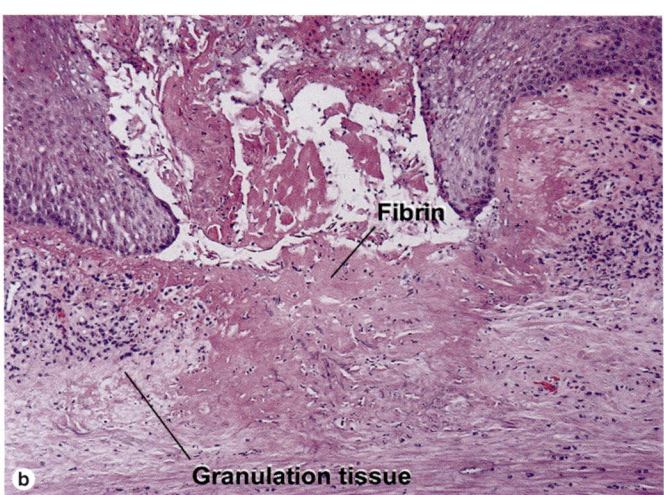

Fig 13-27 Chondrodermatitis nodularis helicis

Acrodermatitis chronica atrophicans

Key features

- Early lesions show a diffuse lymphoplasmacytic infiltrate resembling "polka dots"
- Late lesions show epidermal and dermal atrophy with attenuated wispy collagen fibers

Borrelial spirochetes may be found with silver stains. This is a late manifestation of infection by *Borrelia*. It is most frequently reported in Europe, where *B. afzelii* is endemic.

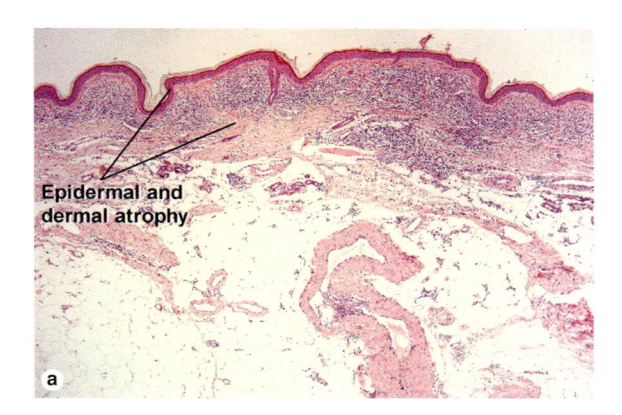

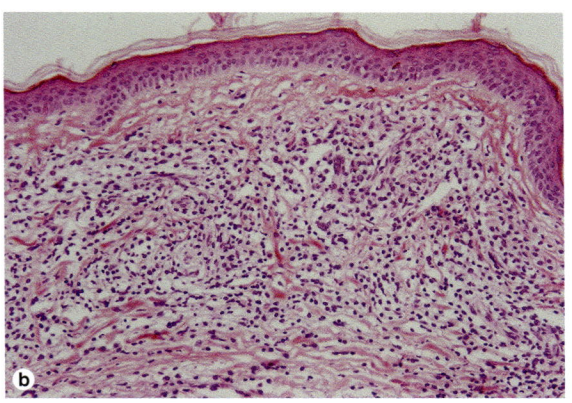

Fig 13-28 Acrodermatitis chronica atrophicans

Ochronosis

Key features

- Glassy yellow-brown (ochre-colored) banana-shaped deposits in the dermis

The inherited form, also known as alkaptonuria, is an autosomal-recessive disorder due to homogentisic acid oxidase deficiency. Exogenous ochronosis occurs as a result of application of hydroquinone or contact with phenol (carbolic acid).

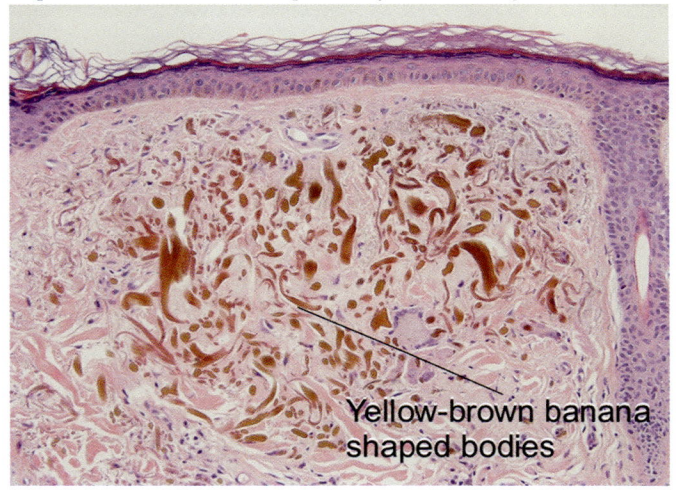

Fig 13-29 Ochronosis

Colloid milium

Key features

- Pale pink, fissured deposits that fill and expand the dermal papillae

The adult type develops in the setting of severe sun damage, on the face, neck, and dorsal hands. This material represents the final product of severe solar degeneration but can stain weakly with amyloid stains (crystal violet, Congo red, thioflavin T). However, it fails to react with pagoda red. The juvenile form develops on the head and neck before the development of sun damage. This type is Congo red-negative but positive with antikeratin antibodies confirming the origin of the material from degenerated keratinocytes.

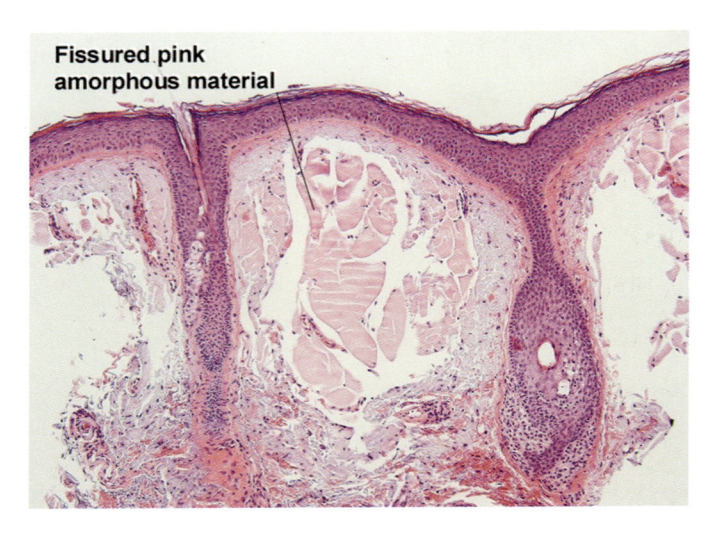

Fig 13-30 Colloid milium

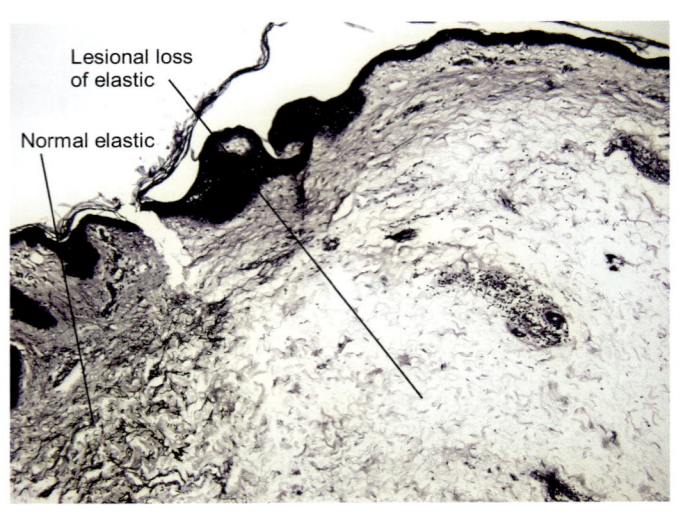

Fig 13-31 Anetoderma (Verhoeff–van Gieson)

Anetoderma

Key features

- Essentially normal hematoxylin and eosin (H&E)-stained sections
- Elastic fibers are sparse to absent in the superficial and mid dermis with elastic tissue stains (Verhoeff–van Gieson)

These oval lesions have an atrophic or wrinkled surface and bulge outward or are slightly depressed and herniate inward with pressure. The upper trunk and upper arms of young adults are typically affected. Primary lesions have been reported with (Jadassohn–Pellizzari type) and without (Schweninger–Buzzi type) a preceding inflammatory stage. Clinically inflamed lesions may have a perivascular and sometimes interstitial infiltrate but established lesions look like normal skin on H&E-stained sections and reveal minimal to no elastic fibers with special stains. Secondary anetoderma can occur from various processes including syphilis, other infectious processes, granulomatous diseases, lupus, and lymphoma.

Atrophoderma

Key features

- Hematoxylin and eosin-stained features are subtle unless compared with normal adjacent skin when the dermal thickness appears reduced
- Collagen shows varying degrees of homogenization

Lesions typically are sharply demarcated gray-brown, atrophic, round to oval, depressed areas with a "cliff-drop" border. Some have suggested that atrophoderma is an atrophic abortive variant of morphea. In contrast to morphea, there is no violaceous border or induration, and lesions tend to be chronic. A superficial perivascular and interstitial inflammatory infiltrate consisting of lymphocytes and histiocytes can be seen. Elastic fibers appear normal.

Connective tissue nevus

Key features

- Collagenoma: thickened dermis due to broad haphazard bundles of collagen that are less well packed than normal collagen and widely spaced elastic fibers likely due to a dilution phenomenon
- Elastoma: H&E-stained sections show a normal or slightly thickened dermis but accumulation of broad, branching and interlacing elastic fibers in the mid and lower dermis with elastic tissue stains

Connective tissue nevi are hamartomas of the extracellular connective tissue, whether it is collagen, elastic, or glycosaminoglycans, that is present in abnormal amounts. Collagenomas can be inherited in an autosomal dominant pattern or associated with Proteus syndrome and tuberous sclerosis (shagreen patches). They present as skin-colored papules, nodules or plaques. Elastomas are associated with Buschke–Ollendorff syndrome.

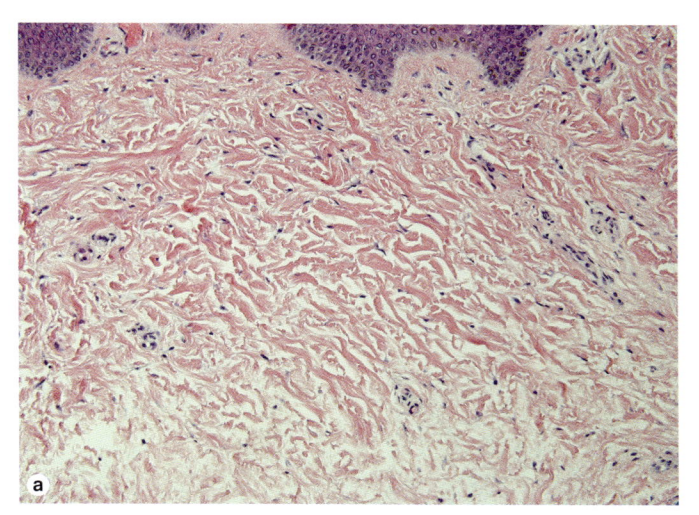

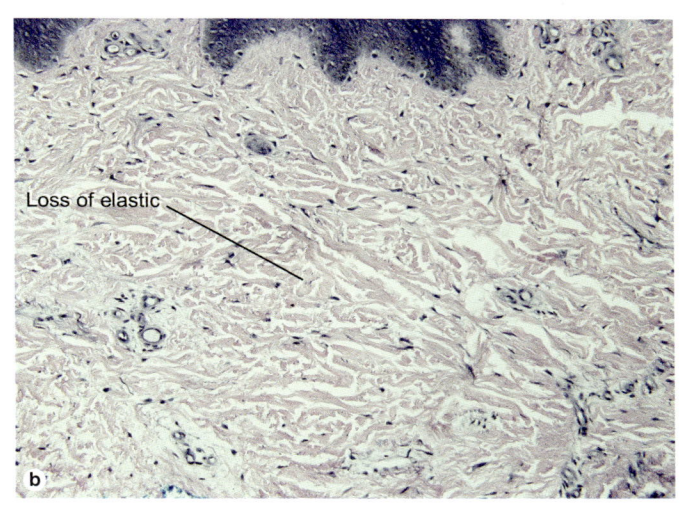

Fig 13-32 (a,b) Collagenoma. (b) Elastic stain (Verhoeff–van Gieson)

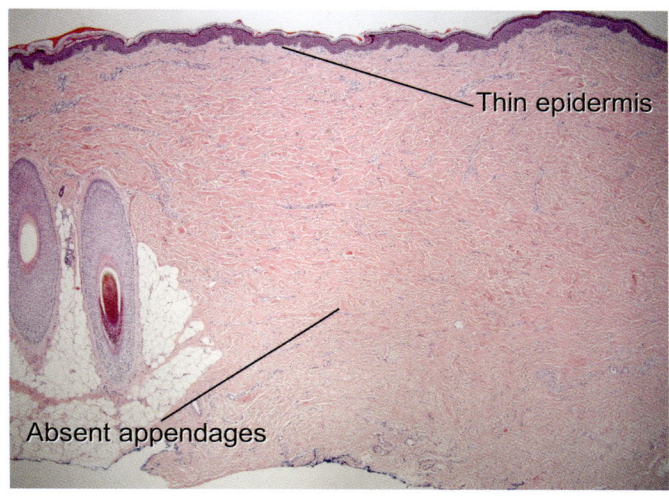

Fig 13-33 Aplasia cutis congenita

Aplasia cutis congenita

> **Key features**
> - Epidermis is absent or thin
> - Appendages are absent or rudimentary

Aplasia cutis is due to congenital absence of skin. It may present as an ulceration, membranous lesion, or atrophic scarring, most commonly on the vertex of the scalp. It may be associated with limb defects (Adams–Oliver syndrome), mental retardation, epidermal nevi, epidermolysis bullosa (Bart syndrome), chromosomal abnormalities, fetus papyraceus, or focal dermal hypoplasia.

Further reading

Aberer E, Klade H, Hobisch G. A clinical, histological, and immunohistochemical comparison of acrodermatitis chronica atrophicans and morphea. Am J Dermatopathol 1991;13(4):334–341.

Aiba S, Tabata N, Ohtani H, et al. CD34+ spindle-shaped cells selectively disappear from the skin lesion of scleroderma. Arch Dermatol 1994;130(5):593–597.

Blackburn WR, Cosman B. Histologic basis of keloid and hypertrophic scar differentiation. Clinicopathologic correlation. Arch Pathol 1966;82(1):65–71.

Choi YJ, Lee SJ, Choi CW, et al. Multiple unilateral zosteriform connective tissue nevi on the trunk. Ann Dermatol 2011;23(Suppl 2):S243–S246.

de Feraudy S, Fletcher CD. Fibroblastic connective tissue nevus: a rare cutaneous lesion analyzed in a series of 25 cases. Am J Surg Pathol 2012;36(10):1509–1515.

Fretzin DF, Beal DW, Jao W. Light and ultrastructural study of reactive perforating collagenosis. Arch Dermatol 1980;116(9):1054–1058.

Gebhart W, Bardach H. The "lumpy-bumpy" elastic fiber. A marker for long-term administration of penicillamine. Am J Dermatopathol 1981;3(1):33–39.

Graham JH, Marques AS. Colloid milium: a histochemical study. J Invest Dermatol 1967;49(5):497–507.

Handfield-Jones SE, Atherton DJ, Black MM, et al. Juvenile colloid milium: clinical, histological and ultrastructural features. J Cutan Pathol 1992;19(5):434–438.

Rahbari H. Histochemical differentiation of localized morphea-scleroderma and lichen sclerosus et atrophicus. J Cutan Pathol 1989;16(6):342–347.

Uitto J, Santa Cruz DJ, Bauer EA, et al. Morphea and lichen sclerosus et atrophicus. Clinical and histopathologic studies in patients with combined features. J Am Acad Dermatol 1980;3(3):271–279.

Wienecke R, Schlupen EM, Zochling N, et al. Staining of amyloid with cotton dyes. Arch Dermatol 1984;120(9):1184–1185.

Chapter 14

Metabolic disorders

Tammie Ferringer

Mucinoses

The mucinoses are a group of disorders characterized by mucin deposition in the dermis. The mucin is typically non-sulfated acid mucopolysaccharide (hyaluronic acid) that appears as wispy, faint blue threads on routine sections. It can be better appreciated with colloidal iron, Alcian blue, and toluidine blue staining.

Scleredema (of Buschke)

Key features

- Thickened dermis
- Widened spaces with mucin between normal collagen bundles
- The mucin is most prominent in the deep dermis
- No inflammatory infiltrate or increased fibroblasts
- The histologic features can be subtle and mimic normal skin at scan, but there is increased space between collagen fibers in the deep dermis

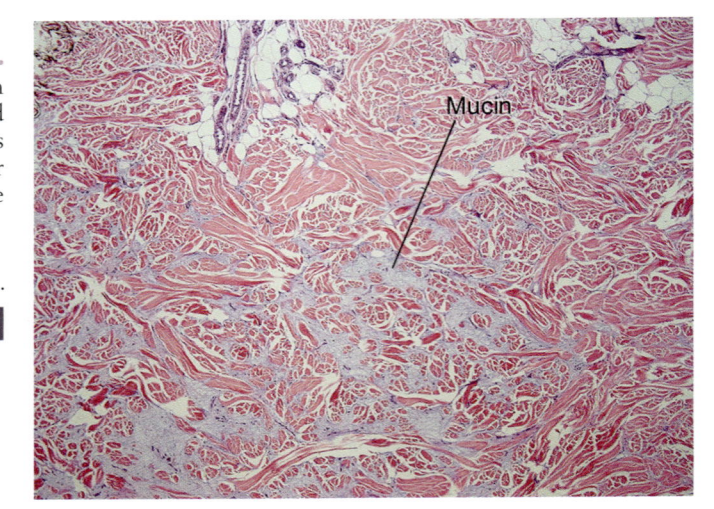

Fig 14-2 Scleredema

Scleredema most often occurs in the setting of insulin-dependent, adult-onset diabetes on the upper back, an area that normally displays a thick dermis. Scleredema can also occur suddenly following a streptococcal infection or in association with a monoclonal gammopathy.

Pretibial myxedema

Key features

- Large amounts of mucin throughout the dermis
- Collagen bundles separated by mucin and reduced to thin wisps

Pretibial myxedema is found in patients with Graves' disease, especially those with exophthalmos. It may not develop until after correction of the hyperthyroidism.

Differential Diagnosis

The mucin deposition in pretibial myxedema involves the full thickness of the dermis while the mucin in stasis is restricted to the papillary dermis. Nodular angioplasia and hemosiderin deposition are also features of stasis. Scleredema lacks attenuation of collagen fibers.

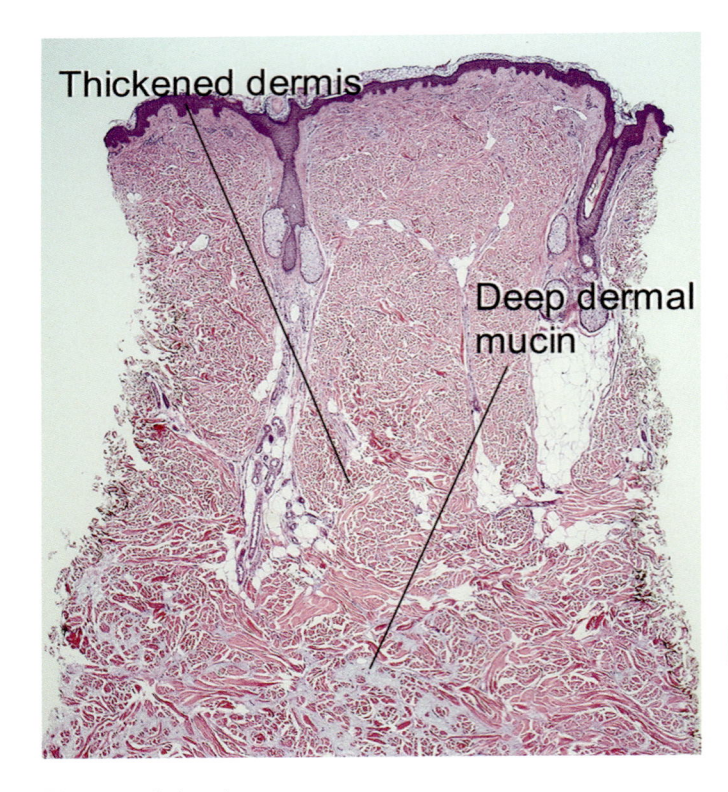

Fig 14-1 Scleredema

Metabolic disorders Chapter 14 225

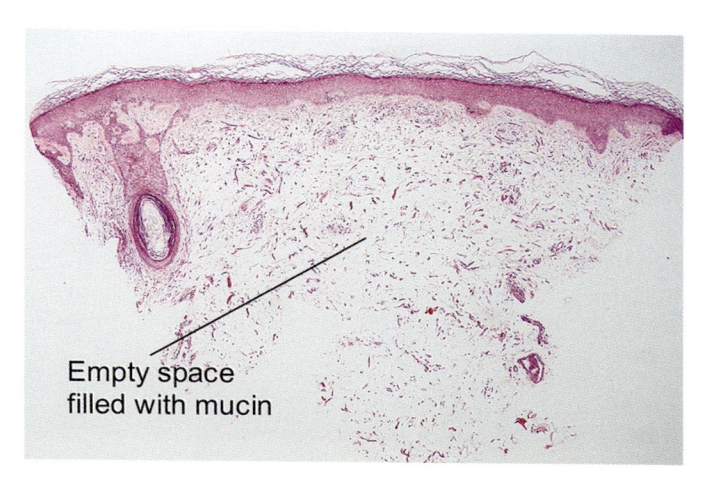

Fig 14-3 Pretibial myxedema

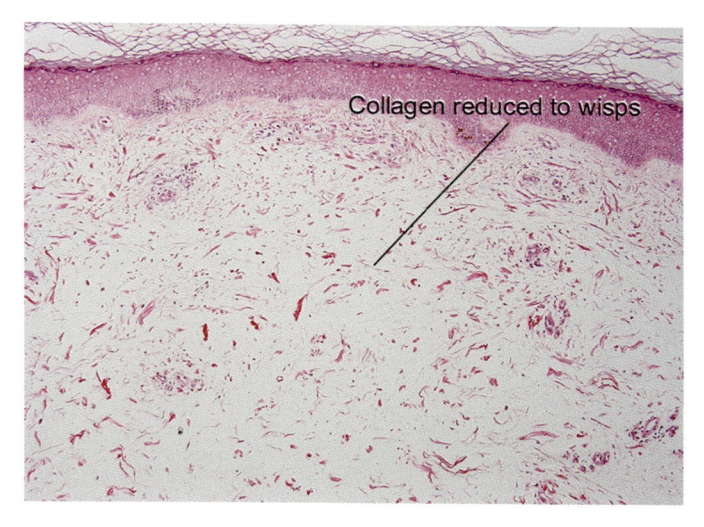

Fig 14-4 Pretibial myxedema

Differential Diagnosis

Histologically, scleromyxedema resembles nephrogenic systemic fibrosis. The clinical setting varies in that nephrogenic systemic fibrosis occurs in patients with renal failure with involvement of the distal extremities, whereas scleromyxedema is associated with IgG paraproteinemia and typically involves the face.

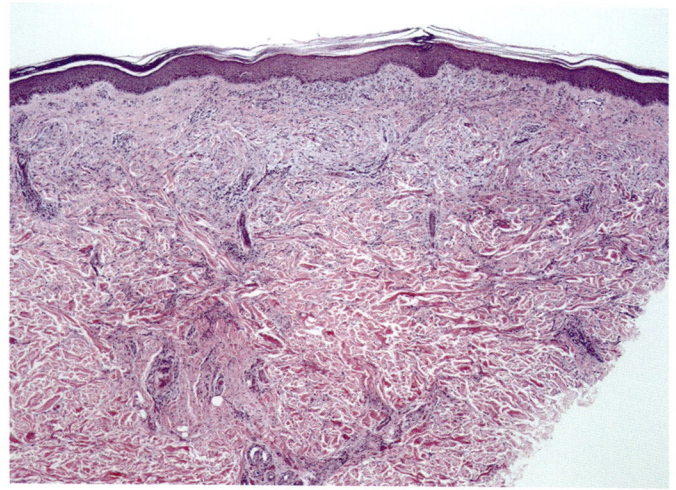

Fig 14-5 Scleromyxedema

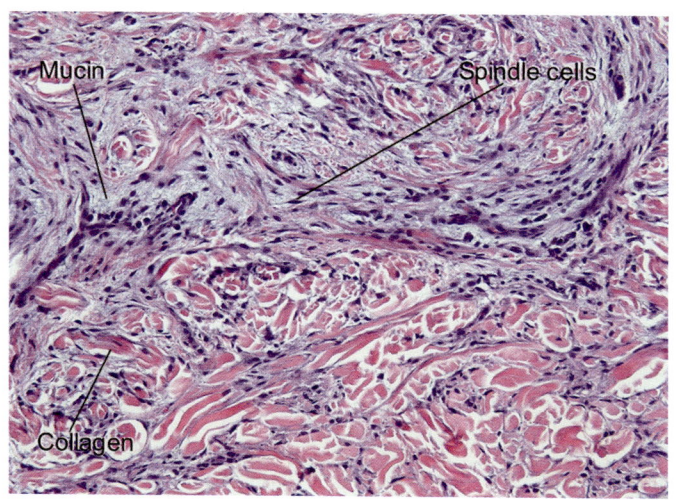

Fig 14-6 Scleromyxedema

Scleromyxedema

Key features

- Increase in dermal fibroblasts, fine collagen fibers, and interstitial mucin

Papular mucinosis (lichen myxedematosus) is composed of linear arrays of waxy papules. Scleromyxedema is a variant in which the papules coalesce with diffuse sclerosis of the skin. An immunoglobulin (Ig) G lambda gammopathy is associated with scleromyxedema and many cases of papular mucinosis.

Dermatopathology

Tumid lupus

Key features

- Interface damage is subtle or absent
- Superficial and deep perivascular and periadnexal lymphocytic infiltrate
- Infiltrate typically involves the eccrine coil
- Abundant mucin is present in the reticular dermis

Reticular erythematous mucinosis is indistinguishable histologically from tumid lupus. Many consider it a variant of tumid lupus.

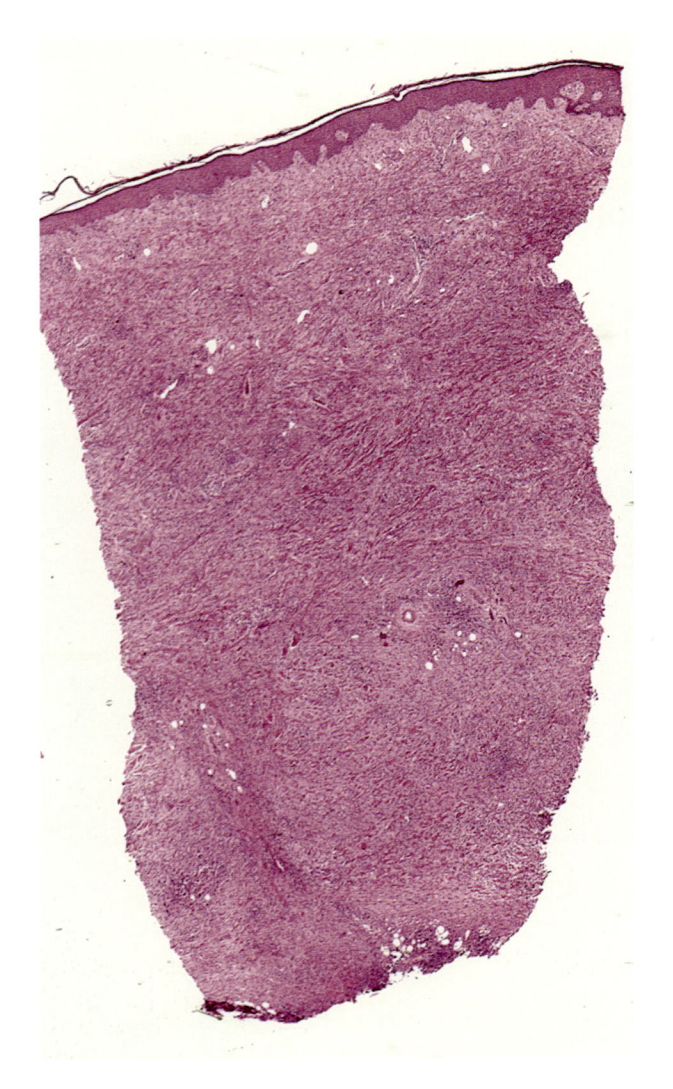

Fig 14-7 Nephrogenic systemic fibrosis

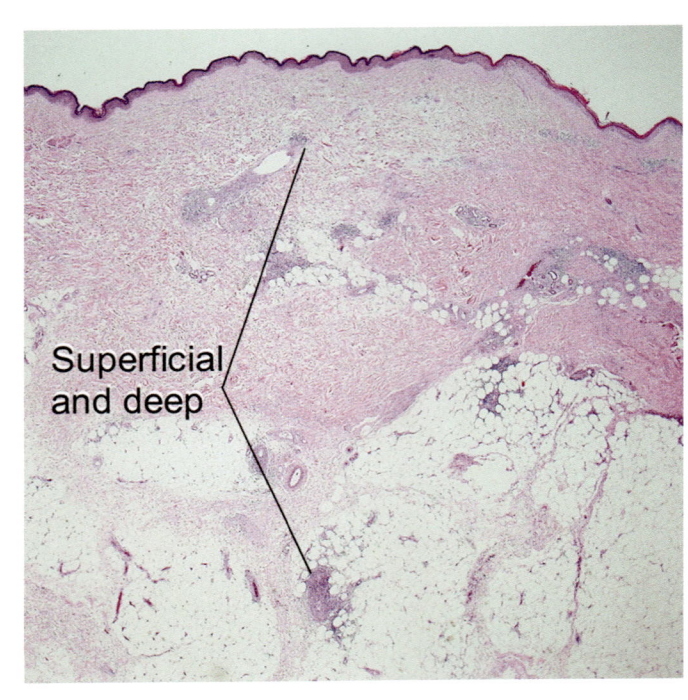

Fig 14-9 Tumid lupus

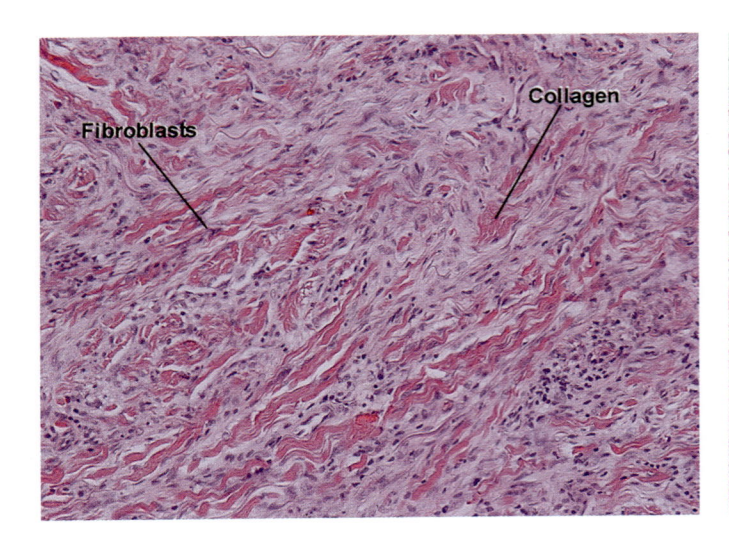

Fig 14-8 Nephrogenic systemic fibrosis

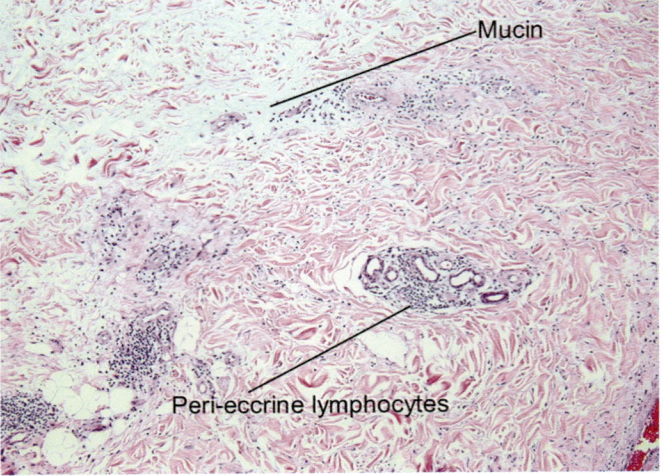

Fig 14-10 Tumid lupus

Focal mucinosis

Key features

- Dome-shaped papule containing a pool of mucin

Digital myxoid cyst resembles focal mucinosis but on acral skin.

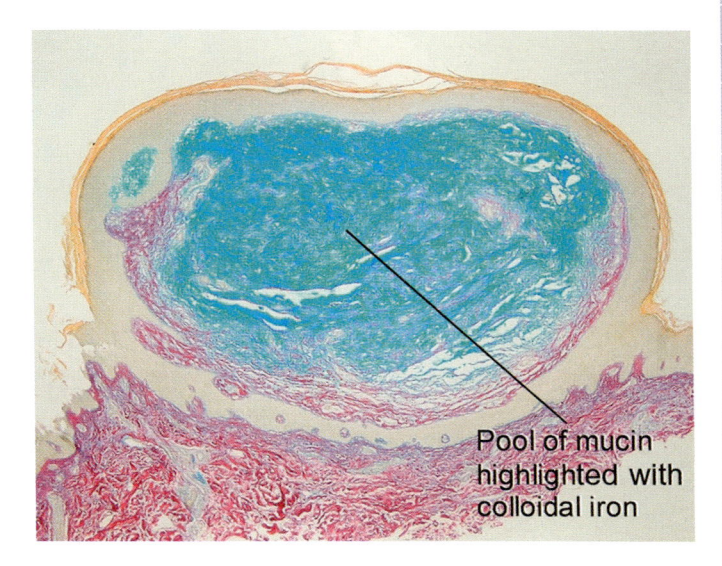

Fig 14-11 Focal mucinosis (colloidal iron)

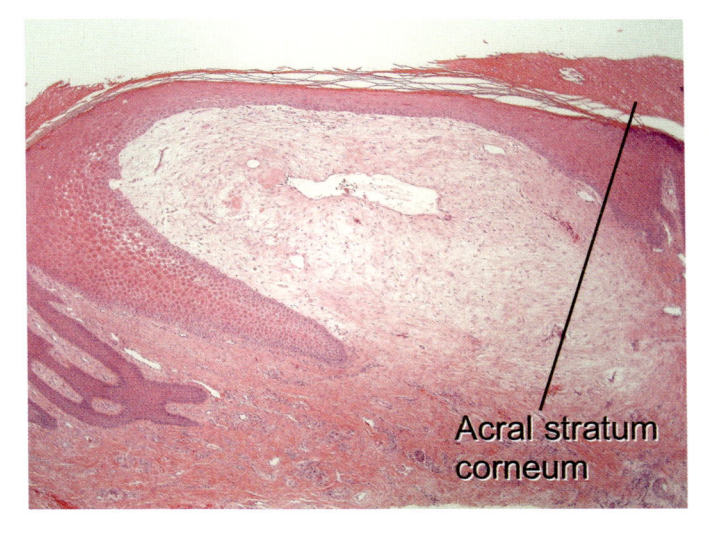

Fig 14-12 Digital myxoid cyst

Amyloidosis

Primary systemic amyloidosis is due to deposition of light chains. Skin lesions may occur but, in those with no obvious lesions, a blind biopsy of salivary glands or abdominal fat can be examined for the presence of amyloid. Light-chain-derived nodular cutaneous amyloidosis is produced locally by plasma cells and may or may not be associated with systemic amyloidosis. Secondary systemic amyloidosis lacks clinical skin lesions, but may demonstrate amyloid deposits in minor salivary glands or abdominal fat. Epidermal (keratin)-derived forms of amyloidosis include macular and lichen amyloidosis. Amyloid is brick red with Congo red stain and apple green with polarization. The cotton dye pagoda red is most specific for amyloid. Staining with thioflavin T is very sensitive but requires examination with a fluorescent microscope, resulting in yellow-green fluorescence of amyloid deposits. Crystal violet is a metachromatic stain that is very sensitive for epidermal-derived amyloid.

The clinical types of amyloidosis and their associated amyloid protein are listed in Table 14.1. In addition to the specific fibrillar component, amyloid P, a non-fibrillar glycoprotein, binds to all types of amyloid fibrils. Antisera to these proteins can be used immunohistochemically to identify the amyloid deposition.

Table 14-1 Clinical types of amyloidosis and their associated amyloid protein

Clinical type	Amyloid fibril protein	Precursor substance
Localized cutaneous		
Macular	AK	Altered keratin
Lichenoid	AK	Altered keratin
Nodular	AL (Aλ and Aκ)	Immunoglobulin light chain
Systemic		
Primary/myeloma-associated	AL (Aλ and Aκ)	Immunoglobulin light chain
Secondary	AA	Serum amyloid A
Familial Mediterranean fever	AA	Serum amyloid A
Muckle–Wells' syndrome	AA	Serum amyloid A
Familial amyloid polyneuropathy	Prealbumin (transthyretin)	
Hemodialysis-associated	β2-microglobulin	

Nodular amyloidosis

Key features

- Large fissured pale pink masses
- Plasma cells usually prominent

Nodular amyloid consists of light chains (AL) and may be a purely cutaneous lesion or occur in association with primary systemic amyloidosis. Lesions may be a manifestation of a localized plasmacytoma.

Dermatopathology

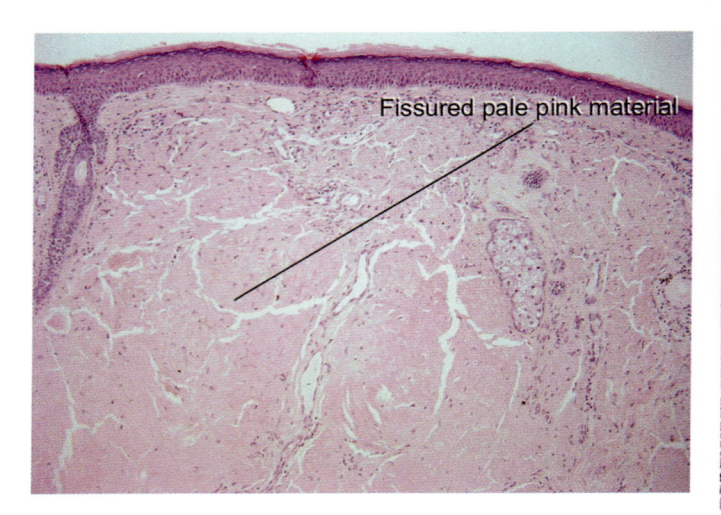

Fig 14-13 Nodular amyloid

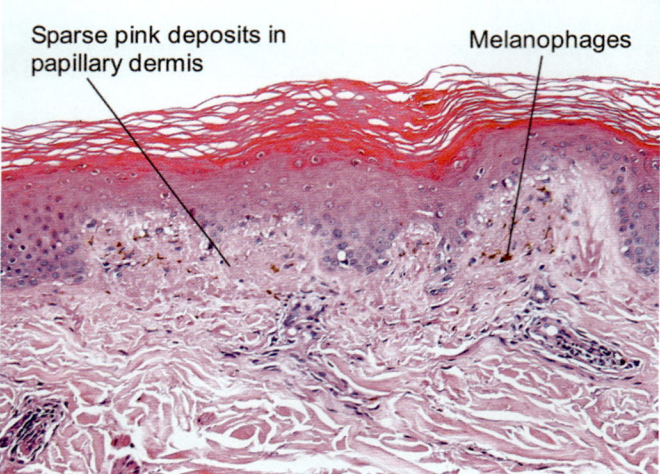

Fig 14-15 Macular amyloid

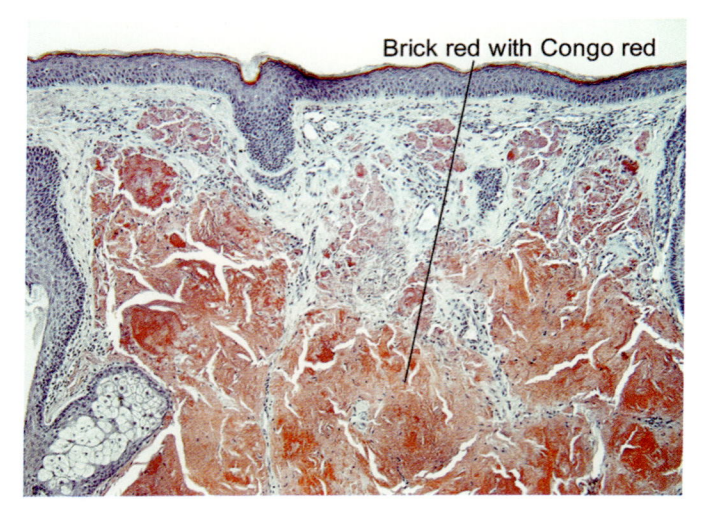

Fig 14-14 Nodular amyloid (Congo red)

Macular amyloid

Key features

- Sparse pink deposits in the papillary dermis
- Amyloid is outlined by a fine network of melanophages

Macular amyloid is a keratin-derived deposition produced by chronic scratching. Clinically, there is mottled hyperpigmentation of the interscapular area. This sparse deposition can be easily overlooked and may mimic normal skin.

Differential Diagnosis

At scan, some biopsies mimic normal skin and require closer inspection or clinical history to determine the diagnosis. Joe English's mnemonic "I vacuum dog pus" includes many of these subtle histologic entities:

- *I*chthyosis vulgaris
- *V*itiligo
- *A*rgyria
- *C*andida
- *U*rticaria
- *U*rticaria pigmentosa (especially telangiectasia macularis eruptiva perstans)
- *M*acular amyloid
- *D*ermatophyte
- *O*nchocerciasis (microfilaria)
- *G*old (chrysiasis)
- *P*seudoxanthoma elasticum and psoriasis (guttate)
- *U*lerythema ophryogenes
- *S*eborrheic dermatitis and scleredema

Alternatively, what initially appears to be normal skin at scan can be approached systematically, starting in the stratum corneum looking for organisms, then moving deeper to look for absence of granular layer, followed by the epidermal pattern, alteration in pigmentation, deposition in the dermal papillae, perivascular or interstitial infiltrate, and down to the eccrine glands looking for silver granules.

Lichen amyloid

Key features

- Hyperkeratosis and acanthosis
- Pink amorphous deposits in the papillary dermis outlined by a network of melanophages

Lichen amyloid is a keratin-derived deposition that histologically resembles macular amyloid with superimposed changes of lichen simplex chronicus. Clinically, it presents as intensely pruritic papules in rows, usually on the anterior shins.

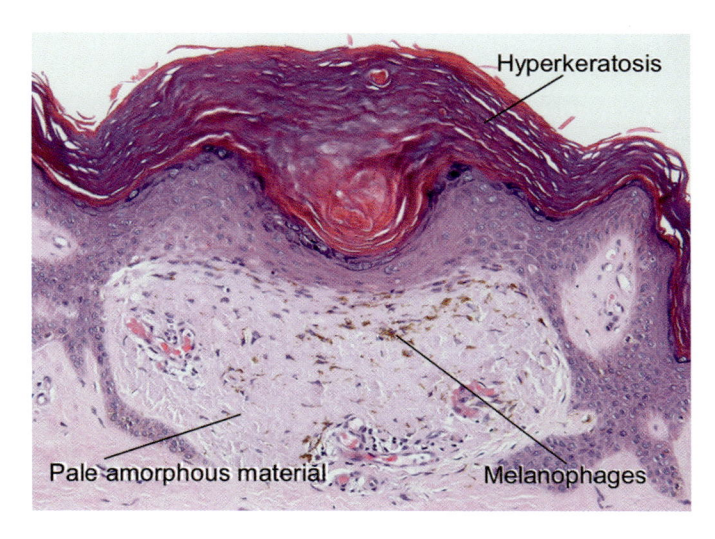

Fig 14-16 Lichen amyloid

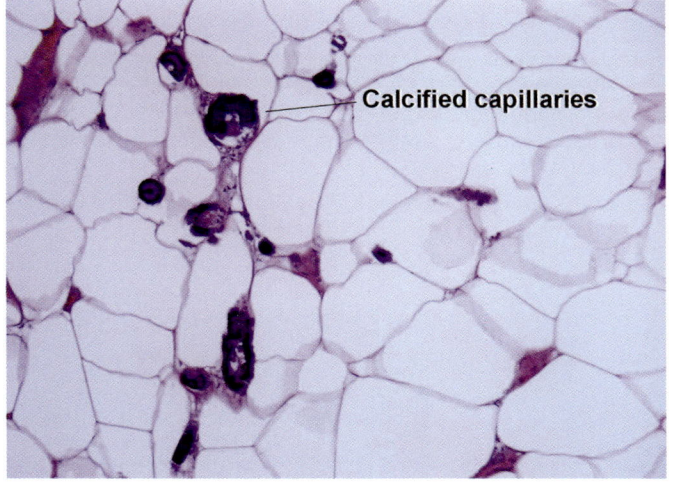

Fig 14-17 Calciphylaxis

Cutaneous calcification

The cutaneous deposition of calcium, calcinosis cutis, has been divided into dystrophic, metastatic, and idiopathic forms. Dystrophic calcium deposition occurs in the presence of normal calcium levels, with the deposits forming in damaged tissue as in dermatomyositis, scleroderma, or in scars. Scrotal calcinosis represents calcified epidermoid cysts. Metastatic calcifications occur in normal tissue and are associated with elevated serum calcium or phosphate or both. Calciphylaxis is a unique form of metastatic calcification. Subepidermal calcified nodules are of unknown pathogenesis and belong to the category of idiopathic calcifications. Calcium typically appears basophilic on hematoxylin and eosin-stained sections, and stains black with von Kossa's silver stain and red with alizarin red.

Calciphylaxis

Key features

- Calcified small vessels in the subcutaneous fat
- Necrosis

Calciphylaxis occurs most frequently in the setting of chronic renal failure and/or hyperparathyroidism, usually in patients with diabetes.

Subepidermal calcified nodule

Key features

- Pseudoepitheliomatous hyperplasia with transepidermal elimination of calcium

This is an idiopathic process most common on the chin of a child or heel of a newborn.

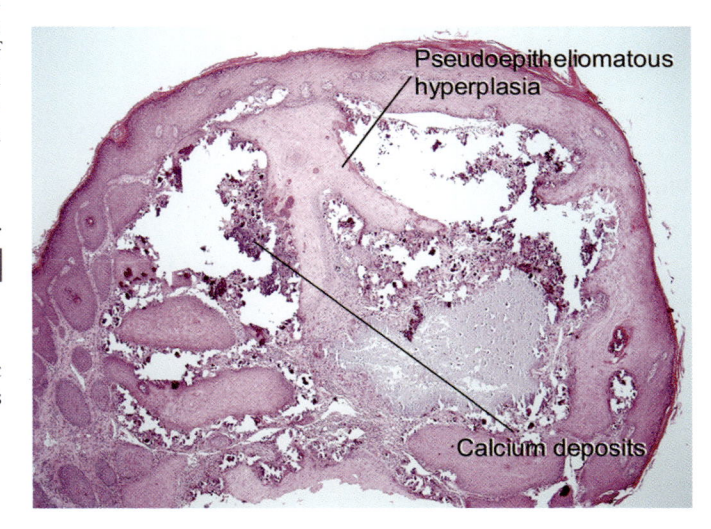

Fig 14-18 Subepidermal calcified nodule

Scrotal calcinosis

Key features

- Amorphous masses of calcium
- Smooth muscles scattered through the dermis indicate genital site

Although considered "idiopathic" by some, the condition appears to represent calcification of epidermoid cysts.

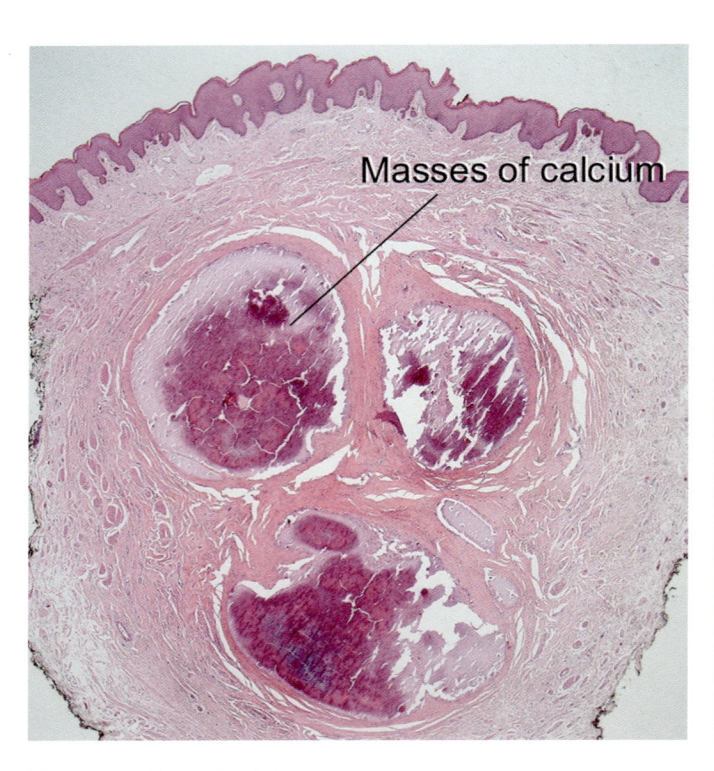

Fig 14-19 Scrotal calcinosis

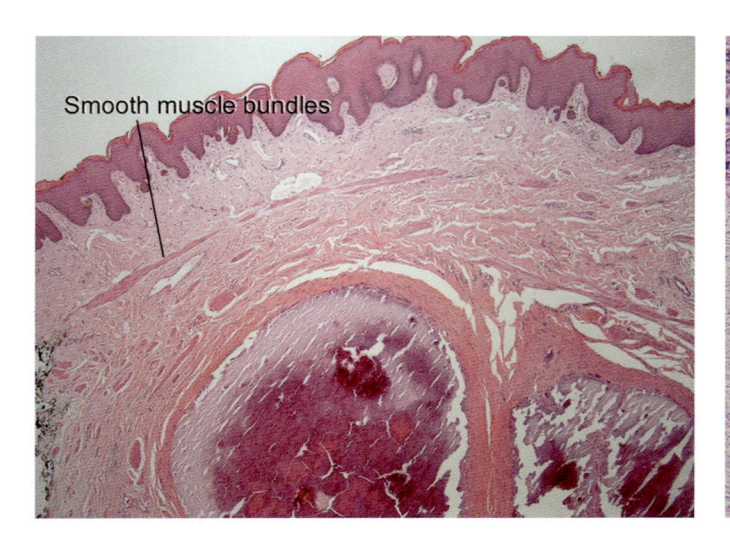

Fig 14-20 Scrotal calcinosis

Gout

Key features

- Palisaded granuloma surrounding amorphous gray material with a feathery appearance

Formalin fixation destroys the uric acid crystals, leaving feathery clefts. Brown crystals that are doubly refractile with polarization are present if the tissue was fixed in ethanol or was incompletely fixed in formalin.

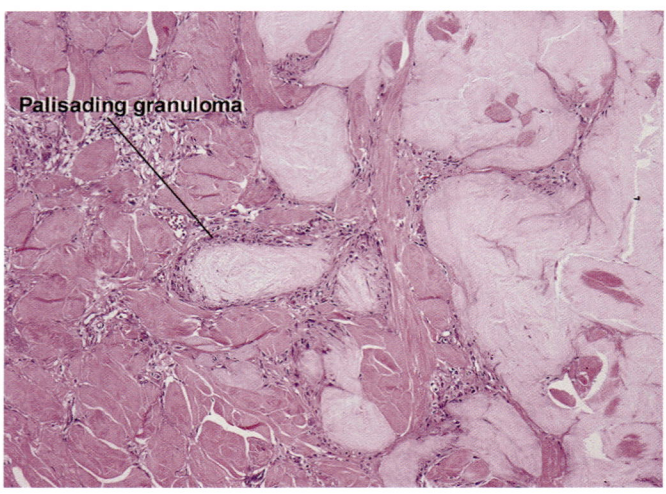

Fig 14-21 Gout

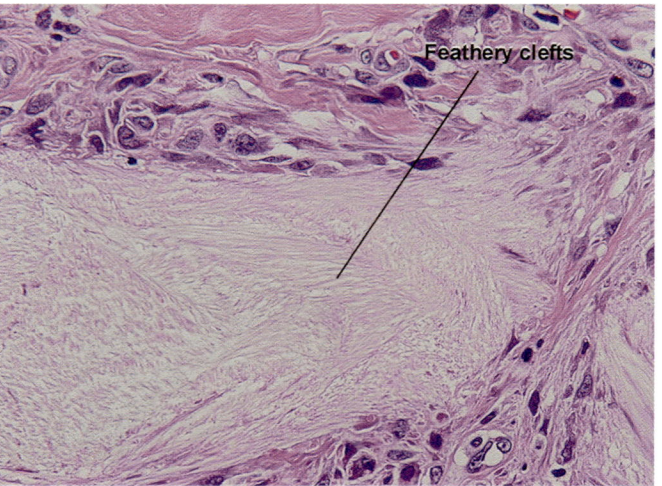

Fig 14-22 Gout

Erythropoietic protoporphyria (EPP)

Key features

- Hyaline cuff (reduplicated basement membrane) around post-capillary venules
- No solar elastosis is present, because patients avoid the burning sensation associated with sun exposure

EPP is associated with a deficiency of ferrochelatase. EPP is the only disorder of porphyrin metabolism with normal urine porphyrins (EPP stands for *empty pee pee*). There are increased protoporphyrins in the feces and blood.

Differential Diagnosis

The hyaline material in EPP affects the superficial vessels, whereas lipoid proteinosis involves the superficial and deeper vessels as well as eccrine glands. Porphyria cutanea tarda demonstrates much smaller hyaline cuffs around superficial vessels, as well as solar elastosis in the surrounding skin. It often also demonstrates caterpillar bodies, subepidermal bullae, and festooning.

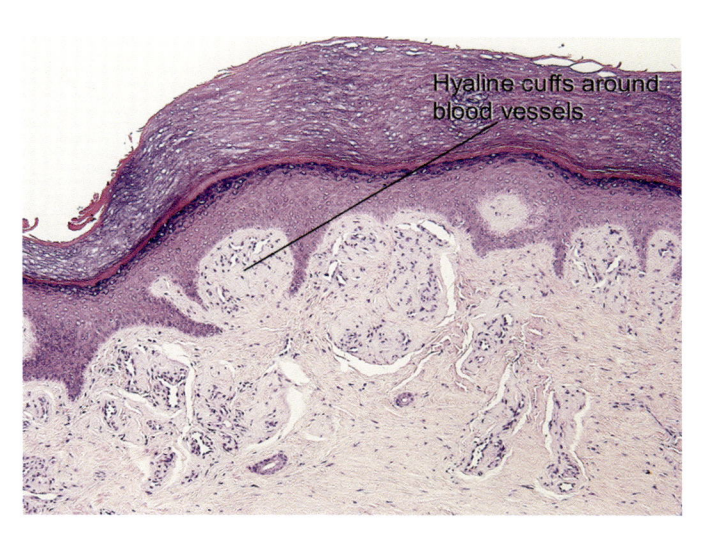

Fig 14-23 Erythropoietic protoporphyria (EPP)

Colloid milium

Key features

- Pale pink, fissured deposits that fill and expand the dermal papillae

The adult type develops in the setting of severe sun damage, on the face, neck, and dorsal hands. This material represents the final product of severe solar degeneration but can stain weakly with amyloid stains (crystal violet, Congo red, thioflavin T). However, it fails to react with pagoda red. The juvenile form develops on the head and neck before the development of sun damage. This type is Congo red negative but positive with antikeratin antibodies, confirming the origin of the material from degenerated keratinocytes.

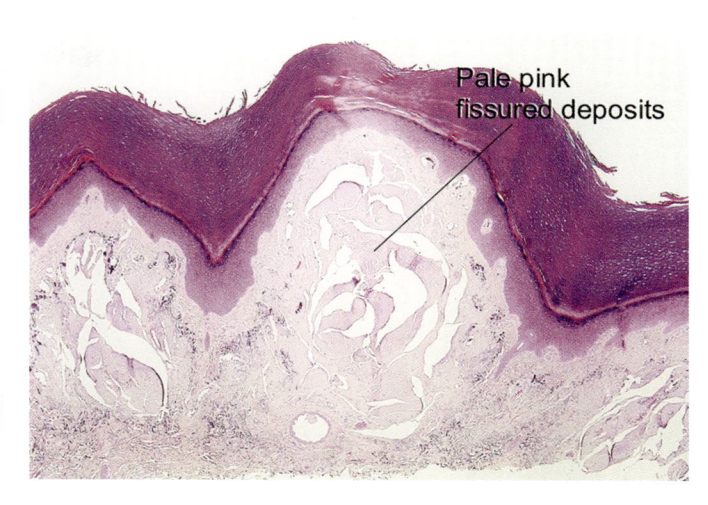

Fig 14-24 Colloid milium

Lipoid proteinosis (hyalinosis cutis et mucosae, Urbach–Wiethe disease)

Key features

- Eosinophilic hyaline deposits around blood vessels, sweat glands, and in thick bundles perpendicular to the surface
- Onion skin concentric pattern around vessels and adnexal structures
- Much deeper and more extensive than in EPP

Lipoid proteinosis is an autosomal-recessive disorder resulting in hoarseness, pitted scars, beaded nodules along the eyelids, verrucous lesions, and seizures due to calcifications of the hippocampus. The material is periodic acid-Schiff-positive and diastase-resistant reduplicated basement membrane (type IV collagen). Stains for amyloid and mucin are unpredictable.

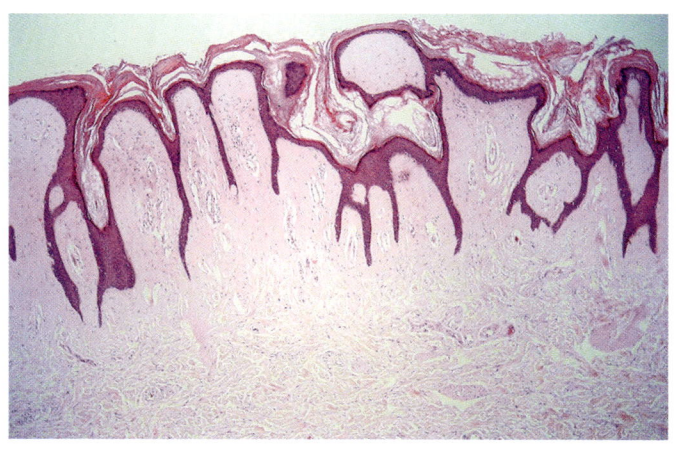

Fig 14-25 Lipoid proteinosis

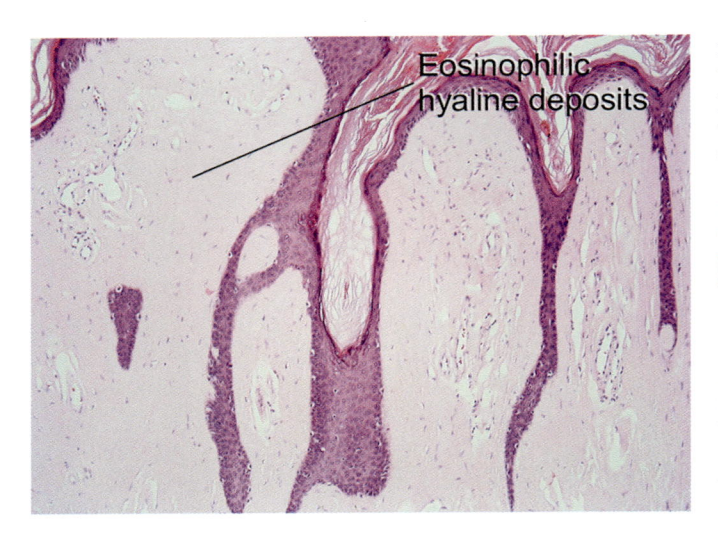

Fig 14-26 Lipoid proteinosis

Nutritional dermatoses

Key features

- Pallor of the superficial third of the epidermis with or without necrosis
- Confluent parakeratosis and psoriasiform epidermal hyperplasia

Pellagra, acrodermatitis enteropathica, and necrolytic migratory erythema (glucagonoma syndrome) share this histologic pattern. Pellagra is caused by niacin deficiency, resulting in the "3 Ds": *d*iarrhea, *d*ementia, and a collar-like *d*ermatitis around the neck known as Casal's necklace. Abnormalities of tryptophan metabolism, carcinoid syndrome, and Hartnup's syndrome cause a pellagra-like state. Acrodermatitis enteropathica is an inherited or acquired zinc deficiency. Clinically, these patients have a periorificial and acral dermatitis with diarrhea. Necrolytic migratory erythema is a marker for a glucagon-secreting tumor of the pancreatic alpha cells. The cutaneous lesions appear as a figurate erythema with flaccid bullae that rupture, leaving an eroded surface and peripheral scale.

Mucocele

Key features

- Pseudocystic space containing mucin
- Muciphages and granulation tissue surround the space

Mucoceles occur due to disruption in the excretory duct of minor salivary glands with mucin extravasation into the connective tissue. The lower labial and buccal mucosa are most commonly affected. Involvement of the floor of the mouth is referred to as ranula.

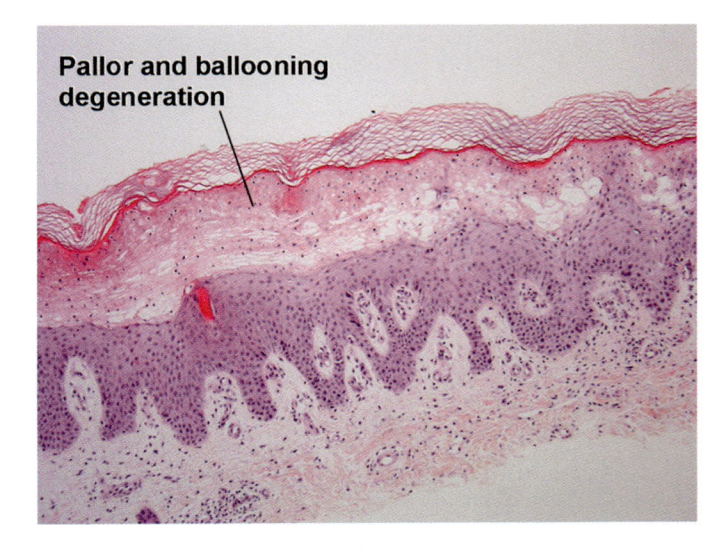

Fig 14-27 Nutritional deficiency

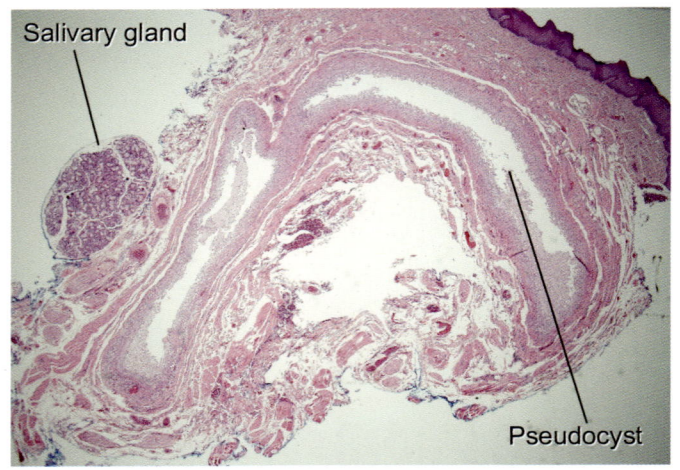

Fig 14-28 Mucocele

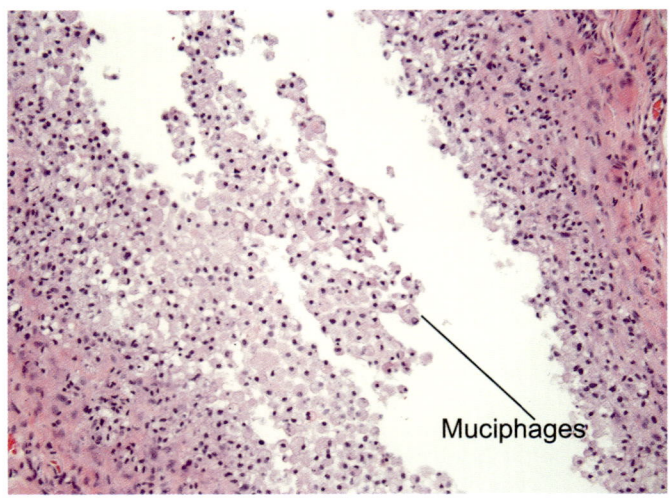

Fig 14-29 Mucocele

Oxalosis

Key features

- Yellow-brown radially arranged refractile needle-shaped crystals
- Vascular involvement and thrombi may be seen, especially in primary disease

Primary oxalosis is an autosomal recessive disorder associated with overproduction of serum oxalate. These patients present with recurrent calcium oxalate stones and renal failure. Vascular deposition of oxalate produces livedo reticularis, acrocyanosis, distal gangrene, and ulcerations.

Secondary oxalosis occurs with ethylene glycol poisoning, excessive intake of ascorbic acid, pyridoxine deficiency, various intestinal diseases, repeated oral antibiotic use leading to elimination of oxalate-degrading bacteria in the intestine, and chronic hemodialysis. Skin manifestations in patients with secondary oxalosis occur as the result of extravascular deposition.

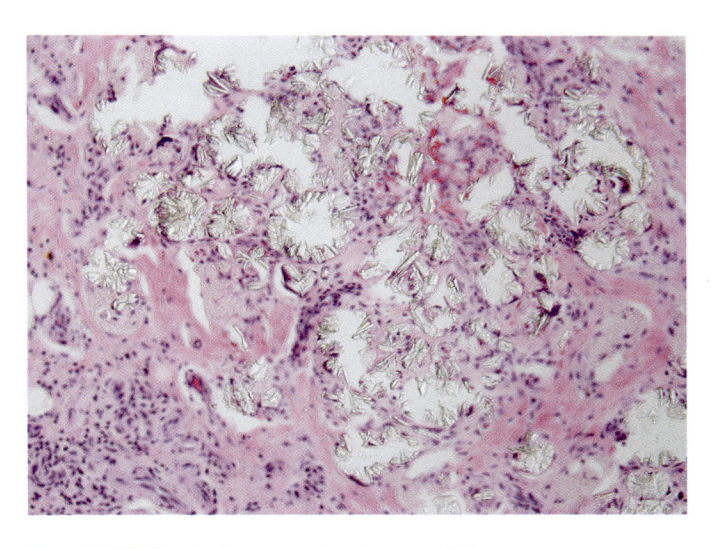

Fig 14-30 Oxalosis secondary to renal failure

Further reading

Blackmon JA, Jeffy BG, Malone JC, et al. Oxalosis involving the skin: case report and literature review. Arch Dermatol 2011;147(11):1302–1305.

Girardi M, Kay J, Elston DM, et al. Nephrogenic systemic fibrosis: clinicopathological definition and workup recommendations. J Am Acad Dermatol 2011;65(6):1095–1106.e7.

Hashimoto K, Nakayama H, Chimenti S, et al. Juvenile colloid milium: Immunohistochemical and ultrastructural studies. J Cutan Pathol 1989;16(3):164–174.

Kövary PM, Vakilzadeh F, Macher E, et al. Monoclonal gammopathy in scleredema. Observations in three cases. Arch Dermatol 1981;117(9):536–539.

Kucher C, Xu X, Pasha T, et al. Histopathologic comparison of nephrogenic fibrosing dermopathy and scleromyxedema. J Cutan Pathol 2005;32(7):484–490.

Markova A, Lester J, Wang J, et al. Diagnosis of common dermopathies in dialysis patients: a review and update. Semin Dial 2012;25(4):408–418.

Masuda C, Mohri S, Nakajima H. Histopathological and immunohistochemical study of amyloidosis cutis nodularis atrophicans – comparison with systemic amyloidosis. Br J Dermatol 1988;119(1):33–43.

Saad AG, Zaatari GS. Scrotal calcinosis: is it idiopathic? Urology 2001;57(2):365.

Yanagihara M, Mehregan AH, Mehregan DR. Staining of amyloid with cotton dyes. Arch Dermatol 1984;120(9):1184–1185.

Chapter 15

Disorders of skin appendages

Dirk M. Elston

Non-inflammatory alopecia

Transverse (horizontal) sections are generally best for evaluation of non-inflammatory alopecia. Vertical sections may be used if serial ribbons of sections are cut from the block. A combination of vertical and transverse sections is always acceptable.

Pattern alopecia (androgenetic balding)

Key features

- Miniaturization of follicular units
- Variability in diameter of follicles (anisotrichosis)
- In vertical sections, hairs extend to variable depths, in proportion to their diameter
- Decreased anagen/telogen ratio
- Many fibrous tract remnants with normal diameter and vascularity

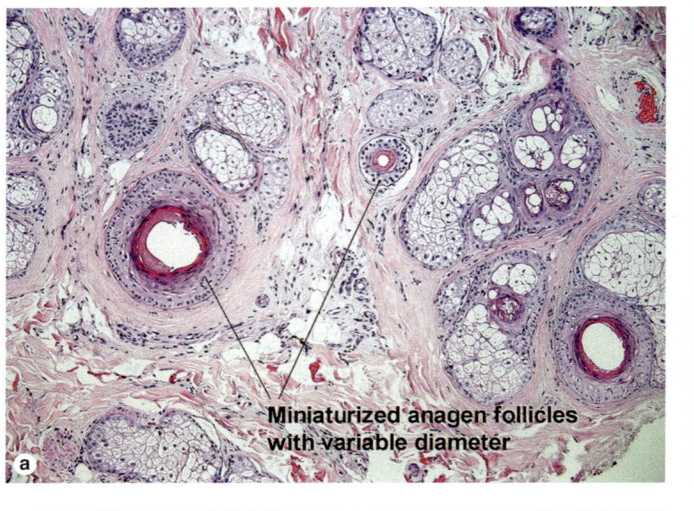

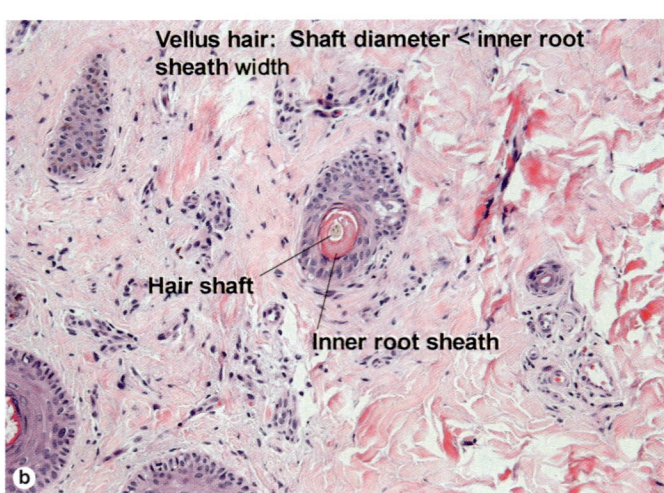

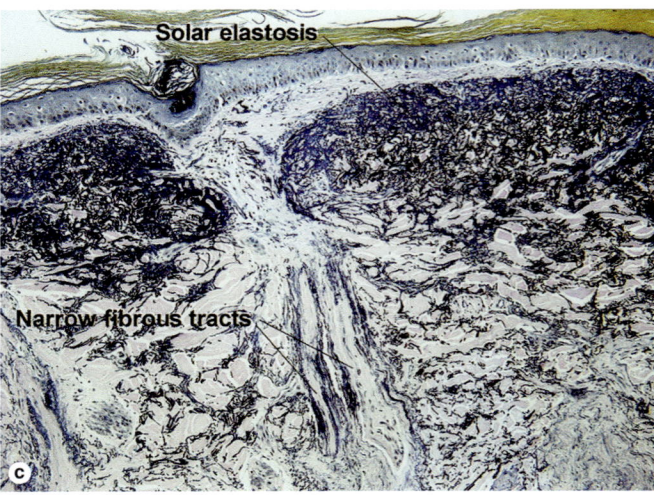

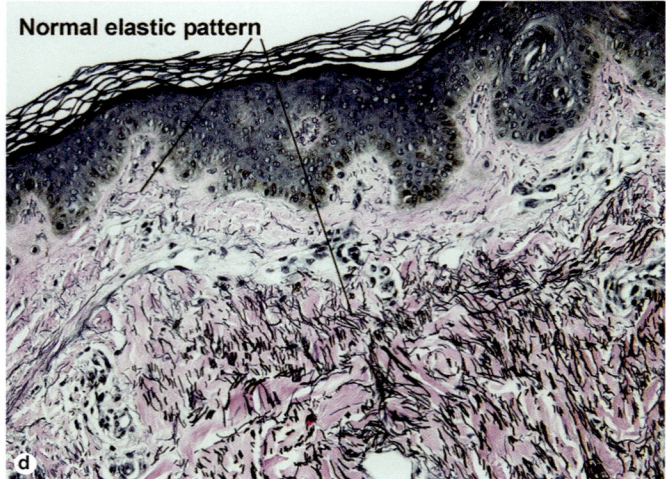

Fig 15-1 (a,b) Pattern alopecia. (c) Solar elastosis and narrow fibrous tract remnants in pattern alopecia (Verhoeff–van Gieson stain). (d) Normal elastic tissue pattern for comparison (Verhoeff–van Gieson stain)

Disorders of skin appendages

The essential histologic finding in pattern alopecia is progressive miniaturization of the follicular unit. This occurs predominantly in the central scalp, and in an asynchronous fashion. The biopsy will demonstrate variability in hair diameter. Focal spongiotic infundibulofolliculitis is common (mild seborrheic folliculitis). In long-standing cases, solar elastosis as well as elastotic degeneration of the fibrous tract remnants may be seen. Advanced pattern alopecia demonstrates a marked increase in vellus hairs (hair shaft diameter < inner root sheath diameter). Large sebaceous glands may be present, especially in males.

Telogen effluvium

Key features
- Many telogen hairs

Telogen effluvium has many telogen hairs. Telogen effluvium caused by premature interruption of anagen growth (such as by a febrile illness or crash diet) lacks the miniaturization of pattern alopecia. The shortened anagen cycle of pattern alopecia results in an altered anagen/telogen ratio, but not to the extent seen after febrile illness or crash dieting.

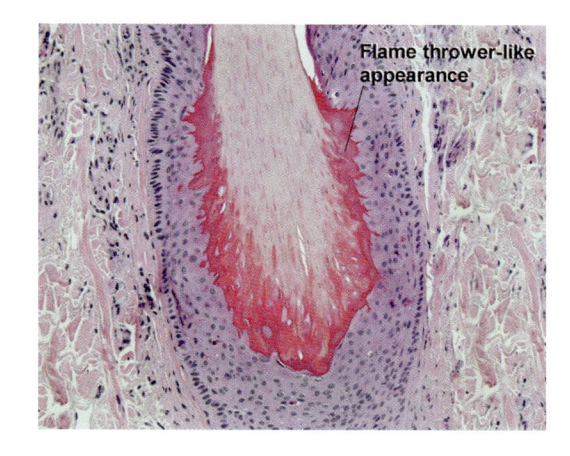

Fig 15-2 Telogen effluvium: telogen hair

Trichotillomania (trichotillosis)

Key features
- Empty anagen follicles
- Many catagen hairs characterized by apoptotic keratinocytes (Figure 15.3c)
- Melanin casts within the follicular canal
- Trichomalacia

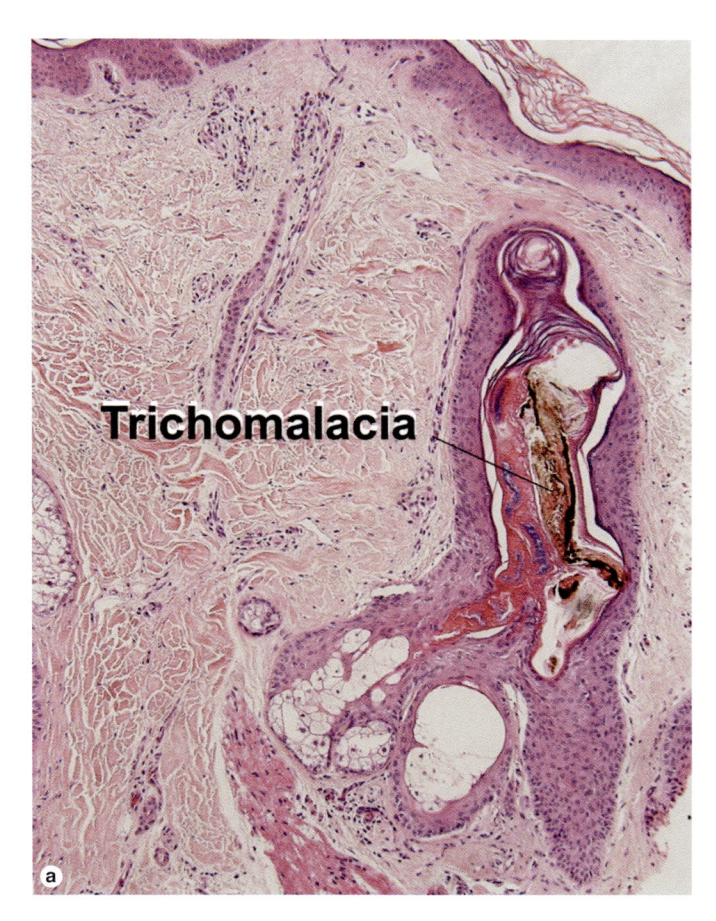

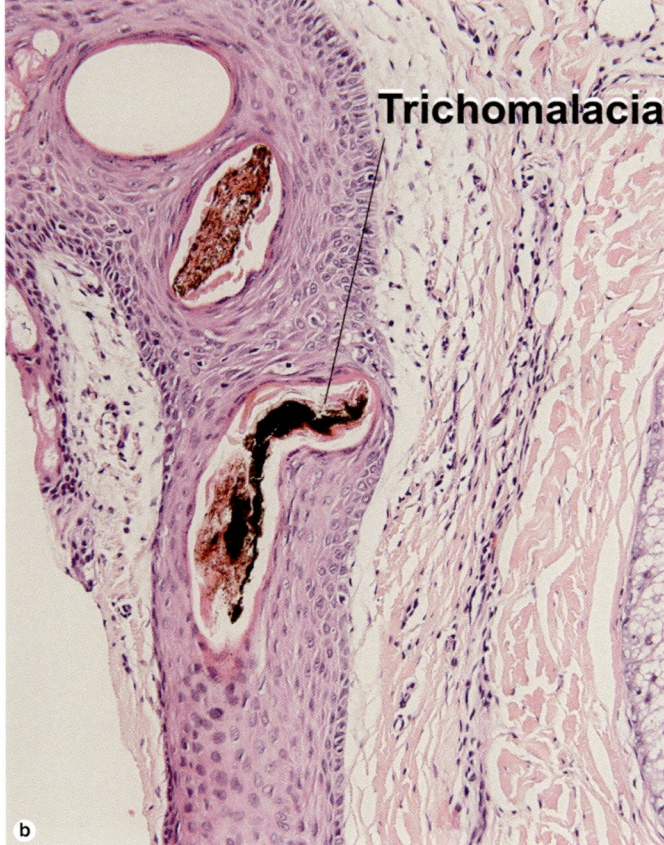

Fig 15-3 Trichotillomania

Continued

236 Dermatopathology

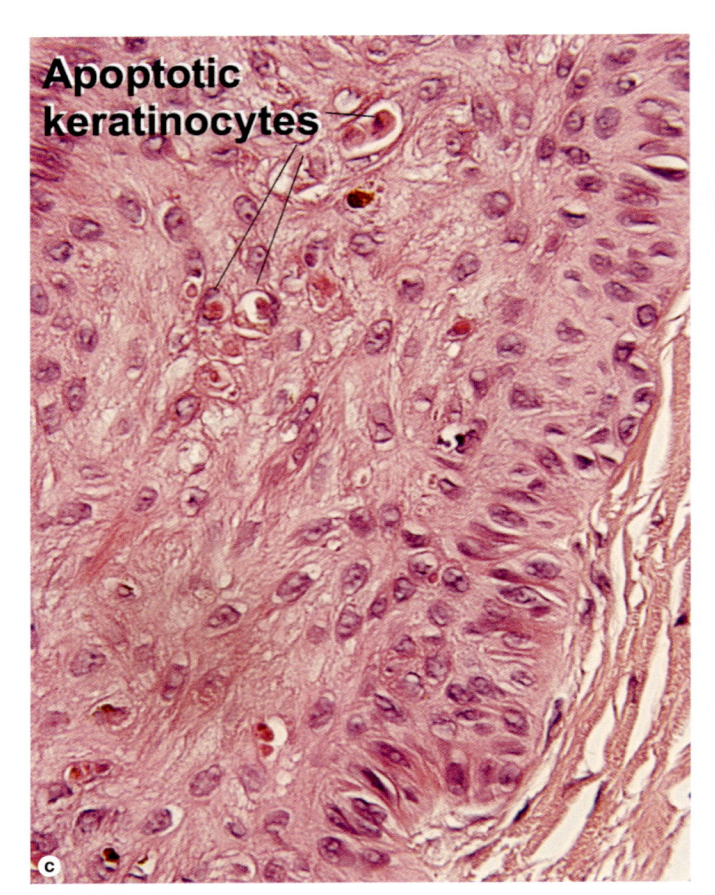

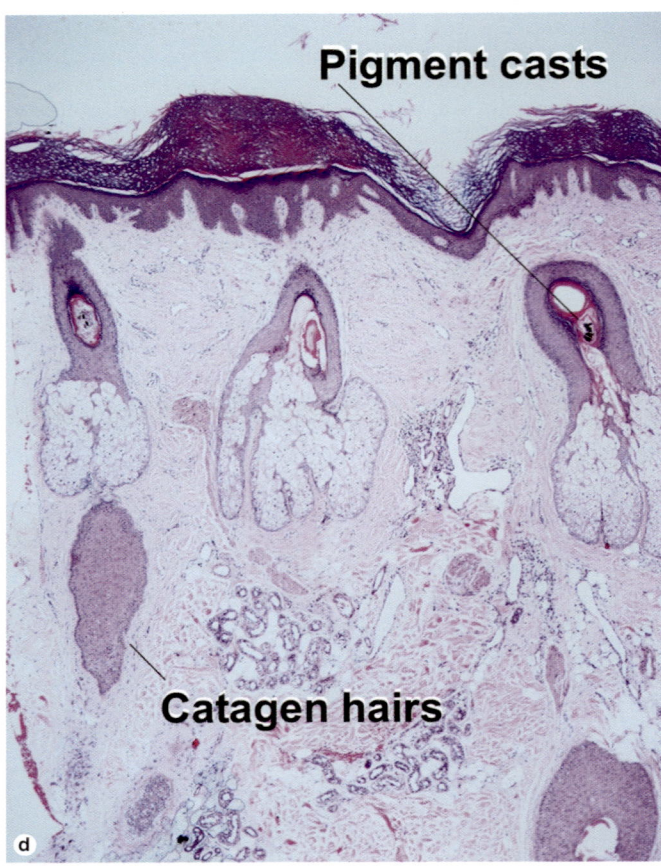

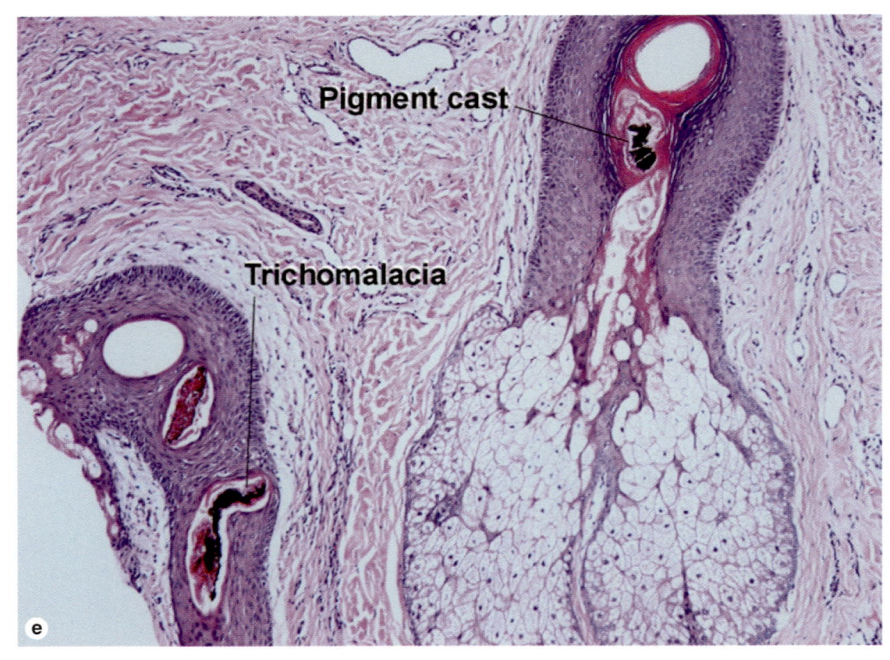

Fig 15-3, cont'd

Traction alopecia

Key features

- Resembles trichotillomania histologically

Inflammatory non-scarring alopecia

Either vertical or transverse (horizontal) sections may be used, but serial ribbons of sections should always be cut from the block. A combination of vertical and transverse sections is always acceptable.

Alopecia areata

Key features

- Lymphoid inflammation at the level of the hair bulb
- Lymphocytes within fibrous tract remnants
- Eosinophils within fibrous tract remnants
- Melanin within fibrous tract remnants
- Follicular miniaturization
- Decreased anagen/telogen ratio
- Increase in catagen hairs
- Melanin casts within the follicular channel
- Dilation of follicular infundibula

The lymphocytes appear to target melanocytes within the hair bulb. White hairs are spared. The inflammation results in damage to the hair matrix, tapered hair shafts with fracture, and miniaturization of the follicular unit.

Differential Diagnosis

Pattern alopecia

- Shares follicular miniaturization, decreased anagen/telogen ratio, and many fibrous tract remnants
- Lacks catagen hairs, melanin casts in follicular channels, lymphoid inflammation at the level of the hair bulb, lymphocytes within fibrous tract remnants, eosinophils within fibrous tract remnants, melanin within fibrous tract remnants

Trichotillomania

- Shares catagen hairs and melanin casts in follicular channels
- Lacks follicular miniaturization, lymphoid inflammation at the level of the hair bulb, lymphocytes within fibrous tract remnants, eosinophils within fibrous tract remnants, melanin within fibrous tract remnants

Table 15-1 Comparison between alopecia areata, pattern alopecia, and trichotillomania

Characteristic	Alopecia areata	Pattern alopecia	Trichotillomania
Miniaturization	Yes	Yes	No
Anagen/telogen ratio	Decreased	Decreased	Variable
Fibrous tract remnants	Increased	Increased	Normal
Catagen hairs	Common	Rare	Common
Pigment in hair canal	Common	No	Common
Pigment in fibrous tract	Common	No	No
Lymphs around bulb	Common	No	No
Lymphs in fibrous tracts	Common	No	No
Eosinophils in fibrous tracts	Common	No	No

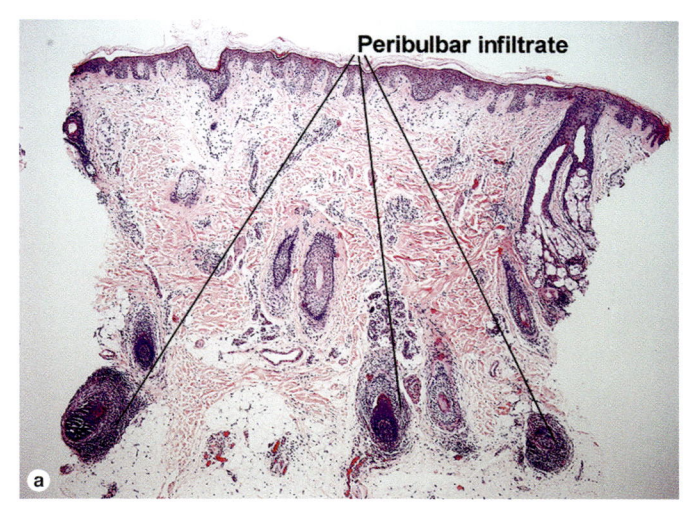

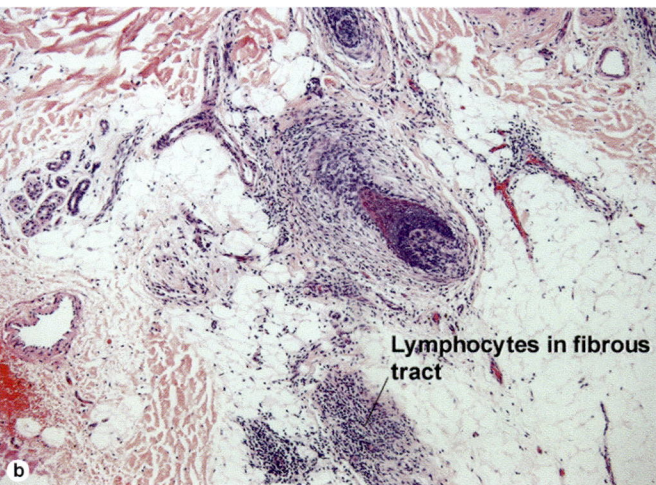

Fig 15-4 Alopecia areata

Continued

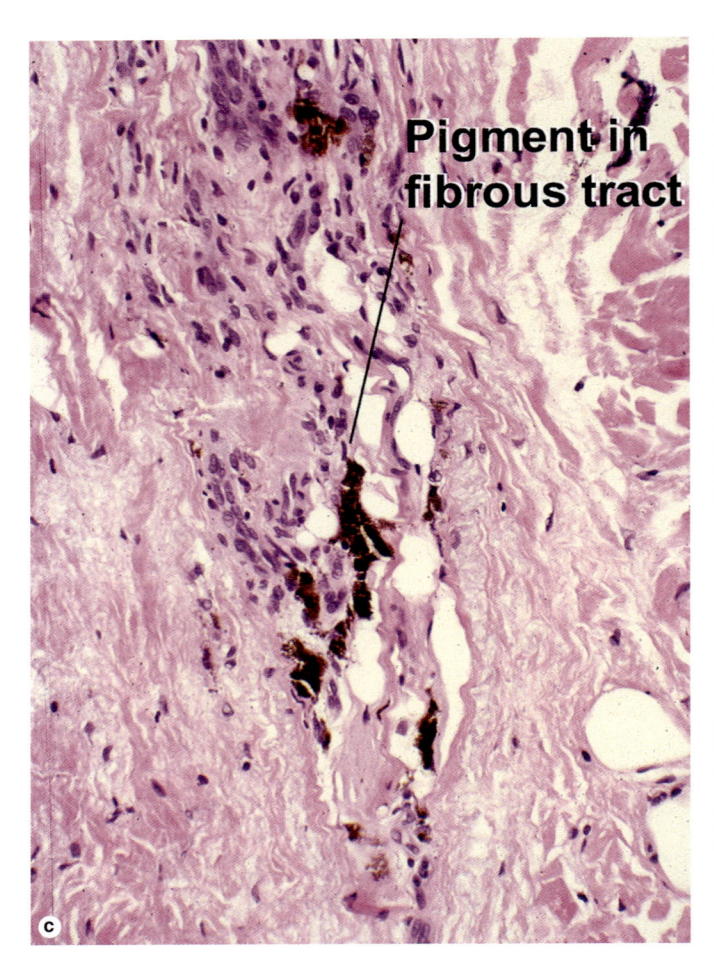

Fig 15-4, cont'd

Syphilitic alopecia

Key features
- May be identical to alopecia areata
- May contain plasma cells (lacking in about one-third of cases)

Alopecia mucinosa

Key features
- Mucin within follicular epithelium
- Variable surrounding lymphoid infiltrate
- May be associated with mycosis fungoides (cutaneous T-cell lymphoma)

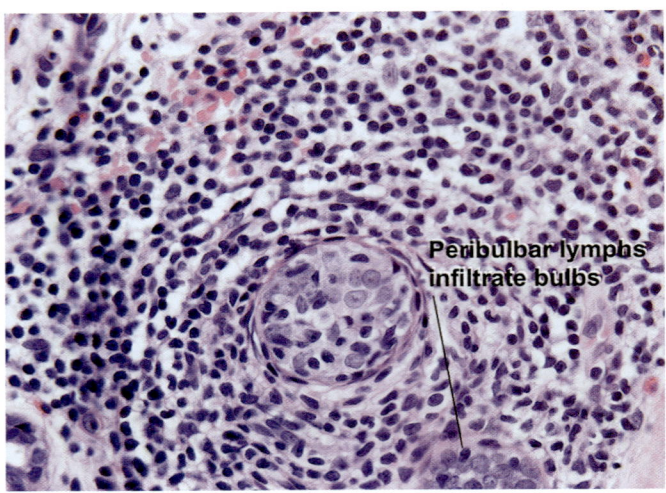

Fig 15-5 Syphilitic alopecia

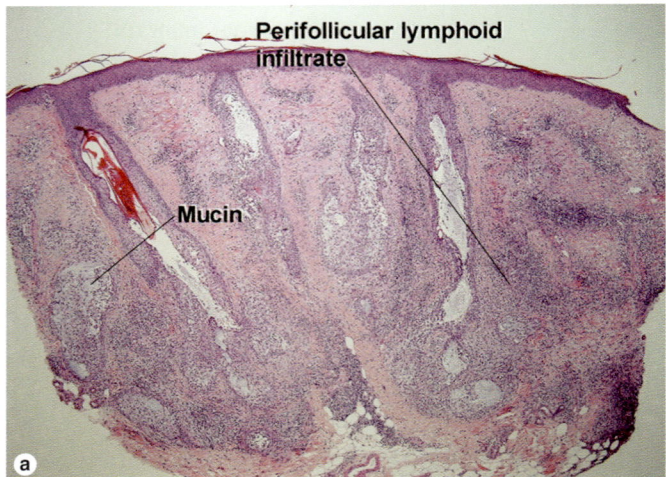

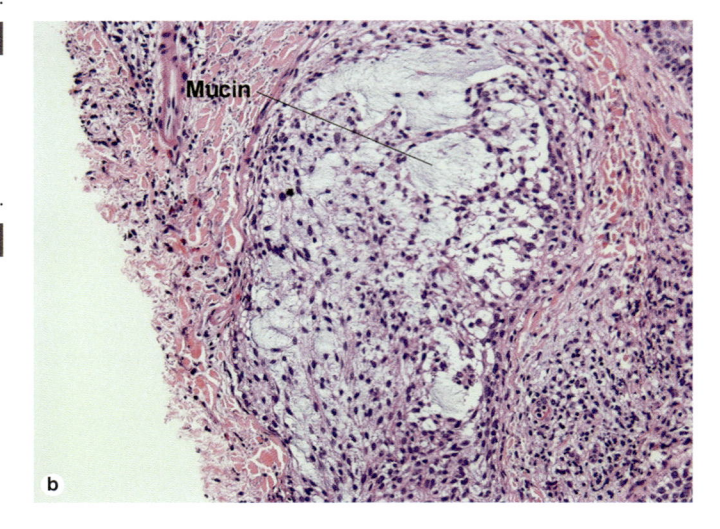

Fig 15-6 Alopecia mucinosa

Disorders of skin appendages

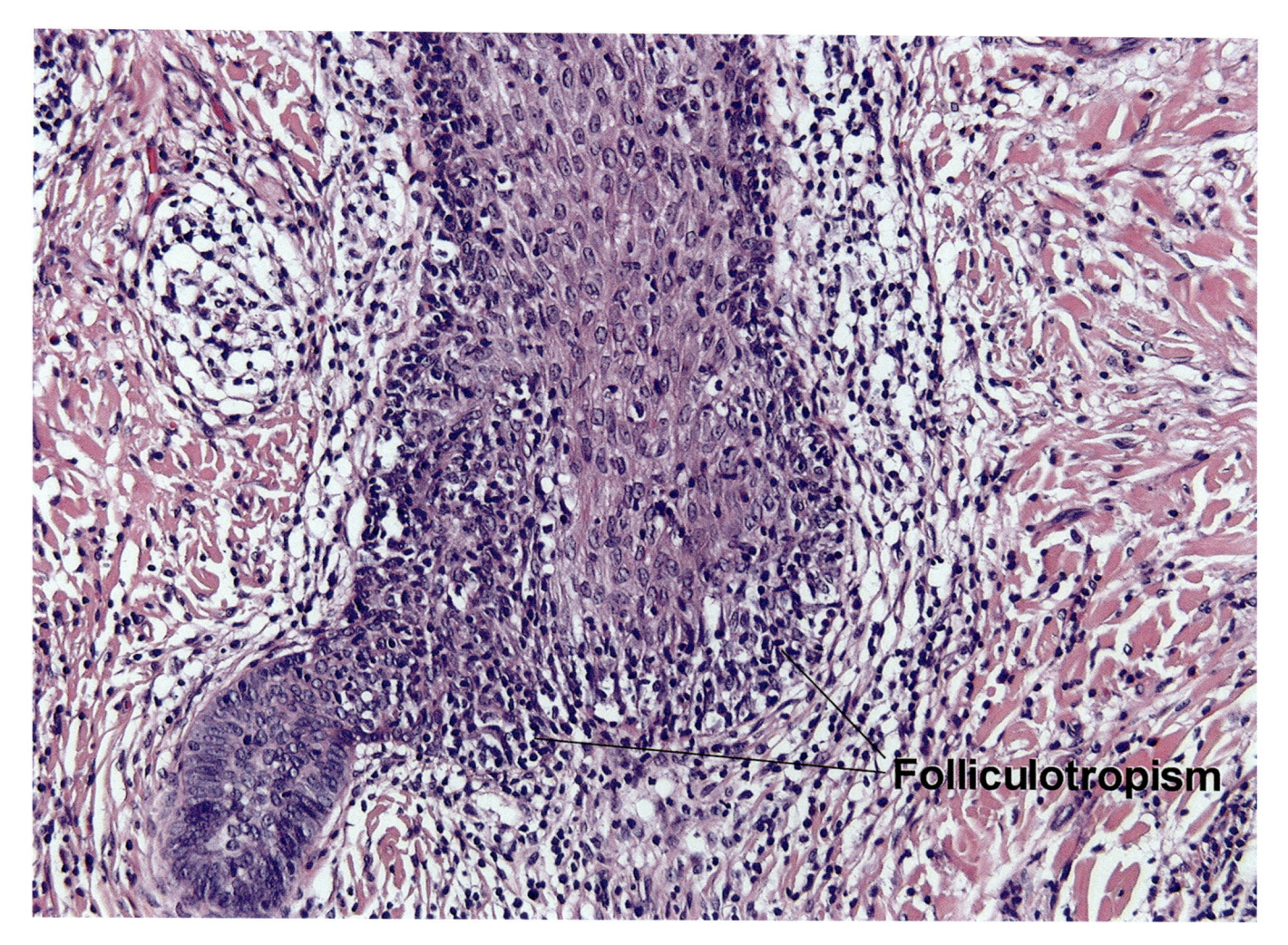

Fig 15-7 Folliculotropic mycosis fungoides

Folliculotropic mycosis fungoides (cutaneous T-cell lymphoma)

Key features

- Large, hyperchromatic, angulated lymphocytes within the follicular epithelium
- Lymphocytes tend to line up along the epithelial side of the dermal–epidermal junction
- Dark lymphocytes are surrounded by a white space (lump of coal on a pillow), but little surrounding spongiosis

Papillary dermal fibrosis is often prominent. Immunostaining may demonstrate deletion of pan-T markers such as CD7, and gene rearrangements can often be demonstrated.

Tinea capitis and Majocchi's fungal folliculitis

Key features

- Mixed inflammatory infiltrate, neutrophils present, eosinophils variable
- Fungal spores within or surrounding hair shaft

Acne vulgaris

Key features

- Infundibulum filled with laminated keratin and debris
- Suppurative inflammation may be present

Cicatricial alopecia

Serial vertical sections are generally superior to transverse (horizontal) sections in the setting of cicatricial alopecia, although the combination of vertical and transverse sections is better than either alone.

Lupus erythematosus

Key features

- Lymphoid infiltrate at the level of the isthmus
- Interface change may be vacuolar or lichenoid
- Compact hyperkeratosis
- Follicular hyperkeratosis
- Basement membrane zone thickening

240 Dermatopathology

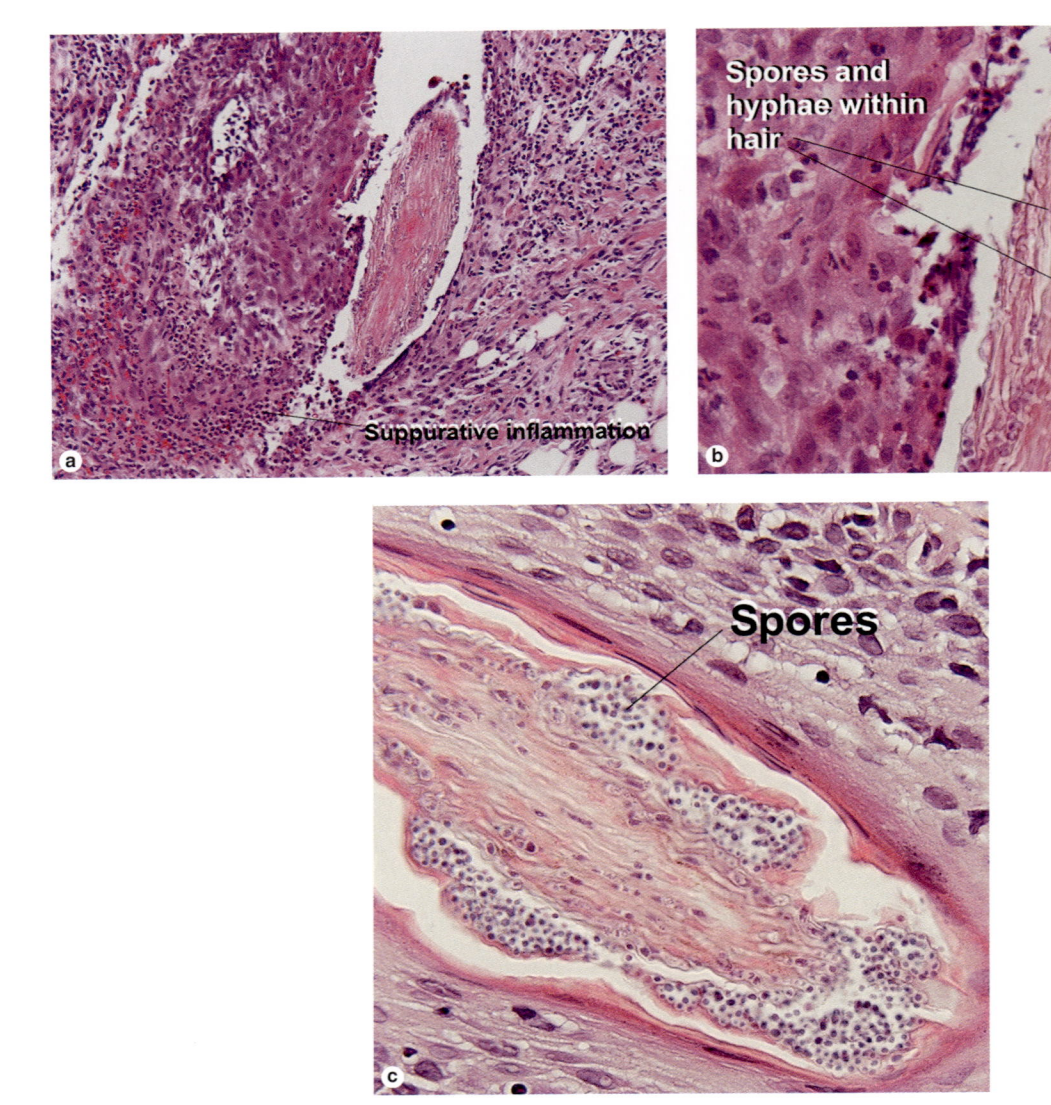

Fig 15-8 Majocchi's granuloma

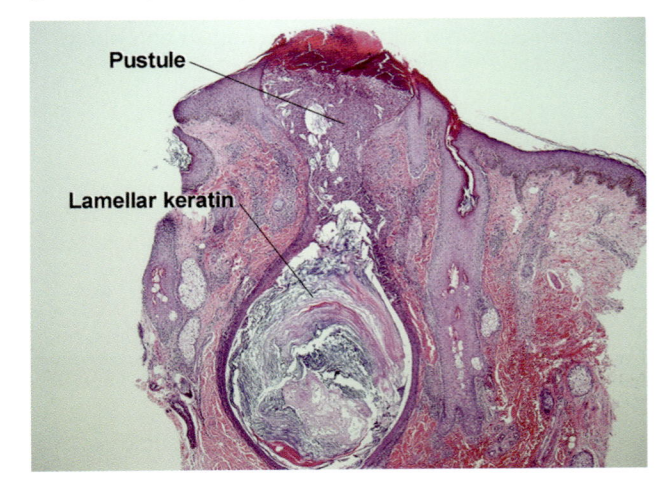

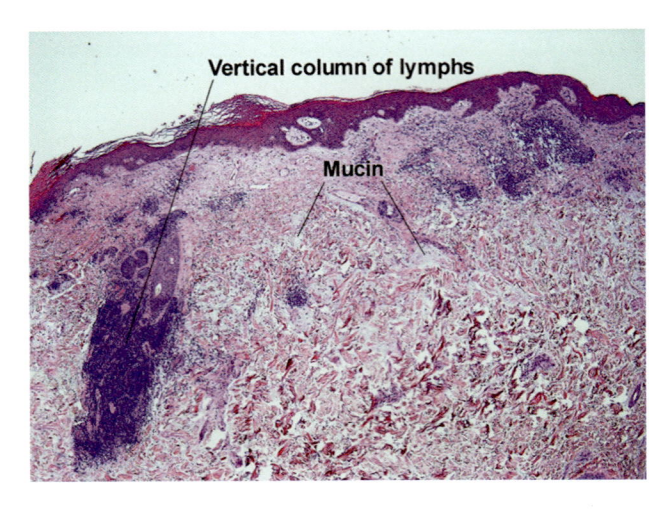

Fig 15-9 Acne

Fig 15-10 Lupus erythematosus

- Melanin pigment incontinence (melanoderma) underlying the dermal–epidermal junction
- Vertical columns of lymphocytes
- Perivascular lymphoid aggregates
- Lymphoid aggregates within the eccrine coil
- Dermal mucin between collagen bundles
- Underlying lupus panniculitis may be present
- Direct immunofluorescence (DIF): continuous granular band of immunoglobulin (Ig) G/A/M and C3 (full house) at the follicular basement membrane zone (see Chapter 7)

The features of discoid lupus erythematosus appear in a time-dependent fashion. Biopsies of early patches will show only perifollicular mucinous fibrosis and focal interface change. DIF will usually be negative at this stage. The biopsy should always be taken from an active lesion, of at least 3 months' duration. Burnt-out patches demonstrate scarring throughout the dermis in elastic tissue-stained sections.

Lichen planopilaris (LPP)

Key features

- Lymphoid infiltrate at the level of the infundibulum
- Lichenoid interface dermatitis
- Entire fibrous tract remnant may be filled with Civatte bodies
- DIF: shaggy linear fibrin and cytoid bodies

As with lupus erythematosus, the features of lichen planopilaris appear in a time-dependent fashion. Biopsies of early patches will show only perifollicular mucinous fibrosis and focal lymphoid inflammation. These changes are most notable about the infundibulum, whereas lupus erythematosus affects the isthmus preferentially. DIF will usually be negative in the early stages, but will often show shaggy linear fibrin and cytoid bodies in more advanced lesions. Burnt-out patches demonstrate wedge-shaped scars at the level of the infundibulum.

Table 15-2 Characteristics of discoid lupus erythematosus versus lichen planopilaris

Characteristic	Discoid lupus erythematosus	Lichen planopilaris
Hyperkeratosis	Yes	Yes
Interface dermatitis	Vacuolar or lichenoid	Lichenoid
Pigment incontinence	Yes	Yes
Lymphoid infiltrate	Centered at isthmus	Centered at the infundibulum
Basement membrane zone thickening	Common	No
Dermal mucin	Common	No
Lymphocytes in eccrine coil	Common	No
Lobular panniculitis with fibrin	Sometimes	No
Direct immunofluorescence	"Full house" common in established lesions, may have cytoid bodies	Negative or shaggy fibrin and cytoid bodies
Scar in late lesions	Throughout dermis	Superficial wedges

242 Dermatopathology

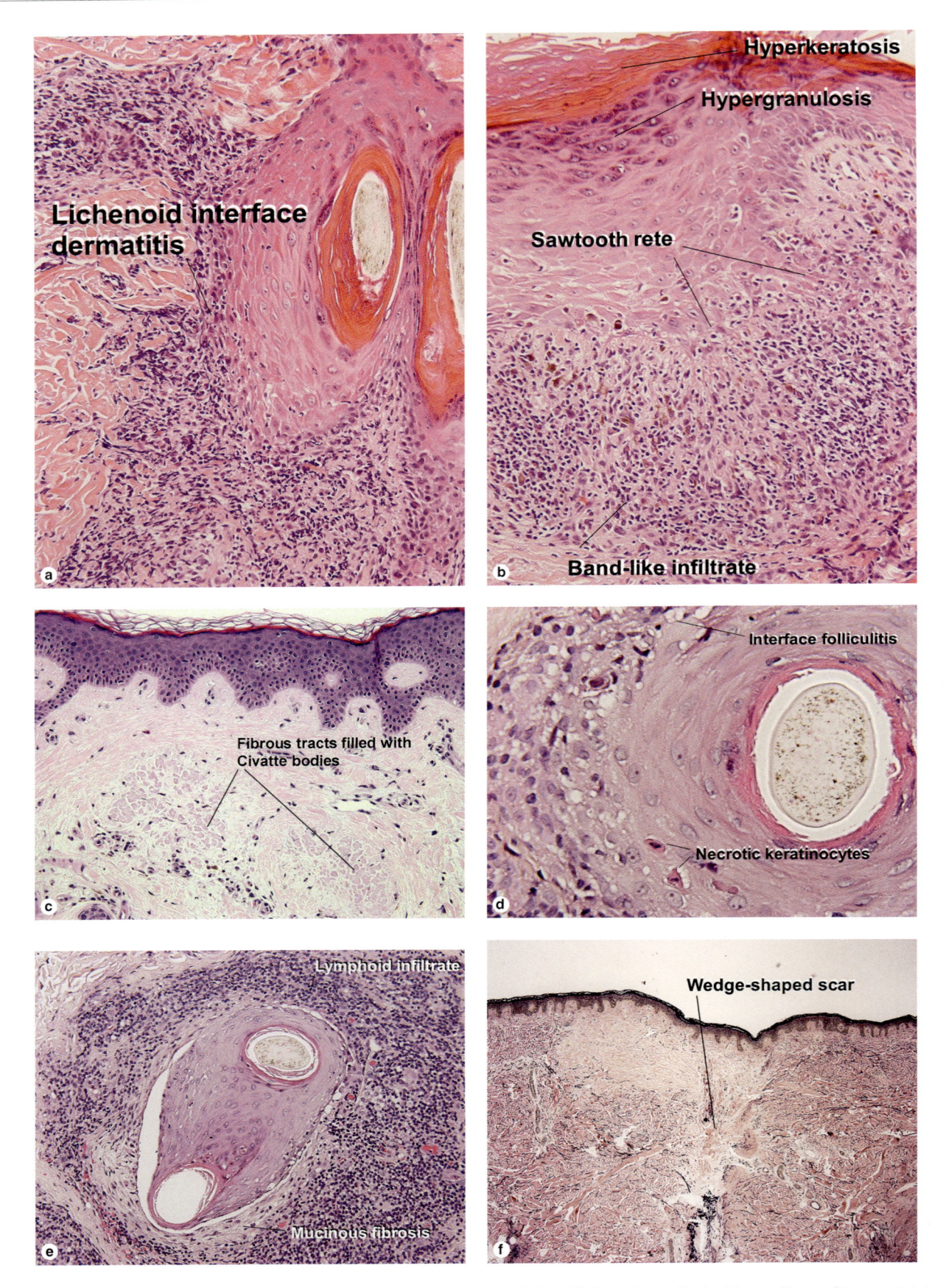

Fig 15-11 (a–e) Lichen planopilaris. (f) Wedge-shaped scar characteristic of lichen planopilaris (Verhoeff–van Gieson stain)

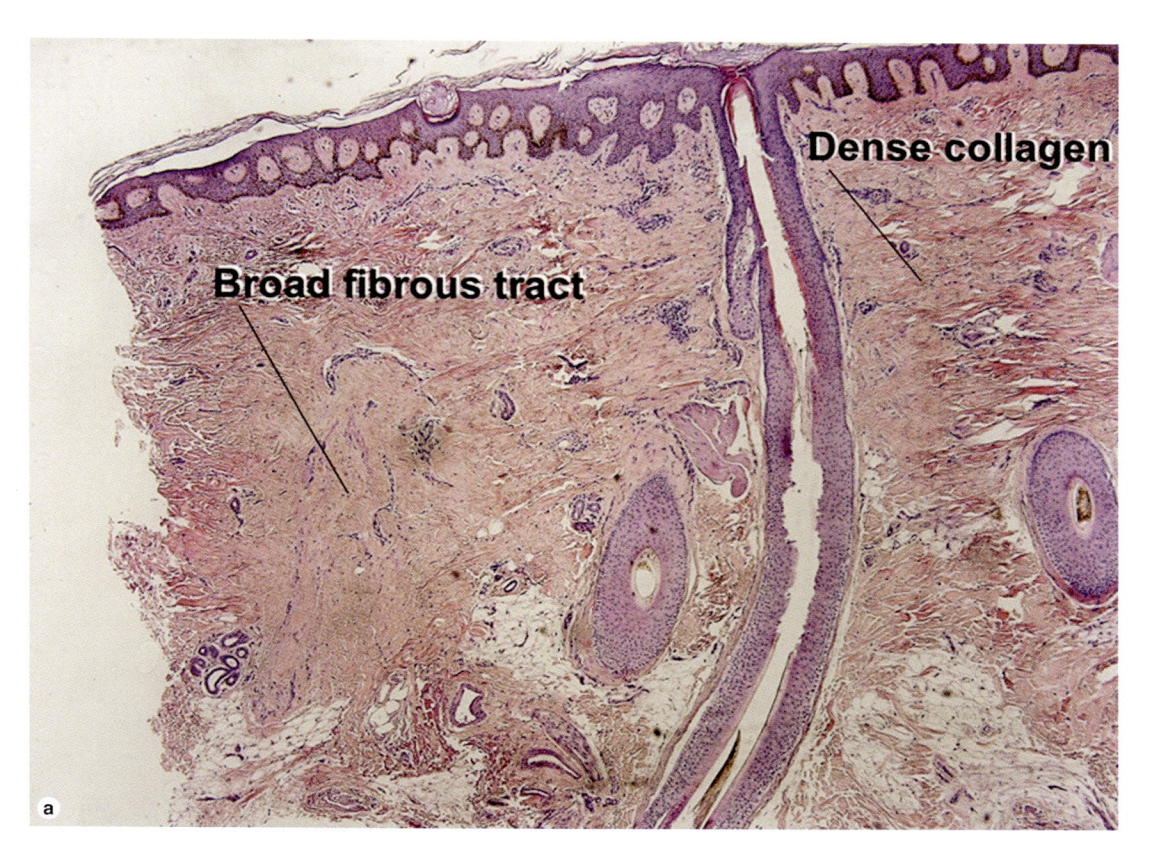

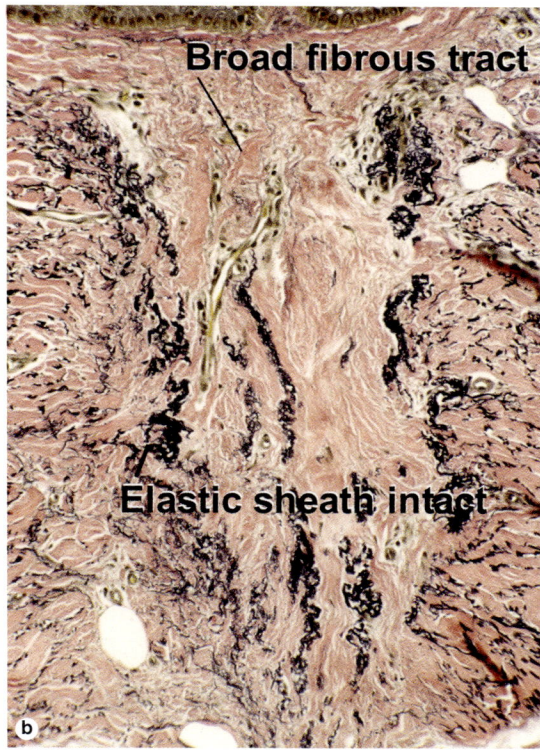

Idiopathic pseudopelade

Key features

- Shrunken deep red dermis
- Broad "tree trunk" fibrous tract remnants
- Preserved elastic sheath
- Thick elastic fibers in dermis

Most patients with ivory white scarring and spared terminal hairs have lichen planopilaris. About 10% of patients with the same clinical features have a unique histology distinct from other forms of alopecia. The dermis is shrunken and deeply eosinophilic with loss of the spaces between collagen bundles. This appearance has been likened to a sweater shrunken in the dryer. Fibrous tract remnants are broad and hyalinized, but the surrounding elastic sheath is intact. Hair granulomas may be noted in fibrous tract remnants. Elastic fibers in the surrounding dermis are thick and "recoiled" because of the contraction of the dermis.

Fig 15-12 (a) Idiopathic pseudopelade. (b) Idiopathic pseudopelade (Verhoeff–van Gieson stain)

244 Dermatopathology

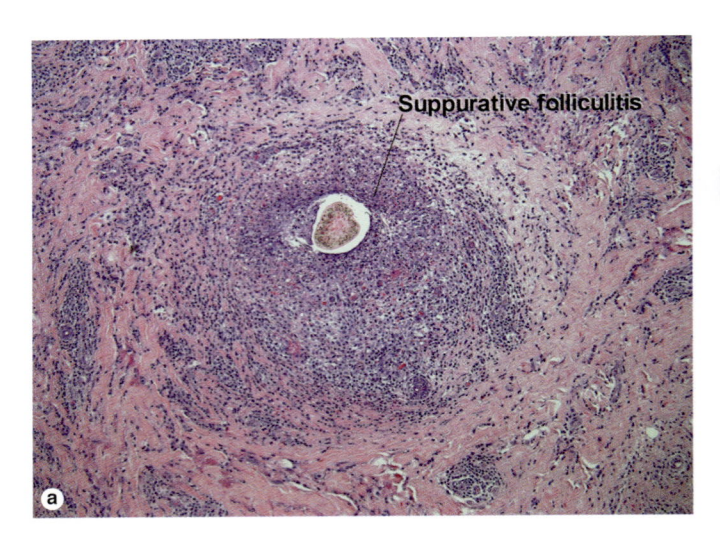

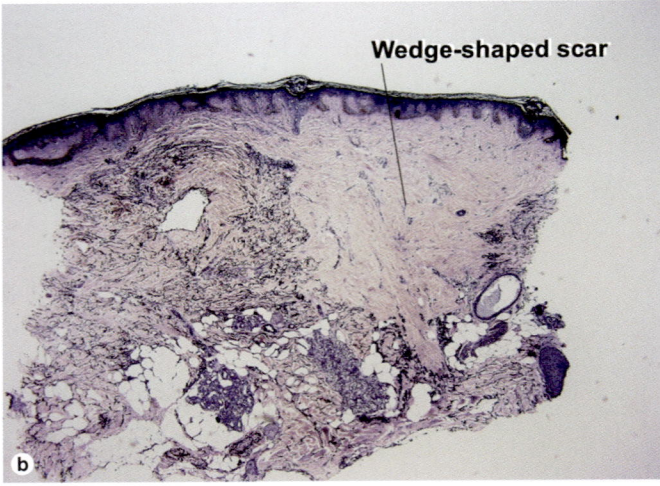

Fig 15-13 (a) Folliculitis decalvans. (b) Wedge-shaped scar of folliculitis decalvans (Verhoeff–van Gieson stain)

Central centrifugal cicatricial alopecia (CCCA)

Key features
- Central alopecia
- Mixed etiologies (including idiopathic pseudopelade, lichen planopilaris, late-stage folliculitis decalvans)

Dissecting cellulitis

Key features
- Clinically similar to nodulocystic acne
- Deep dermal and subcutaneous abscesses, sinus tracts and granulation tissue

Folliculitis decalvans

Key features
- Suppurative folliculitis
- Wedge-shaped scar with elastic stain (similar to LPP)
- "Six pack" tufting of hairs

Patients with folliculitis decalvans present with recurrent crops of epilating follicular pustules. The histologic changes resemble those of a staphylococcal folliculitis. *Staphylococci* are sometimes cultured, and patients respond to prolonged courses of antistaphylococcal therapy.

Patients with Acne keloidalis and progressive alopecia usually demonstrate overlap with folliculitis decalvans.

Acne Keloidalis

See Chapter 13, page 220.

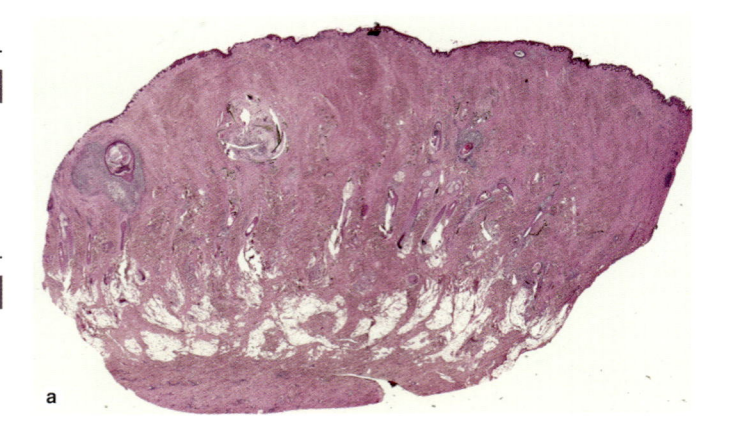

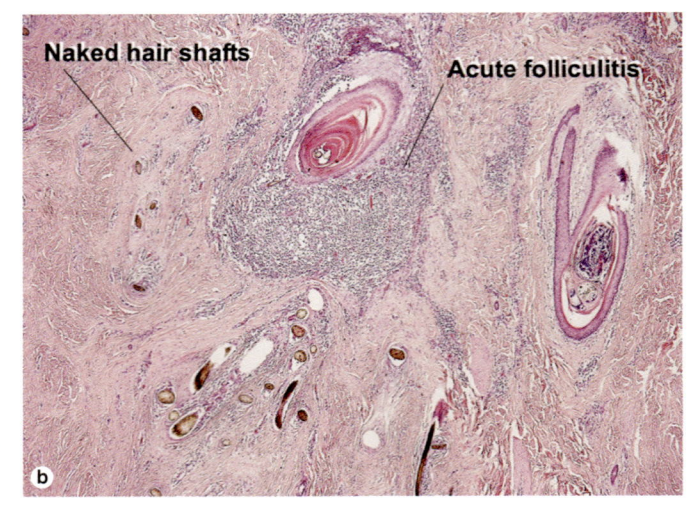

Fig 15-14 Acne keloidalis

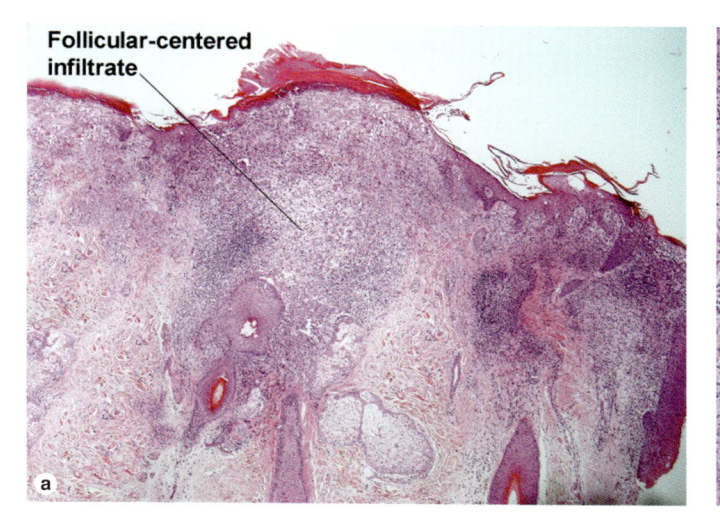

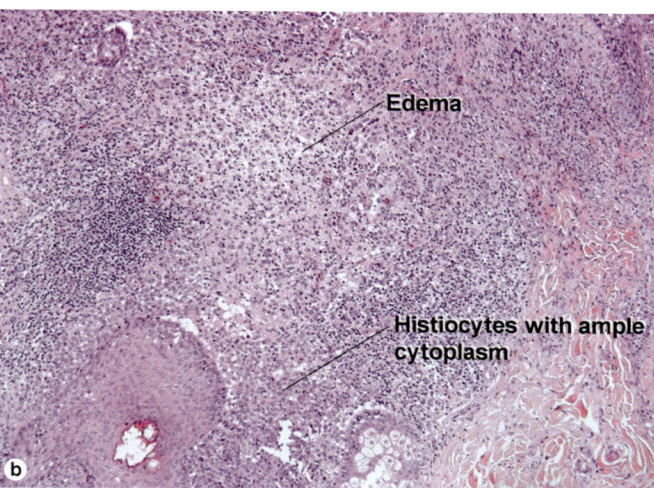

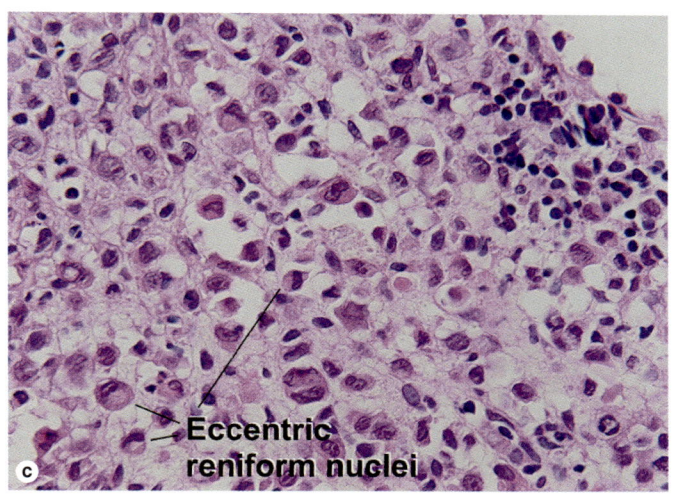

Fig 15-15 Acute Langerhans cell histiocytosis

Acute Langerhans cell histiocytosis (histiocytosis X)

Key features

- Perifollicular epithelioid histiocytes at the level of the infundibulum
- Overlying inflammatory crust common above the infundibulum
- Surrounding edema and erythrocyte extravasation
- Scattered eosinophils common
- Histiocytes stain with S100, CD-1a, peanut agglutinin, langerin
- Electron microscopy: Birbeck granules

At scanning power, acute Langerhans cell histiocytosis has the appearance of a folliculitis at the level of the infundibulum. Instead of lymphocytes, the cells surrounding the follicle are histiocytes with ample cytoplasm and an eccentric pale gray vesicular nucleus. Kidney-shaped nuclei may be present. The surrounding dermis is pale and edematous with erythrocyte extravasation.

Chondrodermatitis nodularis helicis

Key features

- Central crust or ulcer
- Underlying fibrin core within dermis
- Granulation tissue and stellate fibroblasts adjacent to fibrin core

Biopsies do not need to demonstrate cartilage. The primary pathologic change is a small pressure sore on the helical rim. The histologic changes are identical to those of a decubitus ulcer, but on a smaller scale.

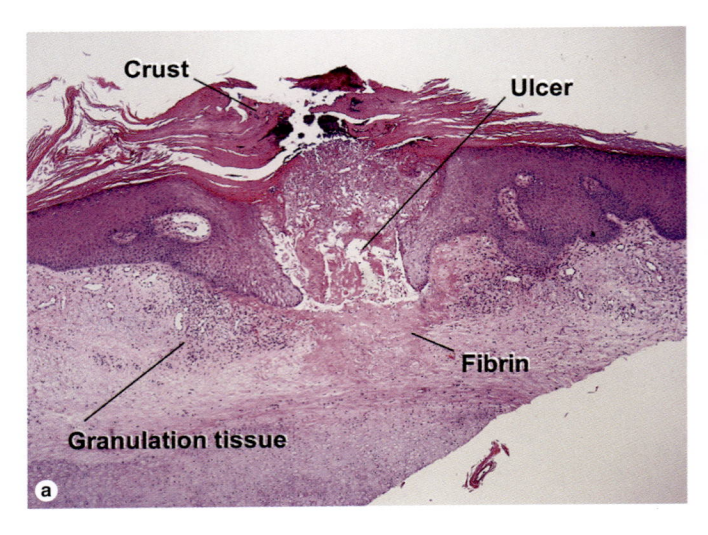

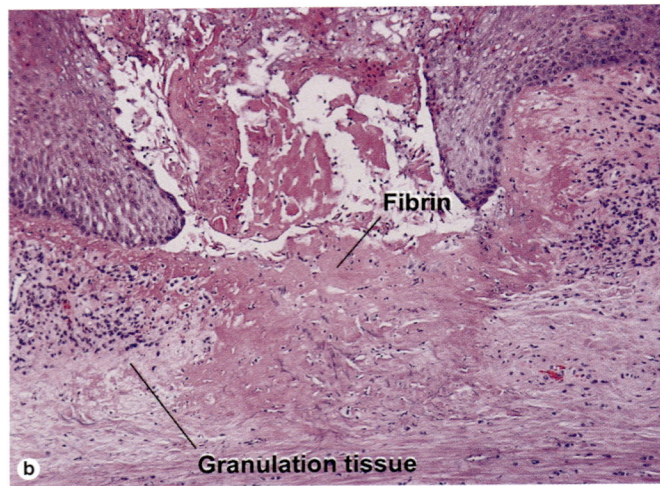

Fig 15-16 Chondrodermatitis nodularis helices

Neutrophilic eccrine hidradenitis

Key features

- Neutrophils within eccrine coil

Neutrophilic eccrine hidradenitis is commonly noted during induction chemotherapy for leukemia. It has also been reported prior to the diagnosis of leukemia, suggesting that it may occur as a paraneoplastic syndrome. In children, idiopathic eccrine hidradenitis may occur on the soles. *Pseudomonas* has been cultured from some of these patients.

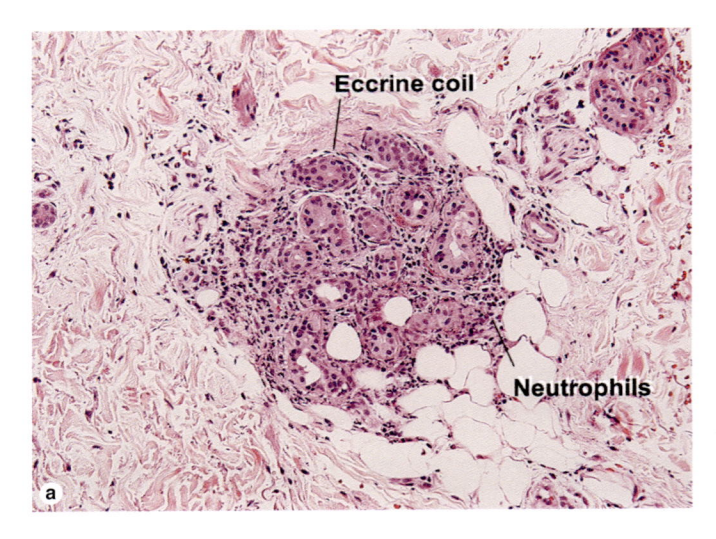

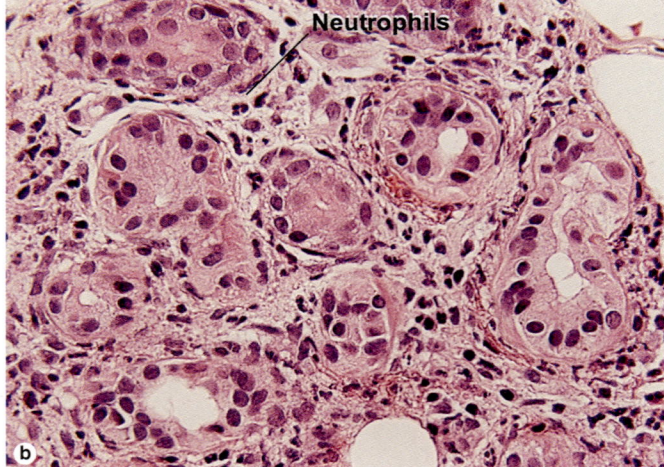

Fig 15-17 Neutrophilic eccrine hidradenitis

Disorders of skin appendages Chapter 15

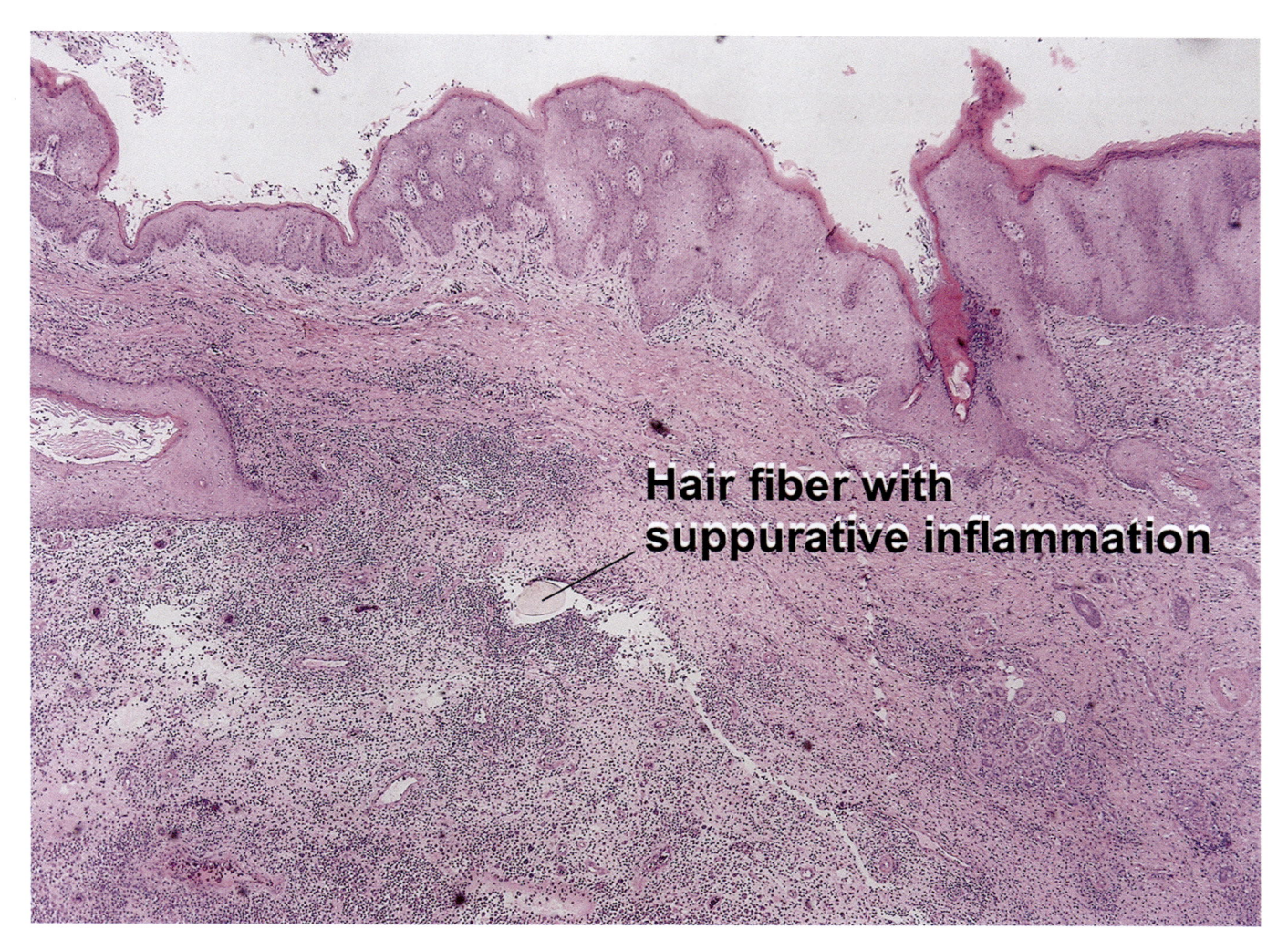

Fig 15-18 Hidradenitis suppurativa

Hidradenitis suppurativa

Key features

- Skin has features of axillary or anogenital skin
- Apocrine glands often present
- Suppurative folliculitis with abscess formation
- Sinus tracts with suppurative and granulomatous inflammation
- Granulation tissue
- Inflammation "spills over" to involve apocrine glands

Mucocele

Key features

- Pooled mucin adjacent to minor salivary gland
- Variable granulomatous response

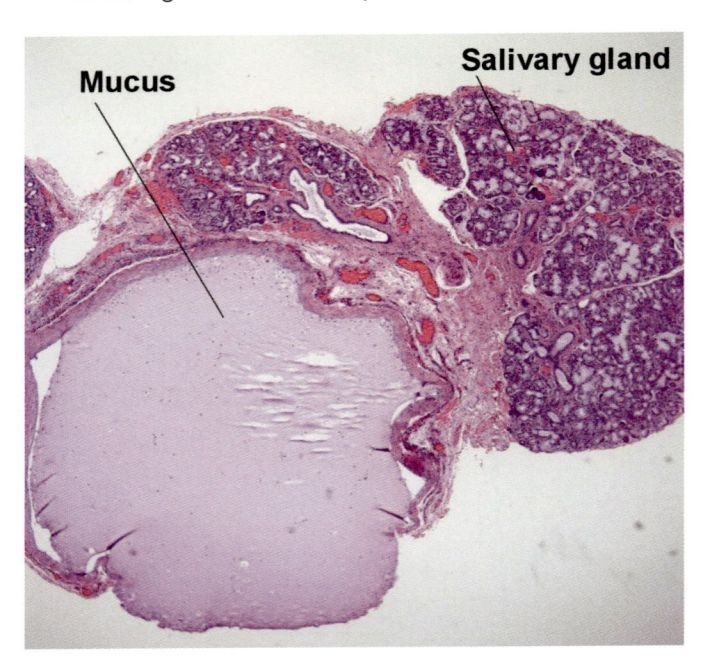

Fig 15-19 Mucocele

Further reading

Böer A, Hoene K. Transverse sections for diagnosis of alopecia? Am J Dermatopathol 2005;27(4):348–352.

Childs JM, Sperling LC. Histopathology of scarring and nonscarring hair loss. Dermatol Clin 2013;31(1):43–56.

Elston DM. What's new in the histologic evaluation of alopecia and hair-related disorders? Dermatol Clin 2012;30(4):685–694.

Elston DM. Vertical vs. transverse sections: both are valuable in the evaluation of alopecia. Am J Dermatopathol 2005;27(4):353–356.

Elston DM, Ferringer T, Dalton S, et al. A comparison of vertical versus transverse sections in the evaluation of alopecia biopsy specimens. J Am Acad Dermatol 2005;53(2):267–272.

Elston DM, McCollough ML, Warschaw KE, et al. Elastic tissue in scars and alopecia. J Cutan Pathol 2000;27(3):147–152.

Elston DM, McCollough ML, Bergfeld WF, et al. Eosinophils in fibrous tracts and near hair bulbs: a helpful diagnostic feature of alopecia areata. J Am Acad Dermatol 1997;37(1):101–106.

Jackson AJ, Price VH. How to diagnose hair loss. Dermatol Clin 2013;31(1):21–28.

Olsen EA, Bergfeld WF, Cotsarelis G, et al. Summary of North American Hair Research Society (NAHRS)-sponsored Workshop on Cicatricial Alopecia, Duke University Medical Center, February 10 and 11, 2001. J Am Acad Dermatol 2003;48(1):103–110.

Peckham SJ, Sloan SB, Elston DM. Histologic features of alopecia areata other than peribulbar lymphocytic infiltrates. J Am Acad Dermatol 2011;65(3):615–620.

Templeton SF, Santa Cruz DJ, Solomon AR. Alopecia: histologic diagnosis by transverse sections. Semin Diagn Pathol 1996;13(1):2–18.

Trachsler S, Trueb RM. Value of direct immunofluorescence for differential diagnosis of cicatricial alopecia. Dermatology 2005;211(2):98–102.

Whiting DA. Histopathologic features of alopecia areata: a new look. Arch Dermatol 2003;139(12):1555–1559.

Panniculitis

Dirk M. Elston

Chapter 16

The inflammatory infiltrate in septal panniculitis spills over into the lobule. The inflammation in lobular panniculitis often involves the septum, therefore, septal and lobular panniculitis are best differentiated by the architecture of the lobule. In septal panniculitis, the lobule is intact; lipocytes are similar in size and shape, and the scan appearance resembles a bowl of toasted oat cereal. In lobular panniculitis, the lobule is necrotic; lipophages are common, and in most instances free lipid accumulates in pools that vary in size and shape. The scan appearance resembles the surface of a bowl of chicken soup. Important exceptions to this rule include conditions that result in solidification of fat (sclerema, subcutaneous fat necrosis of the newborn, and steroid-induced fat necrosis). In each of these conditions, the solidified fat cannot coalesce. Pancreatic panniculitis results in calcification of the necrotic membranes, and also prevents coalescence of lipid.

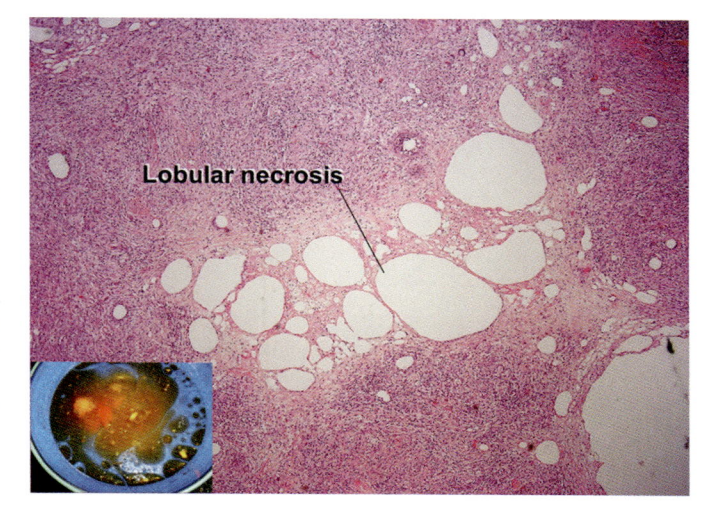

Fig 16-2 Lobular panniculitis

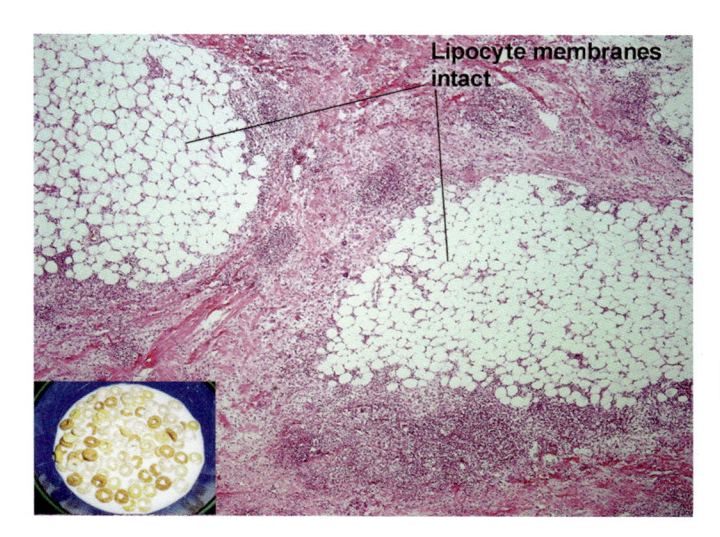

Fig 16-1 Septal panniculitis

Septal panniculitis

Erythema nodosum is the major form of septal panniculitis. Infections can occasionally produce necrosis and inflammation within the septum, without necrosis of the fat lobule. Alpha$_1$-antitrypsin deficiency can occasionally result in liquefactive necrosis of the septum without necrosis of the lobule.

Erythema nodosum

Key features

- Septal panniculitis (little to no necrosis of lobule)
- Neutrophils in septum in acute phase
- Mononuclear cells and granulomatous inflammation in chronic phase
- Miescher's granuloma: central cleft within granuloma

Dermatopathology

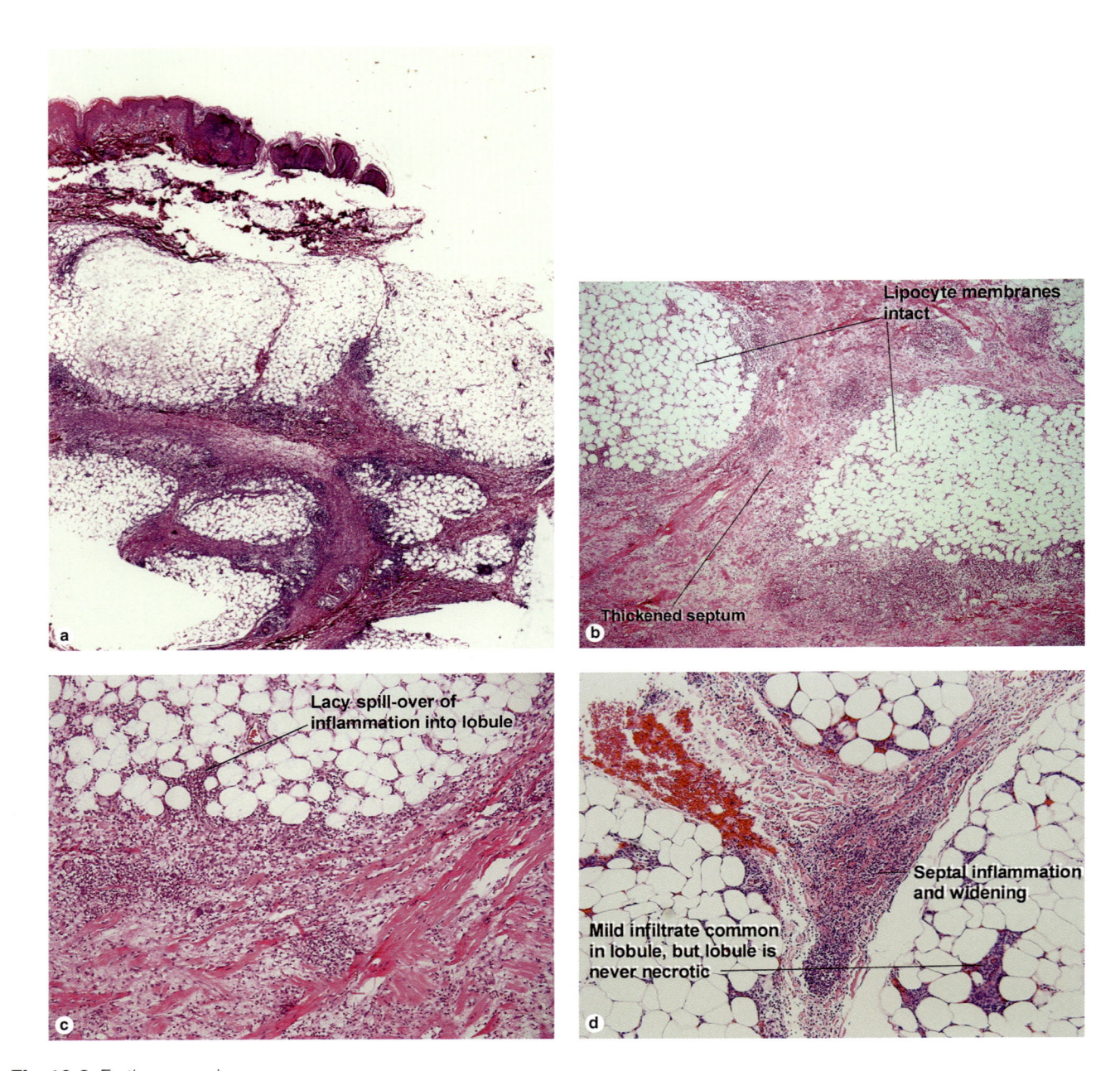

Fig 16-3 Erythema nodosum

Lobular panniculitis

Lupus panniculitis (lupus profundus)

Key features

- Necrosis of fat lobule ("chicken soup")
- Fibrin and hyaline rings around fat
- Nodular lymphoid infiltrates

Although connective tissue disease can produce less specific patterns of granulomatous panniculitis, the features noted above are highly characteristic of lupus panniculitis. Plasma cells are common in the nodular lymphoid foci. Overlying features of lupus erythematosus may be present. The overlying dermis may be sclerotic. Lipomembranous changes may be present (eosinophilic "frost on the windowpane" or "ferning" pattern at the edge of the lipid vacuole).

> **PEARL**
>
> Subcutaneous panniculitis-like lymphoma may have an identical histologic appearance. Features that favor lupus include: interface dermatitis, lymphoid follicles with reactive germinal centers, mixed cellular infiltrate with plasma cells, and lack of T-cell receptor-gamma gene rearrangement. It should, however, be noted that interface change and dermal mucin have been noted in some patients with lymphoma.

Panniculitis Chapter 16 251

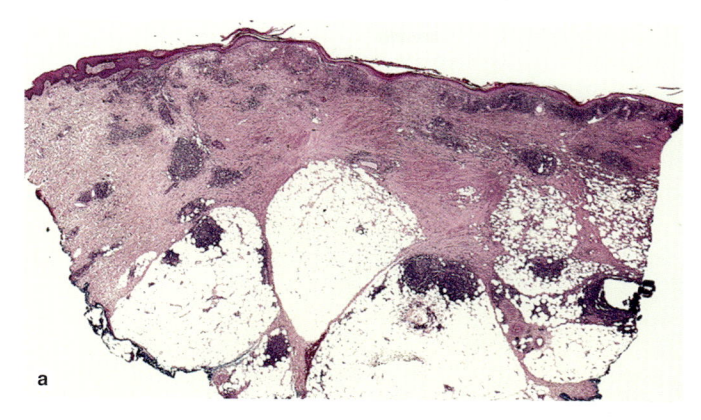

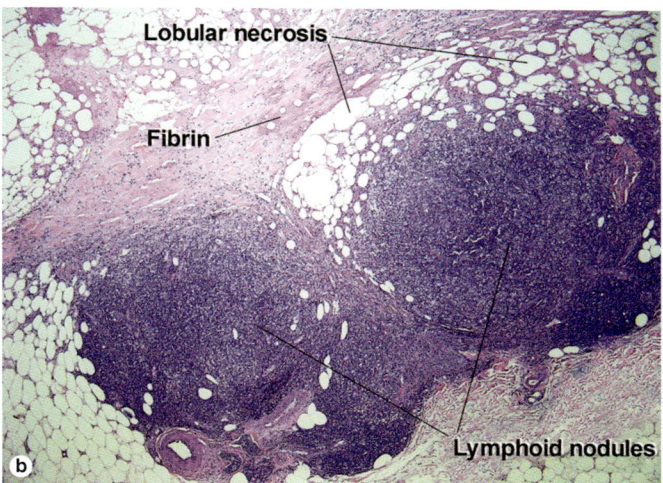

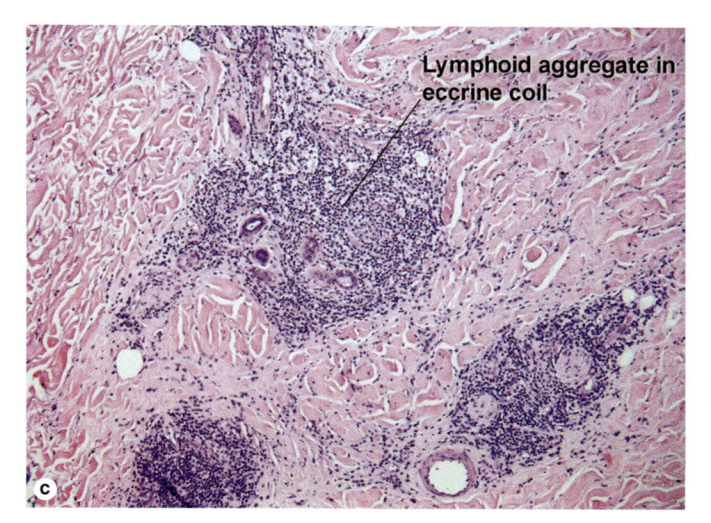

Fig 16-4 Lupus panniculitis

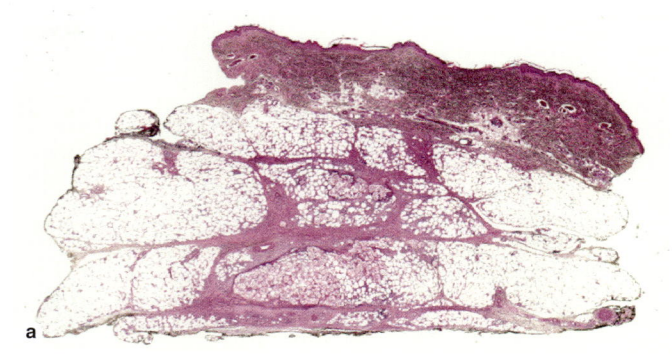

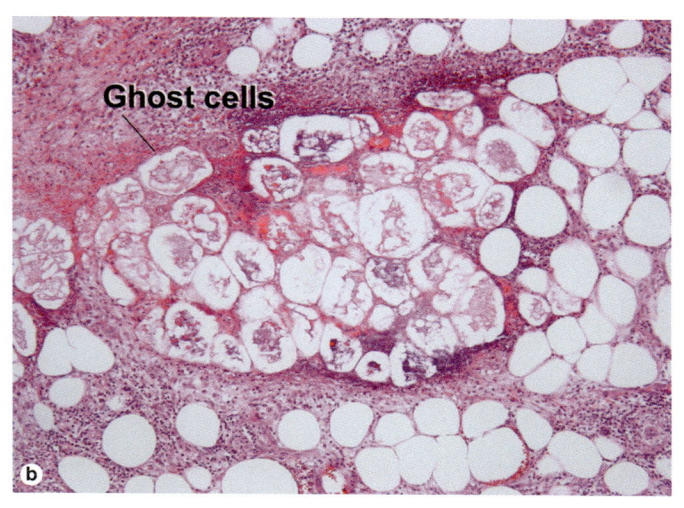

Fig 16-5 Pancreatic panniculitis

Pancreatic panniculitis

Key features

- Necrosis of the fat lobule with calcium soap outlining necrotic lipocytes

Pancreatic panniculitis may occur in the setting of pancreatitis or pancreatic neoplasm.

Subcutaneous fat necrosis of the newborn

Key features

- Necrosis of the fat lobule with crystallization of fat (solid fat cannot coalesce like "chicken soup")
- Radial crystals in lipocytes
- Granulomatous inflammation

Differential Diagnosis

- Steroid-induced fat necrosis (*aka* post-steroid panniculitis) looks identical
- Sclerema neonatorum has identical crystals, but no inflammation

252 Dermatopathology

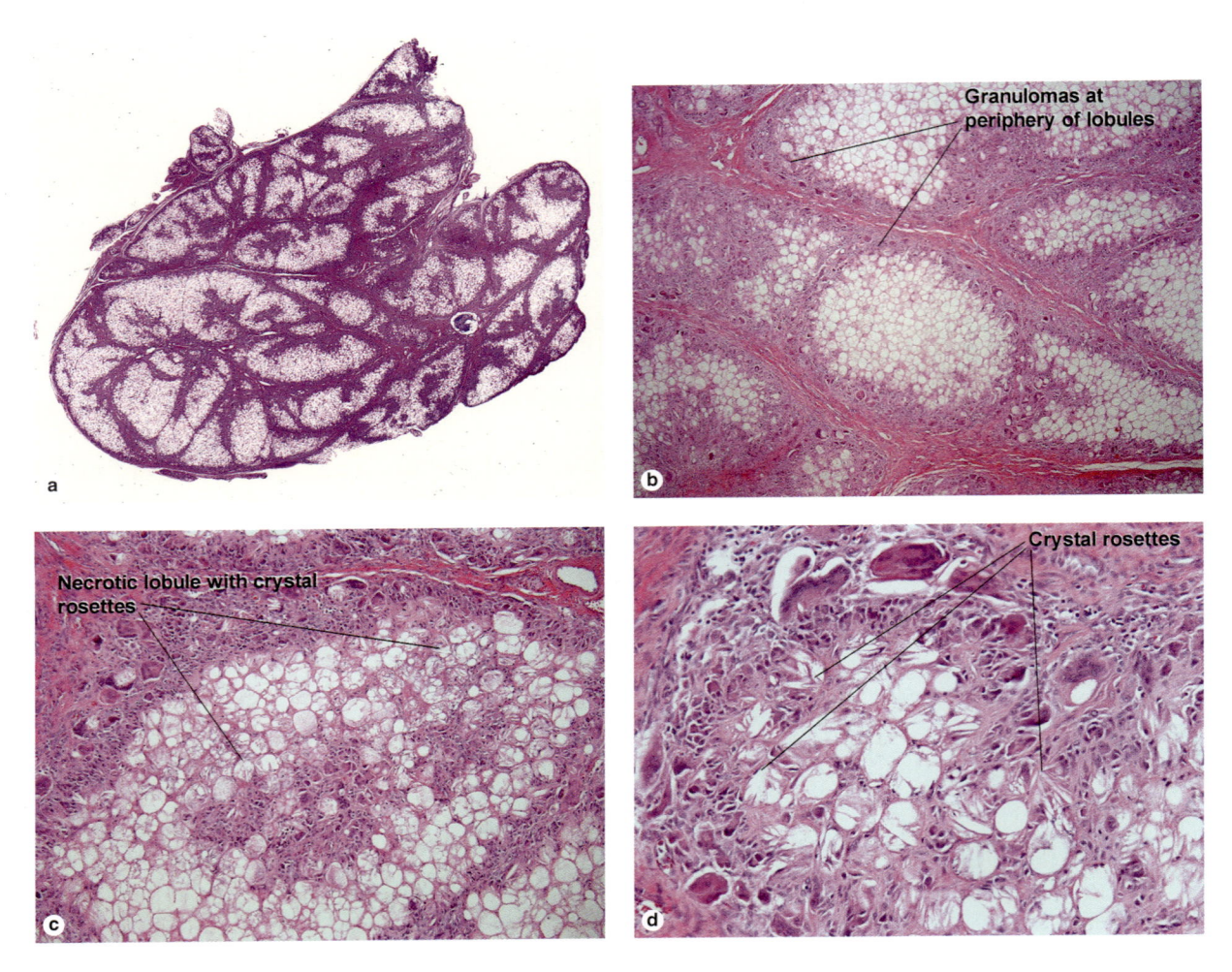

Fig 16-6 Subcutaneous fat necrosis of the newborn

Eosinophilic panniculitis

Key features

- Eosinophils in septum and lobule
- Necrosis variable

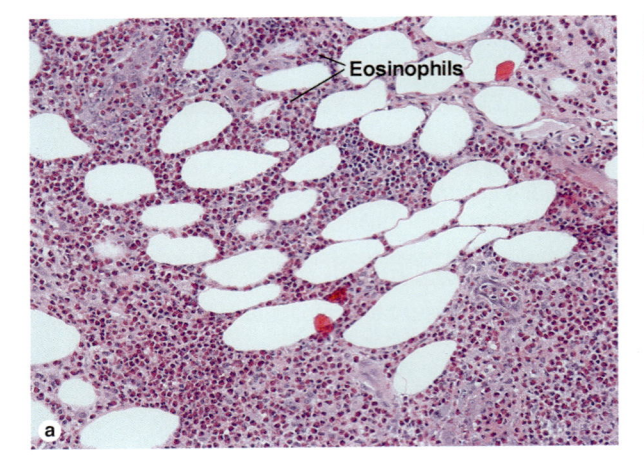

Causes

- Churg–Strauss syndrome
- Helminthic parasite
- Arthropod
- Hypereosinophilic syndrome

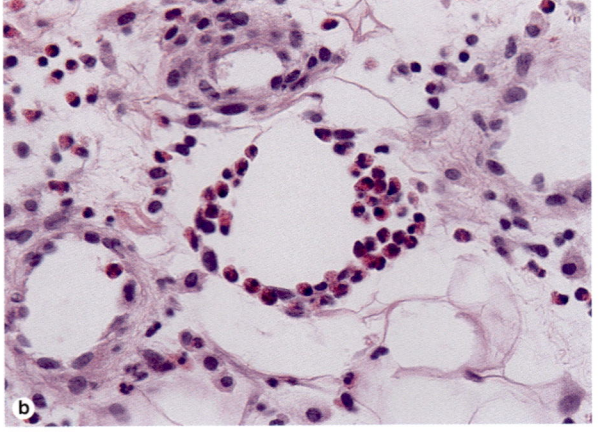

Fig 16-7 Eosinophilic panniculitis

Suppurative and granulomatous panniculitis

Key features
- Lobular panniculitis
- Suppurative and granulomatous infiltrate
- Usually infectious etiology
- May be factitial

Predominantly granulomatous lesions may be associated with lipodystrophy or connective tissue disease.

Nodular vasculitis/erythema induratum (EI) of Bazin

Key features
- Necrosis of the fat lobule ("chicken soup")
- Multinucleated giant cells
- Nodular neutrophilic vasculitis often present in septum
- Caseation necrosis common

EI commonly involves the calves. Liquefied fat may drain from the lesions. Some authorities use the term "nodular vasculitis" when patients are purified protein derivative (PPD) negative, and EI when they are PPD positive. Polymerase chain reaction has been used to identify mycobacterial antigens within lesional tissue.

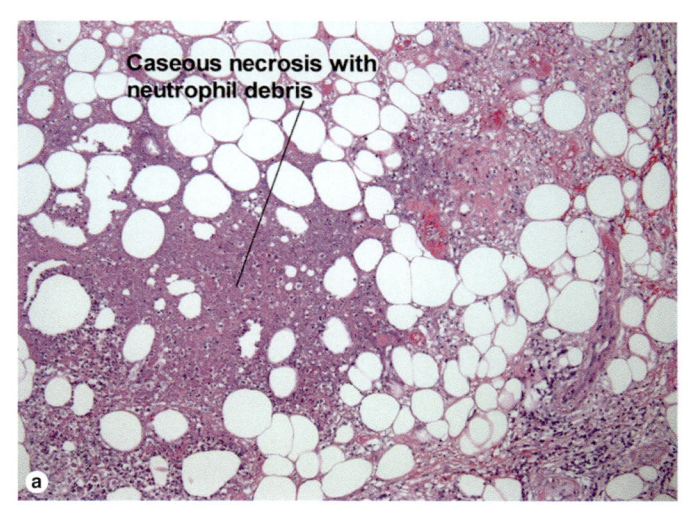

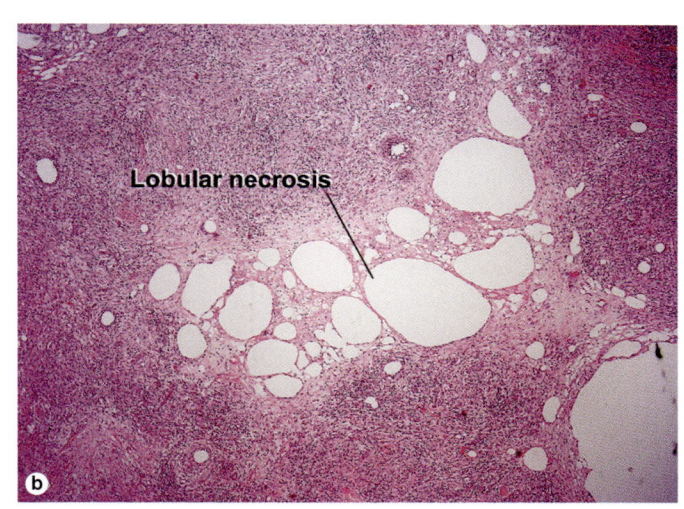

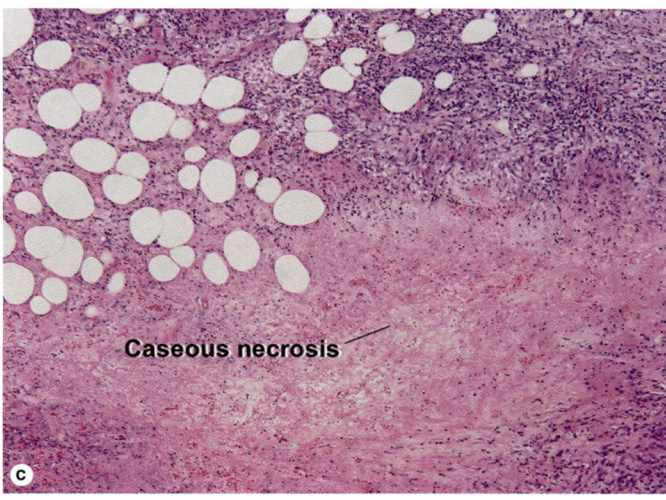

Alpha$_1$-antitrypsin deficiency

Key features
- Neutrophilic infiltrate
- Fat necrosis and granulomatous infiltrate variable
- Liquefactive necrosis of the septum may be seen

Differential Diagnosis

Infectious etiologies should be excluded. Neutrophilic panniculitis may also occur in myelodysplastic syndromes.

Fig 16-8 Erythema induratum

254 Dermatopathology

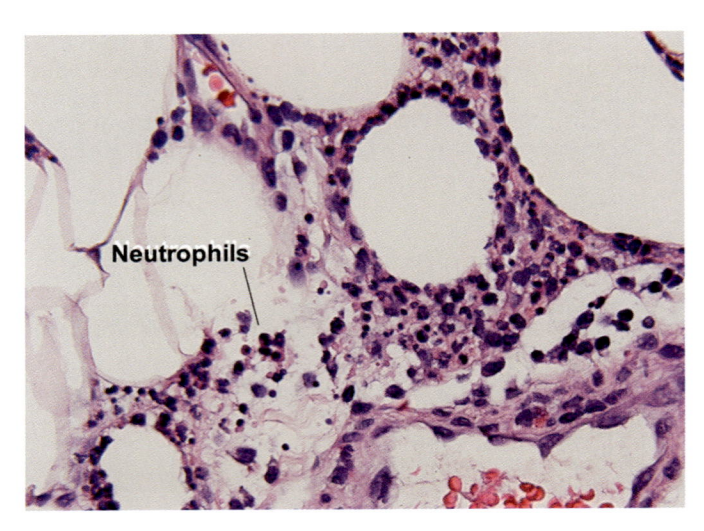

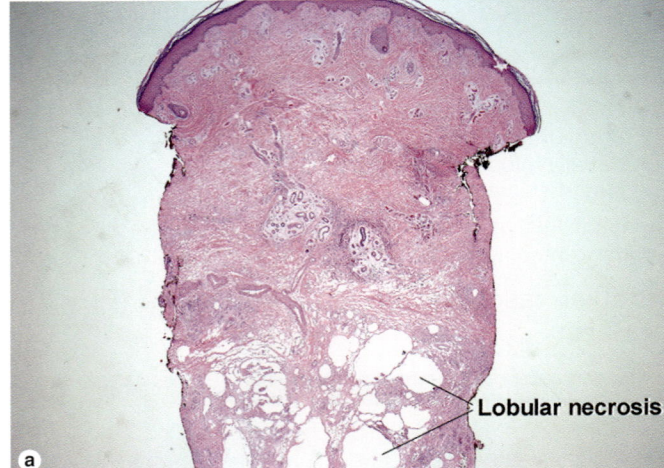

Fig 16-9 Alpha₁-antitrypsin deficiency

Lipodermatosclerosis (stasis panniculitis)

Key features
- Necrosis of the fat lobule ("chicken soup")
- Lipomembranous change ("frost on the windowpane")
- Overlying stasis change

PEARL
Lipomembranous change may be noted in many forms of lobular panniculitis, including lupus panniculitis.

Cytophagic histiocytic panniculitis

Key features
- Lobular panniculitis
- "Beanbag cells"

Cytophagic histiocytic panniculitis may follow infection or may be induced by lymphoma. The patient often dies of a hemorrhagic diathesis. Beanbag cells are histiocytes that have engulfed inflammatory cells and erythrocytes.

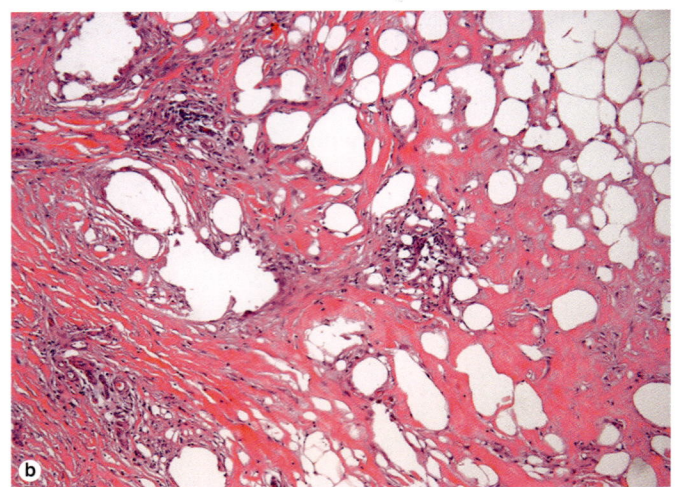

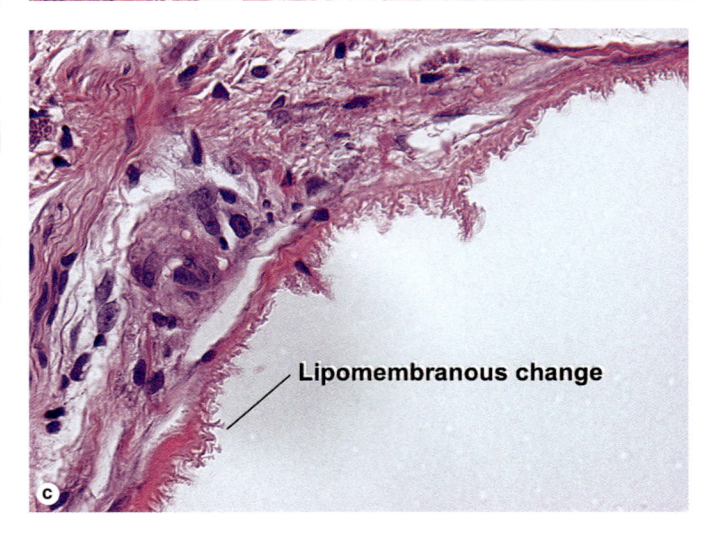

Fig 16-10 Lipodermatosclerosis

Panniculitis | Chapter 16 | 255

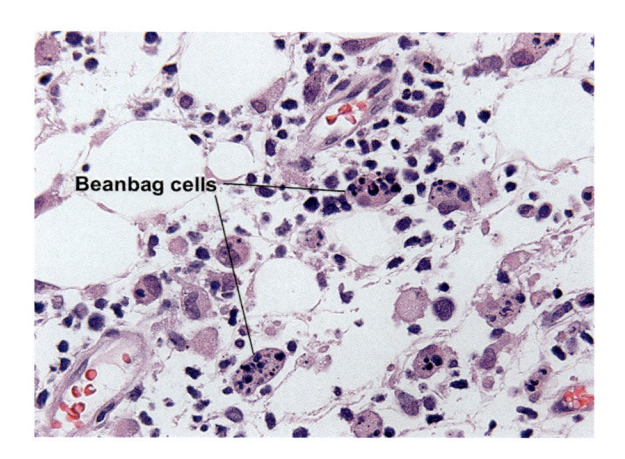

Fig 16-11 Cytophagic histiocytic panniculitis

Traumatic fat necrosis ("mobile encapsulated lipoma")

Key features

- Resembles lobular panniculitis
- Fibrous capsule

Subcutaneous panniculitis-like lymphoma

Key features

- Resembles lobular panniculitis
- May closely resemble lupus panniculitis
- Atypical lymphocytes rimming lipocytes
- Natural killer and gamma–delta phenotypes may be seen

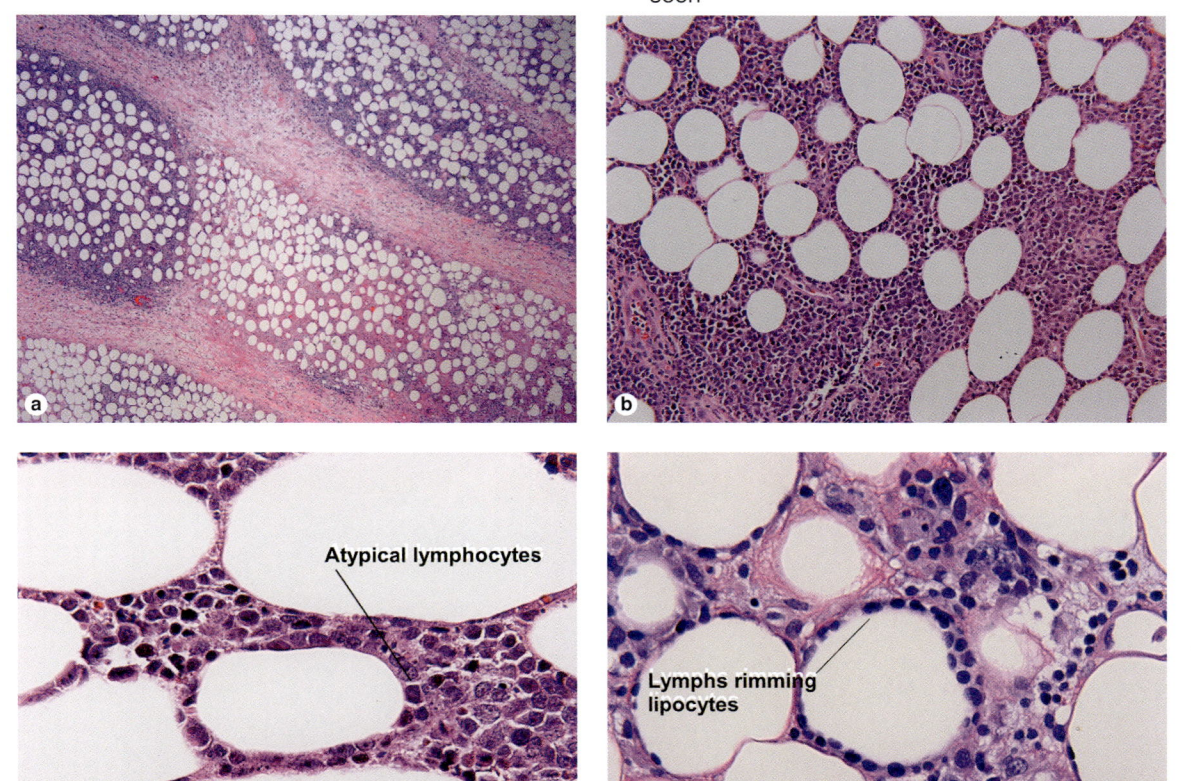

Fig 16-12 Subcutaneous panniculitis-like lymphoma

Further reading

Geraminejad P, DeBloom JR 2nd, Walling HW, et al. Alpha-1-antitrypsin associated panniculitis: the MS variant. J Am Acad Dermatol 2004;51(4):645–655.

Gonzalez EG, Selvi E, Lorenzini S, et al. Subcutaneous panniculitis-like T-cell lymphoma misdiagnosed as lupus erythematosus panniculitis. Clin Rheumatol 2006;26(2):244–246.

Heymann WR. Panniculitis. J Am Acad Dermatol 2005;52(4):683–685.

Ma L, Bandarchi B, Glusac EJ. Fatal subcutaneous panniculitis-like T-cell lymphoma with interface change and dermal mucin, a dead ringer for lupus erythematosus. J Cutan Pathol 2005;32(5):360–365.

Massone C, Kodama K, Salmhofer W, et al. Lupus erythematosus panniculitis (lupus profundus): clinical, histopathological, and molecular analysis of nine cases. J Cutan Pathol 2005;32(6):396–404.

McBean J, Sable A, Maude J, et al. Alpha1-antitrypsin deficiency panniculitis. Cutis 2003;71(3):205–209.

Phelps RG, Shoji T. Update on panniculitis. Mt Sinai J Med 2001;68(4–5):262–267.

Requena L, Sánchez Yus E. Panniculitis. Part II. Mostly lobular panniculitis. J Am Acad Dermatol 2001;45(3):325–361.

Schneider JW, Jordaan HF. The histopathologic spectrum of erythema induratum of Bazin. Am J Dermatopathol 1997;19(4):323–333.

Sutra-Loubet C, Carlotti A, Guillemette J, et al. Neutrophilic panniculitis. J Am Acad Dermatol 2004;50(2):280–285.

Bacterial, spirochete, and protozoan infections

Dirk M. Elston

Chapter 17

An infectious disease atlas can be found in the on-line content for this book.

Bacterial diseases

Impetigo

Key features
- Neutrophilic crust
- Chains or clusters of cocci

Impetigo recruits neutrophils to the stratum corneum. Organisms are commonly visible in hematoxylin and eosin sections. Gram stain and culture may be required.

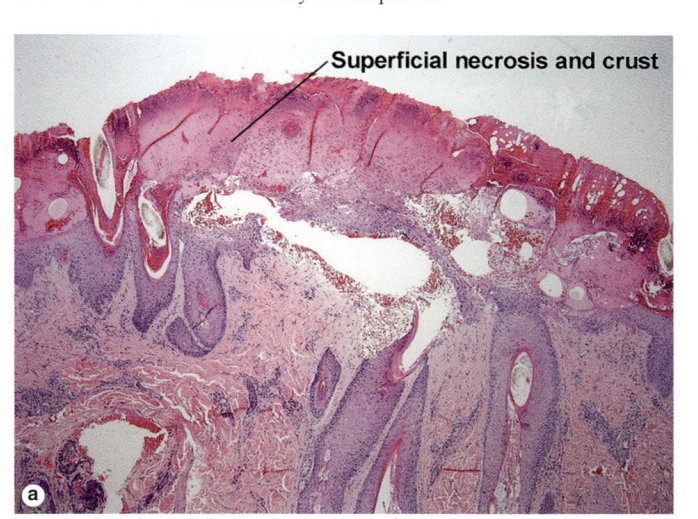

Differential Diagnosis
Collections of neutrophils within the stratum corneum: psoriasis, tinea, impetigo, *Candida*, seborrheic dermatitis, syphilis (PTICSS)

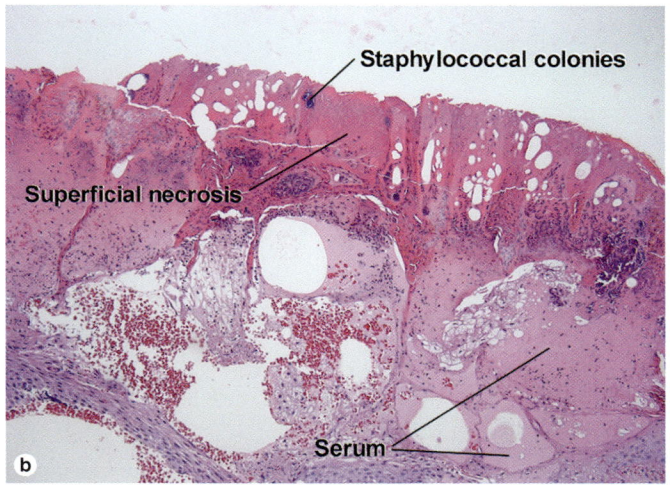

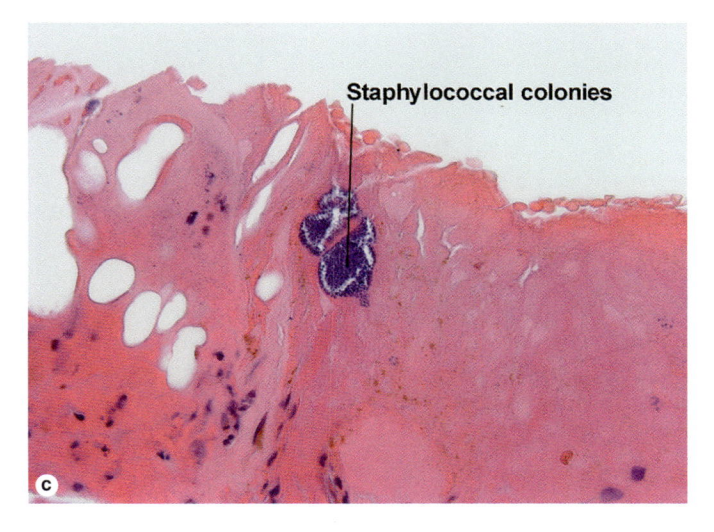

Fig 17-1 Impetigo

Dermatopathology

Bullous impetigo

Key features
- Subcorneal bulla
- Acantholysis in granular layer

Differential Diagnosis
Staphylococcal scalded-skin syndrome and pemphigus foliaceus demonstrate acantholysis at the same level.

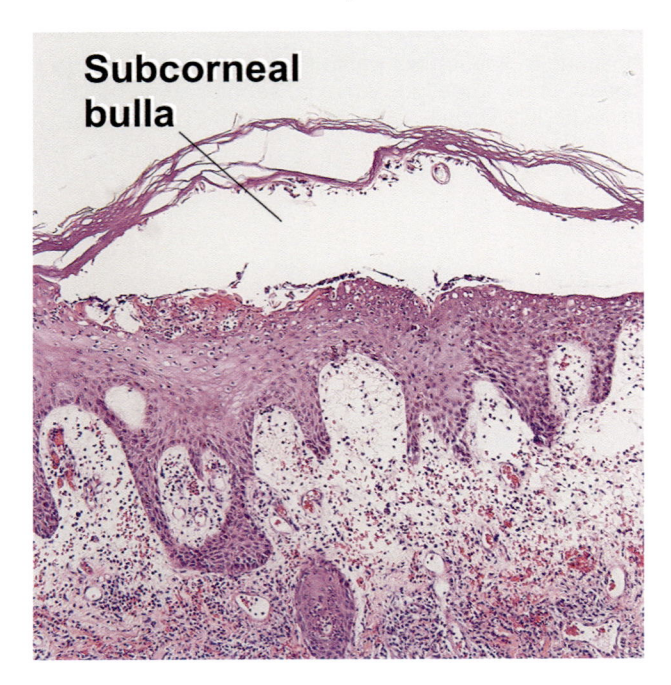

Fig 17-2 Bullous impetigo

Suppurative folliculitis

Key features
- Suppurative inflammation in or around a follicle
- Focal crusts in the stratum corneum
- Vertical column of suppurative inflammation in the dermis

The follicle may not be visible in every plane of section. In some sections, only a focus of inflammatory cells may be noted in the dermis. The microscopic differential diagnosis includes bacterial infection (including furunculosis and hot-tub folliculitis), fungal infection, chemical folliculitis, acne, rosacea, and pustular drug eruption.

Botryomycosis

Key features
- Large staphylococcal grains in tissue
- Abscesses and sinus tracts

Clinically, botryomycosis may resemble a mycetoma. The grains represent huge staphylococcal colonies.

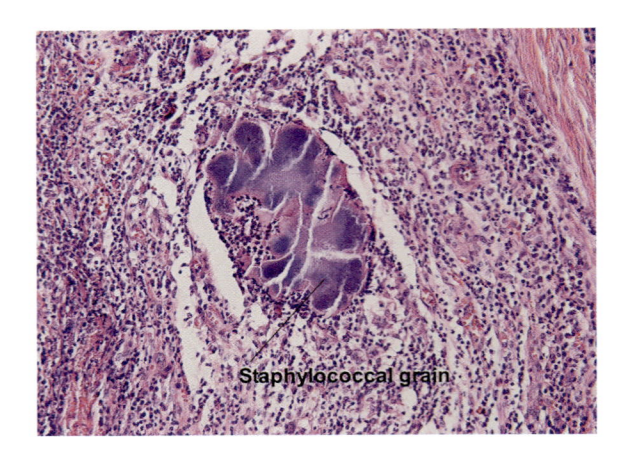

Fig 17-3 Botryomycosis

Pitted keratolysis

Key features
- Acral skin
- Dell or pit in stratum corneum
- Rods and cocci at base of dell

Pitted keratolysis is rarely biopsied because it is readily distinguished by its appearance and smell (so-called "toxic sock syndrome"). Both micrococci and diphtheroids are generally present (*Kytococcus sedentarius* and *Corynebacterium*).

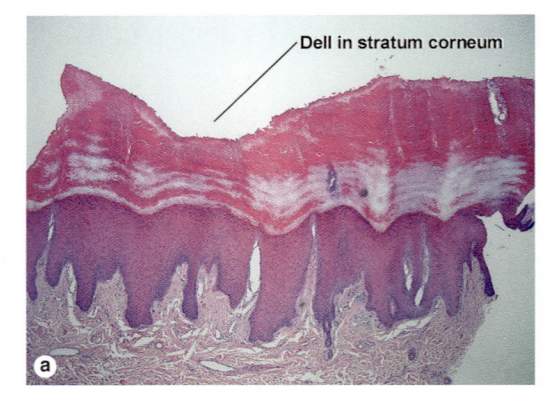

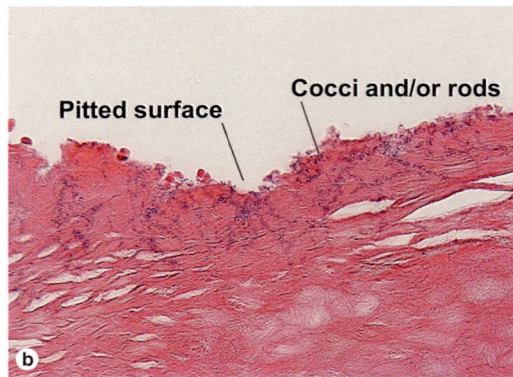

Fig 17-4 Pitted keratolysis

Erythrasma

Key features

- Rods forming vertical filaments in stratum corneum
- Inflammation variable

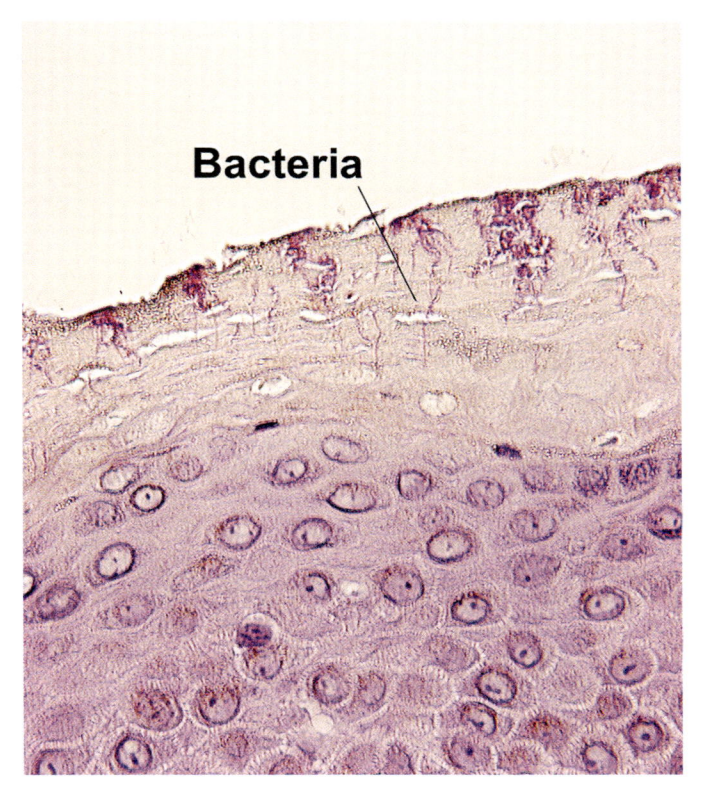

Fig 17-5 Erythrasma

Ecthyma gangrenosum

Key features

- Necrosis of deep dermal vessels
- Amphophilic bacilli surrounding vessels (light blue haze)
- Lack of inflammatory infiltrate around vessels
- Variable hemorrhage and cutaneous necrosis

Ecthyma gangrenosum is usually a manifestation of *Pseudomonas* sepsis.

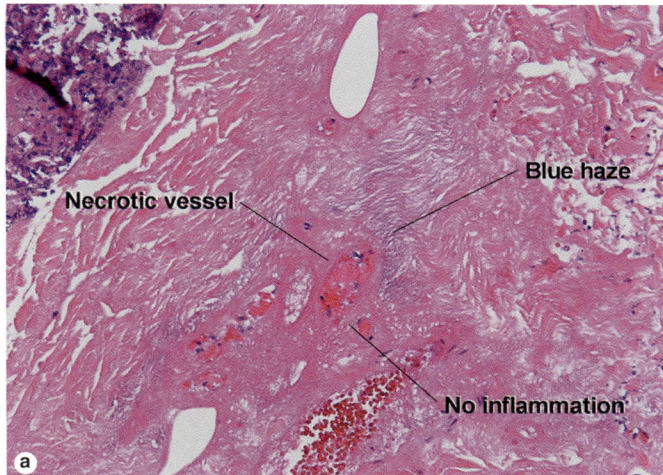

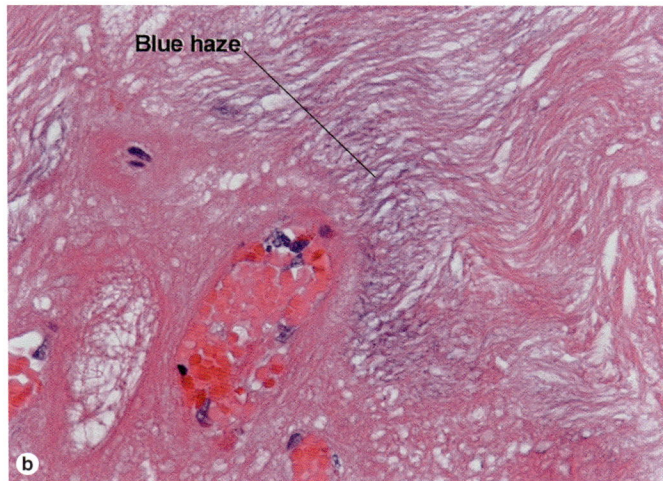

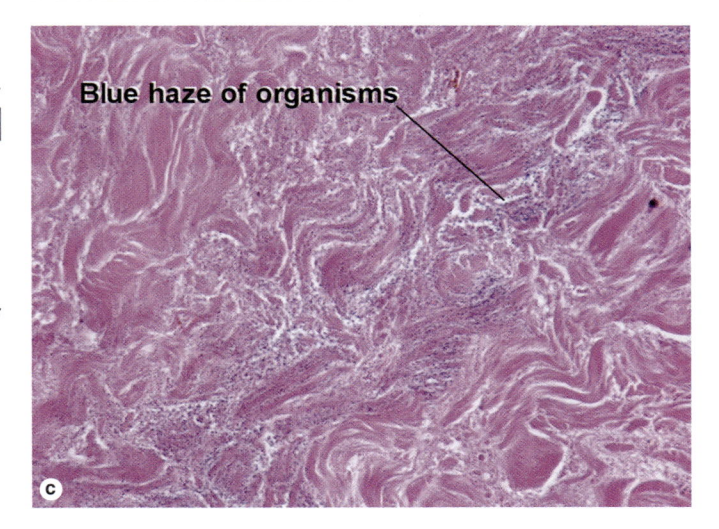

Fig 17-6 Ecthyma gangrenosum

Rhinoscleroma

Key features

- Sheets of plasma cells
- Russell bodies
- Mikulicz cells (resemble globi of leprosy)

Rhinoscleroma is caused by *Klebsiella rhinoscleromatis*. The inflammatory infiltrate is mixed, and contains many plasma cells. Russell bodies are plasma cells filled with bright pink immunoglobulin ("pregnant plasma cells"). The nucleus may no longer be visible. Mikulicz cells are histiocytes containing large round collections of bacilli.

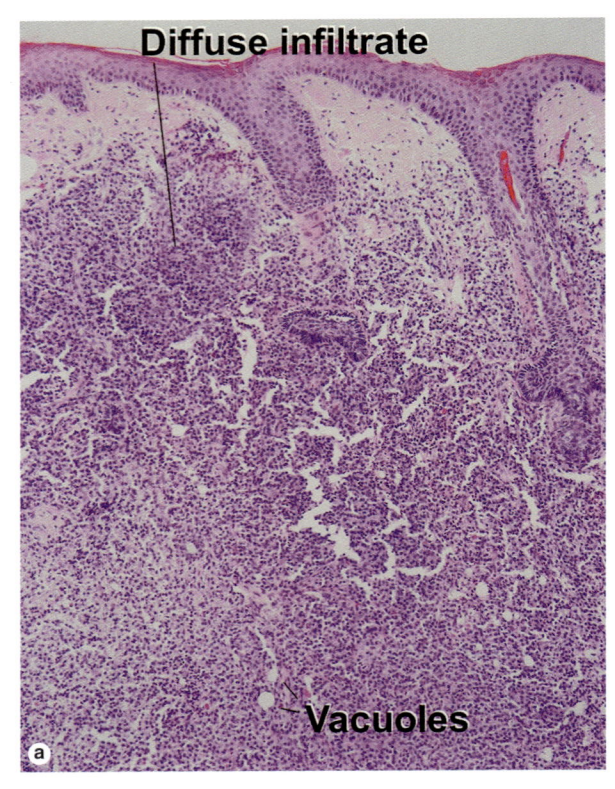

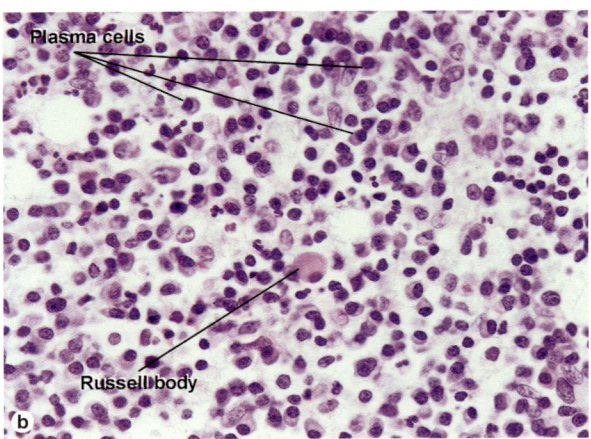

Fig 17-7 Rhinoscleroma

Chancroid

Key features

- Ulcer
- Zone of necrosis, fibrin, and neutrophils at surface
- Granulation tissue
- Many plasma cells below granulation tissue
- Gram stain and culture may demonstrate bacteria

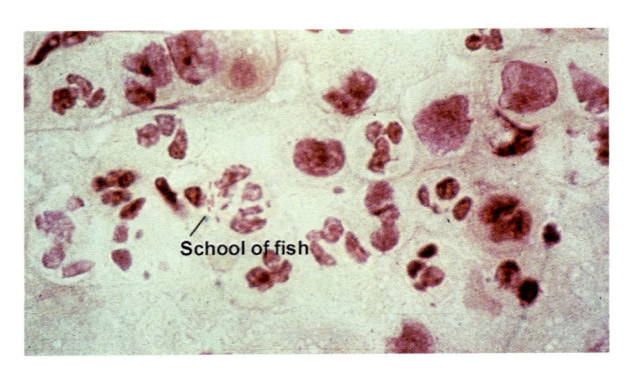

Fig 17-8 Chancroid

Granuloma inguinale

Key features

- Pseudoepitheliomatous hyperplasia with neutrophilic abscesses
- Organisms within histiocytes (Donovan bodies)

The organism may be seen best in very thin, plastic-embedded sections, processed as for electron microscopy.

Differential Diagnosis

Pseudoepitheliomatous hyperplasia with intraepidermal pustules (PEH and pus): "Here come big green leafy veggies":

- Here – **h**alogenoderma
- Come – **c**hromomycosis
- Big   – **b**lastomycosis
- Green – **g**ranuloma inguinale
- Leafy – **l**eishmaniasis
- Veggies – pemphigus **v**egetans

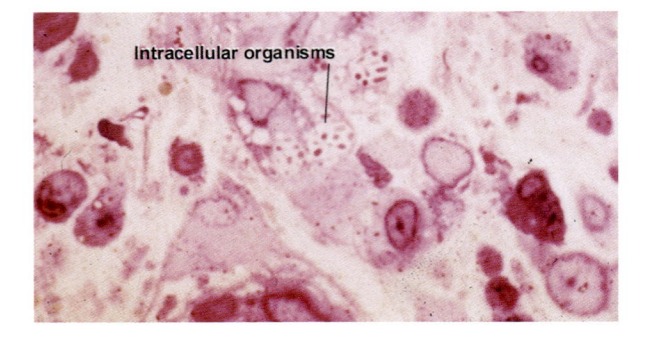

Fig 17-9 Granuloma inguinale

Leprosy

Indeterminate leprosy may only demonstrate mild inflammation and onion skin fibrosis around nerves. Borderline leprosy shows features intermediate between lepromatous and tuberculoid disease. New classification systems often divide disease into multibacillary (lepromatous end of spectrum) and paucibacillary (tuberculoid end) forms.

Lepromatous leprosy

Key features

- Perivascular lymphohistiocytic infiltrate
- Ample amphophilic cytoplasm
- May form sheets of histiocytes with grenz zone
- Globi

Globi are amphophilic collections of mycobacteria. The organisms stain strongly with a Fite stain.

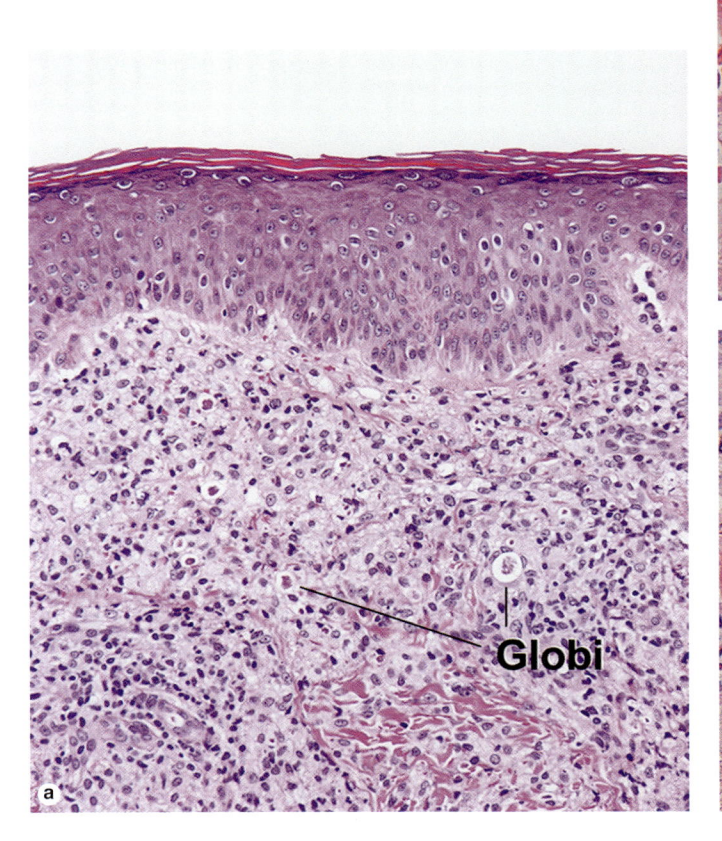

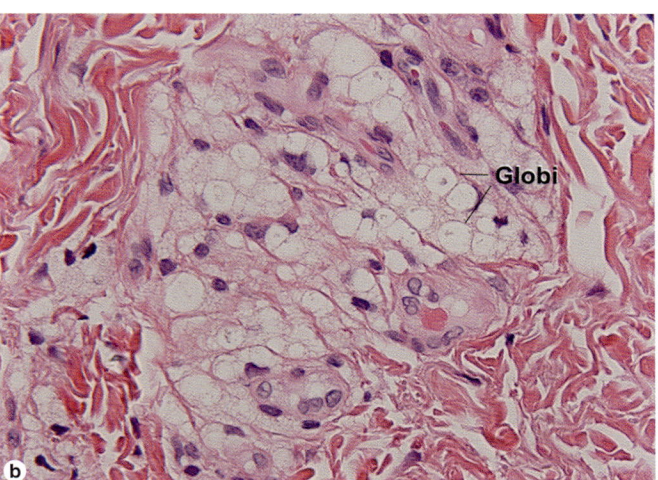

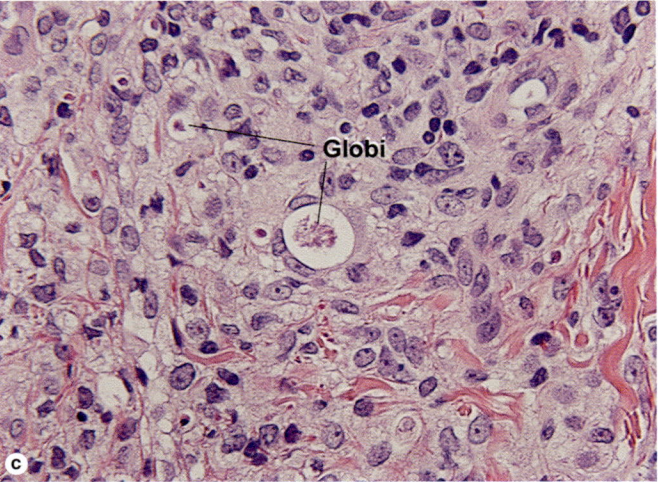

Fig 17-10 Lepromatous leprosy

Dermatopathology

Tuberculoid leprosy

> **Key features**
> - Epithelioid granulomas running east–west in the dermis ("lavender sausages")
> - Unlikely to find organisms with Fite stain

Tuberculoid leprosy is characterized by a high degree of cell-mediated immunity. Organisms are rare. The granulomatous infiltrate follows deep neurovascular bundles. Lesions are commonly anesthetic.

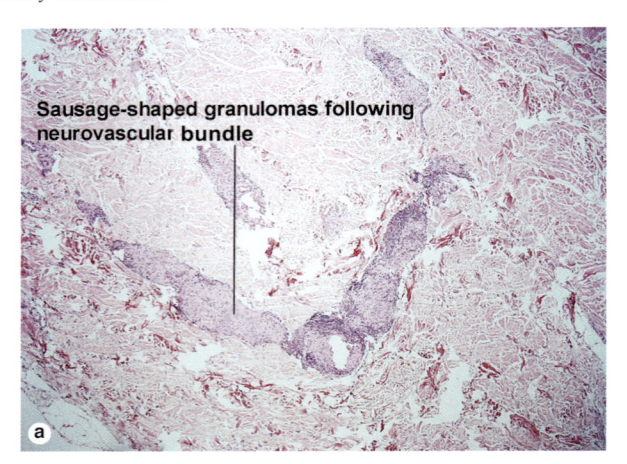

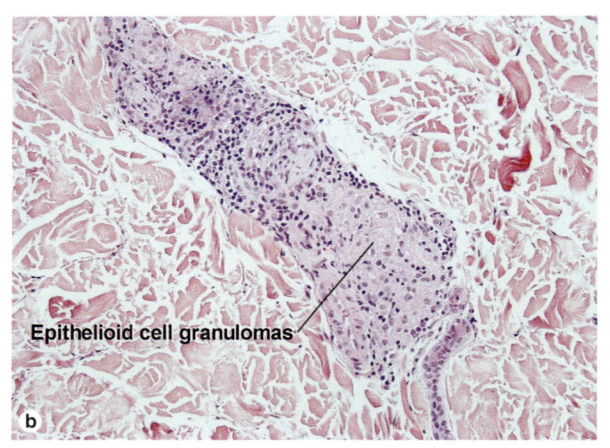

Fig 17-11 Tuberculoid leprosy

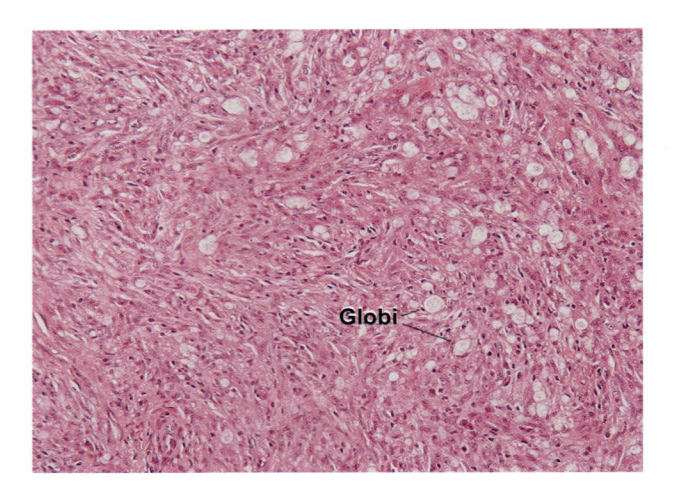

Fig 17-12 Histoid leprosy

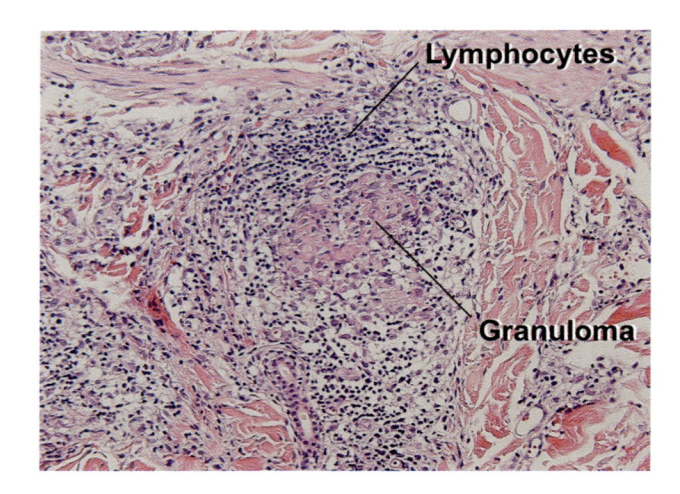

Fig 17-13 Reversal reaction

Histoid leprosy

> **Key features**
> - Usually the result of long-acting dapsone
> - Fibrous nodules
> - Globi present

Leprosy reactions

Type 1: reversal or downgrading reaction

> **Key features**
> - Lymphoid and granulomatous inflammation
> - Centered about neurovascular bundle

Reversal reactions commonly occur after antibiotic therapy is initiated. In response to antibiotic treatment, the patient regains a greater degree of cellular immunity. The increased type IV immune response inflicts damage on the neurovascular bundle.

Type 2: erythema nodosum leprosum

> **Key features**
> - Leukocytoclastic vasculitis superimposed upon pre-existing lesions of leprosy
> - Onion skin fibrosis around nerves
> - Globi

Erythema nodosum leprosum represents a type III immune response. There are no circulating immune complexes. Instead, the antigen–antibody complexes form locally within lesions.

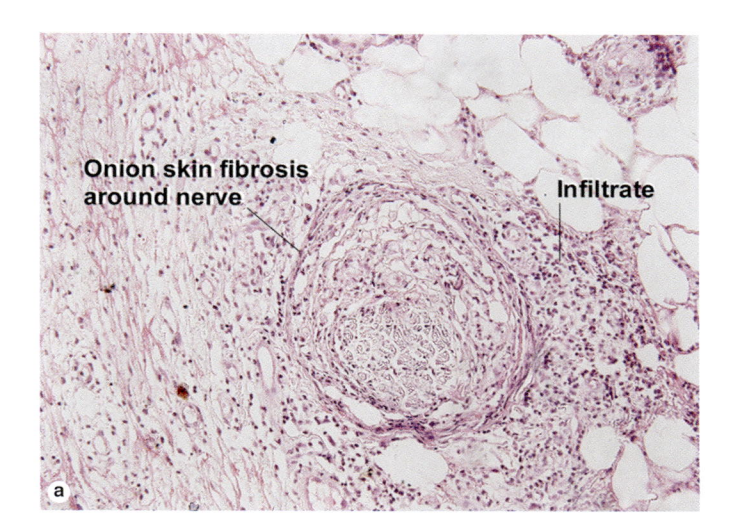

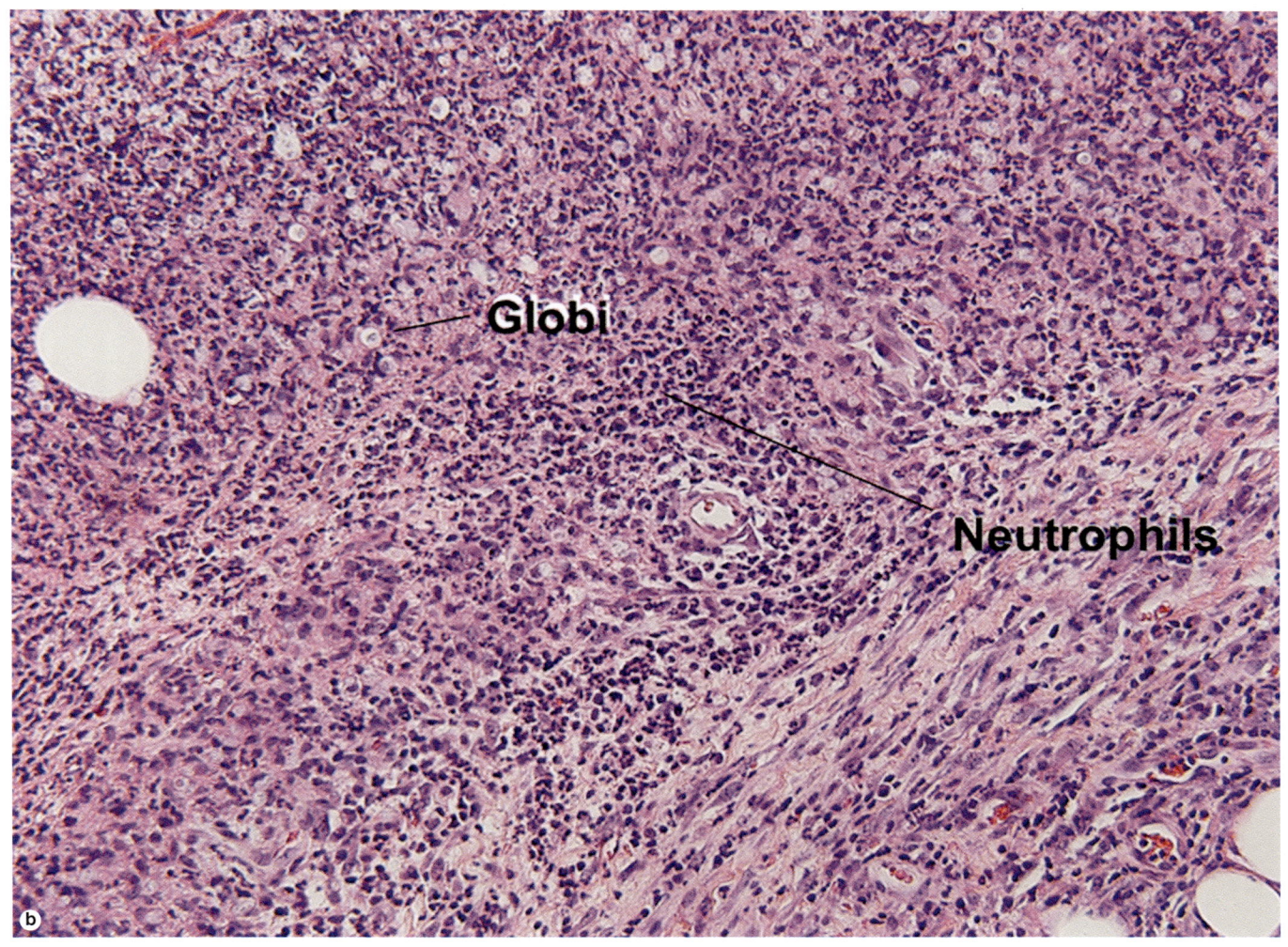

Bacterial, spirochete, and protozoan infections

Fig 17-14 Erythema nodosum leprosum

Dermatopathology

Type 3: Lucio's phenomenon

Key features

- Usual setting is diffuse lepromatous leprosy (lepra bonita) where the skin is tau without wrinkles, but nodules are absent
- Massive load of organisms, inflammation, thrombosis in arterioles
- Stellate infarcts

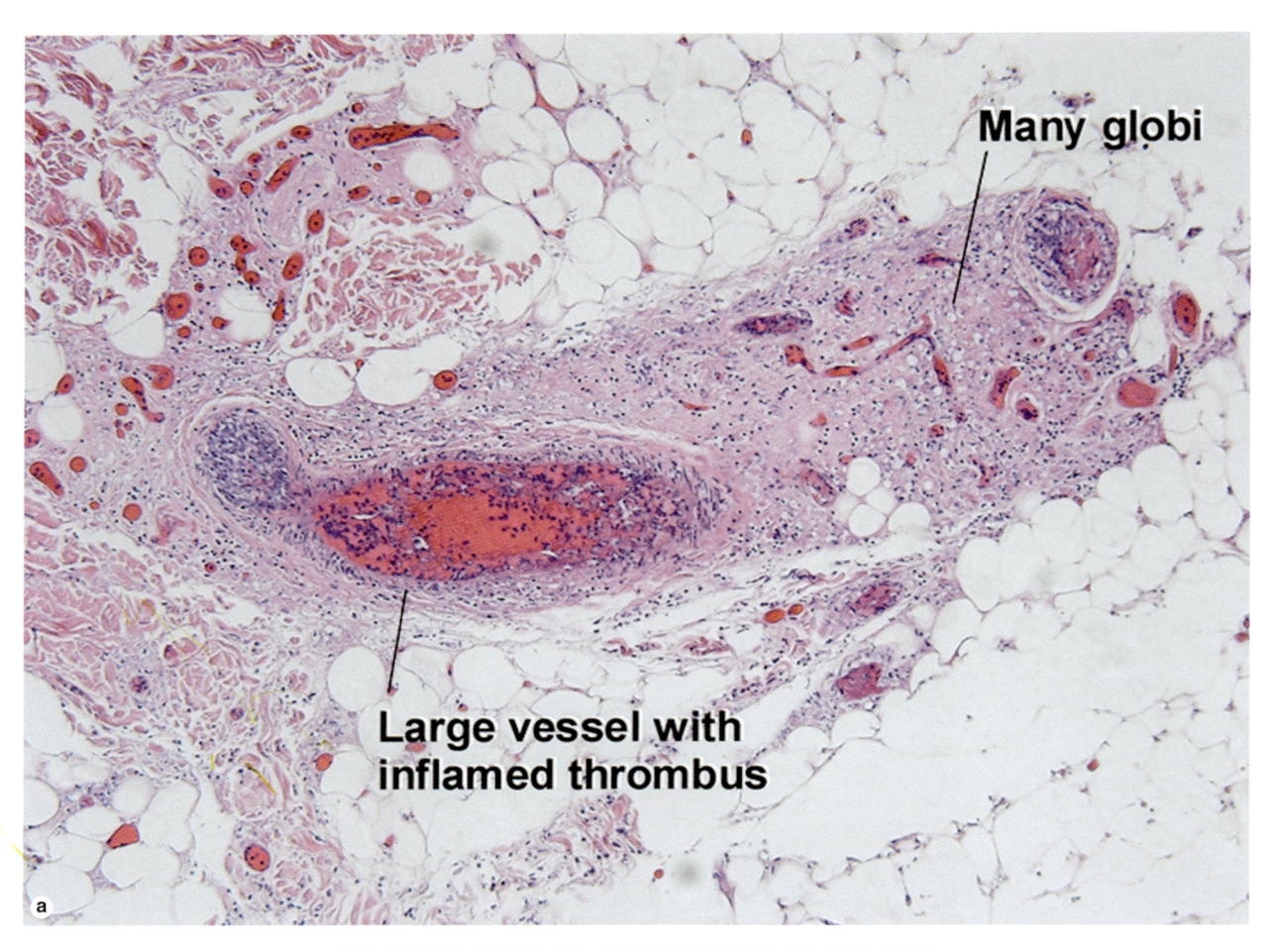

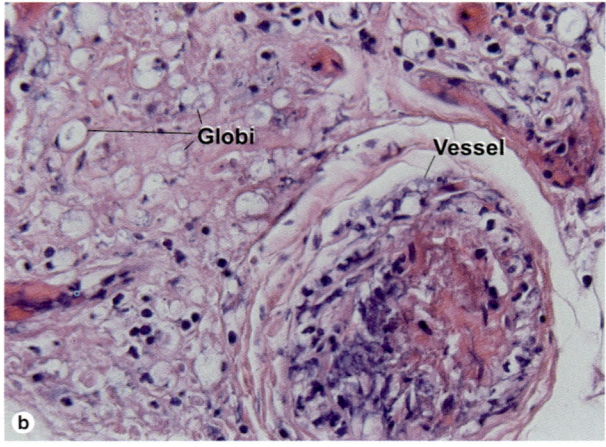

Fig 17-15 Lucio's phenomenon (courtesy of David M. Scollard, MD, PhD)

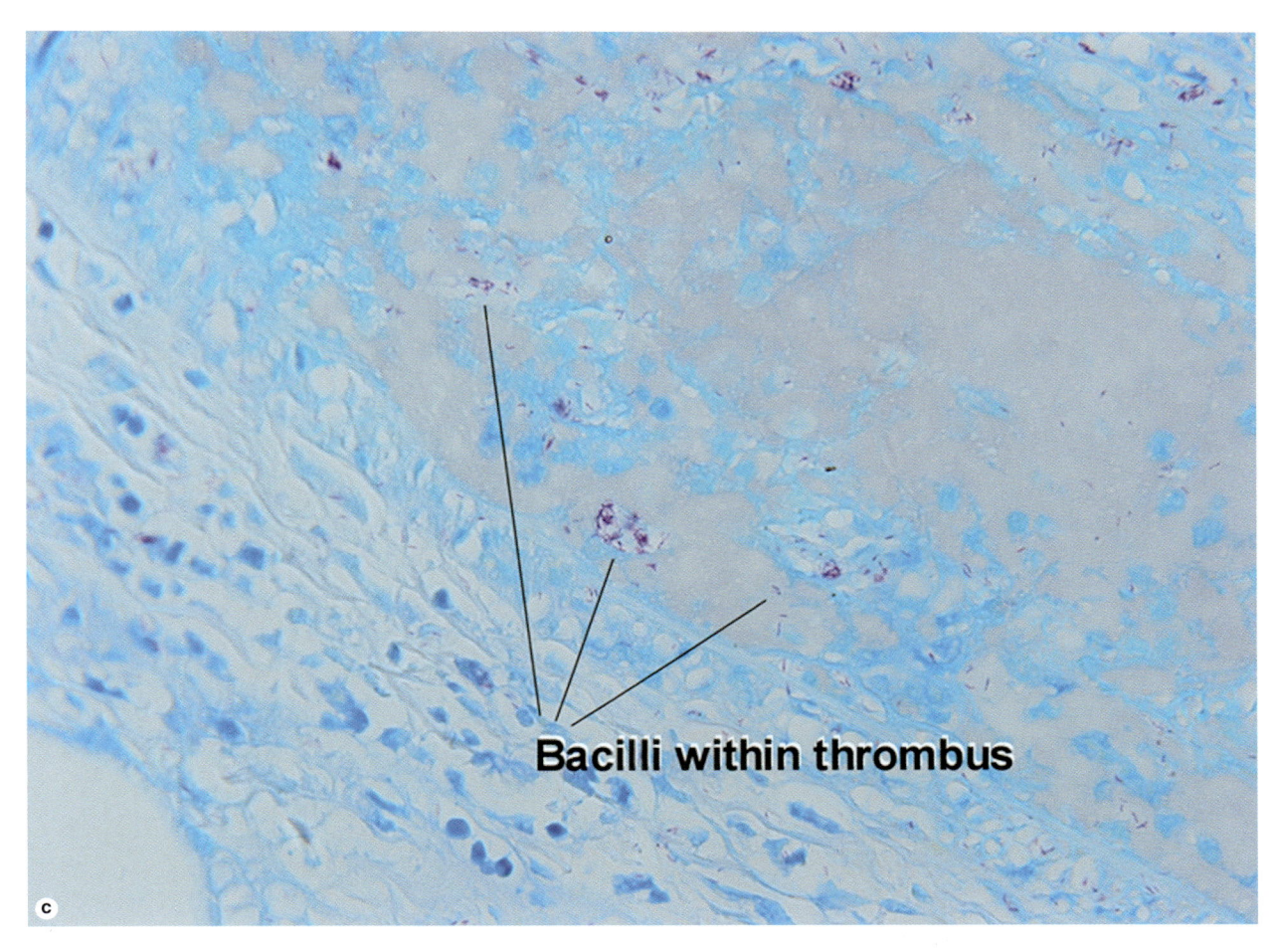

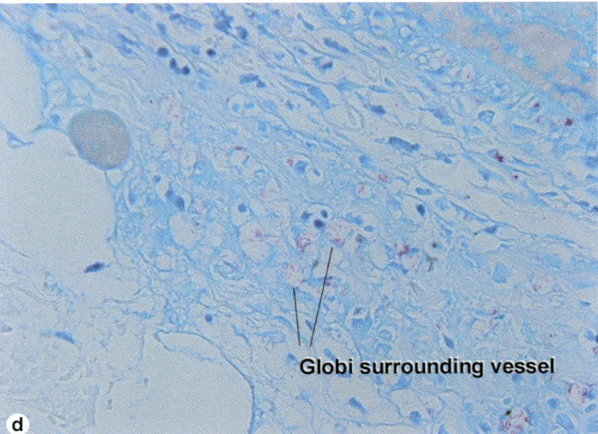

Bacterial, spirochete, and protozoan infections

Bacilli within thrombus

Globi surrounding vessel

Fig 17-15, cont'd

Tuberculosis

Key features

- Early reactions suppurative
- Become granulomatous with central caseous necrosis

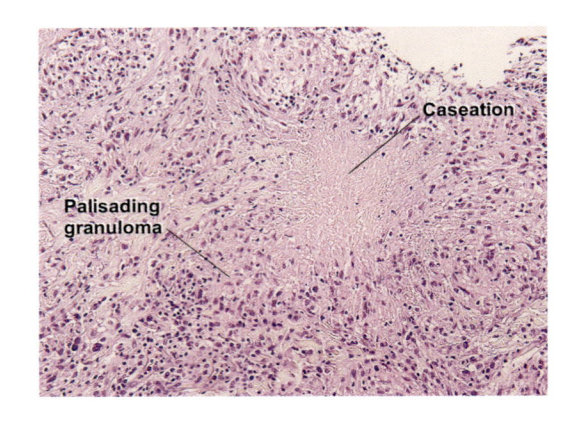

Fig 17-16 Primary inoculation tuberculosis

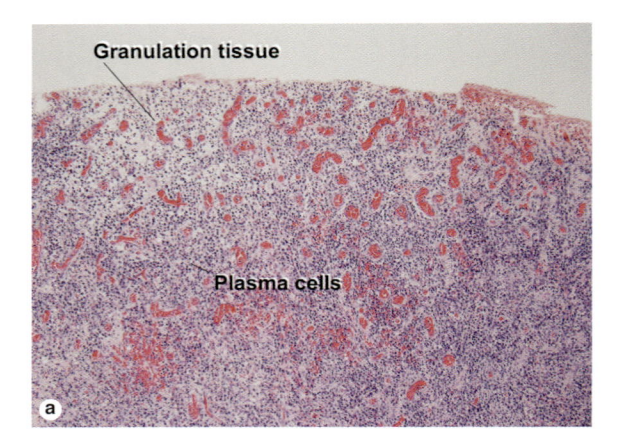

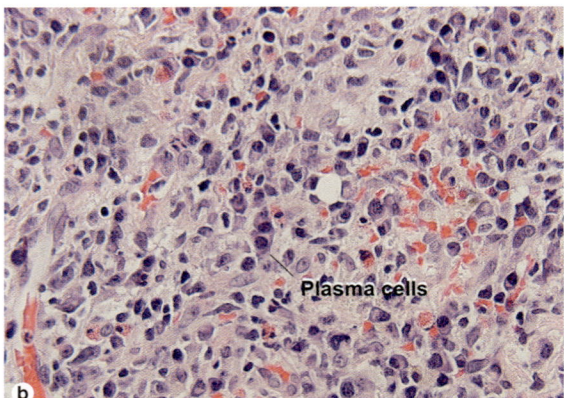

Fig 17-17 (a,b) Chancre H&E stain.

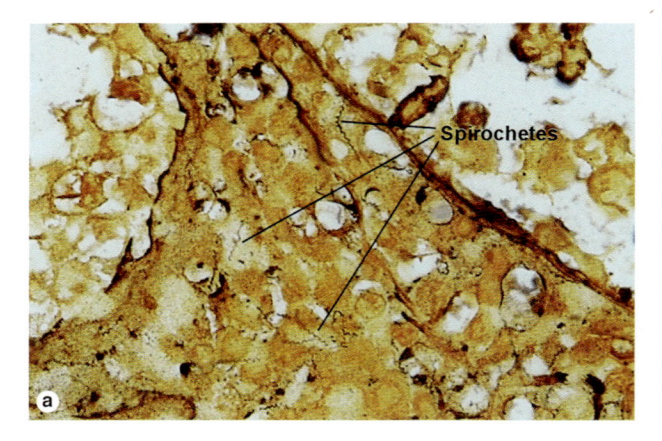

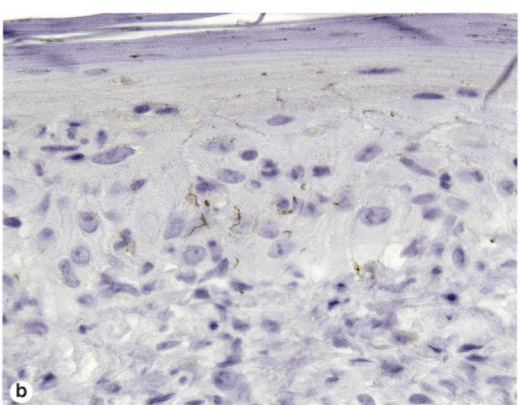

Fig 17-18 *Treponema pallidum.* (a) Steiner stain. (b) Immunostain.

Spirochete-mediated diseases

Syphilitic chancre

Key features

- Ulcer
- Zone of necrosis, fibrin, and neutrophils at surface
- Granulation tissue
- Many plasma cells below granulation tissue
- Immunostain or silver stains may demonstrate spirochetes

Syphilitic chancres and chancroid have a similar histology. Chancroid typically produces a deeper, softer, more painful ulcer, as well as suppurative lymphadenitis. Stains, culture, and serology are typically required.

Secondary syphilis

Key features

- Vacuolar interface dermatitis together with slender psoriasiform acanthosis
- Neutrophils in the stratum corneum
- Plasma cells present in about two-thirds of cases
- Endothelial swelling obliterates the lumen of small vessels
- Perivascular lymphocytes and histiocytes with visible cytoplasm

Secondary syphilis is highly variable in its clinical presentation, and almost as variable in its histologic appearance. Any suspicious feature should prompt an immunostain or silver stain, clinical evaluation, and serologic studies. False-negative prozone reactions are the result of massive antibody excess. Antigen–antibody complexes form most efficiently with mild antigen excess and can be inhibited by massive antibody excess. The serum may need to be diluted many-fold in order to test positive.

A biopsy frequently suggests the diagnosis. While most other forms of vacuolar interface dermatitis are associated with effacement of the rete, secondary syphilis characteristically demonstrates a combination of vacuolar interface dermatitis and acanthosis with long slender rete. This pattern has been referred to as an "icicle" or "icepick" pattern of acanthosis. Some students have found it helpful to remember that syphilis (a sexually transmitted disease) produces long, slender, "sexy" rete ridges with associated vacuolar interface dermatitis. Neutrophils are commonly present in the stratum corneum. Plasma cells are present in about two-thirds of cases. Small dermal blood vessels appear to have no lumen because of endothelial swelling. Another helpful feature is the presence of perivascular lymphocytes and histiocytes with visible cytoplasm. It may be difficult to decide at scanning power whether the infiltrate is granulomatous or lymphoid. A subtle interstitial infiltrate is often present as well.

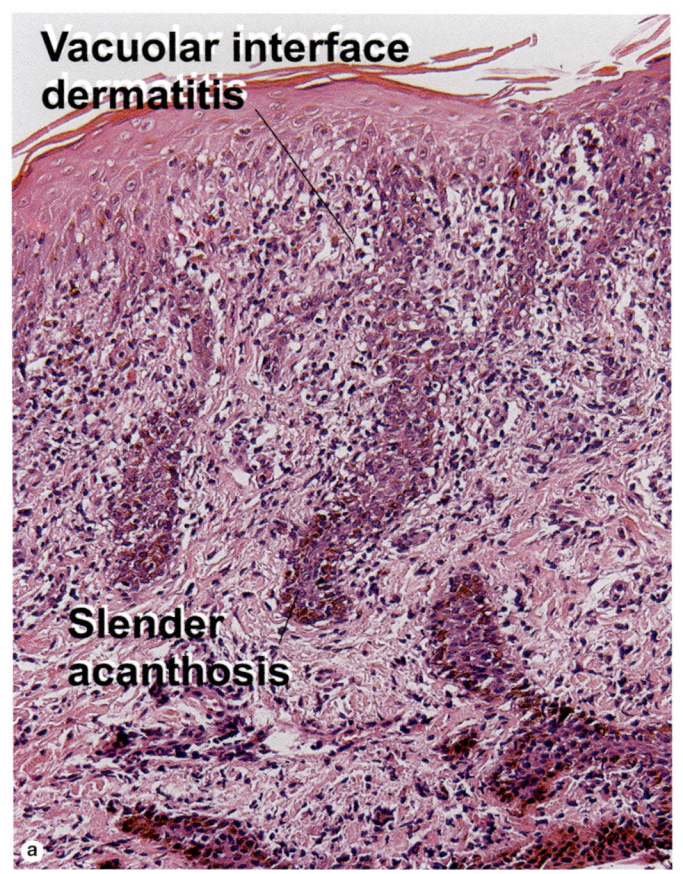

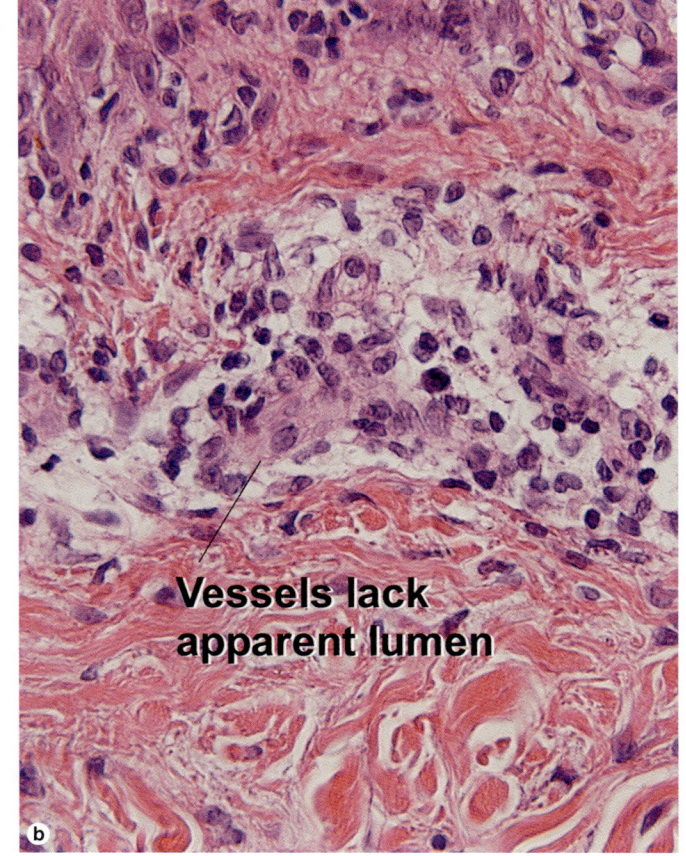

Fig 17-19 Secondary syphilis

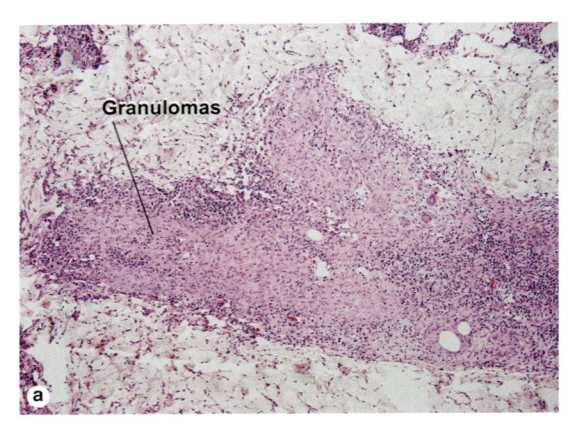

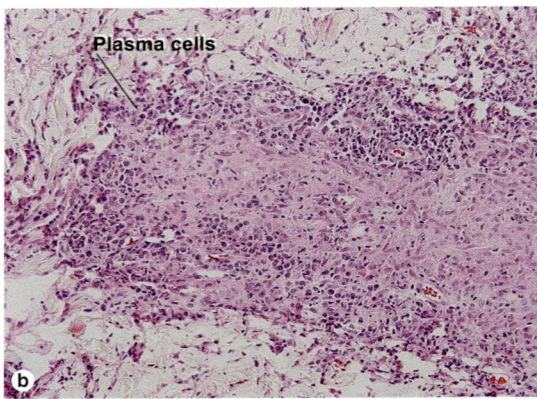

Fig 17-20 Tertiary syphilis

Tertiary syphilis

Key features

- Granulomatous
- Organisms not generally visible

Lyme disease

Erythema migrans

Key features

- Highly variable perivascular infiltrate (often superficial and deep lymphoid, but many variations occur)
- May contain plasma cells
- May contain eosinophils
- Spirochetes may be present around superficial dermal vessels in silver-stained sections

The histologic features are non-specific. The diagnosis is usually made clinically or by culture.

Acrodermatitis chronica atrophicans

Key features

- Dermal atrophy with thin attenuated collagen bundles
- Fat and large subcutaneous vessels appear close to surface
- Sparse lymphohistiocytic band throughout the dermis

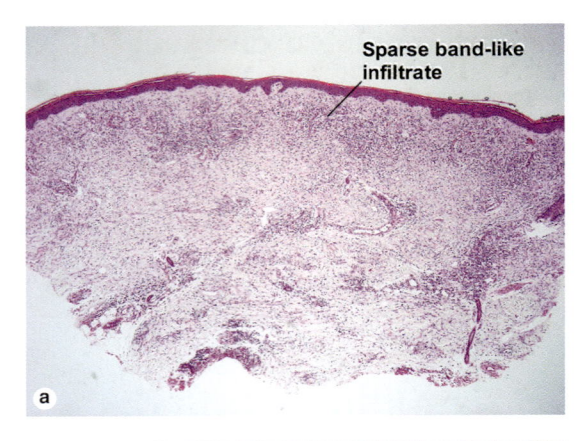

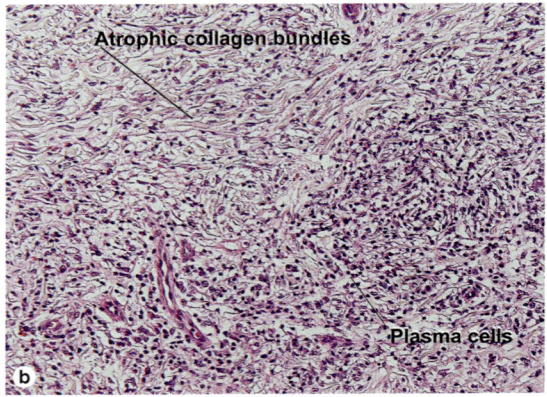

Fig 17-21 Acrodermatitis chronica atrophicans

In the evolving stage, lesions with a morphea-like appearance may show an interstitial granulomatous infiltrate, resembling granuloma annulare.

Protozoan diseases

Leishmaniasis

Key features

- Granulomatous dermatitis
- Plasma cells common
- Intracellular organisms
- Organisms often line up at periphery of vacuole

The organisms are similar in size and shape to histoplasmosis. A kinetoplast is present, but may be difficult to see. The distribution of the organisms within the histiocyte is helpful. *Histoplasma* organisms are evenly spaced and surrounded by a pseudocapsule. In contrast, *Leishmania* organisms lack a pseudocapsule. They may be randomly spaced, or lined up at the periphery of a vacuole, like light bulbs on a make-up mirror or movie marquee. Culture, polymerase chain reaction, and quantitative nucleic acid sequence-based amplification are sensitive techniques used to detect, type, and quantify *Leishmania* in tissue.

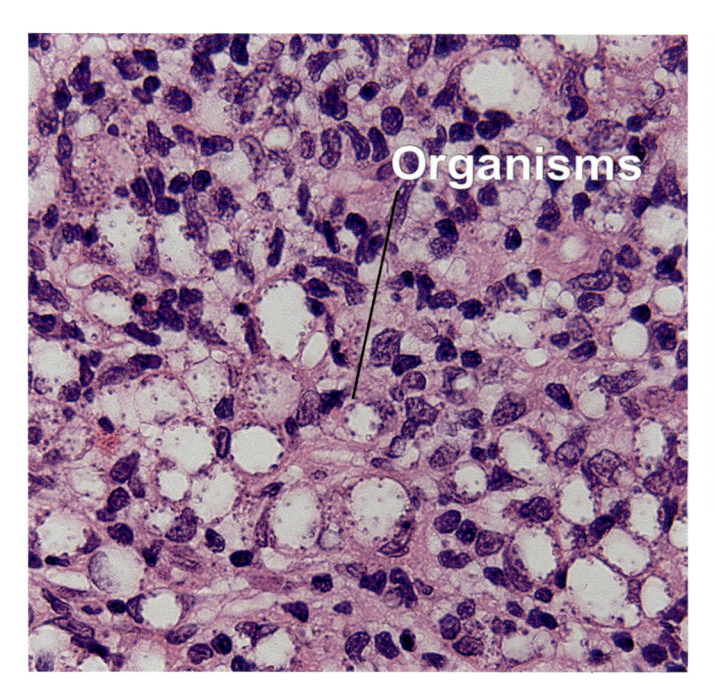

Fig 17-22 Leishmaniasis

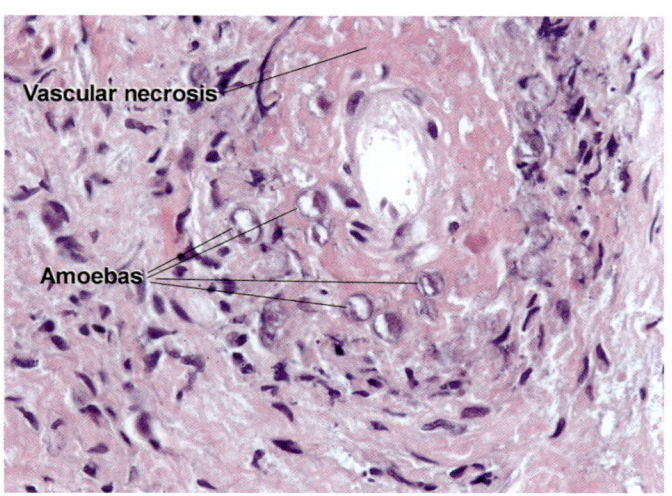

Fig 17-23 *Acanthamoeba* infection

Acanthamoeba

Key features

- Necrosis of deep vessels
- Organisms in vessel wall

At first glance, amoeba trophozoites may look like large histiocytes with somewhat refractile nuclei. Glance again. They have a characteristic appearance, as noted in Figure 17.23. Vascular invasion and necrosis are typical. Lobular fat necrosis has been reported. Disseminated disease is frequently associated with human immunodeficiency virus (HIV) infection or immunosuppressive drugs. Cultures on an agar plate seeded with a lawn of *Escherichia coli* will demonstrate characteristic tracks.

Further reading

Baughn RE, Musher DM. Secondary syphilitic lesions. Clin Microbiol Rev 2005;18(1):205–216.

Blonski KM, Blödorn-Schlicht N, Falk TM, et al. Increased detection of cutaneous leishmaniasis in Norway by use of polymerase chain reaction. APMIS 2012;120(7):591–596.

de Almeida HL Jr, de Castro LA, Rocha NE, et al. Ultrastructure of pitted keratolysis. Int J Dermatol 2000;39(9):698–701.

Engelkens HJ, ten Kate FJ, Vuzevski VD, et al. Primary and secondary syphilis: a histopathological study. Int J STD AIDS 1991;2(4):280–284.

Kaur C, Thami GP, Mohan H. Lucio phenomenon and Lucio leprosy. Clin Exp Dermatol 2005;30(5):525–527.

Lockwood DN, Nicholls P, Smith WC, et al. Comparing the clinical and histological diagnosis of leprosy and leprosy reactions in the INFIR cohort of Indian patients with multibacillary leprosy. PLoS Negl Trop Dis 2012;6(6):e1702.

Mathur MC, Ghimire RB, Shrestha P, et al. Clinicohistopathological correlation in leprosy. Kathmandu Univ Med J (KUMJ) 2011;9(36):248–251.

McBroom RL, Styles AR, Chiu MJ, et al. Secondary syphilis in persons infected with and not infected with HIV-1: a comparative immunohistologic study. Am J Dermatopathol 1999;21(5):432–441.

Moreno C, Kutzner H, Palmedo G, et al. Interstitial granulomatous dermatitis with histiocytic pseudorosettes: a new histopathologic pattern in cutaneous borreliosis. Detection of Borrelia burgdorferi DNA sequences by a highly sensitive PCR-ELISA. J Am Acad Dermatol 2003;48(3):376–384.

Pandhi RK, Singh N, Ramam M. Secondary syphilis: a clinicopathologic study. Int J Dermatol 1995;34(4):240–243.

Raval RC. Various faces of Hansen's disease. Indian J Lepr 2012;84(2):155–160.

Vargas-Ocampo F. Analysis of 6000 skin biopsies of the national leprosy control program in Mexico. Int J Lepr Other Mycobact Dis 2004;72(4):427–436.

Wilson TC, Legler A, Madison KC, et al. Erythema migrans: a spectrum of histopathologic changes. Am J Dermatopathol 2012;34(8):834–837.

Wohlrab J, Rohrbach D, Marsch WC. Keratolysis sulcata (pitted keratolysis): clinical symptoms with different histological correlates. Br J Dermatol 2000;143(6):1348–1349.

Chapter 18

Fungal infections

Dirk M. Elston

Tinea

Key feature

- Non-pigmented hyphae in stratum corneum

The stratum corneum may be basket-weave or compact and eosinophilic. It may contain parakeratosis or clusters of neutrophils.

PEARL

The stratum corneum in tinea is commonly basket-weave, but a narrow zone of compact eosinophilic stratum corneum is present just above the granular layer. Round hyphae cut on end are often visible in this compact layer.

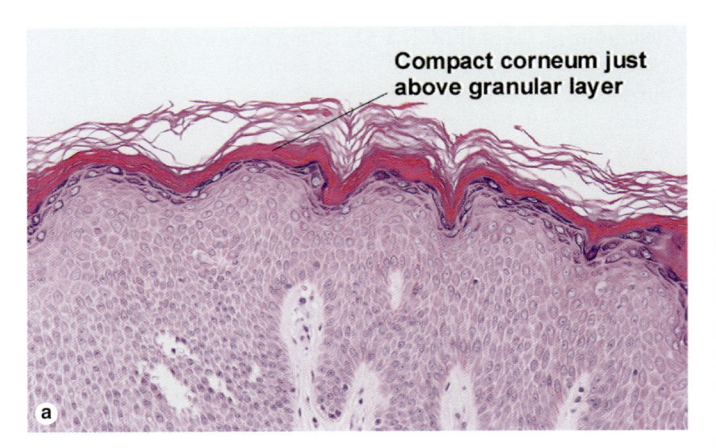

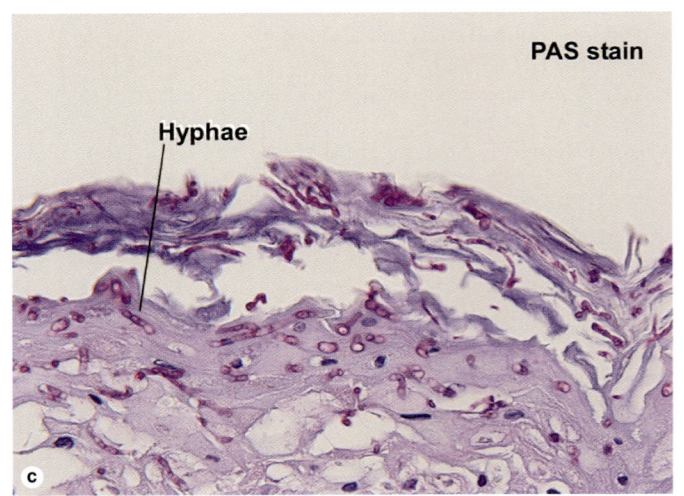

PEARL

If it scales, scrape it. If it scales and you don't know what it is, PAS it.

Differential Diagnosis

Collections of neutrophils within the stratum corneum: psoriasis, tinea, impetigo, *Candida*, seborrheic dermatitis, syphilis (PTICSS).

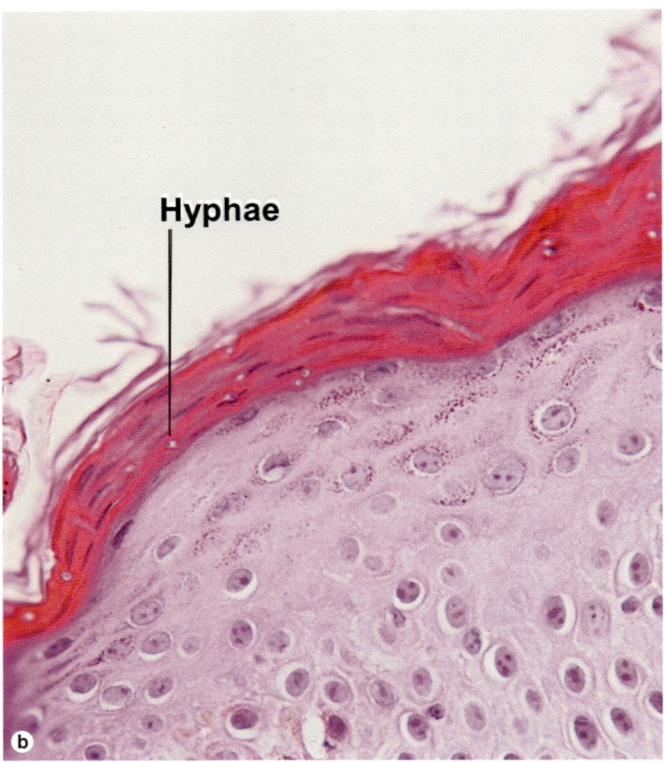

Fig 18-1 Tinea

Bullous tinea

Key features

- Massive papillary dermal edema
- Nonpigmented hyphae in stratum corneum

Reticular (net-like) degeneration of the epidermis is typically present. The infiltrate is typically polymorphous (predominantly lymphoid, with some neutrophils and eosinophils).

Differential Diagnosis

The massive papillary dermal edema resembles that of polymorphous light eruption, perniosis or Sweet's syndrome. Bullous tinea lacks the nodular and diffuse neutrophilic infiltrate and karyorrhexis of Sweet's syndrome.
Polymorphous light eruption and perniosis typically have a purely lymphoid infiltrate and perniosis demonstrates edema surrounding lymphocytes in vessels.

Onychomycosis

Key features

- Periodic acid-Schiff (PAS)-positive hyphae in subungual debris

Tinea versicolor

Key features

- Loose lamellar or basket-weave hyperkeratosis
- Groups of round spores and short curved hyphae in the stratum corneum ("ziti and meatballs")

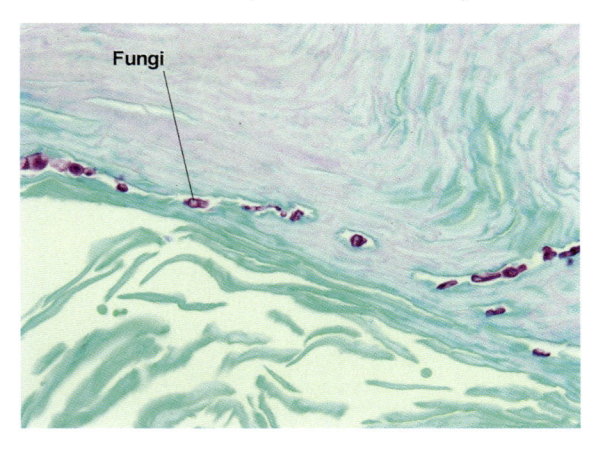

Fig 18-3 Onychomycosis (periodic acid-Schiff)

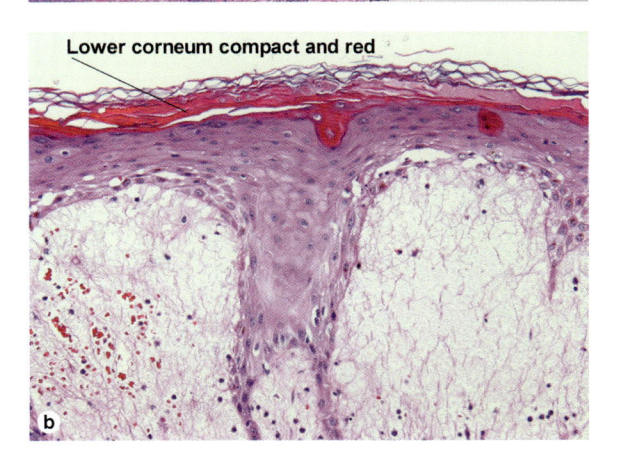

Fig 18-2 Bullous tinea

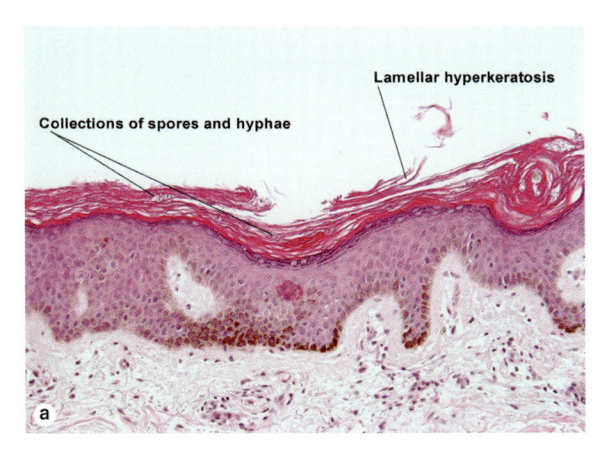

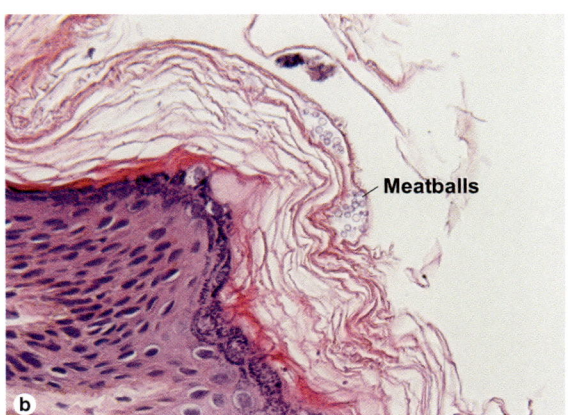

Fig 18-4 Tinea versicolor

Candidiasis

Key features
- Pseudohyphae in stratum corneum
- Often vertically oriented
- Neutrophils common in stratum corneum
- Hyperkeratosis and crusting common

Differential Diagnosis
Collections of neutrophils within the stratum corneum: PTICSS (see above)

Budding yeast may sometimes be seen, or the pseudohyphae may resemble dermatophyte hyphae. Dermatophyte hyphae tend to be oriented east–west within the stratum corneum, whereas *Candida* pseudohyphae are often oriented north–south.

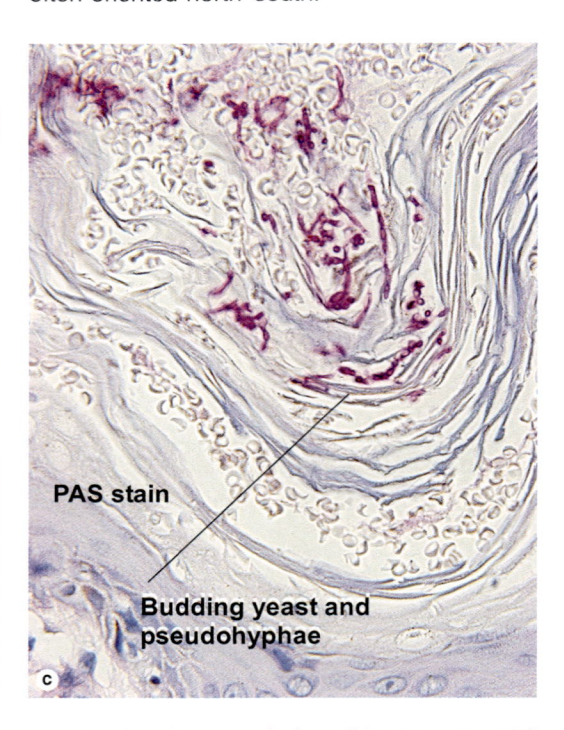

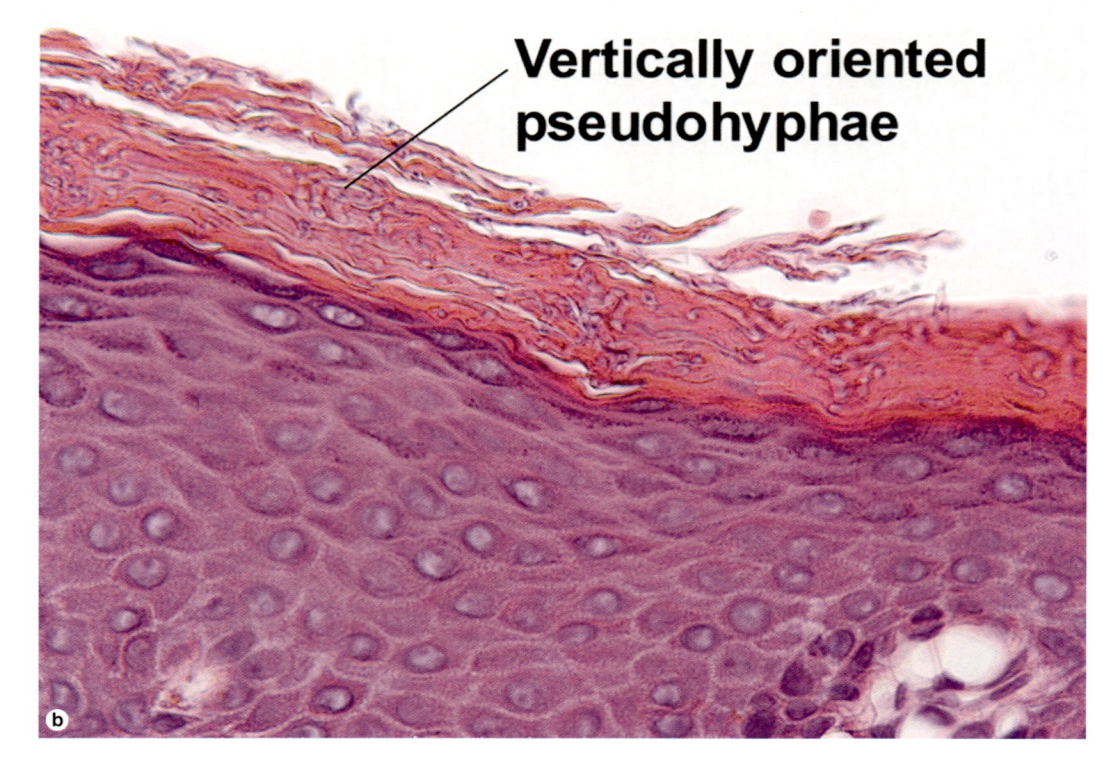

Fig 18-5 Candidiasis

Fungal infections Chapter 18 273

Coccidioidomycosis

Key features

- Large spherules with gray lacy and granular cytoplasm
- Uniform in size and shape
- Refractile wall
- Endospores sometimes present

Coccidioidomycosis is endemic to southwestern USA and California. The organism grows easily on agar at room temperature. As such cultures are highly infectious; deep fungal infections should never be cultured in the office setting.

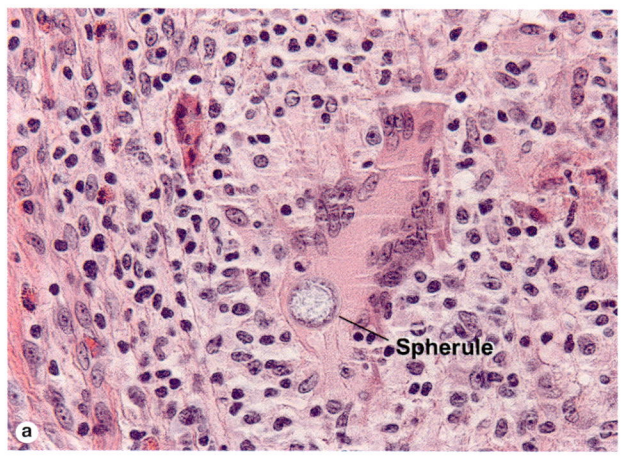

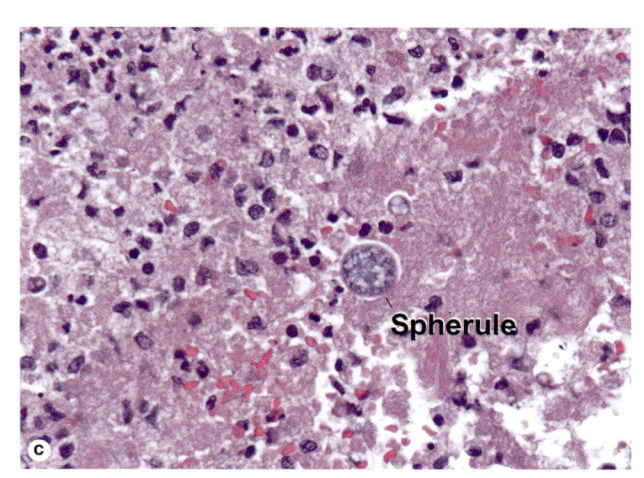

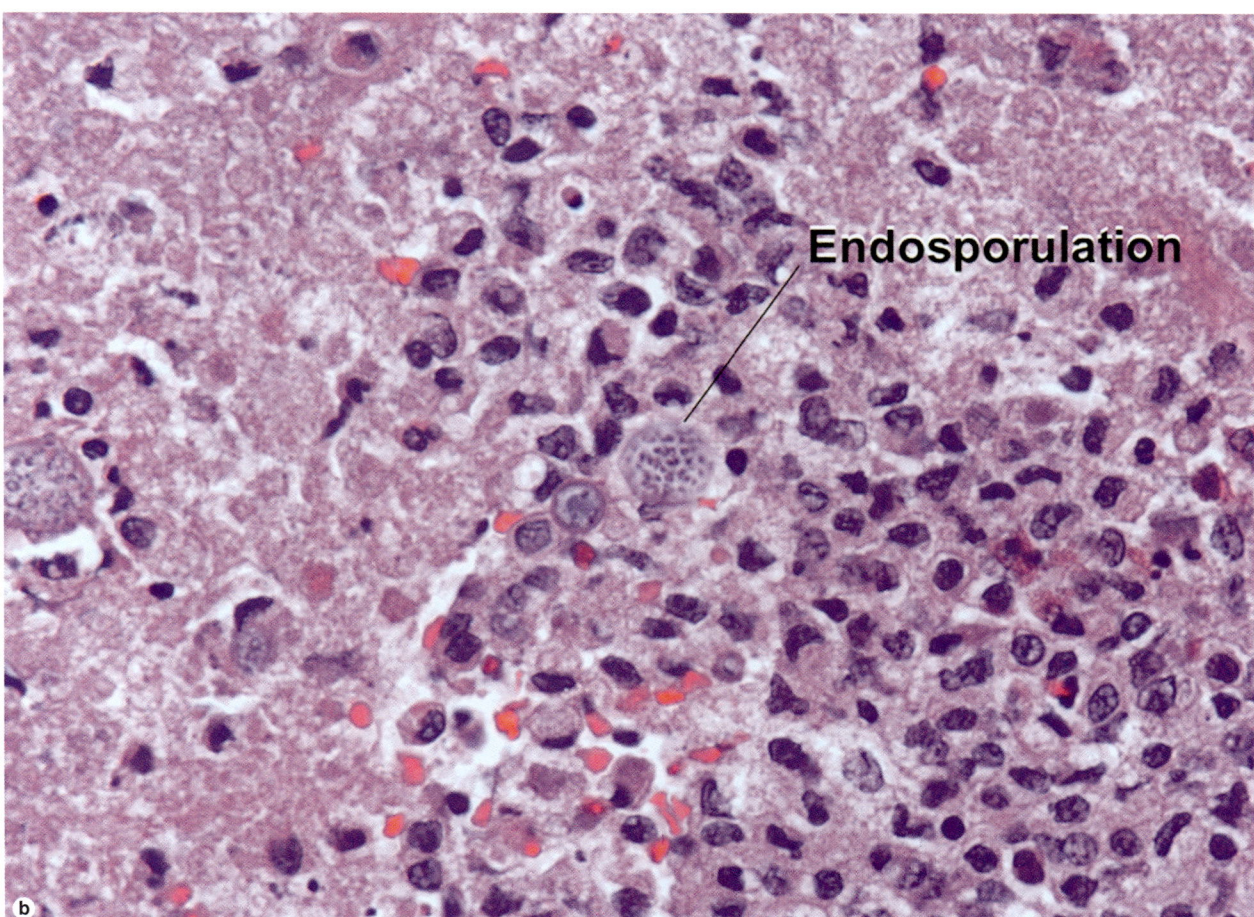

Fig 18-6 Coccidioidomycosis

Dermatopathology

Cryptococcosis

Key features

- Pleomorphic yeast, varies markedly in size and shape
- Clear gelatinous capsules containing small groups of organisms ("gelatinous condominiums")
- Amount of capsular material is inversely proportional to granulomatous infiltrate

While most other deep fungal organisms have a characteristic size and shape, *Cryptococcus* varies markedly in size and shape. The organisms are "gregarious" and cluster within clear spaces that correspond to the mucinous capsule. The capsule stains red with mucicarmine. Although they never appear brown in tissue, the organisms stain with a Fontana–Masson melanin stain. Umbilicated, molluscum-like lesions are often associated with human immunodeficiency virus (HIV).

Blastomycosis

Key features

- Pseudoepitheliomatous hyperplasia with intraepidermal pustules
- Organisms are few in number, usually within giant cells, uniform in size and shape
- Thick refractile, asymmetrical wall
- Dark nucleus
- If budding is seen, it is broad-based

Blastomycosis is caused by *Blastomyces dermatitidis*. Skin lesions are typically slowly advancing verrucous plaques, with central scarring and a heaped edge.

Differential Diagnosis

Pseudoepitheliomatous hyperplasia with intraepidermal pustules (PEH and pus): "Here come big green leafy veggies":

- Here   – *h*alogenoderma
- Come   – *c*hromomycosis
- Big   – *b*lastomycosis
- Green   – *g*ranuloma inguinale
- Leafy   – *l*eishmaniasis
- Veggies – pemphigus *v*egetans

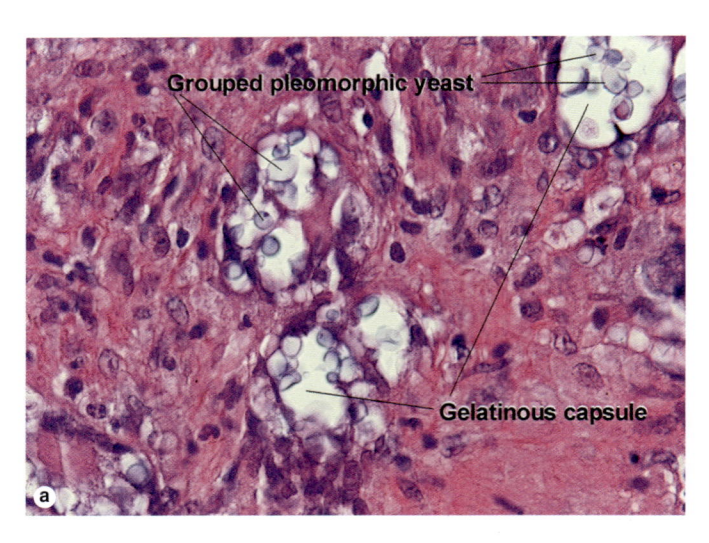

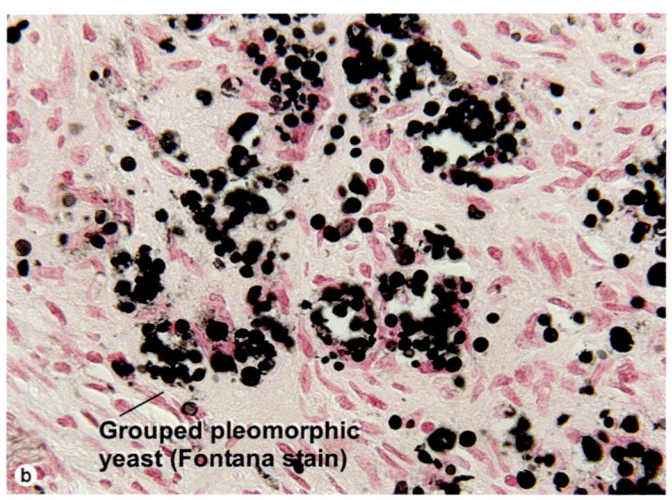

Fig 18-7 Cryptococcosis

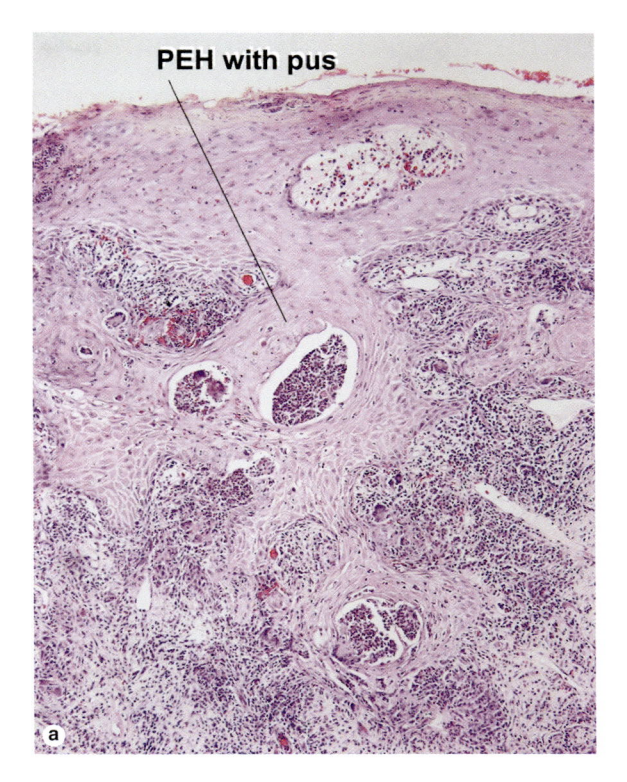

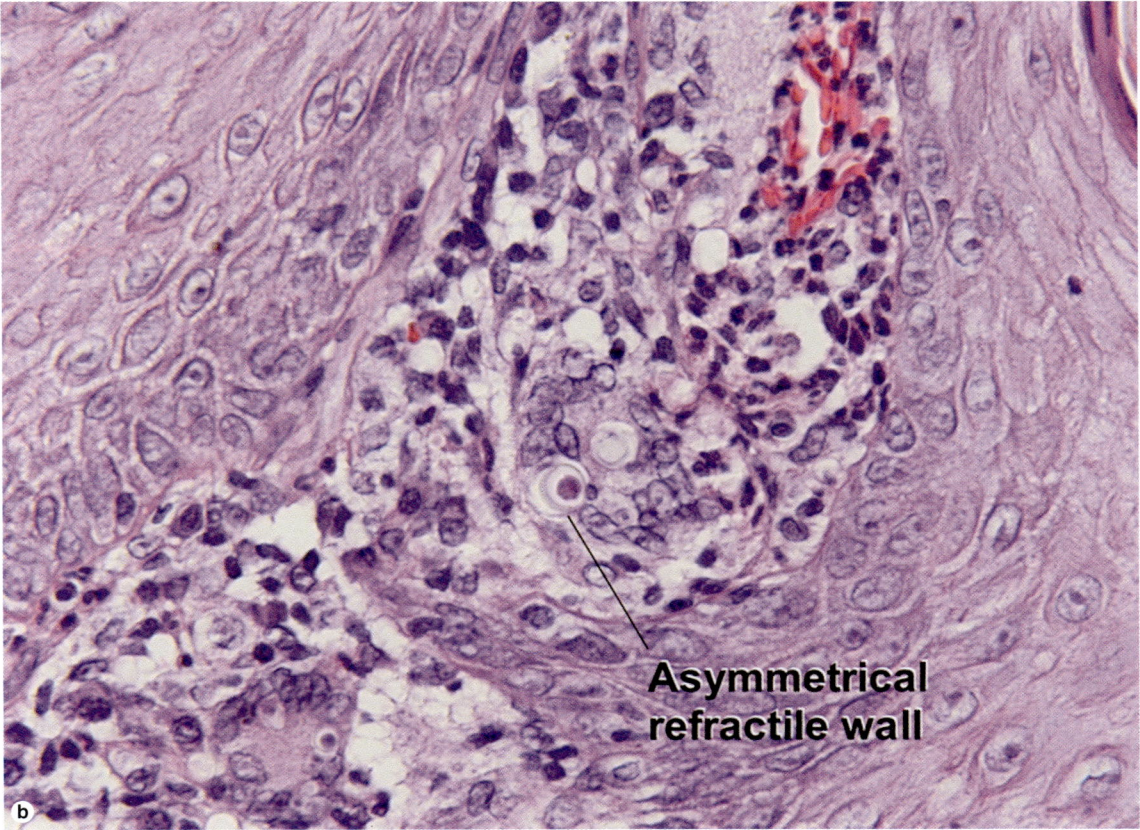

Fig 18-8 Blastomycosis pseudoepitheliomatous hyperplasia (PEH)

Paracoccidioides infection (South American "blastomycosis")

Key features

- Small yeast (*Paracoccidioides braziliensis*)
- Lacks the thick refractile wall and eccentric nucleus of *Blastomyces dermatitidis*
- Narrow-based budding
- Mariner's wheel pattern of budding occasionally

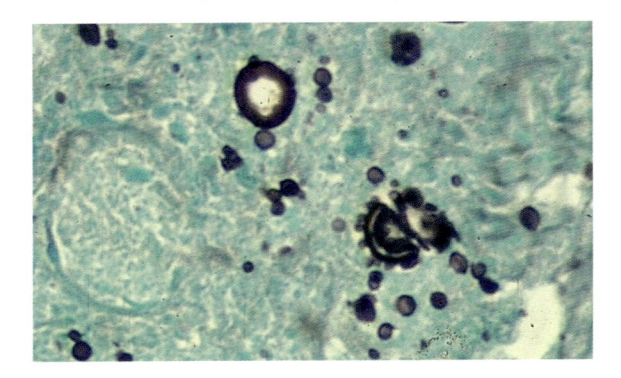

Fig 18-9 *Paracoccidioides* infection (Grocott's methenamine silver)

Histoplasmosis

Key features

- Small uniform dots within histiocytes
- Each surrounded by a pseudocapsule
- Evenly spaced within histiocyte

Despite the name, *Histoplasma capsulatum* lacks a true capsule. The organisms are similar in size and shape to *Leishmania*, but lack a kinetoplast. The distribution of the organisms within the histiocyte is helpful. *Histoplasma* organisms are evenly spaced and surrounded by a pseudocapsule. In contrast, *Leishmania* organisms lack a pseudocapsule. They may be randomly spaced, or lined up at the periphery of a vacuole like light bulbs on a make-up mirror or movie marquee. In cavitary lesions or within vascular spaces, histoplasmosis may grow in a mycelial (hyphal) phase.

Differential Diagnosis

"pH girl"

Differential of parasitized histiocytes

- *Penicillium marneffei* (looks strikingly similar to histoplasmosis)
- *H*istoplasmosis
- *G*ranuloma inguinale
- *R*hinoscleroma
- *L*eishmaniasis

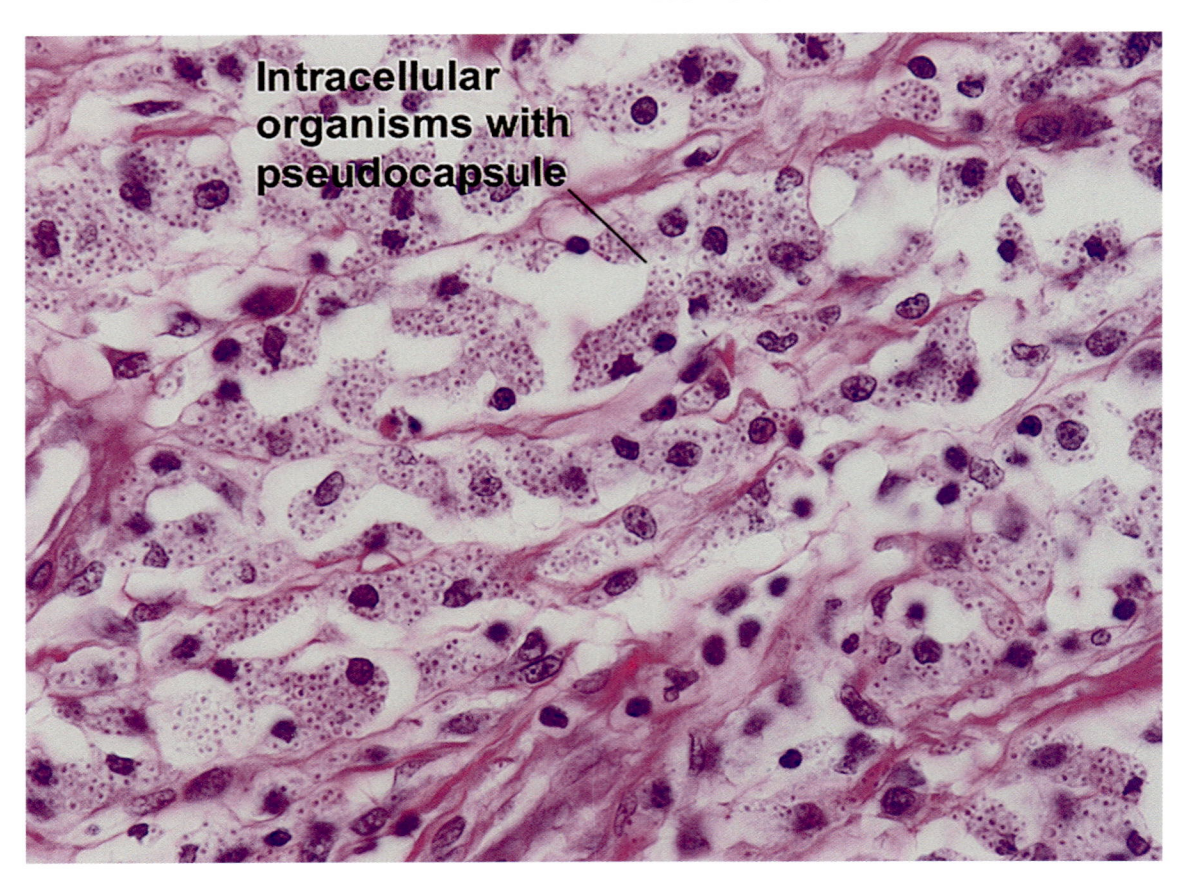

Fig 18-10 Histoplasmosis

African histoplasmosis

Key features

- Numerous large intracellular organisms in histiocytes and multinucleated giant cells
- Evenly spaced distribution of organisms in giant cells

Histoplasma duboisii infection differs from the usual *H. capsulatum* infection by the size of the organism, and the presence of multinucleated giant cells. The organism is similar in size and shape to the lobomycosis organism, but lacks the characteristic "pop-bead" chains of lobomycosis.

Lobomycosis (keloidal blastomycosis)

Key features

- Large organisms (similar in size to African histoplasmosis)
- Often within histiocytes and multinucleated giant cells
- Characteristic pop-bead chains

Lobomycosis is caused by *Lacazia loboi*. The organism is similar in size and shape to African histoplasmosis, but chains are present, resembling a child's pop-beads. In biopsies from dolphins, the organism is significantly smaller than in human tissue.

Sporotrichosis

Key features

- Stellate abscess, surrounded by granuloma
- Rare cigar-shaped yeasts

Sporotrichosis forms characteristic stellate abscesses. Pseudoepitheliomatous hyperplasia is sometimes present. Some cases from Japan have numerous organisms, but generally, the organisms are few in number and culture is more sensitive than special stains. Among the organisms that form stellate abscesses, some demonstrate lymphangitic spread (nodules along lymph vessels), whereas others demonstrate ulceroglandular spread (ulcer with suppurative lymph node). Clinicopathologic correlation can narrow the differential diagnosis.

Differential Diagnosis

Stellate abscesses in skin: "CLATS"

- *C*at scratch
- *L*ymphogranuloma venereum
- *A*typical mycobacteria (usually *Mycobacterium marinum*)
- *T*ularemia
- *S*porotrichosis

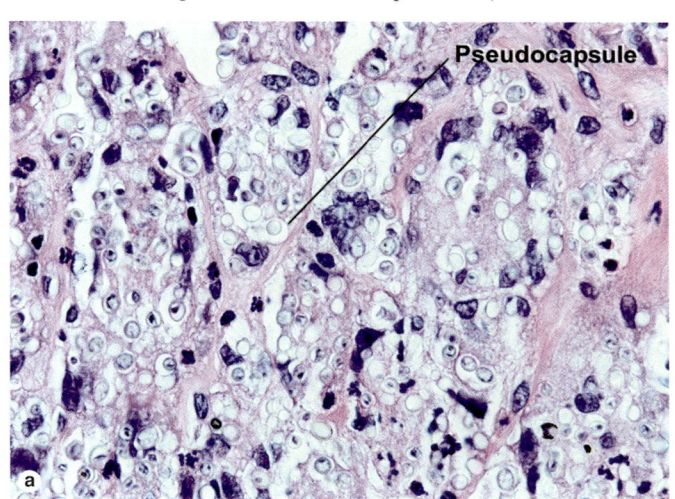

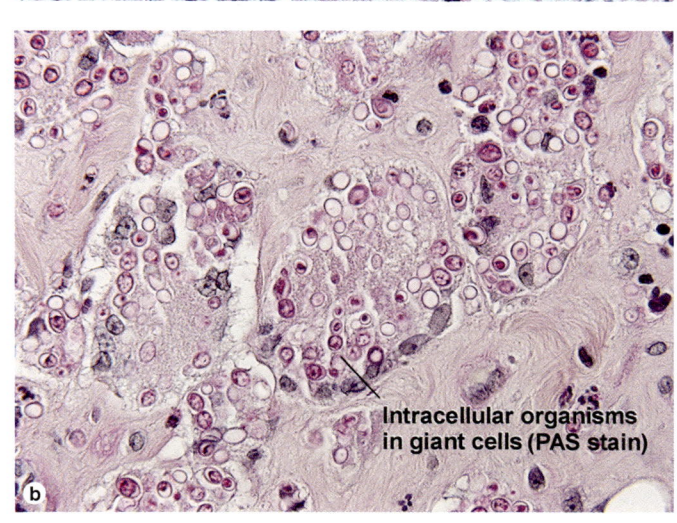

Fig 18-11 African histoplasmosis

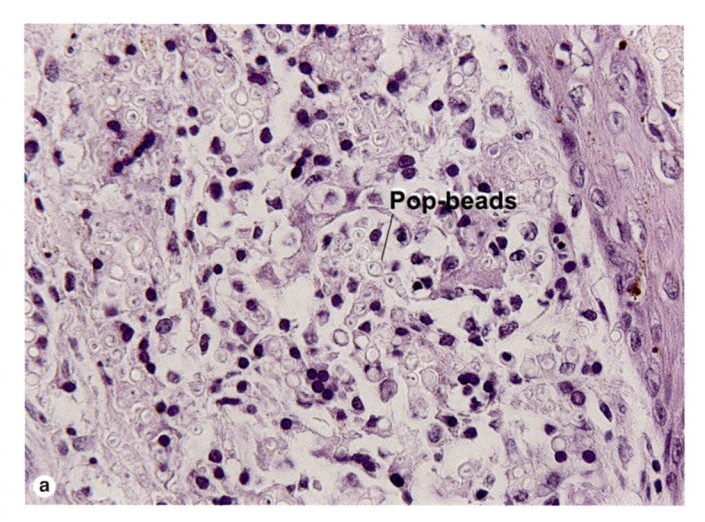

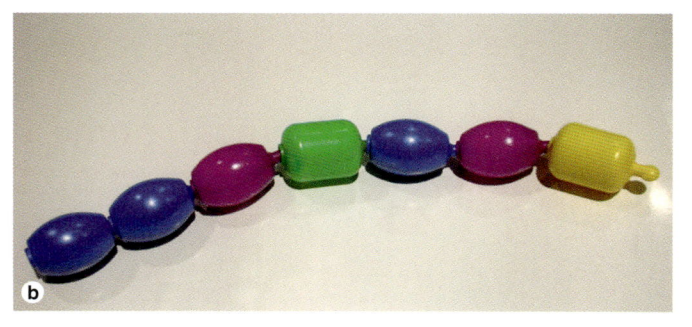

Fig 18-12 (a) Lobomycosis. (b) Pop-beads for comparison

Dermatopathology

PEARL

Lymphangitic syndromes	Ulceroglandular syndromes
Sporotrichosis	Tularemia
Leishmaniasis	Lymphogranuloma venereum
Atypical mycobacteria	Cat scratch
Nocardia	Glanders
Blastomyces	Melioidosis
	Chancroid
	Plague
	Tuberculosis

Mycetomas

Eumycetoma

Key features

- Sinus tracts filled with neutrophils (resemble stellate abscesses)
- Grains within suppurative foci
- Grains made up of fungal hyphae
- Club-shaped Splendore–Hoeppli phenomenon at periphery of grain

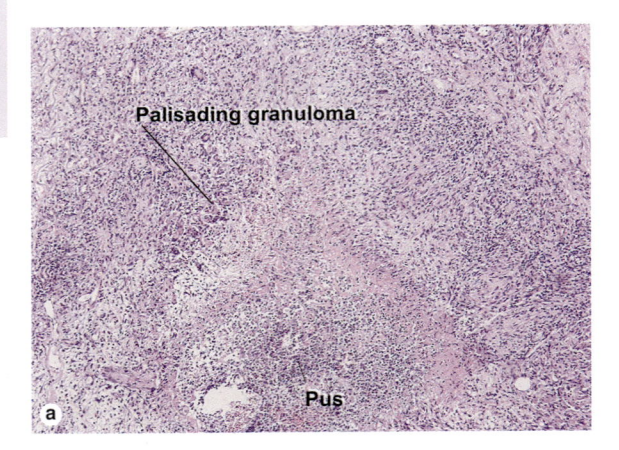

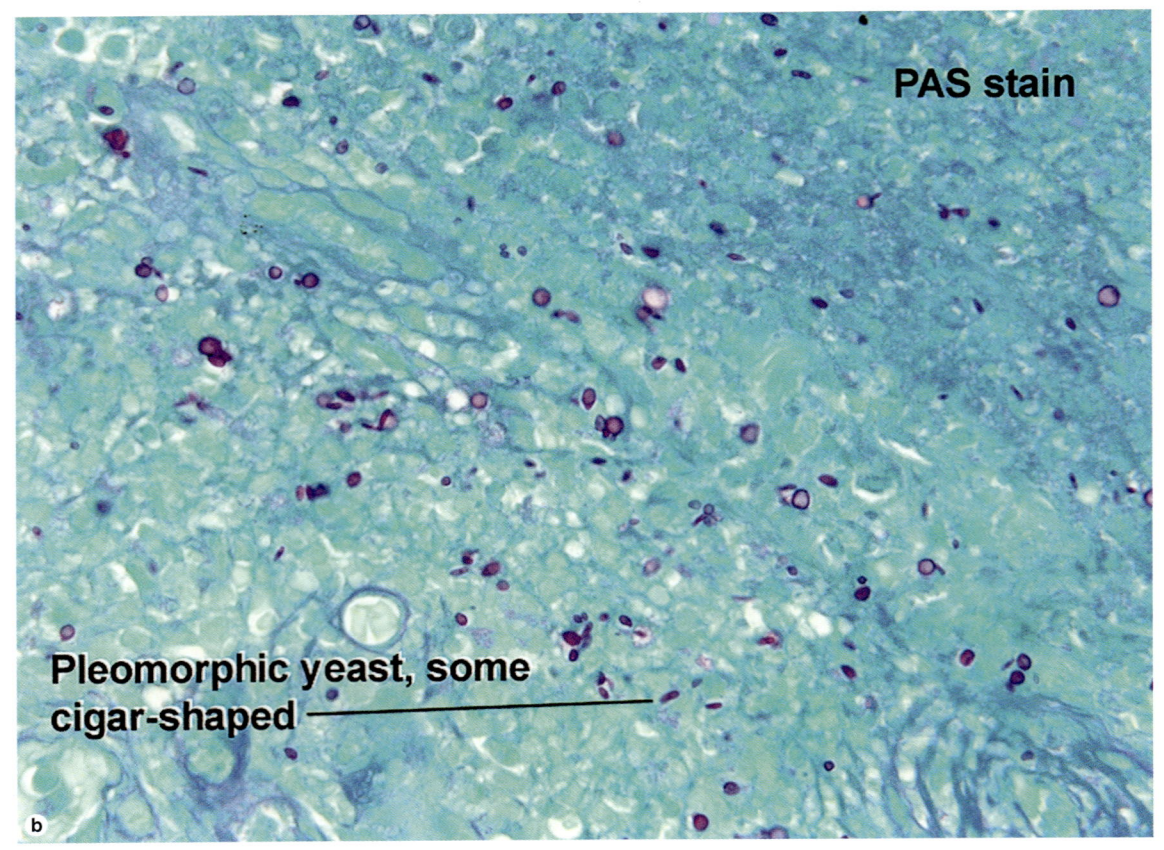

Fig 18-13 Sporotrichosis

Eumycetomas are true fungal mycetomas. The grains are composed of fungal hyphae, which may be pigmented. At the periphery of the grain, red club-shaped accumulations of immunoglobulin appear as the Splendore–Hoeppli phenomenon.

PEARL

Dark grain eumycetoma organisms are sometimes remembered by the mnemonic: "My lousy greasy jeans are black":
- My — Madurella mycetomatis
- Lousy — Leptosphaeria spp.
- Greasy — M. grisea
- Jeans — Exophiala jeanselmei
- are black — pigmented

Actinomycetomas

Key features

- Sinus tracts filled with neutrophils (resemble stellate abscesses)
- Grains within suppurative foci
- Grains made up of filamentous bacteria
- Smooth Splendore–Hoeppli phenomenon at periphery of grain

Actinomycetomas are caused by filamentous bacteria but are discussed in this chapter because of their resemblance to fungal mycetomas. The grains are typically light in color. *Actinomadura* species commonly cause pink to red grain mycetomas, although some *A. madurae* grains are white or yellow.

Dark grain eumycetoma	Non-pigmented eumycetoma	Actinomycetoma
Madurella mycetomatis	Pseudoallescheria boydii	Nocardia brasiliensis
Leptosphaeria sp–.	Acremonium sp–.	N. asteroides
M. grisea	Fusarium sp–.	N. transvalensis
Exophiala jeanselmei	Cylindrocarpon destructans	Actinomyces israelii
	Neotestudina sp–.	Streptomyces somaliensis
	Dermatophytes	Actinomadura pelletieri
		A. madurae

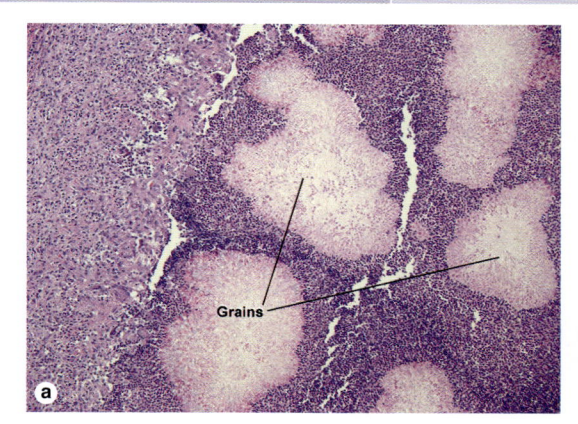

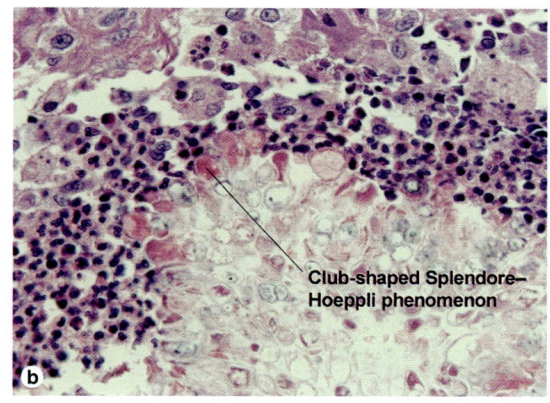

Fig 18-14 Eumycetoma

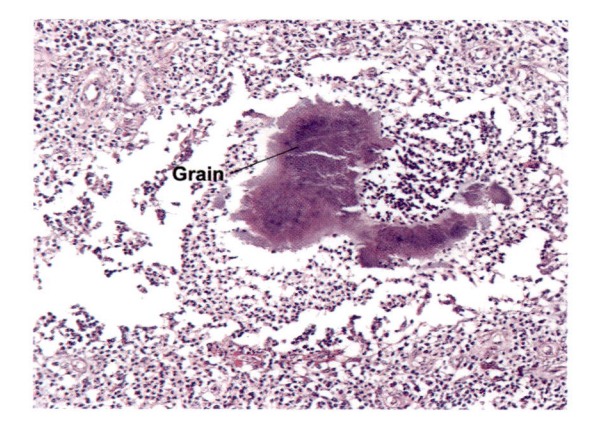

Fig 18-15 Actinomycetoma

Tinea nigra

Key features

- Acral skin
- Gold to brown hyphae in stratum corneum

Tinea nigra is usually caused by *Hortaea werneckii*. It is more common in hot, humid climates, and typically occurs on a palm or sole.

Phaeohyphomycosis

Key features

- Pigmented hyphae in tissue
- Commonly thick-walled with vesicular swellings and visible bubbly cytoplasm

Phaeohyphomycosis is caused by a wide variety of black molds (dematiaceous fungi, mildew organisms). A cavity surrounded by histiocytes and giant cells may be seen. This pattern is referred to as a phaeomycotic "cyst." Most patients with phaeomycotic cysts are immunocompetent, and the most common organism is *Exophiala jeanselmei*. Most patients with invasive phaeohyphomycosis are immunocompromised, and the most common organism is *Bipolaris spicifera*.

PEARL

Pigment can sometimes be inconspicuous in the hyphal wall. Clues that the organism is a black mold include the combination of a thick refractile wall and bubbly cytoplasm. Some black mold hyphae form characteristic round swellings. Using a Fontana–Masson melanin stain to identify lightly pigmented dematiaceous fungi is problematic, as some non-pigmented molds (including zygomycetes and dermatophytes) will stain.

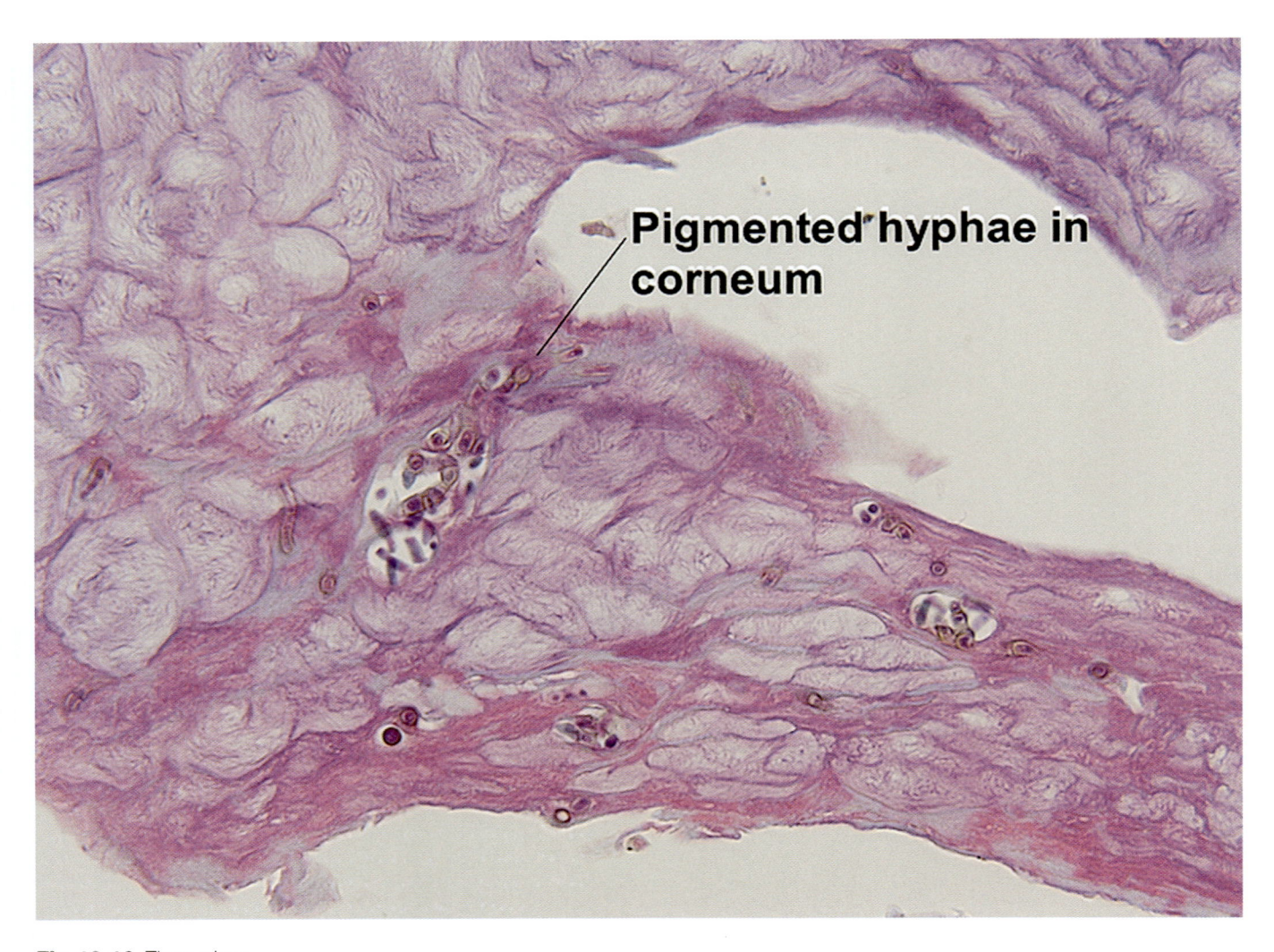

Fig 18-16 Tinea nigra

Fungal infections Chapter 18

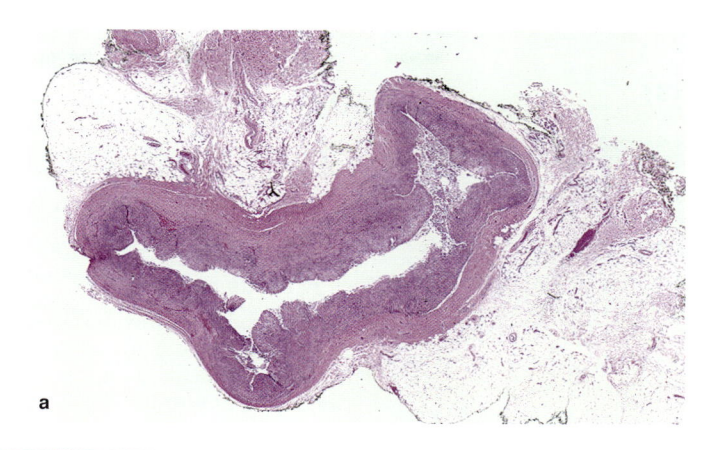

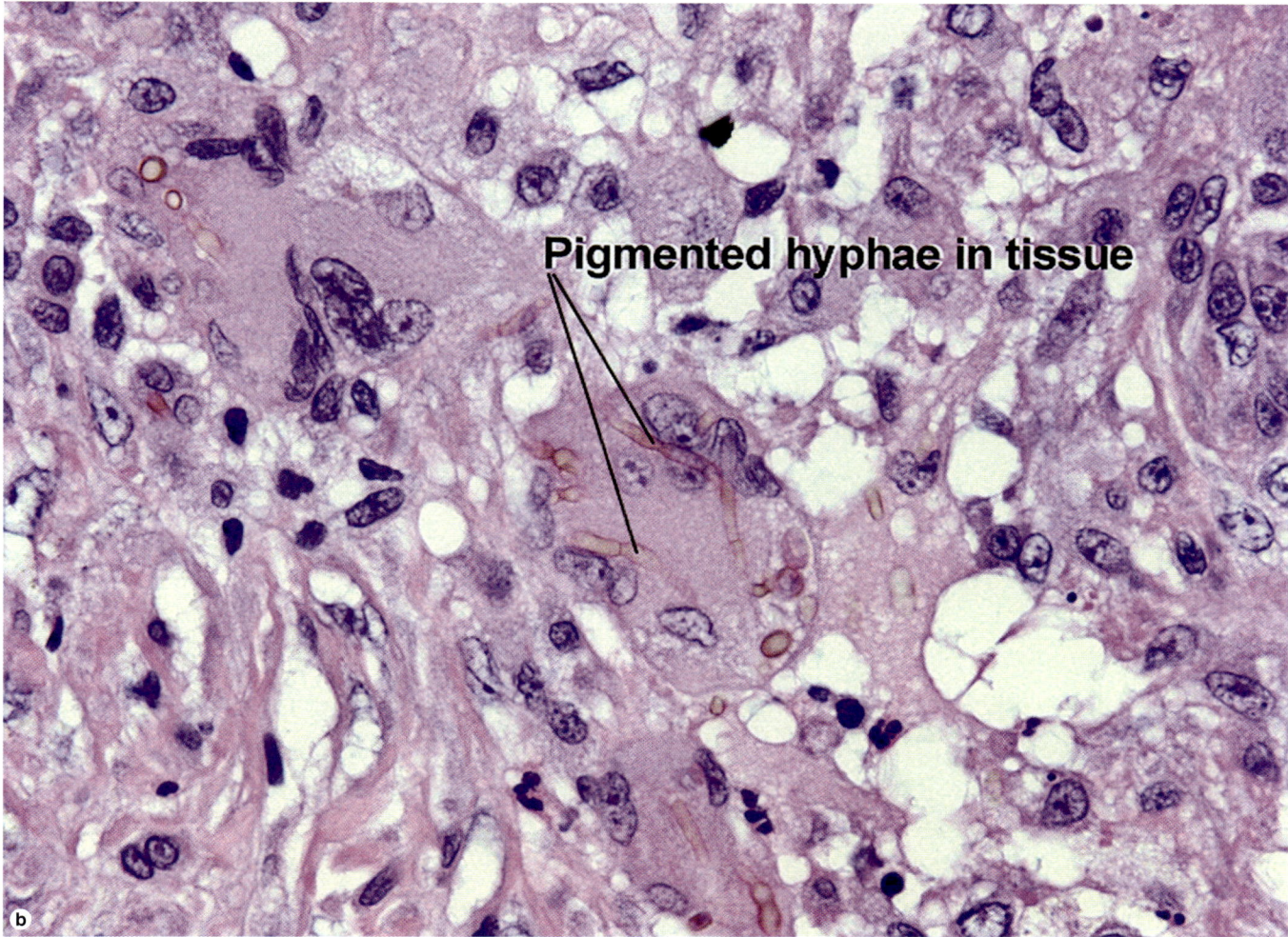

Fig 18-17 Phaeohyphomycosis

Chromomycosis (chromoblastomycosis)

Key features
- Pseudoepitheliomatous hyperplasia with intraepidermal pustules
- Medlar bodies: "copper pennies," "sclerotic bodies"

Round copper-colored Medlar bodies are often seen in groups within giant cells or suppurative foci. Sometimes, they are noted within a wood splinter. Internal septation may be noted.

PEARL
Chromomycosis is caused by:
- Compact – *Fonsecaea compacta*
- Dead – *Cladosporium carrionii*
- Wet – *Rhinocladiella aquaspersa*
- Warty – *Phialophora verrucosa*
- Feet – *Fonsecaea pedrosoi*

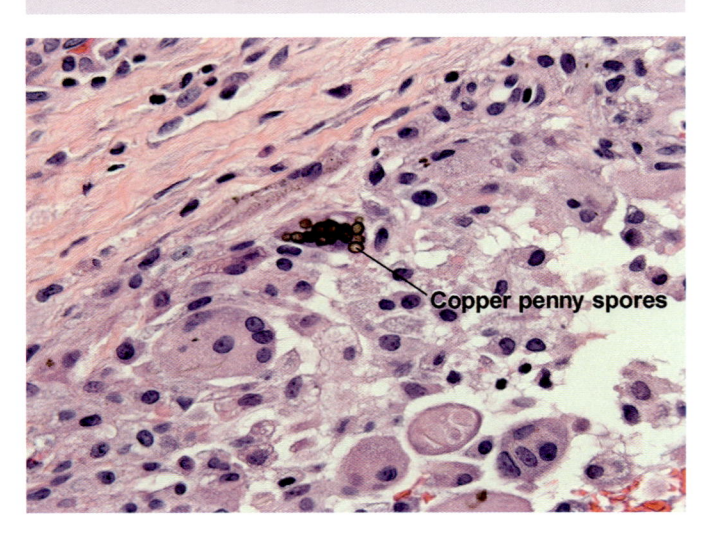

Fig 18-18 Chromomycosis

Zygomycosis

Mucorales infection (mucormycosis)

Key features
- Broad, hollow-appearing, lumpy bumpy, refractile hyphae
- Blood vessel invasion
- Tissue necrosis

Although 90° branching is typical, some hyphae will appear to branch at more acute angles. The hyphae are non-septate, but twists and bends in the wall commonly mimic a septum. An excellent clue to the non-septate nature of the organism is that the hyphae appear hollow, as there are no septa to retain cytoplasm. Tissue sent for culture must be diced carefully, as homogenization easily renders the non-septate hyphae non-viable. Causative organisms include *Rhizopus*, *Absidia*, *Mucor*, *Cunninghamella*, *Apophysomyces*, *Rhizomucor*, *Saksenaea*, *Mortierella*, and *Cokeromyces* species. They stain poorly with fungal stains such as PAS and Gomori methenamine silver (GMS: Grocott), but may stain well with a Gram stain.

Entomophthorales infection (entomophthoromycosis)

Key features
- Indolent infections
- Resemble zygomycetes in tissue

Conidiobolus coronatus causes perinasal disease. *Basidiobolus ranarum* causes broader subcutaneous lesions in non-facial skin. The Splendore–Hoeppli phenomenon is commonly seen as an eosinophilic sleeve around the hyphae. *Pythiosis*, an aquatic hyphal organism, has a similar appearance.

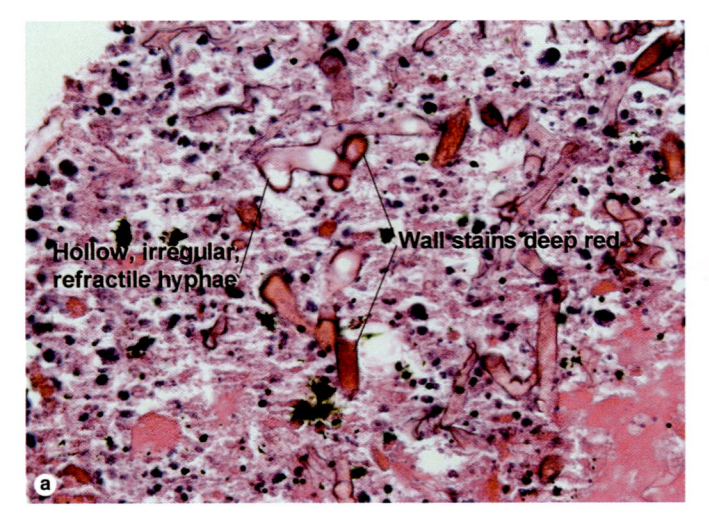

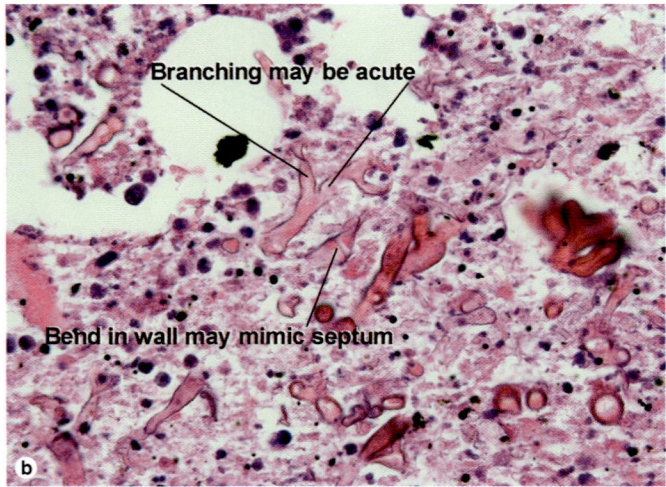

Fig 18-19 *Rhizopus* infection

Hyalohyphomycosis (including aspergillosis and fusariosis)

Key features

- Narrow, non-pigmented hyphae in tissue
- Prominent blue bubbly cytoplasm
- Inconspicuous, delicate wall
- Septate
- 45° angle branching
- Invade vessels causing tissue necrosis
- *Fusarium* may demonstrate vesicular swellings like a black mold, but lacks the thick refractile wall characteristic of *Bipolaris* (the most common invasive black mold)

The term "hyalohyphomycosis" is used for invasive infections by any non-pigmented mold, excluding zygomycetes. As a group, they tend to be vasculotropic and cause tissue necrosis. They are septate organisms, and the septa typically retain bubbly blue cytoplasm within the delicate hyphal walls. The blue cytoplasm is always more conspicuous than the nearly invisible wall. The only exception is when a Splendore–Hoeppli phenomenon (eosinophilic immunoglobulin) coats the fungal wall. The immunoglobulin is never refractile like chitin. Dead hyphae will swell to the diameter of a zygomycete, but the dead wall will be pale-staining and will never be thick and refractile like a zygomycete.

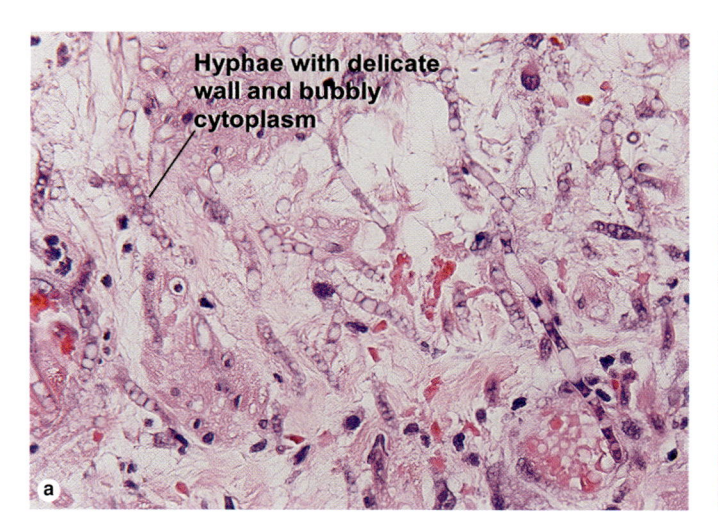

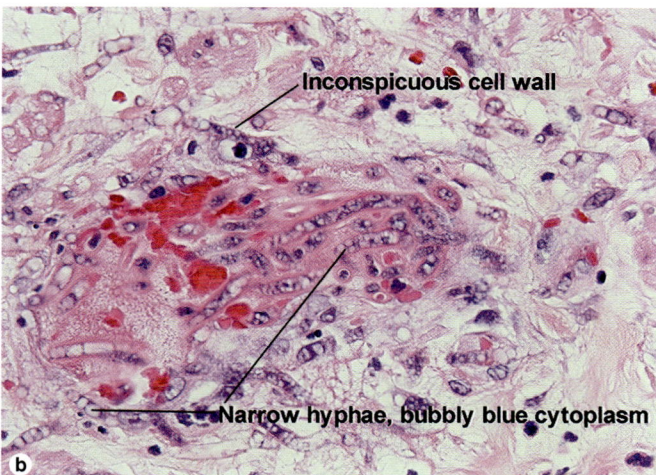

Fig 18-20 Aspergillosis

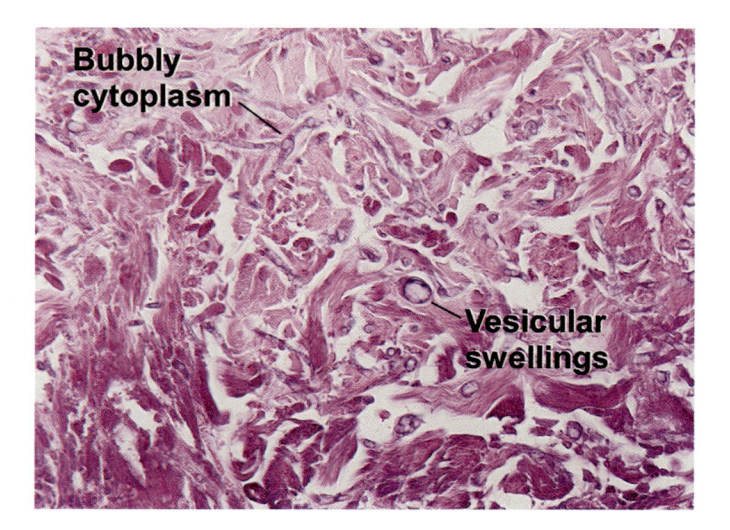

Fig 18-21 Fusariosis

Protothecosis

Key features

- Morula (soccer ball-like)
- Non-morulating forms have characteristic "eyeball" appearance

The organism (genus *Prototheca*) is found in tree slime, and generally classified as an achloric (non-pigmented) algae.

Rhinosporidiosis

Key features

- Huge sporangia with many endospores
- Non-sporulating trophocyte form resembles *Coccidioides*, but with a central small nucleus

Rhinosporidium has been classified as a fungus or protist. Granulomas are present in about 50% of cases. A suppurative response

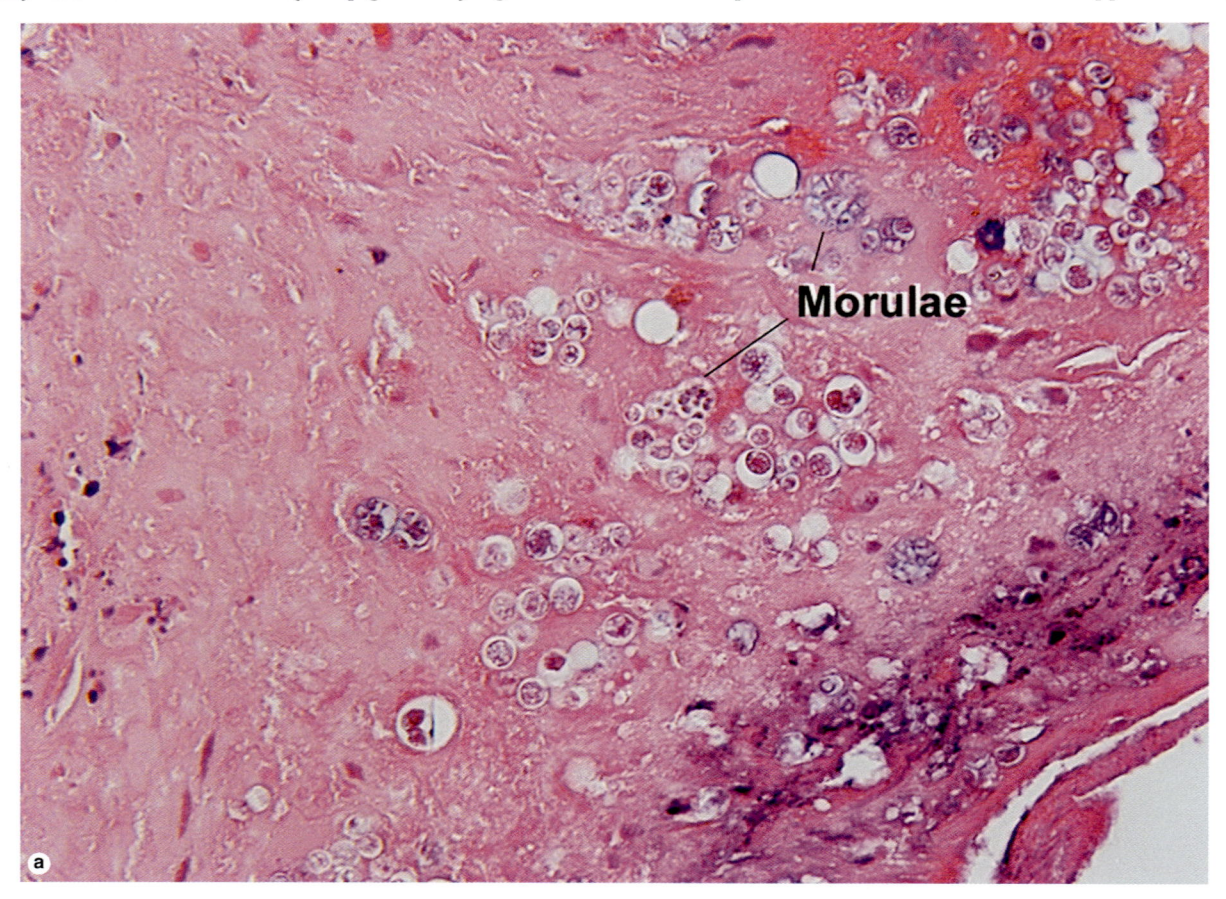

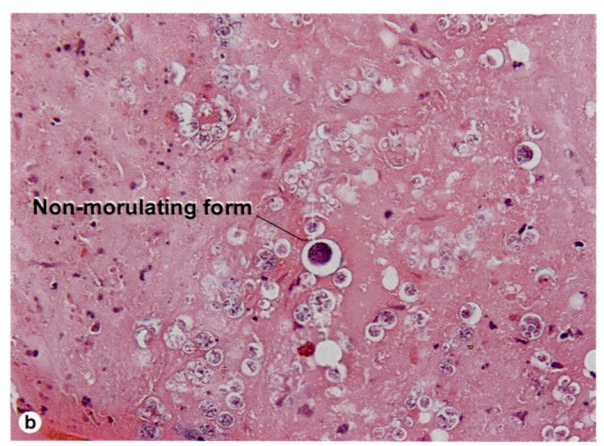

Fig 18-22 Protothecosis

may be present when sporangia rupture. Transepithelial elimination of sporangia may be seen. The organism requires synergistic bacteria for growth. Culture of the organism has been accomplished when it is grown with the cyanobacterium *Microcystis aeruginosa*. The organisms are naturally found together in pond water.

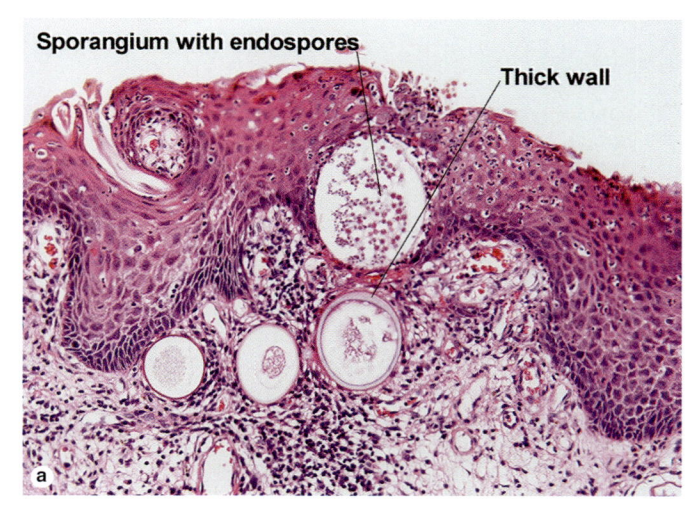

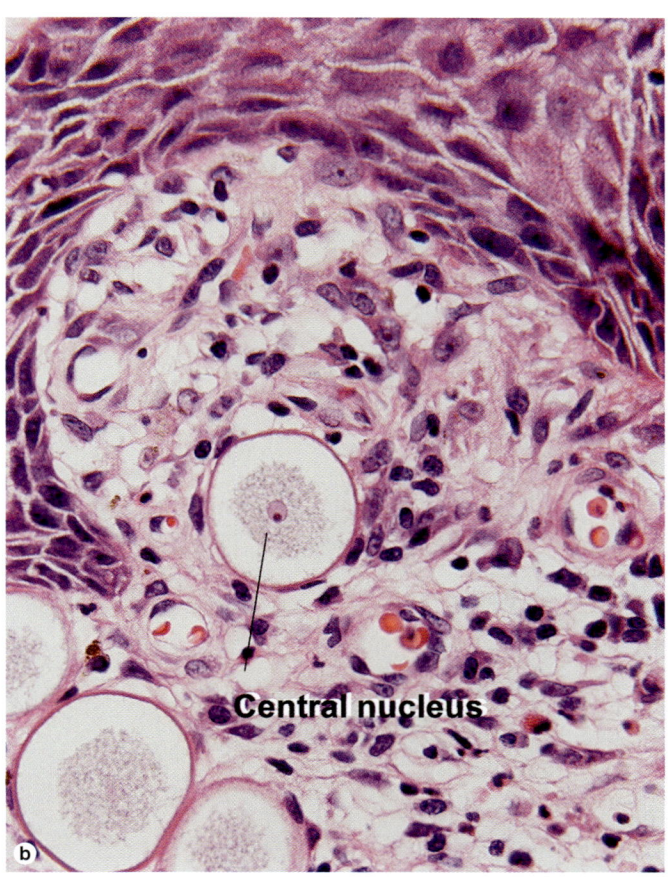

Fig 18-23 Rhinosporidiosis

Further reading

Arseculeratne SN, Panabokke RG, Atapattu DN. Lymphadenitis, trans-epidermal elimination and unusual histopathology in human rhinosporidiosis. Mycopathologia 2002;153(2):57–69.

Bracca A, Tosello ME, Girardini JE, et al. Molecular detection of Histoplasma capsulatum var. capsulatum in human clinical samples. J Clin Microbiol 2003;41(4):1753–1755.

Haubold EM, Cooper CR Jr, Wen JW, et al. Comparative morphology of Lacazia loboi (syn. Loboa loboi) in dolphins and humans. Med Mycol 2000;38(1):9–14.

Hu S, Chung WH, Hung SI, et al. Detection of Sporothrix schenckii in clinical samples by a nested PCR assay. J Clin Microbiol 2003;41(4):1414–1418.

Husain S, Alexander BD, Munoz P, et al. Opportunistic mycelial fungal infections in organ transplant recipients: emerging importance of non-Aspergillus mycelial fungi. Clin Infect Dis 2003;37(2):221–229.

Kantrow SM, Boyd AS. Protothecosis. Dermatol Clin 2003;21(2):249–255.

Makannavar JH, Chavan SS. Rhinosporidiosis – a clinicopathological study of 34 cases. Indian J Pathol Microbiol 2001;44(1):17–21.

Minotto R, Bernardi CD, Mallmann LF, et al. Chromoblastomycosis: a review of 100 cases in the state of Rio Grande do Sul, Brazil. J Am Acad Dermatol 2001;44(4):585–592.

Perfect JR. The triple threat of cryptococcosis: it's the body site, the strain, and/or the host. MBio 2012;3(4):pii: e00165-12.

Ramesh A, Deka RC, Vijayaraghavan M, et al. Entomophthoromycosis of the nose and paranasal sinus. Indian J Pediatr 2000;67(4):307–310.

Revankar SG, Patterson JE, Sutton DA, et al. Disseminated phaeohyphomycosis: review of an emerging mycosis. Clin Infect Dis 2002;34(4):467–476.

Shinozaki M, Okubo Y, Sasai D, et al. Development and evaluation of nucleic acid-based techniques for an auxiliary diagnosis of invasive fungal infections in formalin-fixed and paraffin-embedded (FFPE) tissues. Med Mycol J 2012;53(4):241–245.

Talhari S, Talhari C. Lobomycosis. Clin Dermatol 2012;30(4):420–424.

Chapter 19

Viral infections, helminths, and arthropods

Dirk M. Elston

Viral infections

Warts

Verruca vulgaris

Key features

- Exophytic
- Papillomatosis
- Compact eosinophilic hyperkeratosis
- Coarse hypergranulosis in dells
- Vertical tiers of round parakeratosis common above peaks
- Blood and serum common above peaks
- Koilocytes variable

The biopsy will demonstrate a compact stratum corneum, coarse hypergranulosis, and papillomatosis. The papillomatosis often curves inward. Vascular ectasia is common. Koilocytes (vacuolated cells with hyperchromatic shriveled nuclei) may be present. Red cytoplasmic inclusions may sometimes be present.

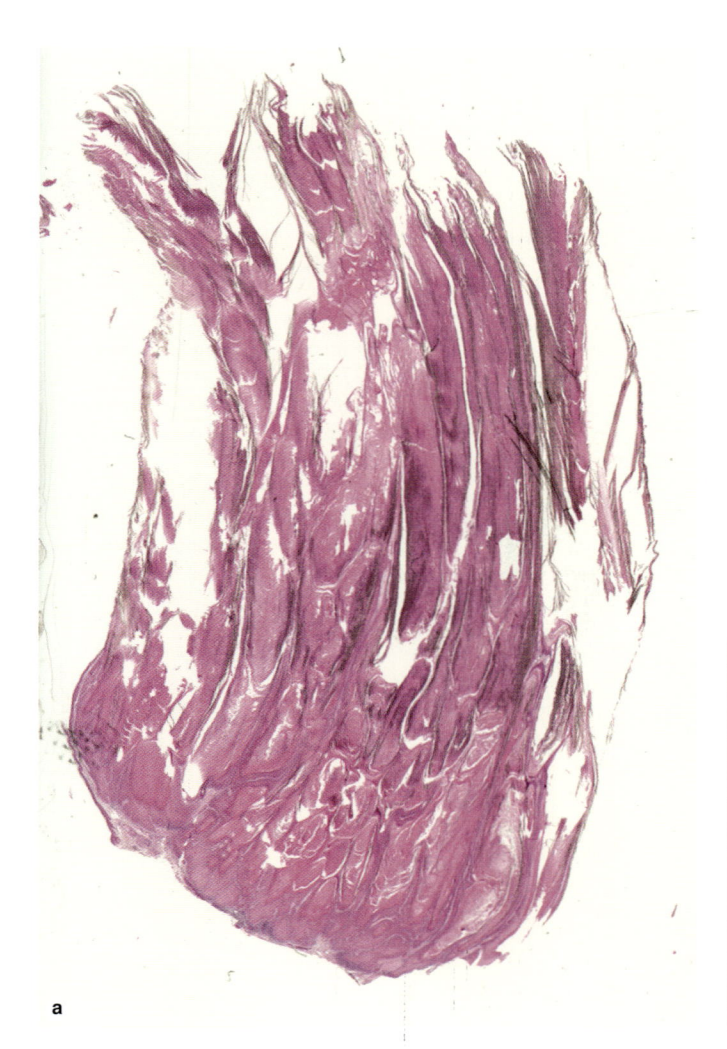

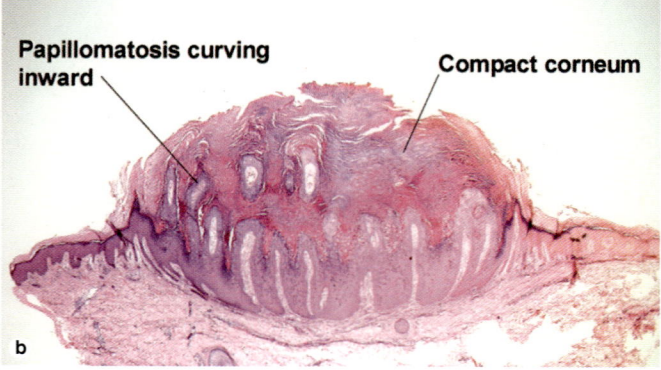

Fig 19-1 Verruca vulgaris

Viral infections, helminths, and arthropods Chapter **19**

Myrmecia

Key features
- Deep palmoplantar wart with anthill-like appearance clinically
- Endophytic
- Coarse red cytoplasmic inclusions

Myrmecia are associated with human papillomavirus 1 (HPV-1).

Verruca plana (flat wart)

Key features
- Coarse basket-weave hyperkeratosis
- Hypergranulosis common
- "Bird's eye" cells (like koilocytes but lack shriveled nuclei)

Epidermodysplasia verruciformis (EDV)

Key feature
- Widespread flat warts with foamy blue cytoplasm

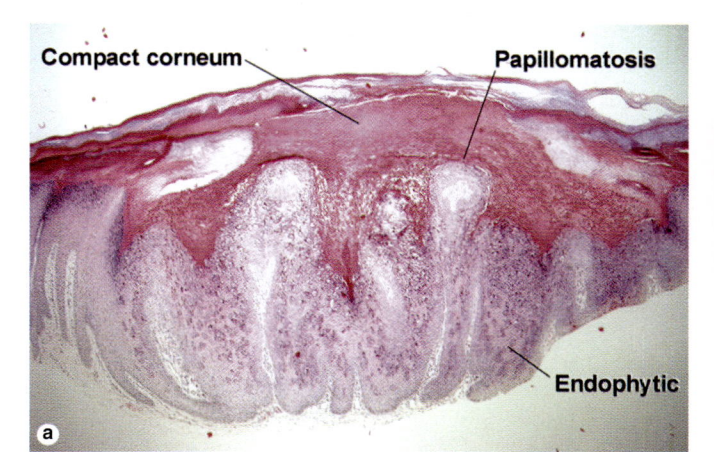

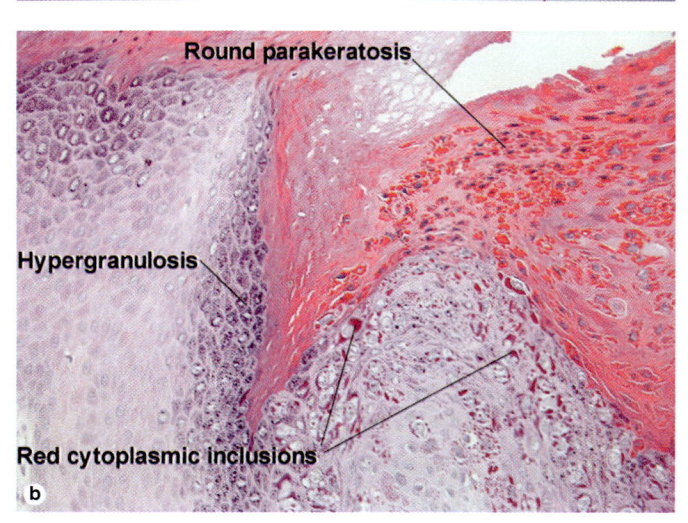

Fig 19-2 Myrmecia

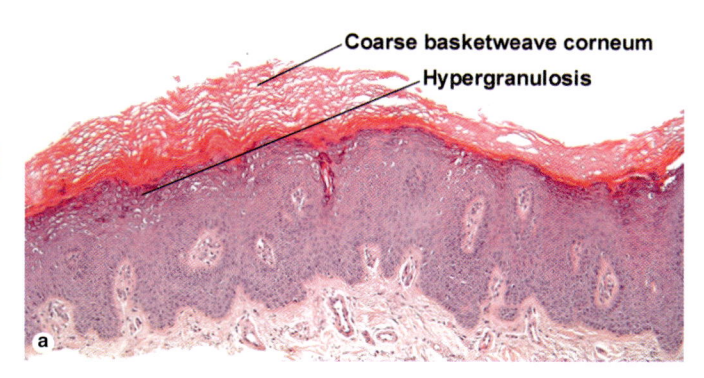

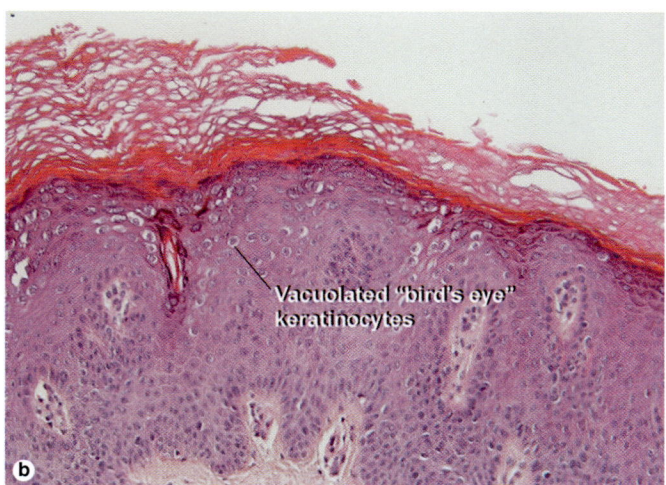

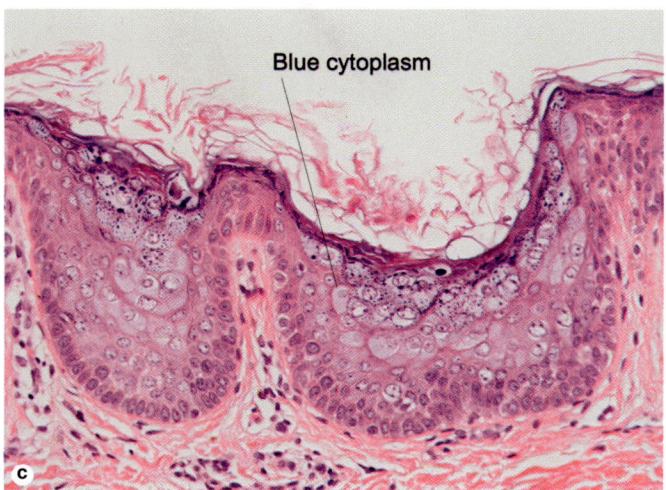

Fig 19-3 (a,b) Verruca plana. (c) Verruca plana with changes characteristic of epidermodysplasia verruciformis

Condyloma acuminatum

Key features
- Benign acanthoma on genital skin
- Areas of compact stratum corneum, round parakeratosis and coarse hypergranulosis generally present
- Vacuolated keratinocytes, typically with large gray nuclei
- True koilocytes rare

Condylomata acuminata commonly have horn cysts and resemble seborrheic keratoses. The two are differentiated by areas of compact stratum corneum, round parakeratosis, coarse hypergranulosis, and vacuolated keratinocytes with large gray nuclei. *In situ* hybridization can identify the human papillomavirus (HPV) type.

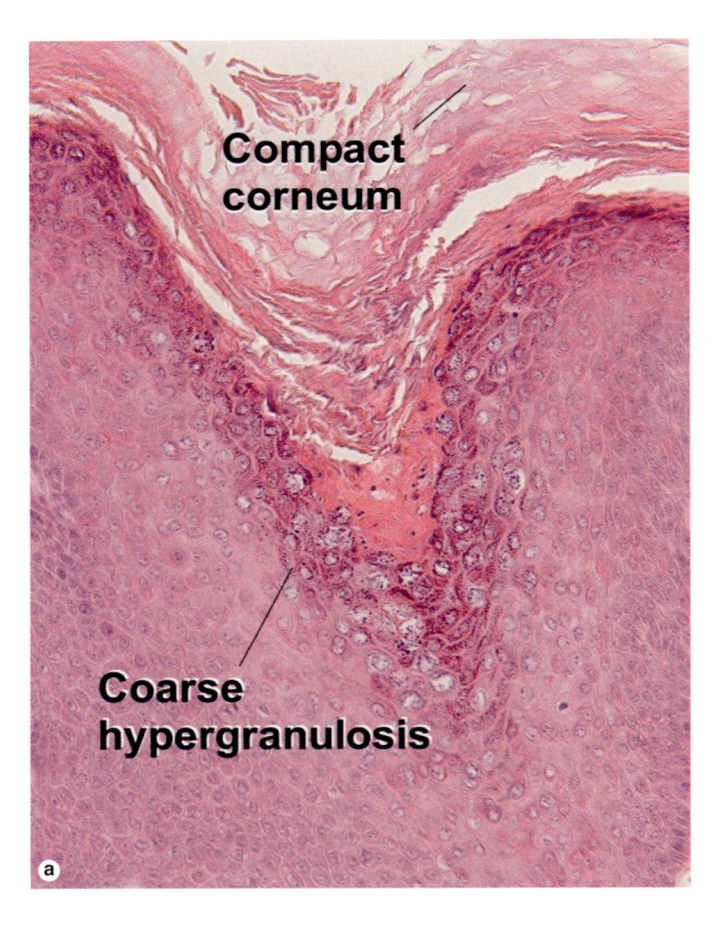

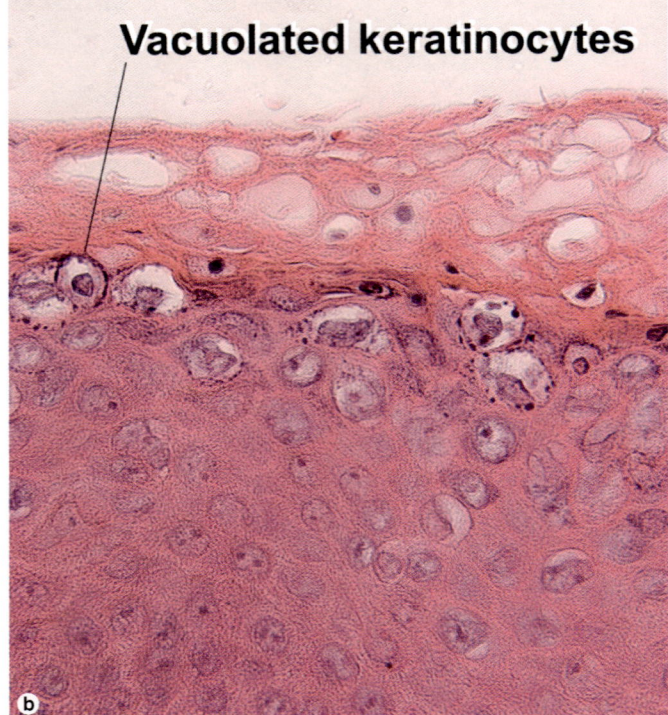

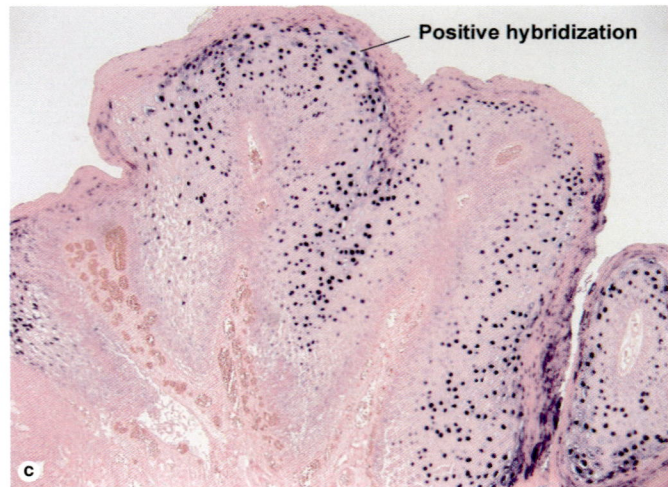

Fig 19-4 (a,b) Condyloma accuminatum. (c) Condyloma accuminatum *in situ* hybridization for low risk HPV (types 6 and 11)

Bowenoid papulosis

Key features

- HPV-16 most commonly
- Atypia

Bowenoid papulosis presents as discrete pink, brown, or gray lesions in the genitalia. They are typically sessile, rather than papillomatous or cauliflower-like. The histologic spectrum ranges from that of a condyloma with buckshot scatter of atypical cells to full-thickness atypia, indistinguishable from Bowen's disease.

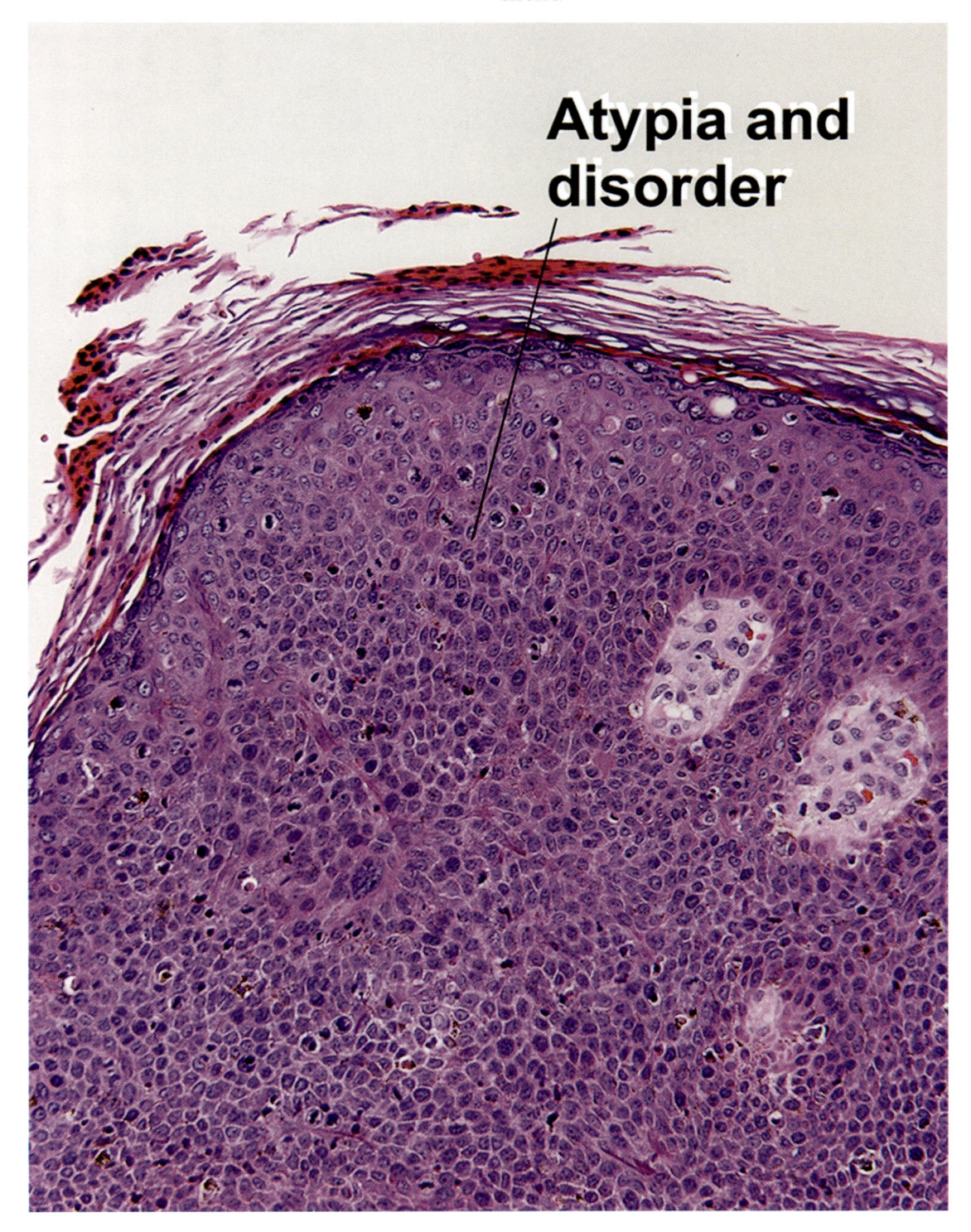

Fig 19-5 Bowenoid papulosis

Heck's disease

Key features
- Focal oral hyperplasia
- Hyperkeratosis with round parakeratosis
- Epithelial pallor
- HPV-13 and -32

PEARL

Type of wart	HPV type
Common	1, 2, 4
Flat (verruca plana)	3, 5
Plantar	1 (myrmecia), 2, 4 (mosaic)
Epidermodysplasia verruciformis	5, 8, and many others
Buschke–Löwenstein tumor	6, 11
Butcher's	7 and others
Laryngeal papillomas	6, 11
Genital dysplasia	16, 18, 31, 33, 35, and others
Heck's focal oral hyperplasia	13, 32
Subungual squamous cell carcinoma	16

Verrucous cyst (cystic papilloma)

Key features
- Cyst with wart-like lining

Verrucous cysts may arise as a result of papillomavirus infection of a hair follicle. On plantar surfaces, they may arise from eccrine ducts and the lining is more likely to resemble myrmecia.

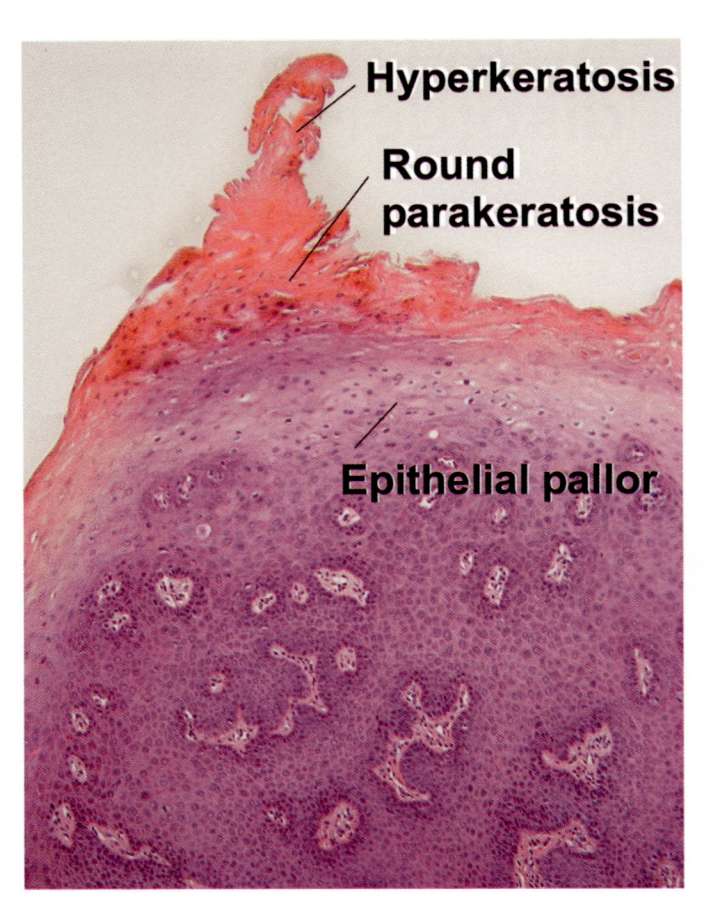

Fig 19-6 Heck's disease

Viral infections, helminths, and arthropods

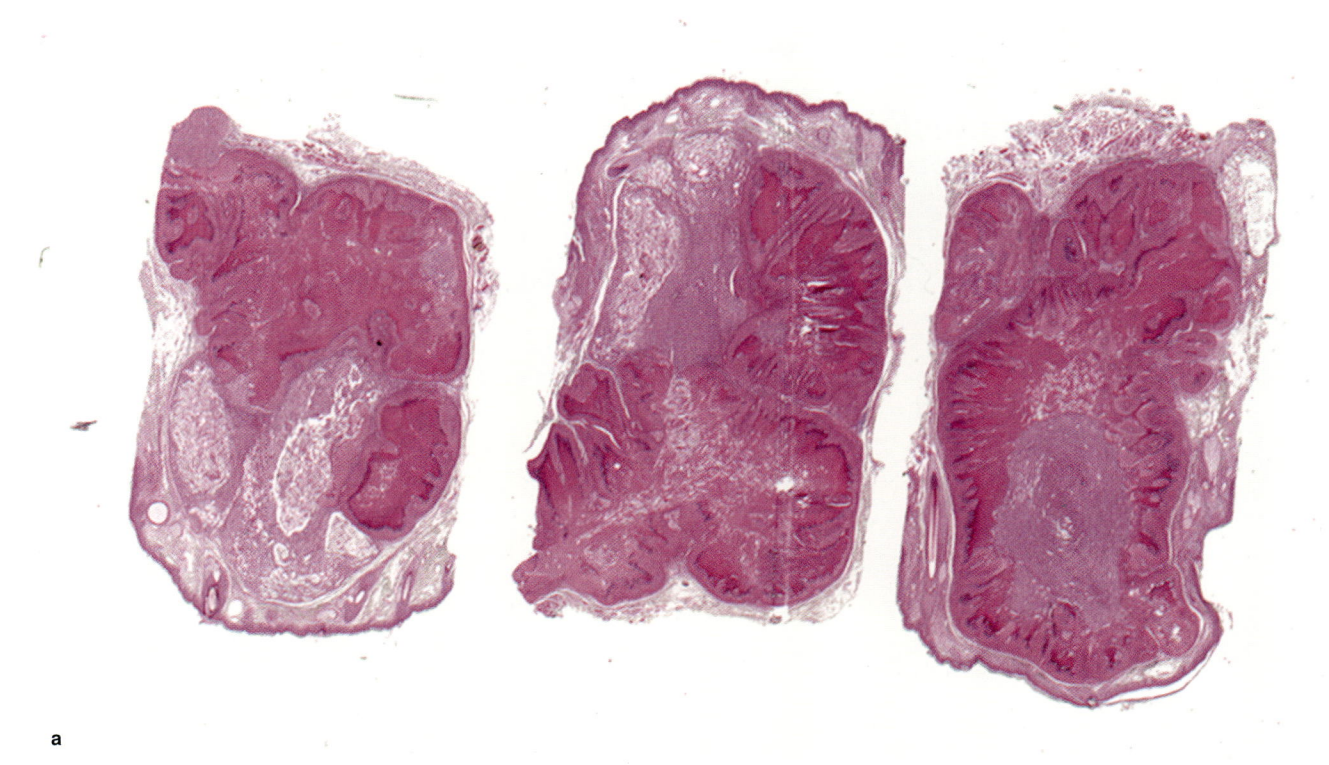

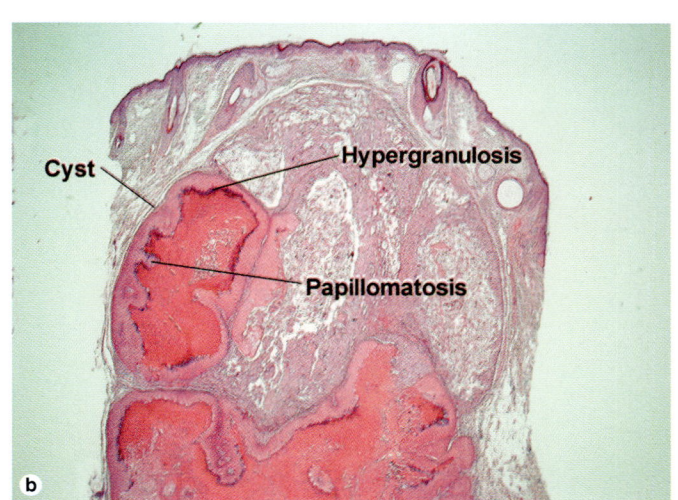

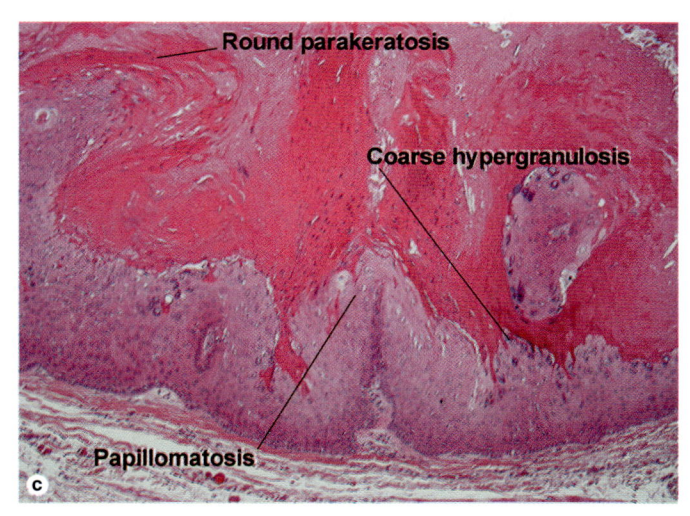

Fig 19-7 Verrucous cyst

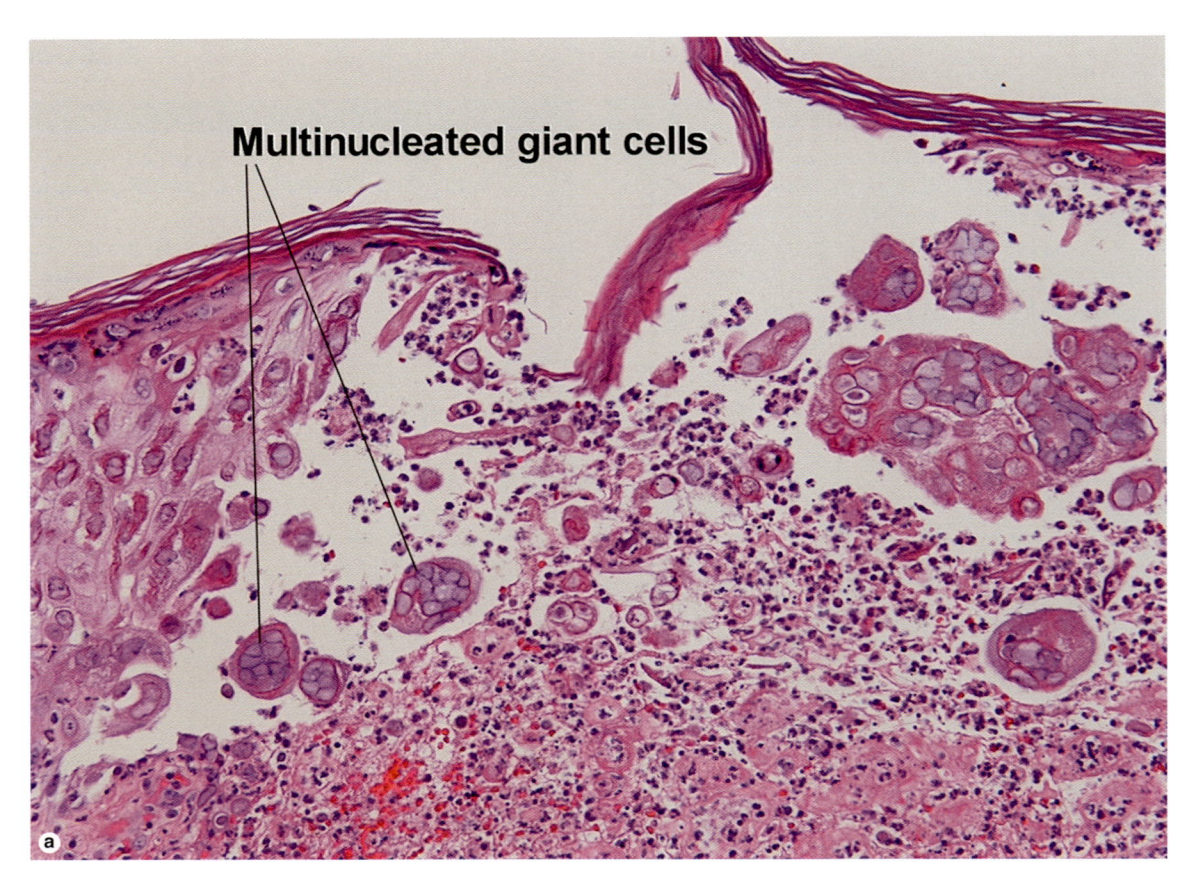

Herpetic infections

Herpes simplex

Key features
- Ballooning degeneration of keratinocytes
- Multinucleated keratinocytes with nuclear molding
- Herpetic cytopathic effect (basophilic eggshell of chromatin at the periphery of the nucleus)
- Mild features of leukocytoclastic vasculitis may be present

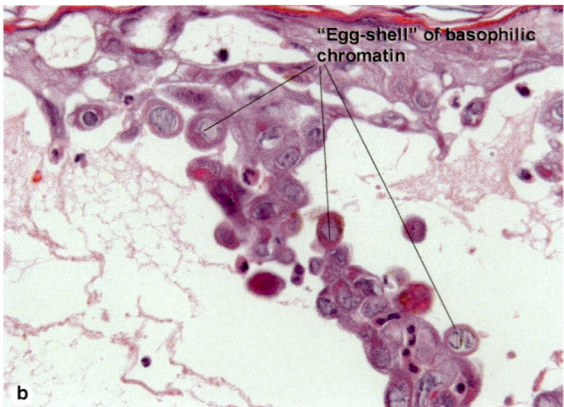

Fig 19-8 Herpes simplex

Herpes zoster (varicella-zoster virus: VZV)

Key features
- Ballooning degeneration of keratinocytes
- Multinucleated keratinocytes with nuclear molding
- Herpetic cytopathic effect (basophilic eggshell of chromatin at the periphery of the nucleus)
- Dramatic leukocytoclastic vasculitis typical

Chicken pox (VZV)

Key features
- Ballooning degeneration of keratinocytes
- Multinucleated keratinocytes with nuclear molding
- Herpetic cytopathic effect (basophilic eggshell of chromatin at the periphery of the nucleus)
- Mild features of leukocytoclastic vasculitis may be present

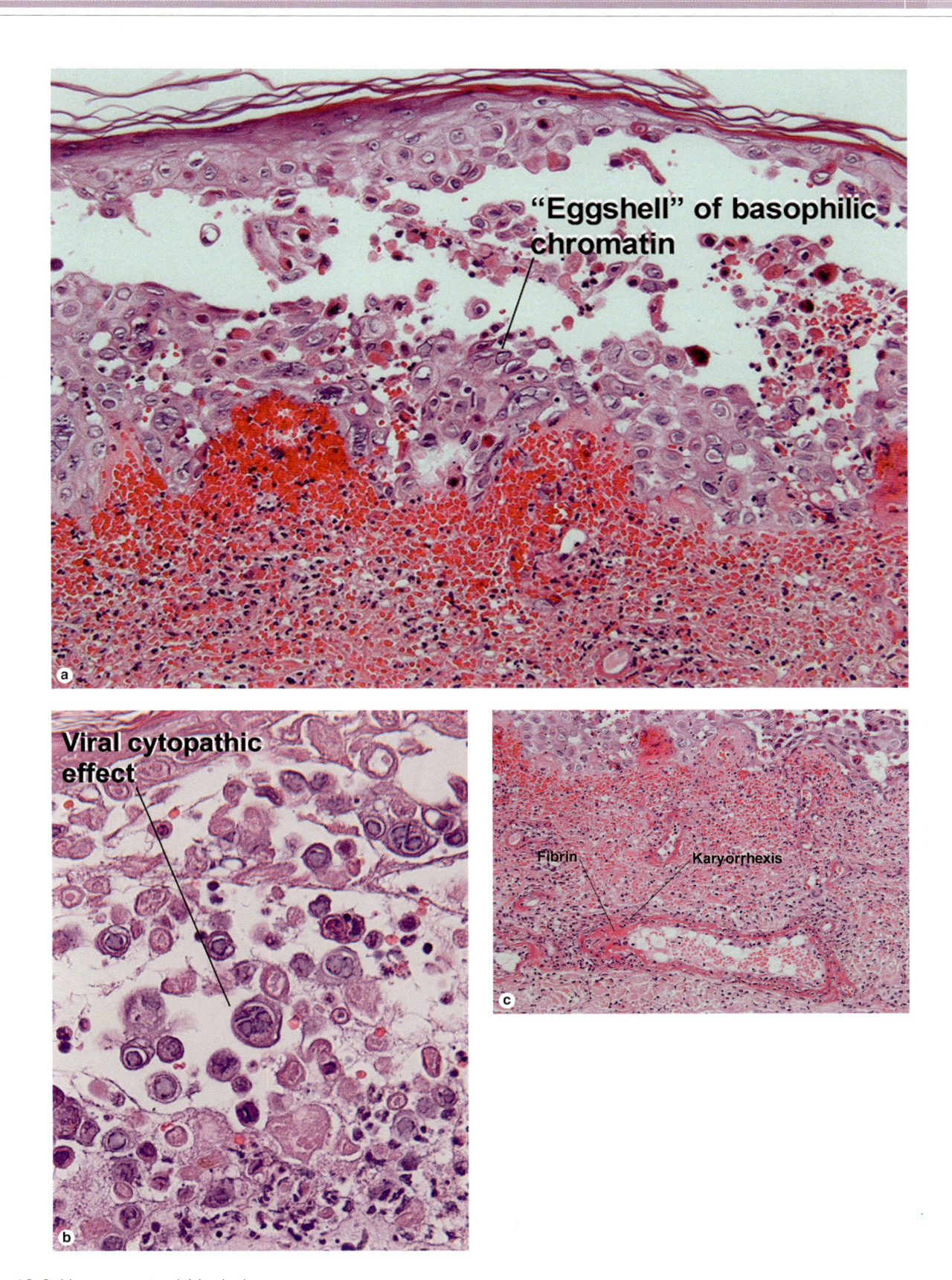

Viral infections, helminths, and arthropods **Chapter 19** 293

Fig 19-9 Herpes zoster (shingles)

Dermatopathology

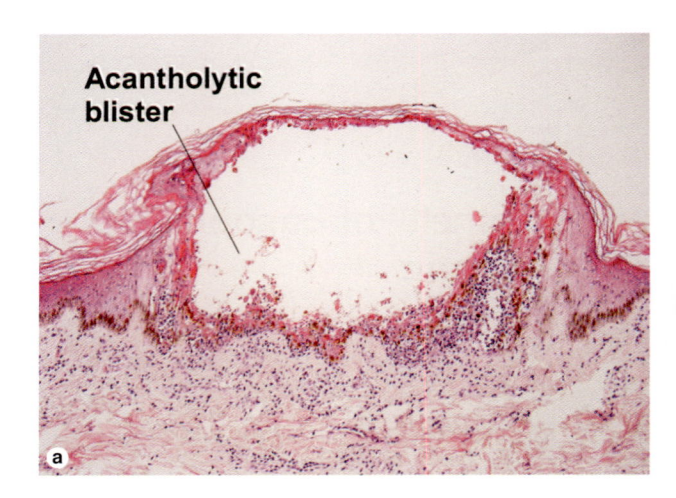

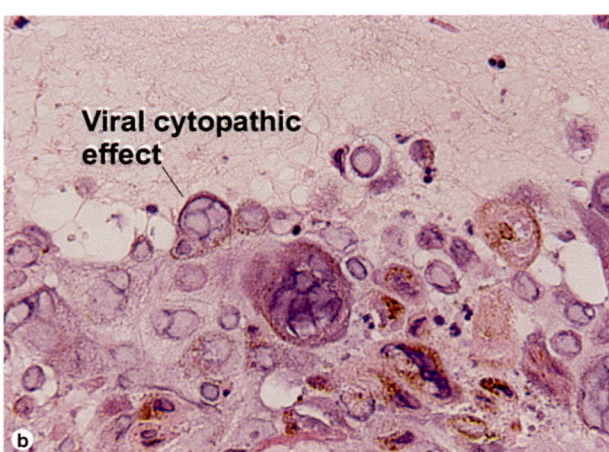

Fig 19-10 Varicella (chicken pox)

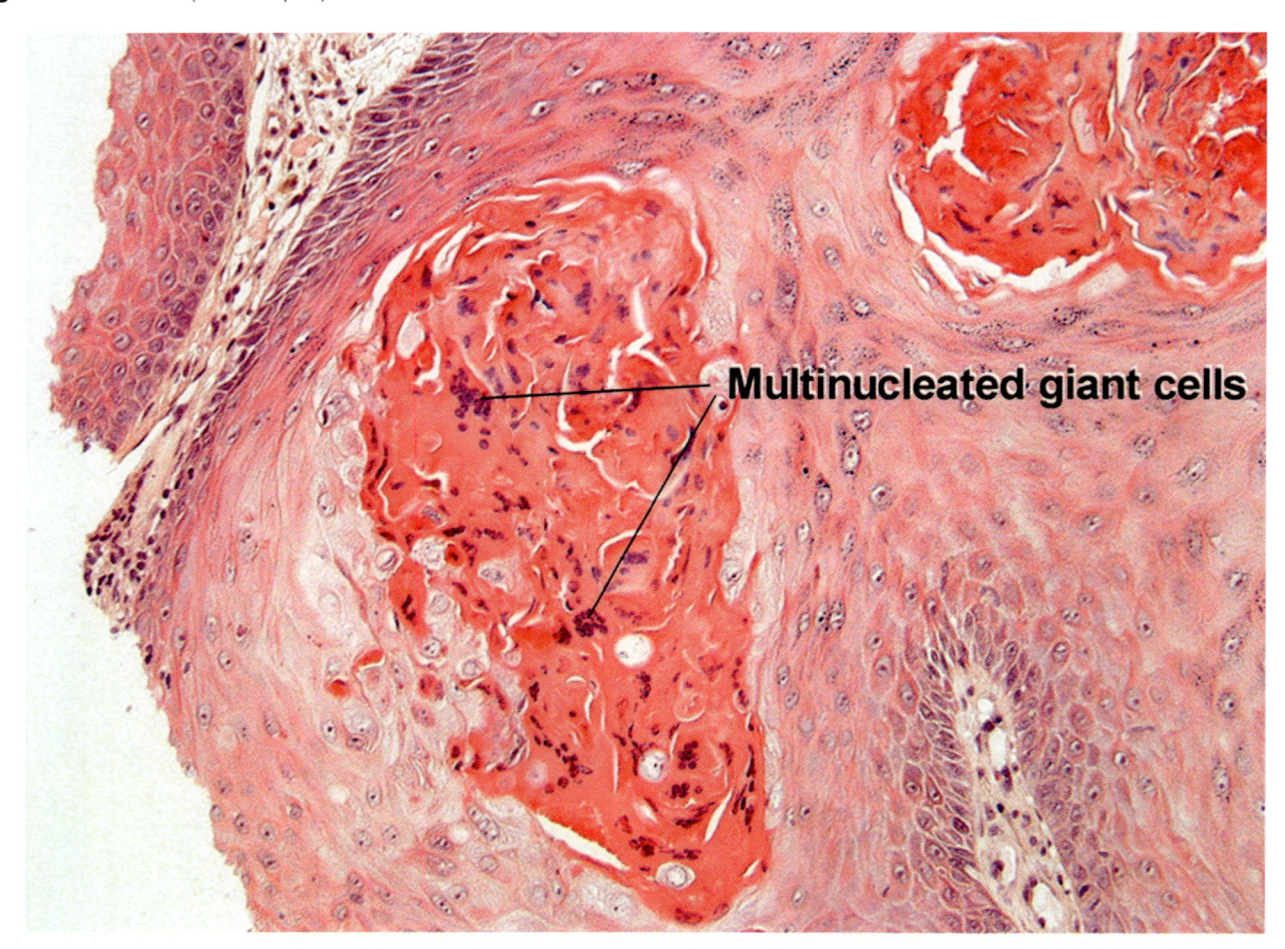

Fig 19-11 Verrucous zoster

Verrucous VZV infection

Key features
- Compact hyperkeratosis
- Variable papillomatosis
- Follicular herpetic cytopathic effect

Multinucleated giant cells with basophilic nuclear rims and nuclear molding are noted within follicular epithelium. This pattern is typically seen in immunosuppressed patients, especially in the setting of human immunodeficiency virus (HIV) infection.

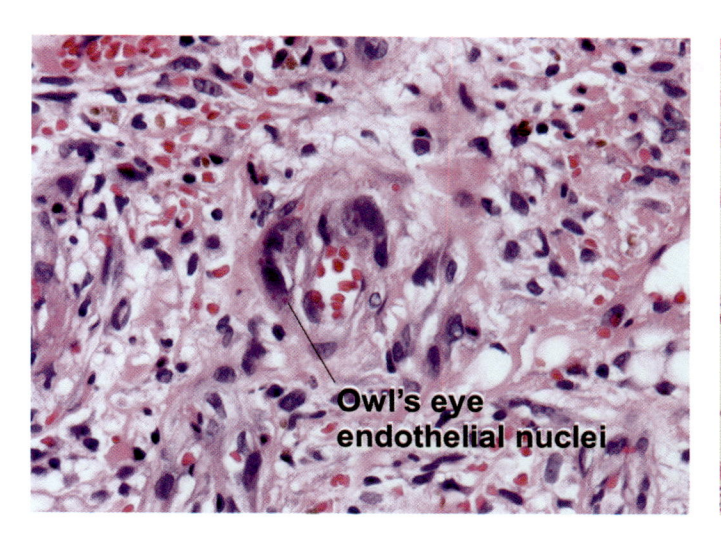

Fig 19-12 Cytomegalovirus infection

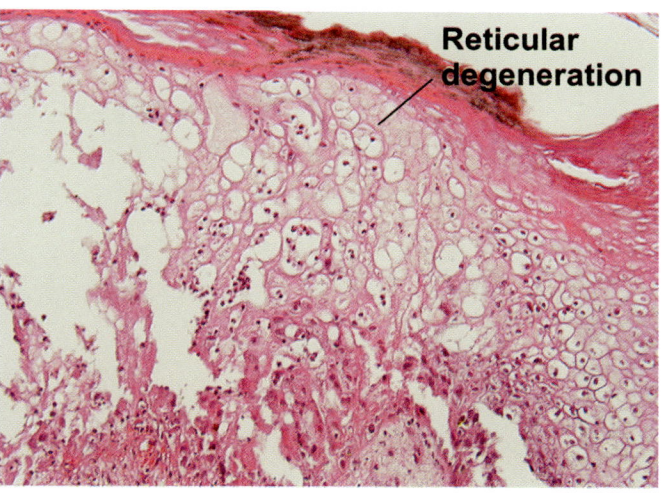

Fig 19-13 Smallpox

Cytomegalovirus

Key features

- Large endothelial cells with owl's-eye nuclei
- Cytoplasm may be ample or scant

In HIV patients, cytomegalovirus probably does not cause ulcers, but reactivates within ulcers. Viral cytopathic changes may be found in ulcers of various causes. This alerts the clinician to look for evidence of cytomegalovirus retinal involvement.

Pox and parapox infections

Smallpox (variola)

Key features

- Epidermal necrosis, often with reticular degeneration
- Eosinophilic cytoplasmic inclusions
- Nuclear inclusions may also be seen

In scrapings, Guarnieri bodies appear black with Gispen's modified silver stain. Guarnieri bodies are aggregations of the smaller Paschen bodies.

296　Dermatopathology

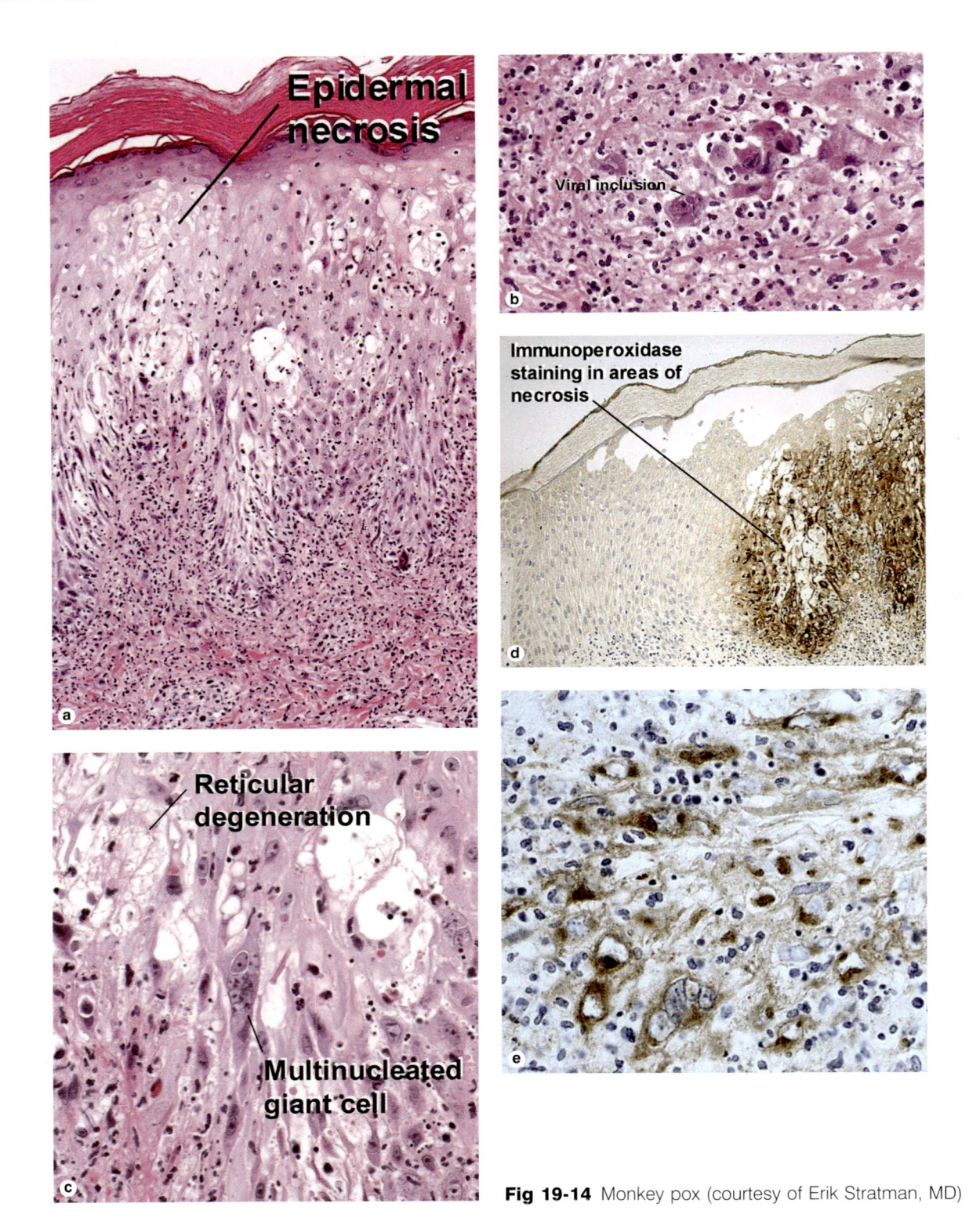

Fig 19-14 Monkey pox (courtesy of Erik Stratman, MD)

Monkey pox

Key features

- Ballooning degeneration of basal keratinocytes
- Epidermal necrosis
- Spongiosis
- Band-like polymorphous infiltrate
- Superficial and deep perivascular and periadnexal infiltrate
- Multinucleated syncytial keratinocytes
- Animal contact

Viral infections, helminths, and arthropods

Molluscum contagiosum

Key features

- Cup-shaped lesion with scalloped border
- Henderson–Paterson bodies (molluscum bodies)

Molluscum contagiosum is readily recognized by the characteristic cytoplasmic inclusions. These vary from eosinophilic to basophilic as the inclusion bodies mature.

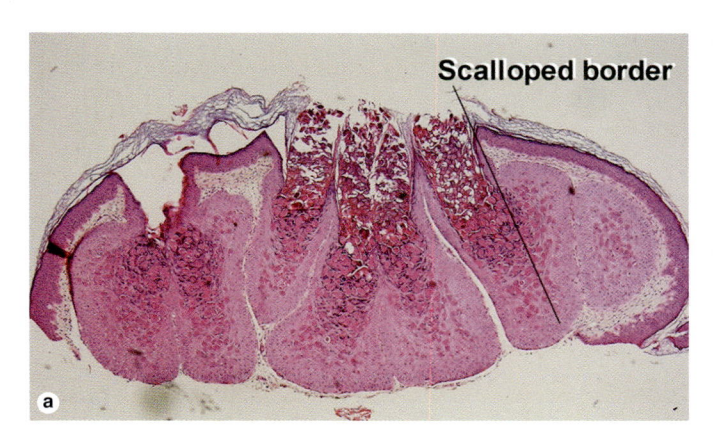

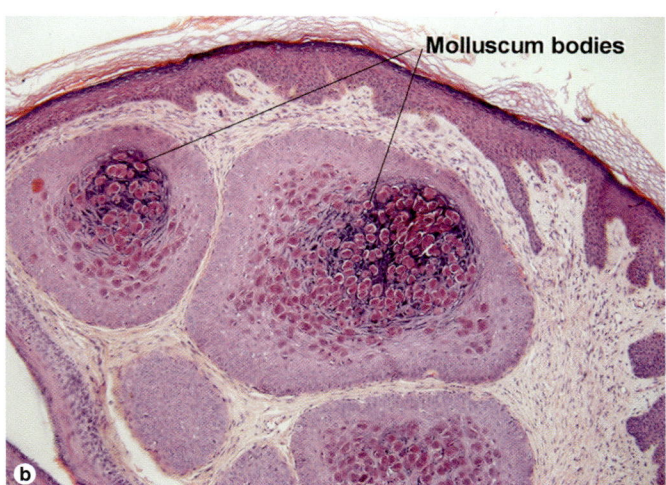

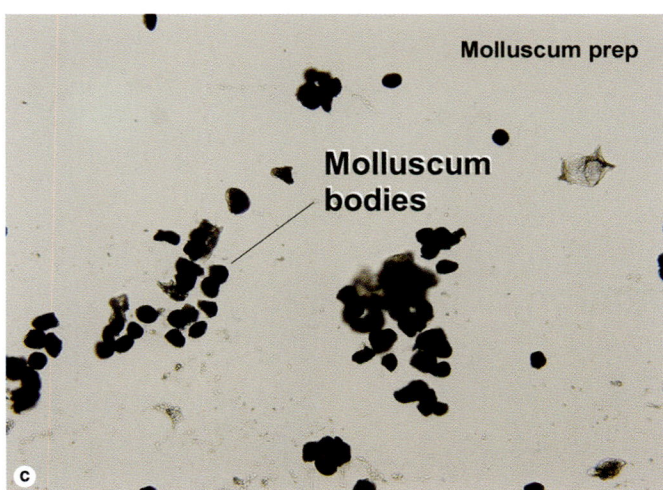

Fig 19-15 Molluscum contagiosum

Dermatopathology

Orf and milker's nodules

> **Key features**
> - Epidermal necrosis
> - Viral inclusion bodies (may be both cytoplasmic and intranuclear)
> - Animal contact

Orf and milker's nodules are caused by distinct viruses, but have a similar histologic appearance. Each lesion evolves through a series of clinical stages, and the histologic appearance varies by stage. During the verrucous phase, the epidermis demonstrates endophytic strand-like proliferations. The dermal papillae are edematous with dilated vessels. A dense, predominantly lymphoid infiltrate is present. Plasma cells and histiocytes are often present. Viral inclusion bodies, clumping of keratohyalin, and cytoplasmic vacuolation may still be seen.

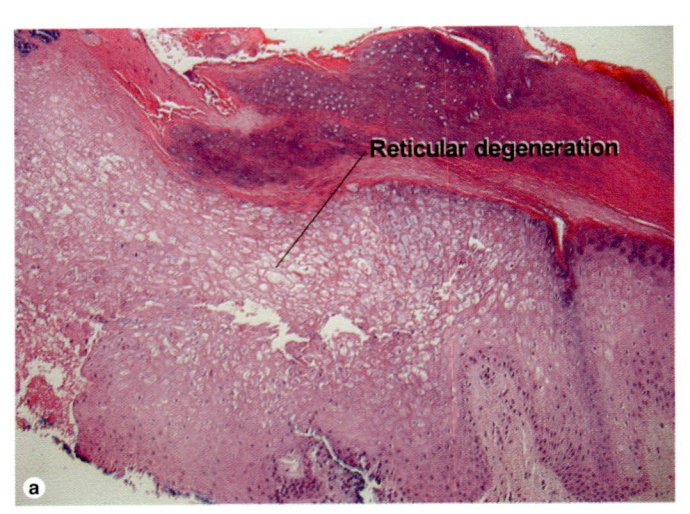

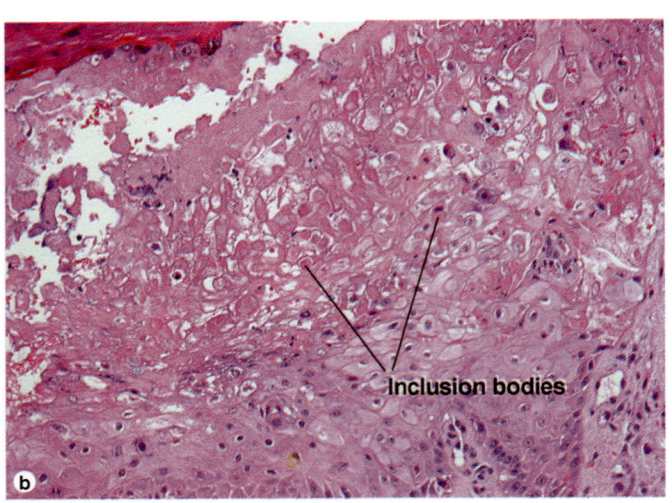

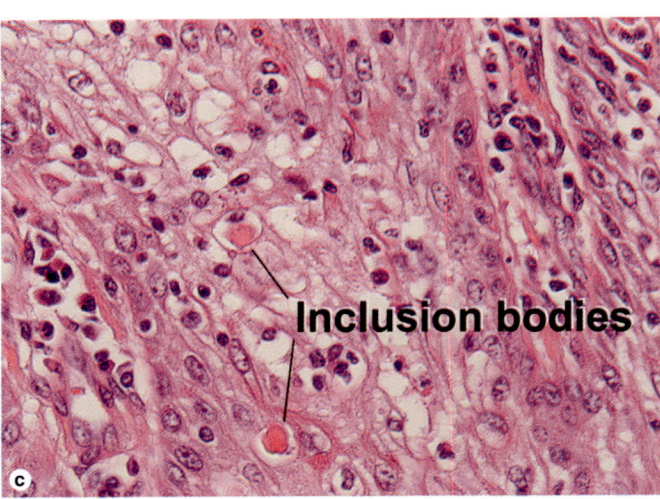

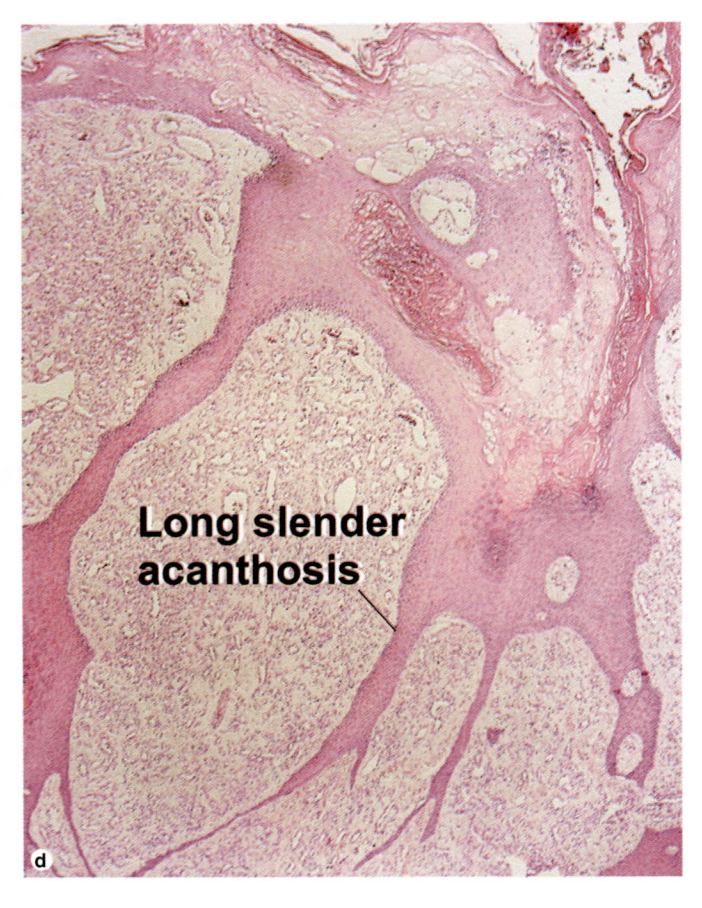

Fig 19-16 Orf nodules

Viral infections, helminths, and arthropods

Gianotti–Crosti syndrome

Key features

- Papular acrolocated syndrome
- Associated with various viruses, notably hepatitis B (HBV) in Italy
- In the USA, papulovesicular acrolocated syndrome is rarely associated with HBV
- Minor crusting
- Spongiosis
- Papillary dermal edema
- Superficial perivascular lymphoid infiltrate

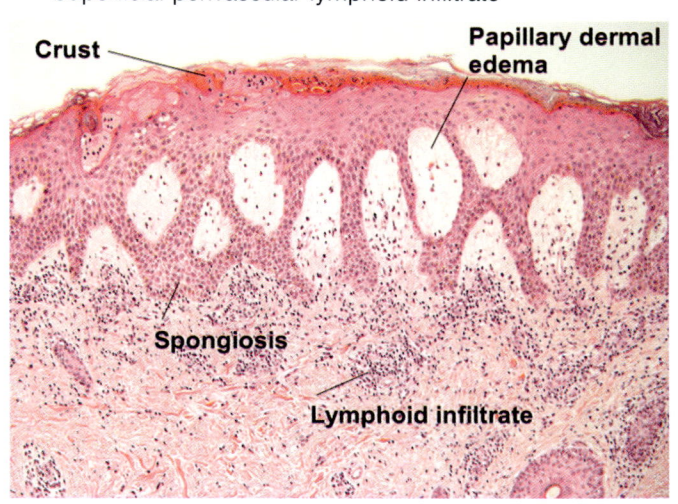

Fig 19-17 Gianotti–Crosti syndrome

Hand, foot, and mouth syndrome

Key features

- Oval vesicles or ulcers on the sides of the digits, palms, soles, mouth, and buttocks
- Coxsackie A16 and others
- Reticular and ballooning degeneration of keratinocytes

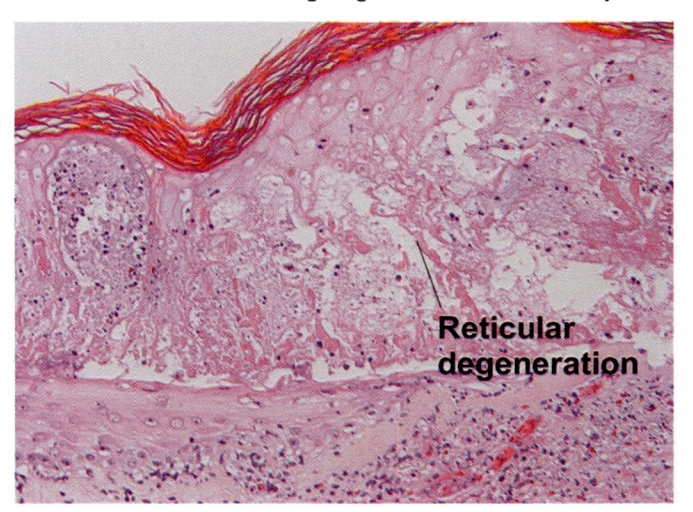

Fig 19-18 Hand, foot, and mouth syndrome

Flukes, tapeworms and roundworms

Schistosomiasis

Key features

- Ova with stippled contents
- Mixed inflammatory response, commonly granulomatous

Schistosomes are trematodes (flukes). When cutaneous involvement occurs, it usually involves genital skin. *Schistosoma haematobium* is typically implicated.

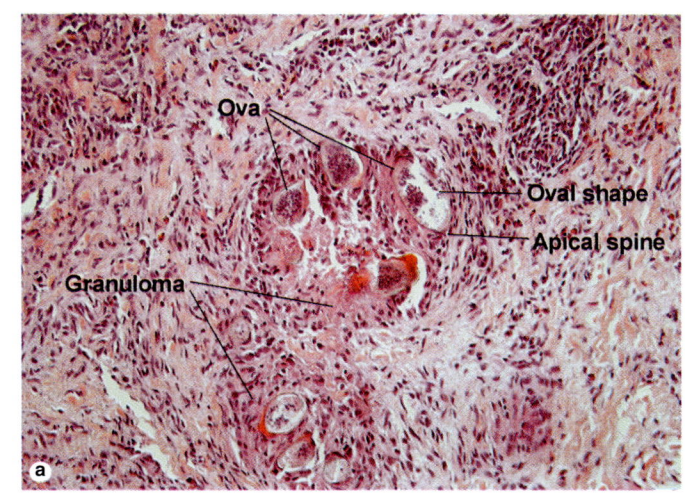

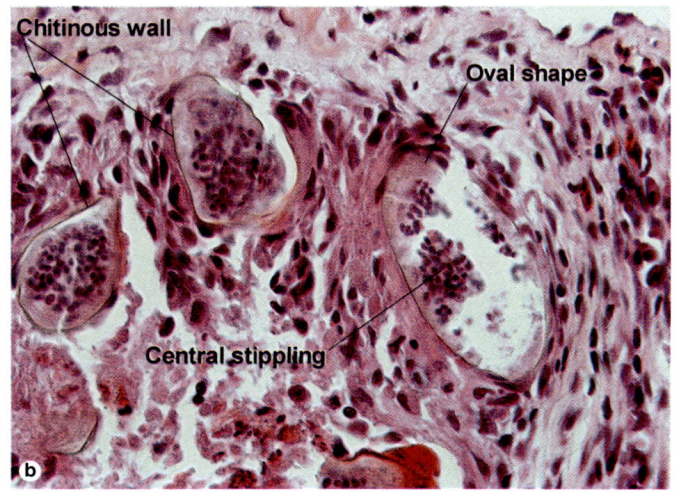

Fig 19-19 Cutaneous schistosomiasis

Dermatopathology

> **PEARL**
> Identification of schistosome ova:
> - *S. haematobium* – thin wall with thin vertical spine (Figure 19.20)
> - *S. mansoni* – thick refractile wall with thick angular spine (Figure 19.21)
> - *S. japonicum* – round with refractile wall and no visible spine (Figure 19.22)

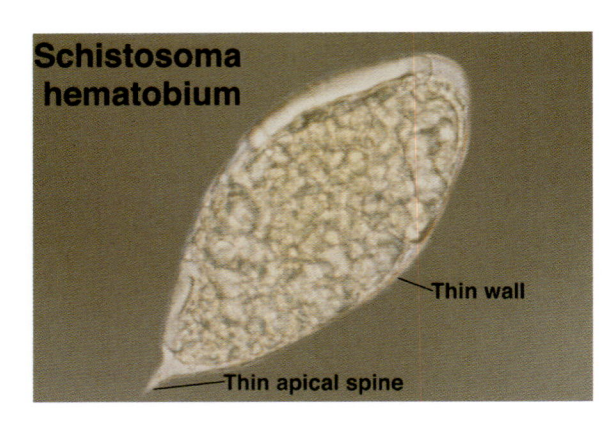

Fig 19-20 Schistosoma hematobium

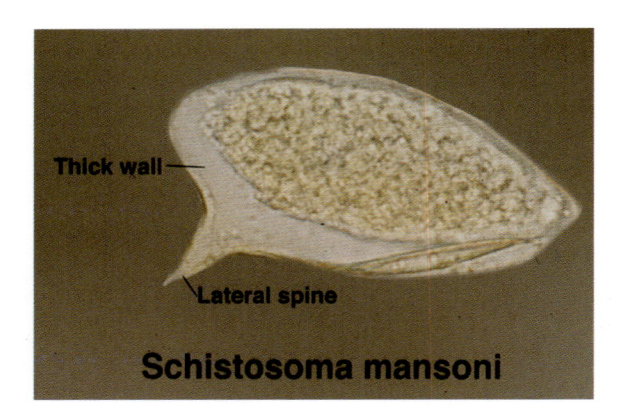

Fig 19-21 Schistosoma mansoni

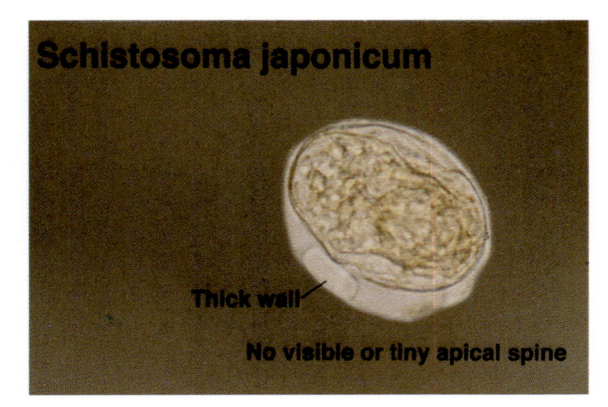

Fig 19-22 Schistosoma japonicum

Flatworms

Key features
- Secretory tegument, rows of subtegumental cells
- Calcareous bodies
- Smooth muscle
- No gut

Spirometra worms, the cause of sparganosis, are typical cestodes. They lack a gut, and must absorb nutrients through the tegumental cells. They cannot excrete waste, and so calcify it internally as calcareous bodies.

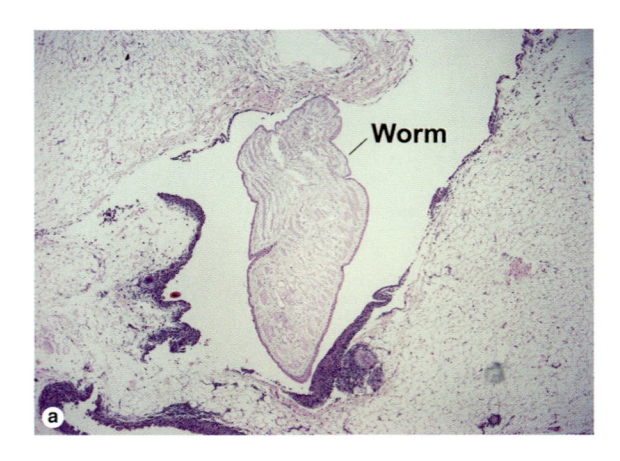

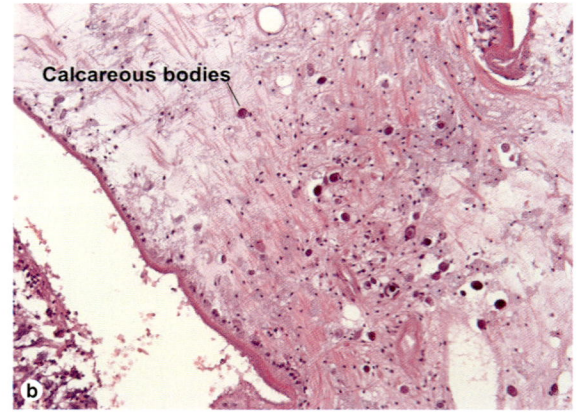

Fig 19-23 Sparganosis

Sparganum proliferum

Key features
- Multilocular cyst
- High-power views show features of a flatworm

Differential Diagnosis

The features of other tapeworm cysts are similar. Some tapeworms demonstrate scolices (rings of hooks). The cysts can degenerate to little more than a rim of epithelium.

Viral infections, helminths, and arthropods Chapter 19 301

Fig 19-24 *Sparganum proliferum* (Courtesy of Richard Bernert, MD)

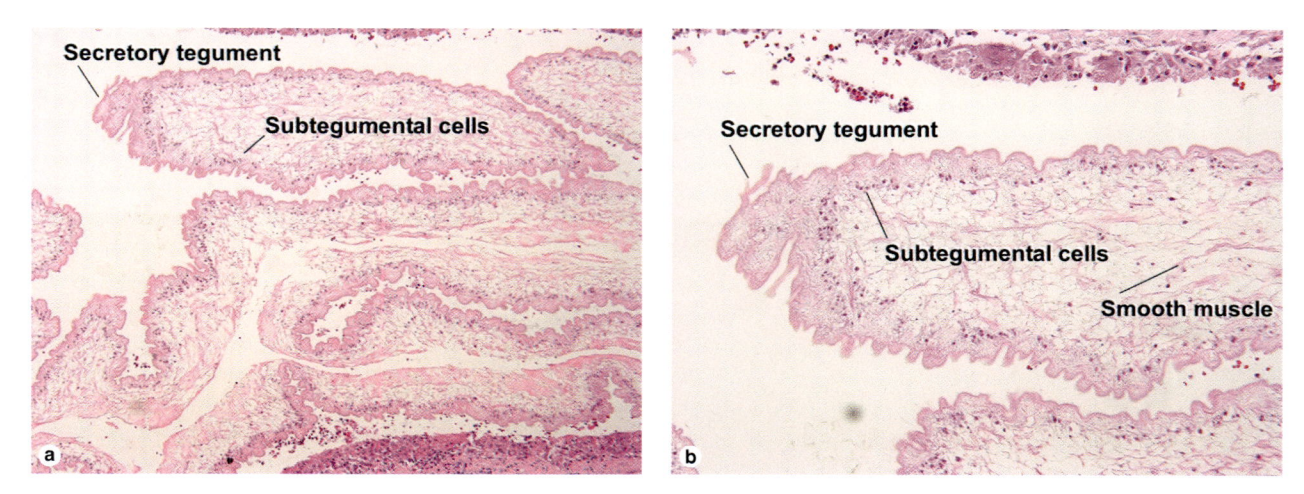

Fig 19-25 Cysticercosis for comparison

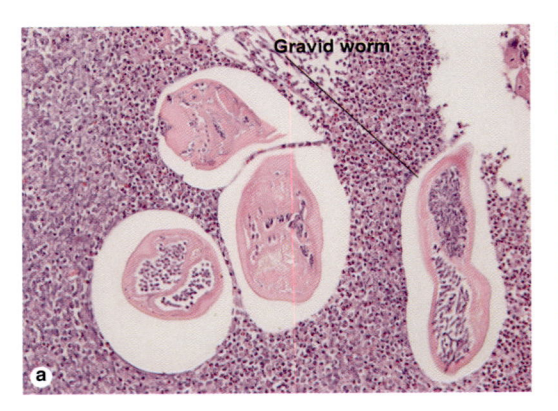

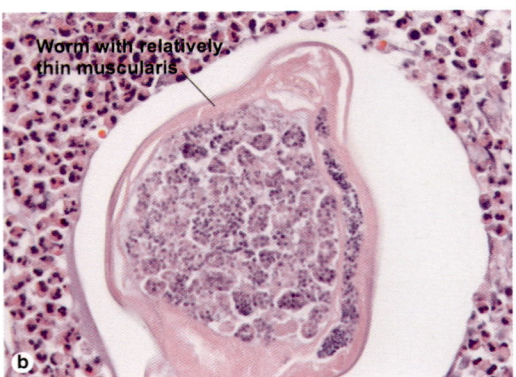

Fig 19-26 Elephantiasis (courtesy of Brooke Army Medical Center teaching file)

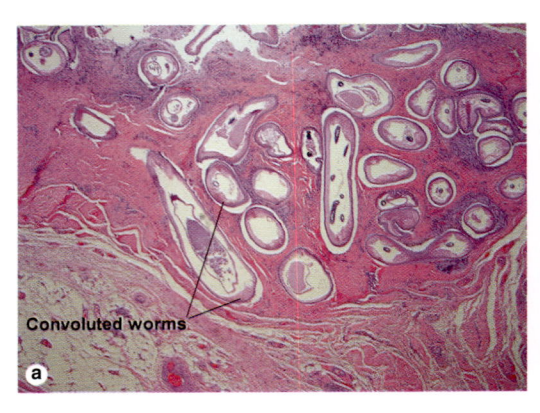

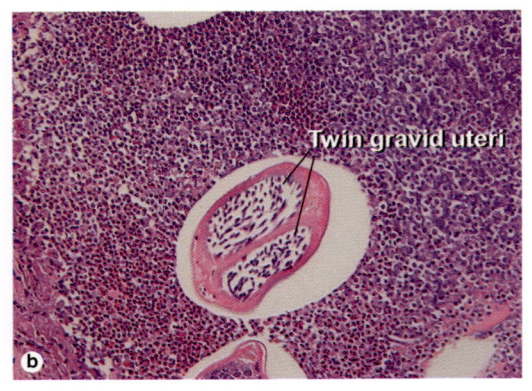

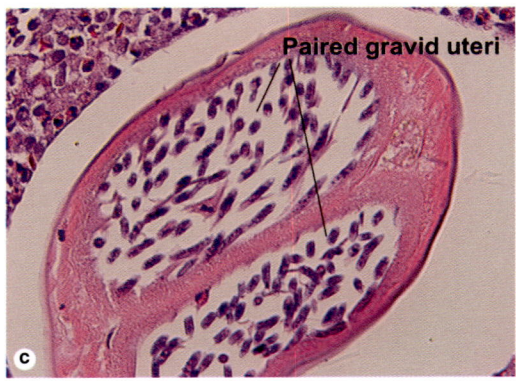

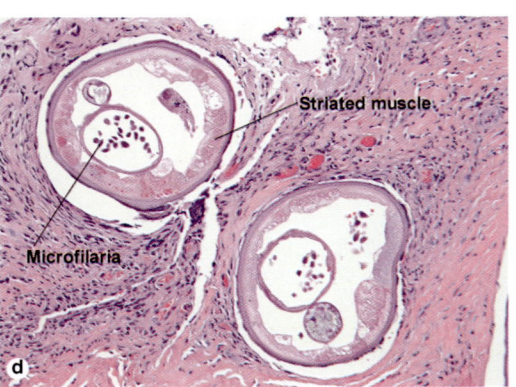

Fig 19-27 Onchocercoma

Elephantiasis

Key features

- Filarial roundworm within lymphatic vessel
- Inflammatory response leads to lymphedema

Onchocerciasis

Onchocerciasis is caused by *Onchocerca volvulus*, an obligate human pathogen spread by *Simulium* blackflies.

Onchocercoma

Key features

- Well-defined ball of convoluted worms
- Male and female
- Females gravid
- Thin layer of striated muscle
- Corrugated cuticle

An onchocercoma represents a "mating ball" of convoluted worms. The females demonstrate microfilaria within the paired uteri. Because of their thin musculature they have been likened to married adults who no longer go to the gym and have "gone

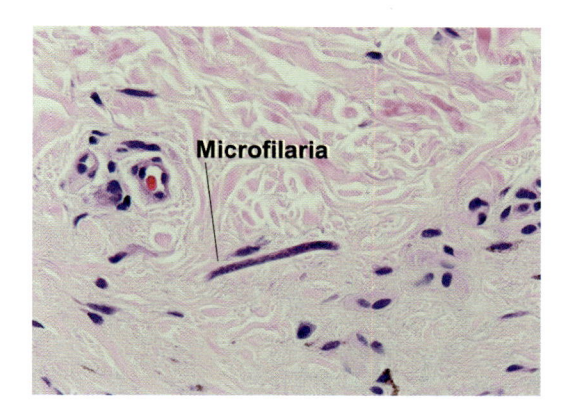

Viral infections, helminths, and arthropods Chapter **19** 303

Fig 19-28 *Onchocerca* microfilaria

to flab." This is in stark contrast to zoonotic dirofilarial worms that possess a thick muscular layer. In human dirofilarial infestations, a solitary "bachelor" worm is typically identified. Like other bachelors (with little to do besides work out at the gym) the musculature is well developed.

Onchocerca microfilaria

> **Key features**
> - Large microfilaria in lymphatics and free in the dermis
> - Large cephalic and caudal spaces
> - Paired oval terminal nuclei

Dirofilariasis

> **Key features**
> - Thick muscular layer interrupted by lateral cords
> - Internal chitinous ridge

Early lesions may demonstrate abscesses with a mix of neutrophils and eosinophils. Later biopsies show a 1–3 cm

Table 19-1 Ridge patterns of *Dirofilaria* species

Species	Ridge pattern
D. tenuis	Wide/broken
D. repens	Narrow/sharp
D. ursi	Spaced far apart/round
D. immitis	None

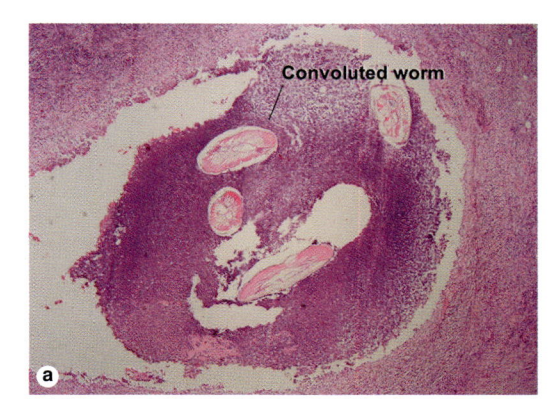

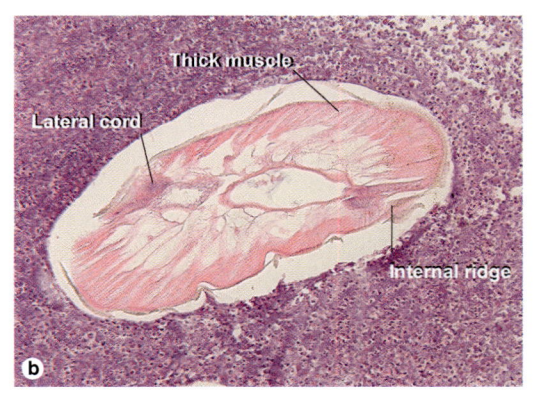

Fig 19-29 Subcutaneous dirofilariasis

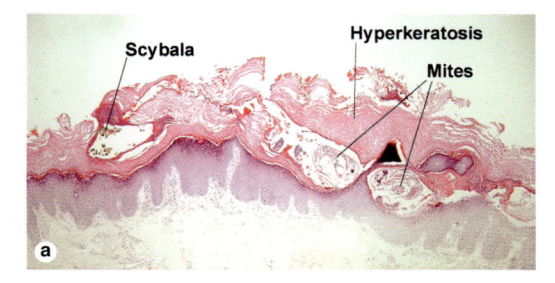

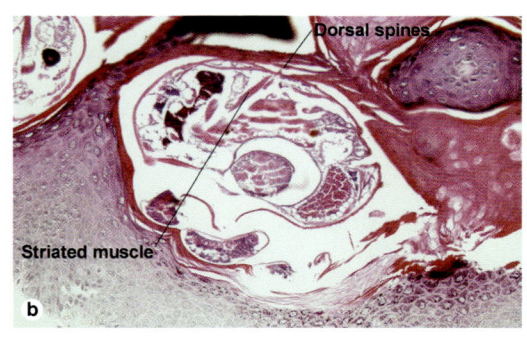

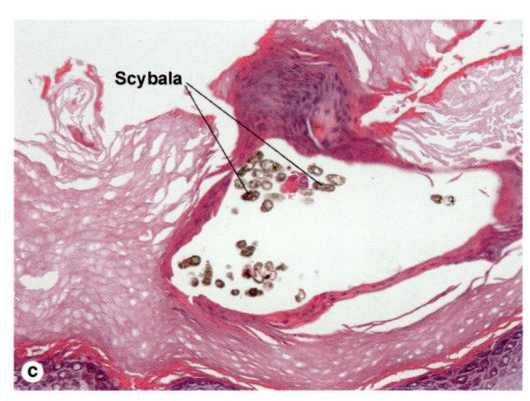

Fig 19-30 Scabies

Dermatopathology

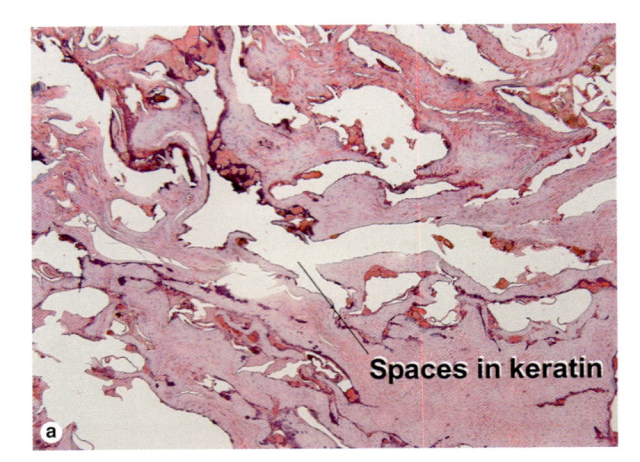

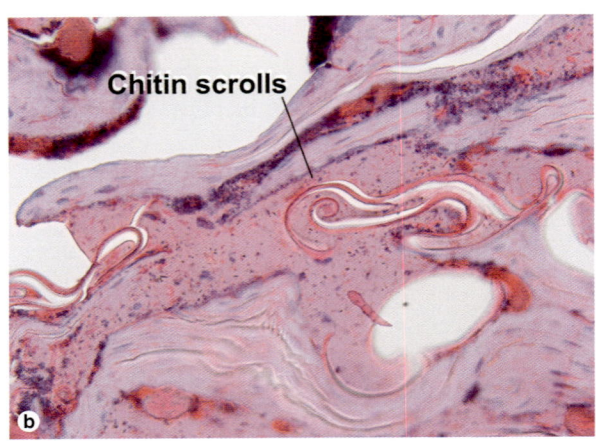

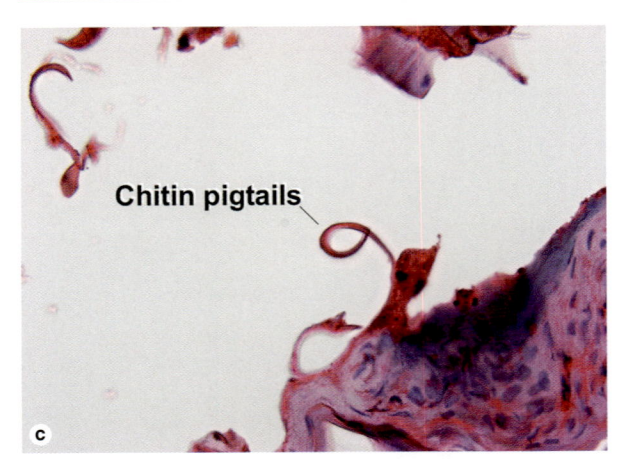

Fig 19-31 Crusted ("Norwegian") scabies

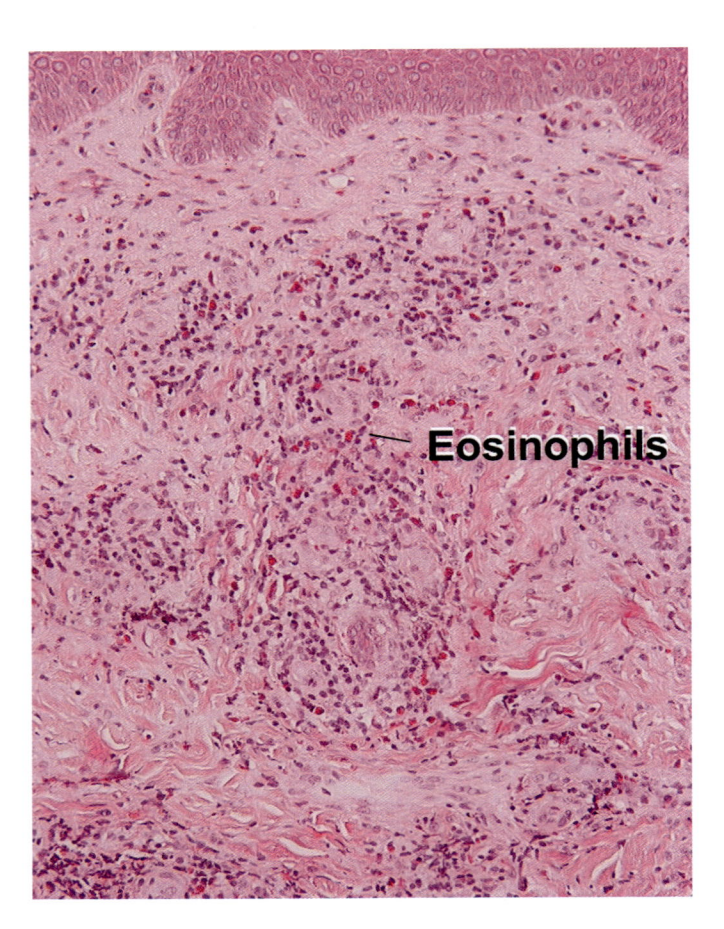

(a) Spaces in keratin
(b) Chitin scrolls
(c) Chitin pigtails

Fig 19-32 Insect bite — Eosinophils

granulomatous nodule surrounded by dense eosinophilic fibrin. Because humans are accidental hosts, there is only a single adult worm, and reproduction cannot occur. Microfilaria are not seen. Most human cases are associated with *Dirofilaria tenuis*. *Aedes*, *Anopheles*, and *Culex* mosquitoes act as vectors for most *Dirofilaria*. *D. ursi* is transmitted by *Simulium* blackflies.

All *Dirofilaria* demonstrate an internal lateral thickening of the cuticle in the area of the lateral cords. In *D. tenuis*, it appears as a prominent 10 μm pointed ridge. The cuticle is multilayered with criss-cross fibers at right angles. A gut is present, and twin non-gravid uteri are noted in females. At the ends of the worm, longitudinal ridges are absent. In this area, the uteri form loops, with four or more seen in cross-section.

Arthropods

Scabies

> **Key features**
> - Mite, ova, or scybala in stratum corneum
> - Chitin scrolls and pigtails
> - Dermal infiltrate may resemble an insect bite
> - Subepidermal bulla with eosinophils occasionally present

The dermal host response to scabies mites often resembles an insect bite reaction. There may be a wedge-shaped perivascular lymphoid infiltrate with eosinophils. The diagnosis rests on demonstration of the mite, eggs, or feces. Oval spaces in the stratum corneum should prompt deeper sections looking for an intact mite. Fragmented mites and ova curl inward, forming scrolls in the stratum corneum. Intact mites have internal striated muscle and dorsal spines. In crusted scabies, many mites are seen within a thick and crusted stratum corneum.

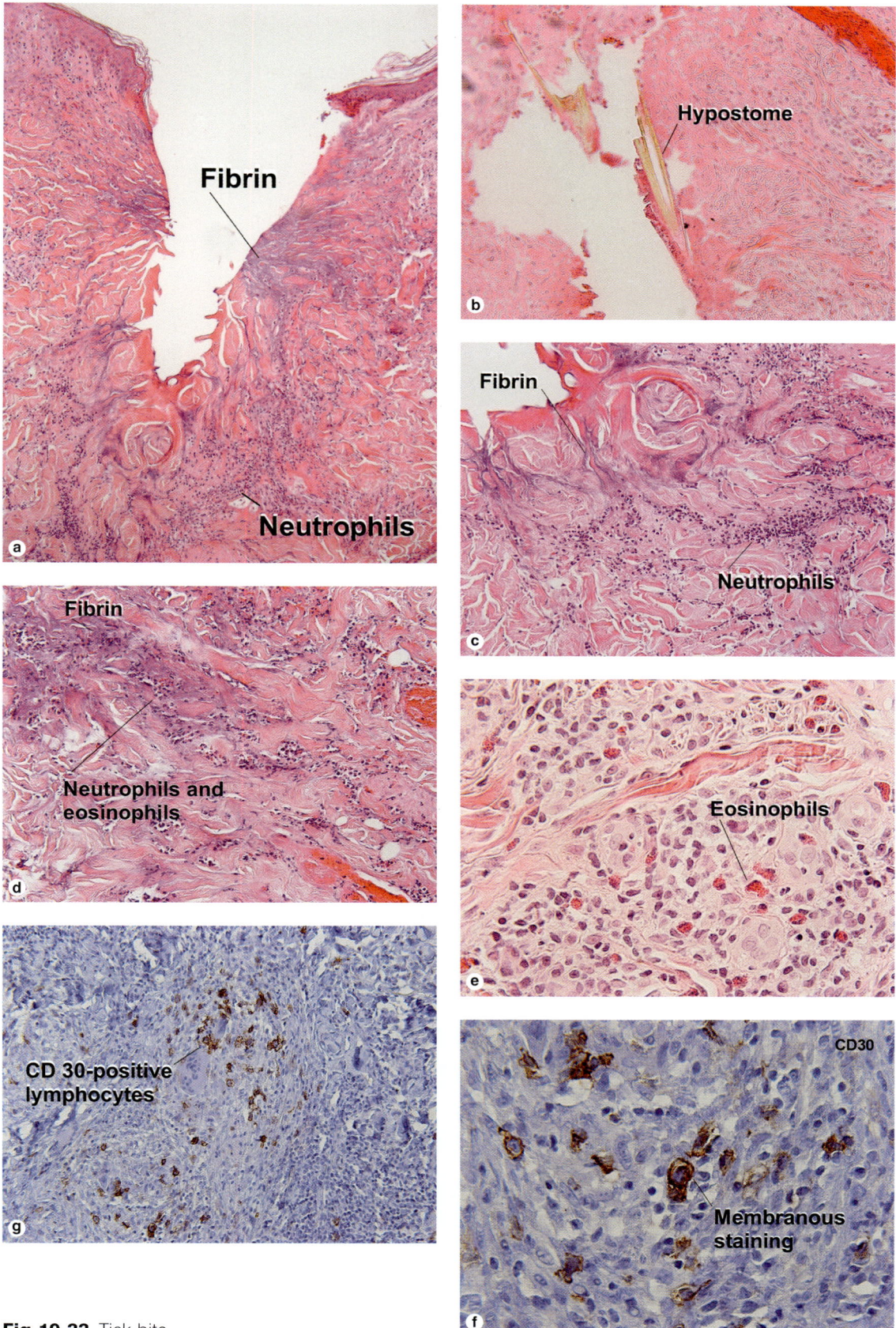

Viral infections, helminths, and arthropods   Chapter 19   305

Fig 19-33 Tick bite

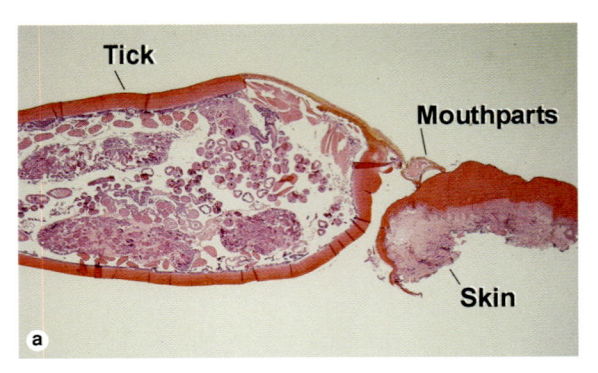

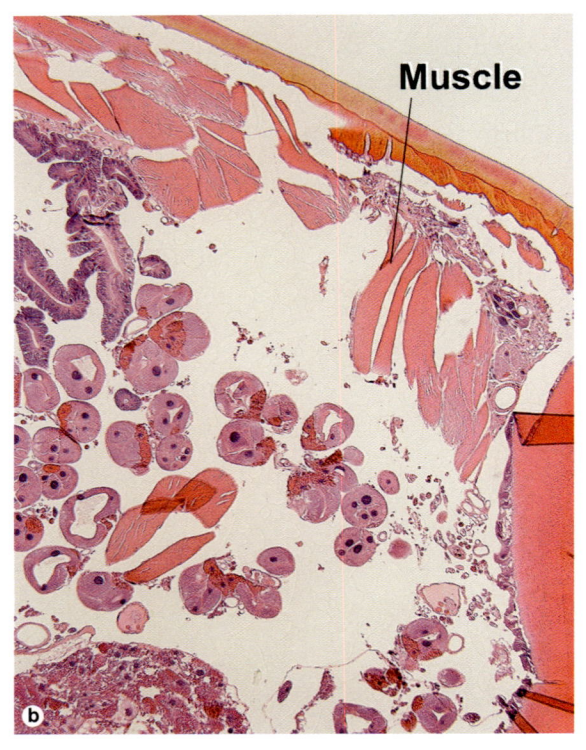

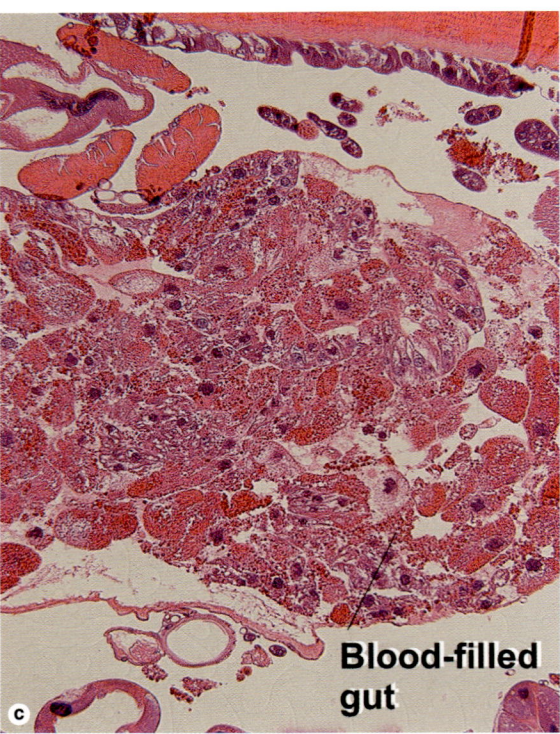

Fig 19-34 Tick

PEARL
Scabies can mimic bullous pemphigoid with eosinophil-filled bullae and positive immunofluorescence. In children, scabies can induce a Langerhans cell infiltrate and mimic Langerhans cell histiocytosis. Cases with CD30+ cells can mimic lymphomatoid papulosis.

Bites and stings
Insect bite
Key features
- Dense wedge-shaped perivascular lymphoid infiltrate
- Eosinophils
- Variable vascular damage
- Variable atypical lymphocytes

Insect sting
Key features
- Findings are highly variable
- Fire ant stings produce an urticarial reaction, followed by a late-phase reaction with fibrin and eosinophils or a neutrophil-filled pustule

Tick bite
Key features
- Wedge-shaped area of necrosis
- Early-stage neutrophilic
- Late-stage polymorphous with variable eosinophils and atypical lymphocytes
- CD30+ cells may be numerous
- Variable vascular damage

Viral infections, helminths, and arthropods   Chapter 19

Tick

Key features

- Pigmented mouthparts embedded in skin
- Neutrophilic inflammation and necrosis of the dermis
- Thick chitinous wall
- Striated muscle
- Blood-filled gut

Spider bite

Key features

- Findings are highly variable
- Brown recluse bites demonstrate cutaneous necrosis with an underlying neutrophilic band, and variable small and large vessel vasculitis

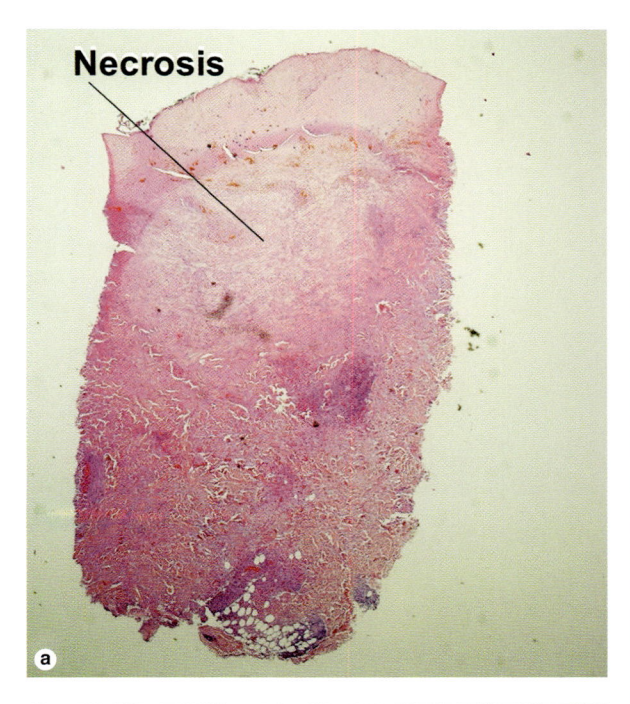

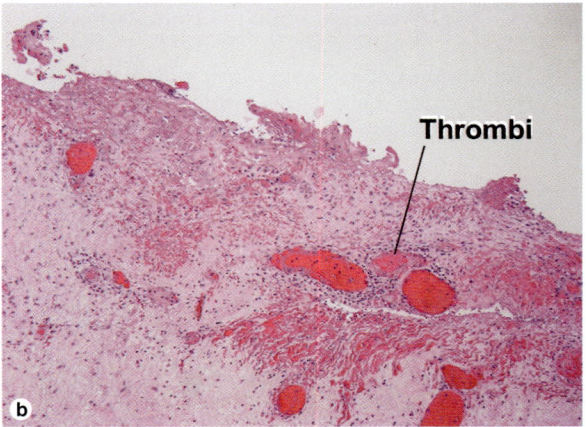

Myiasis

Key features

- Fly larva with thick corrugated chitinous wall
- Pigmented setae
- Striated muscle
- Gut

Tungiasis

Key features

- Acral skin
- Embedded organism near surface
- Gravid female flea
- Red hollow tubules
- Blood in gut
- Striated muscle

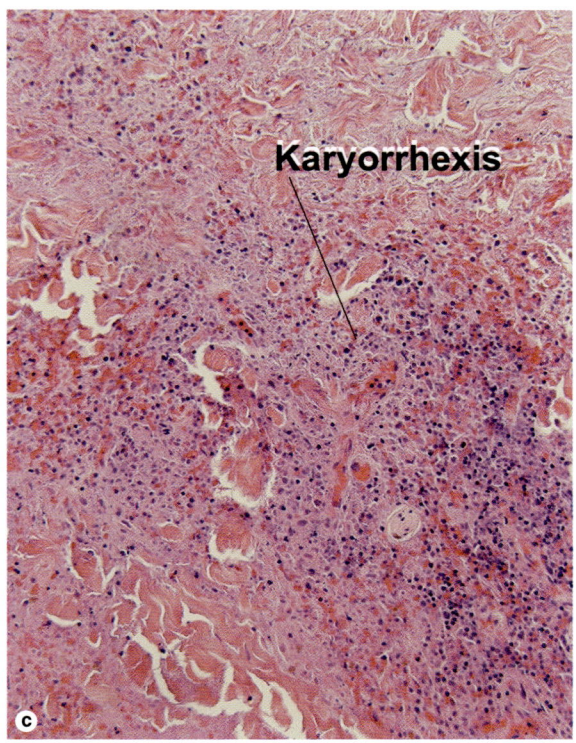

Fig 19-35 Brown recluse bite

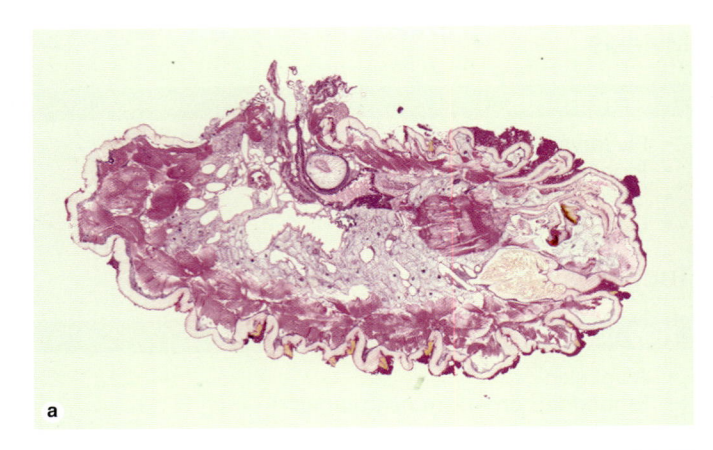

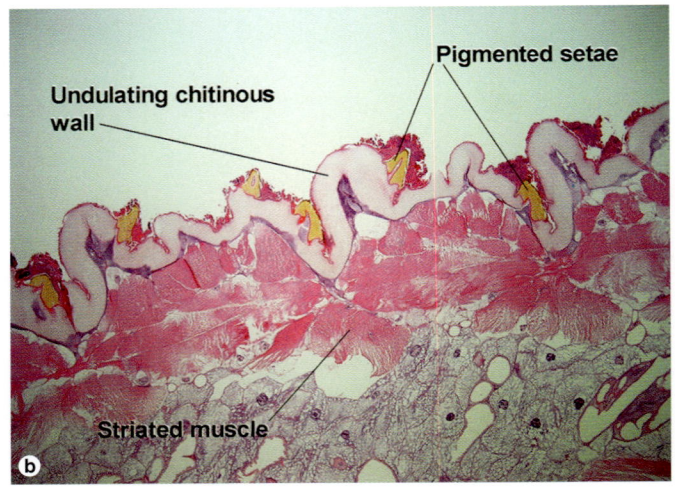

Fig 19-36 Myiasis

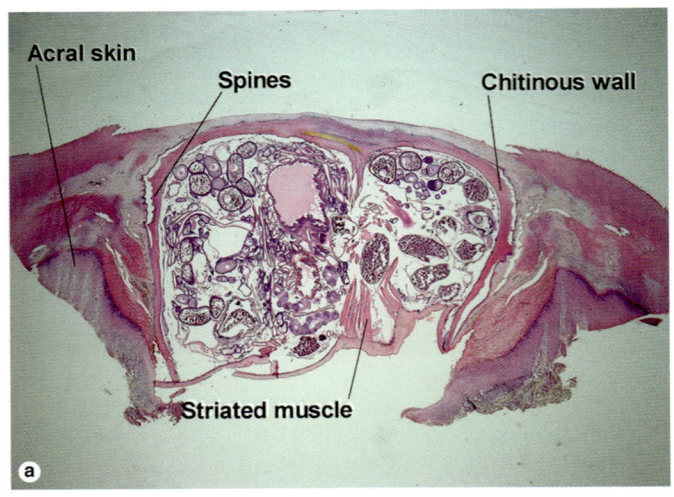

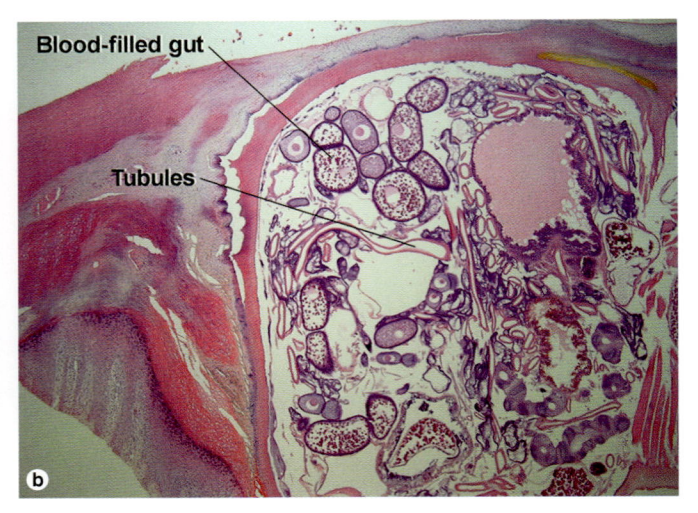

Fig 19-37 Tungiasis

Further reading

Bayer-Garner IB. Monkeypox virus: histologic, immunohistochemical and electron-microscopic findings. J Cutan Pathol 2005;32(1):28–34.

Brar BK, Pall A, Gupta RR. Bullous scabies mimicking bullous pemphigoid. J Dermatol 2003;30(9): 694–696.

Burch JM, Krol A, Weston WL. Sarcoptes scabiei infestation misdiagnosed and treated as Langerhans cell histiocytosis. Pediatr Dermatol 2004;21(1):58–62.

Burroughs RF, Elston DM. What's eating you? Human Dirofilaria infections. Cutis 2003;72(4):269–272.

Elston DM, Eggers JS, Schmidt WE, et al. Histological findings after brown recluse spider envenomation. Am J Dermatopathol 2000;22(3):242–246.

Fagan WA, Collins PC, Pulitzer DR. Verrucous herpes virus infection in human immunodeficiency virus patients. Arch Pathol Lab Med 1996;120(10):956–958.

Groves RW, Wilson-Jones E, MacDonald DM. Human orf and milkers' nodule: a clinicopathologic study. J Am Acad Dermatol 1991;25(4):706–711.

Mukherjee A, Ahmed NH, Samantaray JC, et al. A rare case of cutaneous larva migrans due to Gnathostoma sp. Indian J Med Microbiol 2012;30(3):356–358.

Nikkels AF, Snoeck R, Rentier B, et al. Chronic verrucous varicella zoster virus skin lesions: clinical, histological, molecular and therapeutic aspects. Clin Exp Dermatol 1999;24(5):346–353.

Soyer HP, Schadendorf D, Cerroni L, et al. Verrucous cysts: histopathologic characterization and molecular detection of human papillomavirus-specific DNA. J Cutan Pathol 1993;20(5):411–417.

Uthida-Tanaka AM, Sampaio MC, Velho PE, et al. Subcutaneous and cerebral cysticercosis. J Am Acad Dermatol 2004;50:S14.

Yang Y, Ellis MK, McManus DP. Immunogenetics of human echinococcosis. Trends Parasitol 2012;28(10):447–454.

Fibrous tumors

Dirk M. Elston

Chapter 20

Many additional entities are included in the on-line atlas of fibrous and soft tissue tumors that accompanies this book.

Dermatofibroma

Key features

- Interstitial spindle cell proliferation
- Collagen trapping
- Overlying plate-like acanthosis
- Follicular induction common
- Ringed lipidized siderophages may be present
- Factor XIIIa+
- CD34−

All dermatofibromas demonstrate a proliferation of fibrohistiocytic cells. A curlicue pattern is typical. Another typical feature is that some areas of the tumor will be densely cellular, while others are sclerotic and hypocellular. The overlying epidermis is acanthotic and often demonstrates primitive follicular germs or sebaceous follicles. At the periphery of the tumor, collagen trapping (collagen balls) can be seen. The tumor may extend into the superficial fat in a lacy pattern.

When present, ringed lipidized siderophages are pathognomonic for dermatofibroma. These cells are like Touton giant cells with hemosiderin. They have central pink cytoplasm surrounded by a wreath of nuclei. There is both lipid and hemosiderin peripheral to the ring of nuclei.

Immunostaining can be helpful to separate cellular dermatofibromas from dermatofibrosarcoma protuberans. Large stellate cells within a dermatofibroma stain for factor XIIIa. The surrounding stroma will stain for CD34, but the central tumor is negative (except for endothelial cells).

Differential Diagnosis

- Densely cellular tumors are suspicious for dermatofibrosarcoma protuberans, even if overlying acanthosis and collagen trapping are present. CD34 and factor XIIIa staining should be performed
- Long fascicles of parallel nuclei suggest a melanocytic tumor. Nodular lymphoid aggregates suggest desmoplastic malignant melanoma. S100 staining should be performed
- Corkscrew nuclei running parallel to the epidermis suggest a dermatomyofibroma

PEARLS

- Factor XIIIa is positive in dermatofibromas, fibrous papules of the face, angiofibromas, acquired digital fibrokeratomas, and pleomorphic undifferentiated sarcoma
- CD34 is positive in dermatofibrosarcoma protuberans, pleomorphic fibromas, sclerotic fibroma, spindle cell lipoma, and nephrogenic systemic fibrosis
- CD34 expression is lost in morphea

310 Dermatopathology

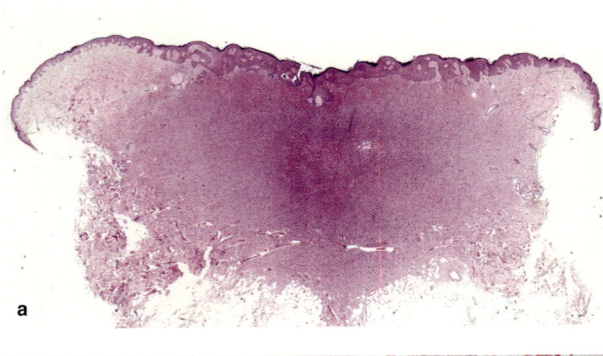

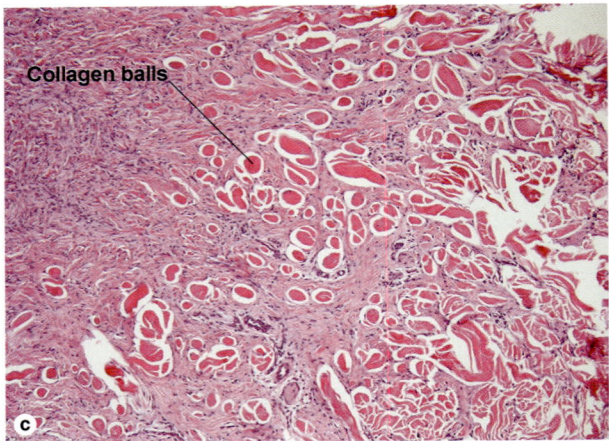

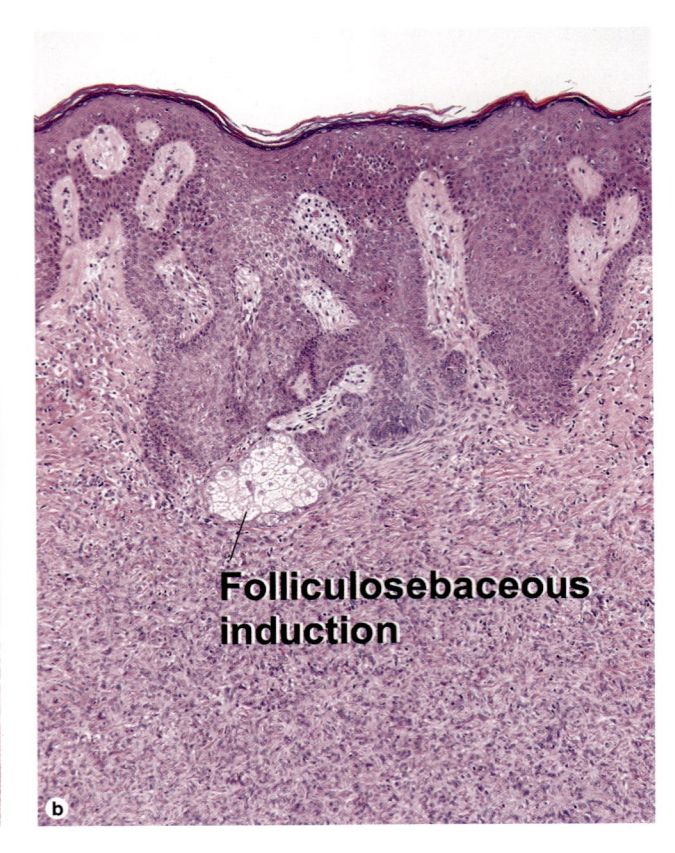

Fig 20-1 Dermatofibroma

Aneurysmal dermatofibroma (sclerosing hemangioma)

Key features

- Type of dermatofibroma
- Aneurysmal dilatation of vessels

Fibrous histiocytoma

Key features

- Type of dermatofibroma
- Large histiocytoid vesicular nuclei with prominent nucleoli

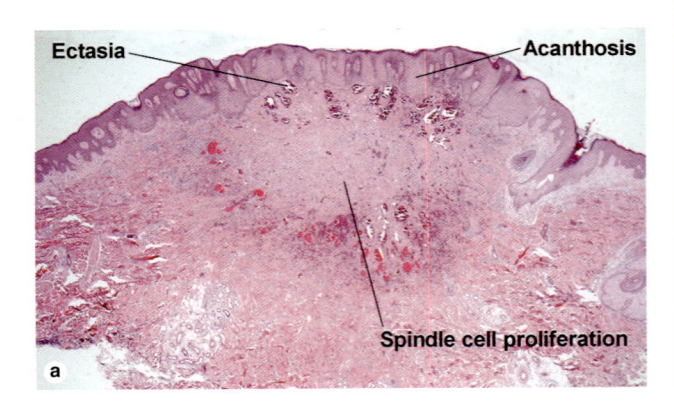

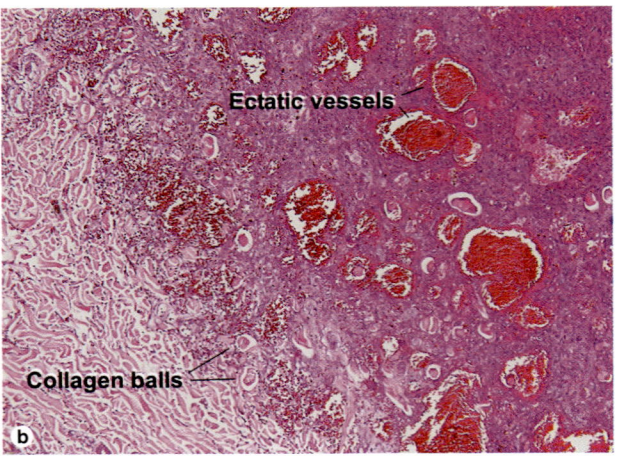

Fig 20-2 Aneurysmal dermatofibroma

Fibrous tumors Chapter 20 311

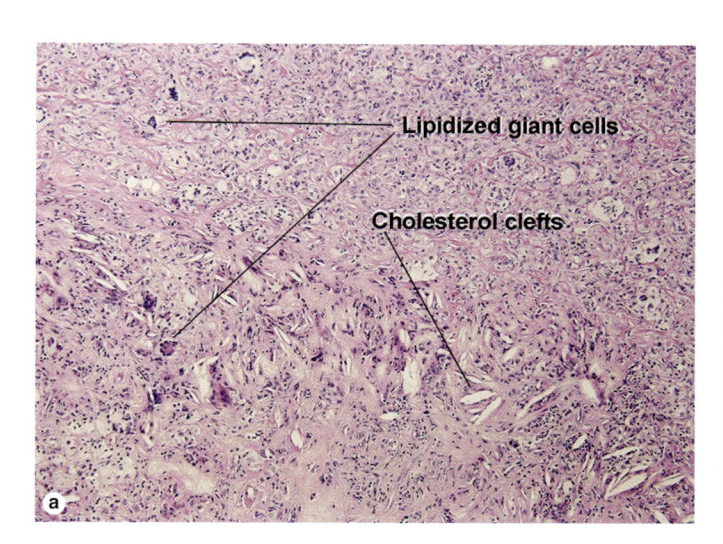

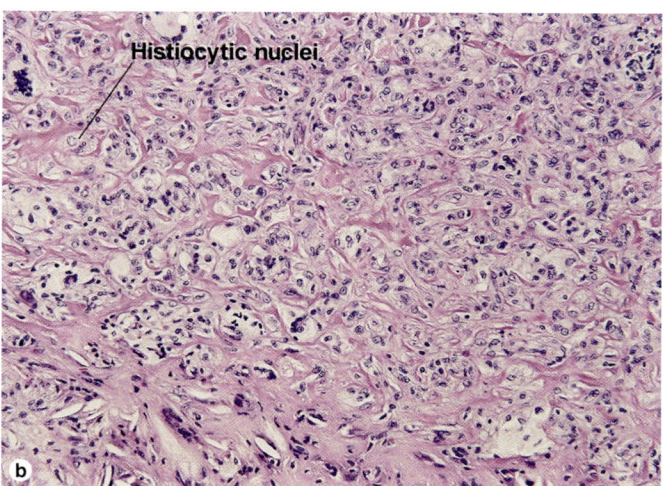

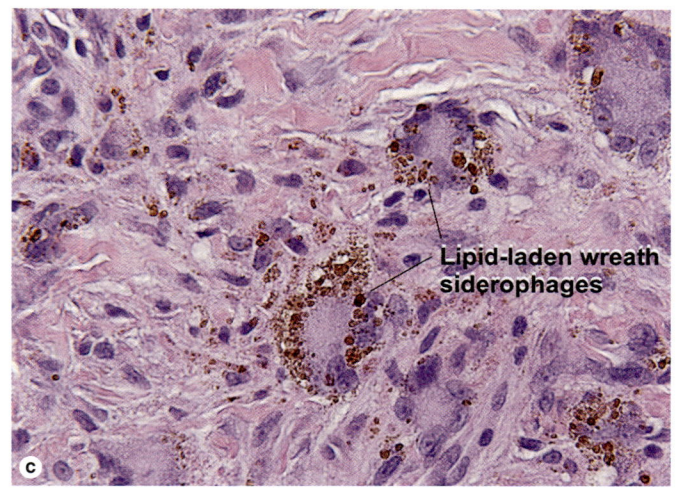

Fig 20-3 Fibrous histiocytoma

Dermatofibroma with monster cells

Key features

- Very large cells with vesicular nuclei and prominent nucleoli
- Sometimes hyperchromatic
- Despite large alarming cells, these are completely benign lesions

Adult myofibroma

Key features

- Nodules with blue centers
- Myofibroblasts
- Peripheral fibrovascular proliferation

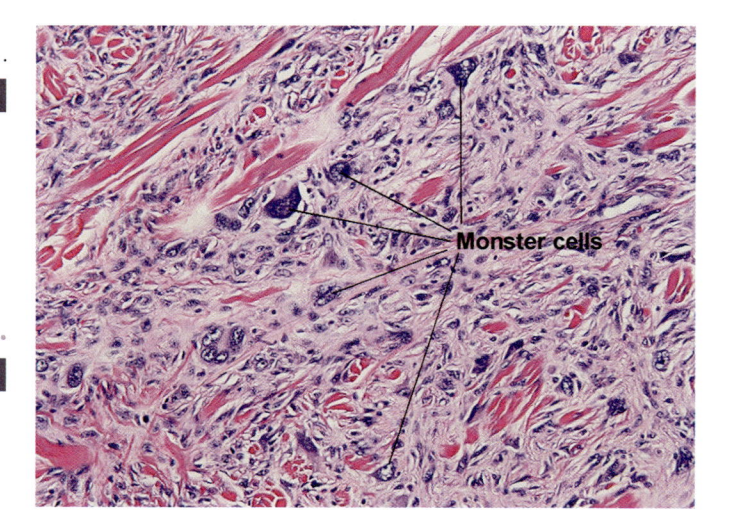

Fig 20-4 Dermatofibroma with monster cells

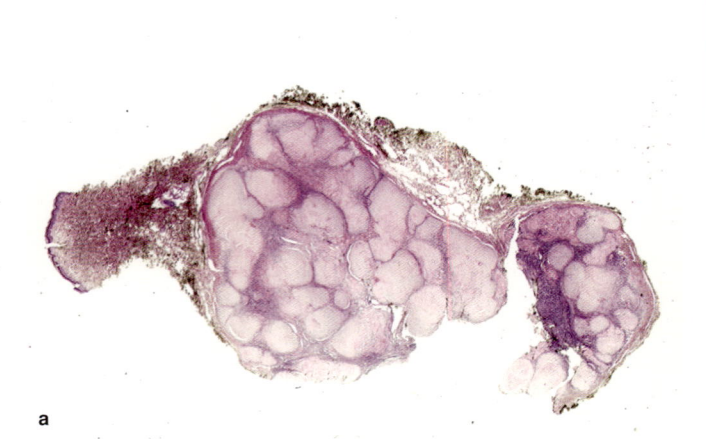

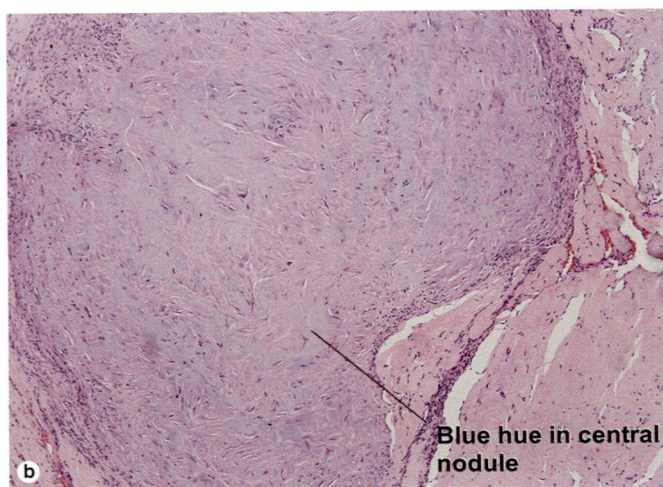

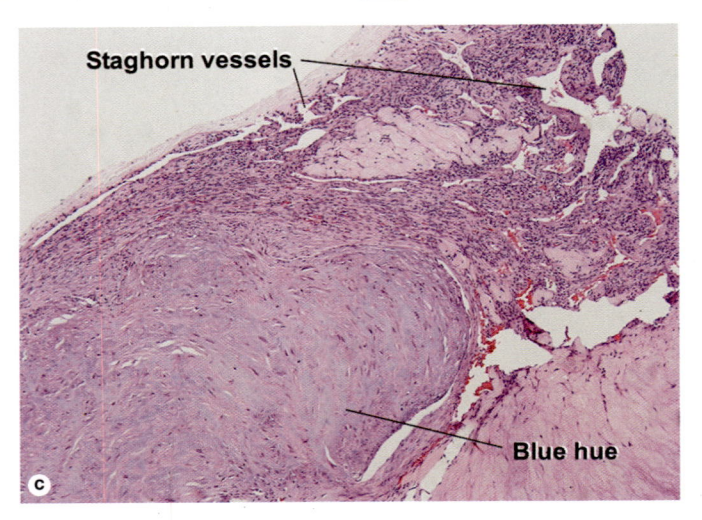

Fig 20-5 Adult myofibroma

The shade of blue in the center of the nodule resembles that of cartilage. The peripheral vascular proliferation may have staghorn vessels and resemble hemangiopericytoma.

Dermatomyofibroma

Key features

- Plaque-like tumor
- Spindle cells with east–west orientation
- Proliferation "respects" adnexal structures
- Corkscrew appearance of some myofibroblast nuclei
- Thick elastic fibers visible with Verhoeff–van Gieson stain

At scanning magnification, the most striking features of a dermatomyofibroma are the horizontal orientation of the spindle cell nuclei and the pattern of the proliferation with respect to the adnexal structures, especially hair follicles. The follicles are normal in appearance, and the proliferation extends up to each follicle, then continues on the other side without any displacement of the follicle.

Fibrous tumors | Chapter 20

Does not displace follicle

East - West orientation

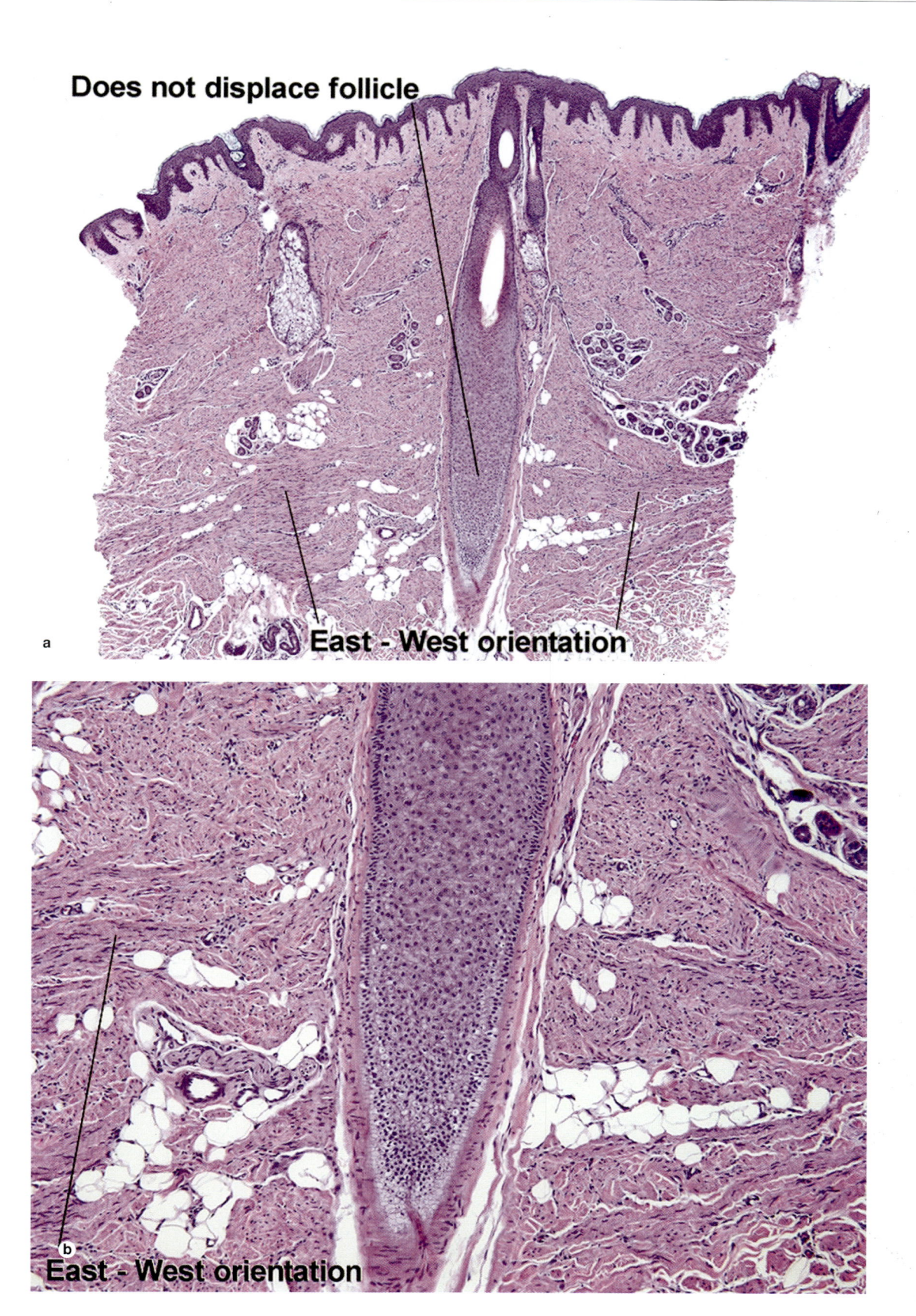

Fig 20-6 Dermatomyofibroma. (d) Elastic stain or Verhoeff-van Gieson

Continued

314　Dermatopathology

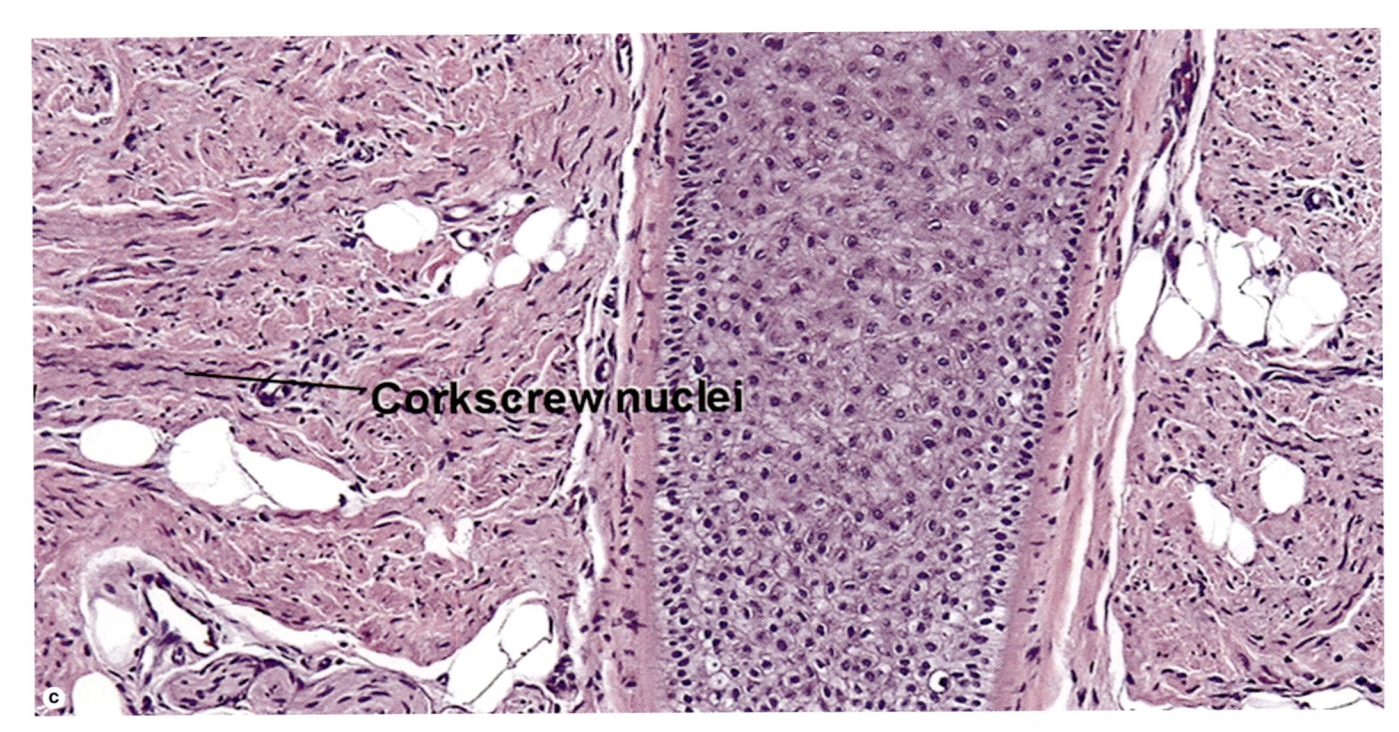

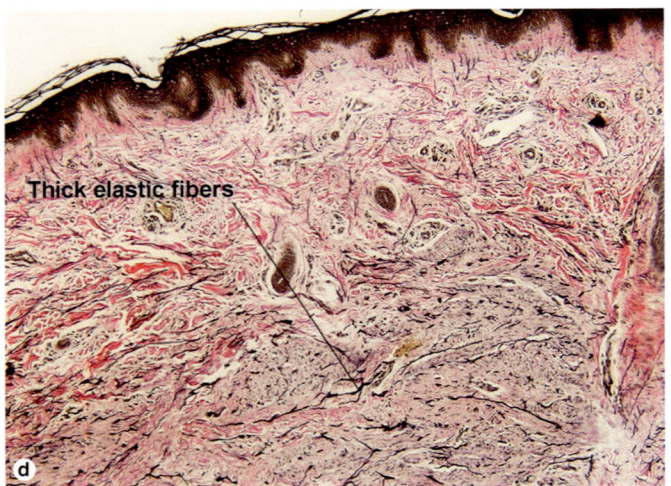

Fig 20-6, cont'd

Fibromatosis

Key features
- Myofibroblastic proliferation
- Locally infiltrative, but does not metastasize
- Corkscrew-shaped myofibroblasts

The fibromatoses include Dupuytren's (hand) contracture, Peyronie's (penis) disease and Ledderhose (foot) plantar fibromatosis. All forms demonstrate corkscrew-shaped myofibroblasts and collagen. Ledderhose disease tends to form large whorled nodules.

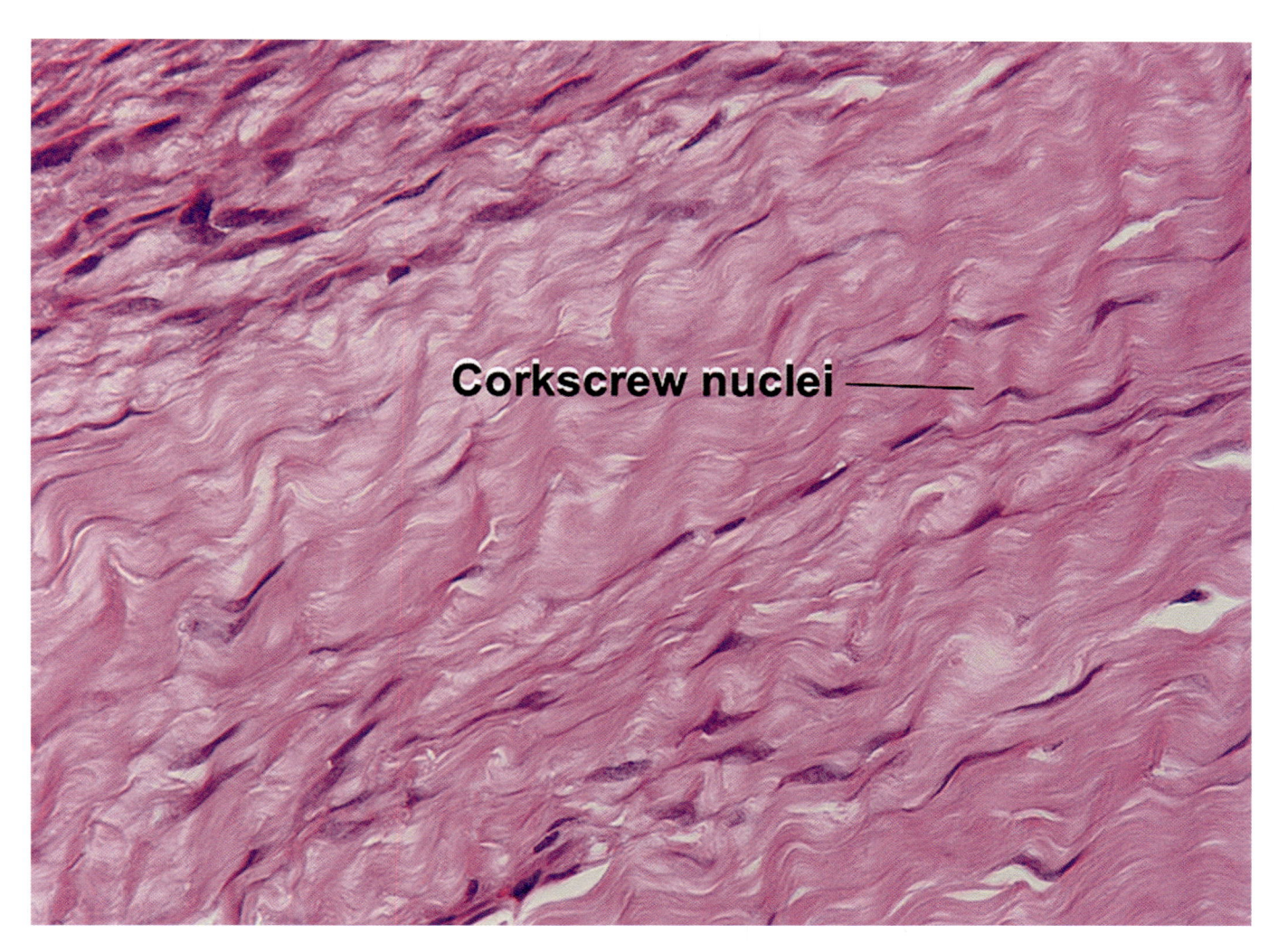

Fig 20-7 Dupuytren's contracture

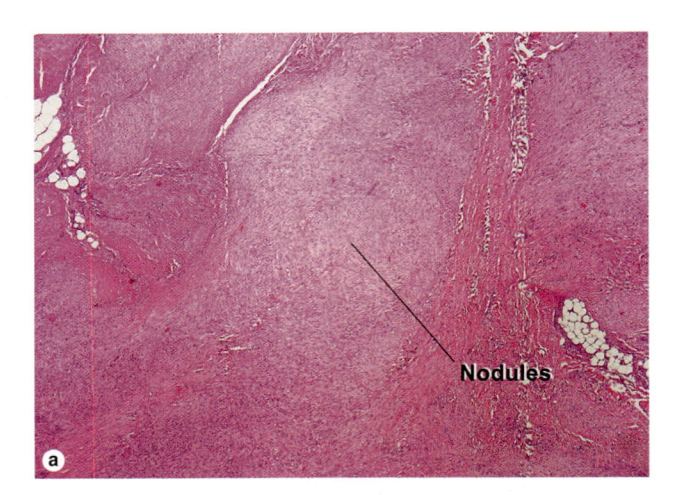

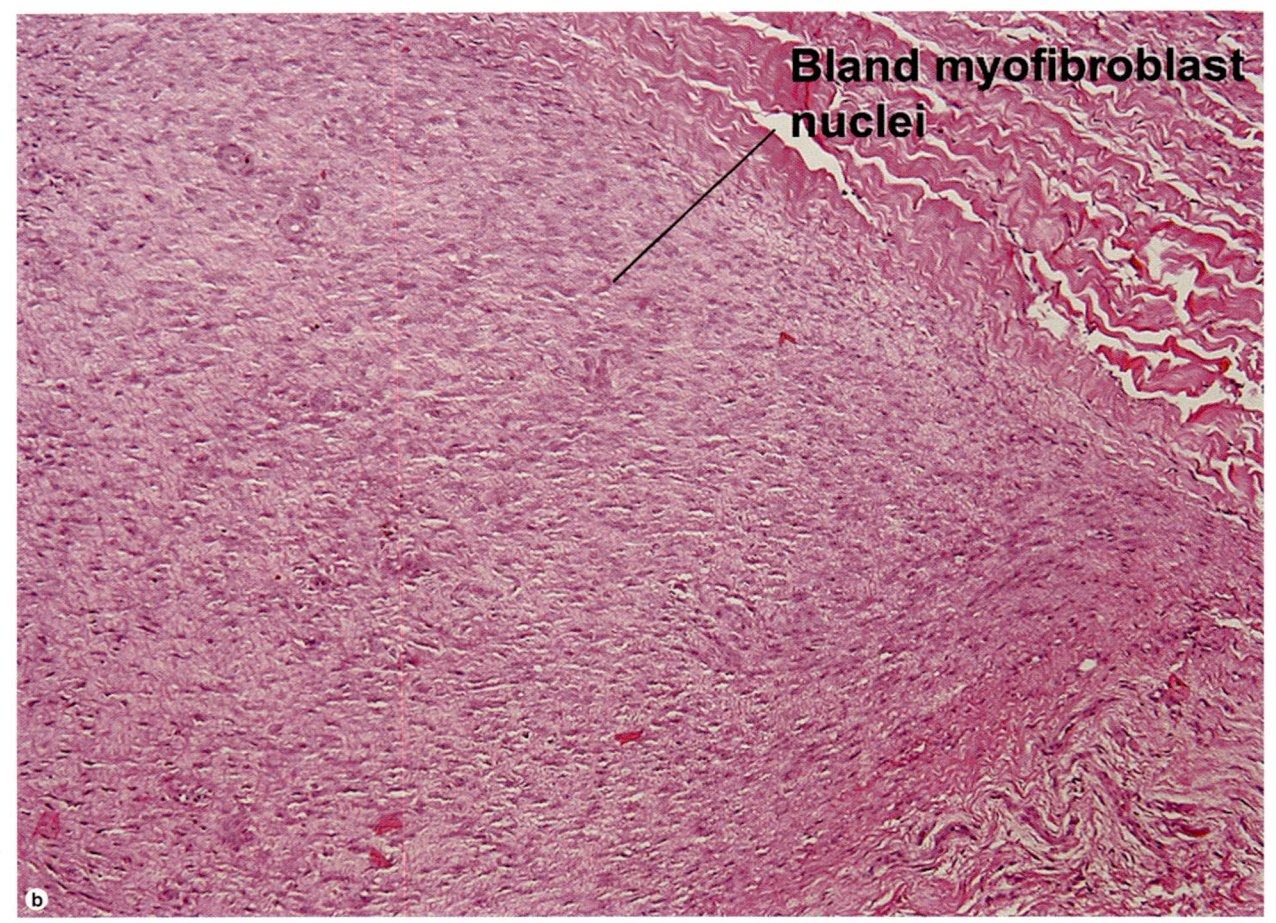

Fig 20-8 Ledderhose disease

Infantile myofibromatosis

Key features

- Myofibroblastic proliferation
- Locally infiltrative, but does not metastasize
- Corkscrew-shaped myofibroblasts

There is a tendency towards spontaneous regression. Superficial disease has an excellent prognosis. Visceral involvement may be fatal in some cases. In one series, more than half of the lesions were present at or soon after birth, approximately 80% were solitary, and 50% involved the head and neck. In the early stage, undifferentiated immature histiocytic cells may predominate. As the lesion matures, they develop characteristics of myofibroblasts. Regressing lesions become progressively less cellular and more fibrous.

Fibrous tumors Chapter 20 317

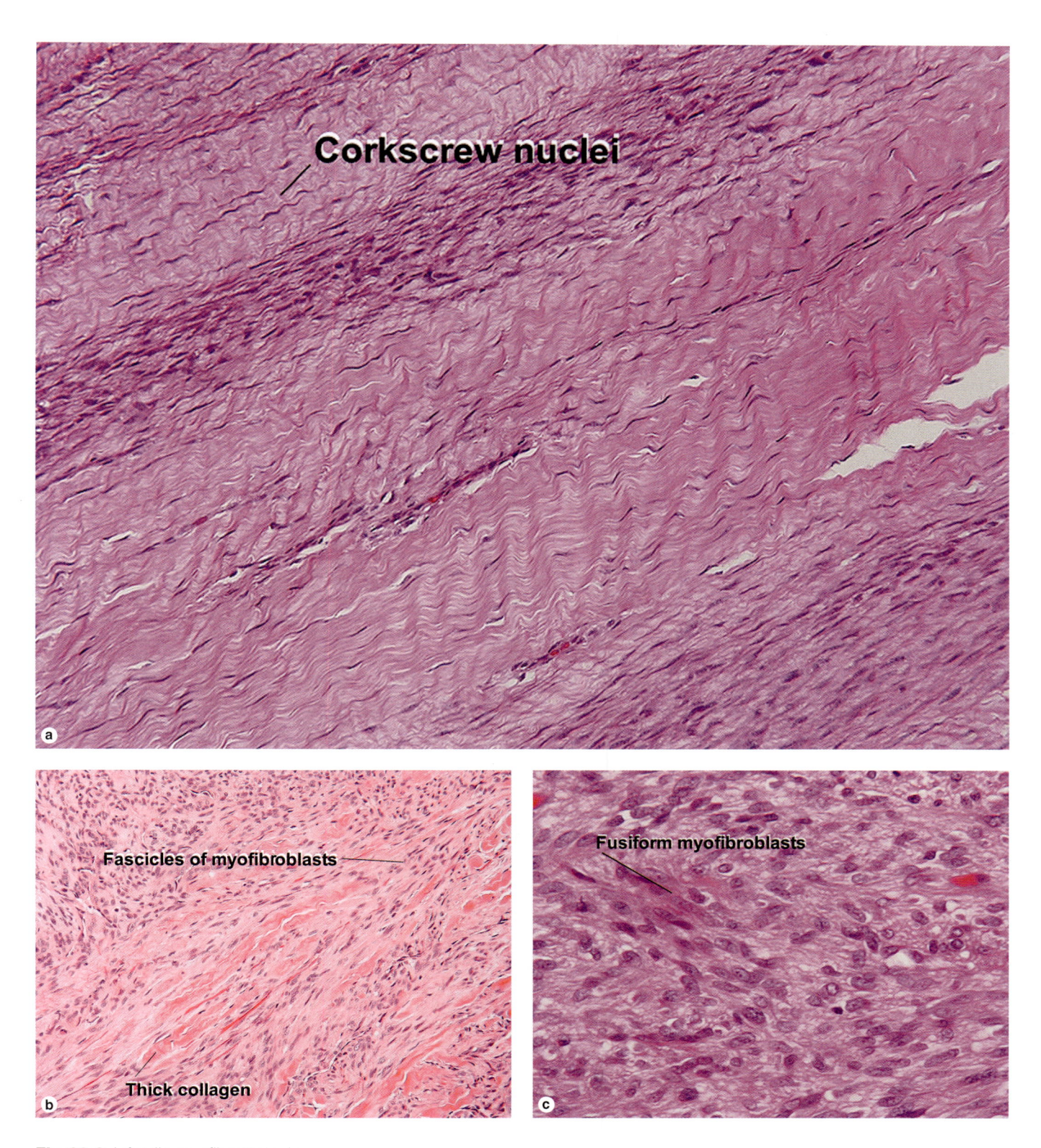

Fig 20-9 Infantile myofibromatosis

Dermatopathology

Juvenile hyaline fibromatosis

Key features

- Autosomal recessive
- Nodular skin lesions of the hands, scalp, ears, and central face
- Gingival hypertrophy
- Joint contractures and osteopenia
- Nodular hyaline fibrosis in the dermis
- Linked to *CMG2* or *ANTXR2* mutations (gene encoding capillary morphogenesis protein-2 on chromosome 4q21)

Scar

Key features

- Fibroblasts with east–west orientation
- Blood vessels with north–south orientation
- Loss of elastic tissue (see Chapter 13)

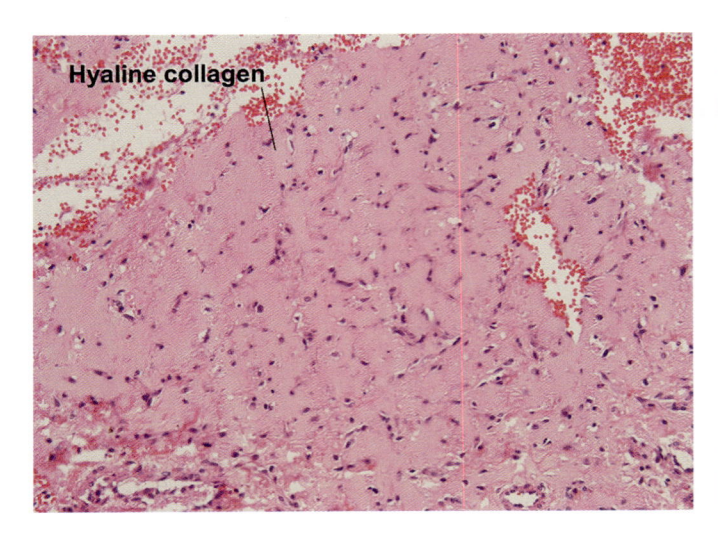

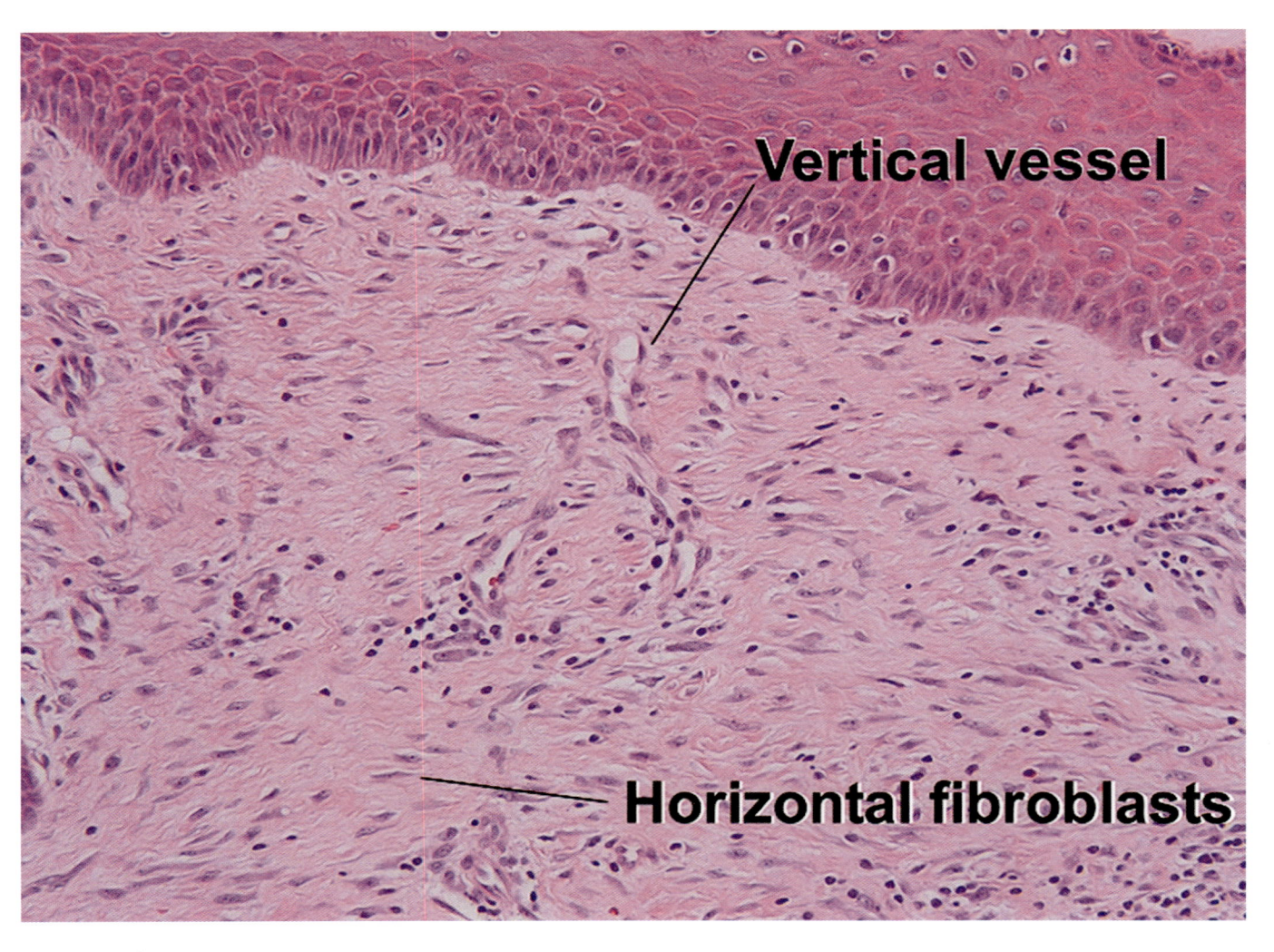

Fig 20-10 Juvenile hyaline fibromatosis

Fig 20-11 Scar

Hypertrophic scar

Key features

- Whorled proliferation of fibroblasts and blood vessels

Keloid

Key features

- Whorled proliferation of fibroblasts and blood vessels
- Central bundles of amorphous "bubble gum" collagen

Fibrous hamartoma of infancy

Key features

- Disorderly growth of benign tissues
- Myxoid areas, mature fibrous areas, and fat
- Organoid (compartmentalized) appearance
- Surrounding skin has features of "kid" skin

A young child's skin ("kid" skin) is characterized by delicate collagen bundles that stain deeply red. Many fibroblast nuclei are present. Lipocytes and adnexal structures tend to be small.

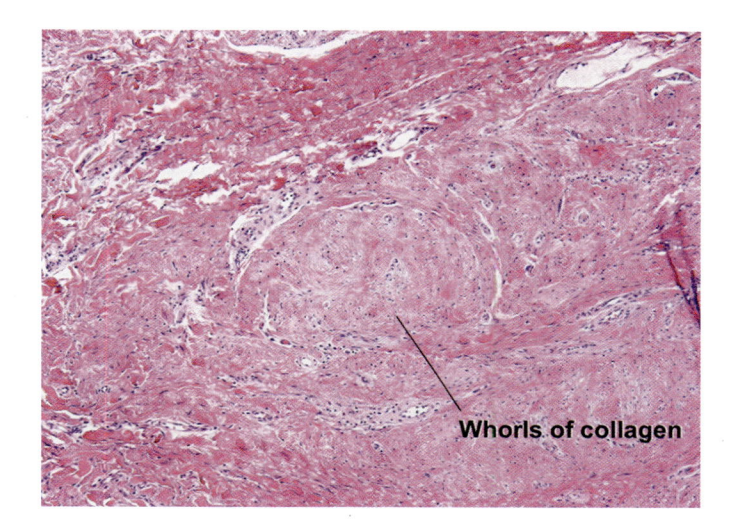

Fig 20-12 Hypertrophic scar

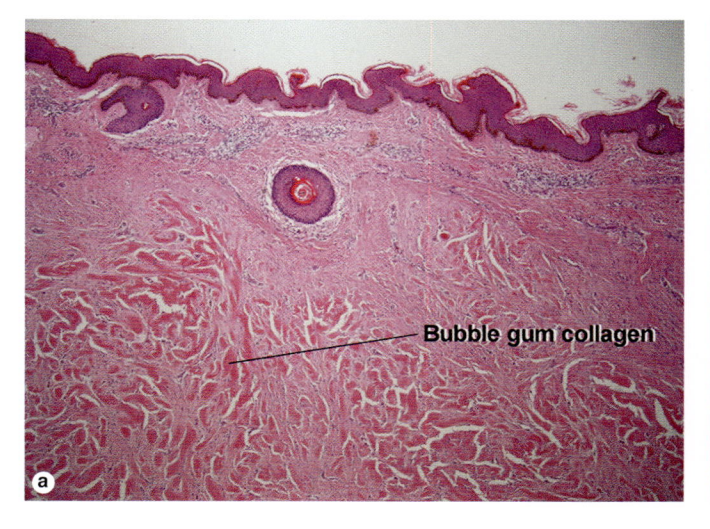

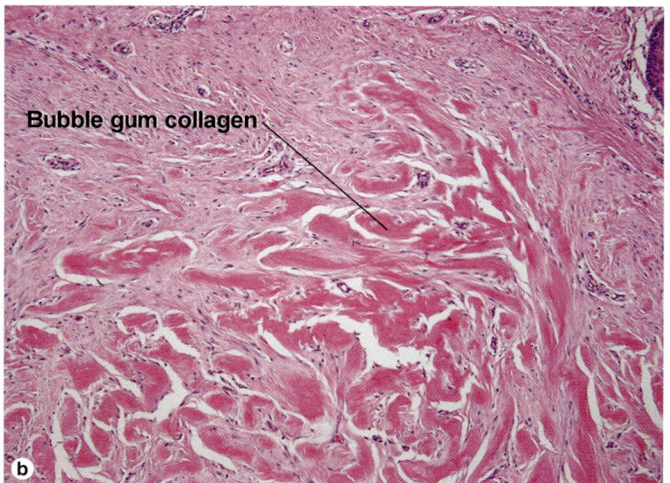

Fig 20-13 Keloid

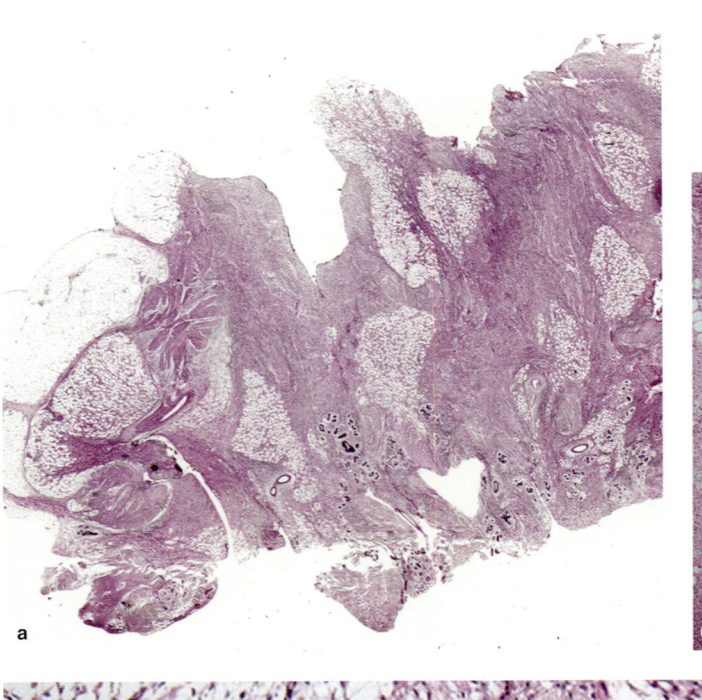

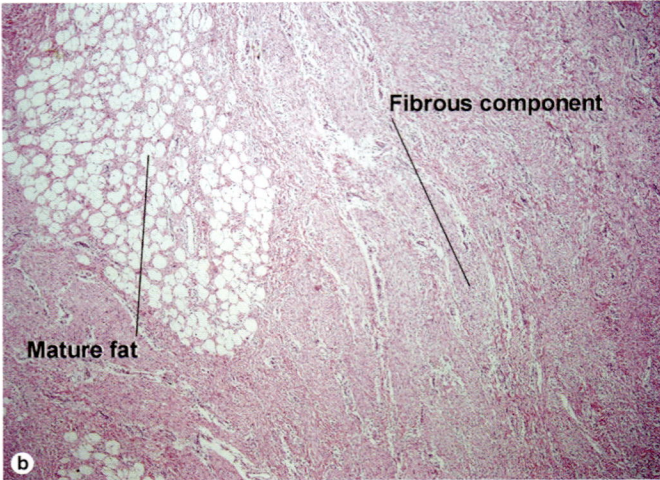

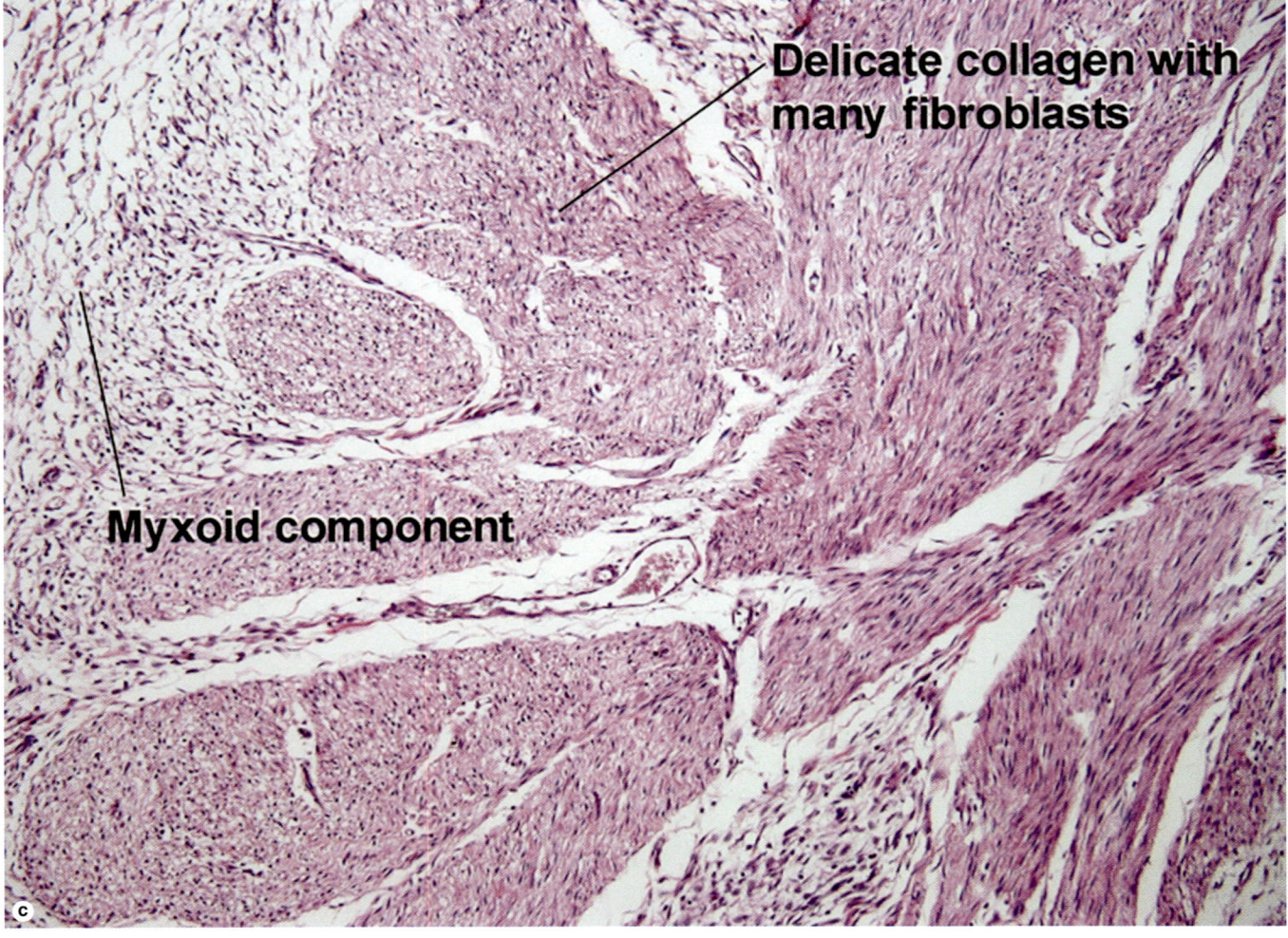

Fig 20-14 Fibrous hamartoma of infancy

Infantile digital fibroma (inclusion body fibroma)

Key features
- Acral skin
- Criss-cross fascicles
- Spindle cells with red inclusion bodies

Infantile digital fibroma is also called recurrent infantile digital fibroma or aggressive digital fibromatosis. It is benign, but often extends deeply and has a high recurrence rate after excision. The inclusions stain purple with phosphotungstic acid hematoxylin (PTAH) and red with both H&E and Masson's trichrome. They are actin positive.

Giant cell tumor of the tendon sheath

Key features
- Osteoclast-like giant cells
- Plump fibroblasts
- Focal dense collagen
- Hemosiderin pigment common

Osteoclast-like giant cells have randomly distributed nuclei. The cytoplasm stains deeply pink to amphophilic and has scalloped edges where the cell exhibits molding against adjoining tissue.

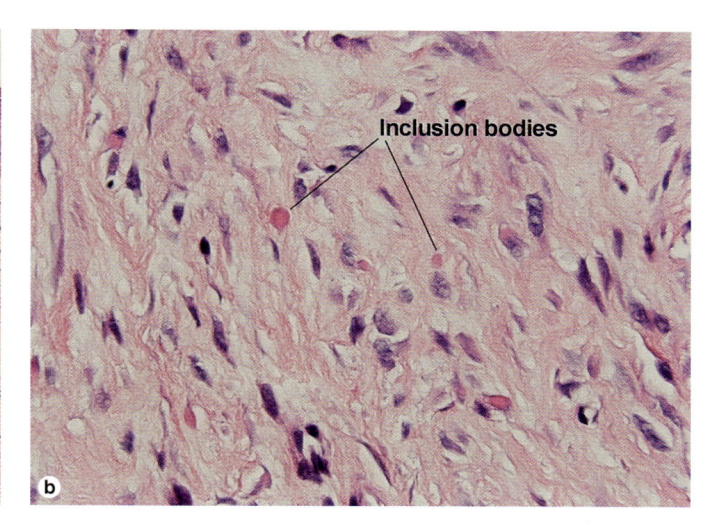

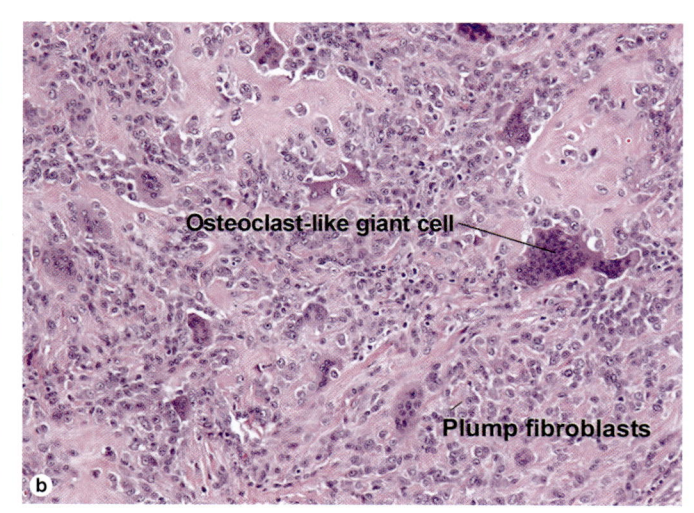

Fig 20-15 Infantile digital fibroma

Fig 20-16 Giant cell tumor of tendon sheath

Fibroma of tendon sheath

Key features

- Giant cell tumor of tendon sheath without the giant cells
- Characteristic plump fibroblasts often present

Elastofibroma dorsi

Key features

- Large fibrous tumor
- Elastin deposits throughout tumor
- Beaded elastic fibers

As the name implies, elastofibroma dorsi is typically found on the back.

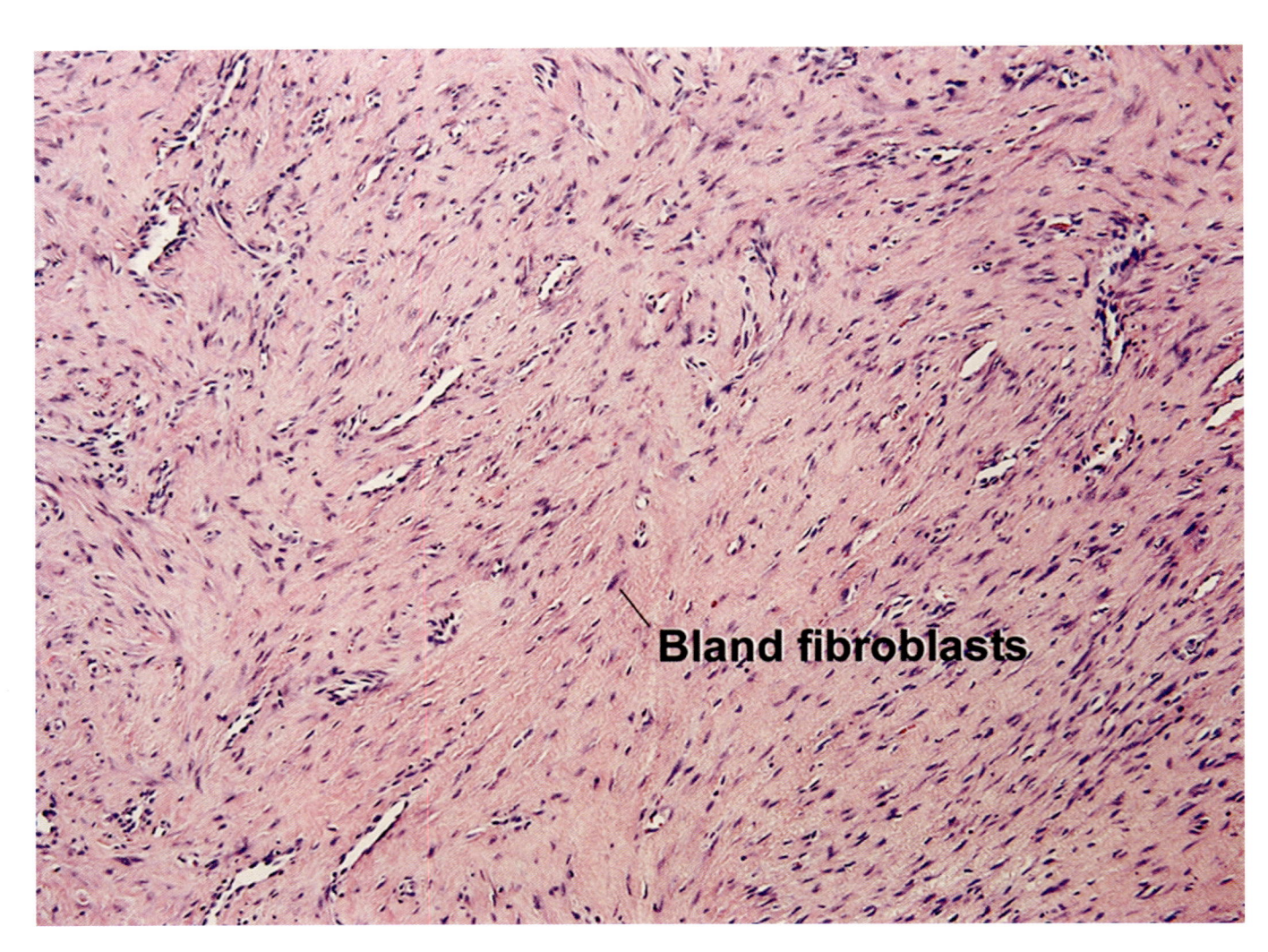

Fig 20-17 Fibroma of tendon sheath

Sclerotic fibroma

Key features

- Collagen pattern resembles van Gogh's "Starry night"
- Hypocellular
- May be a marker for Cowden's syndrome

Because of the association with Cowden's syndrome, sclerotic fibromas should be considered a distinct entity. Similar hypocellular areas have been seen in other fibrous tumors, especially dermatofibromas.

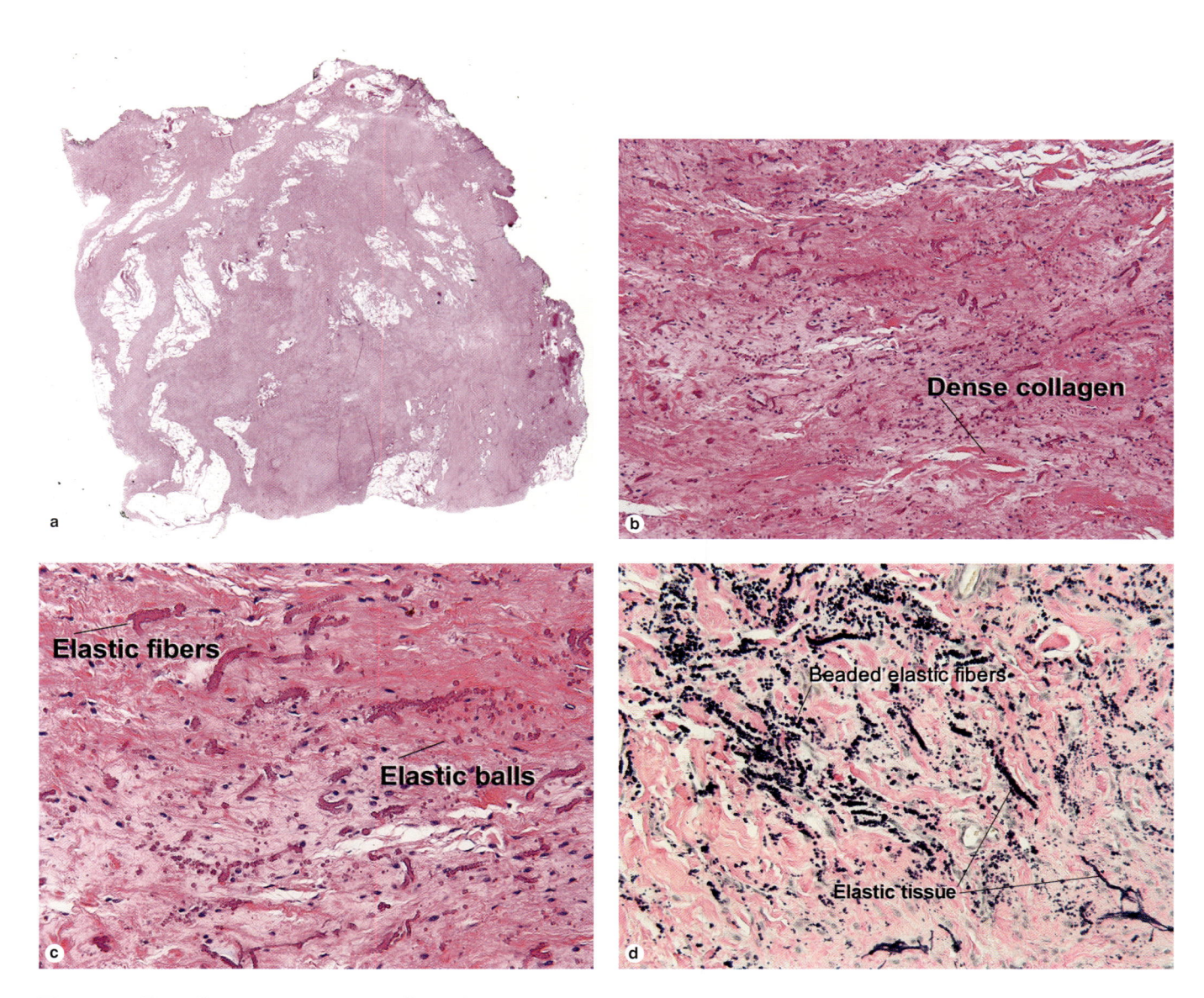

Fig 20-18 Elastofibroma dorsi, D Verhoeff-van Gieson

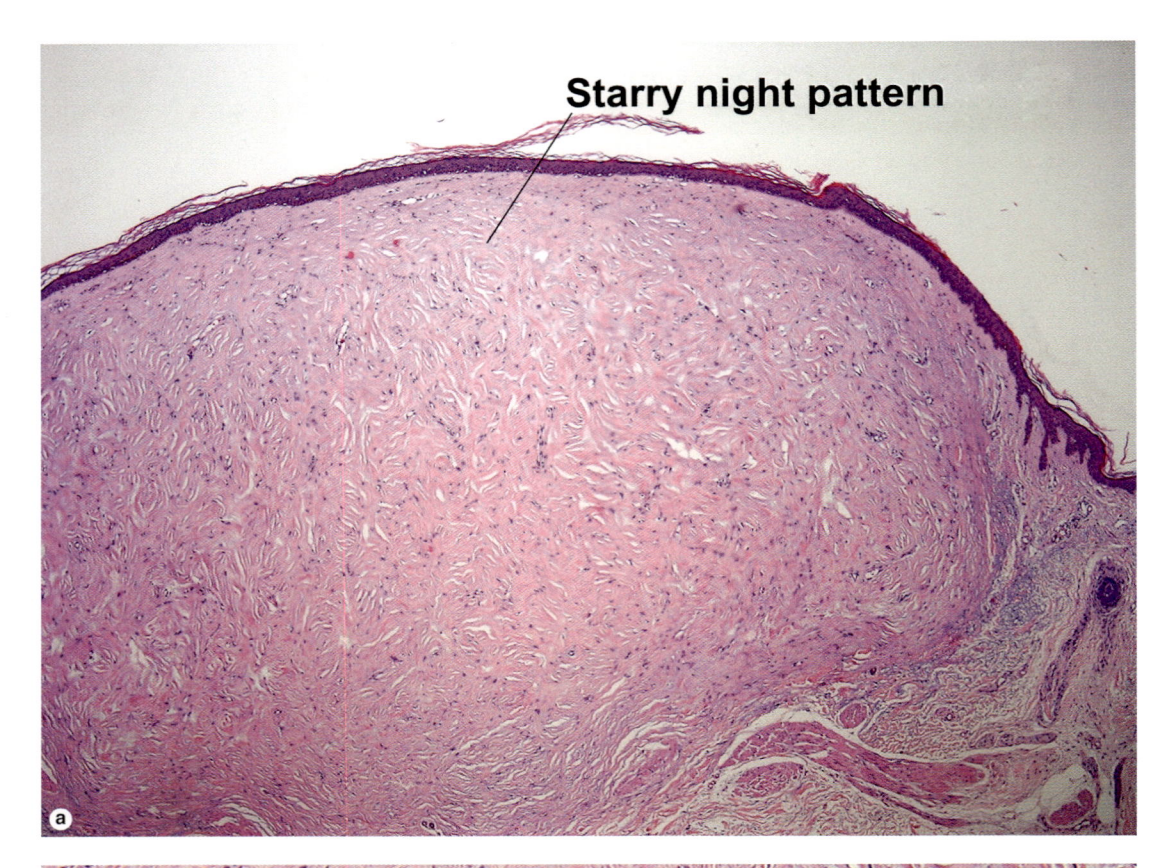

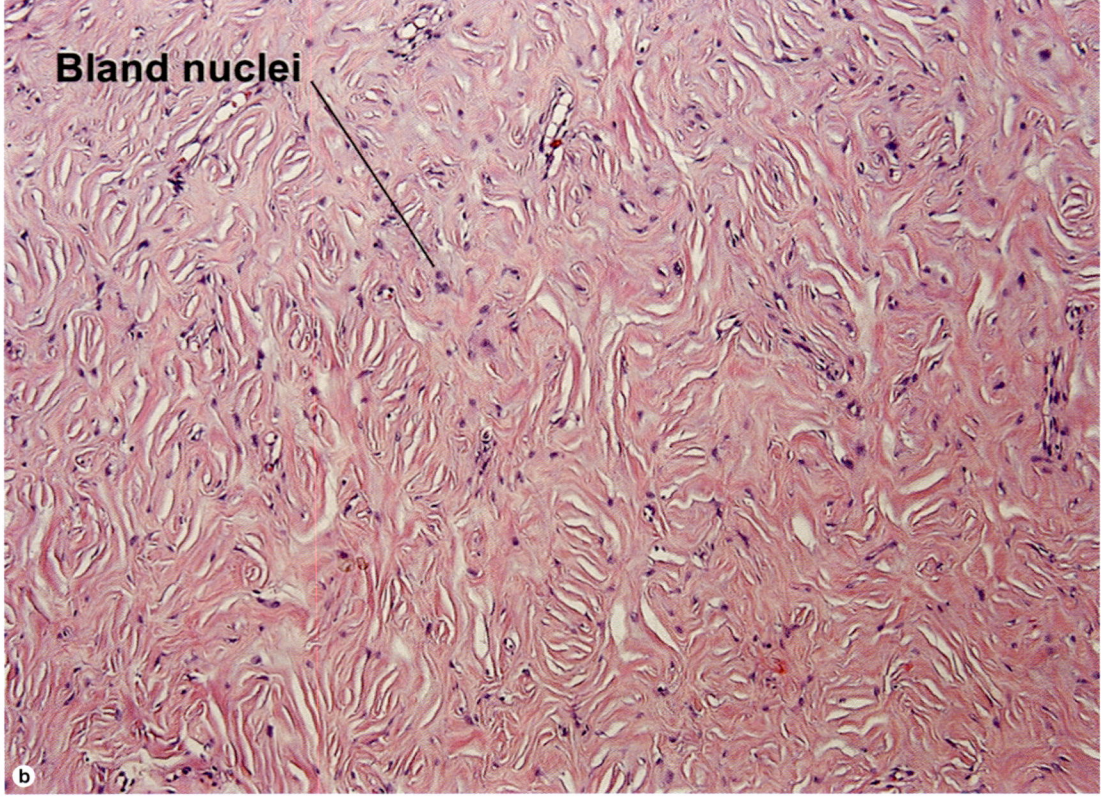

Fig 20-19 Sclerotic fibroma

Pleomorphic fibroma

Key features

- Scattered large hyperchromatic stellate nuclei
- Never hypercellular
- No mitoses

Despite the large hyperchromatic nuclei, pleomorphic fibromas are benign. They are peppered with hyperchromatic stellate nuclei that resemble the stellate nuclei in fibrous papules. Although the stellate cells resemble those of a fibrous papule, they are usually CD34 positive. Multinucleated cells may be present, but mitoses are absent. Tumors with overlapping features of sclerotic and pleomorphic fibroma have been described.

Sclerosing perineurioma

Key features

- Whorled, nodular, or storiform appearance
- Epithelial membrane antigen+

Angiofibromas

Key features

- Concentric perivascular fibrosis
- Stellate, factor XIIIa+ stromal cells

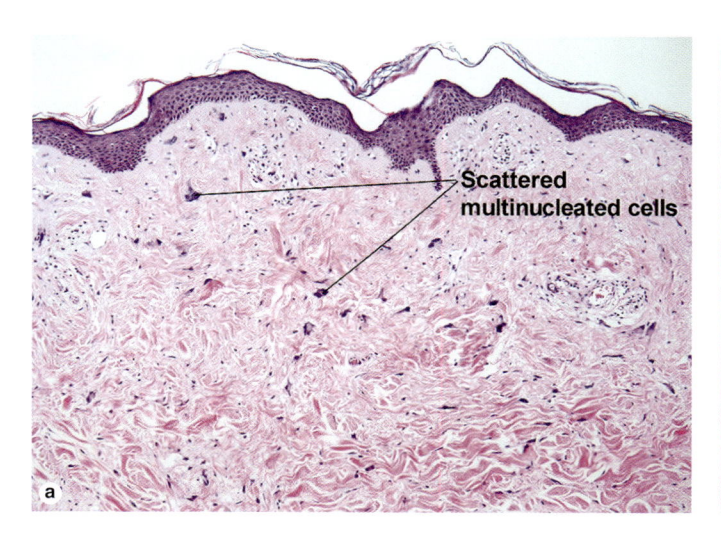

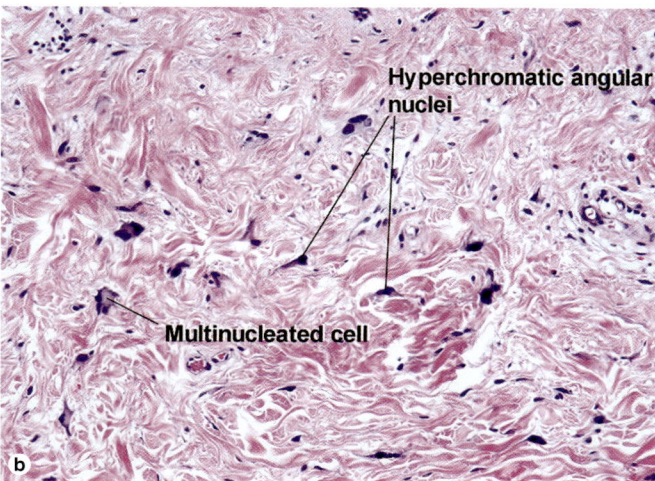

Fig 20-20 Pleomorphic fibroma

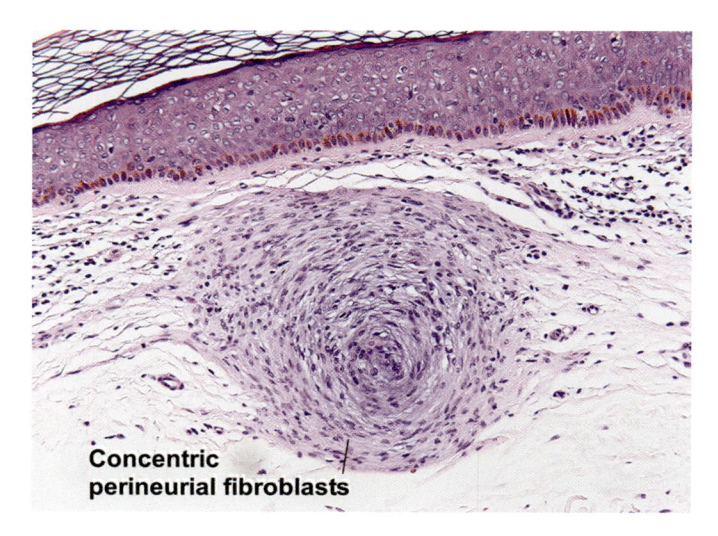

Fig 20-21 Sclerosing perineurioma

Dermatopathology

In tuberous sclerosis, we call them adenoma sebaceum or Koenen's periungual fibromas. Multiple angiofibromas may also be seen in multiple endocrine neoplasia type I (MEN 1) and in type II neurofibromatosis.

On the face, we refer to the most common variant of solitary angiofibroma as fibrous papule of the face. On the penis, we call them *pearly penile papules*. Acquired digital fibrokeratoma is a closely related lesion.

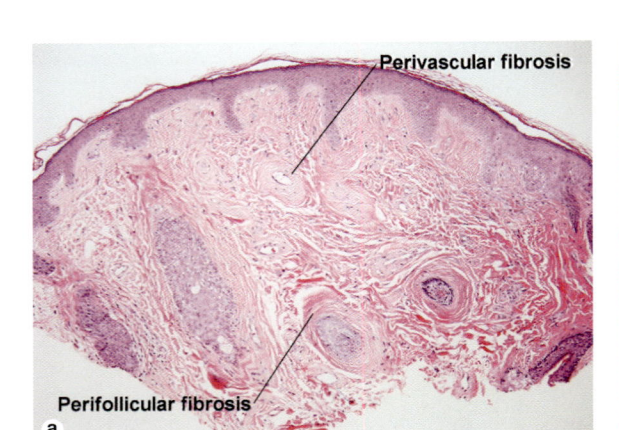

Fibrous papule of the face (benign fibrous papule, solitary angiofibroma)

Key features
- Common variant of angiofibroma
- Concentric perivascular fibrosis
- Stellate, factor XIIIa+ stromal cells
- Large pyramid-shaped melanocytes may be present at the dermal–epidermal junction

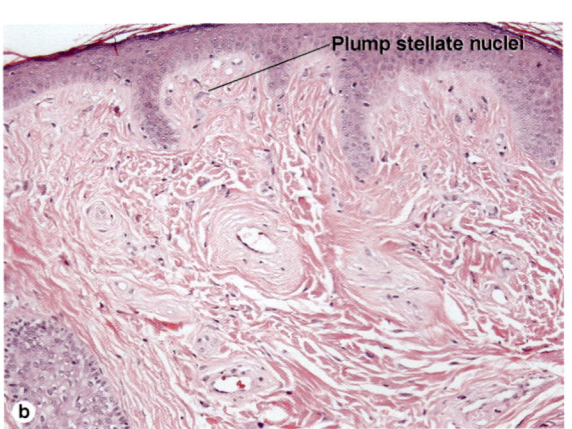

Fig 20-22 Angiofibroma

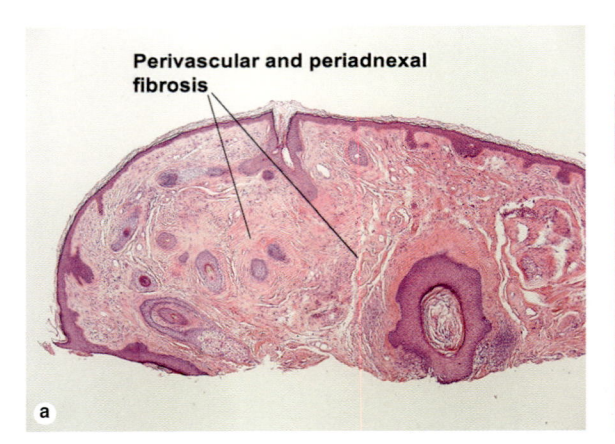

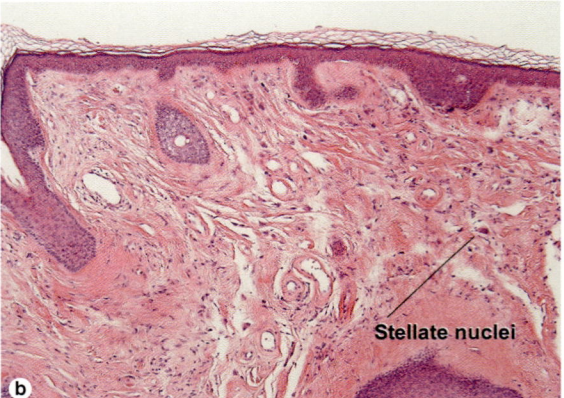

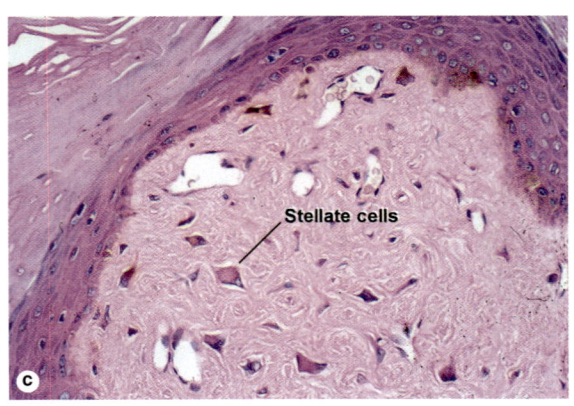

Fig 20-23 Fibrous papule of the face

Fibrous tumors **Chapter 20** 327

A superficial shave biopsy of a fibrous papule may suggest a melanocytic lesion, because of the large melanocytes at the dermal–epidermal junction. Before the advent of immunostains, the stellate dermal cells were thought to be degenerated melanocytes.

Acquired digital fibrokeratoma

Key features

- Acral skin
- Hyperkeratosis, acanthosis, hypergranulosis
- Spindle cells and collagen often perpendicular to the surrounding skin surface
- Stellate, factor XIIIa+ stromal cells may be present

Nodular fasciitis

Key features

- "Tissue culture" fibroblasts
- Erythrocyte extravasation
- Loose myxoid pattern
- Foci of inflammatory cells

With time, nodular fasciitis develops thick red collagen bundles, but young lesions appear loose and myxoid, with erythrocyte extravasation and nodular aggregates of inflammatory cells. The stellate fibroblasts look like those in tissue culture.

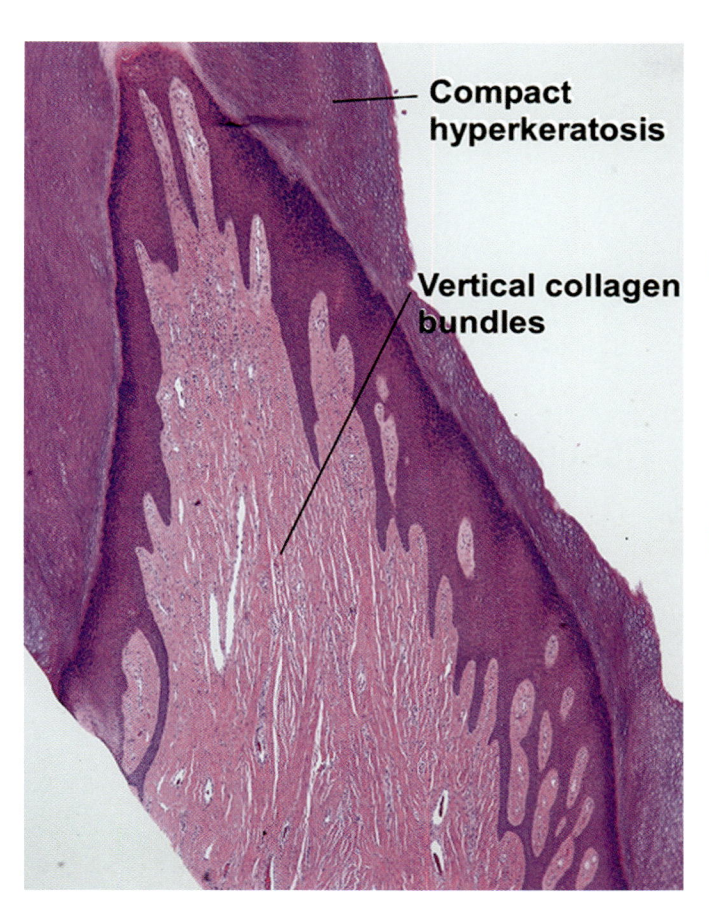

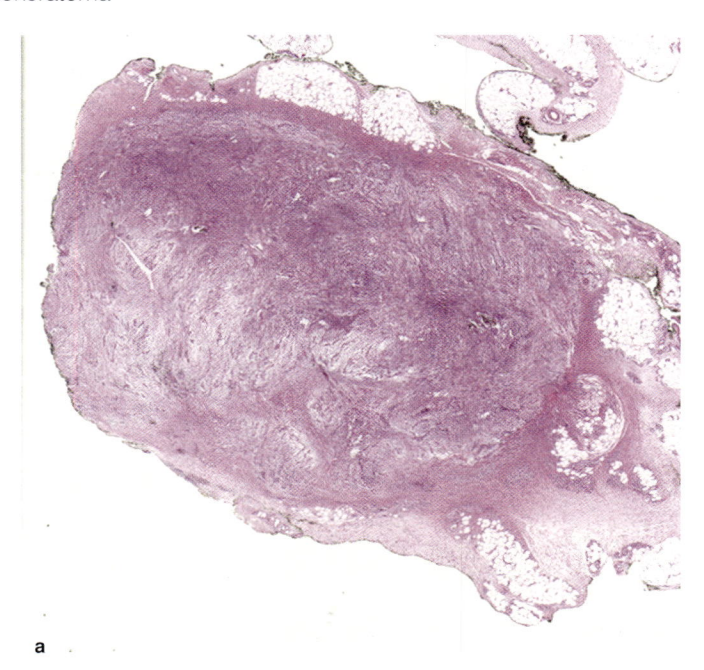

Fig 20-24 Acquired digital fibrokeratoma

Fig 20-25 Nodular fasciitis

Continued

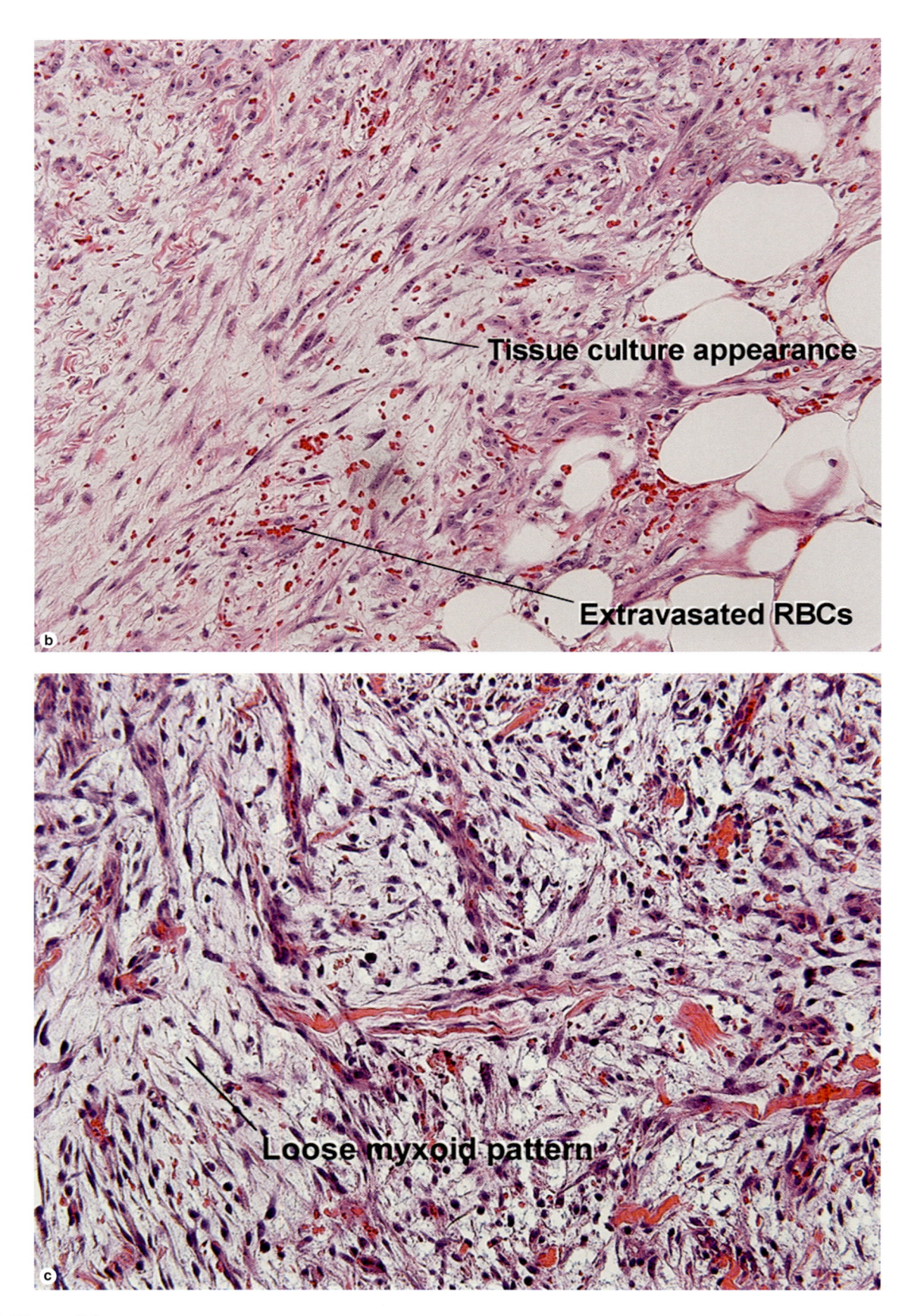

Fig 20-25, cont'd

Cranial fasciitis

Key features

- Variant of nodular fasciitis that occurs on the head of a child

Proliferative fasciitis

Key features

- Variant of nodular fasciitis
- Ganglion-like giant cells
- Collagen trapping at periphery

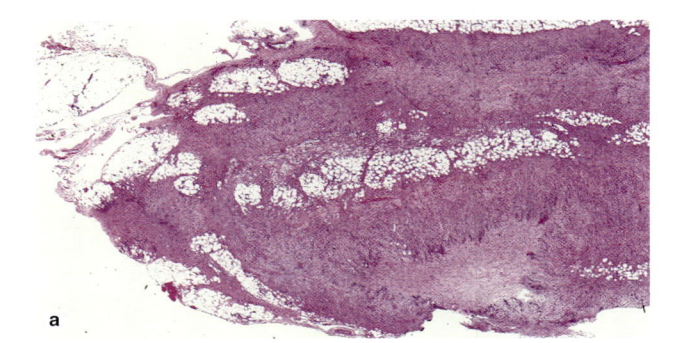

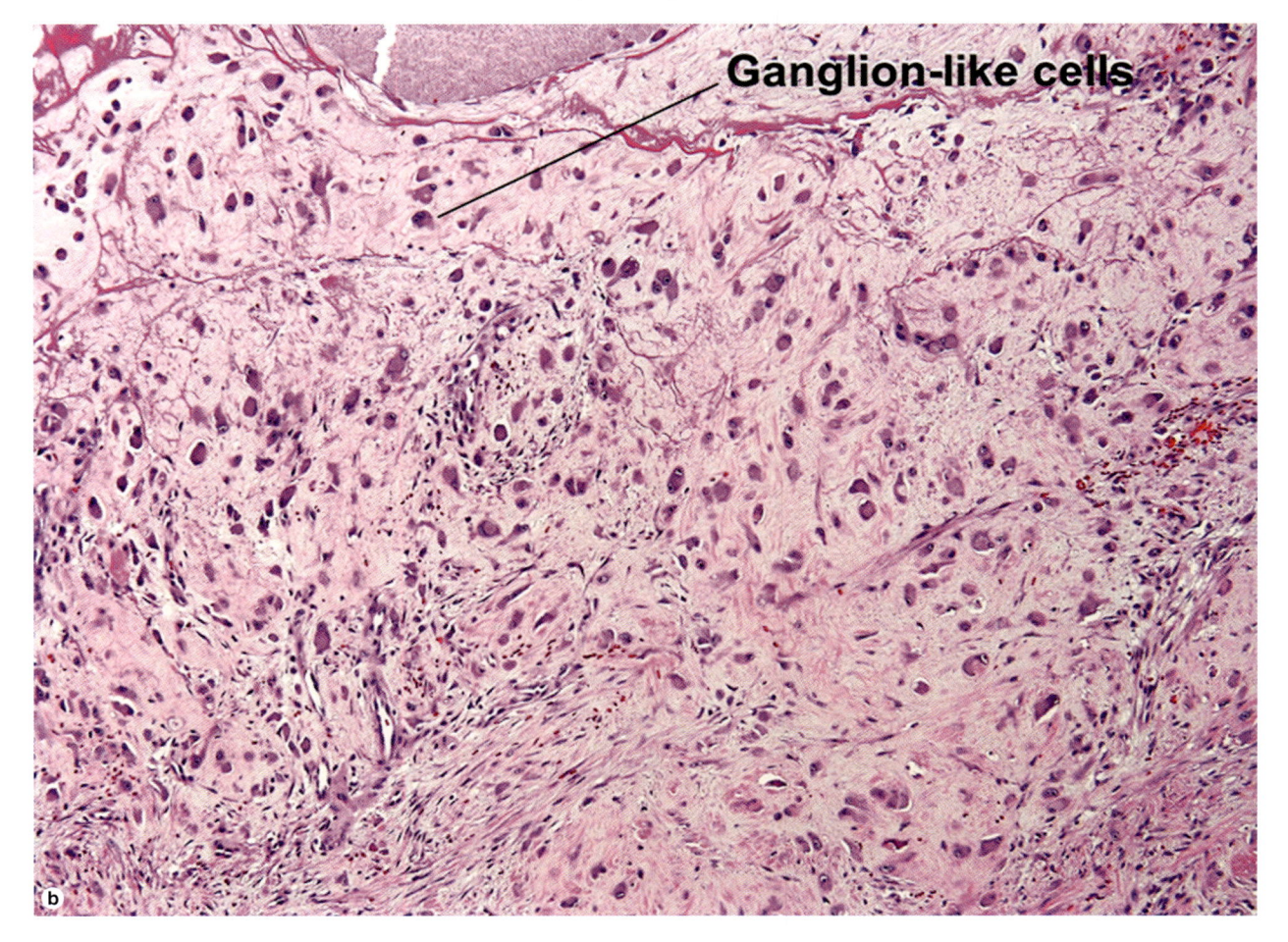

Calcifying aponeurotic fibroma

Key features

- Plump, epithelioid fibroblasts palisading around chondroid foci with or without calcification, occasionally with osteoclast-like cells
- Distal extremities
- Commonly found in children and adolescents

Fig 20-26 Proliferative fasciitis

Dermatopathology

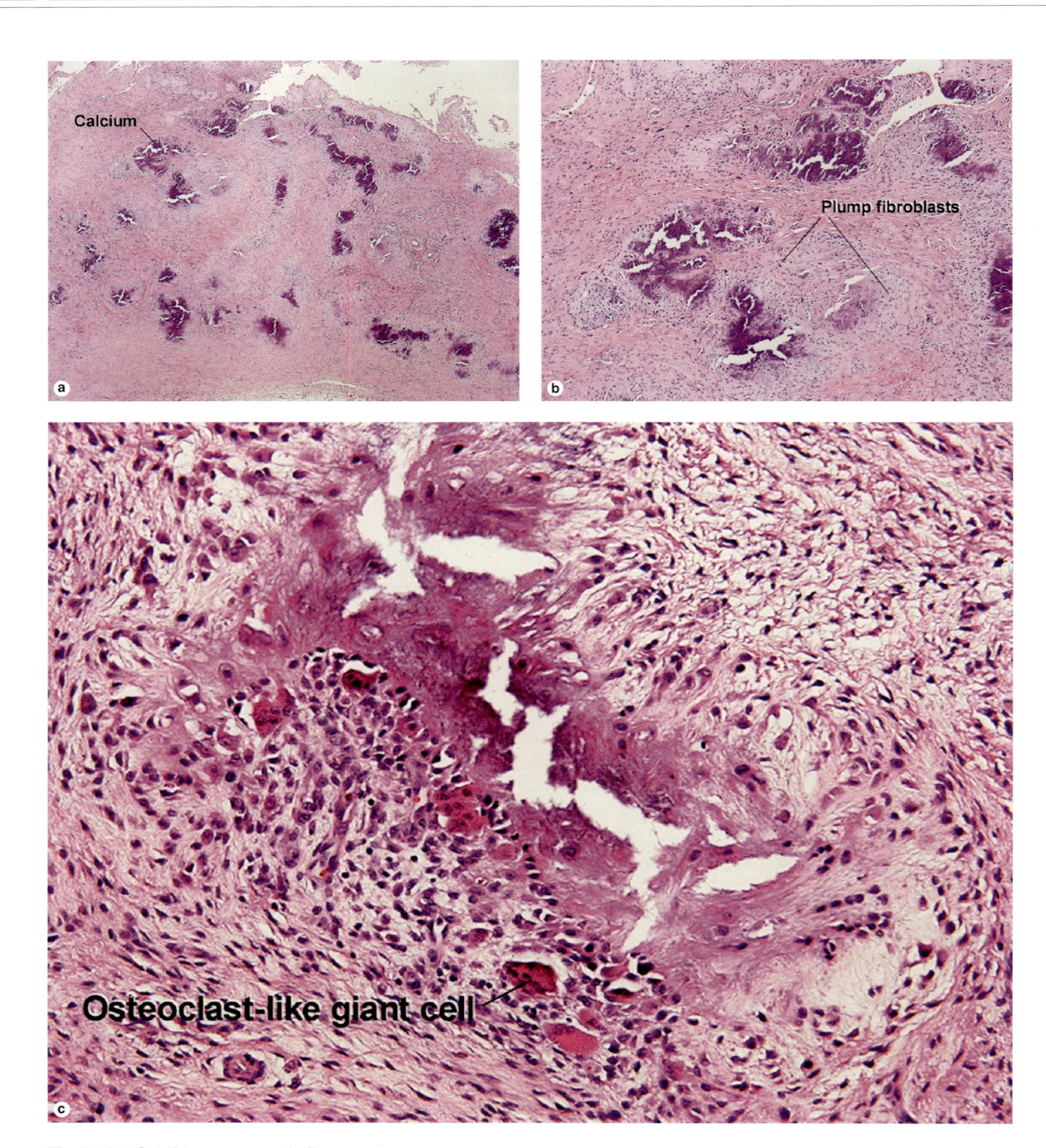

Fig 20-27 Calcifying aponeurotic fibroma

Borderline tumors

Desmoid tumor (aggressive fibromatosis)

Key features

- Myofibroblastic proliferation
- Bland nuclei
- Tendency for deep infiltration and recurrence
- Beta catenin expressed
- Most are sporadic but can be associated with Gardner's syndrome

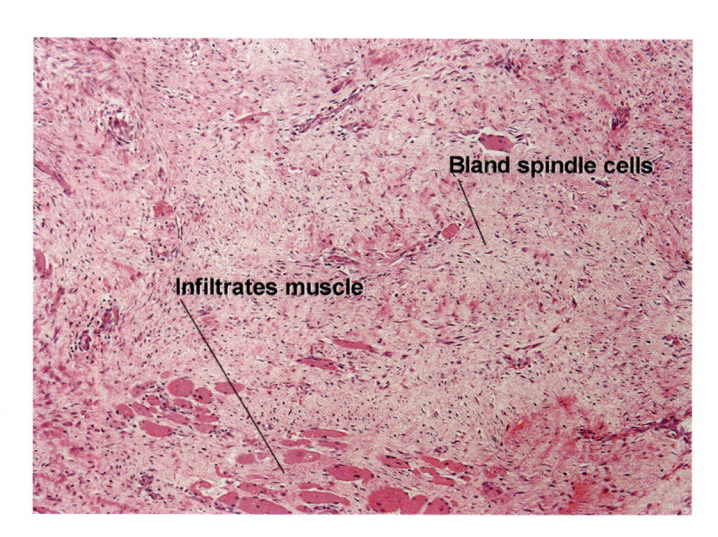

Fig 20-28 Desmoid tumor

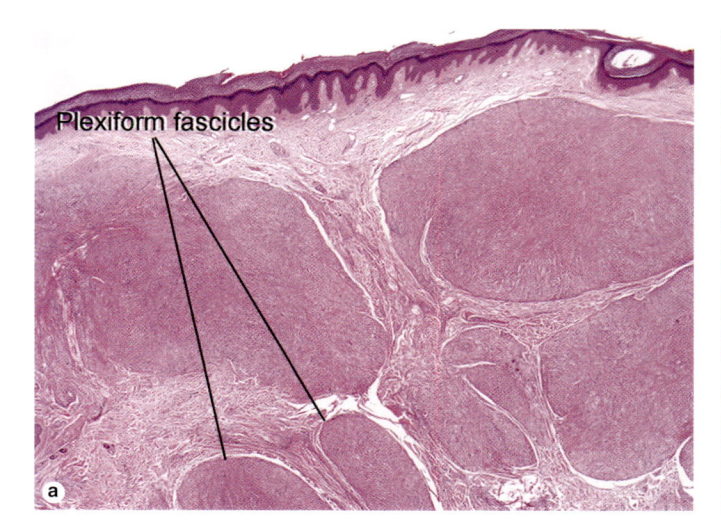

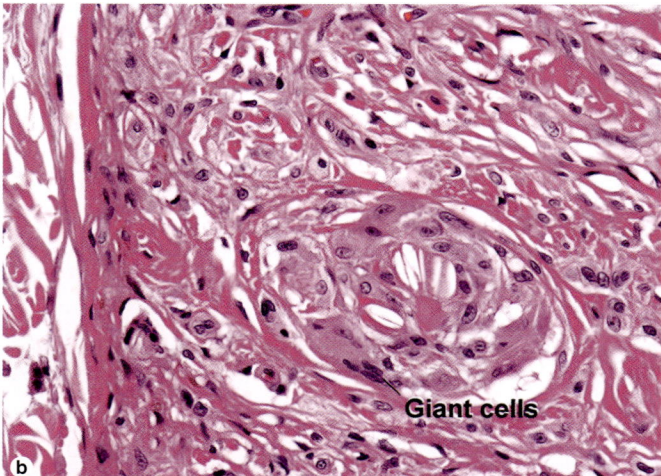

Plexiform fibrohistiocytic tumor

Key features

- Plexiform fascicles of myofibroblast-like fusiform and spindle cells
- Nodules of histiocytic cells and osteoclast-like giant cells (biphasic tumor)
- Variable pleomorphism and mitotic rate

Fig 20-29 Plexiform fibrohistiocytic tumor

Continued

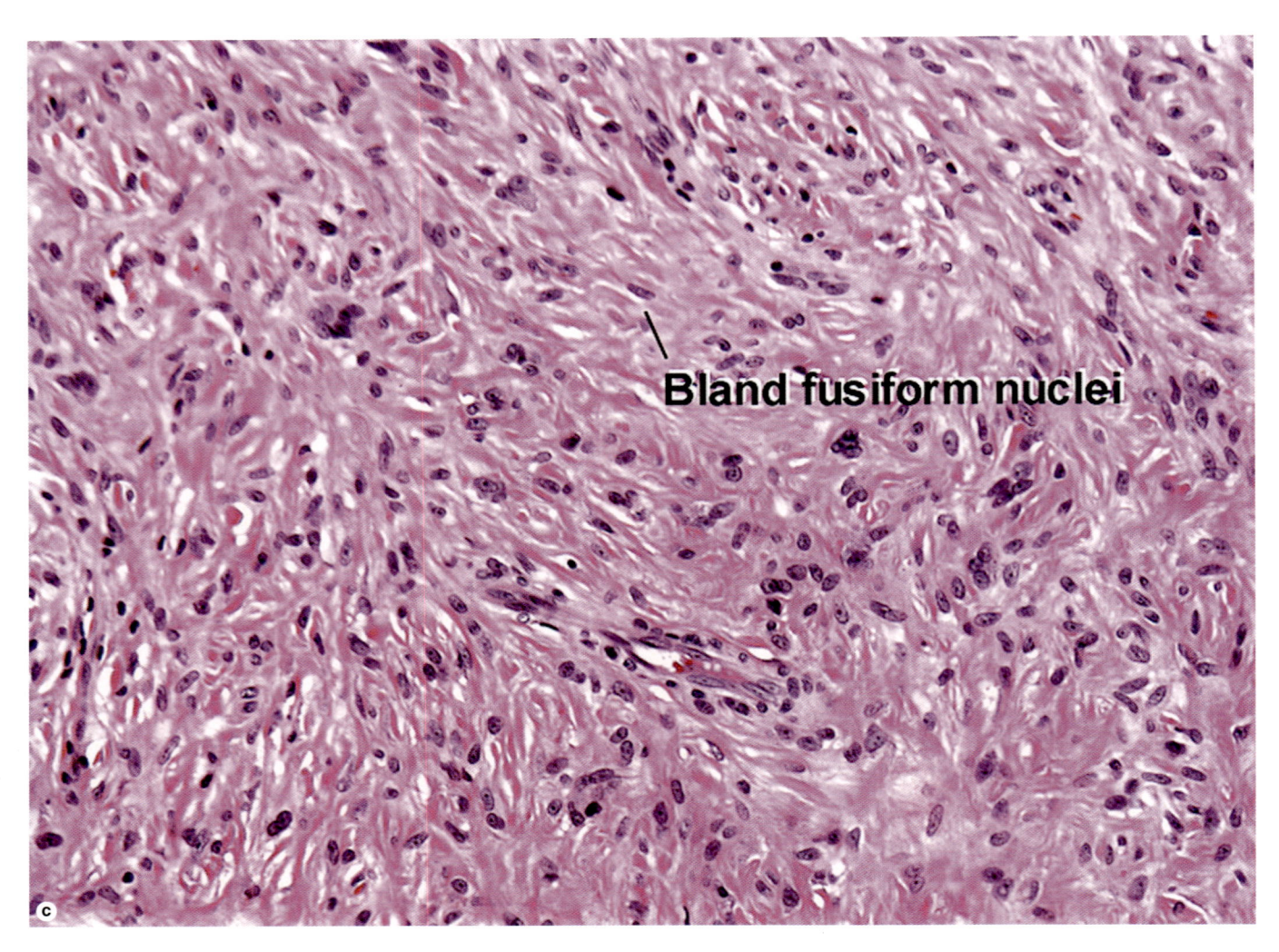

Fig 20-29, cont'd

Plexiform fibrohistiocytic tumor is a tumor of intermediate malignant behavior that occurs in children and young adults. It commonly involves an arm.

Malignant tumors

Dermatofibrosarcoma protuberans (DFSP)

> **Key features**
> - Densely hypercellular
> - Storiform (woven) pattern
> - Infiltrates fat in a honeycomb pattern
> - Forms fibrous layers in the fat, parallel to the surface epidermis
> - Epidermal rete pattern usually effaced
> - CD34+, factor XIIIa–

Dermatofibrosarcoma protuberans infiltrates the fat in a honeycomb pattern. As the tumor progresses, parallel layers of tumor form in the fat, like a layer cake with lipocytes (frosting) in between the layers. The nuclei appear as dark spindle cells when cut across, and as pale gray oval nuclei when cut en face. Chromosomal translocations, especially t(17;22) sometimes present. A pigmented dermatofibrosarcoma protuberans is referred to as a Bednar tumor.

> **PEARL**
>
> Occasionally, overlying acanthosis and collagen trapping may be present in a dermatofibrosarcoma protuberans. If the tumor is densely hypercellular and infiltrates fat, CD34 staining should be performed.

Fibrous tumors Chapter 20 333

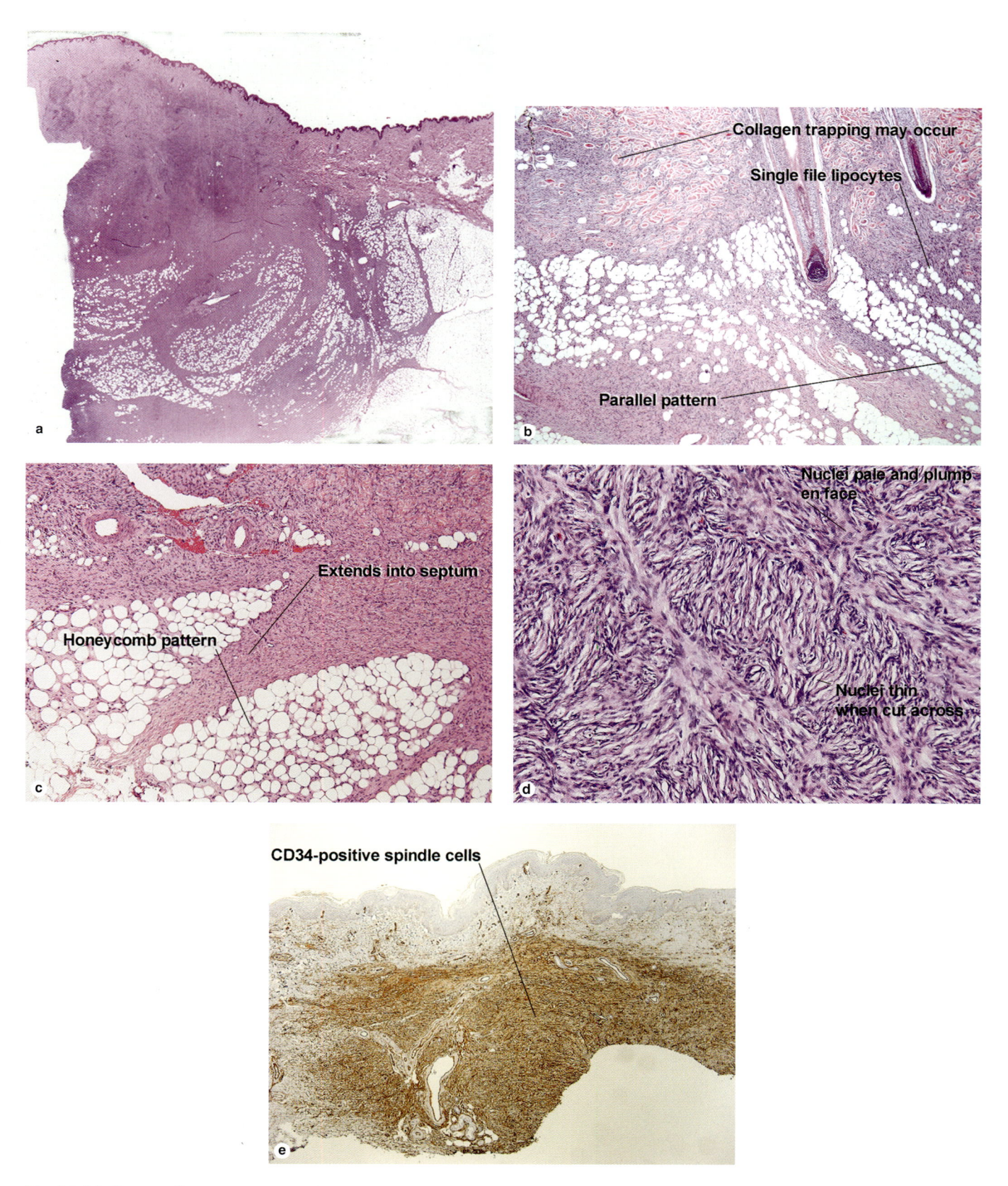

Fig 20-30 Dermatofibrosarcoma protuberans

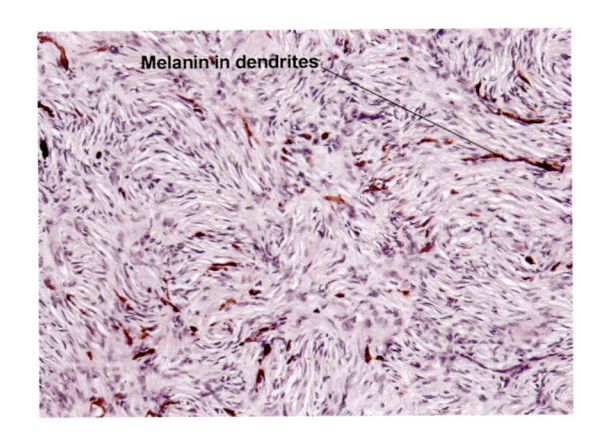

Dermatopathology

Fig 20-31 Bednar tumor

Giant cell fibroblastoma

Key features

- Juvenile variant of dermatofibrosarcoma protuberans
- Multinucleated giant cells lining vascular-like spaces

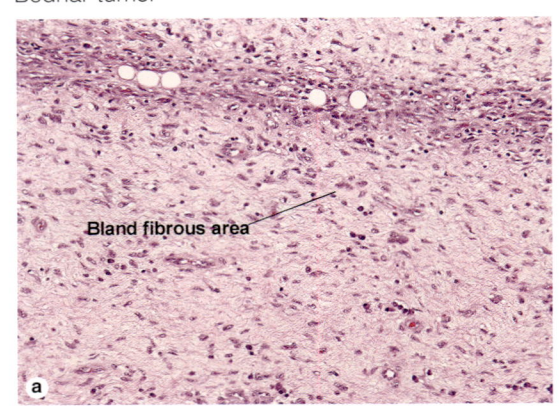

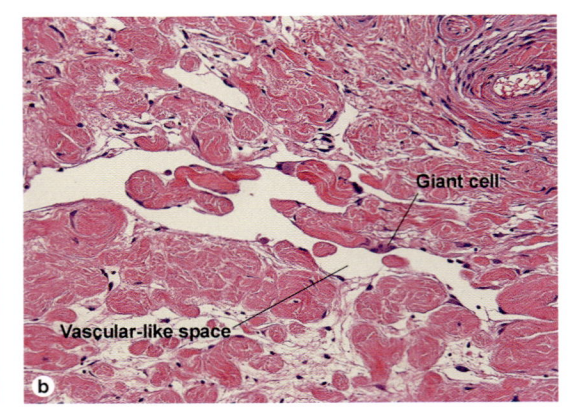

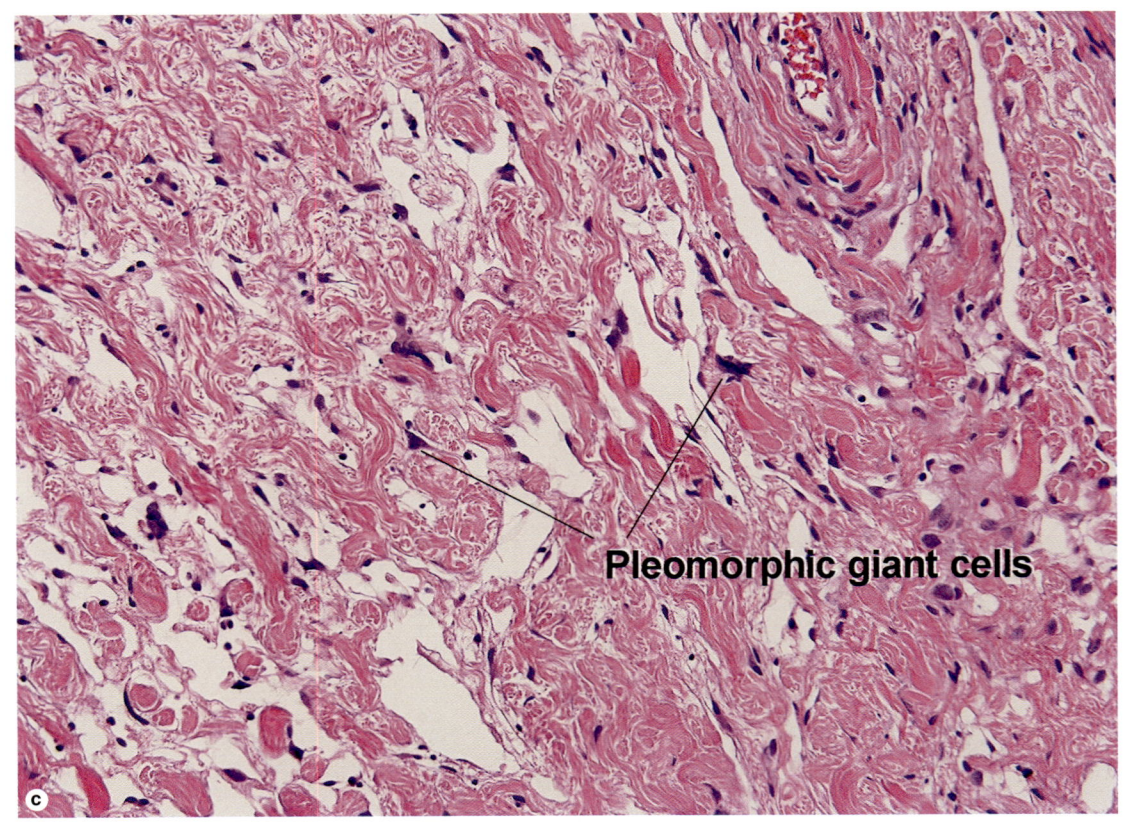

Fig 20-32 Giant cell fibroblastoma

Fibrous tumors   20   335

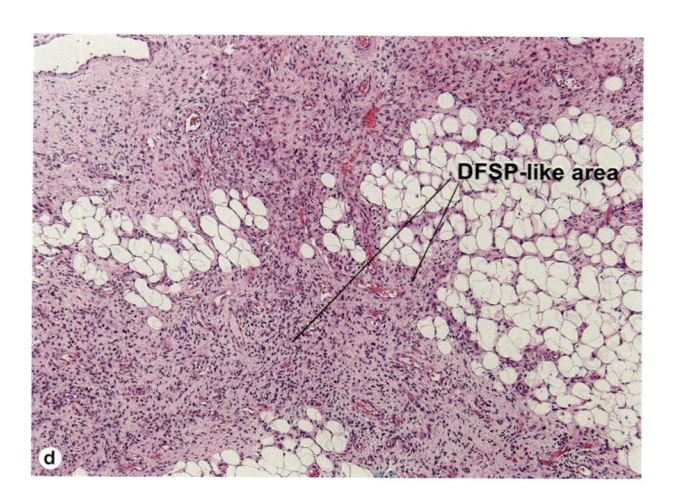

DFSP-like area

Fig 20-32, cont'd

Fibrosarcoma

Key features

- Densely hypercellular
- Herringbone or fir tree pattern common
- Variable mitotic rate
- Nuclei may be large and hyperchromatic

Many fibrosarcomas tend to have a herringbone or fir tree pattern. Dermatofibrosarcoma protuberans is a type of fibrosarcoma with a characteristic storiform and honeycomb pattern. In contrast, dermatofibromas and hemangiopericytomas have a curlicue pattern.

Herringbone pattern

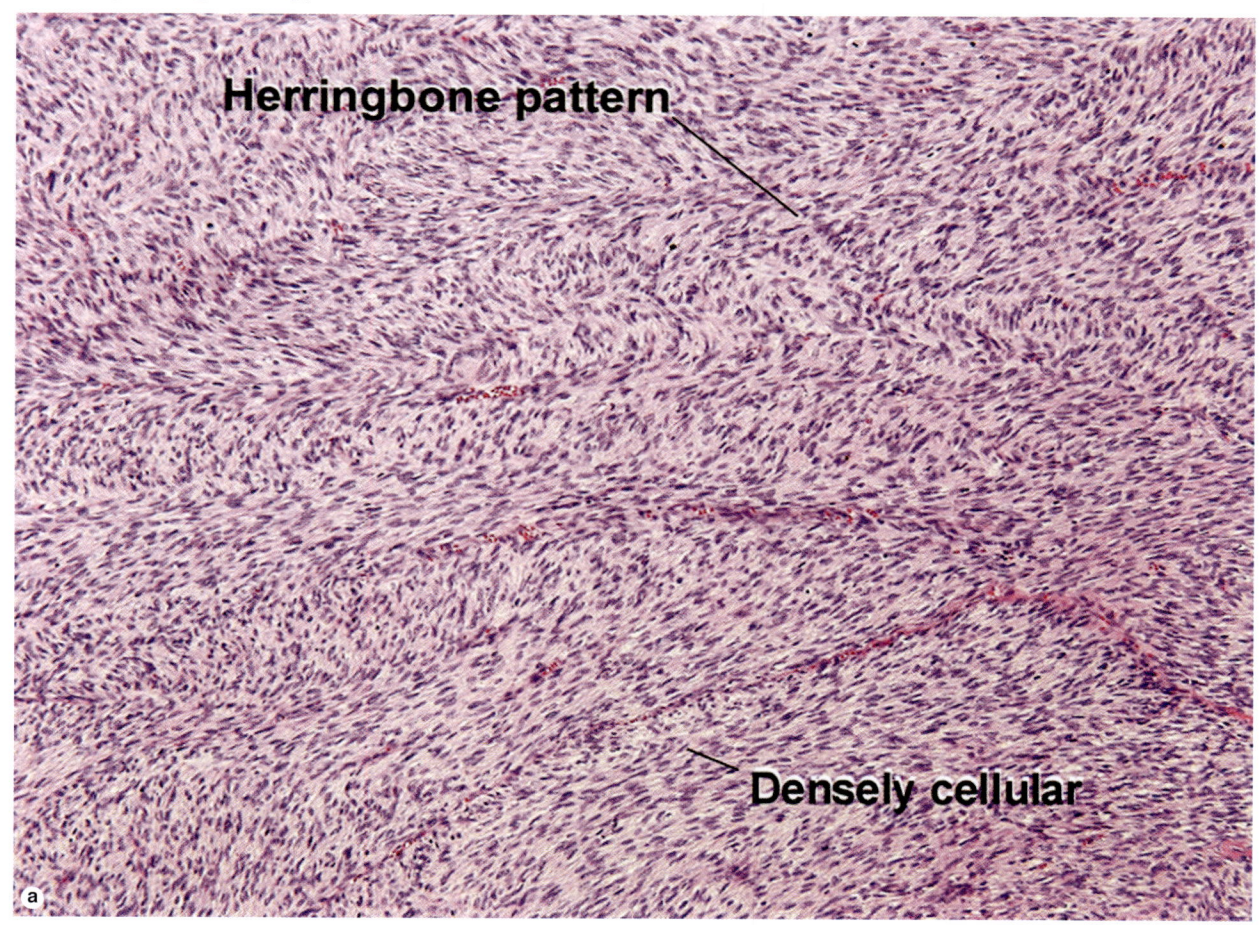

Densely cellular

Fig 20-33 Fibrosarcoma

Continued

Fig 20-33, cont'd

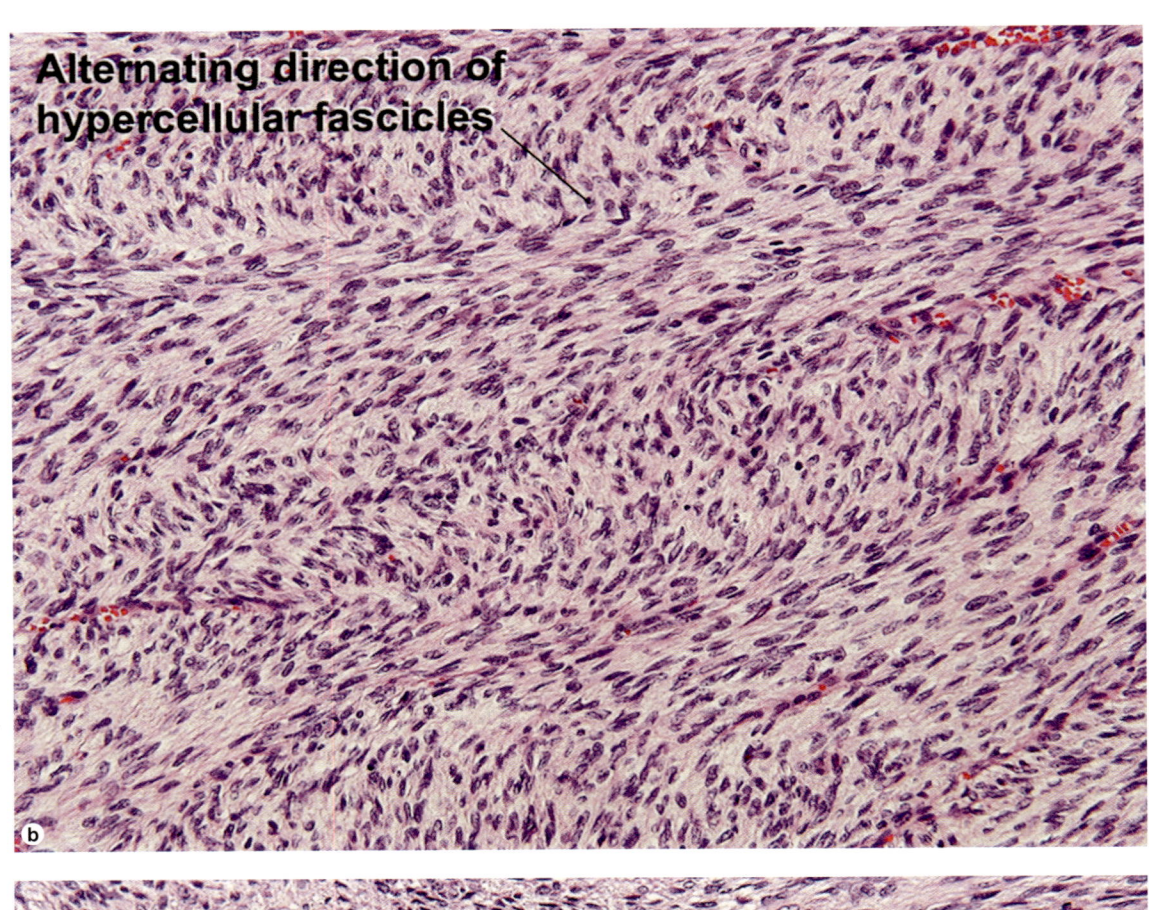

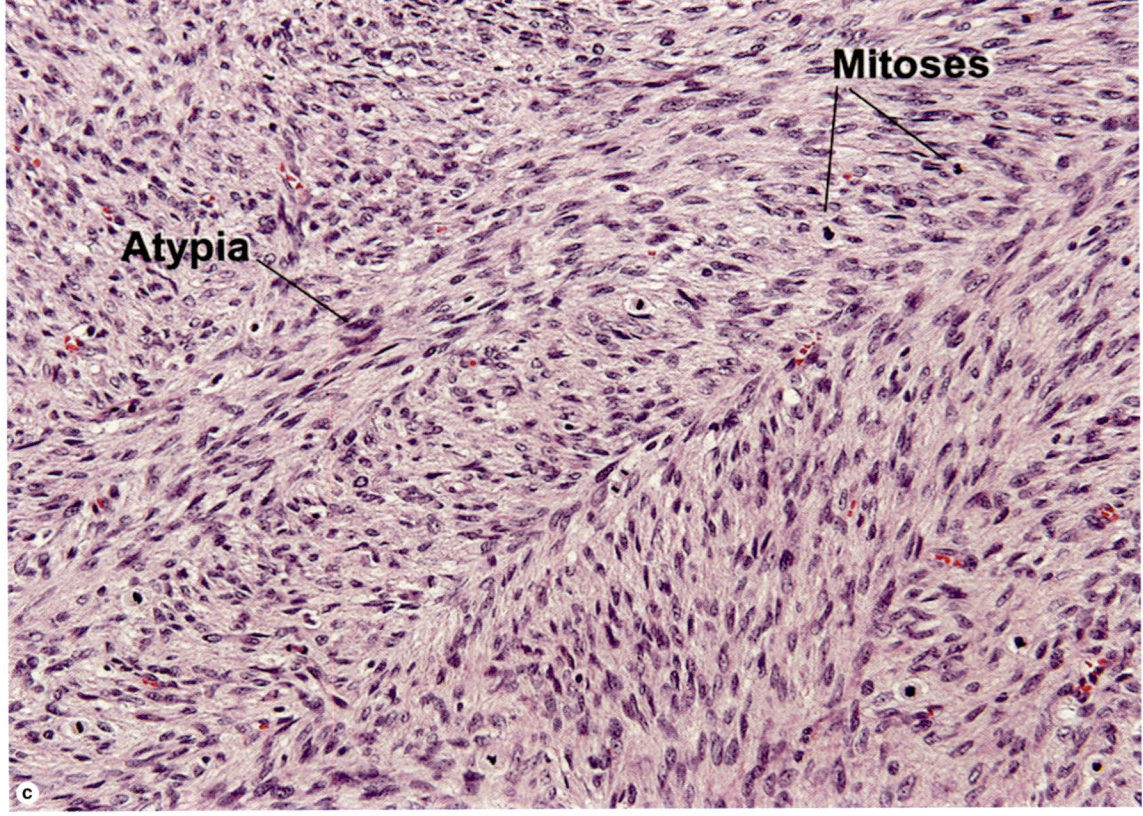

Atypical fibroxanthoma (AFX)

Key features

- CD10+, S100A6+, and procollagen+ but none of these stains is specific; it remains a diagnosis of exclusion
- Atypical pleomorphic or spindle cells

Some consider atypical fibroxanthoma to be a superficial variant of pleomorphic undifferentiated sarcoma.

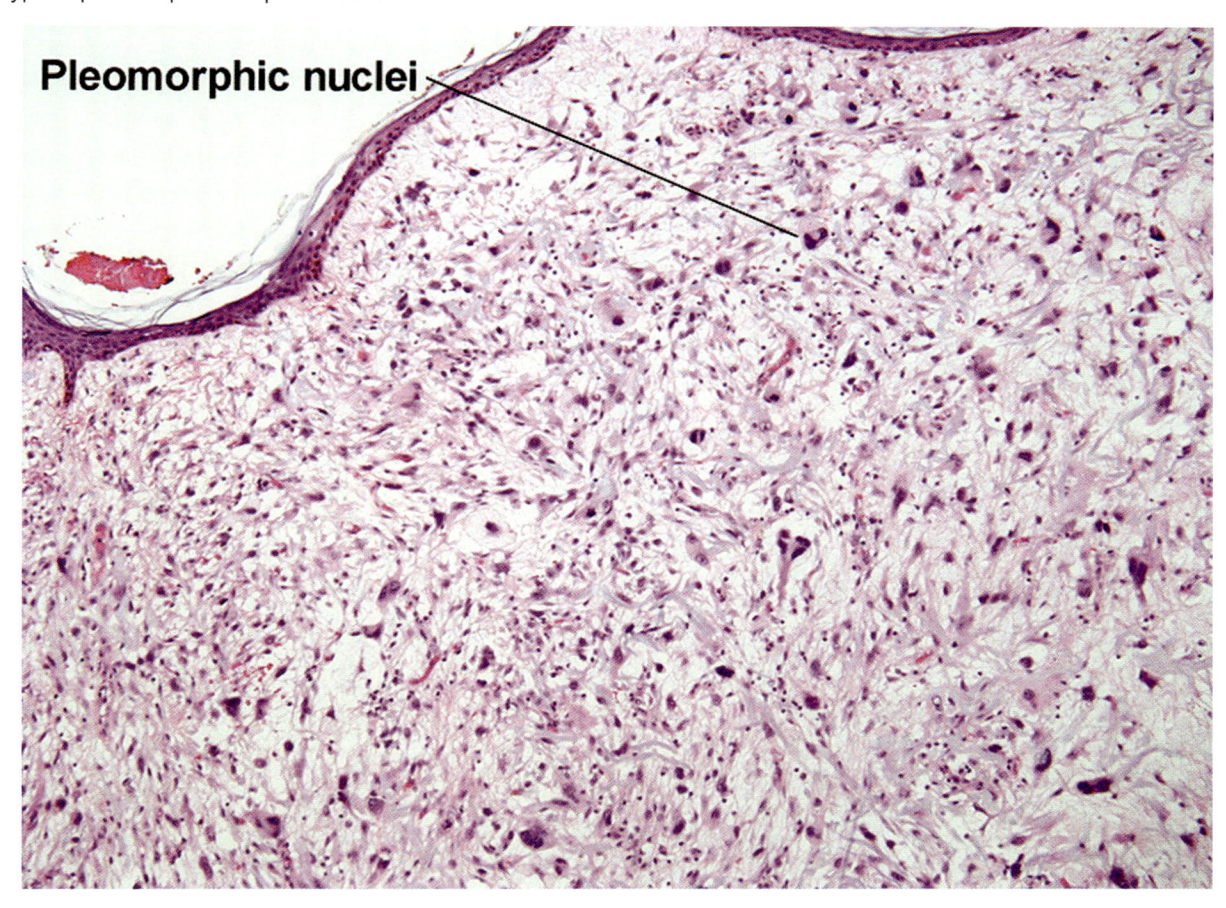

Fig 20-34 Pleomorphic atypical fibroxanthoma (AFX)

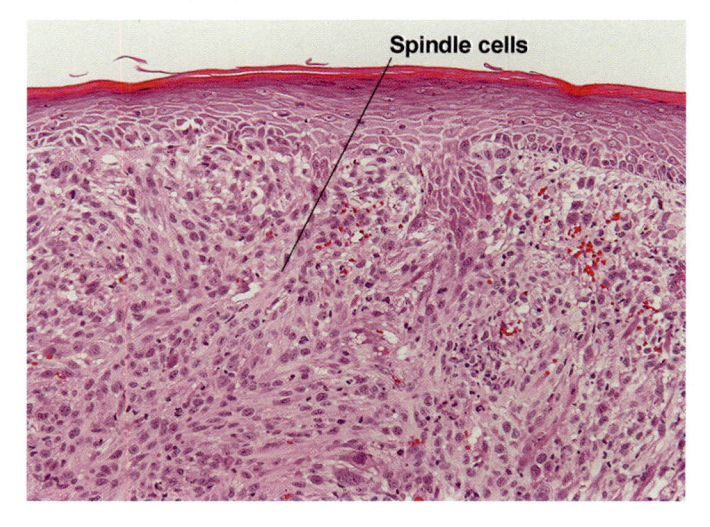

Fig 20-35 Spindled atypical fibroxanthoma (AFX)

Dermatopathology

Pleomorphic undifferentiated sarcoma

Key features

- Heterogeneous group of soft-tissue sarcomas
- Pleomorphic, myxoid, inflammatory, and other variants

Newer classifications no longer include malignant fibrous histiocytoma (MFH) as a distinct diagnosis, but rather as subtypes of pleomorphic undifferentiated sarcoma. Superficial dermal tumours formerly called superficial MFH mostly fall into the category of myxofibrosarcoma.

Epithelioid sarcoma

Key features

- Mimics a palisaded granuloma
- Biphasic (transition between epithelioid and spindle cells)
- Central necrosis
- Stains for both keratin and vimentin

Epithelioid sarcomas tend to occur on the extremity.

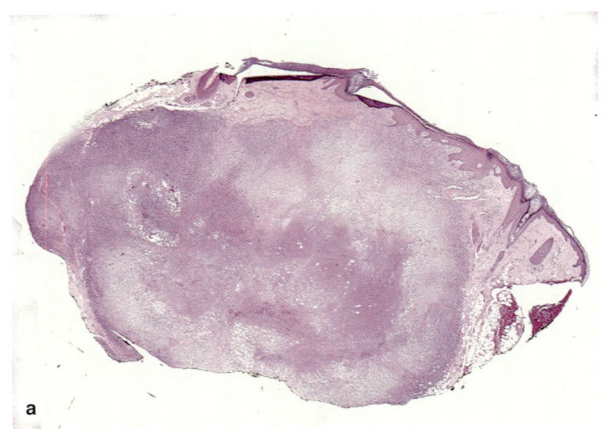

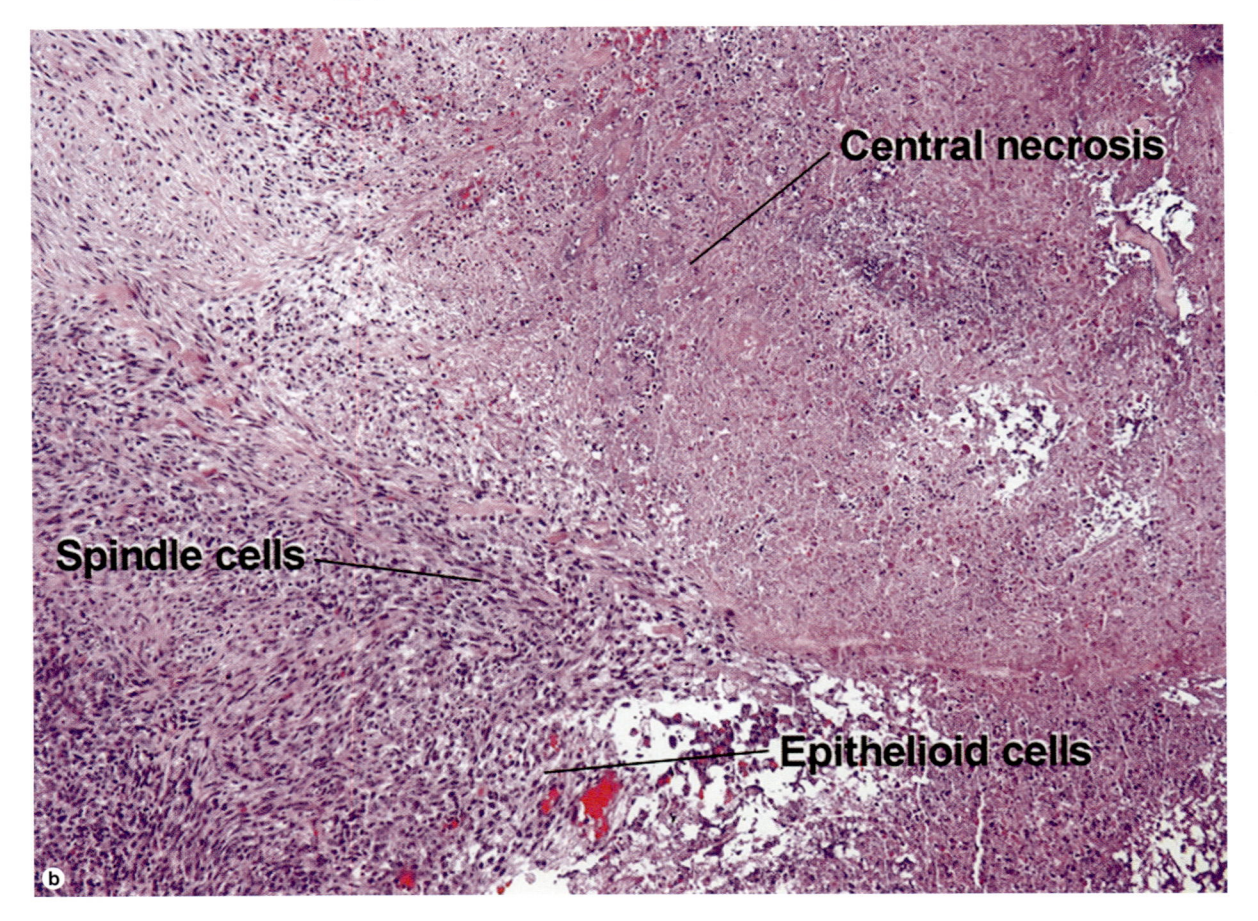

Fig 20-36 Epithelioid sarcoma

Fibrous tumors

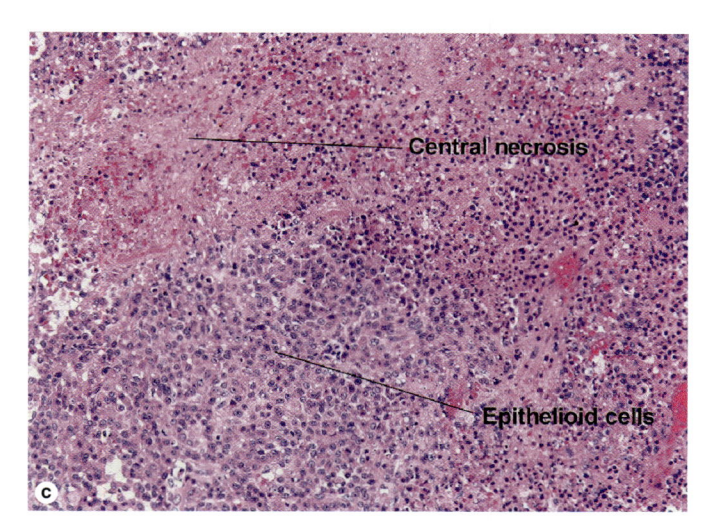

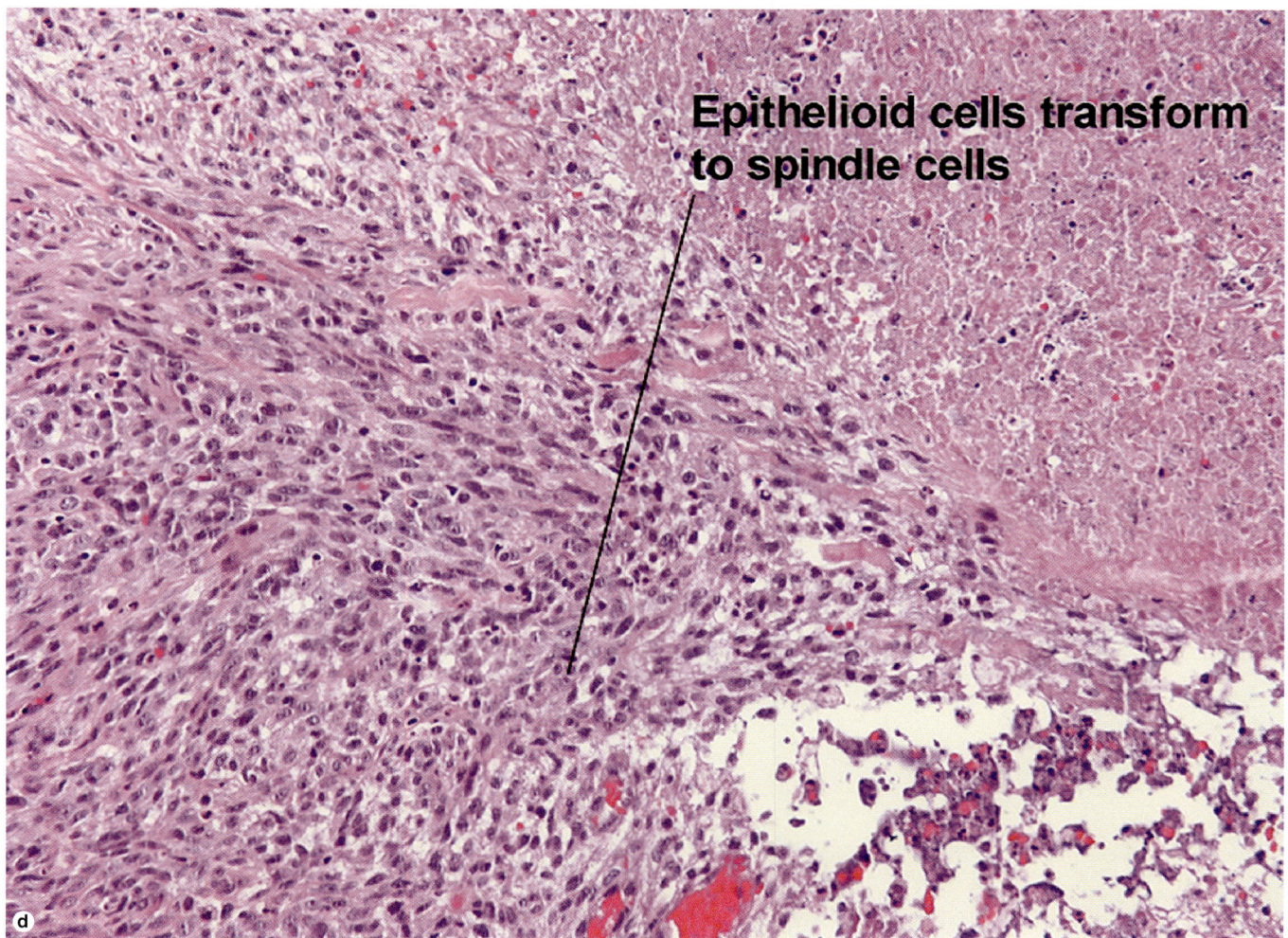

Fig 20-36, cont'd

Further reading

Baerg J, Murphy JJ, Magee JF. Fibromatoses: clinical and pathological features suggestive of recurrence. J Pediatr Surg 1999;34(7):1112–1114.

Billings SD, Folpe AL. Cutaneous and subcutaneous fibrohistiocytic tumors of intermediate malignancy: an update. Am J Dermatopathol 2004;26(2):141–155.

Clarke LE. Fibrous and fibrohistiocytic neoplasms: an update. Dermatol Clin 2012;30(4):643–656.

Franchi A, Santucci M. The contribution of electron microscopy to the characterization of soft tissue fibrosarcomas. Ultrastruct Pathol 2013;37(1):9–14.

Iijima S, Suzuki R, Otsuka F. Solitary form of infantile myofibromatosis: a histologic, immunohistochemical, and electron microscopic study of a regressing tumor over a 20-month period. Am J Dermatopathol 1999;21(4):375–380.

Mahmood MN, Salama ME, Chaffins M, et al. Solitary sclerotic fibroma of skin: a possible link with pleomorphic fibroma with immunophenotypic expression for O13 (CD99) and CD34. J Cutan Pathol 2003;30(10):631–636.

Martín-López R, Feal-Cortizas C, Fraga J. Pleomorphic sclerotic fibroma. Dermatology 1999;198(1):69–72.

Parish LC, Yazdanian S, Lambert WC, et al. Dermatofibroma: a curious tumor. Skinmed 2012;10(5):268–270.

Stanford D, Rogers M. Dermatological presentations of infantile myofibromatosis: a review of 27 cases. Australas J Dermatol 2000;41(3):156–161.

Tani M, Komura A, Ichihashi M. Dermatomyofibroma (Plaqueformige Dermale Fibromatose). J Dermatol 1997;24(12):793–797.

Terrier-Lacombe MJ, Guillou L, Maire G, et al. Dermatofibrosarcoma protuberans, giant cell fibroblastoma, and hybrid lesions in children: clinicopathologic comparative analysis of 28 cases with molecular data – a study from the French Federation of Cancer Centers Sarcoma Group. Am J Surg Pathol 2003;27(1):27–39.

Tumors of fat, muscle, cartilage, and bone

Tammie Ferringer

Chapter 21

Lipoma

Key features
- Well-circumscribed tumor with a thin capsule
- Mature lipocytes

Lipomas typically present as asymptomatic, mobile soft nodules in the deep soft tissue or subcutis. Histologically, they are thinly encapsulated tumors composed of sheets of mature adipocytes that are indistinguishable from the fat cells in the subcutaneous tissue. Each adipocyte has a single vacuole and an eccentric nucleus. The thin fibrous septa, which contain sparse blood vessels, are delicate and inconspicuous. Intramuscular lipomas, commonly of the forehead, consist of mature fat cells that displace muscle, splaying the fibers.

There are several rare syndromes in which multiple lipomas occur. Hundreds of slow-growing subcutaneous and deep or visceral lipomas develop in early adulthood in the autosomal-dominant condition familial multiple lipomatosis. Benign symmetric lipomatosis (Madelung's disease) has a predilection for middle-aged men with a propensity to develop multiple lesions, especially in the region of the neck in a "horse-collar" distribution. Tender, circumscribed or diffuse fatty deposits of the lower legs, abdomen, and buttocks in obese patients exemplify adiposis dolorosa (Dercum's disease), sometimes associated with weakness and mental disturbances. Lipomas may also be a component of Gardner's syndrome, Bannayan–Zonana syndrome, Cowden's syndrome, and Proteus syndrome.

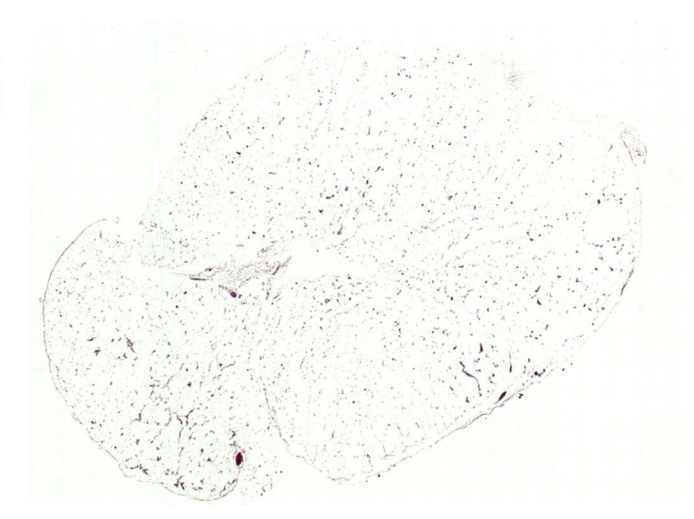

Fig 21-1 Lipoma

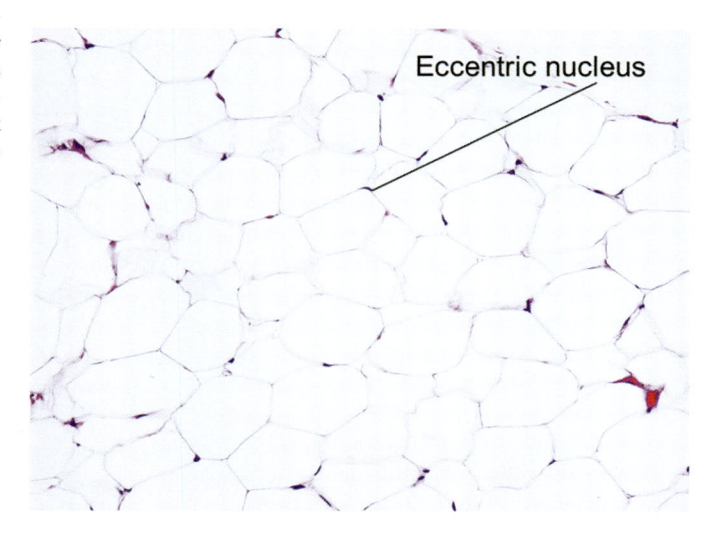

Fig 21-2 Lipoma

Angiolipoma

Key features

- Lipoma with proliferations of capillary-sized blood vessels
- Erythrocytes and scattered fibrin microthrombi are commonly present in the lumens

Clinically, angiolipoma are often tender to palpation. They commonly occur in women, are multifocal, and have a predilection for the forearm.

Differential Diagnosis

The differential diagnosis of painful tumors can be remembered by the mnemonic "BANGLE":

- *B*lue rubber bleb
- *A*ngiolipoma
- *N*euroma
- *G*lomus tumor
- *L*eiomyoma
- *E*ccrine spiradenoma

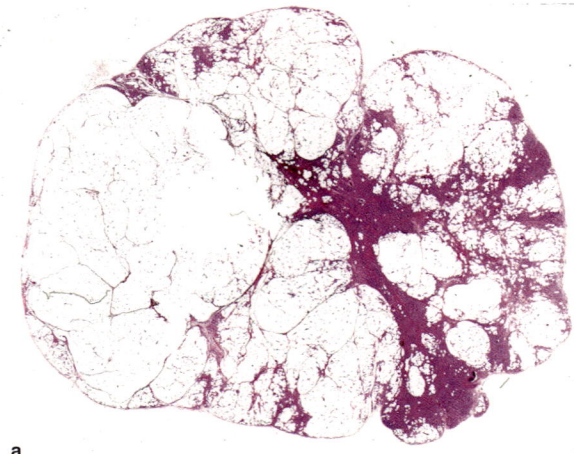

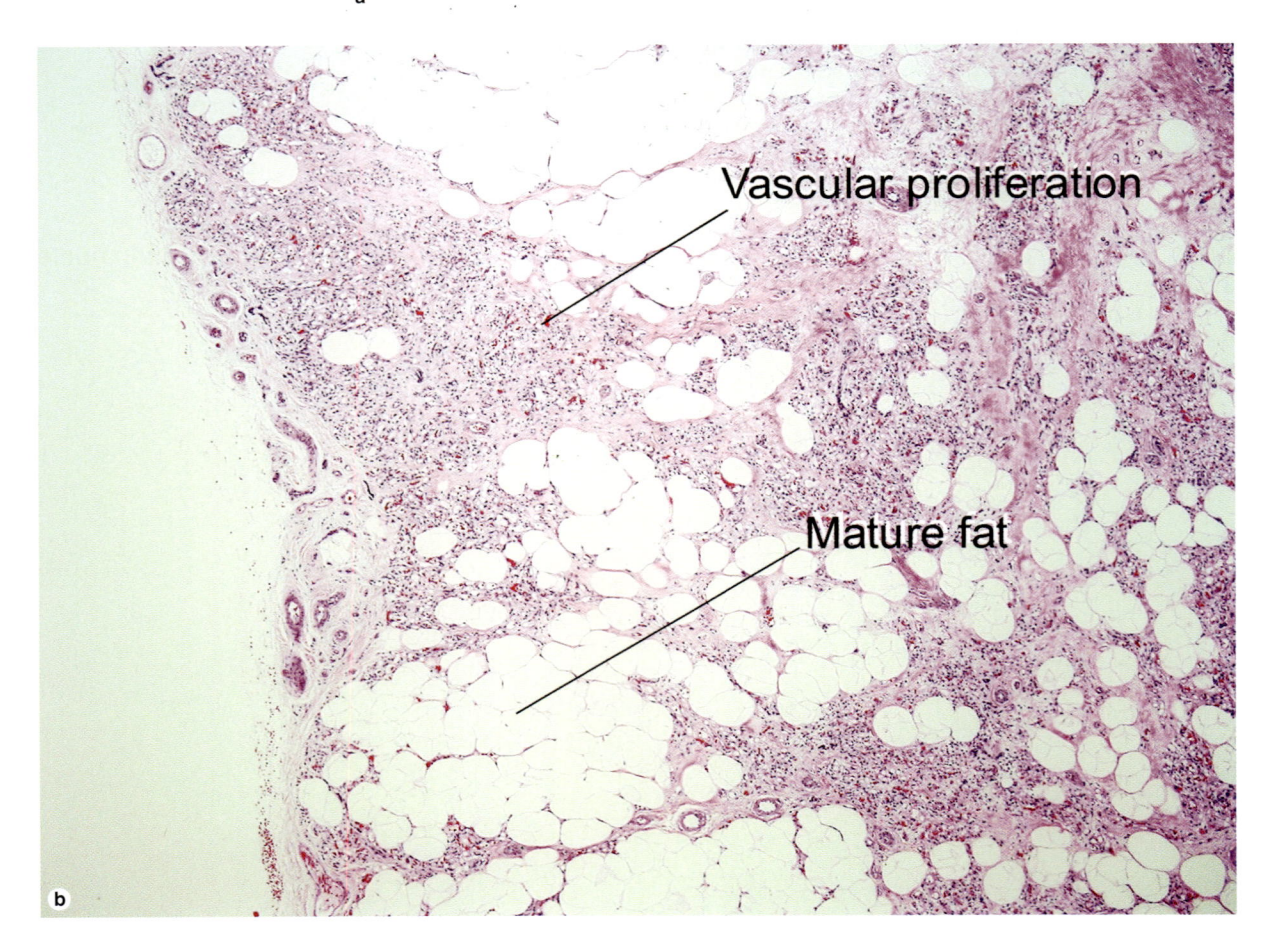

Fig 21-3 Angiolipoma

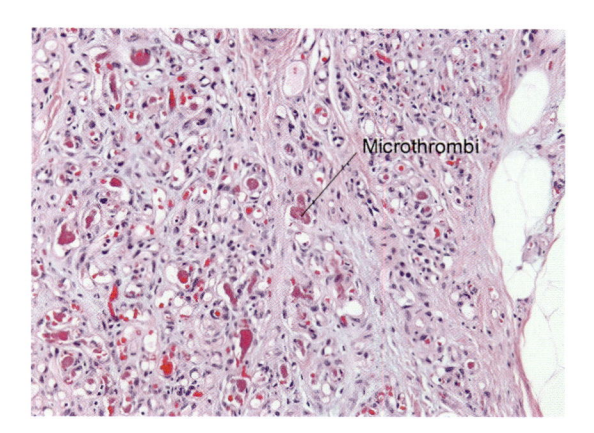

Tumors of fat, muscle, cartilage, and bone Chapter 21 343

Fig 21-4 Angiolipoma

Spindle cell lipoma

Key features

- Well-circumscribed tumor of mature fat with interspersed zones of bland spindle cells and variable amounts of collagen
- In young lesions, the spindle cell areas are myxoid, with many mast cells
- No lipoblasts or mitotic figures
- CD34+ spindle cells
- Ropey collagen bundles

The most common presentation is a solitary lesion at the base of the neck, shoulder, or upper back in an older man. These lesions are generally firmer and more fixed to surrounding tissue than the usual lipoma.

Differential Diagnosis

When spindle cell and myxoid components predominate, there may be confusion with neural or fibroblastic proliferations, especially diffuse neurofibroma.

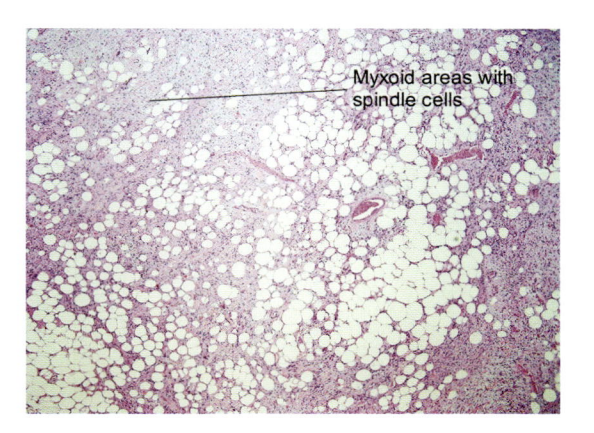

Fig 21-5 Spindle cell lipoma

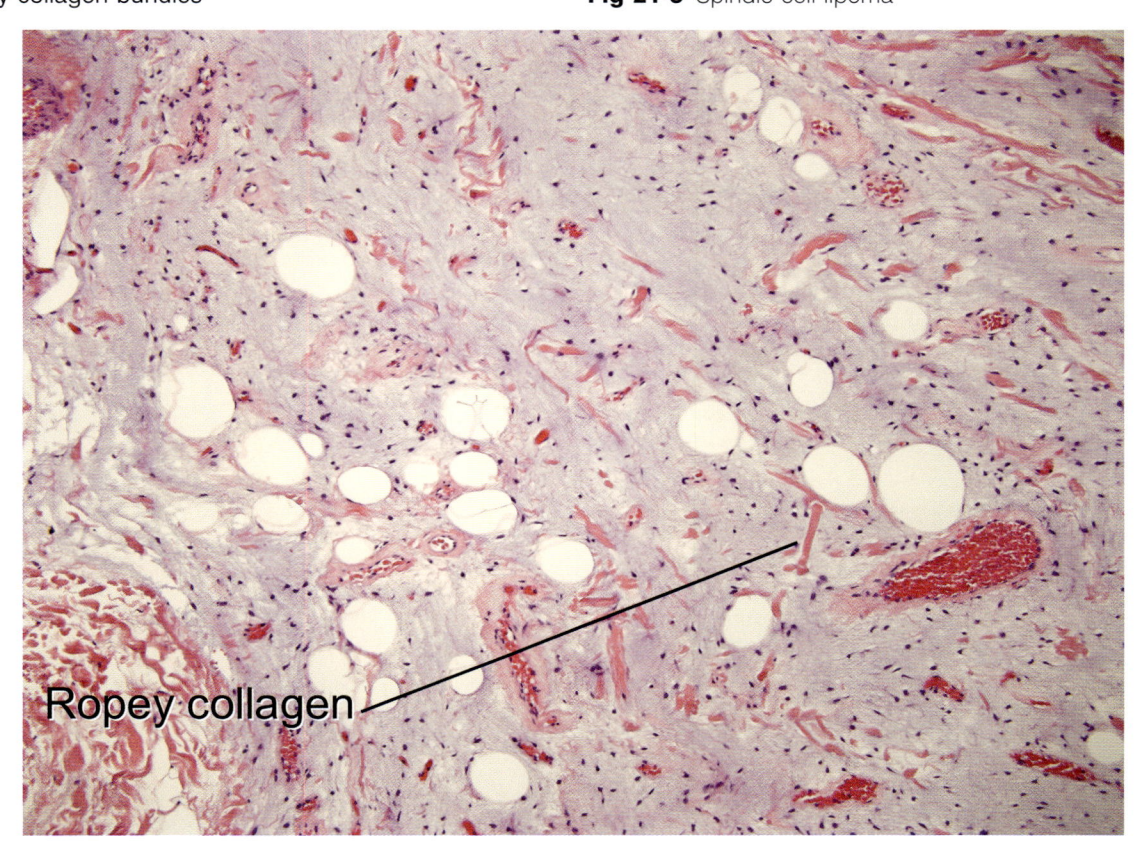

Fig 21-6 Spindle cell lipoma

Fibrolipoma

> **Key features**
> - Well-circumscribed tumor of mature lipocytes containing large bundles of mature collagen

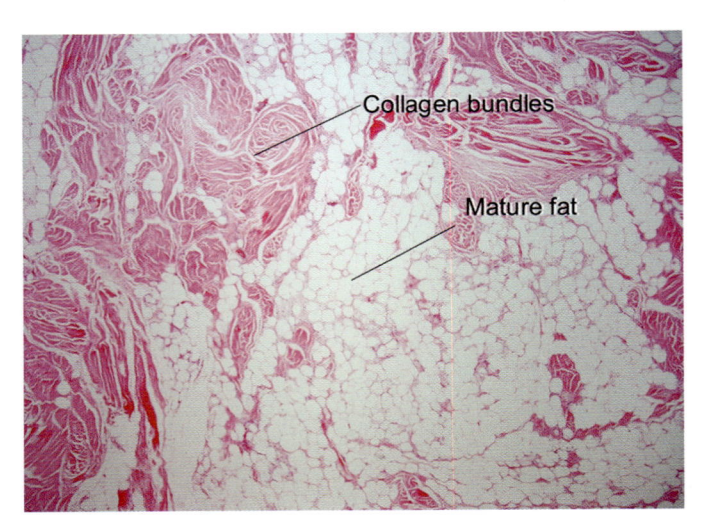

Fig 21-7 Fibrolipoma

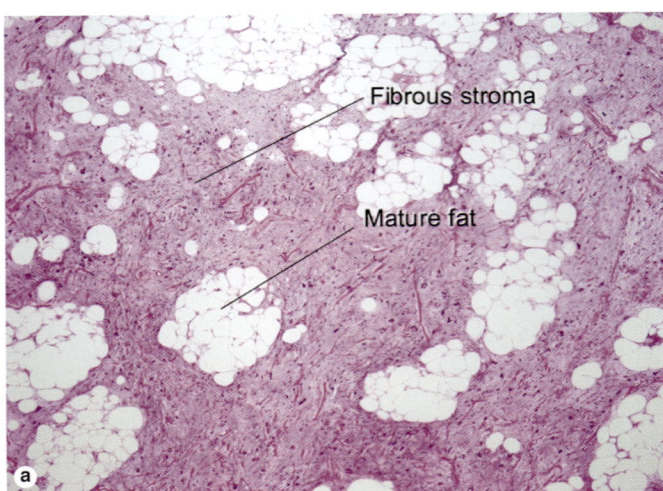

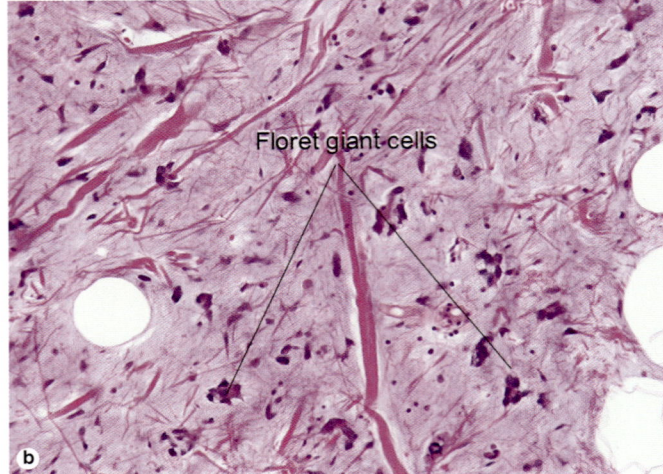

Fig 21-8 Pleomorphic lipoma

Pleomorphic lipoma

> **Key features**
> - Well-circumscribed tumor of lipocytes containing multinucleate floret cells with overlapping nuclei arranged at the periphery like the petals of a flower
> - Hyperchromatic nuclei may be present
> - Myxoid areas and ropey collagen bundles may be present, as in spindle cell lipoma

Pleomorphic lipomas have a firm consistency and similar distribution to spindle cell lipomas on the neck and shoulder girdle of older men.

> **Differential Diagnosis**

The sharp circumscription, superficial location, floret cells, paucity of mitotic activity, and absence of lipoblasts distinguish pleomorphic lipoma from pleomorphic liposarcoma. Lipoblasts are immature fat cells that may have an eccentric nucleus (signet-ring lipoblasts) or have a central scalloped nucleus indented by lipid vacuoles (mulberry lipoblasts). Liposarcoma typically arises in deep soft tissue, especially the retroperitoneum, but may involve the skin. Liposarcomas demonstrate an arborizing pattern of blood vessels that resembles "chicken wire." More information on liposarcoma and other soft tissue neoplasms is available in the on-line component of this text.

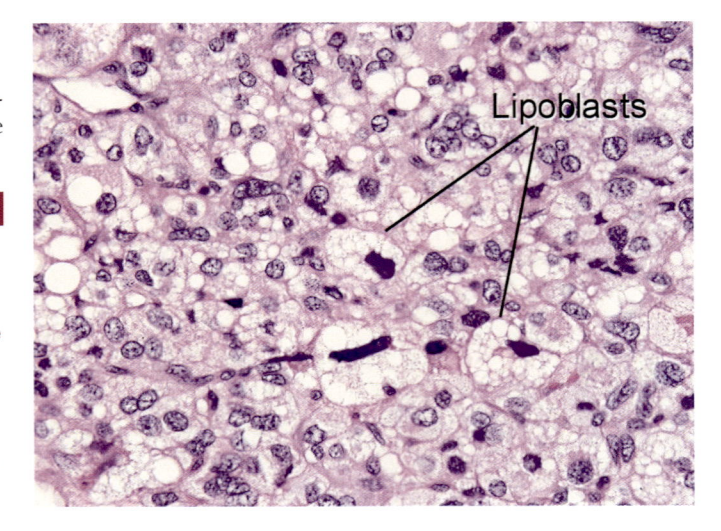

Fig 21-9 Pleomorphic liposarcoma

Angiomyolipoma

Key features

- Well-circumscribed tumor
- Smooth muscle radiating in a pinwheel fashion from the walls of muscular vessels
- Mature fat

Cutaneous angiomyolipomas are rare, solitary, painless subcutaneous nodules most commonly on the extremity of middle-aged men. Unlike renal angiomyolipomas, cutaneous lesions are not associated with tuberous sclerosis. Some consider these lesions to be angioleiomyomas with admixed mature fat.

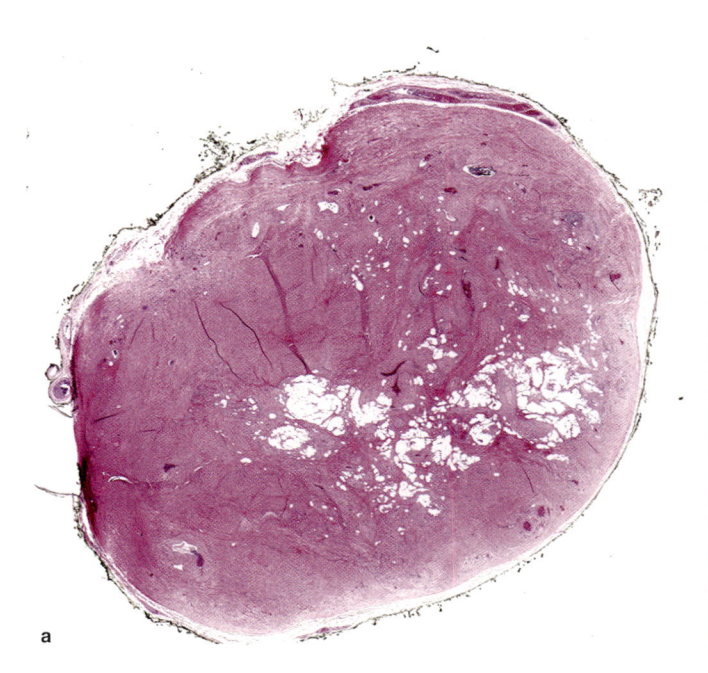

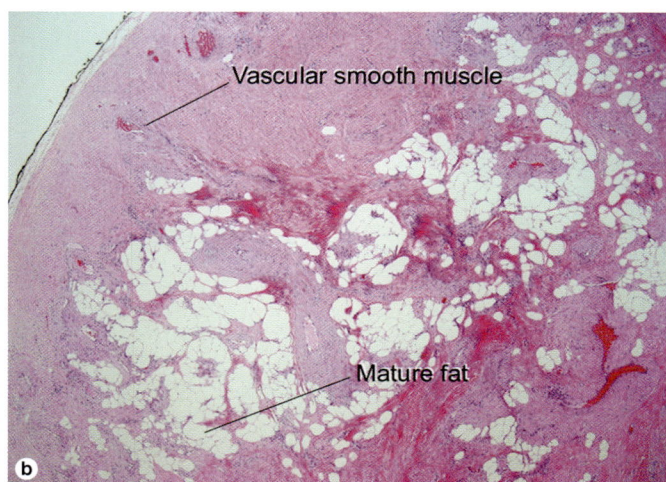

Fig 21-10 Angiomyolipoma

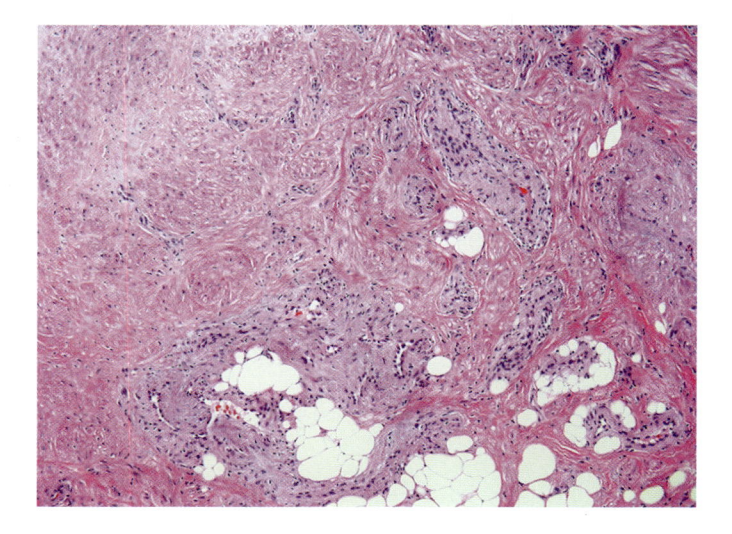

Fig 21-11 Angiomyolipoma

Hibernoma

Key features
- Well-circumscribed tumor
- Multivacuolated "mulberry cells"

Hibernomas are rare tumors that demonstrate differentiation toward brown (fetal) fat. While brown fat occurs anywhere in a fetus, hibernomas in adults most frequently arise in the subcutis of the shoulder girdle, posterior neck, and axilla. The gross brown color is a result of the prominent vascularity and many mitochondria within the tumor cells.

Mulberry cells with central nuclei predominate in most hibernomas. Smaller cells with granular cytoplasm and univacuolated cells may sometimes be seen.

Differential Diagnosis

Lipoblasts of liposarcoma have hyperchromatic scalloped nuclei. The tumors are large, poorly circumscribed, and have an arborizing vascular pattern.

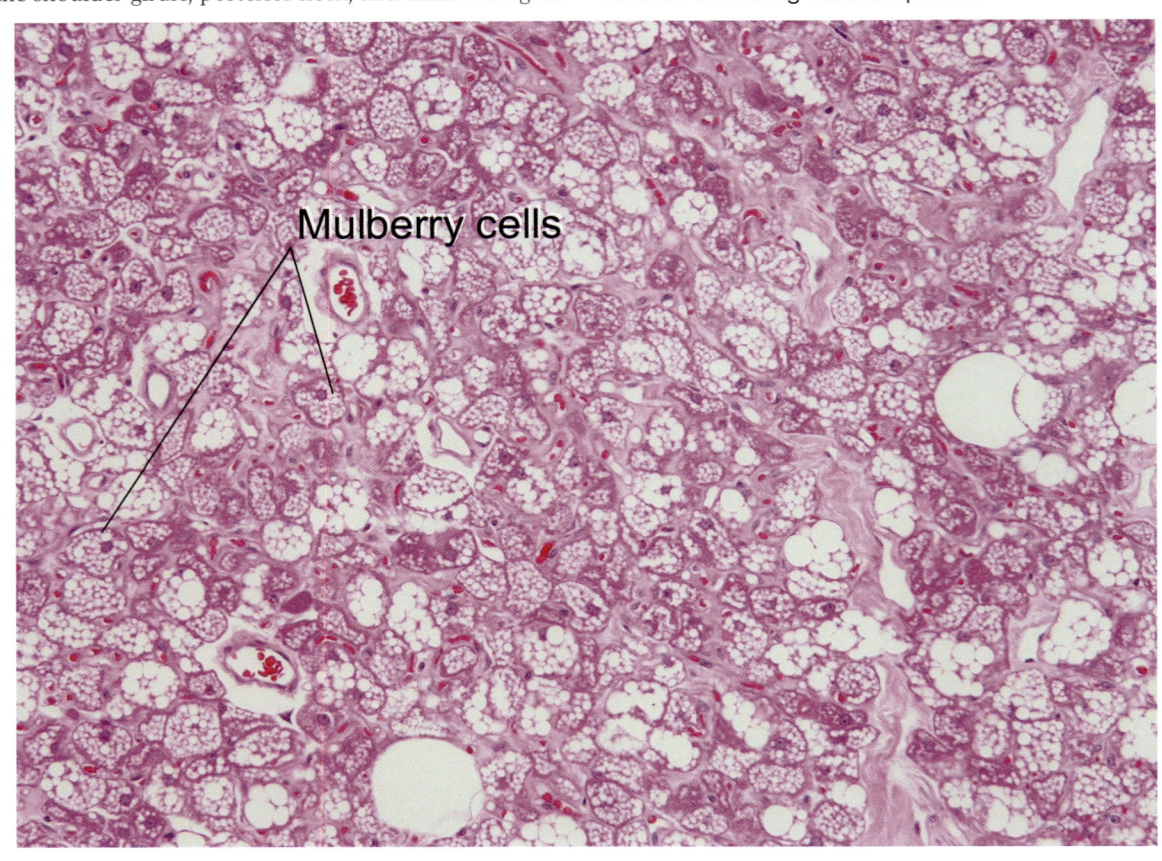

Fig 21-12 Hibernoma

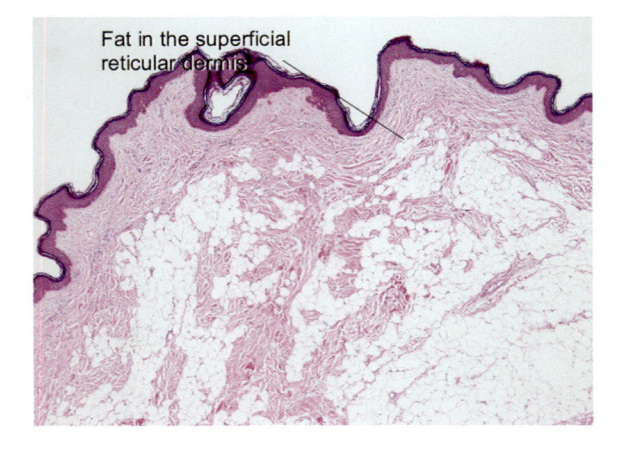

Fig 21-13 Nevus lipomatosis superficialis

Tumors of fat, muscle, cartilage, and bone

Nevus lipomatosis superficialis of Hoffmann and Zurhelle

Key features
- Mature adipocytes replacing much of the dermis

Nevus lipomatosis superficialis presents as multiple soft yellow-tan papules or nodules on the hip or buttock that coalesce into plaques or form a linear arrangement. Rarely, there is disseminated body involvement with extensively folded skin ("Michelin tire baby syndrome").

Large acrochordons with a broad base may have a similar appearance.

Differential Diagnosis

The histologic differential diagnosis includes Goltz syndrome (focal dermal hypoplasia), an X-linked dominant syndrome with a Blaschkoid distribution. Long-standing dermal nevi may also undergo extensive fatty degeneration but retain focal residual nevus.

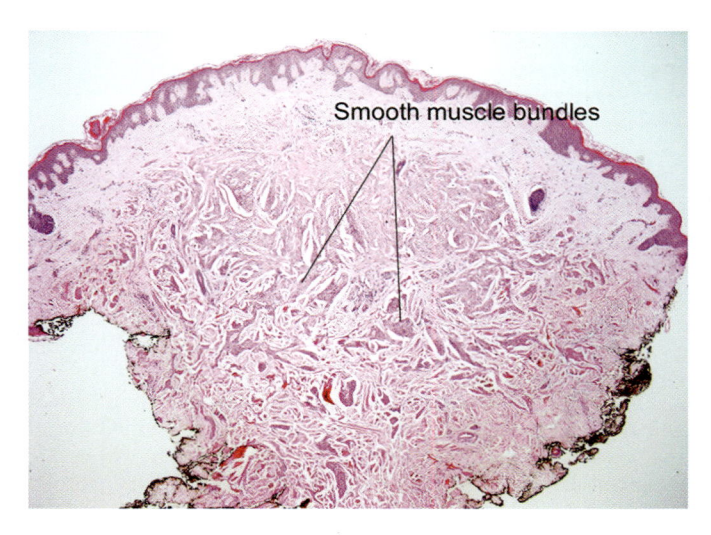

Fig 21-14 Piloleiomyoma

Leiomyoma

Leiomyomas are benign smooth muscle tumors. Smooth muscle is normally found in the skin as arrector pili muscles, in the walls of blood vessels, breast, and genital skin (periareolar or dartos muscle). Smooth muscle tumors can arise from each of these sources and are known as piloleiomyoma, angioleiomyoma, and leiomyoma of the genital skin, respectively.

Smooth muscle cells are characterized by long, thin cigar-shaped nuclei with blunt ends. A paranuclear vacuole, representing a glycogen "snack" for the muscle, is well demonstrated in cross-section.

Piloleiomyoma

Key features
- Circumscribed but non-encapsulated dermal nodule
- Interlacing bundles of smooth muscle fibers resemble arrector pili muscle "on steroids"
- Mitotic activity is negligible
- Nuclear density matches that of normal smooth muscle

Piloleiomyomas, derived from the arrector pili muscle, typically present as multiple firm, red-brown lesions in the third decade. They may be solitary, grouped, or in a linear pattern. Manipulation and exposure to cold result in pain.

Multiple lesions have been associated with papillary renal cell carcinoma and uterine leiomyomas (fibroids) in females. This constellation of findings, known as Reed's syndrome, is inherited in an autosomal-dominant pattern and is due to a mutation in the fumarate hydratase gene.

Differential Diagnosis

Smooth muscle hamartomas consist of smaller bundles that are sparsely distributed in a broad hyperpigmented patch or plaque-like lesion. Terminal hair may be present, and these lesions overlap with Becker's nevi.

The muscle bundles of piloleiomyoma can be distinguished from collagen bundles by the blunt, cigar-shaped nuclei with adjacent vacuole rather than the short tapered nuclei of the fibroblasts in collagen. The cytoplasm of smooth muscle cells is more conspicuous than in fibroblasts. A trichrome stain will stain muscle red and collagen green-blue. Immunoperoxidase markers for smooth muscle (smooth muscle actin and desmin) can also be used.

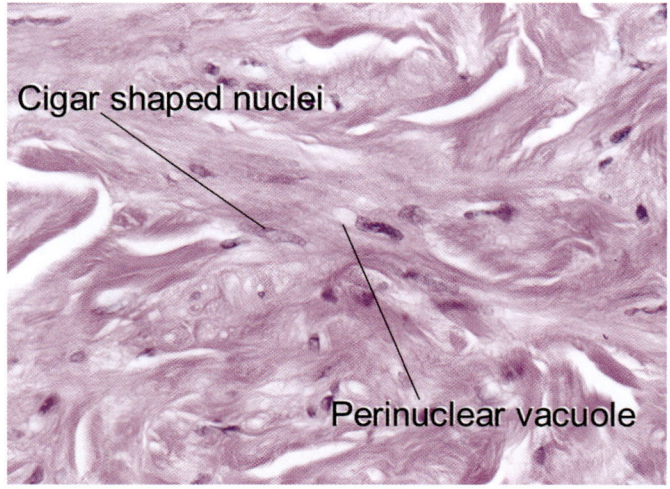

Fig 21-15 Piloleiomyoma

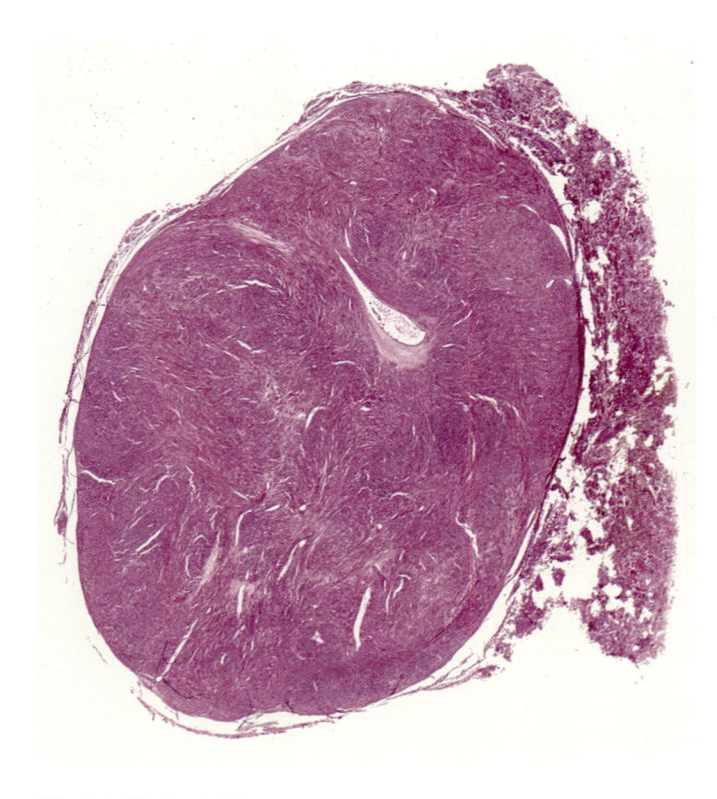

Fig 21-16 Angioleiomyoma

Angioleiomyoma

Key features

- Subcutaneous nodule of smooth muscle containing round and slit-like vascular spaces

Angioleiomyomas are usually tender subcutaneous nodules on the lower extremities of middle-aged adults. More than half of lesions are spontaneously painful. Each vessel has several layers of smooth muscle that merge with the intervascular smooth muscle fascicles.

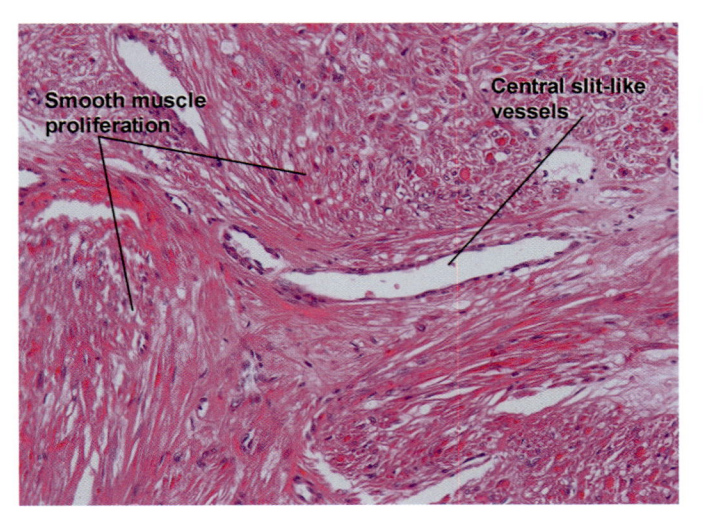

Fig 21-17 Angioleiomyoma

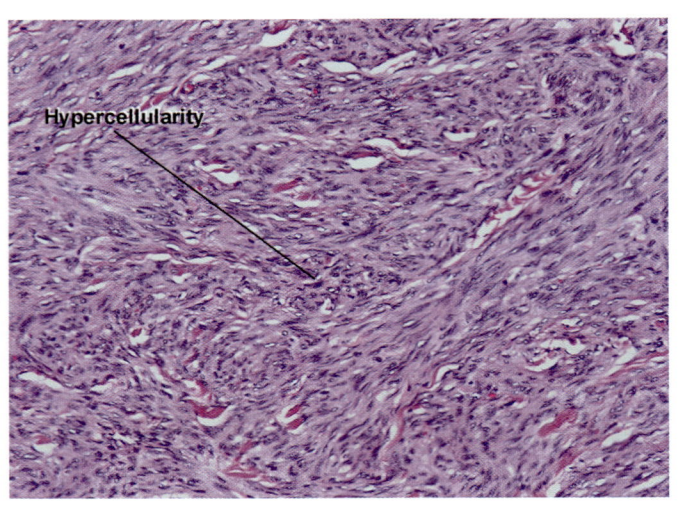

Fig 21-18 Leiomyosarcoma

Leiomyosarcoma

Key features

- High cellularity
- Mitoses and nuclear atypia

Superficial or dermal leiomyosarcomas are neoplasms that arise from the pili or genital smooth muscle. They occur predominantly in middle-aged men on the extensor extremities. Lesions recur in 30% of cases but metastasis is extremely rare.

Subcutaneous leiomyosarcomas, presumably arising from vascular smooth muscle, are larger, and have a greater tendency for metastasis to lung, other soft-tissue sites, and the liver, in one-third of cases.

Similar to leiomyomas, leiomyosarcomas are composed of intertwined fascicles of fusiform cells with blunt-ended nuclei and eosinophilic cytoplasm. Leiomyosarcomas, however, are hypercellular with a high nucleocytoplasmic ratio. Mitotic figures are variable. Subcutaneous leiomyosarcomas have a greater degree of pleomorphism and nuclear atypia, a higher mitotic rate, and may show focal necrosis.

Differential Diagnosis

Although a grenz zone is often present, dermal leiomyosarcomas may be *slam*med up against the epidermis and resemble other spindle cell neoplasms. Immunohistochemistry can aid in the microscopic differential diagnosis.

- *S*pindled squamous cell carcinoma (keratin+)
- *L*eiomyosarcoma (desmin+)
- *A*typical fibroxanthoma (diagnosis of exclusion)
- *M*elanoma (S100+)

Tumors of fat, muscle, cartilage, and bone

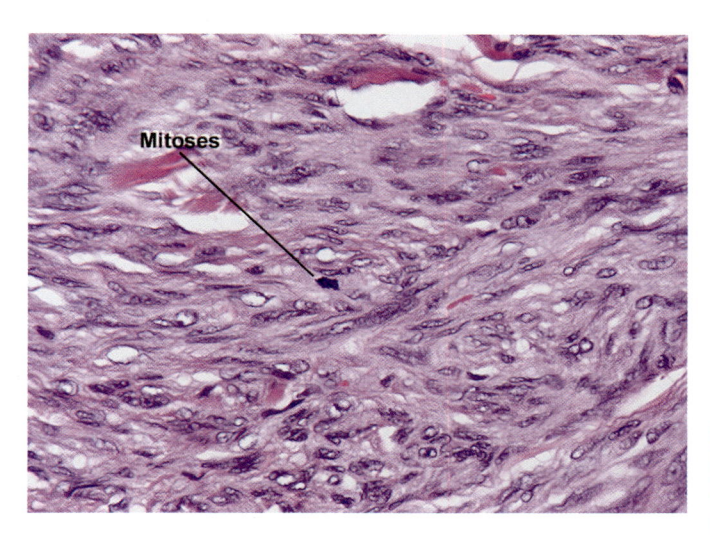

Fig 21-19 Leiomyosarcoma

Cutaneous bone formation may be primary or secondary. It is primary if no preceding cutaneous lesion is present. Primary cutaneous ossification can occur in Albright's hereditary osteodystrophy and as osteoma cutis. Secondary bone formation occurs through metaplasia within a pre-existing lesion such as a pilomatricoma, chondroid syringoma, intradermal nevus (nevus of Nanta), acne scar, scleroderma, or dermatomyositis.

The osteoblasts that form bone in cutaneous ossification originate in pre-existing fibrous connective tissue and result in intramembranous rather than enchondral bone formation. An important exception would be chondroid syringoma in which endochondral bone formation may occur.

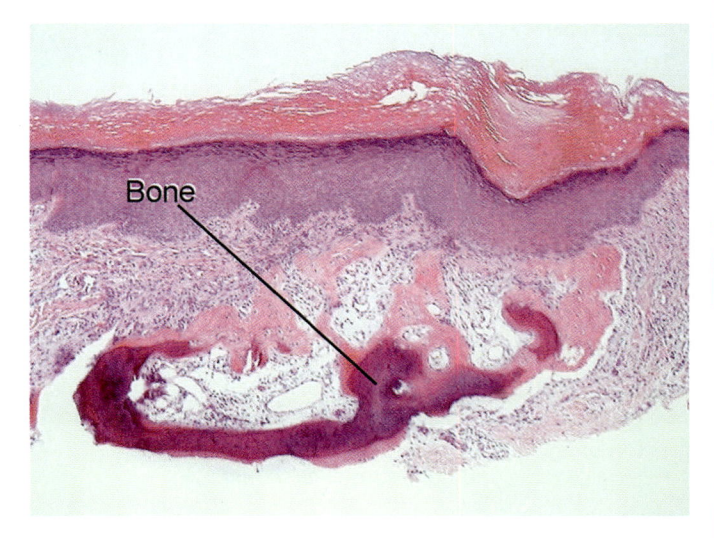

Fig 21-20 Osteoma cutis

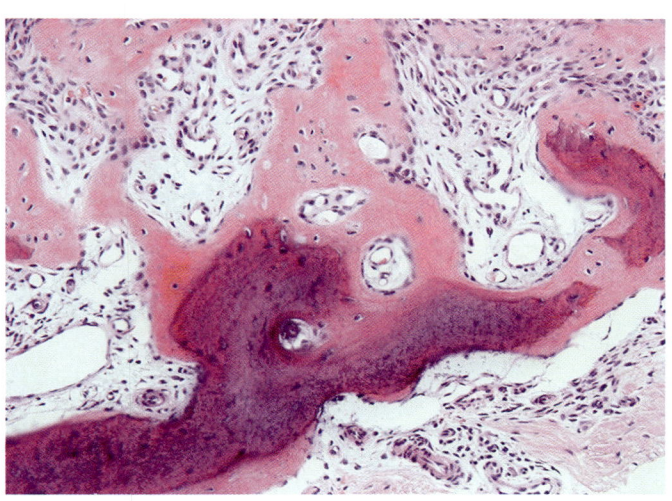

Fig 21-21 Osteoma cutis

Osteoma cutis

Key features

- Dermal or subcutaneous bone
- Haversian canals, osteocytes in lacunae, and osteoclasts similar to normal bone

Relapsing polychondritis

Key features

- Cartilage with neutrophilic infiltrate in the surrounding perichondrium
- Direct immunofluorescence (DIF): continuous granular band of IgG/A/M and C3 (full house) in the perichondrium

Dermatopathology

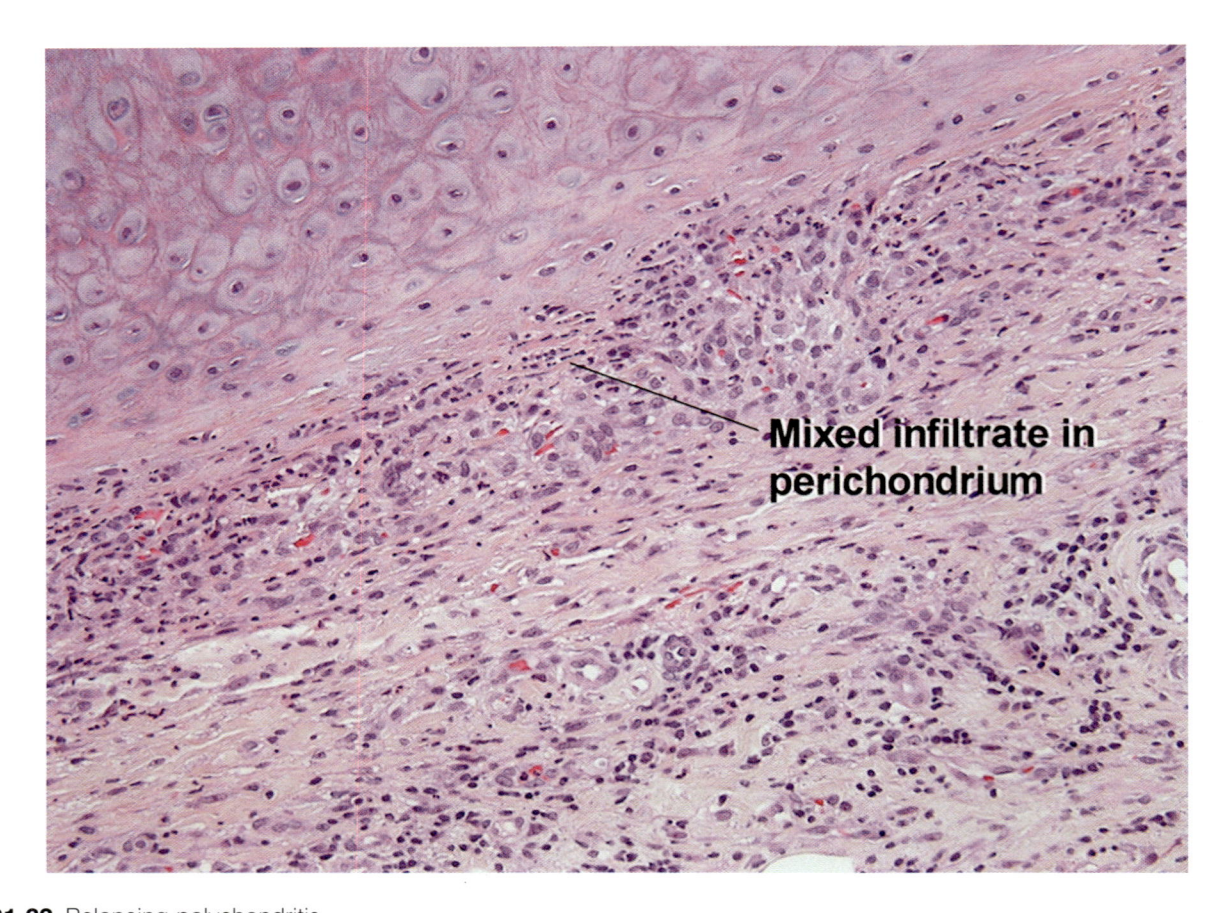

Fig 21-22 Relapsing polychondritis

Accessory tragus (cartilaginous rest)

Key features

- Fibrovascular polyp containing numerous vellus follicles
- Core of adipose tissue and cartilage may be seen

Accessory tragi are congenital lesions, typically in the preauricular area but sometimes involving the neck. Rarely, they are associated with oculo-auriculo-vertebral syndrome (Goldenhar syndrome).

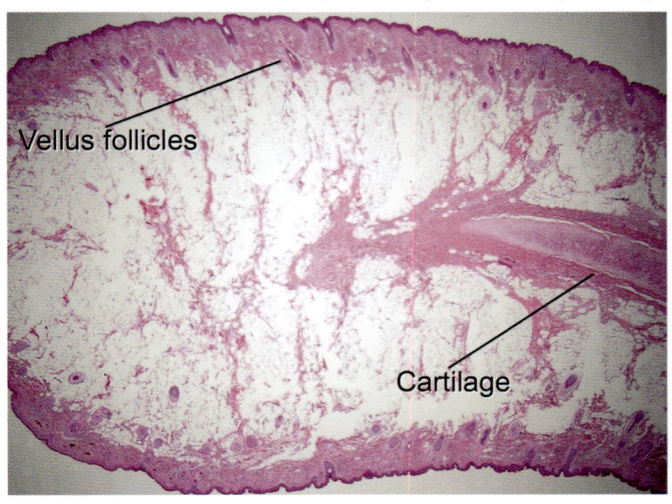

Fig 21-23 Accessory tragus, scanning magnification

Chondroma

Key features

- Circumscribed mass of mature hyaline cartilage
- Single or grouped chondrocytes in lacunae

Soft-tissue chondromas typically occur on the fingers of middle-aged adults. Calcification can be seen.

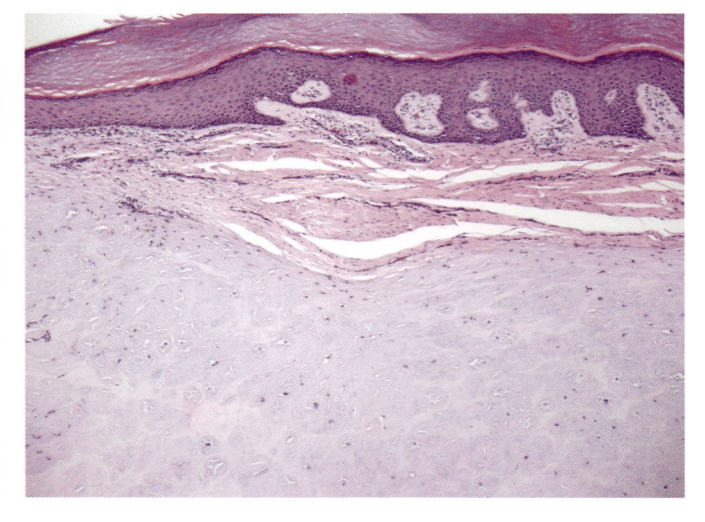

Fig 21-24 Chondroma

Tumors of fat, muscle, cartilage, and bone — Chapter 21

Chordoma

Key features

- Lobules separated by fibrous bands
- Sheets, cords, or individual cells in chondroid stroma
- Abundant pale bubbly cytoplasm (physaliphorous)
- No lacunae-like chondroma or ducts like chondroid syringoma

These tumors originate from a remnant of the notochord and thus are typically seen along the axial spine, especially the sacrococcygeal area. Cutaneous involvement can occur directly or via metastasis. There is triple positivity with S100, vimentin, and keratin. Parachordomas are similar histologically but develop on the extremities adjacent to tendons, synovium, or bone. Cutaneous parachordomas are related to cutaneous myoepitheliomas.

Pseudocyst of the auricle

Key features

- Intracartilaginous space without true lining

Low-grade trauma may be a predisposing factor in development of these lesions and, if untreated, can result in deformity of the ear. There is a predilection for the antihelix of males. There is no significant inflammatory reaction.

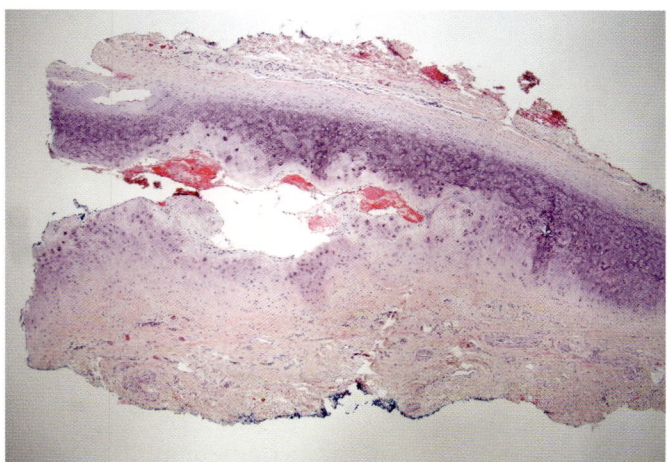

Fig 21-26 Pseudocyst of the auricle

Supernumerary nipple (polythelia)

Key features

- Subtle epidermal thickening with underlying pilosebaceous structures
- Surrounding scattered smooth muscle bundles typical of areola
- Central mammary duct may be visible

This developmental anomaly occurs anywhere along the embryonic milk line but has a predilection for the chest or upper abdomen. Histologically, polythelia resembles the normal nipple. Underlying breast tissue may be present.

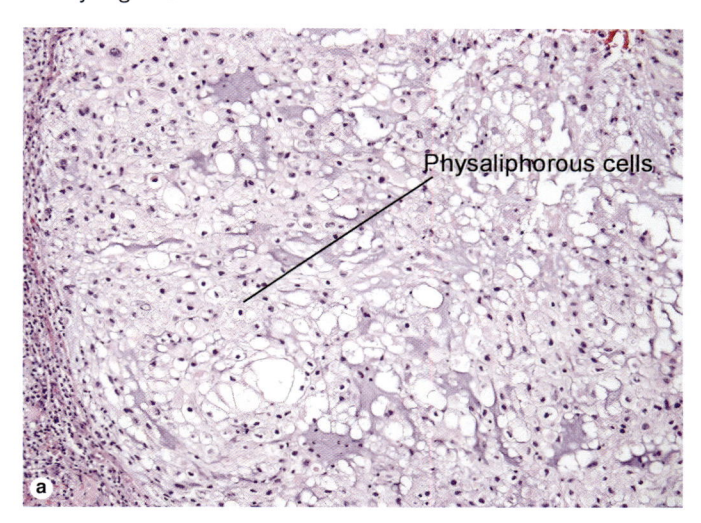

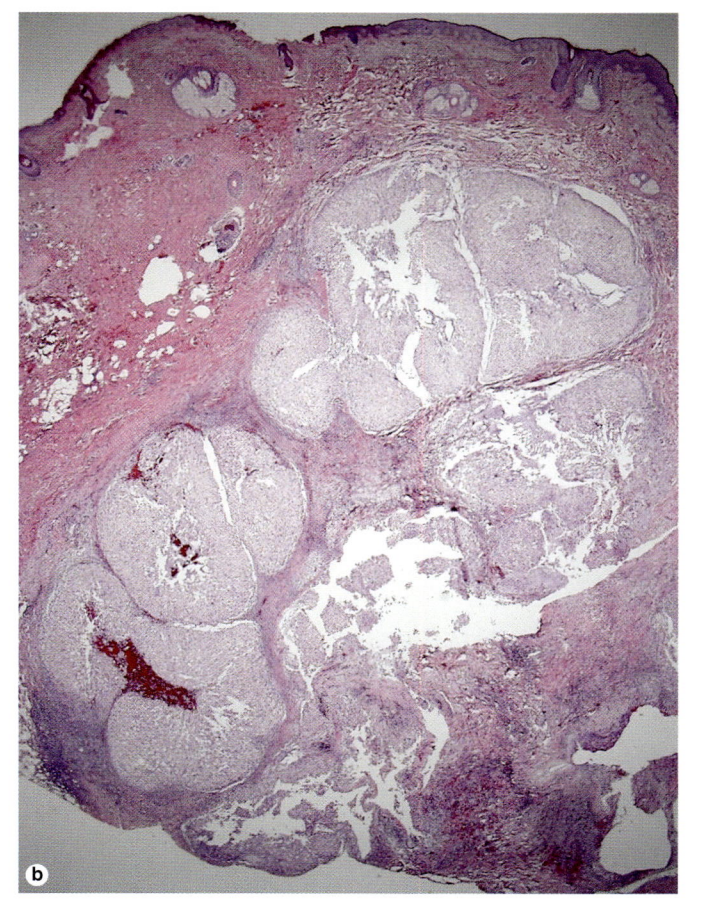

Fig 21-25 Chordoma

352 Dermatopathology

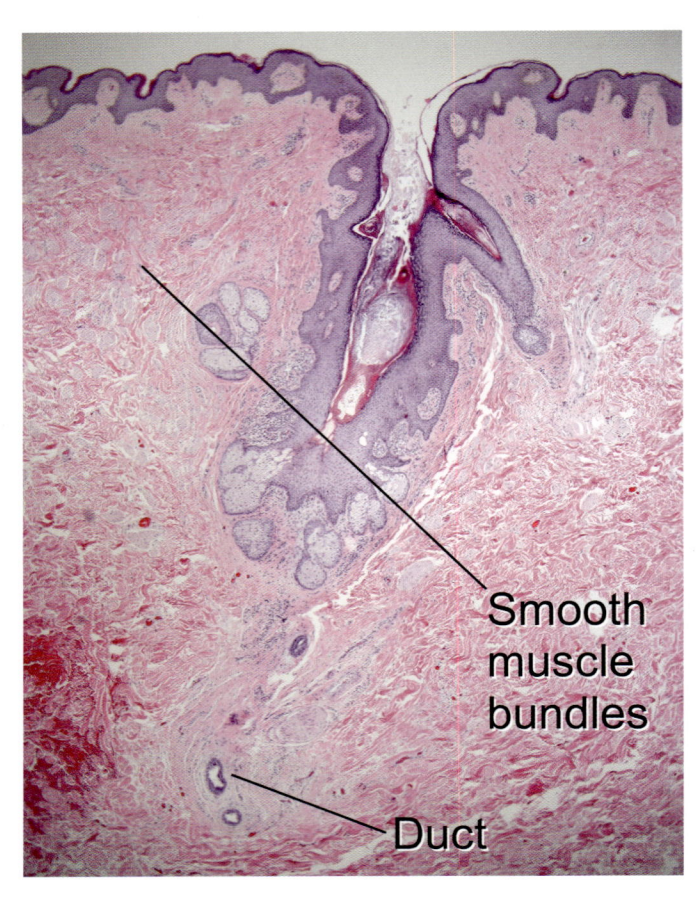

Fig 21-27 Supernumerary nipple

Mobile encapsulated lipoma (encapsulated fat necrosis, nodular–cystic fat necrosis)

Key features
- Lobules of necrotic fat surrounded by fibrous capsule

These clinically mobile lesions are typically associated with prior trauma. The necrosing fat consists of non-nucleated adipocytes.

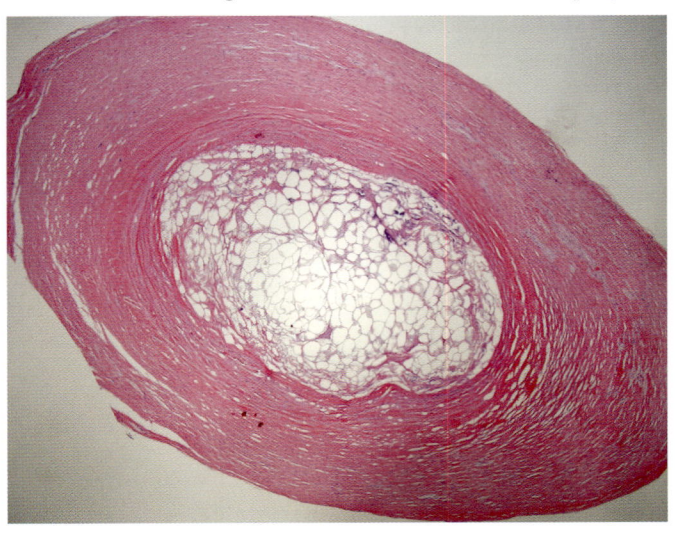

Fig 21-28 Mobile encapsulated lipoma (localized fat necrosis)

Smooth muscle hamartoma

Key features
- Numerous haphazard bundles of smooth muscle in the dermis

Most are congenital plaques of the lumbosacral area or proximal extremity composed of perifollicular papules. Becker's nevus and smooth muscle hamartoma are on the same developmental spectrum but Becker's nevus is hyperpigmented and hypertrichotic.

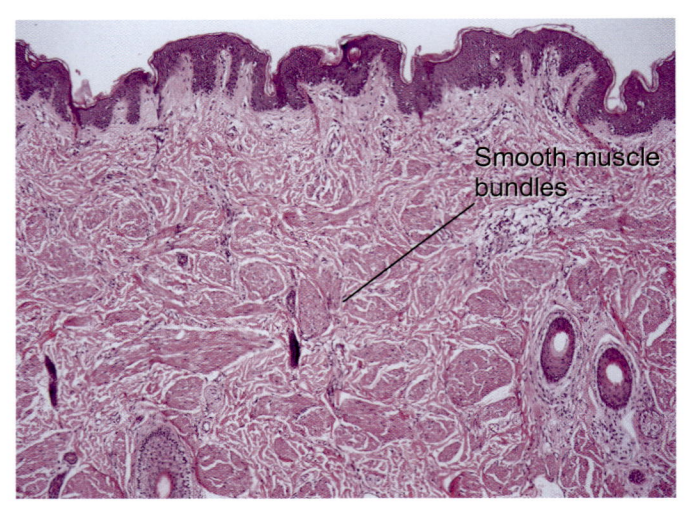

Fig 21-29 Smooth muscle hamartoma

Subungual exostosis

Key features
- Bony stalk with fibrocartilaginous cap

This lesion occurs under the nail plate, resulting in subungual hyperkeratosis, onycholysis or nail deformity. The great toe is the most common site. There is no cortical or medullary continuity with the underlying bone.

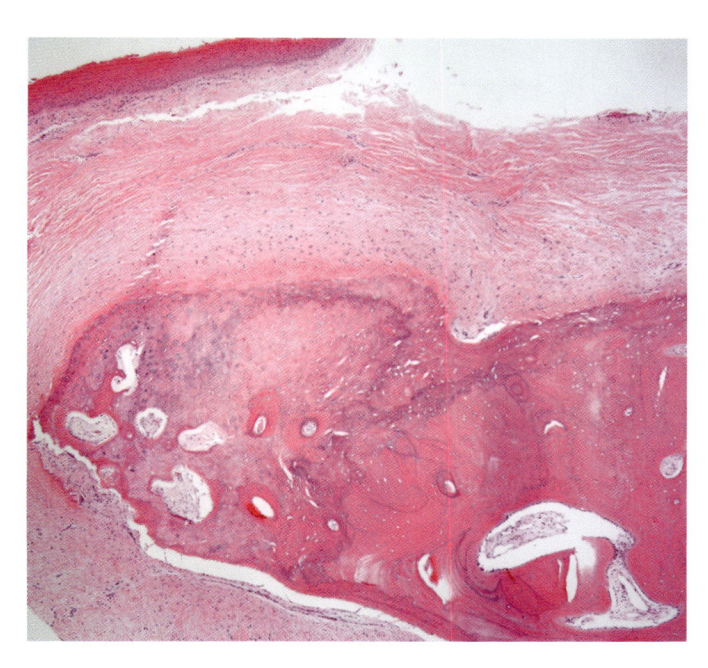

Fig 21-30 Subungual exostosis

Focal dermal hypoplasia (Goltz syndrome)

Key features

- Markedly hypoplastic dermis with adipocytes approaching the papillary dermis

This X-linked dominant disorder is due to a mutation in PORCN. The linear raised or depressed erythematous macules reveal a diminished dermis with fatty replacement. Other findings include verrucous and papillomatous lesions, skeletal defects including "lobster claw" hand, syndactyly, polydactyly, osteopathia striata, colobomata, deafness, and aplasia cutis.

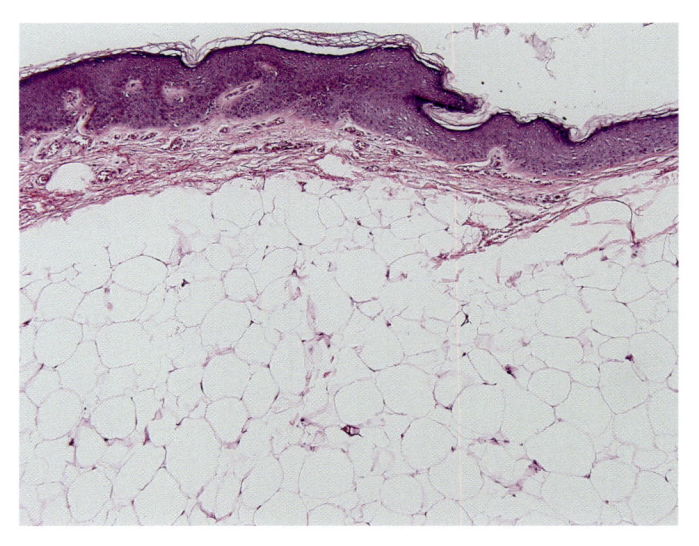

Fig 21-31 Goltz syndrome

Further reading

Burgdorf W, Nasemann T. Cutaneous osteomas: a clinical and histopathologic review. Arch Dermatol Res 1977;260(2):121–135.

Dixon AY, McGregor DH, Lee SH. Angiolipomas: an ultrastructural and clinicopathological study. Hum Pathol 1981;12(8):739–747.

Fields JP, Helwig EB. Leiomyosarcoma of the skin and subcutaneous tissue. Cancer 1981;47(1):156–169.

Fletcher CD, Martin-Bates E. Spindle cell lipoma: a clinicopathological study with some original observations. Histopathology 1987;11(8):803–817.

Hachisuga T, Hashimoto H, Enjoji M. Angioleiomyoma. A clinicopathologic reappraisal of 562 cases. Cancer 1984;54(1):126–130.

Hurt MA, Santa Cruz DJ. Nodular-cystic fat necrosis. A reevaluation of the so-called mobile encapsulated lipoma. J Am Acad Dermatol 1989;21(3 Pt 1):493–498.

Jansen T, Romiti R, Altmeyer P. Accessory tragus: report of two cases and review of the literature. Pediatr Dermatol 2000;17(5):391–394.

Jensen ML, Jensen OM, Michalski W, et al. Intradermal and subcutaneous leiomyosarcoma: a clinicopathological and immunohistochemical study of 41 cases. J Cutan Pathol 1996;23(5):458–463.

Lee SK, Jung MS, Lee YH, et al. Two distinctive subungual pathologies: subungual exostosis and subungual osteochondroma. Foot Ankle Int 2007;28(5):595–601.

Mehregan AH, Tavafoghi V, Ghandchi A. Nevus lipomatosus cutaneus superficialis (Hoffmann-Zurhelle). J Cutan Pathol 1975;2(6):307–313.

Mehregan DA, Mehregan DR, Mehregan AH. Angiomyolipoma. J Am Acad Dermatol 1992;27(2 Pt 2):331–333.

Newman PL, Fletcher CD. Smooth muscle tumours of the external genitalia: clinicopathological analysis of a series. Histopathology 1991;18(6):523–529.

Raj S, Calonje E, Kraus M, et al. Cutaneous pilar leiomyoma: clinicopathologic analysis of 53 lesions in 45 patients. Am J Dermatopathol 1997;19(1):2–9.

Roth SI, Stowell RE, Helwig EB. Cutaneous ossification. Report of 120 cases and review of the literature. Arch Pathol 1963;76:44–54.

Shmookler BM, Enzinger FM. Pleomorphic lipoma: a benign tumor simulating liposarcoma. A clinicopathologic analysis of 48 cases. Cancer 1981;47(1):126–133.

Svoboda RM, Mackay D, Welsch MJ, et al. Multiple cutaneous metastatic chordomas from the sacrum. J Am Acad Dermatol 2012;66(6):e246–e247.

Thompson J, Squires S, Machan M, et al. Cutaneous mixed tumor with extensive chondroid metaplasia: a potential mimic of cutaneous chondroma. Dermatol Online J 2012;18(3):9.

Chapter 22

Neural tumors

Tammie Ferringer

Neurofibroma

Key features

- Loose arrangement with pale myxoid stroma
- Haphazard spindle cells with small wavy or S-shaped nuclei
- Mast cells are numerous

Neurofibromas may occur as solitary lesions. Multiple widespread neurofibromas characterize neurofibromatosis (von Recklinghausen's disease) in which they are seen in association with café-au-lait macules, axillary freckling, and pigmented hamartomas of the iris (Lisch nodules).

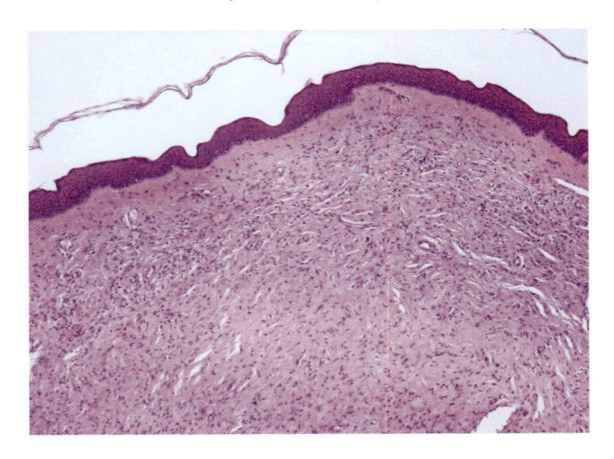

Fig 22-1 Neurofibroma

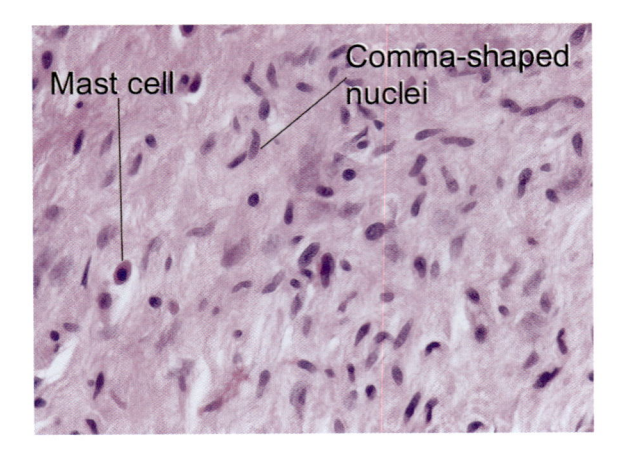

Fig 22-2 Neurofibroma

Diffuse neurofibroma

Key features

- At scanning magnification, diffuse replacement of dermis and infiltration of fat
- Higher magnification shows features typical of neurofibroma

Differential Diagnosis

Dermatofibrosarcoma protuberans has a similar growth pattern and can be myxoid, bearing a considerable resemblance to diffuse neurofibroma. Both may be CD34 positive, but S100 staining of the neurofibroma can distinguish the two. Spindle cell lipoma can appear similar, but occurs as an encapsulated nodule.

Plexiform neurofibroma

Key features

- Large fascicles of neurofibroma surrounded by perineurium
- Often embedded within a diffuse neurofibroma

Plexiform neurofibroma clinically resembles a "bag of worms" and is considered pathognomonic of neurofibromatosis. Both diffuse and plexiform neurofibromas probably result from loss

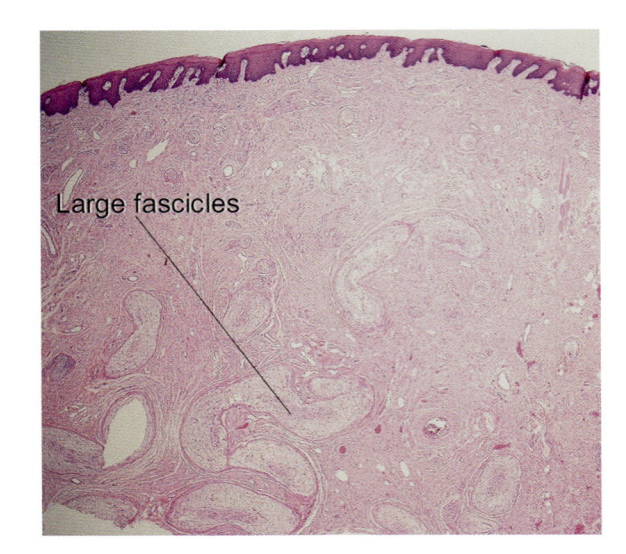

Fig 22-3 Plexiform neurofibroma

Neural tumors   Chapter 22   355

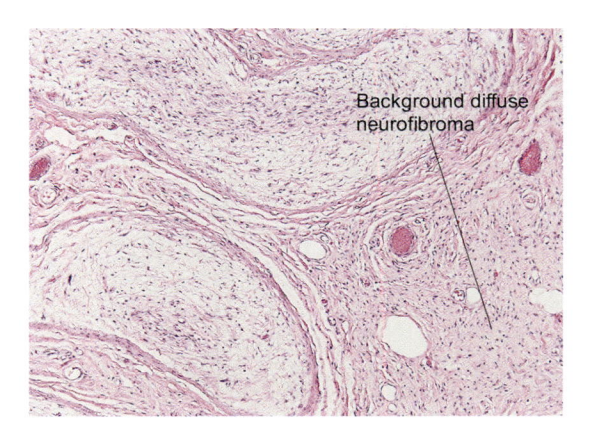

Fig 22-4 Plexiform neurofibroma

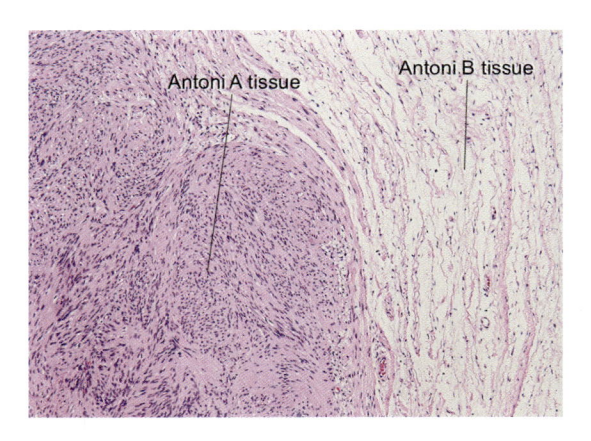

Fig 22-5 Schwannoma

of heterozygosity, where segmental loss of the remaining normal allele for the *NF1* gene results in a localized complete lack of tumor suppressor protein.

Schwannoma (neurilemmoma)

Key features

- Deep dermal or subcutaneous tumors with perineural capsule
- Arise within a nerve, displacing axons to the periphery, causing pain
- Antoni A tissue contains parallel rows of nuclei separated by acellular areas (Verocay bodies)
- Antoni B tissue represents a degenerative change with edematous stroma, typically just below the capsule

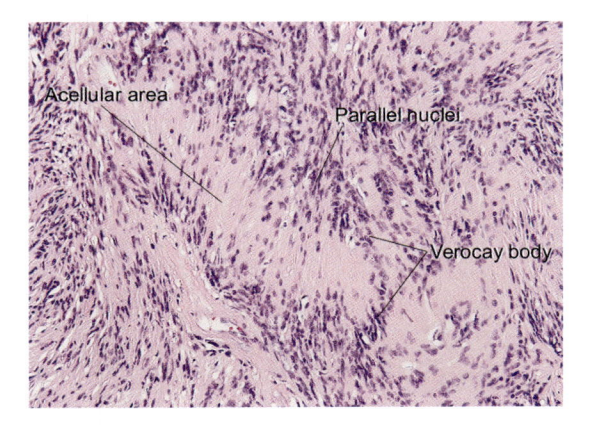

Fig 22-6 Schwannoma (Verocay bodies)

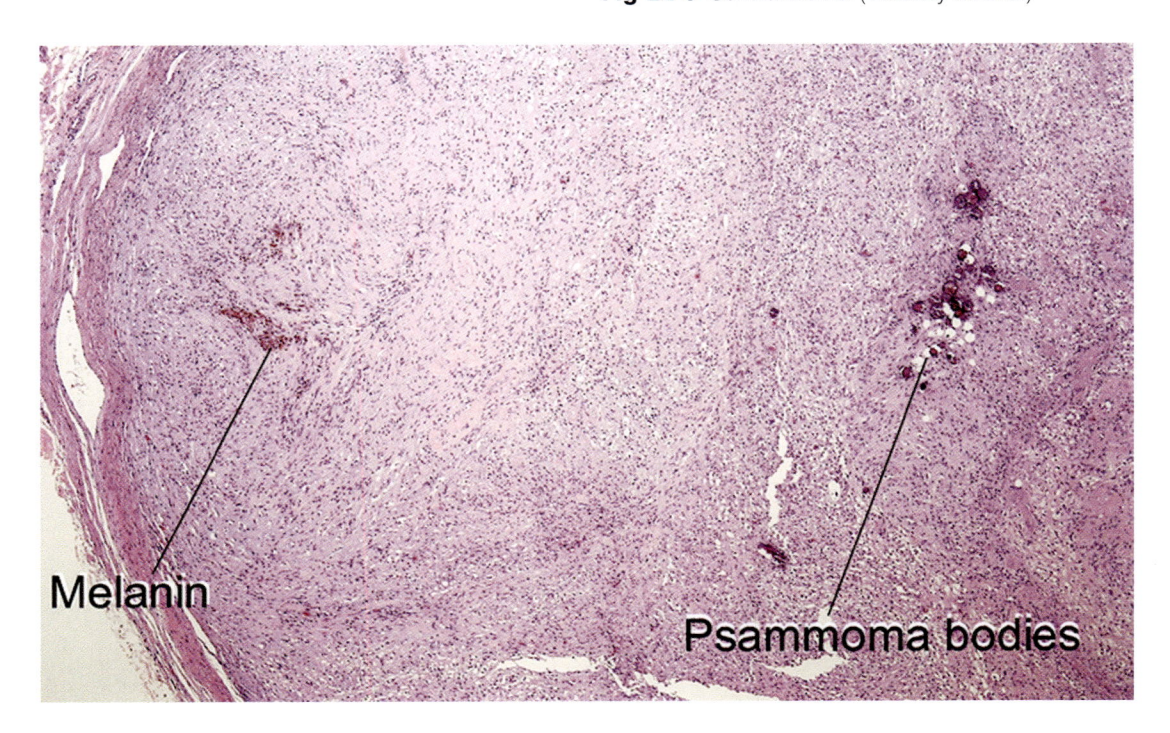

Fig 22-7 Psammomatous melanotic schwannoma

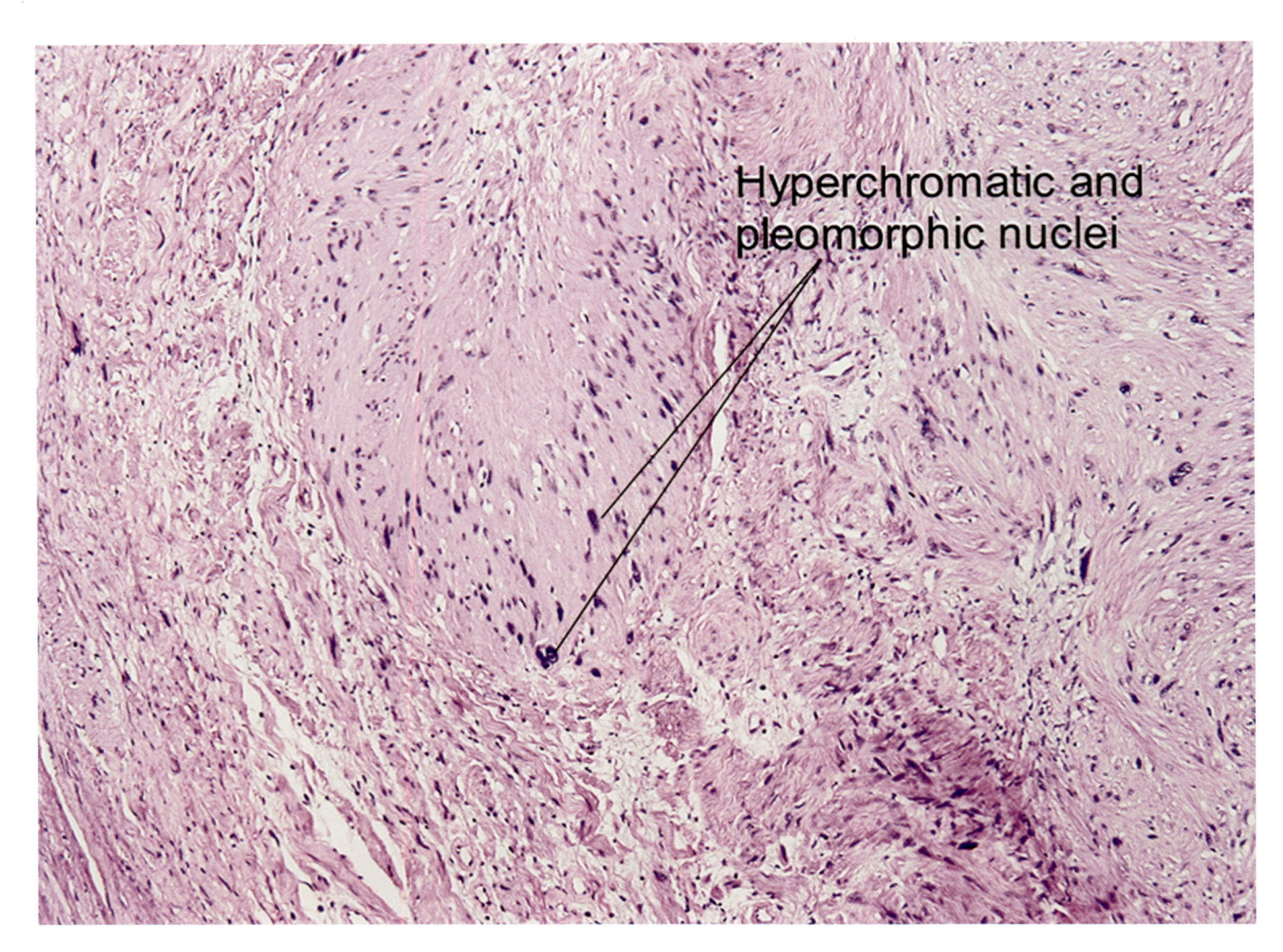

Fig 22-8 Ancient schwannoma

Psammomatous melanotic schwannoma is a variant with psammoma bodies and melanin. It is associated with Carney's complex (myxomas, spotty pigmentation, and endocrinopathy).

"Ancient" schwannoma

Key features

- Benign schwannoma with hyperchromatic pleomorphic nuclei
- No mitoses are present

These "ancient" changes in schwannomas represent a degenerative phenomenon. The absence of mitotic figures and absence of an expansile growth pattern distinguish benign ancient schwannoma from malignant peripheral nerve sheath tumors (MPNST). Typically, MPNSTs arise from neurofibromas, rather than schwannomas.

Neuromas

Neuromas are nerve sheath tumors with a roughly 1:1 ratio of axons to Schwann cells.

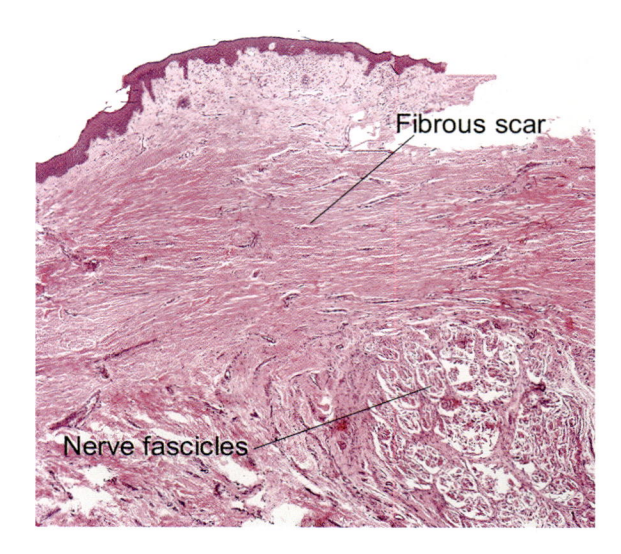

Fig 22-9 Traumatic neuroma

Traumatic neuroma

Key features

- Multiple nerve fascicles embedded within a fibrous scar
- Clefts between fascicles

Traumatic neuromas occur most commonly on the extremities where mechanical injuries are most frequent. Longitudinal growth of the regenerating nerve trunk results in complex folding. In cross-section, this appears as multiple discrete nerve fascicles.

Palisaded encapsulated neuroma

Key features

- Superficial dermal tumors with a thin, delicate capsule
- Fascicles of spindle cells separated by clefts

Palisaded encapsulated neuromas are solitary painless papules that occur most commonly on the lower central face. The name is somewhat of a misnomer, as there is usually no palisading and only an inconspicuous capsule. Histologically, they resemble the mucosal neuromas of multiple endocrine neoplasia syndrome

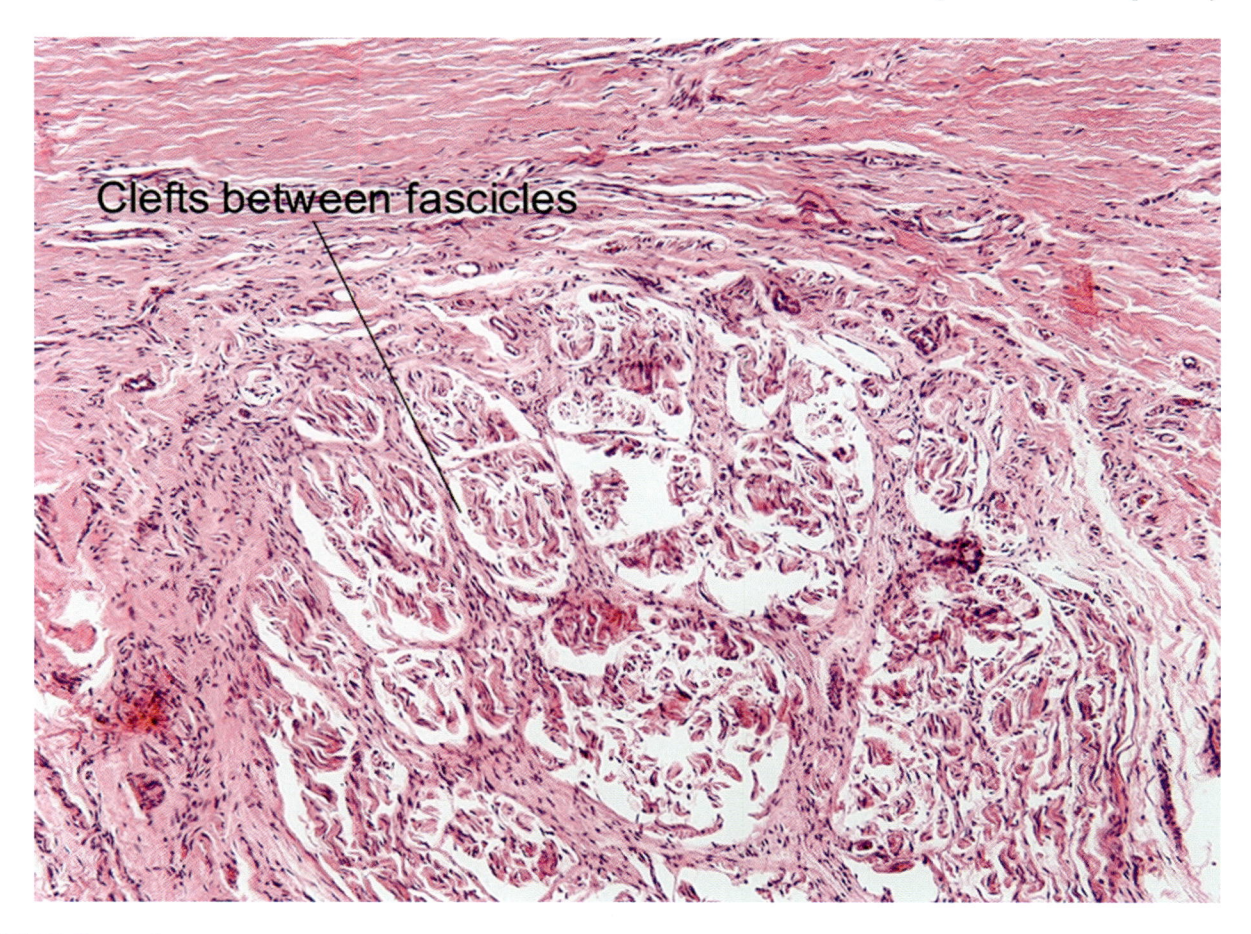

Fig 22-10 Traumatic neuroma

type 2b, an autosomal-dominant syndrome caused by a mutation of the *RET* proto-oncogene. In addition to the multiple mucosal neuromas, the syndrome is characterized by a marfanoid habitus, medullary carcinoma of the thyroid, pheochromocytoma, and hyperparathyroidism.

Differential Diagnosis

Unlike schwannomas, palisaded encapsulated neuromas are superficial tumors with adjacent sebaceous glands and small vellus follicles typical of facial skin. Schwannomas lack the fascicles with clefts seen in palisaded encapsulated neuromas.

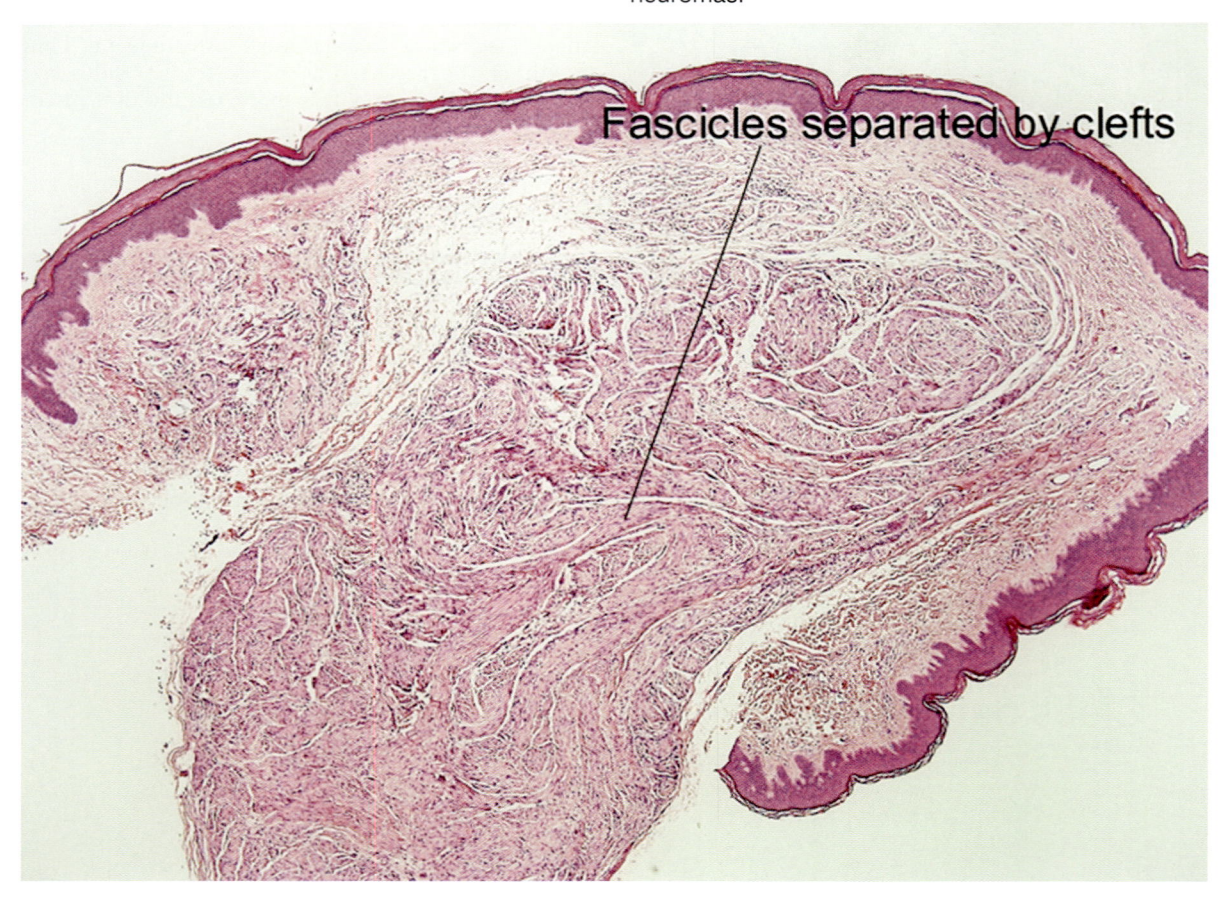

Fig 22-11 Palisaded encapsulated neuroma

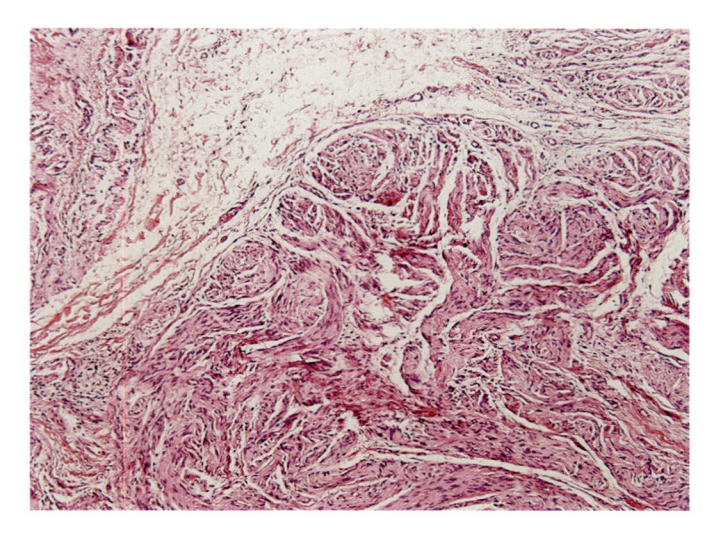

Fig 22-12 Palisaded encapsulated neuroma

Neural tumors Chapter 22 359

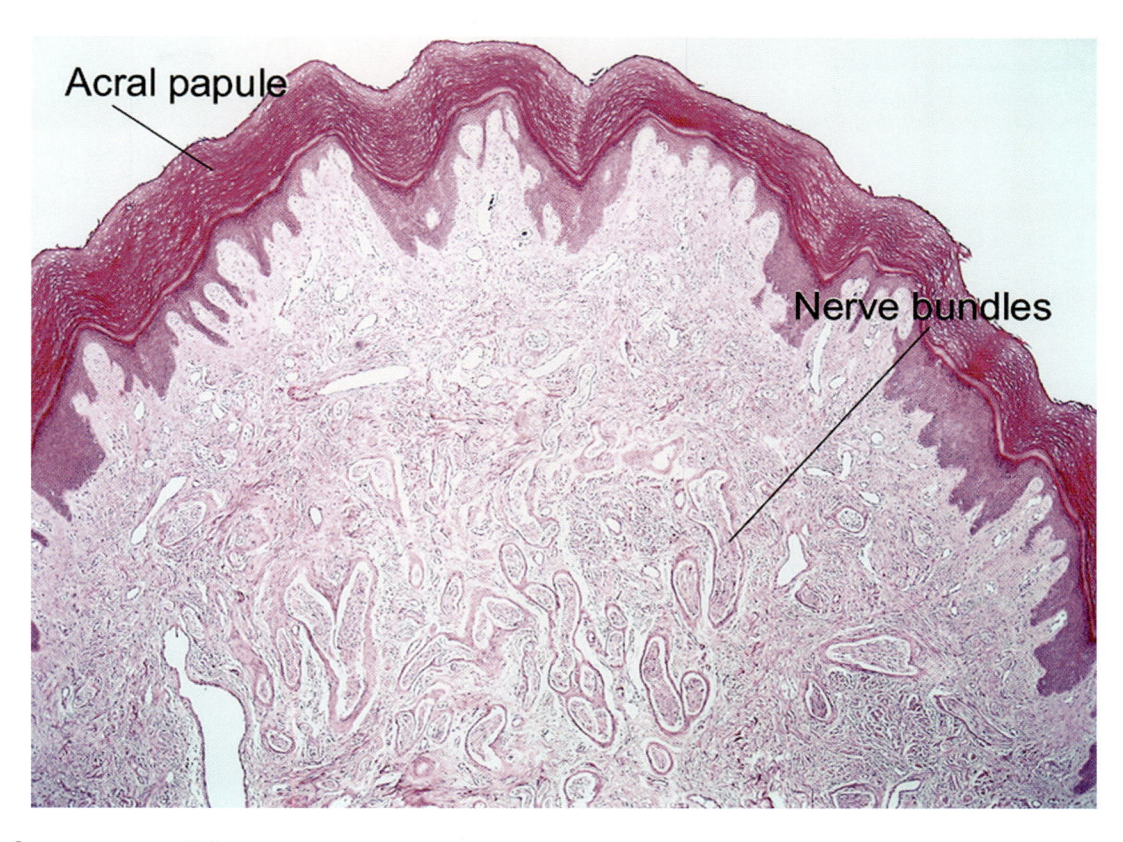

Fig 22-13 Supernumerary digit

Supernumerary digit (rudimentary polydactyly)

Key features

- Acral papule with nerve bundles
- Bone or cartilage may be present

Supernumerary digit presents as a congenital papule, typically located at the base of the fifth digit along the ulnar border.

Differential Diagnosis

Acquired digital fibrokeratoma is also an acral papule; however, there are no nerve bundles and large stellate factor XIIIa-positive dendrocytes may be present. There is often longitudinal streaking of collagen.

Merkel cell carcinoma (primary neuroendocrine carcinoma of the skin, trabecular carcinoma)

Key features

- Composed of small blue cells with scant cytoplasm and tightly packed nuclei in sheets or a trabecular array
- Nuclear molding, apoptotic cells, and mitoses are often present
- Synaptophysin, chromogranin, and neuron-specific enolase+
- CK20+ in a paranuclear dot pattern

Membrane-bound dense core granules on electron microscopy are characteristic. Metastatic small (oat) cell carcinoma of the lung also consists of small blue cells, but CK20 is typically negative and thyroid transcription factor (TTF-1) is positive. Also in the differential diagnosis of small blue cell tumors is lymphoma, which can be distinguished by positivity for hematopoietic markers. Melanoma is S100 positive. Neuroblastoma often demonstrates elongated, angulated "carrot-shaped" blue cells and may form rosettes.

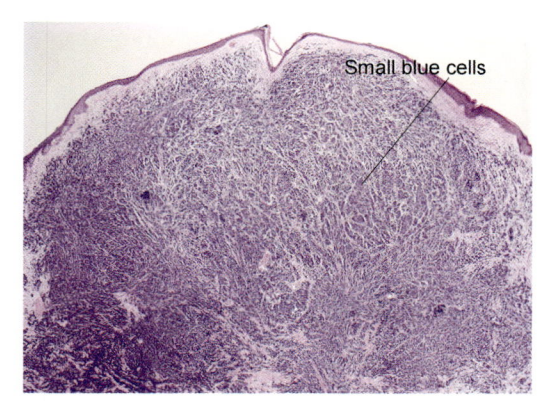

Fig 22-14 Merkel cell carcinoma

Dermatopathology

Differential Diagnosis

The microscopic differential diagnosis for "small blue cell" tumors can be remembered by the mnemonic "LEMONS":

- *L*ymphoma
- *E*wing's sarcoma
- *M*erkel cell carcinoma/melanoma
- *O*at cell carcinoma of the lung
- *N*euroblastoma
- *S*mall cell endocrine carcinoma

Granular cell tumor

Key features

- Sheets of large polygonal cells with abundant eosinophilic granular cytoplasm with central nucleus
- Discrete round eosinophilic giant lysosomal granules (pustulo-ovoid bodies of Milian)
- Overlying pseudoepitheliomatous hyperplasia can be mistaken for squamous cell carcinoma
- S100+

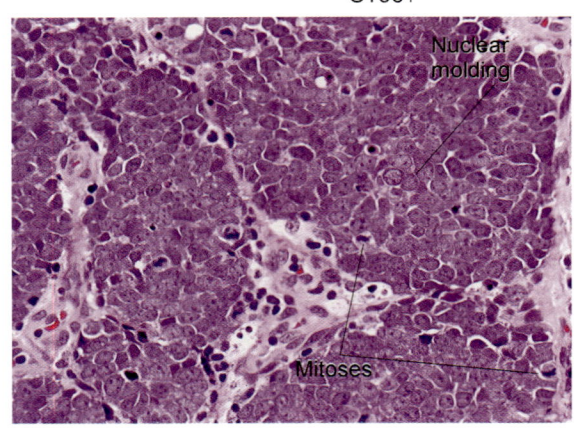

Fig 22-15 Merkel cell carcinoma

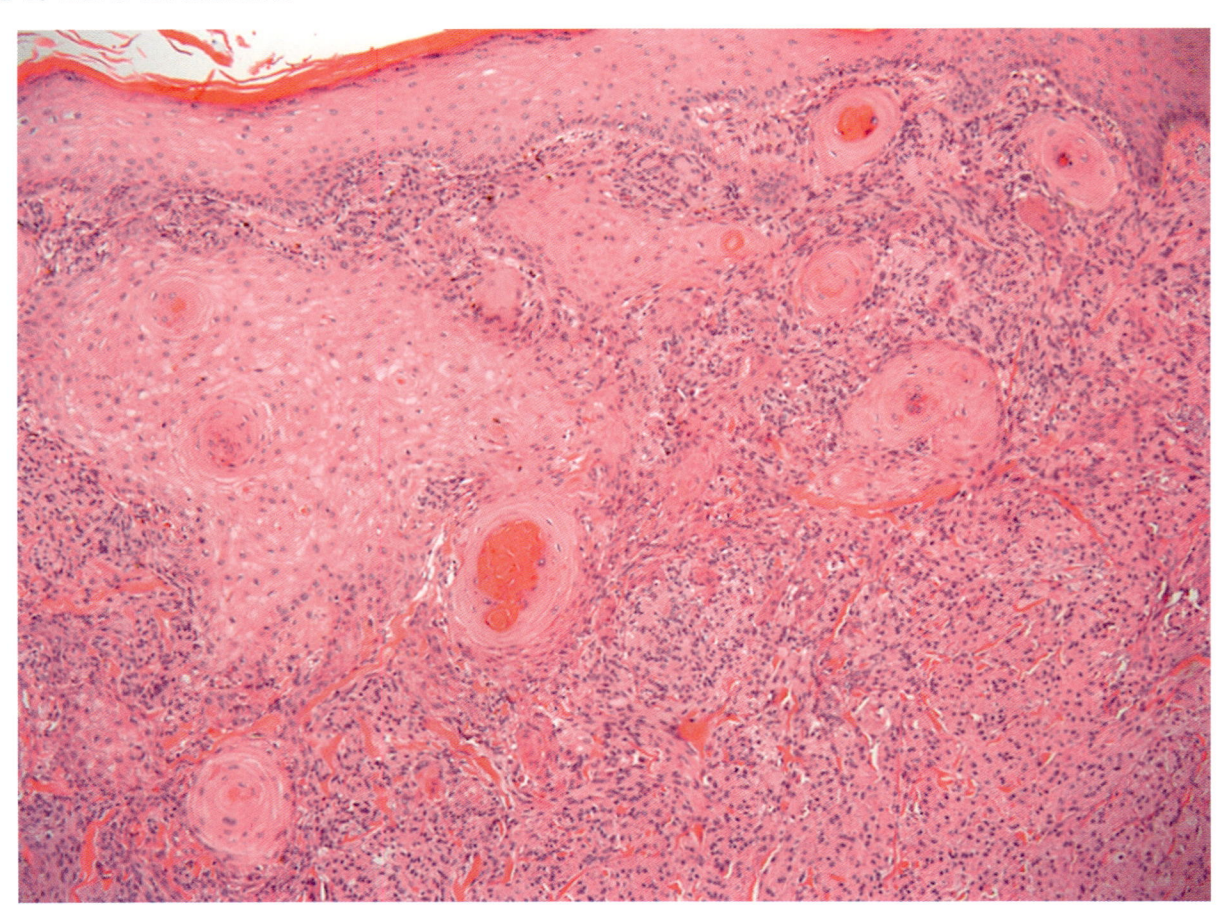

Fig 22-16 Granular cell tumor with pseudoepitheliomatous hyperplasia

Neural tumors   Chapter 22   361

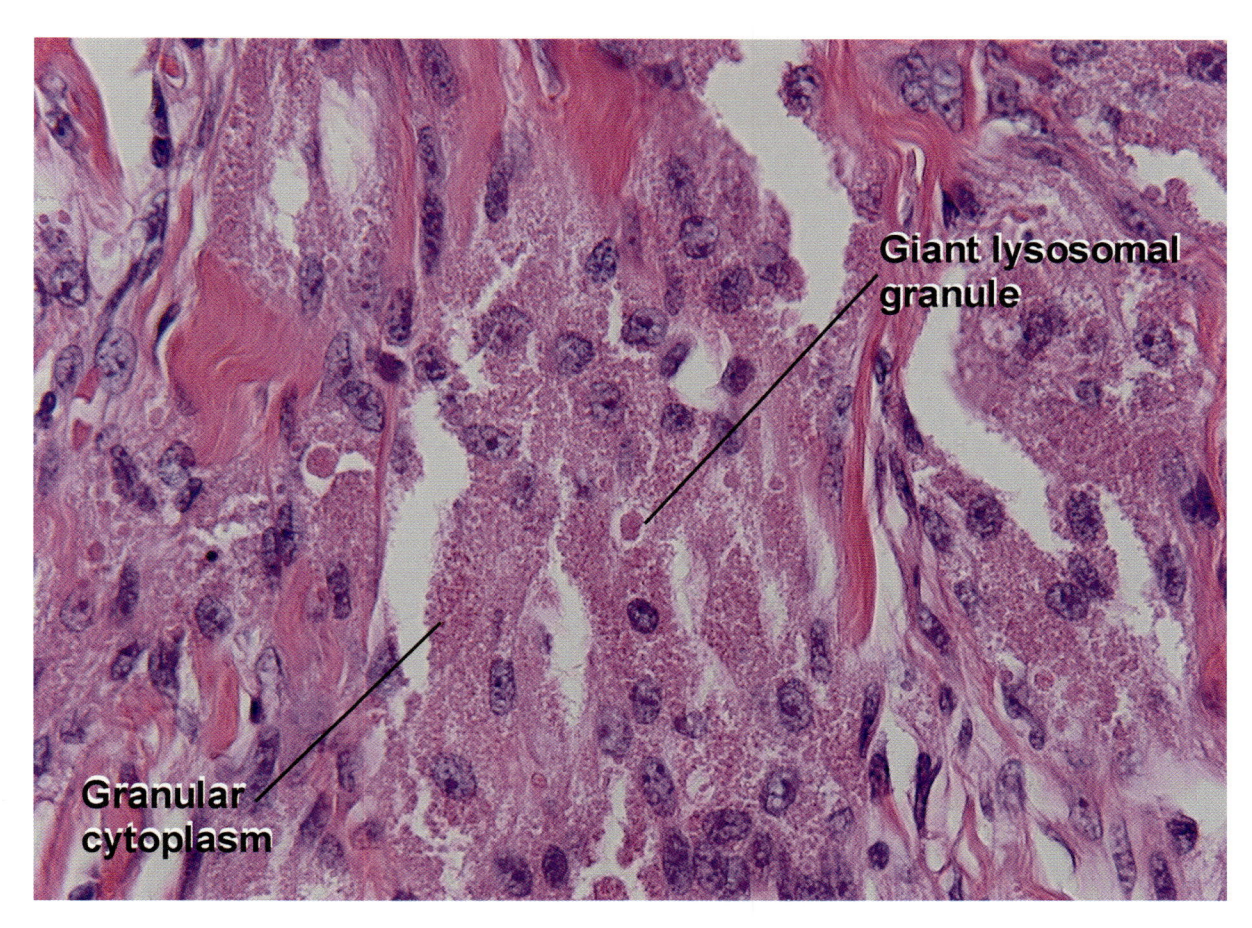

Fig 22-17 Granular cell tumor

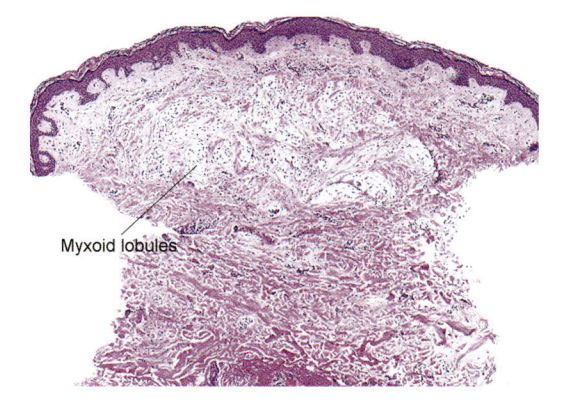

Fig 22-18 Myxoid neurothekeoma

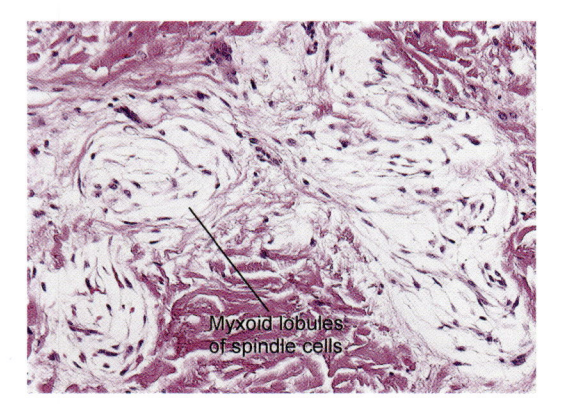

Fig 22-19 Myxoid neurothekeoma

Granular cell tumors are Schwann cell-derived tumors that can occur anywhere, but most commonly on the tongue. The granules within the cytoplasm are phagolysosomes. Bland cytology can be a poor predictor of biologic behavior, and large tumors should be regarded as potentially malignant.

Neurothekeoma

Neurothekeomas are benign neoplasms that are divided into myxoid, mixed, and cellular types. The myxoid type is strongly S100 positive, whereas those on the cellular end of the spectrum are composed of undifferentiated cells with partial features of Schwann cells, smooth muscle cells, myofibroblasts, and fibroblasts.

Myxoid neurothekeoma (nerve sheath myxoma)

Key features

- Multiple myxoid lobules containing sparse stellate cells
- S100+

Cellular neurothekeoma

Key features

- Nests and fascicles of epithelioid or spindled cells
- Myxoid stroma is absent or sparse
- S100– but S100A6+

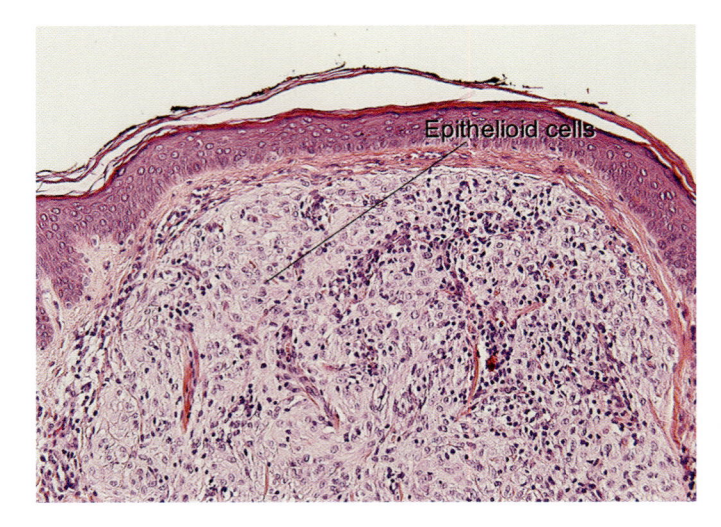

Fig 22-20 Cellular neurothekeoma

The cellular variant is negative for S100 and desmin, but sometimes positive for smooth muscle actin, neuron-specific enolase, and factor XIIIa. It is frequently positive for NK1/C-3, S100A6, and PGP9.5 with antigen retrieval. S100A6 also stains histiocytic tumors, including atypical fibroxanthoma, as well as Spitz nevi.

Differential Diagnosis

Histologically, cellular neurothekeomas may be confused with melanocytic lesions such as dermal Spitz nevi. S100 positivity strongly favors the melanocytic lesion. The variable reactivity for factor XIIIa in cellular neurothekeoma can result in confusion with epithelioid fibrous histiocytoma. S100A6 positivity can lead to confusion with spindled atypical fibroxanthoma. Of the two, atypical fibroxanthoma is less likely to demonstrate fascicles of tumor cells. Epithelioid pilar leiomyomas may also be considered in the differential diagnosis due to the variable smooth muscle actin positivity in cellular neurothekeomas. However, the absence of desmin in cellular neurothekeoma aids in the distinction.

Malignant peripheral nerve sheath tumor (MPNST) (neurofibrosarcoma, malignant schwannoma)

Key features

- Malignant transformation of neurofibromas, especially plexiform neurofibromas
- Intersecting fascicles of spindle cells
- Expansile growth pattern
- Hypercellularity is more characteristic than atypia
- Mitoses are present but not always frequent

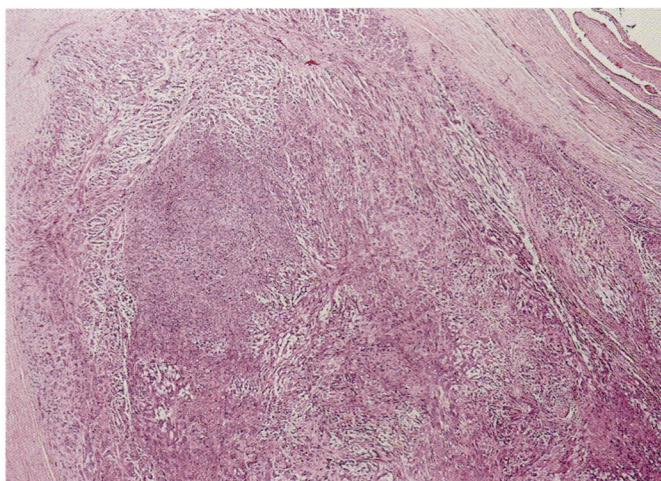

Fig 22-21 Malignant peripheral nerve sheath tumor

Foci of divergent differentiation may be present, including osseous, chondroid, and rhabdoid foci as well as foci of adenocarcinoma or angiosarcoma. Malignant peripheral nerve sheath tumor with focal rhabdomyosarcoma is known as malignant Triton tumor. S100 staining is usually focal and weak in MPNSTs but diffusely positive in its mimicker, desmoplastic melanoma.

Neural tumors   Chapter 22   363

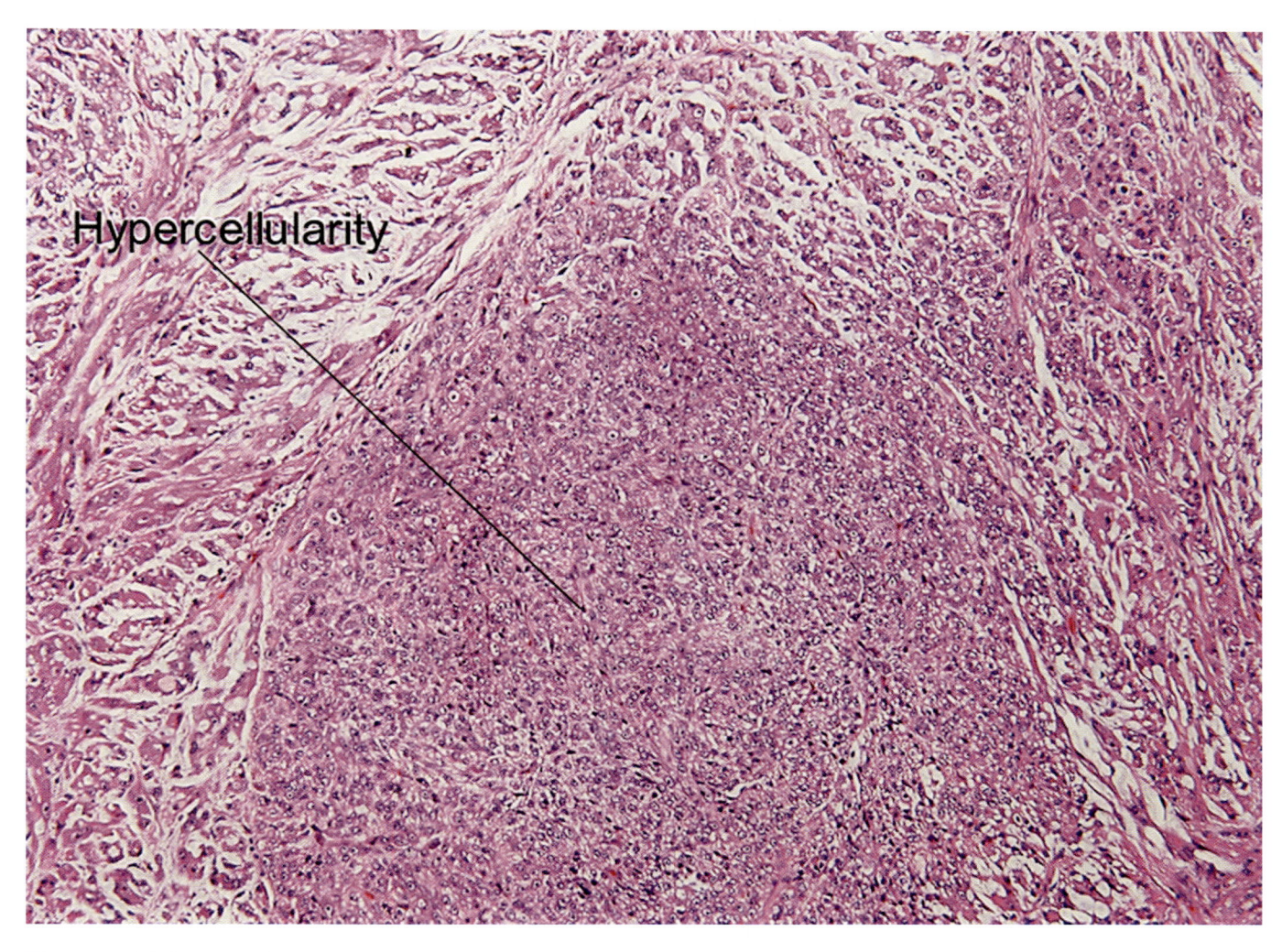

Fig 22-22 Malignant peripheral nerve sheath tumor

Cutaneous ganglioneuroma

Key features

- Localized dermal collection of Schwann cells with uniform wavy buckled nuclei
- Admixed large polygonal ganglion cells with eccentric large round nucleus with prominent nucleolus

The ganglion cells are positive with glial fibrillary acidic protein. Ganglioneuroma has mature ganglion cells scattered in a Schwann cell background, in contrast to ganglion cell choristoma, which contains only a proliferation of ganglion cells without supporting neuromatous elements.

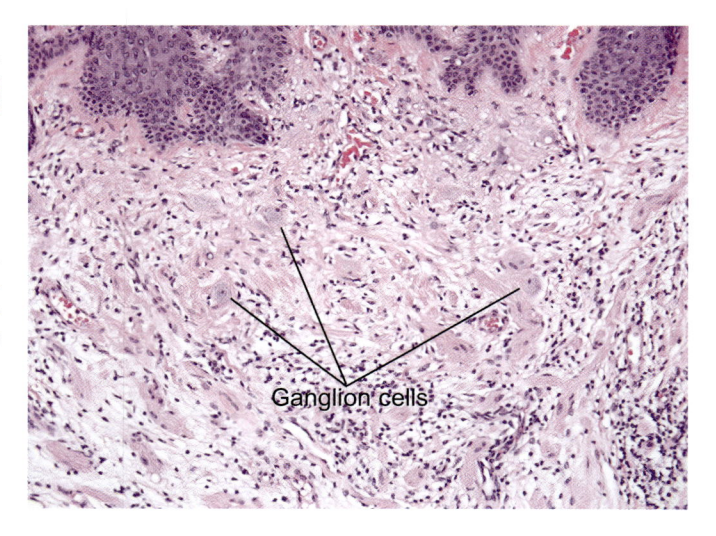

Fig 22-23 Cutaneous ganglioneuroma

Perineurioma

> **Key features**
> - Circumscribed tumor of spindle cells with elongate bipolar cytoplasmic processes
> - Fascicle of cells parallel to each other or in concentric onion skin-like whorls

Variants of perineurioma include: intraneural, soft tissue, sclerosing, and cutaneous. The sclerosing variant, seen most on the hand of young adults, is characterized by prominent hyalinized stroma. Soft-tissue perineuriomas are generally more cellular. Occasionally, the perineural cells are more epithelioid. These tumors are EMA, GLUT1, and claudin-1 positive and S100 negative.

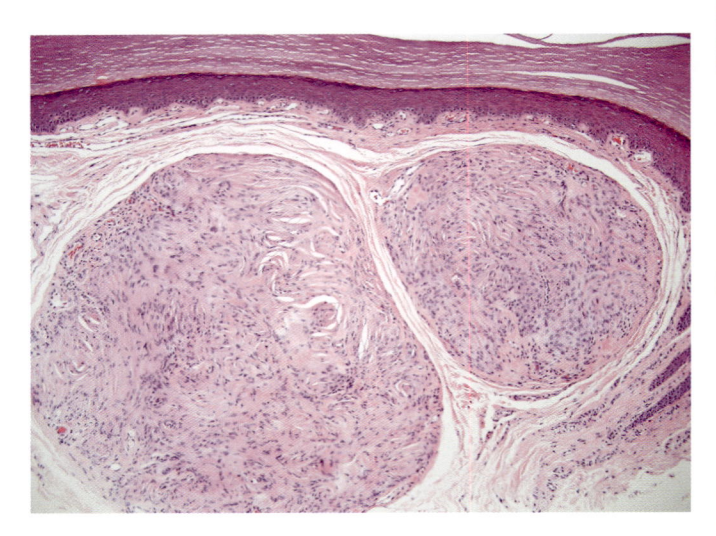

Fig 22-24 Sclerosing perineurioma

Glial heterotopia (nasal glioma)

> **Key features**
> - Astrocytes with round vesicular nuclei in a loose neurofibrillary stroma

This congenital nodule or polyp typically presents in or around the nose, thus the "nasal" designation. Connection with the frontal lobe must be excluded with neuroimaging studies preoperatively. Oligodendrocytes with small hyperchromatic nuclei may be focally identified. S100 and GFAP are positive.

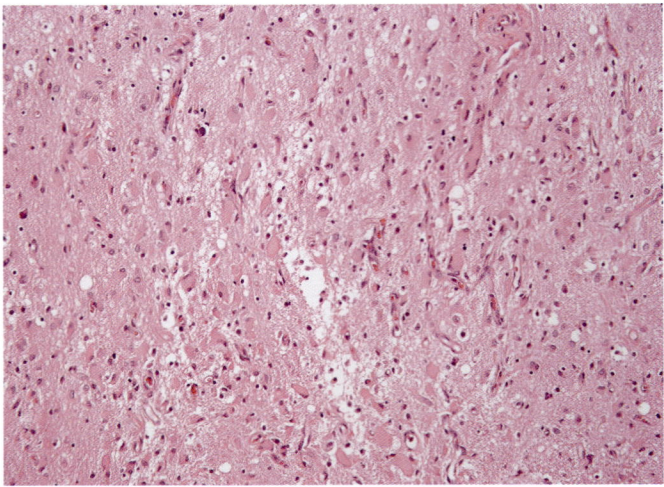

Fig 22-25 Nasal glioma

Meningeal heterotopia (rudimentary meningocele)

> **Key features**
> - Pseudovascular spaces dissect through collagen bundles
> - Spaces are lined by small round epithelioid meningothelial cells
> - Psammoma bodies may be present

Meningeal lesions in the skin are often referred to as cutaneous meningiomas; however, only type III lesions are an extension or metastasis from intracranial meningioma. Type I and type II are probably developmental and lack bone defects. Type I is the most common meningeal heterotopia. It is congenital and is also known as ectopic meningothelial hamartoma and rudimentary or sequestered meningocele. Meningothelial cells are EMA positive.

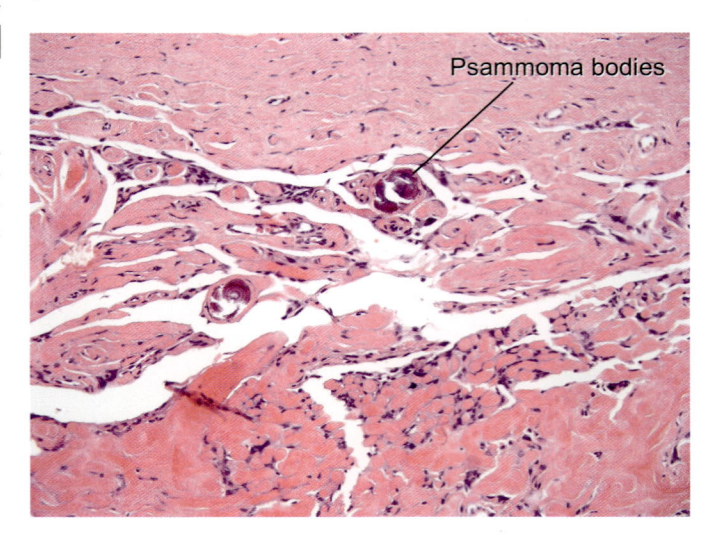

Fig 22-26 Rudimentary meningocele

Further reading

Argenyi ZB. Cutaneous neural heterotopias and related tumors relevant for the dermatopathologist. Semin Diagn Pathol 1996;13(1):60–71.

Argenyi ZB, Balogh K, Abraham AA. Degenerative ("ancient") changes in benign cutaneous schwannoma. A light microscopic, histochemical and immunohistochemical study. J Cutan Pathol 1993;20(2):148–153.

Argenyi ZB, Kutzner H, Seaba MM. Ultrastructural spectrum of cutaneous nerve sheath myxoma/cellular neurothekeoma. J Cutan Pathol 1995;22(2):137–145.

Calonje E, Wilson-Jones E, Smith NP, et al. Cellular "neurothekeoma": an epithelioid variant of pilar leiomyoma? Morphological and immunohistochemical analysis of a series. Histopathology 1992;20(5):397–404.

Carney JA, Stratakis CA. Epithelioid blue nevus and psammomatous melanotic schwannoma: the unusual pigmented skin tumors of the Carney complex. Semin Diagn Pathol 1998;15(3):216–224.

Chambers PW, Schwinn CP Chordoma. A clinicopathologic study of metastasis. Am J Clin Pathol 1979;72(5):765–776.

Dewit L, Albus-Lutter CE, de Jong AS, et al. Malignant schwannoma with a rhabdomyoblastic component, a so-called triton tumor. A clinicopathologic study. Cancer 1986;58(6):1350–1356.

Ducatman BS, Scheithauer BW. Malignant peripheral nerve sheath tumors with divergent differentiation. Cancer 1984;54(6):1049–1057.

Kluwe L, Friedrich RE, Mautner VF. Allelic loss of the NF1 gene in NF1-associated plexiform neurofibromas. Cancer Genet Cytogenet 1999;113(1):65–69.

Macarenco RS, Ellinger F, Oliveira AM. Perineurioma: a distinctive and underrecognized peripheral nerve sheath neoplasm. Arch Pathol Lab Med 2007;131(4):625–636.

Miedema JR, Zedek D Cutaneous meningioma. Arch Pathol Lab Med 2012;136(2):208–211.

Wallace CA, Hallman JR, Sangueza OP. Primary cutaneous ganglioneuroma: a report of two cases and literature review. Am J Dermatopathol 2003;25(3):239–242.

Wang AR, May D, Bourne P, et al. PGP9.5: a marker for cellular neurothekeoma. Am J Surg Pathol 1999;23(11):1401–1407.

Chapter 23
Vascular tumors
Dirk M. Elston

Angiokeratoma

Key features
- Hyperkeratosis
- Acanthosis
- Ectatic thin-walled vessels in contact with the epidermis
- Resembles a "bloody seborrheic keratosis"

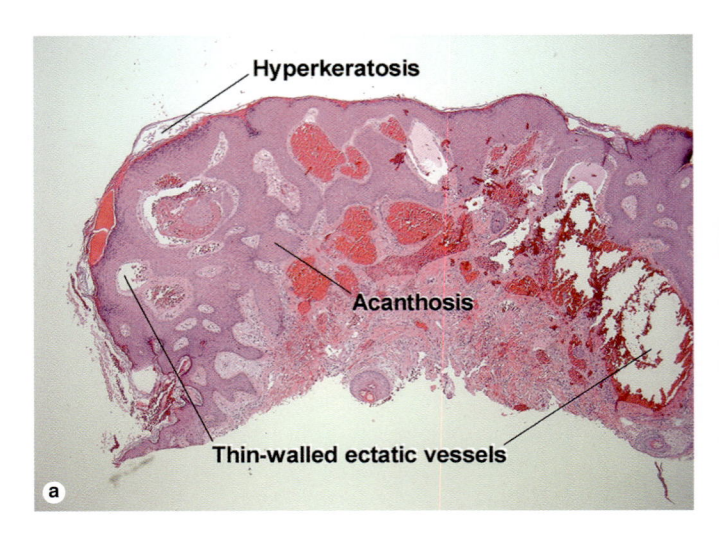

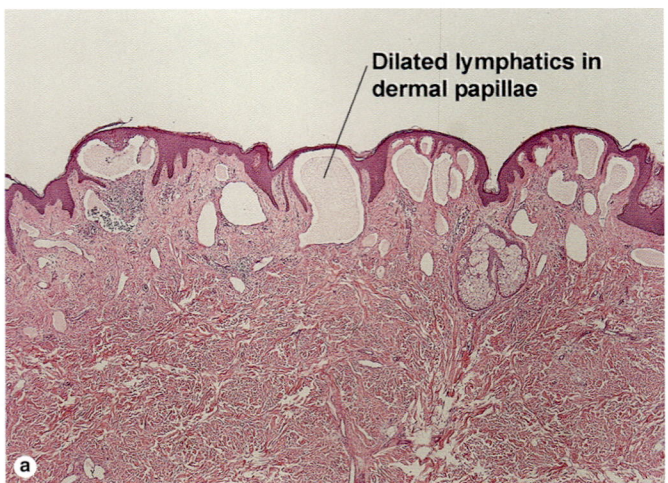

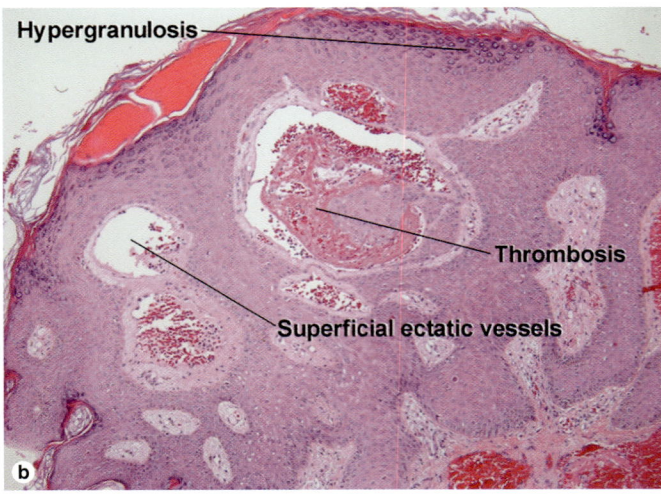

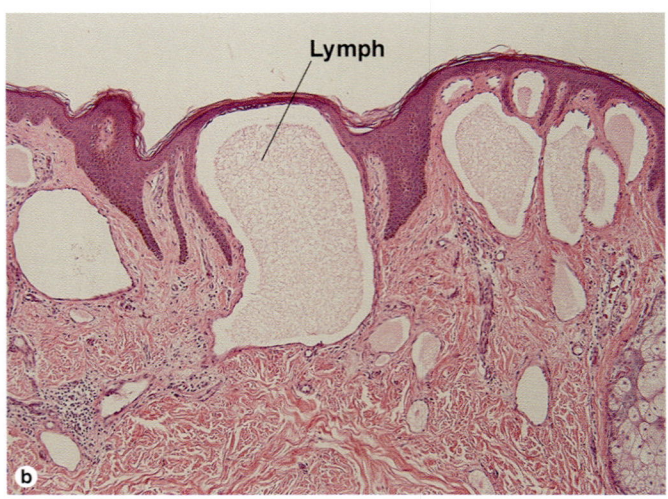

Fig 23-1 Angiokeratoma

Lymphangioma

Key features
- "Frog spawn" clinically
- Similar to angiokeratoma with lymph in vessels, but few erythrocytes
- D2-40+

Fig 23-2 Lymphangioma

Nevus flammeus

Key features
- Dilated capillary-sized vessels

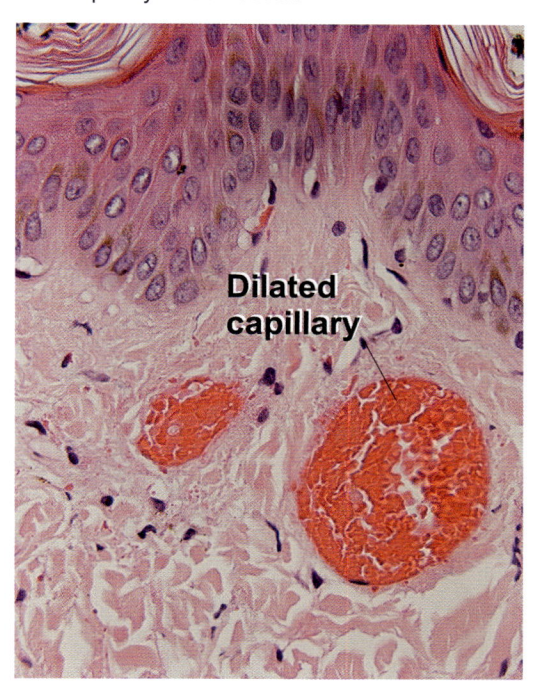

Fig 23-3 Nevus flammeus

Angioma serpiginosum

Key features
- Dilated tortuous capillaries in dermal papillae and the upper dermis
- Vessels lack alkaline phosphatase activity

Angioma serpiginosum presents as a progressive vascular lesion on a woman's leg. The ectatic vessels begin as minute puncta in clusters, but merge to form a serpiginous array. They often bleed freely when traumatized.

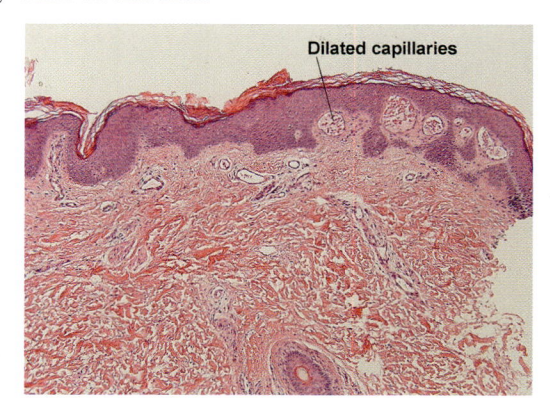

Fig 23-4 Angioma serpiginosum

Venous lake

Key features
- Irregular, thin-walled, ectatic vessel
- Usually collapses after biopsy

Venous lakes are common on the lips and ears of older patients. They may appear very dark, but blanch easily when compressed.

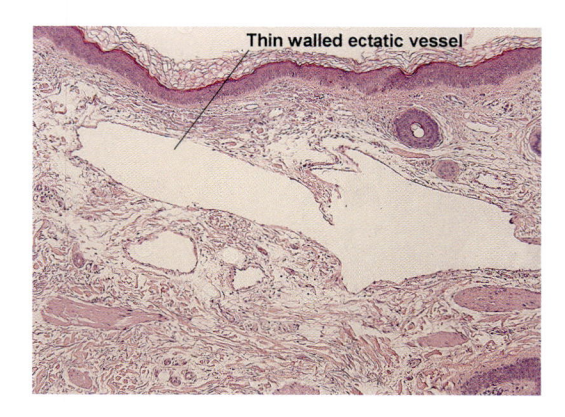

Fig 23-5 Venous lake

Glomus tumor

Key features
- Rows of round dark nuclei with little cytoplasm ("string of black pearls")
- Glomus cells surround delicate vascular spaces
- Commonly tender

PEARL
- Normal glomus bodies are found on the sides of digits. A large physiologic glomus coccygeum is present in the sacral area
- Glomus cells are modified smooth muscle cells (SMA+/CD31−)
- In general, vascular smooth muscle stains reliably with vimentin and smooth muscle actin, but not with desmin.

Glomangioma

Key features
- Commonly multiple
- One to two layers of glomus cells around prominent vessels

The vessels usually have thicker walls than the vessels in a glomus tumor. Glomangiomas have been described as vascular malformations with a few glomus cells, whereas glomus tumors have been described as tumors of glomus cells surrounding inconspicuous vessels.

368 Dermatopathology

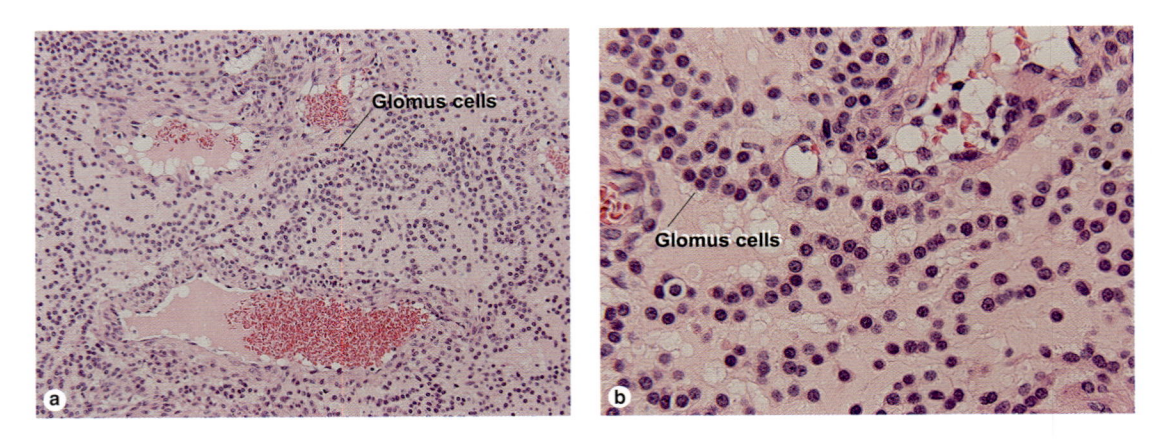

Fig 23-6 Glomus tumor

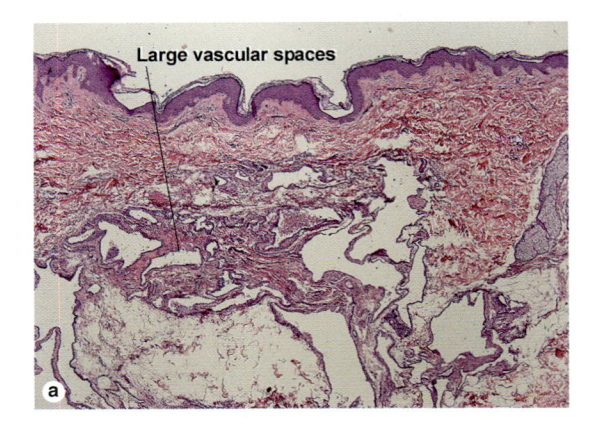

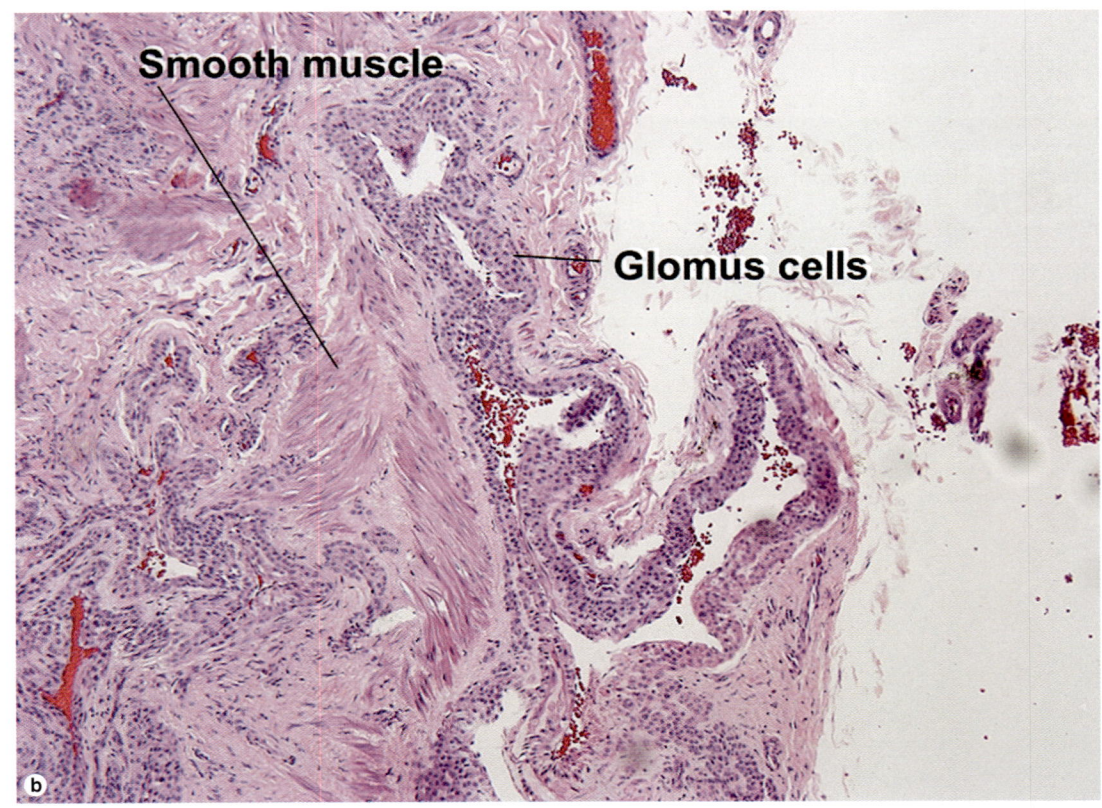

Fig 23-7 Glomangioma

Vascular tumors

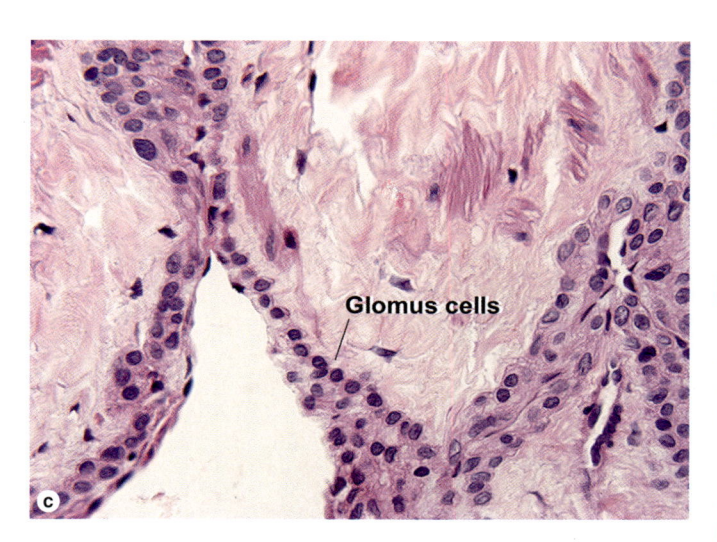

Fig 23-7, cont'd

Pyogenic granuloma

Key features

- Eruptive lobular capillary hemangioma
- Early lesions show solidly packed endothelial cells
- Later lesions show more ectatic vessels, erosion, and crusting
- Epidermal collarette common
- Commonly impetiginized on surface

Bacillary angiomatosis

Key features

- Usually not distinctly lobular
- Clusters of neutrophils within lesion
- Amphophilic collections of organisms

Differential Diagnosis

Pyogenic granulomas are distinctly lobular. Although surface crusting is common in pyogenic granulomas, they lack the deep clusters of neutrophils that characterize bacillary angiomatosis.

Cherry angioma

Key features

- Capillary hemangioma
- Pink hyalinized vessel walls

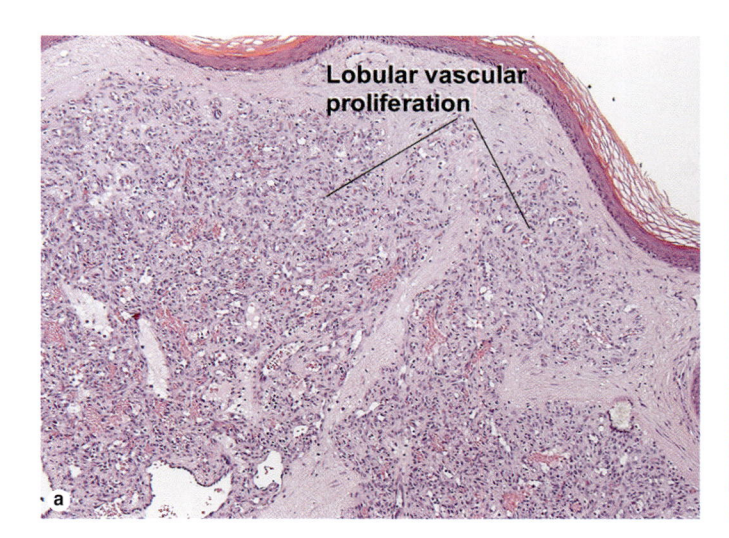

Fig 23-8 Pyogenic granuloma

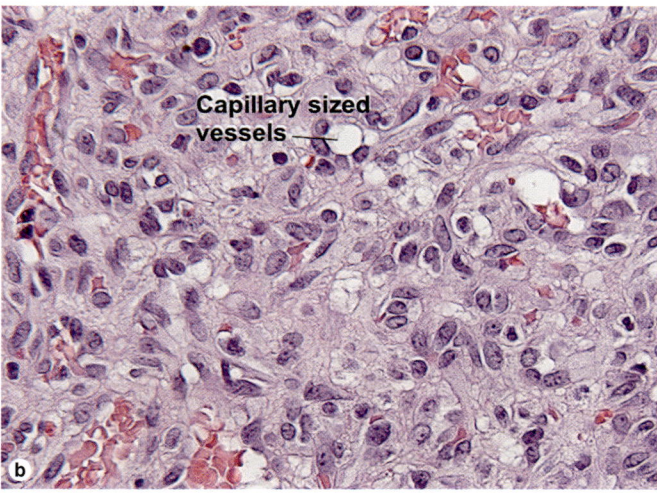

Dermatopathology

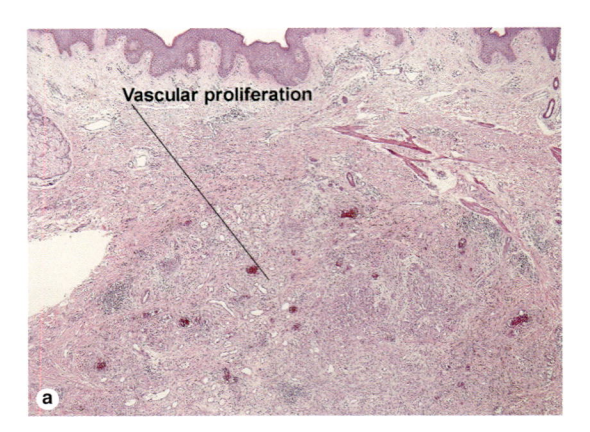

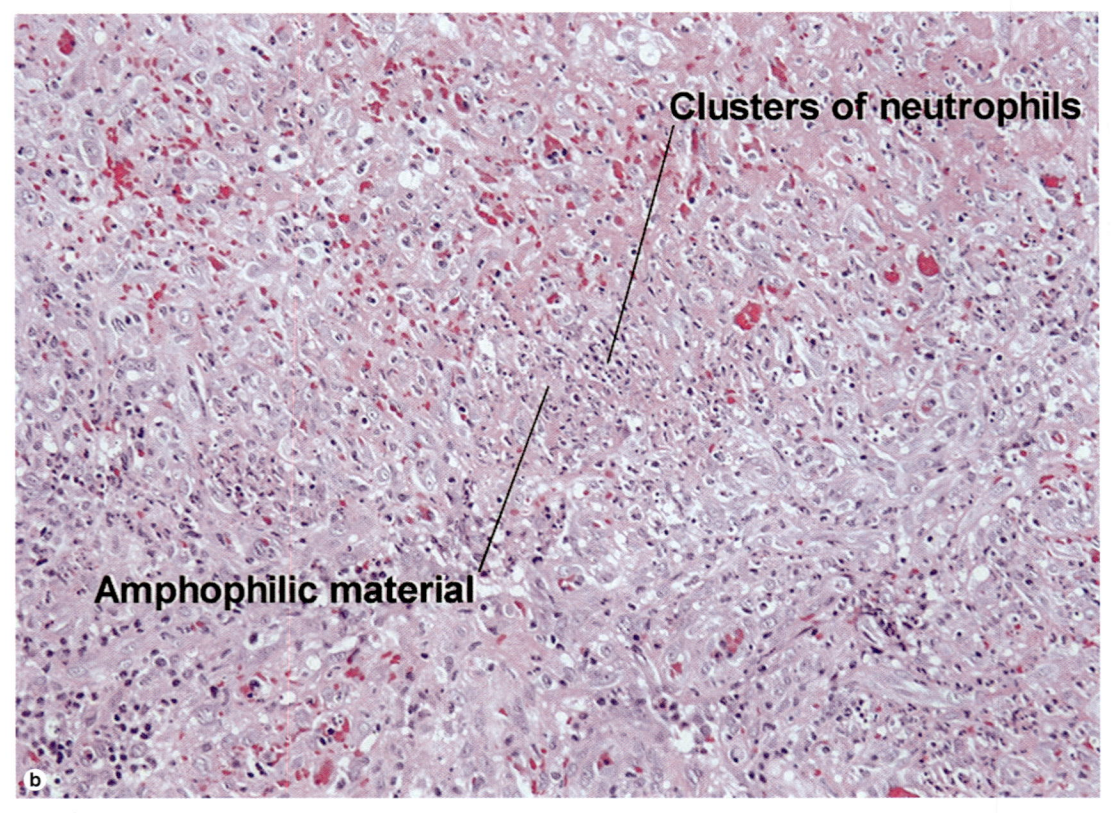

Fig 23-9 Bacillary angiomatosis

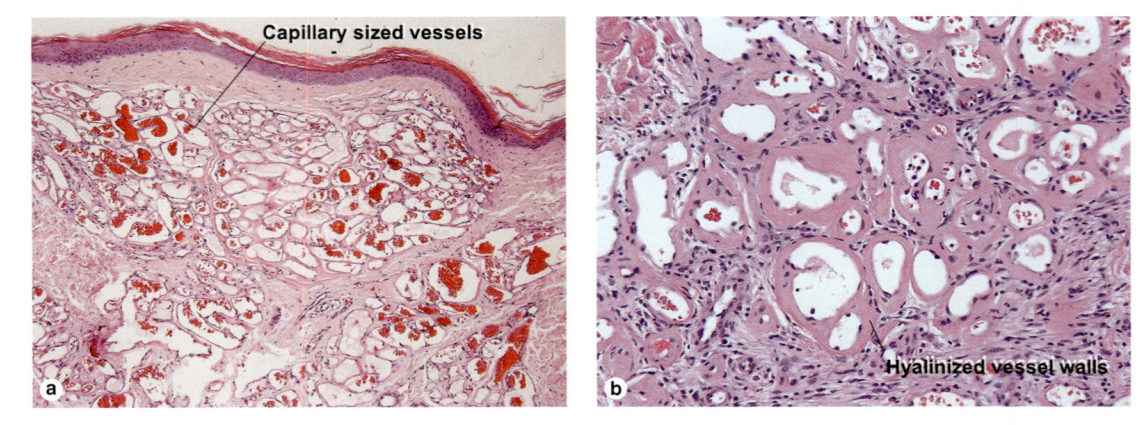

Fig 23-10 Cherry angioma

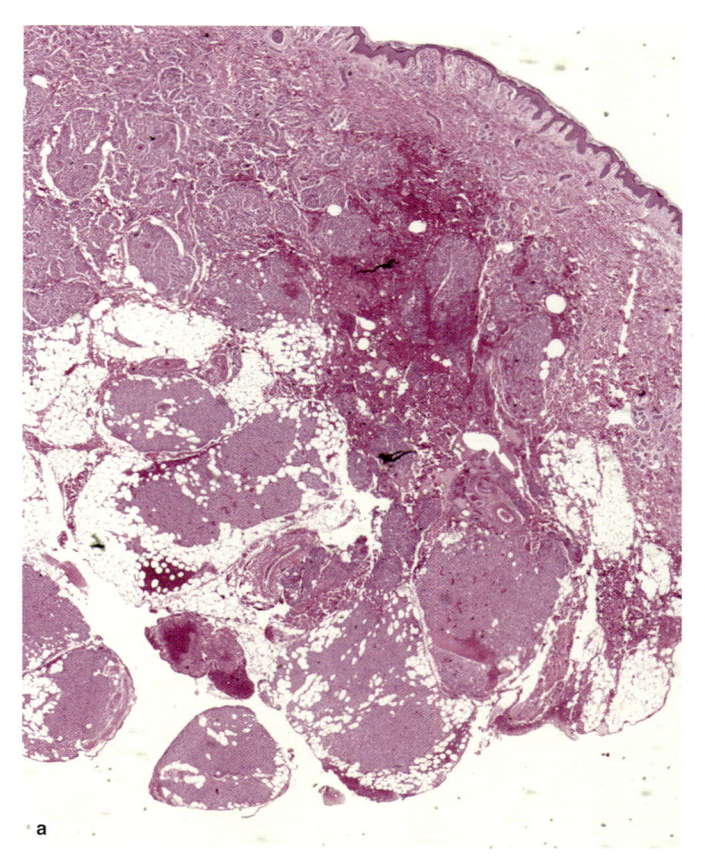

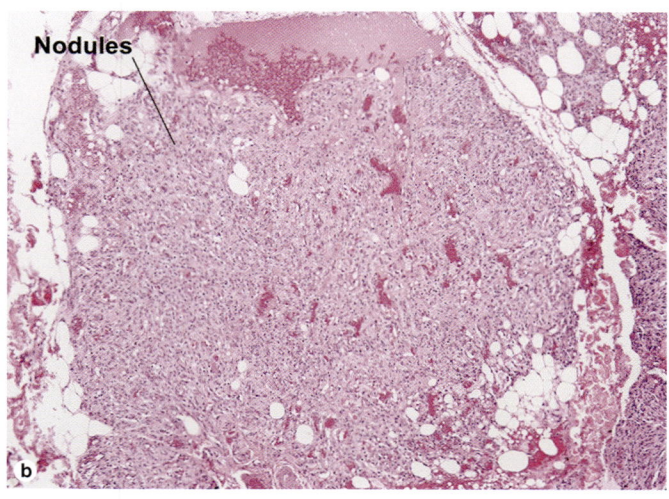

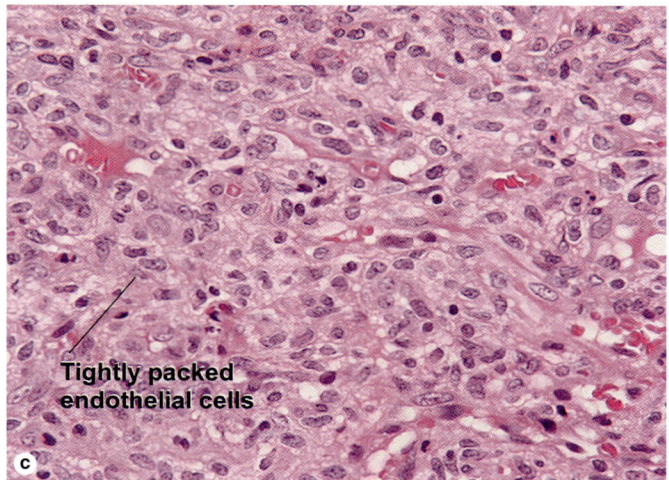

Fig 23-11 Infantile hemangioma

Infantile hemangioma

Key features

- Early lesions show solidly packed endothelial cells
- Later lesions show more ectatic vessels
- Glucose transporter 1 (GLUT1)+

Differential Diagnosis

Rapidly involuting congenital hemangioma (RICH) and non-involuting congenital hemangioma (NICH) are fully grown at birth and are GLUT1 negative.

Angiolymphoid hyperplasia with eosinophilia

Key features

- Central thick-walled vessels with hobnail endothelium
- Peripheral proliferation of smaller vessels
- Nodular lymphoid aggregates with eosinophils

Subtypes include histiocytoid and epithelioid hemangioma. Histiocytoid endothelial cells are common.

Kimura's disease

Key features

- Lacks central thick-walled vessels with hobnail endothelium
- Deep lymphoid nodules with eosinophils
- Peripheral eosinophilia
- Elevated immunoglobulin E
- East and SE Asia
- Large subcutaneous lymphoid nodules
- Lymphadenopathy

372 Dermatopathology

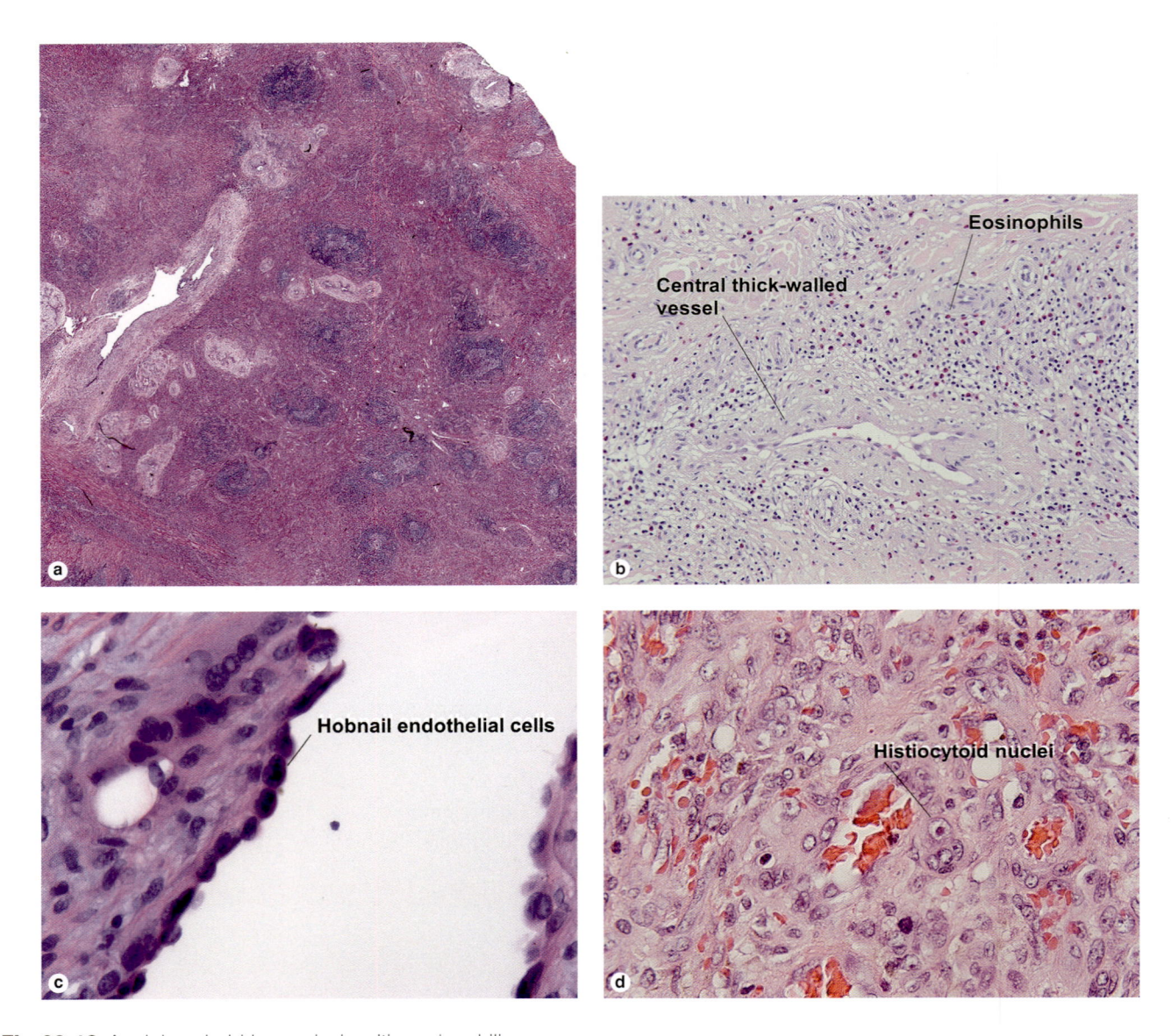

Fig 23-12 Angiolymphoid hyperplasia with eosinophilia

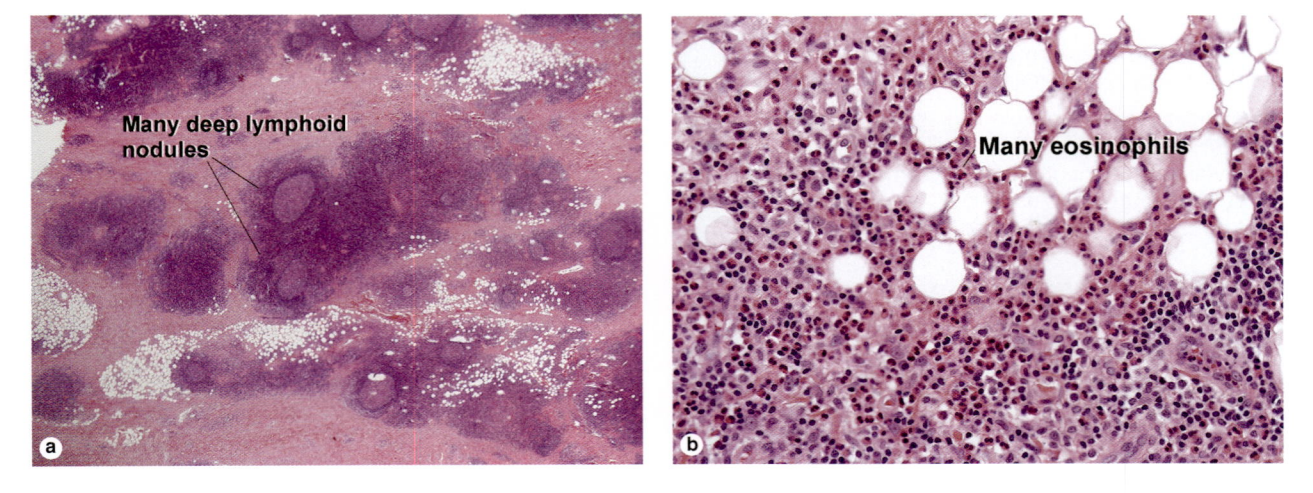

Fig 23-13 Kimura's disease (Courtesy of James Fitzpatrick, MD)

Vascular tumors Chapter 23

Intravascular papillary endothelial hyperplasia of Masson (IPEH)

Key features

- Recanalizing thrombus within a vascular space
- Fibrin in thrombus
- Papillary projections with hyalinized cores

IPEH can occur in any vascular space. It is common in angiokeratomas.

Arteriovenous malformation (arteriovenous hemangioma)

Key features

- Thick- and thin-walled vessels
- Thick-walled vessels tend to be central

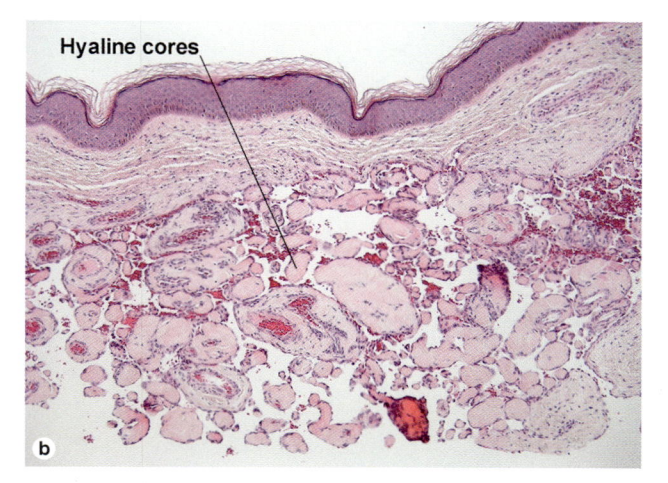

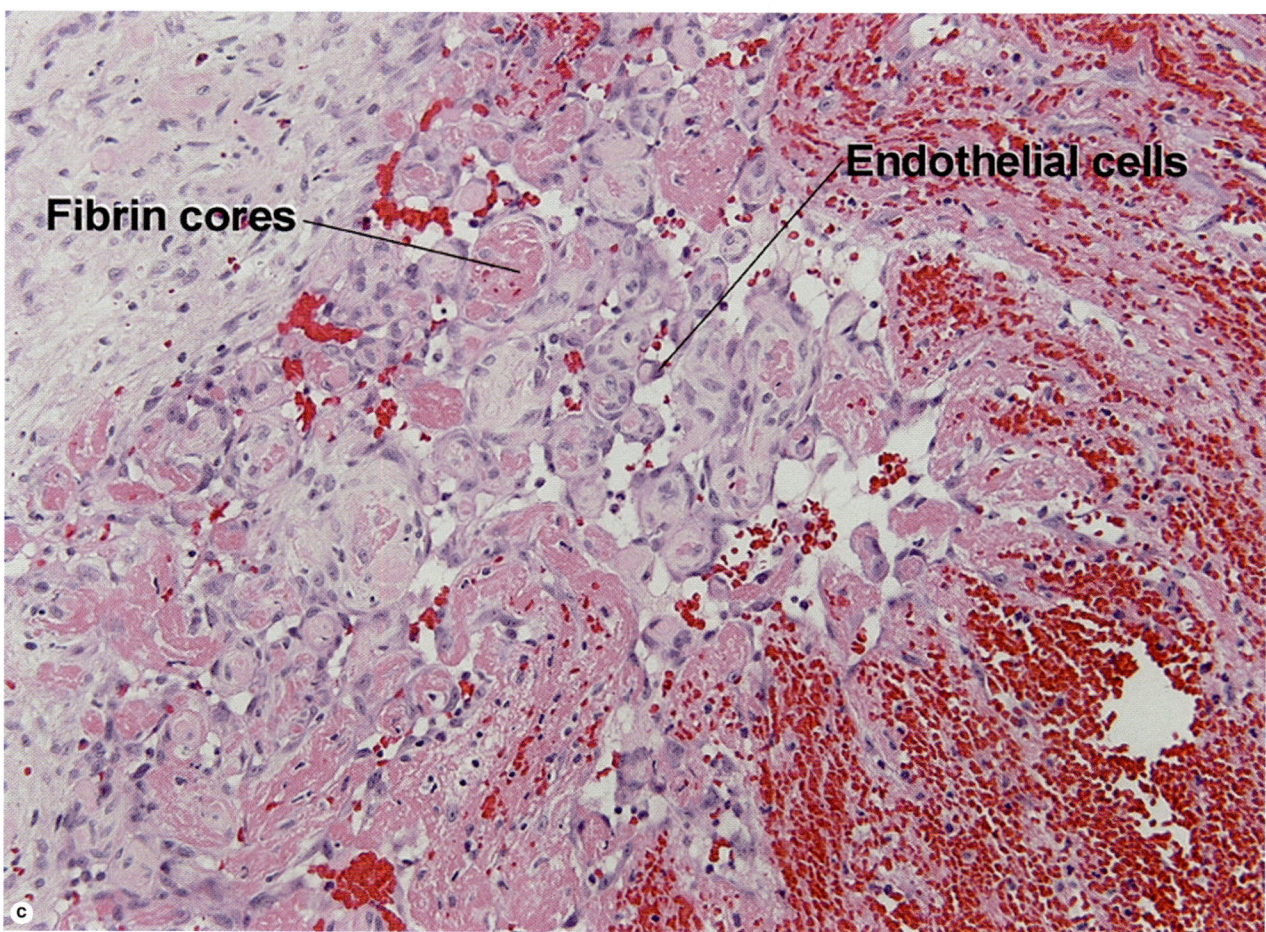

Fig 23-14 Intravascular papillary endothelial hyperplasia

Targetoid hemosiderotic hemangioma (hobnail hemangioma)

Key features

- Central superficial dilated vessels with hobnail nuclei
- Peripheral proliferation of small vessels
- Peripheral vascular proliferation tends to surround pre-existing vessels and adnexae (like Kaposi's sarcoma)
- Hemosiderin

Targetoid hemosiderotic hemangiomas probably arise as a result of trauma to a pre-existing hemangioma.

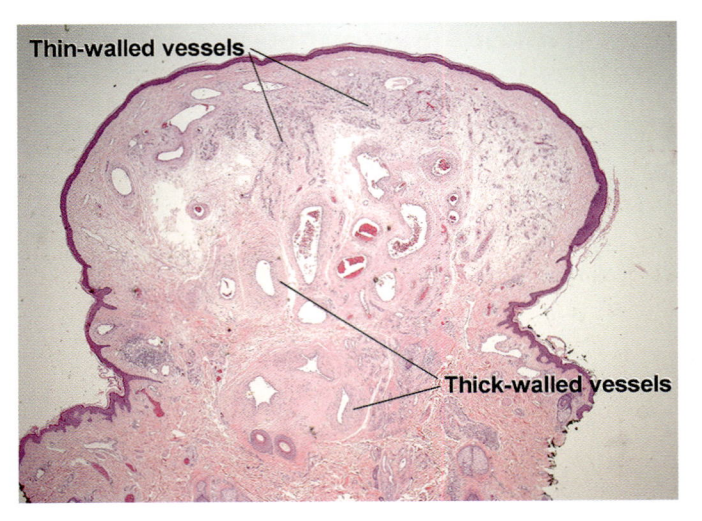

Fig 23-15 Arteriovenous malformation

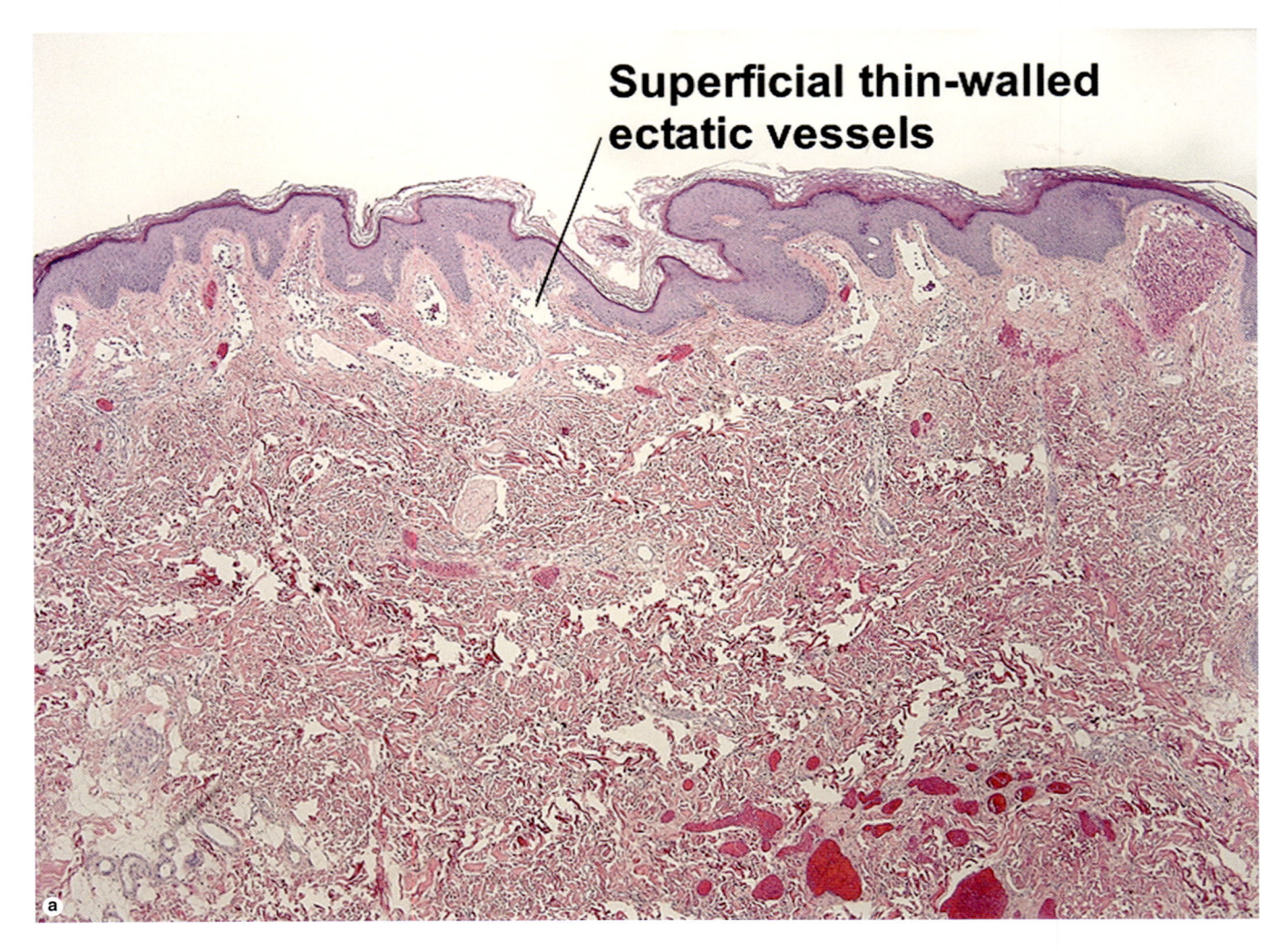

Fig 23-16 Targetoid hemosiderotic hemangioma

Vascular tumors • Chapter 23

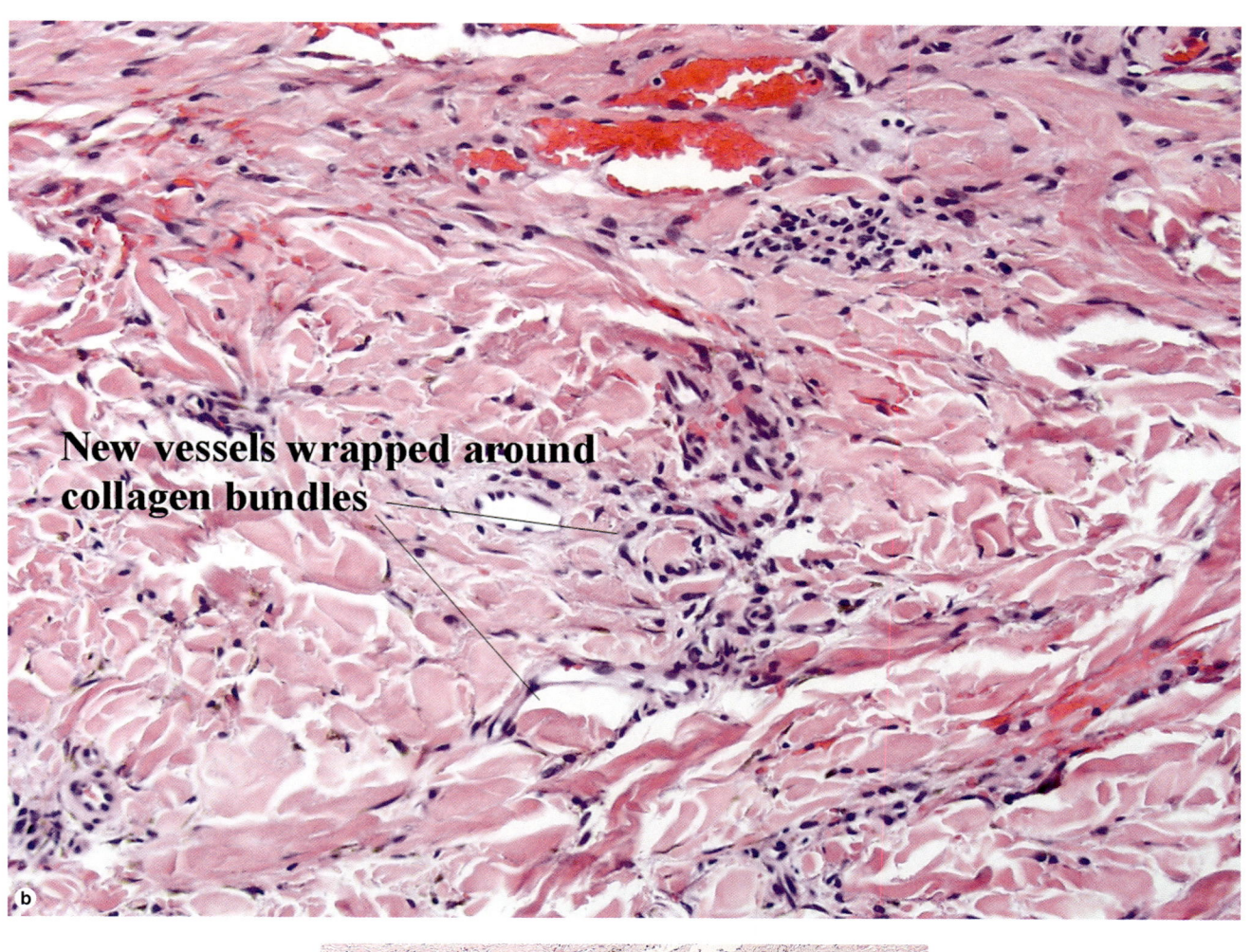

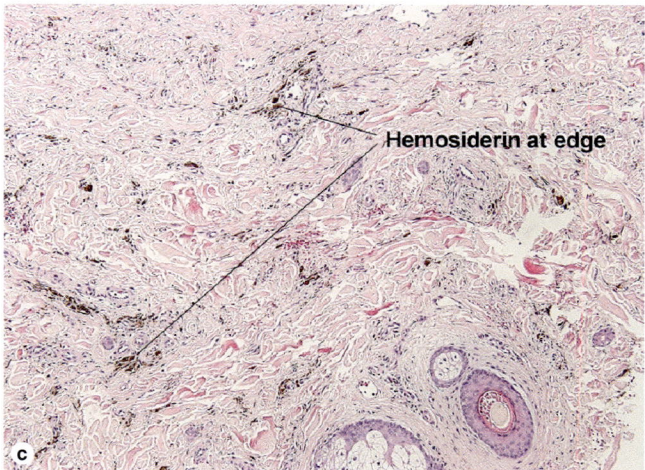

Fig 23-16, cont'd
Eccrine angiomatous hamartoma

Key features
- Discrete lobules
- Each composed of capillaries, mature eccrine glands, and ducts

Usually a solitary bluish nodule. Often involves acral sites, although the example shown was on the back. May be tender.

Glomeruloid hemangioma

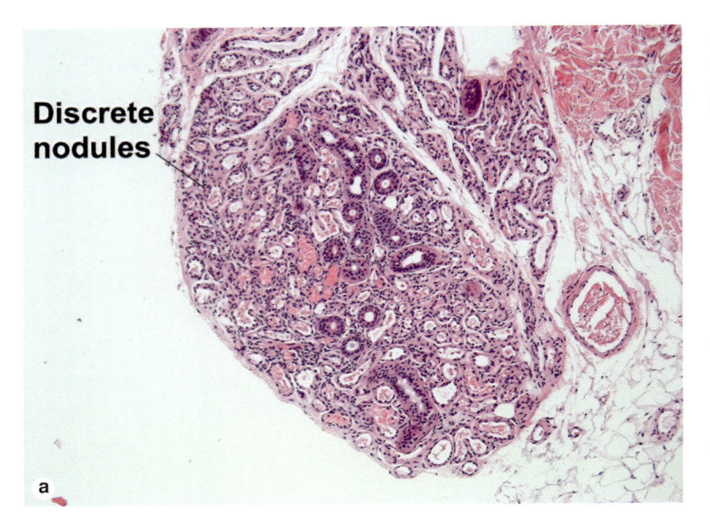

Key features

- Capillary loops within a dilated vascular space, resembling a glomerulus
- Sequestered degenerating erythrocytes

Glomeruloid hemangioma is associated with POEMS syndrome (Crow–Fukase syndrome, polyneuropathy, organomegaly, endocrinopathy, M protein, and skin changes) and Castleman's disease. Two types of endothelial cell have been noted: cells with large vesicular nuclei, an open chromatin pattern, and large amount of cytoplasm, and a second population with small basal nuclei, a dense chromatin pattern, and scant cytoplasm. Lesions not associated with POEMS syndrome have been referred to as papillary hemangioma.

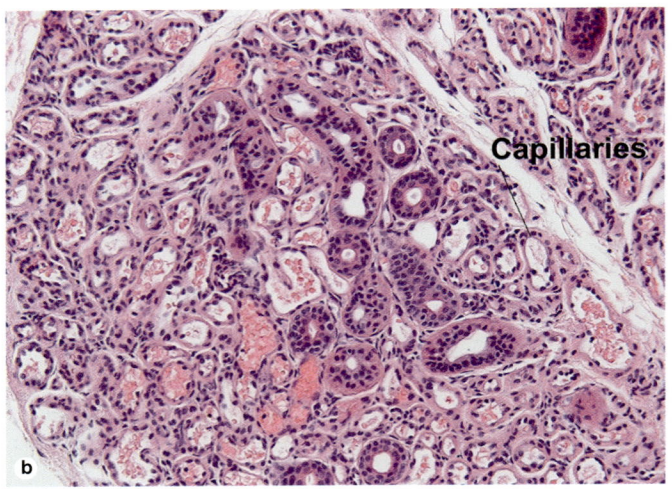

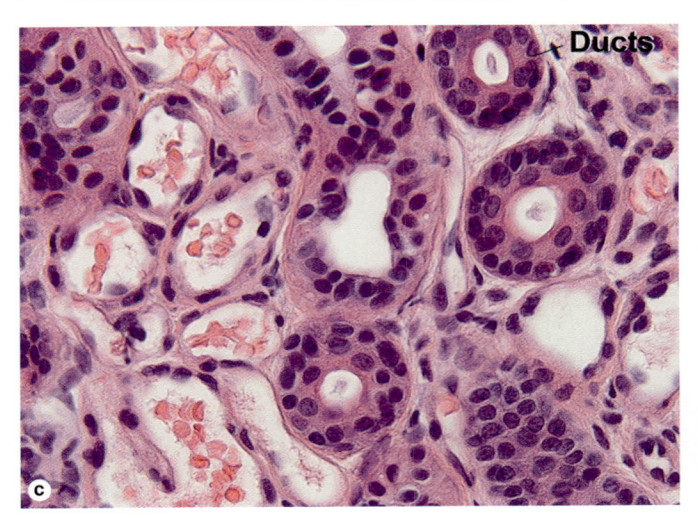

Fig 23-17 Eccrine angiomatous hamartoma

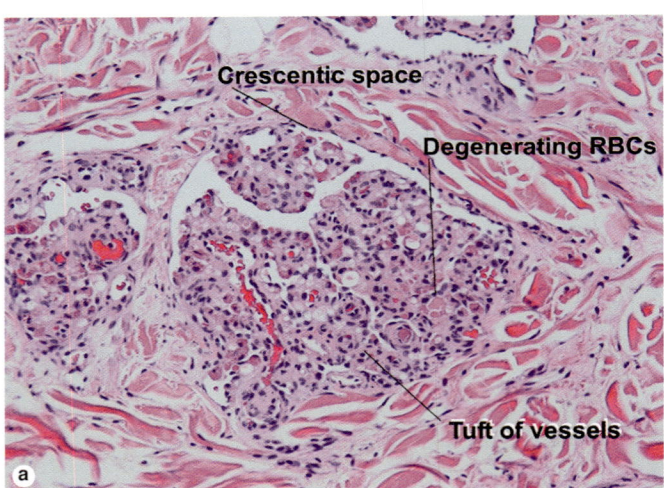

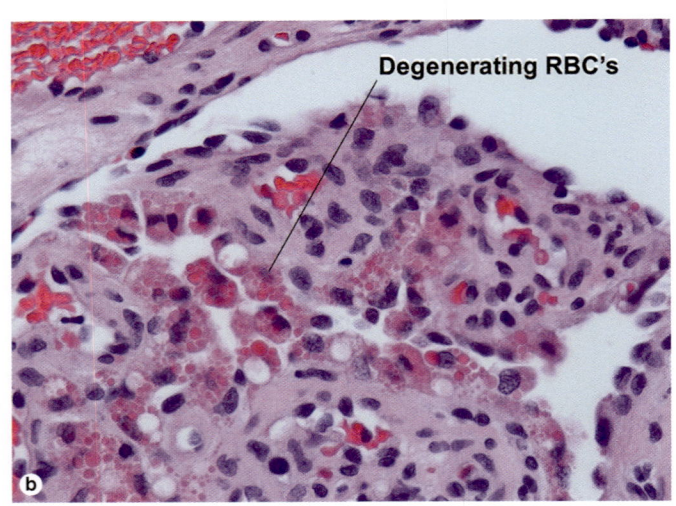

Fig 23-18 Glomeruloid hemangioma

Vascular tumors Chapter 23 377

Microvenular hemangioma

Key features

- Monomorphous, elongated blood vessels with small lumens
- Surrounding pericytes

Sometimes occurs in POEMS syndrome.

Tufted angioma (angioblastoma)

Key features

- "Cannonball" tufts of capillary-sized vessels in the dermis
- Slowly expanding plaque clinically, often on the shoulder of a child

Differential Diagnosis

- Glomeruloid hemangioma has sequestered degenerating erythrocytes and tufts protruding into a crescent-like space
- Dermal pyogenic granuloma has fibrous septae with ropey collagen between lobules

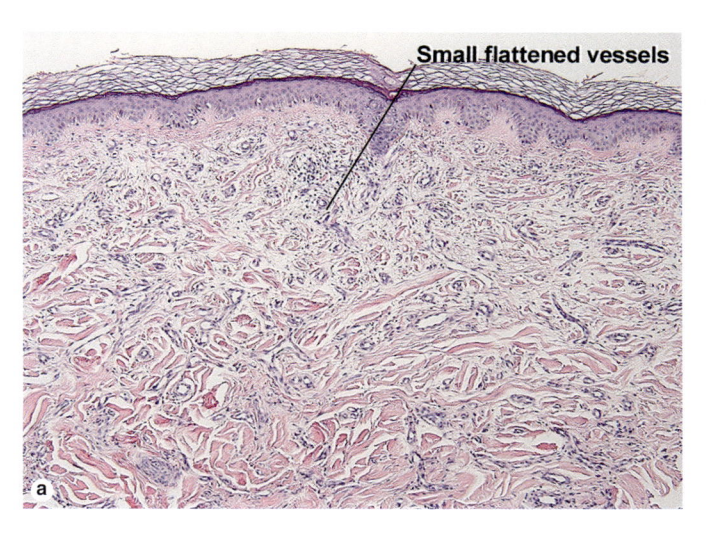

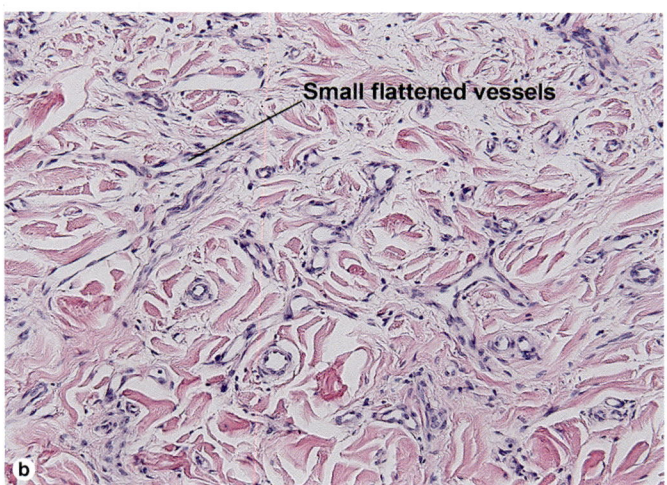

Fig 23-19 Microvenular hemangioma

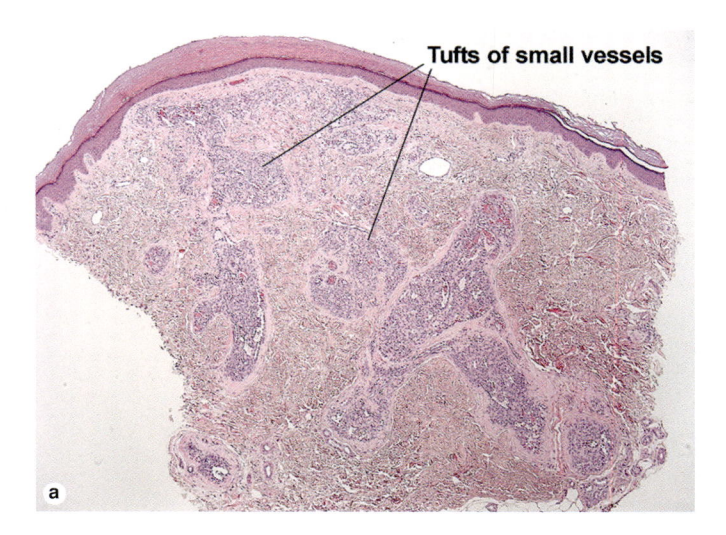

Fig 23-20 Tufted angioma

Continued

Dermatopathology

Tufts of capillary sized vessels

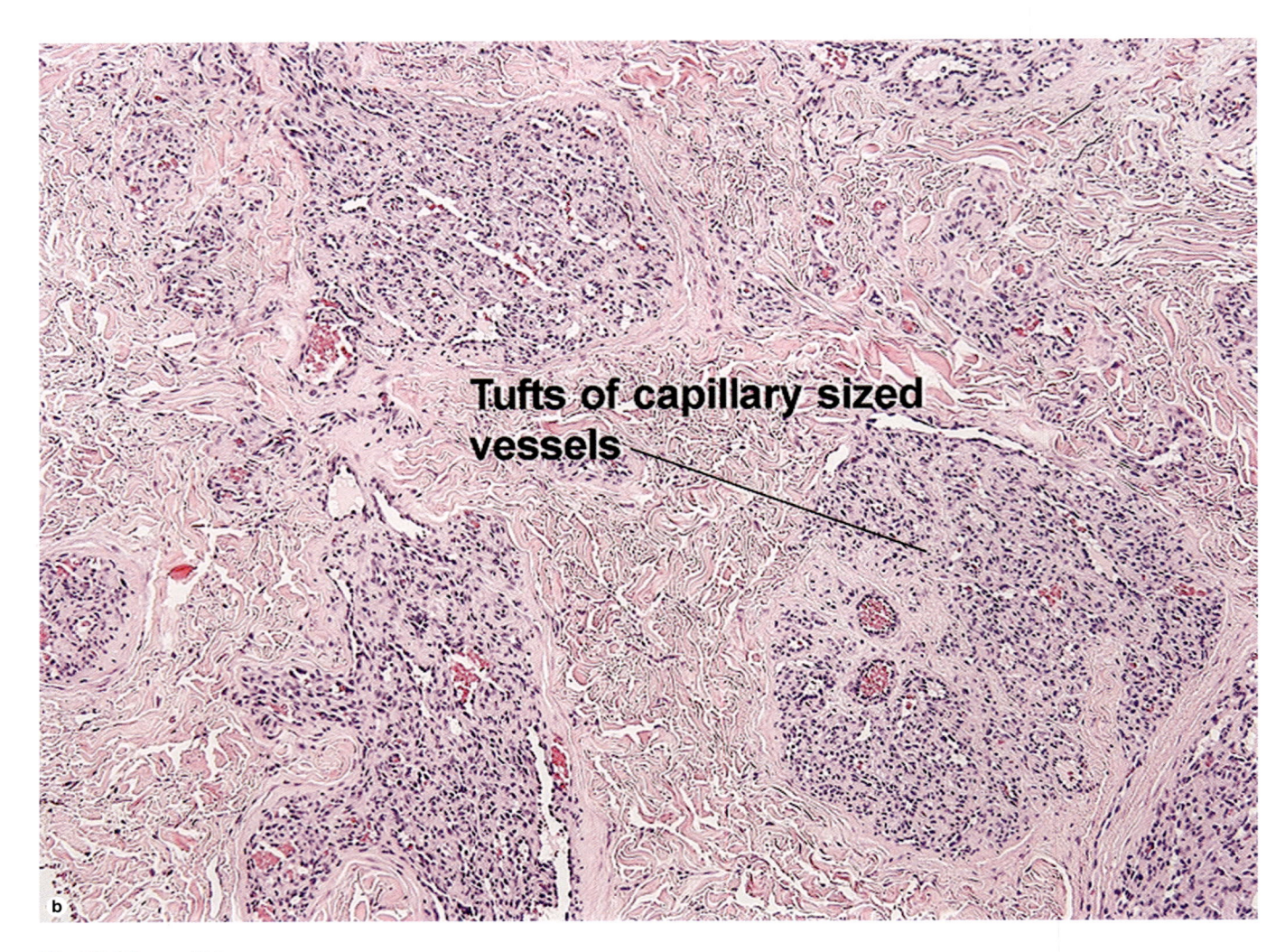

Fig 23-20, cont'd

Kaposiform hemangioendothelioma

Key features

- Large lobules
- Less well circumscribed than tufted angioma
- Involves deeper tissues
- Spindled endothelial cells
- Slit-like, crack-like and staghorn vascular spaces
- Deep extension to soft tissue and bone

Kasabach–Merritt coagulopathy is usually associated with kaposiform hemangioendothelioma or tufted angioma, and hybrid tumors have been described.

PEARL

Kaposiform hemangioendothelioma shows CD34 staining restricted to luminal endothelial cells, tufted angiomas show a proliferation of CD34-positive endothelial cells with few actin-positive cells, and infantile hemangiomas show actin-positive cells outnumbering CD34-positive cells.

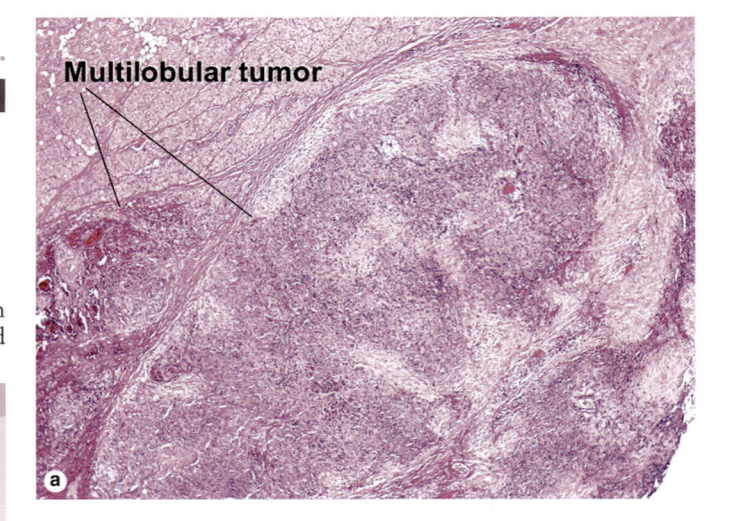

Multilobular tumor

Fig 23-21 Kaposiform hemangioendothelioma

Fig 23-21, cont'd

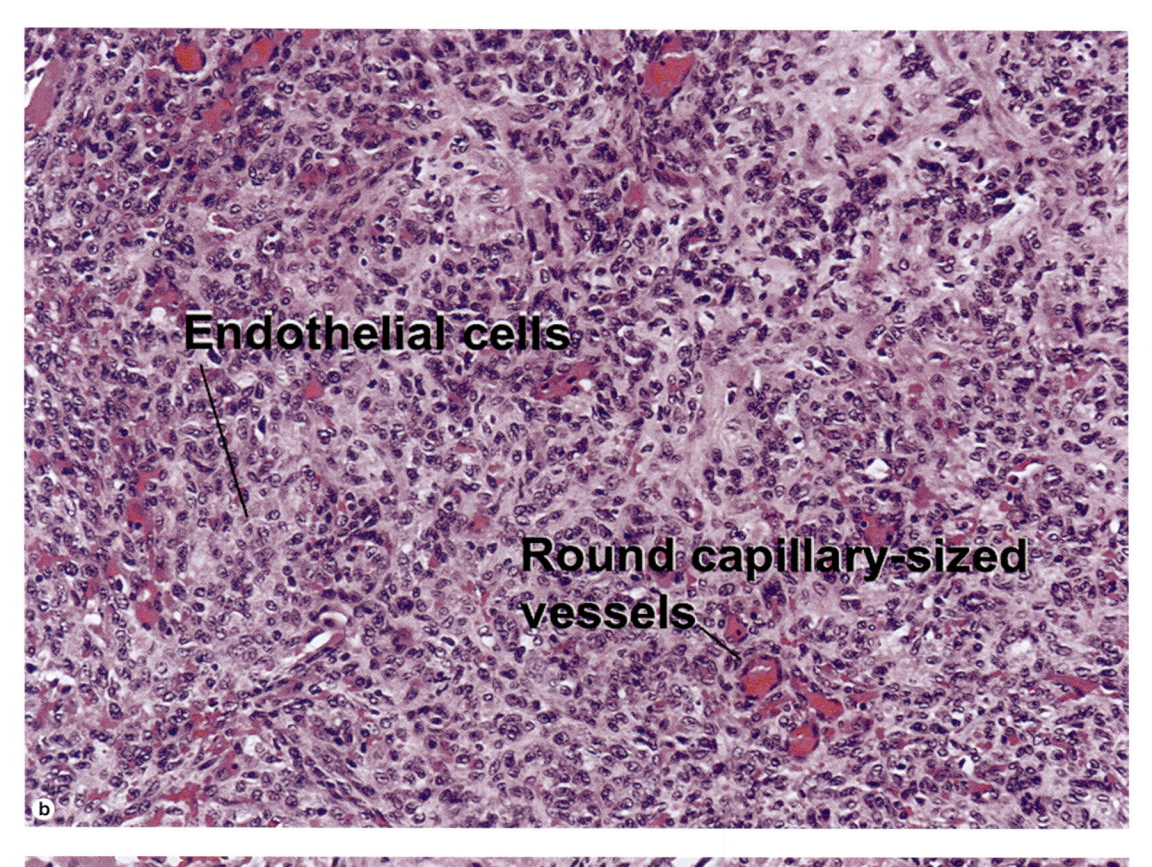

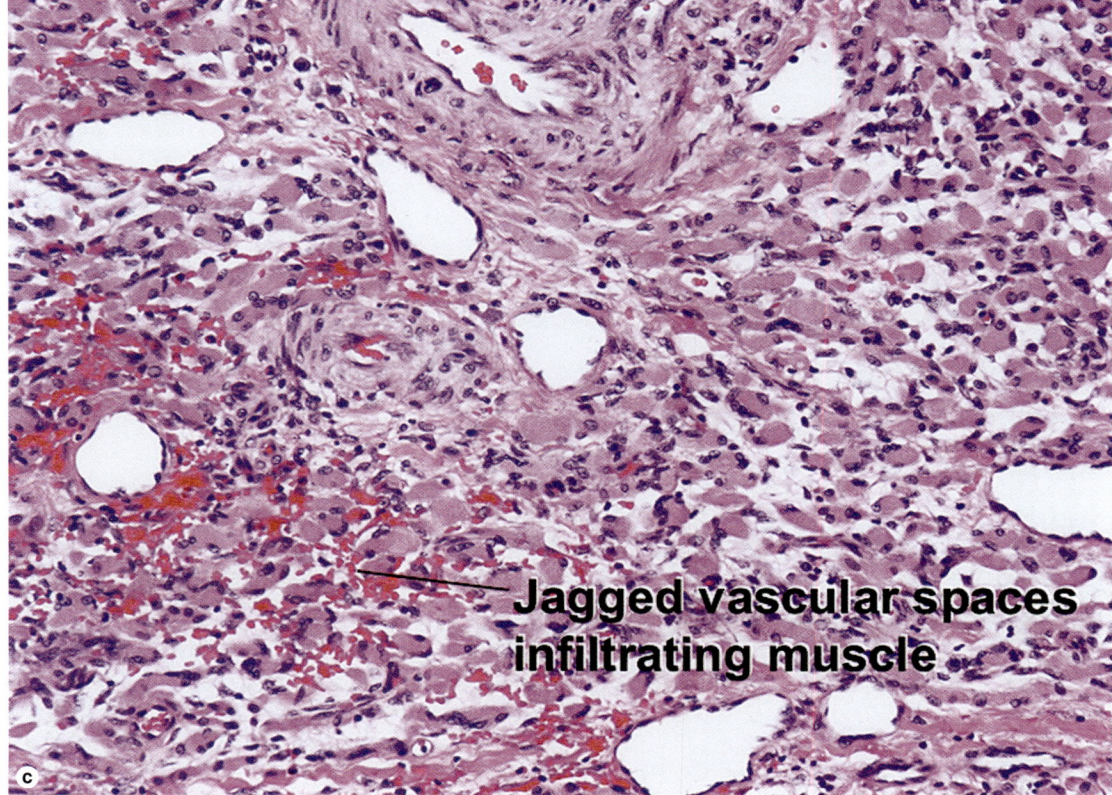

Hemangiopericytoma

Key features

- Endothelial-lined vessels surrounded by a proliferation of pericytes
- Concentric or curlicue pattern of spindle cells
- Stag-horn ectatic vascular spaces
- Most represent examples of solitary fibrous tumor with stag-horn vessels

Hemangiopericytomas occur in the skin and soft tissues. It may be difficult to distinguish between benign and malignant hemangiopericytoma histologically. Large size and higher mitotic rate suggest a malignant potential. Infantile tumors are typically cutaneous, with a good prognosis.

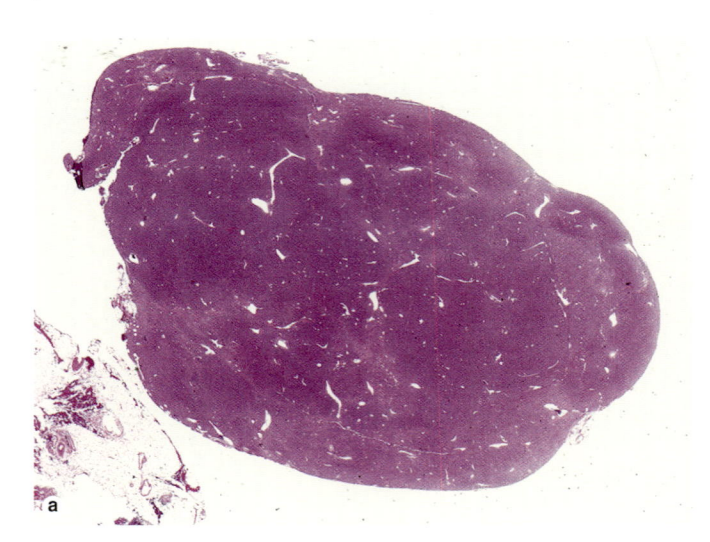

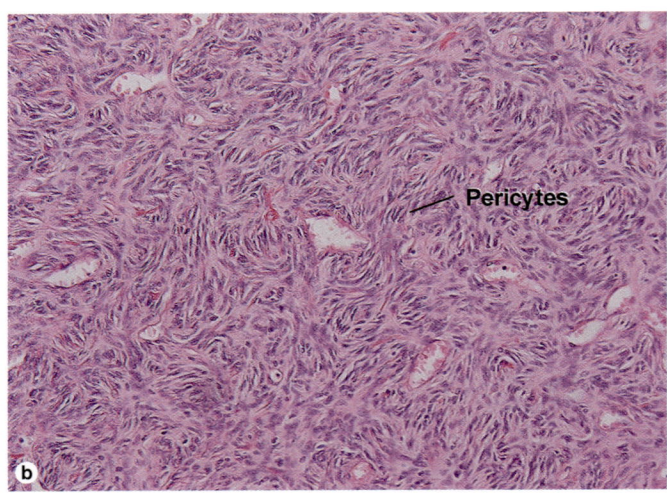

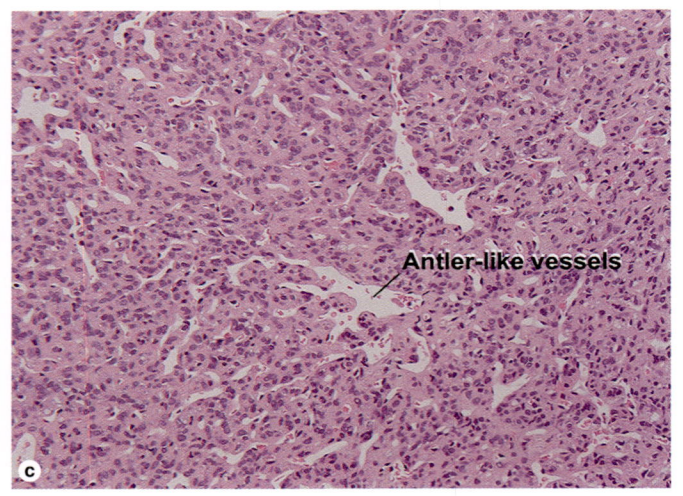

Fig 23-22 Hemangiopericytoma

Spindle cell hemangioma (spindle cell hemangioendothelioma)

Key features

- At scanning power, resembles "hemorrhagic lung" with alveolar spaces
- Solid areas of spindle cells
- Phleboliths

Epithelioid hemangioendothelioma

Key features

- Dilated vascular channels with solid epithelioid and spindle cell areas
- Intracytoplasmic lumens
- Variable pleomorphism and mitotic activity

Epithelioid hemangioendotheliomas tend to occur on the extremities of young people. They are best regarded as low-grade malignancies.

Vascular tumors Chapter 23

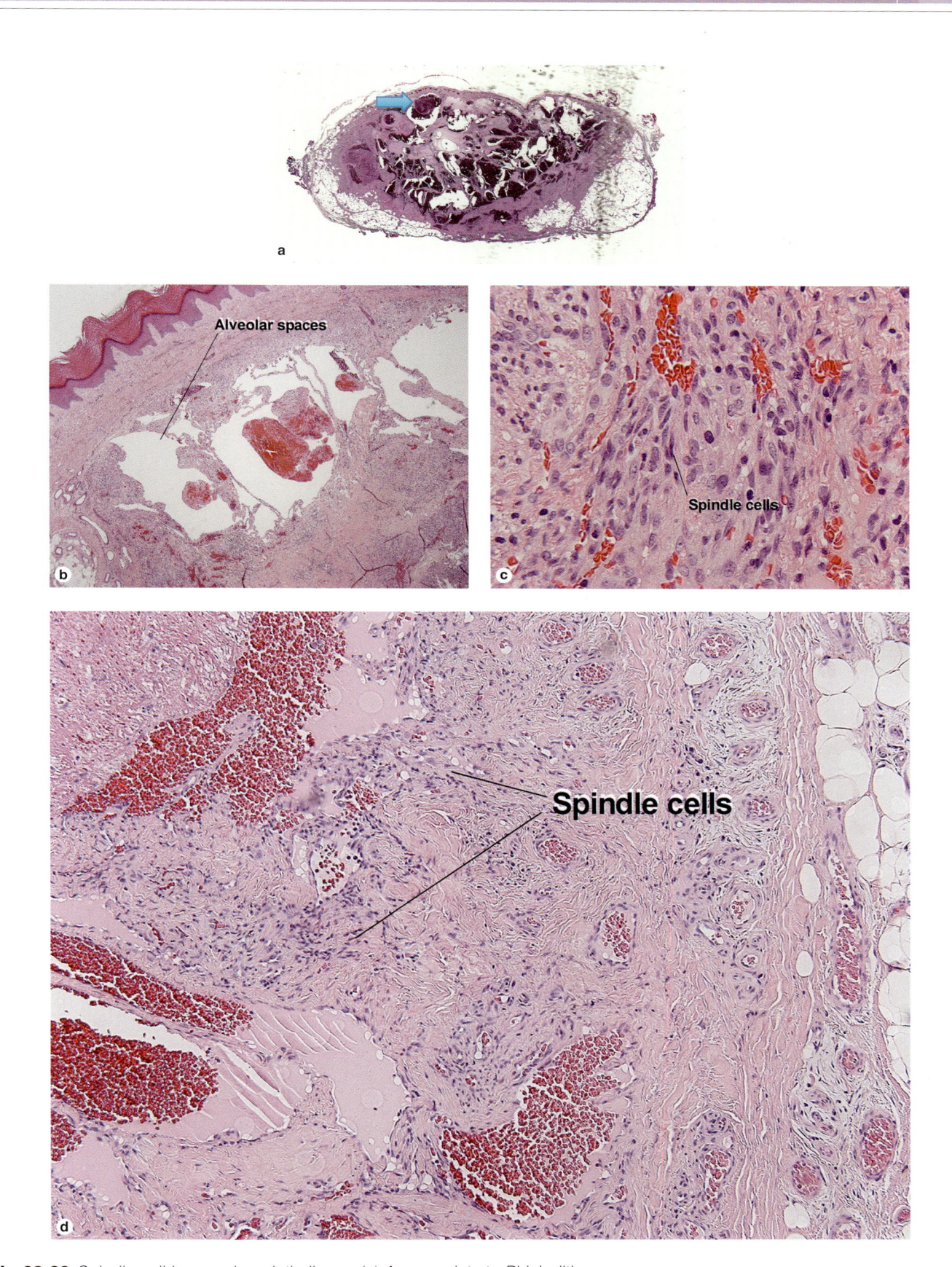

Fig 23-23 Spindle cell hemangioendothelioma. (a) Arrow points to Phlebolith

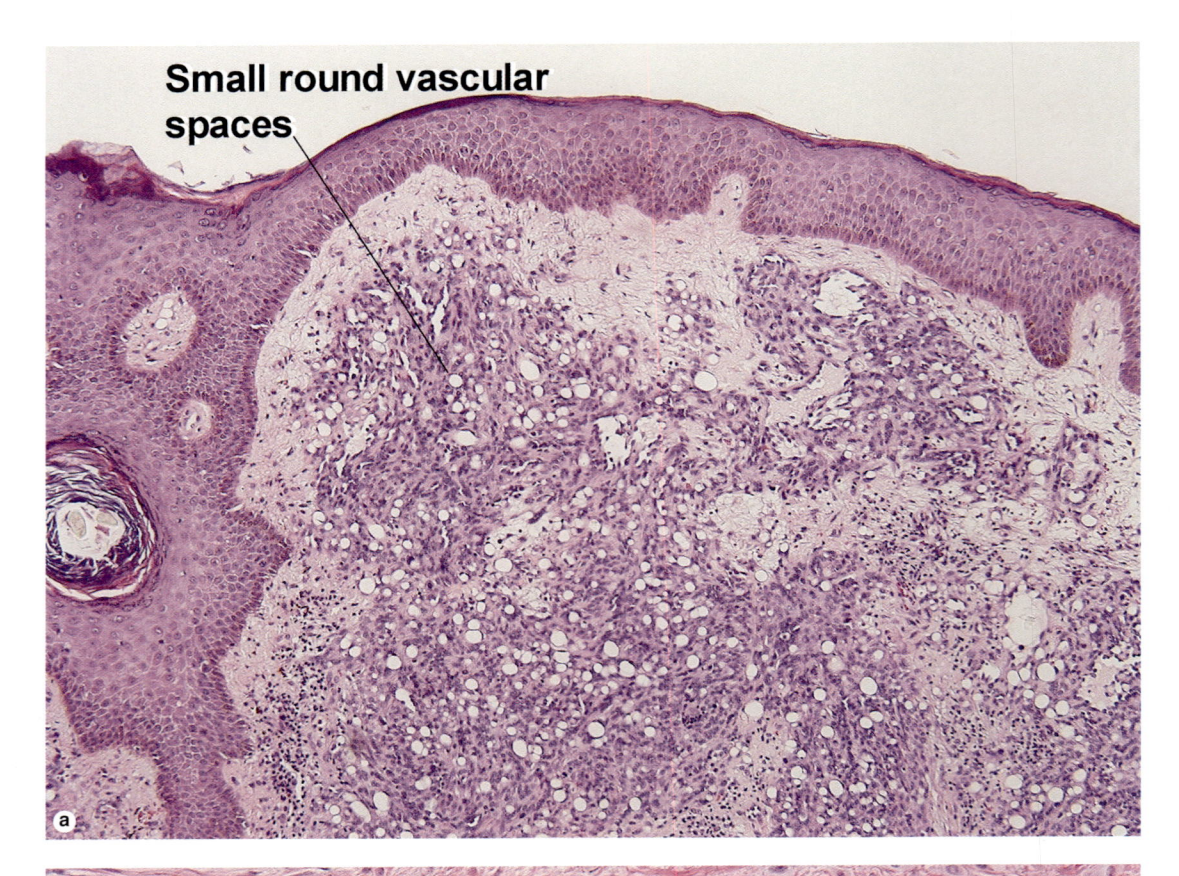

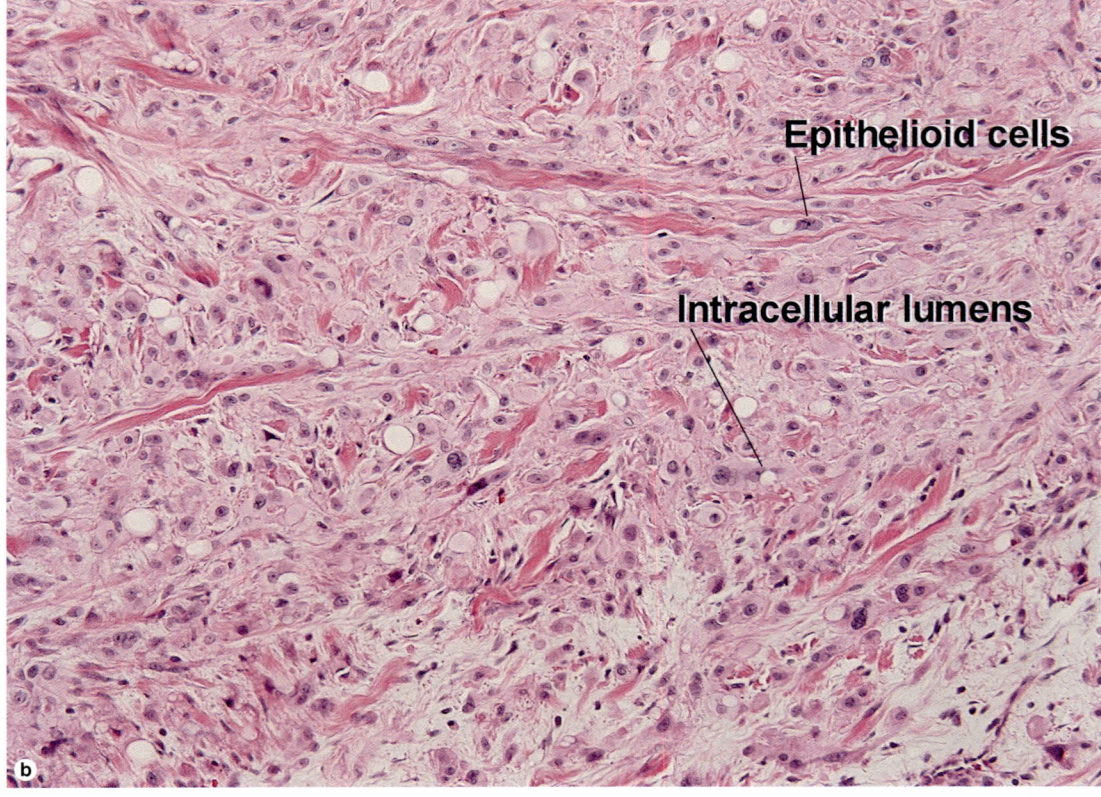

Fig 23-24 Epithelioid hemangioendothelioma

Retiform hemangioendothelioma

Key features
- Arborizing blood vessels reminiscent of rete testis

Retiform hemangioendothelioma is a low-grade angiosarcoma that occurs mostly on the extremities of young adults.

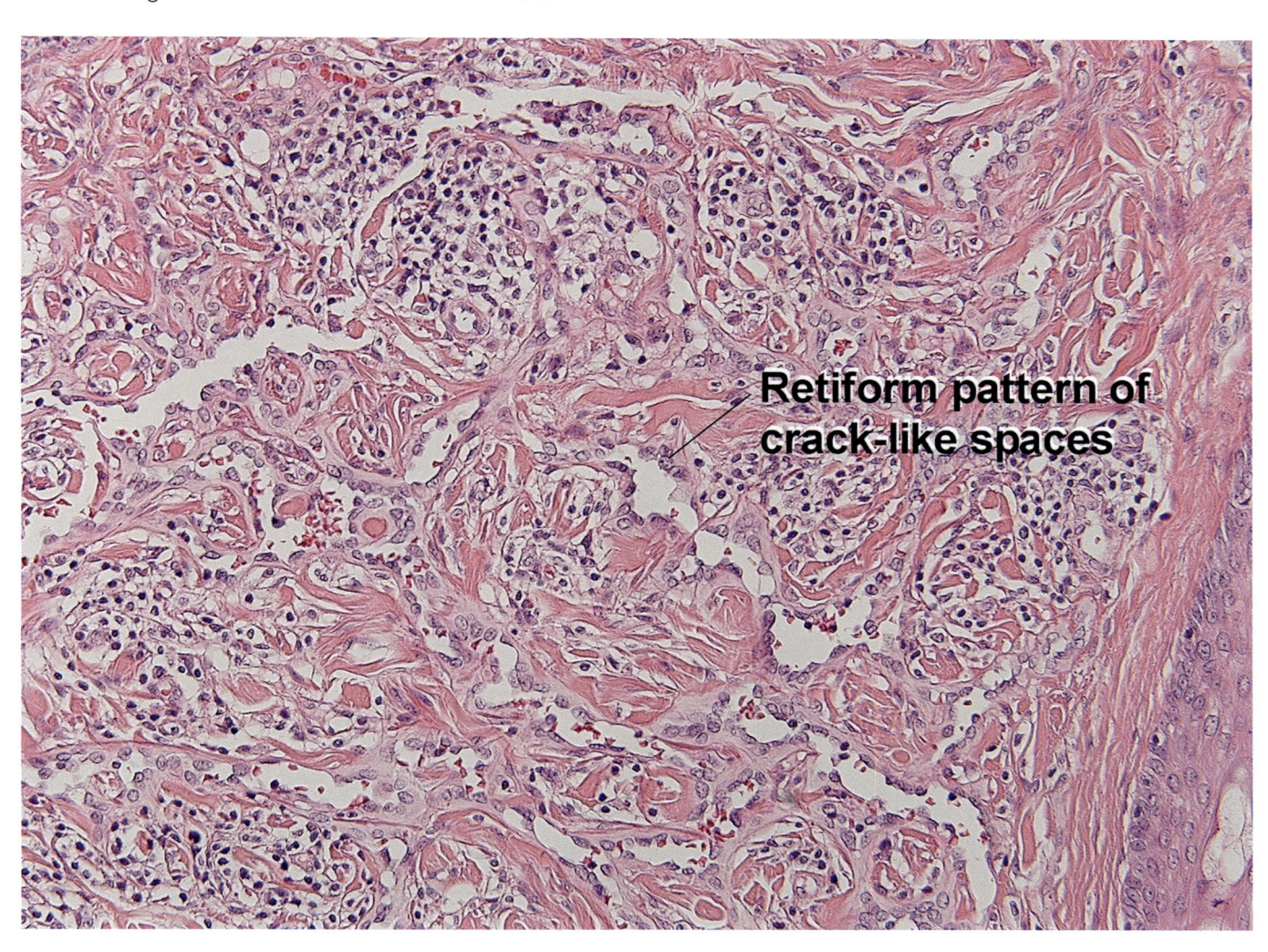

Fig 23-25 Retiform hemangioendothelioma

Angiosarcoma

Key features
- Crack-like spaces between collagen bundles
- Spaces lined by hyperchromatic endothelial cells
- Nodular areas commonly epithelioid with more pronounced atypia

Angiosarcomas typically appear as bruise-like lesions on the forehead or scalp of an older patient. Epithelioid variants may be nodular. Stewart–Treves syndrome is angiosarcoma in the setting of a lymphedematous limb. Often, there is a history of radiation therapy.

PEARL
Markers of angiosarcoma:
- Factor VIII (unreliable)
- CD34 (clean stain, little background, not specific)
- CD31 (very specific, but background staining common)
- Ulex europeus lectin (clean staining, marks endothelium and epithelium)
- D2-40+
- MYC is amplified in post-radiation angiosarcoma, but not in atypical vascular lesion (AVL) occurring after radiation therapy.

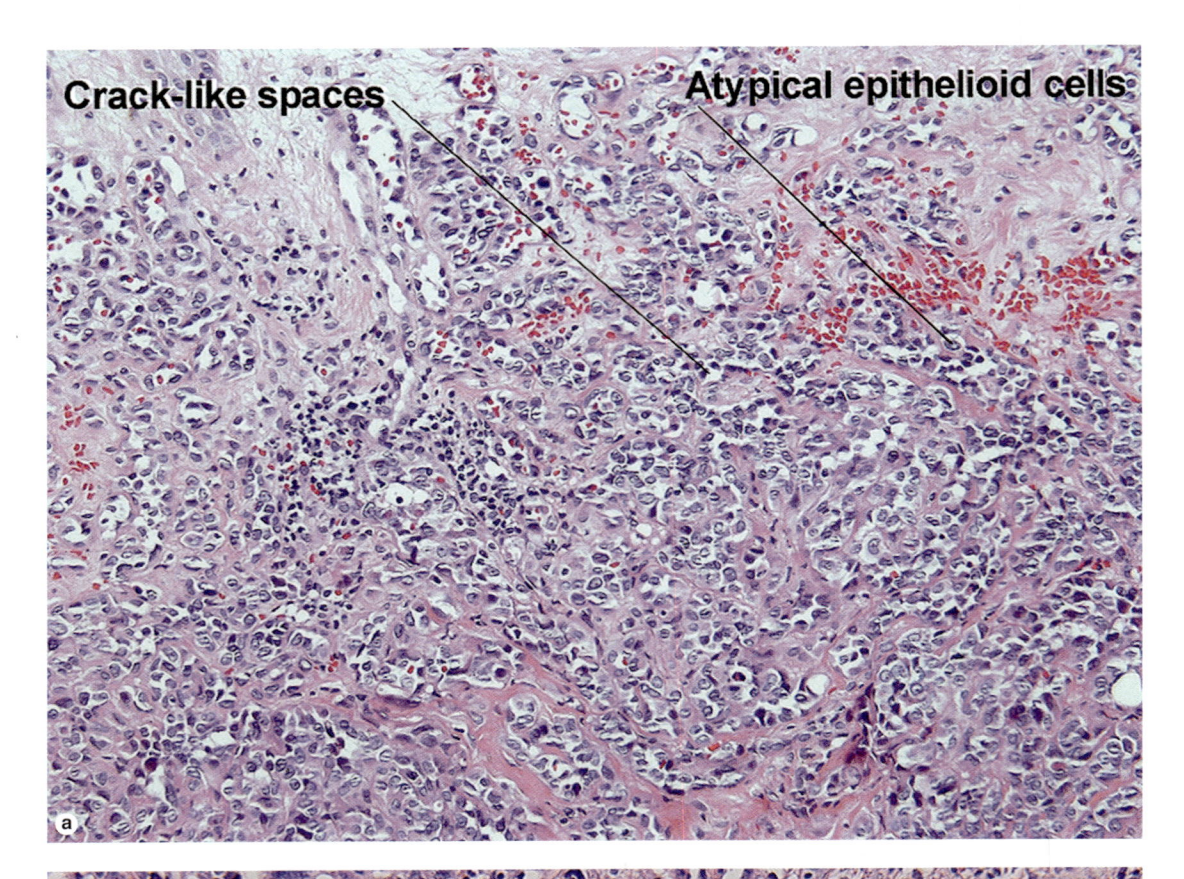

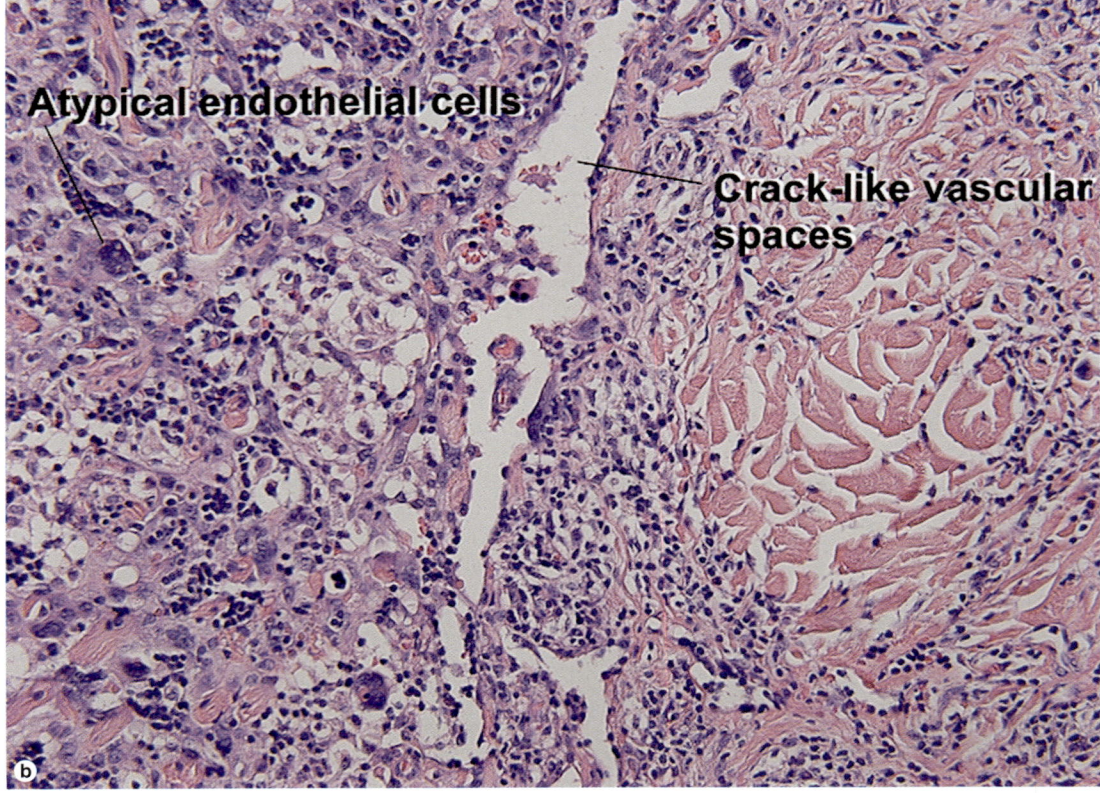

Fig 23-26 Angiosarcoma

Vascular tumors **Chapter 23** 385

Atypical endothelial cells

Crack-like vascular spaces

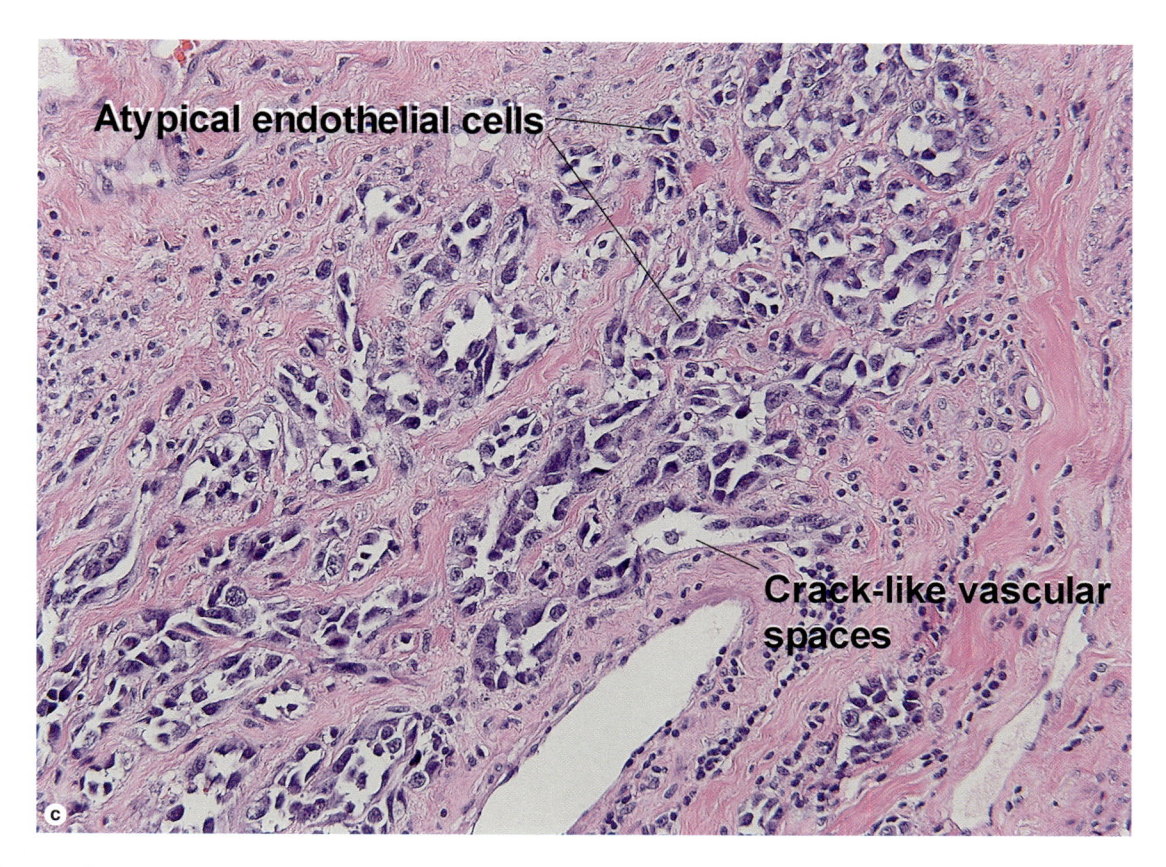

Fig 23-26, cont'd

Differential Diagnosis

Diffuse dermal angiomatosis is an acquired benign vascular proliferation in response to stasis or ischemia. It occurs in association with arteriovenous fistulae or in large pendulous breasts. The patients are often heavy smokers. It is characterized by poorly circumscribed, violaceous plaques with frequent ulceration. New vessels dissect between collagen bundles, but atypia and mitoses are absent.

Kaposi's sarcoma

Key features
- HHV-8 associated
- Patch, plaque, and tumor stages

Early-patch-stage Kaposi's sarcoma

Key features
- Bizarre stag-horn ectatic lymphatic-like vessels
- Plasma cells

386 Dermatopathology

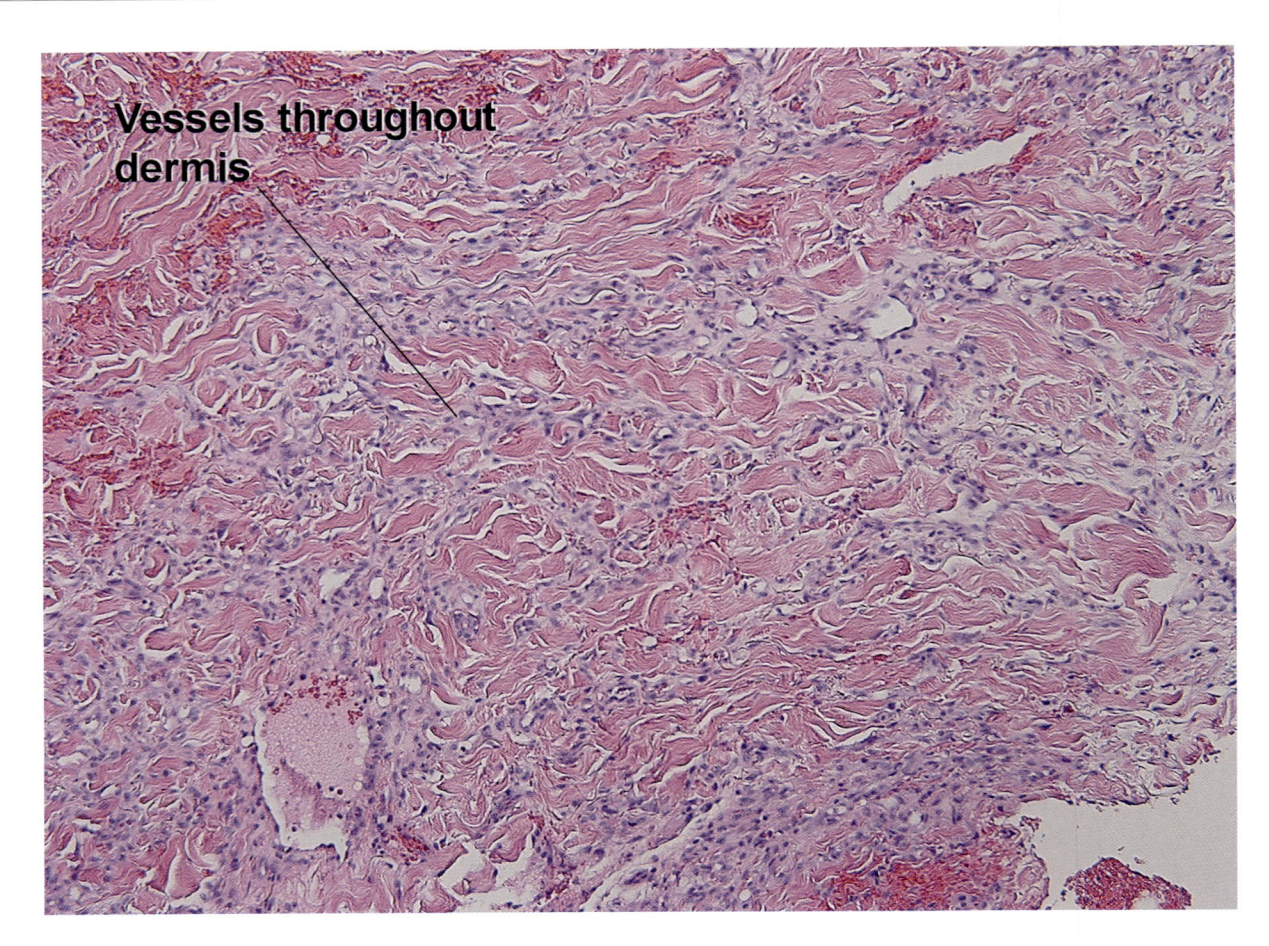

Fig 23-27 Diffuse dermal angiomatosis

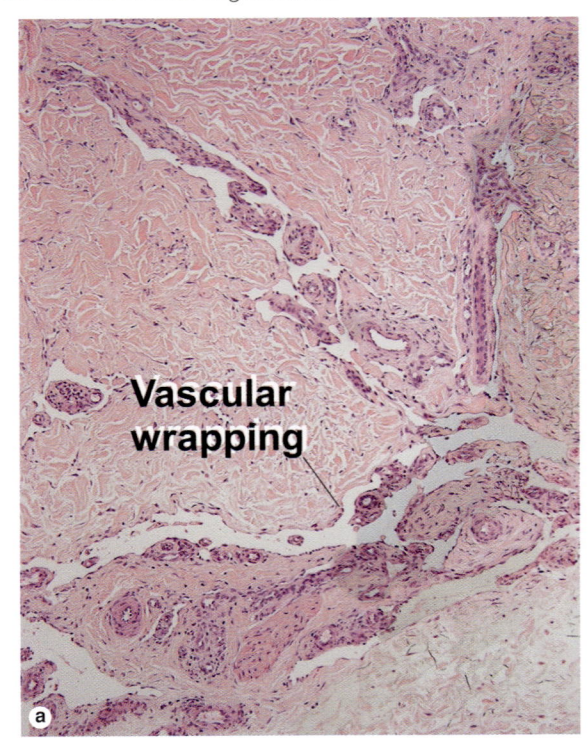

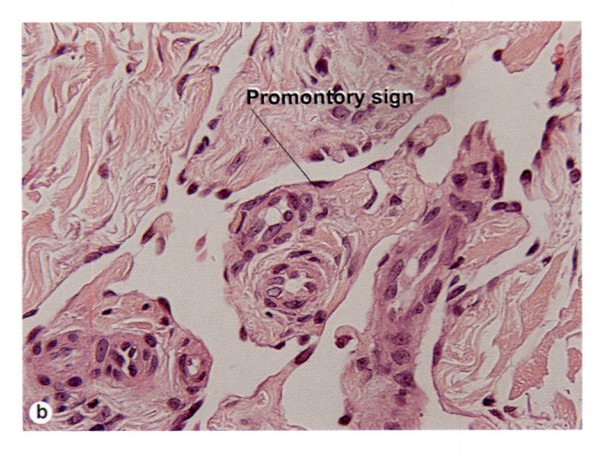

Fig 23-28 Early-patch Kaposi's sarcoma

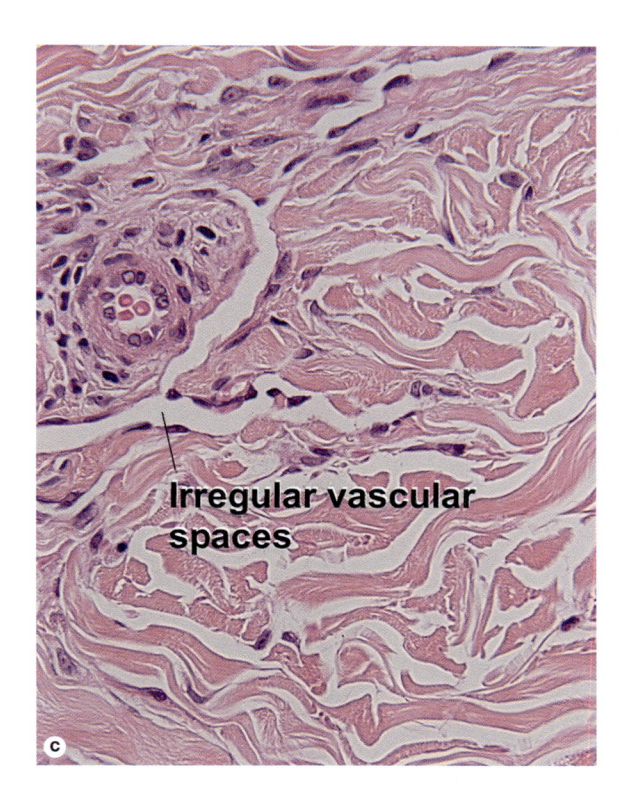

Fig 23-28, cont'd

Later-patch/plaque Kaposi's sarcoma

Key features

- Busy dermis surrounding adnexal structures and pre-existing vessels
- Pale appearance of busy area (appears understained)
- Promontory sign

Plaque lesions of Kaposi's sarcoma are characterized by "vascular wrapping." New vessels wrap and surround pre-existing vascular and adnexal structures. The pre-existing structure commonly protrudes into a lake-like ectatic space (promontory sign).

Nodular Kaposi's sarcoma

Key features

- Nodule composed of fascicles of parallel spindle cells
- Erythrocytes between spindle cells
- Eosinophilic globules
- Mitoses
- Hemosiderin

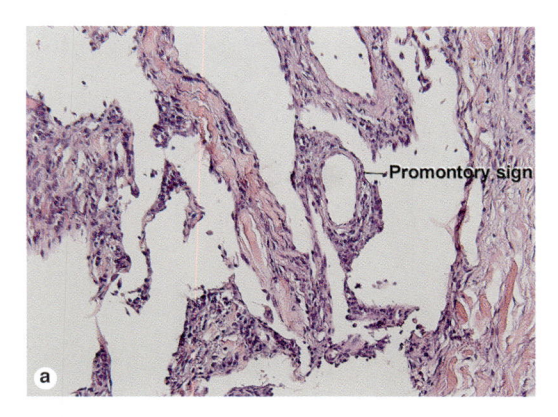

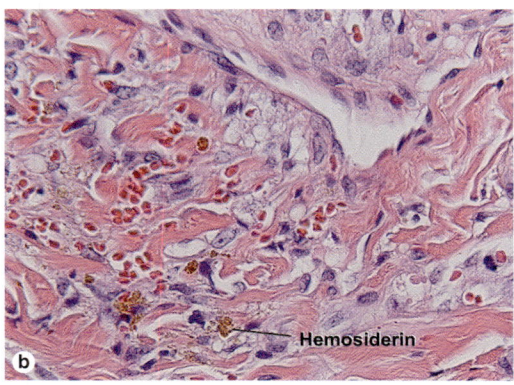

Fig 23-29 Plaque Kaposi's sarcoma

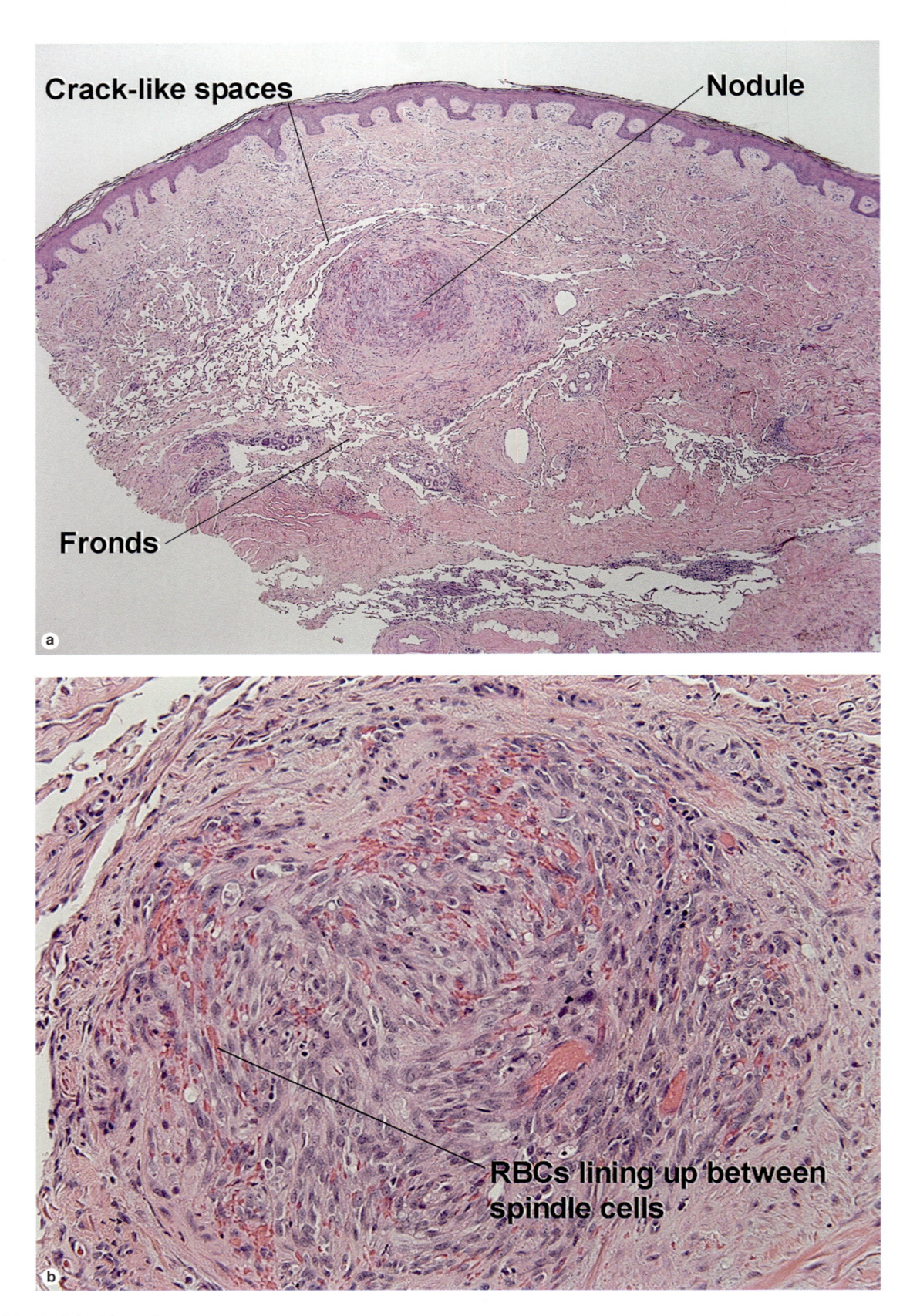

Fig 23-30 Nodular Kaposi's sarcoma

Further reading

Alvarez-Mendoza A, Lourdes TS, Ridaura-Sanz C, et al. Histopathology of vascular lesions found in Kasabach-Merritt syndrome: review based on 13 cases. Pediatr Dev Pathol 2000;3(6):556–560.

Berenguer B, Mulliken JB, Enjolras O, et al. Rapidly involuting congenital hemangioma: clinical and histopathologic features. Pediatr Dev Pathol 2003;6(6):495–510.

Billings SD, Folpe AL, Weiss SW. Epithelioid sarcoma-like hemangioendothelioma. Am J Surg Pathol 2003;27(1):48–57.

Chu CY, Hsiao CH, Chiu HC. Transformation between Kaposiform hemangioendothelioma and tufted angioma. Dermatology 2003;206(4):334–337.

Espat NJ, Lewis JJ, Leung D, et al. Conventional hemangiopericytoma: modern analysis of outcome. Cancer 2002;95(8):1746–1751.

Kishimoto S, Takenaka H, Shibagaki R, et al. Glomeruloid hemangioma in POEMS syndrome shows two different immunophenotypic endothelial cells. J Cutan Pathol 2000;27(2):87–92.

Mentzel T, Partanen TA, Kutzner H. Hobnail hemangioma ("targetoid hemosiderotic hemangioma"): clinicopathologic and immunohistochemical analysis of 62 cases. J Cutan Pathol 1999;26(6):279–286.

Nayler SJ, Rubin BP, Calonje E, et al. Composite hemangioendothelioma: a complex, low-grade vascular lesion mimicking angiosarcoma. Am J Surg Pathol 2000;24(3):352–361.

Pelle MT, Pride HB, Tyler WB. Eccrine angiomatous hamartoma. J Am Acad Dermatol 2002;47(3):429–435.

Pellegrini AE, Drake RD, Qualman SJ. Spindle cell hemangioendothelioma. J Cutan Pathol 1995;22:173.

Reis-Filho JS, Paiva ME, Lopes JM. Congenital composite hemangioendothelioma: case report and reappraisal of the hemangioendothelioma spectrum. J Cutan Pathol 2002;29(4):226–231.

Requena L, Sangueza OP. Cutaneous vascular neoplasms. Part II. J Am Acad Dermatol 1997;37:887.

Requena L, Sangueza OP. Cutaneous vascular neoplasms. Part III. J Am Acad Dermatol 1998;38:143.

Requena L, Kutzner H. Hemangioendothelioma. Semin Diagn Pathol 2013;30(1):29–44.

Sangüeza OP. Update on vascular neoplasms. Dermatol Clin 2012;30(4):657–665.

Chapter 24
Cutaneous T-cell lymphoma, NK-cell lymphoma, and myeloid leukemia

David J. DiCaudo

Cutaneous T-cell lymphoma and NK-cell lymphoma

Mycosis fungoides

Patch stage

Key features

- Lymphocytes "line up" along the dermal–epidermal junction (simulates vacuolar interface dermatitis, with a "lymphocyte in every hole")
- Large dark lymphocytes with irregular nuclear contours and perinuclear haloes ("lump of coal on a pillow")
- *Pautrier's microabscesses* (intraepidermal clusters of atypical lymphocytes, larger than the benign recruited dermal lymphocytes)
- Mild band-like infiltrate in superficial dermis
- Sclerosis of the papillary dermis
- Eosinophils and necrotic keratinocytes are rarely present

Mycosis fungoides (MF) is the most common type of cutaneous lymphoma. In most cases, the disease is indolent and slowly progressive over a period of years or decades. Three main stages of the lymphoma are recognized: patch, plaque, and tumor stages. In the patch stage of mycosis fungoides, patients typically present with broad pink or tan oval-shaped patches with a predilection for the bathing trunk area. The patches may be asymptomatic or pruritic. Both clinically and histopathologically, distinction from eczematous dermatitis is sometimes difficult in the earliest stages of the lymphoma. In the evaluation of patch

Table 24-1 Primary cutaneous T-cell lymphomas, NK-cell lymphomas, and precursor hematologic neoplasm in the 2008 WHO classification

Mature T-cell and NK-cell neoplasms

Mycosis fungoides
Mycosis fungoides variants and subtypes
    Pagetoid reticulosis
    Folliculotropic mycosis fungoides
    Granulomatous slack skin
Sézary syndrome
Adult T-cell leukemia/lymphoma
Primary cutaneous CD30+ T-cell lymphoproliferative disorders
    Lymphomatoid papulosis
    Primary cutaneous anaplastic large cell lymphoma
Subcutaneous panniculitis-like T-cell lymphoma
Extranodal NK/T-cell lymphoma, nasal type
Primary cutaneous peripheral T-cell lymphoma, rare subtypes
    Primary cutaneous aggressive epidermotropic CD8+ cytotoxic T-cell lymphoma[a]
    Primary cutaneous gamma–delta T-cell lymphoma
    Primary cutaneous CD4+ small/medium T-cell lymphoma[a]
Hydroa vacciniforme-like lymphoma

Precursor hematologic neoplasm

Blastic plasmacytoid dendritic cell neoplasm (CD4+/CD56+ hematodermic neoplasm)

[a]Provisional entities.
Adapted from WHO Classification of Tumours of Haematopoietic and Lymphoid Tissues, 4th edn. Lyon, France: IARC; 2008.

Fig 24-1 Patch stage mycosis fungoides

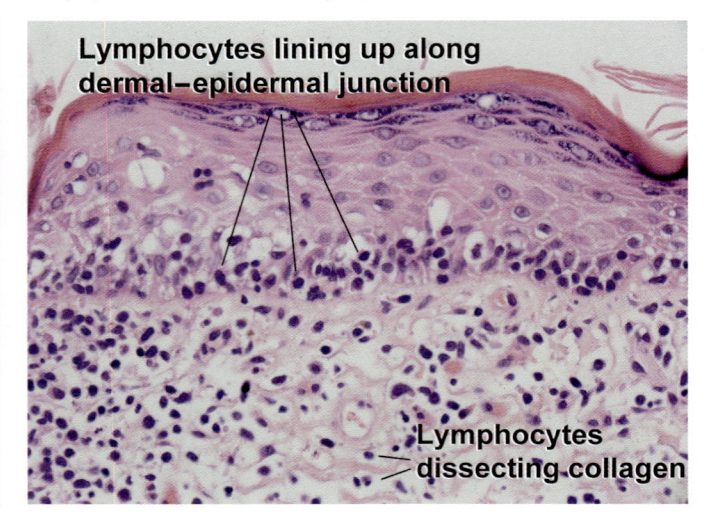

Fig 24-2 Patch stage mycosis fungoides

stage mycosis fungoides, multiple shave biopsies are often helpful, since the shave technique provides a broad area of epidermis for examination. The typical immunophenotype is CD3+, CD4+, CD8–, CD30–. Aberrant immunophenotypes (with loss of normal T-cell markers, such as CD7) can frequently be demonstrated. Clonal rearrangement of the T-cell receptor gene is helpful in supporting the diagnosis, although the earliest cases may sometimes not have a detectable clone.

Differential Diagnosis

- Dermatitis generally has more spongiosis and fewer intraepidermal lymphocytes
- Lichenoid drug eruption typically has more apoptotic keratinocytes
- Lymphomatoid drug eruption may look nearly identical. Pautrier's microabscesses favor mycosis fungoides

Plaque stage

Key features

- Like patch stage, but with a denser, band-like infiltrate in the upper dermis
- Atypical lymphocytes present in the dermal band

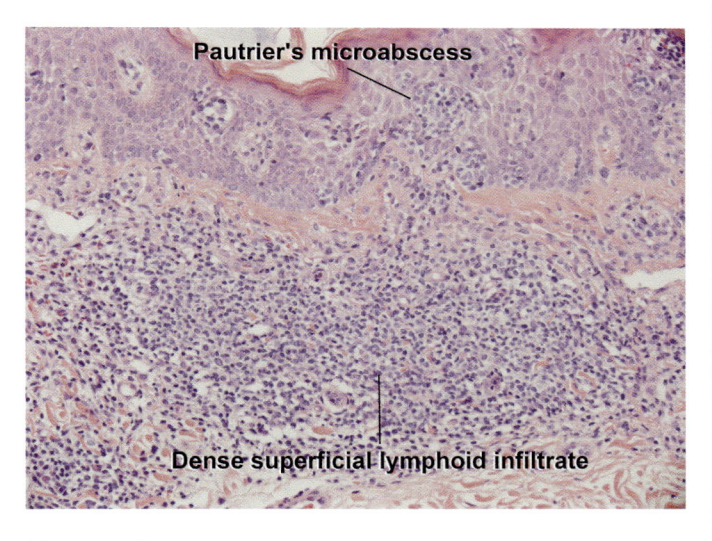

Fig 24-3 Plaque stage mycosis fungoides

Tumor stage

Key features

- Dense, nodular lymphocytic infiltrate in the superficial and deep dermis
- Many atypical lymphocytes present in the dermal infiltrate
- Transformation to large-sized lymphocytes in some cases
- Acquisition of CD30 expression in some cases
- Loss of epidermotropism with progression

Over time, patients with mycosis fungoides may progress to develop thicker plaques and tumors. Whereas patch stage mycosis fungoides is usually associated with long survival, the prognosis is poor for those patients who progress to tumor stage.

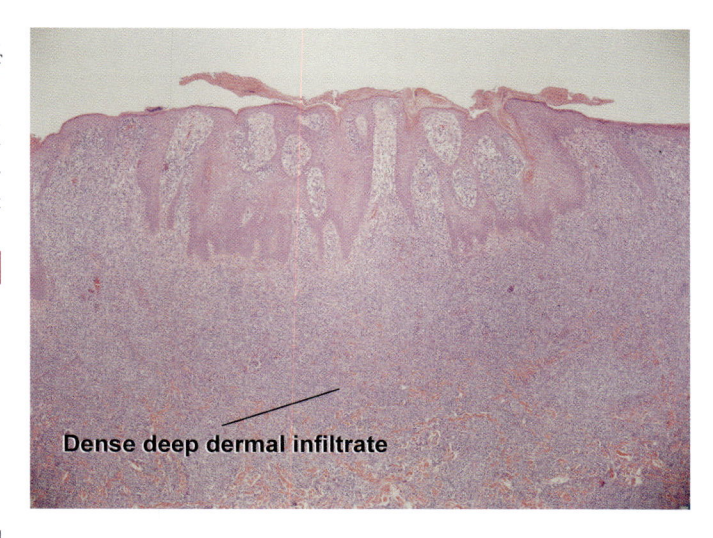

Fig 24-4 Tumor stage mycosis fungoides

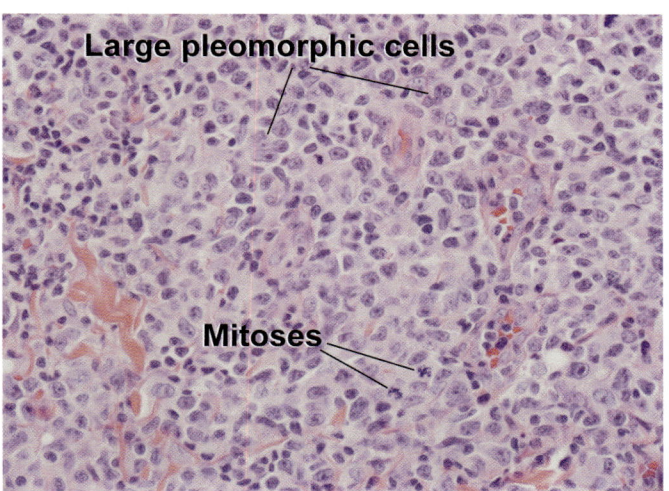

Fig 24-5 Tumor stage mycosis fungoides

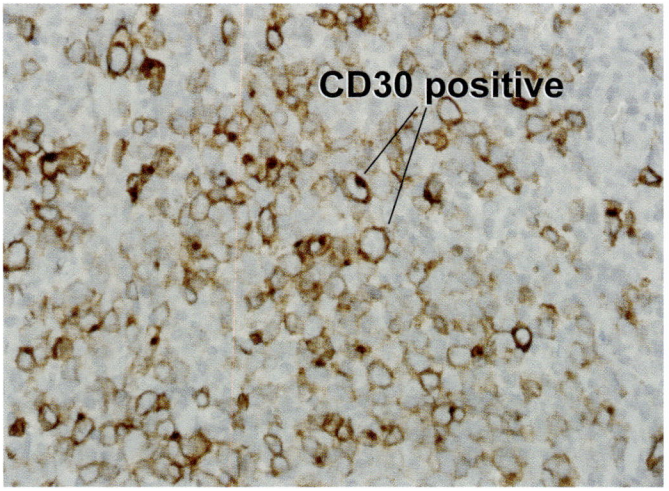

Fig 24-6 Tumor stage mycosis fungoides

Pagetoid reticulosis variant

Key features

- Solitary or multiple patches or plaques on distal extremities
- Atypical large lymphocytes extensively infiltrating the epidermis
- CD3+
- CD4+ CD8– or CD4– CD8+
- Small reactive lymphocytes in papillary dermis

The term *pagetoid reticulosis* is now limited to the *Woringer–Kolopp* type, which presents as one or several patches or plaques on the distal extremities. This type of lymphoma is associated with an excellent prognosis. The disseminated *Ketron–Goodman* type of pagetoid reticulosis has been reclassified into several other types of cutaneous T-cell lymphoma.

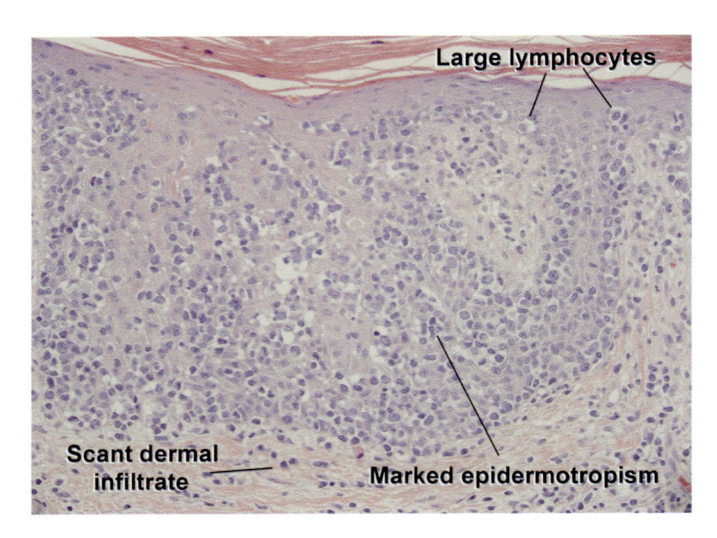

Fig 24-7 Pagetoid reticulosis variant of mycosis fungoides

Folliculotropic variant

Key features

- Atypical lymphocytes infiltrate the follicular epithelium
- Basaloid induction and hyperplasia of follicular epithelium
- Eosinophils common
- *Follicular mucinosis* (pools of mucin in the follicular epithelium)
- Epidermis usually spared
- CD3+ CD4+ CD8– in most cases

The folliculotropic variant of mycosis fungoides presents with follicular papules and boggy plaques, most frequently involving the head and neck. Follicular mucinosis is often associated. This variant of mycosis fungoides is sometimes associated with a more rapidly progressive clinical course.

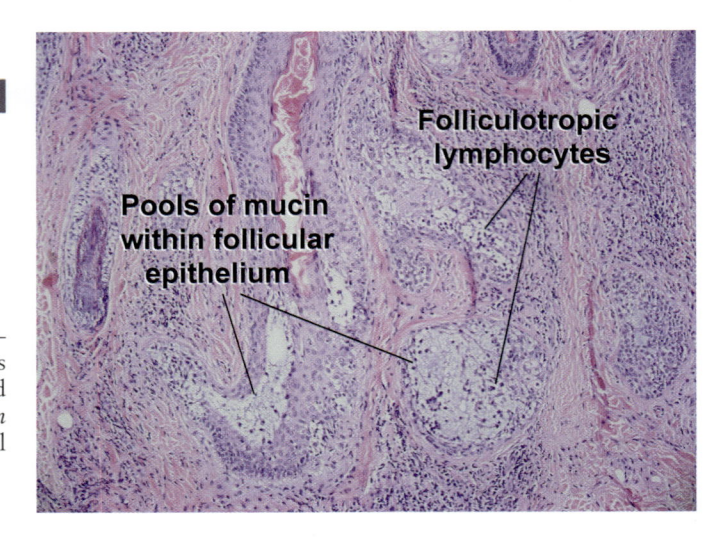

Fig 24-8 Folliculotropic variant of mycosis fungoides

Granulomatous slack skin

Key features

- Pendulous folds in intertriginous regions
- Preceded by insidious onset of patches, papules, and plaques
- Massive dermal and subcutaneous infiltrate ± epidermal involvement
- Small T lymphocytes with epidermotropism and mild cytologic atypia
- Huge multinucleate giant cells with numerous nuclei, often in wreath-like arrangement
- Phagocytosis of lymphocytes by multinucleate cells
- Dermal edema or fibrosis
- Loss of dermal elastic tissue fibers
- CD3+ CD4+ CD8– immunophenotype

Granulomatous slack skin syndrome is an extremely rare variant of mycosis fungoides with a slowly progressive clinical course.

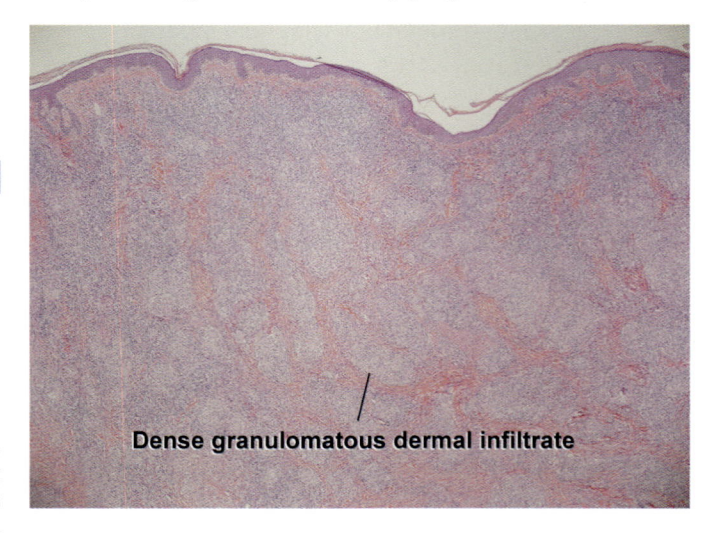

Fig 24-9 Granulomatous slack skin variant of mycosis fungoides

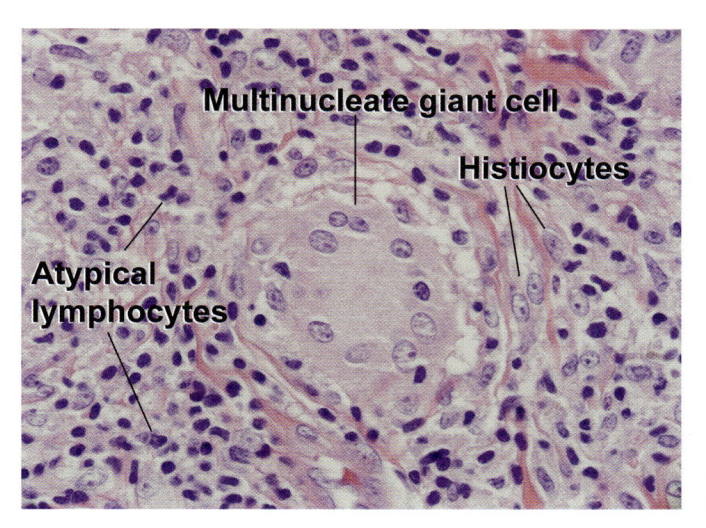

Fig 24-10 Granulomatous slack skin variant of mycosis fungoides

The clinical presentation is striking. In fully developed cases, massive folds of skin extend from flexural areas, such as the axillae or groin. An association with nodal Hodgkin lymphoma has been documented in multiple cases.

Sézary syndrome

> **Key features**
> - Erythroderma with generalized pruritus
> - Palmoplantar keratoderma
> - Generalized lymphadenopathy
> - Peripheral blood Sézary cell count of ≥1000 cells/microliter
> - Peripheral blood lymphocytes with aberrant phenotype or CD4/CD8 ratio >10
> - Clonal rearrangement of T-cell receptor genes in blood and/or skin
> - Histopathology like mycosis fungoides or may show only non-specific dermatitis

Although previously believed to be a leukemic variant of mycosis fungoides, Sézary syndrome is now considered to originate from a different subset of T cells (central memory T cell in Sézary syndrome versus skin resident memory T cell in mycosis fungoides). In contrast to mycosis fungoides, Sézary syndrome has a rapidly progressive clinical course and a poor prognosis. The diagnosis is confirmed by evaluation of the peripheral blood. Skin biopsy is sometimes useful in demonstrating a histopathologic pattern similar to mycosis fungoides. It should be recognized, however, that skin biopsy findings may be non-diagnostic in some cases of Sézary syndrome. In an erythrodermic patient, non-specific biopsy findings (such as spongiotic dermatitis) do not exclude the diagnosis. It is important to evaluate the peripheral blood if there is clinical suspicion for Sézary syndrome.

Adult T-cell leukemia/lymphoma (ATCLL)

> **Key features**
> - Endemic in Japan, Caribbean, southeastern USA, and Central Africa
> - Hypercalcemia
> - Osteolytic bone lesions
> - Organomegaly
> - Lymphadenopathy
> - Dermal and/or subcutaneous lymphoid infiltrates
> - T cells with multilobed nuclei
> - Epidermotropism in some cases
> - CD3+ CD4+ CD8– *CD25+* neoplastic cell population in blood, nodes, and skin
> - Peripheral blood *flower cells* with multilobed nuclei
> - Clonal integration of the HTLV-1 genome within neoplastic cells
> - Clonal rearrangement of T-cell receptor genes

Adult T-cell leukemia/lymphoma is remarkable for its well-established viral etiology, i.e. *human T-cell leukemia virus type 1* (*HTLV-1*). HTLV-1 infection is transmitted by sexual contact, blood transfusion, and by mother-to-child vertical transmission. In areas with the highest rates of HTLV-1 infection, such as southwestern Japan, only a relatively small percentage of infected individuals eventually develop the lymphoma or leukemia. ATCLL may occur as an acute or smoldering disease. The

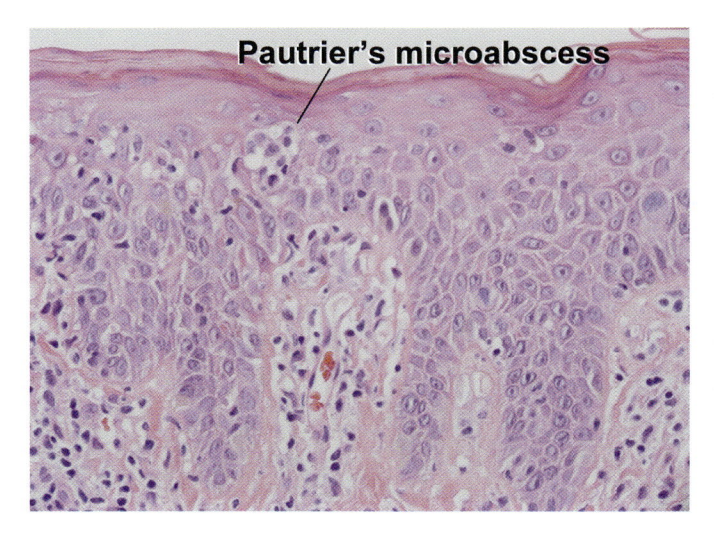

Fig 24-11 Sézary syndrome

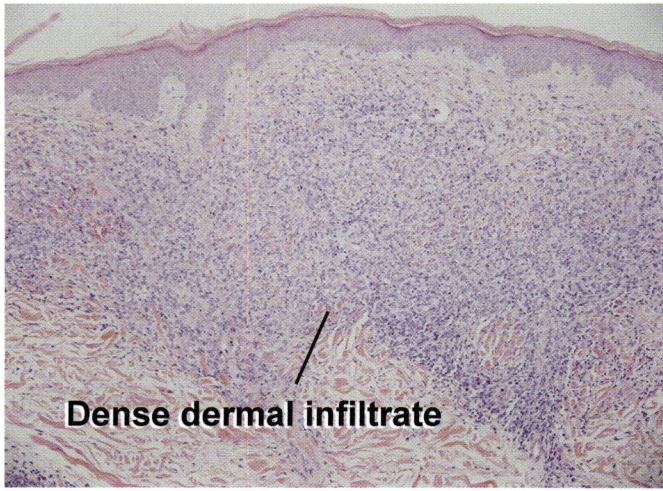

Fig 24-12 Adult T-cell leukemia/lymphoma

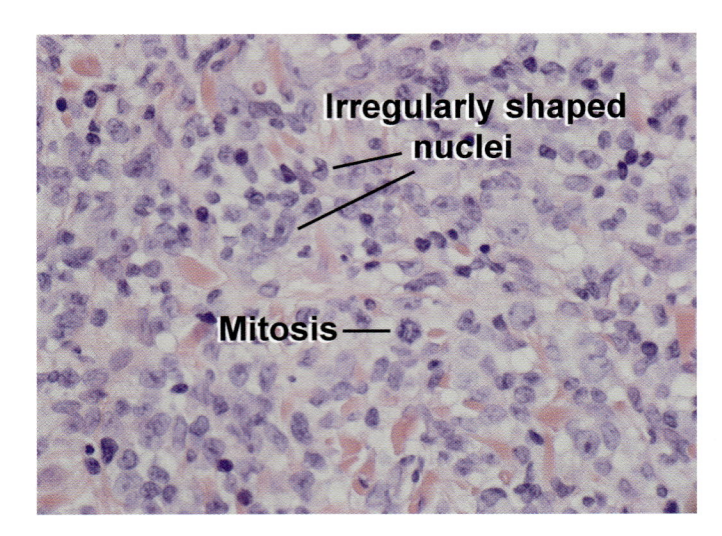

Fig 24-13 Adult T-cell leukemia/lymphoma

skin is involved in up to 50% of patients. Nodules, papules, and plaques may occur. The most specific diagnostic finding is the clonal integration of the HTLV-1 genome within lymphoma cells. This feature is helpful in distinguishing the smoldering variant of ATCLL from mycosis fungoides.

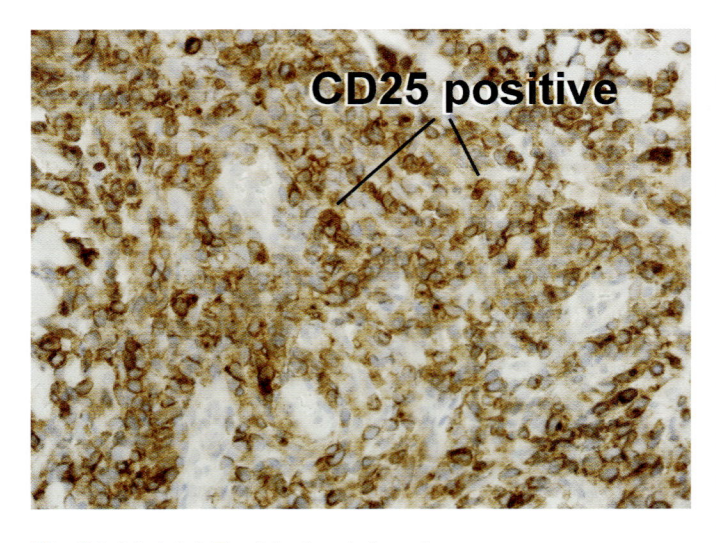

Fig 24-14 Adult T-cell leukemia/lymphoma

Primary cutaneous CD30+ lymphoproliferative disorders

Lymphomatoid papulosis

> **Key features**
>
> **Type A**
> - Wedge-shaped dermal infiltrate with mixed population of cells
> - CD30+ *Reed–Sternberg-like cells* with large nuclei, prominent nucleoli, and abundant cytoplasm
> - Neutrophils, eosinophils, and small lymphocytes in background
>
> **Type B**
> - Epidermotropic infiltrate of CD3+ small lymphocytes, often CD30–
>
> **Type C**
> - Diffuse sheets of CD30+ *Reed–Sternberg-like cells* in dermis
>
> **Type D**
> - Markedly epidermotropic CD8+ CD30+ lymphocytes, often TIA-1+ or granzyme B+
>
> **Type E**
> - Angioinvasive CD30+ Beta F1+ lymphocytes, often CD8+ and/or TIA-1+

Clinicopathologic correlation is particularly important in the diagnosis of lymphomatoid papulosis (LyP). Patients present with crops of ulcerated nodules and papules most frequently involving the trunk and limbs. Lesions regress spontaneously, while new lesions erupt at other sites. Three histologic subtypes (A, B, and C) are recognized in the 2008 WHO classification, and two additional cytotoxic variants (types D and E) have

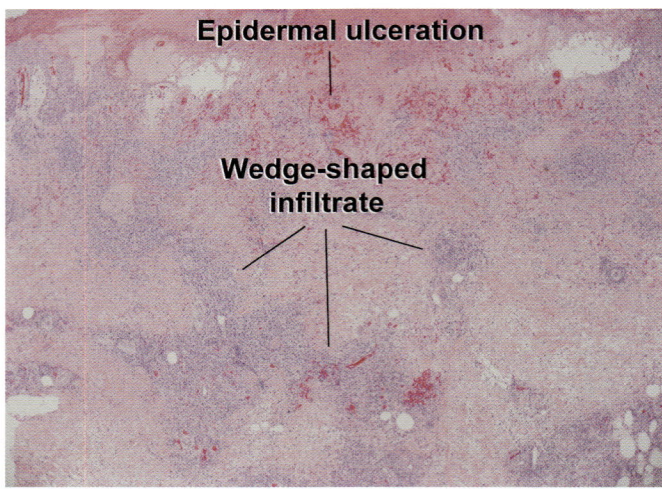

Fig 24-15 Lymphomatoid papulosis

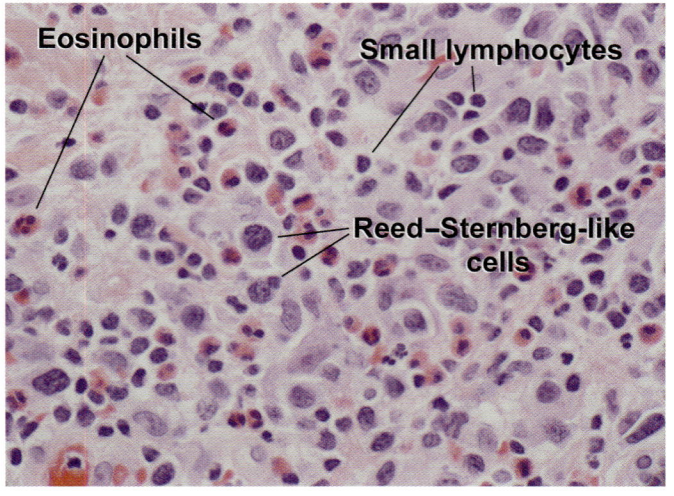

Fig 24-16 Lymphomatoid papulosis, type A

subsequently been described in the literature. Different lesions from an individual patient may simultaneously demonstrate a single or multiple histologic subtypes. Type A is the most common and characteristic type of LyP; type B is uncommon.

LyP is a spontaneously regressing lymphoproliferative disorder. Clonal rearrangement of the T-cell receptor genes is detectable in many cases. LyP itself is a non-fatal disease, but it can be associated with other more aggressive lymphoproliferative disorders. In 10–20% of cases, it is associated with mycosis fungoides, cutaneous or systemic anaplastic large cell lymphoma, or Hodgkin's lymphoma. These associated lymphomas may precede, accompany, or follow the diagnosis of LyP.

PEARLS

Type B LyP may histologically mimic mycosis fungoides. The clinical features distinguish the two entities. Spontaneously regressing papules or nodules favor LyP. Persistent patches or plaques favor MF.

Type C LyP may be histologically indistinguishable from anaplastic large cell lymphoma (ALCL). Crops of spontaneously regressing papules or nodules favor LyP. Persistent, solitary or localized nodules or tumors favor ALCL. The two are closely related and may in fact represent a spectrum of a single disorder.

Type D LyP histologically mimics primary cutaneous aggressive epidermotropic CD8+ cytotoxic T-cell lymphoma, but is CD30 positive and has the typical course of LyP with crops of self-resolving ulcerative papulonodules.

Type E LyP histologically mimics extranodal NK/T-cell lymphoma, nasal type, which is similarly angioinvasive and angiodestructive. The two entities are distinguished by the clinical course and the presence or absence of Epstein–Barr virus (EBV) within the tumor cells. NK/T-cell lymphoma has an aggressive clinical course; lesions of type E LyP regress spontaneously. The tumor cells of NK/T-cell lymphoma are Epstein–Barr virus (EBV) positive by *in situ* hybridization and usually CD56 positive by immunohistochemistry; the cells of type E LyP are EBV negative and usually CD56 negative.

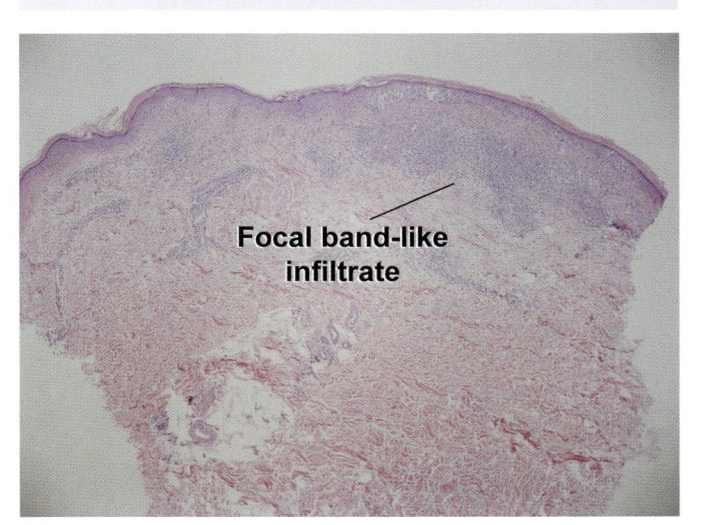

Fig 24-17 Lymphomatoid papulosis, type B

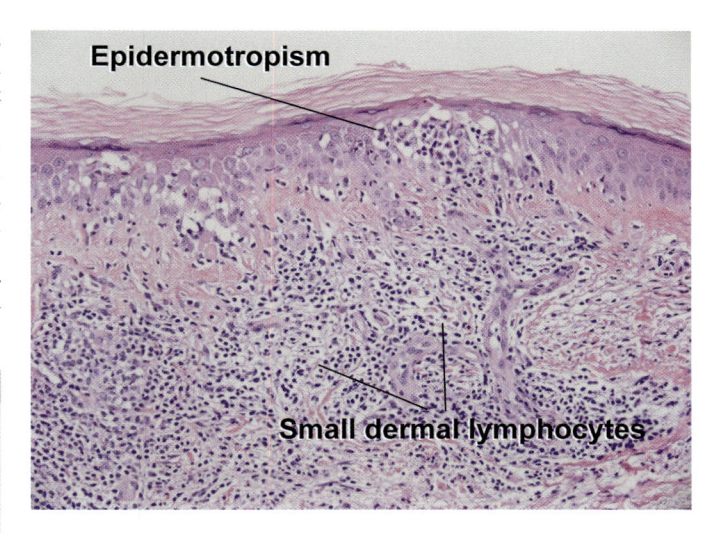

Fig 24-18 Lymphomatoid papulosis, type B

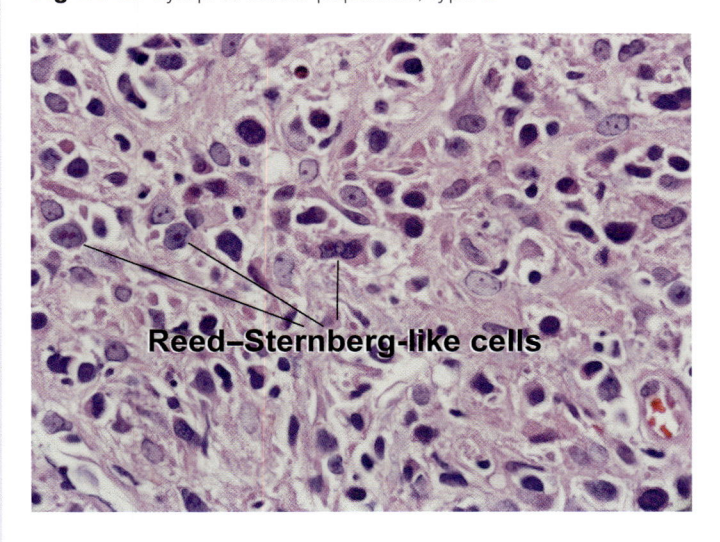

Fig 24-19 Lymphomatoid papulosis, type C

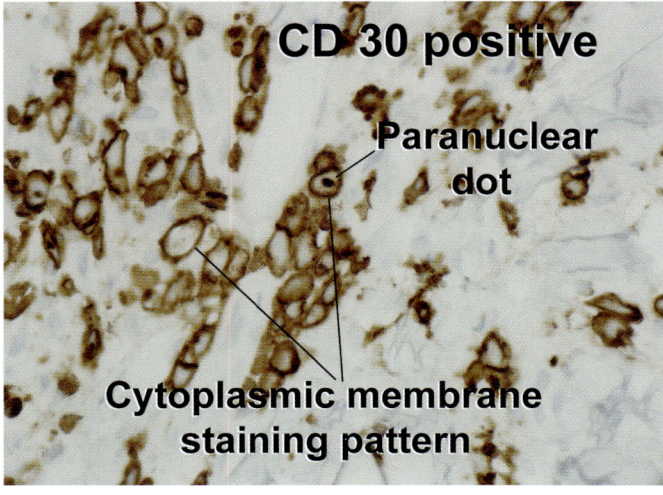

Fig 24-20 Lymphomatoid papulosis

Primary cutaneous anaplastic large cell lymphoma

Key features

- Sheets of large *Reed–Sternberg-like cells* in dermis ± subcutaneous fat
- Reactive small lymphocytes, histiocytes, and eosinophils in background
- CD30 expression by >75% of large cells in infiltrate

Primary cutaneous anaplastic large cell lymphoma (ALCL) most often presents with solitary or localized tumors or nodules. Spontaneous regression occasionally occurs. Extracutaneous dissemination is uncommon. The prognosis is generally favorable with 5-year survival rates of ≥90%.

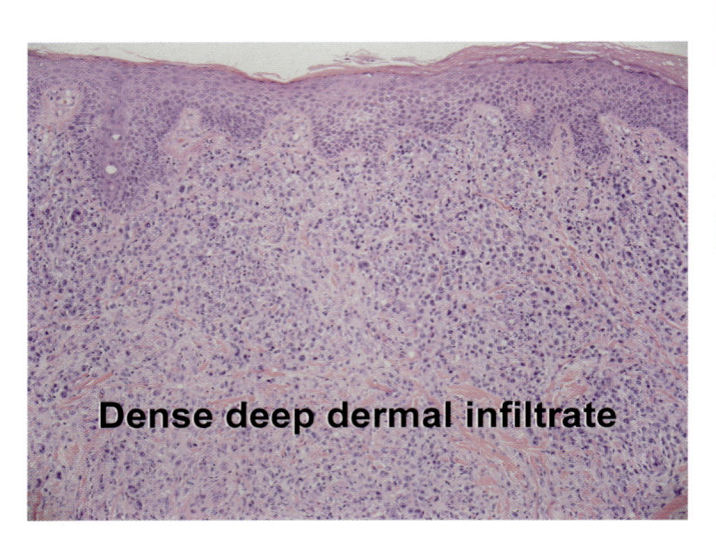

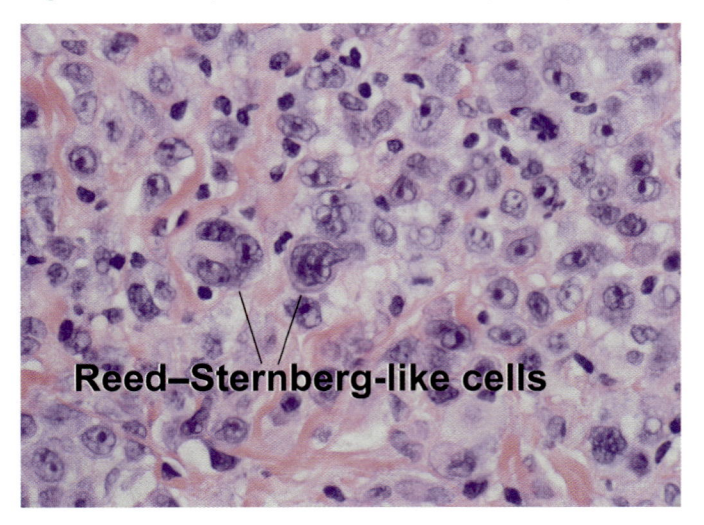

PEARL

ALCL may also originate in lymph nodes and spread secondarily to the skin. By routine microscopy, primary cutaneous ALCL is virtually indistinguishable from nodal ALCL. The distinction is important since nodal ALCL has a much worse prognosis. Immunohistochemistry can provide useful clues in this situation. Nodal ALCL has a chromosomal translocation t(2;5), which results in expression of anaplastic lymphoma-related tyrosine kinase (ALK-1). ALK-1 expression can be demonstrated by immunohistochemistry in most cases of nodal ALCL, but ALK-1 is generally absent in primary cutaneous ALCL. Nevertheless, staging is mandatory in all cases and is ultimately more important than immunohistochemistry in distinguishing primary cutaneous ALCL from its nodal counterpart.

Fig 24-21 Primary cutaneous anaplastic large cell lymphoma

Fig 24-22 Primary cutaneous anaplastic large cell lymphoma

Subcutaneous panniculitis-like T-cell lymphoma

Key features

- Lace-like pattern of infiltration in the fat
- Lymphoid cells rimming the individual adipocytes
- No significant involvement of the dermis or epidermis
- Variable cytologic atypia, minimal to marked
- Cytophagocytosis: *Beanbag cells* – macrophages filled with karyorrhectic debris
- CD8+, alpha/beta T-cell receptor (BF1)+, gamma/delta T-cell receptor–
- Cytotoxic phenotype: granzyme B+ TIA-1+ perforin+

Patients with subcutaneous panniculitis-like T-cell lymphoma (SPTCL) typically present with deep indurated nodules and plaques. The legs are a common site of involvement. Survival rates are approximately 80% at 5 years. SPTCL is sometimes associated with a potentially fatal *hemophagocytic syndrome*, consisting of pancytopenia, hepatosplenomegaly, and fever. In hemophagocytic syndrome, blood cells are engulfed by macrophages in the bone marrow and lymphoid organs.

Differential Diagnosis

Lupus panniculitis may be very difficult to distinguish from early SPTCL. Interface vacuolization, dermal mucin, and hyaline necrosis are all typical of lupus panniculitis but may sometimes be seen in SPTCL. Clonal rearrangement of T-cell receptor genes generally supports the diagnosis of SPTCL.

Cutaneous T-cell lymphoma, NK-cell lymphoma, and myeloid leukemia

Extranodal NK/T-cell lymphoma, nasal type

Key features

- Dense lymphoid infiltrates in dermis, subcutaneous fat, ± epidermis
- Angiocentricity, angiodestruction, and zonal necrosis
- CD2+ CD3epsilon+, usually CD56+ (NK-cell marker)
- CD3 expression variable
- Cytotoxic phenotype: granzyme B+ TIA-1+ perforin+
- *Epstein–Barr virus* detected within lymphoma cells by *in situ* hybridization

Extranodal NK/T-cell lymphoma, nasal type (ENKTCL) develops within the nasal cavity or skin. It is most commonly seen in Asia and Latin America. The nasal cavity and palate can be infiltrated and destroyed by the lymphoma. Cases previously described as *lethal midline granuloma* included some examples of ENKTCL. This lymphoma is associated with a very aggressive clinical course. Hemophagocytic syndrome occurs in a subset of

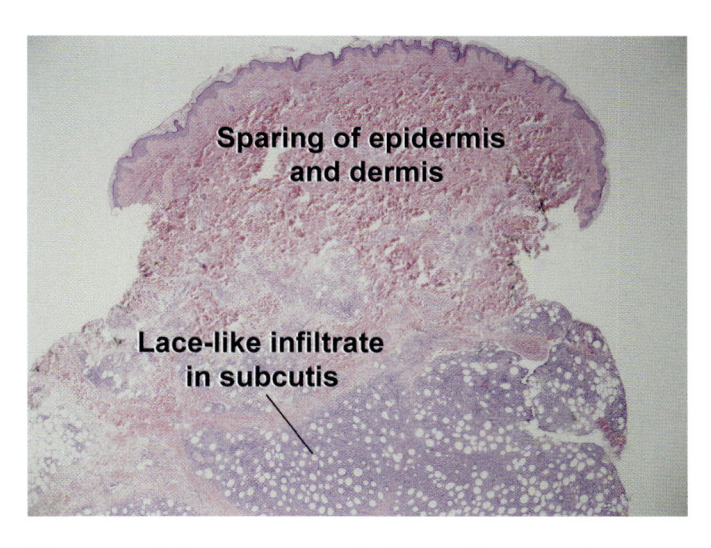

Fig 24-23 Subcutaneous panniculitis-like T-cell lymphoma

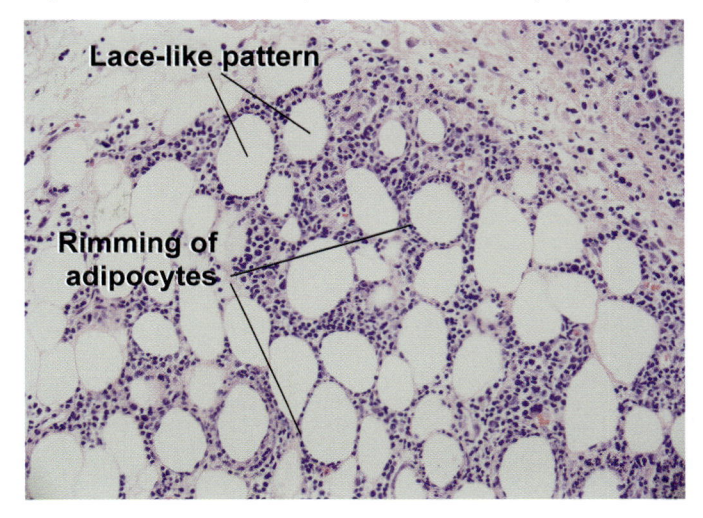

Fig 24-24 Subcutaneous panniculitis-like T-cell lymphoma

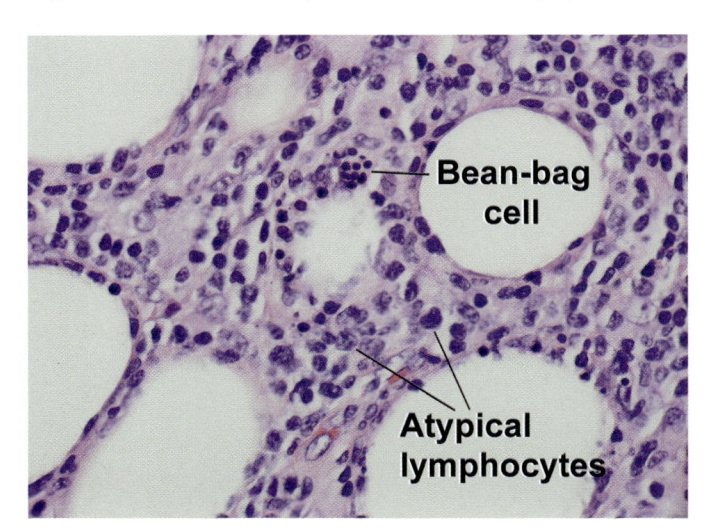

Fig 24-25 Subcutaneous panniculitis-like T-cell lymphoma

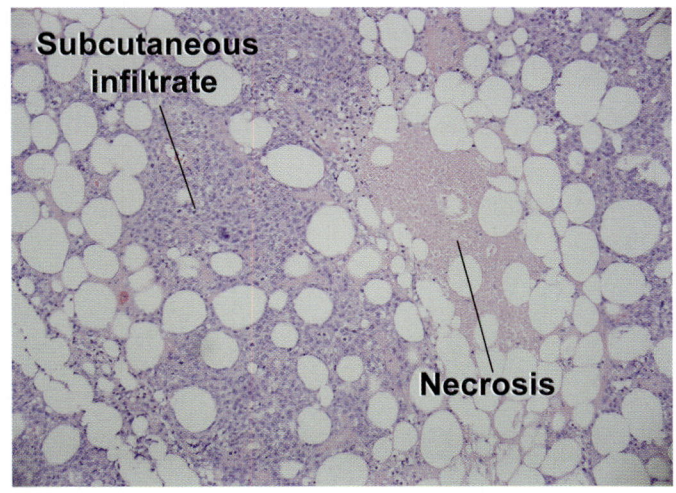

Fig 24-26 Extranodal NK/T-cell lymphoma, nasal type

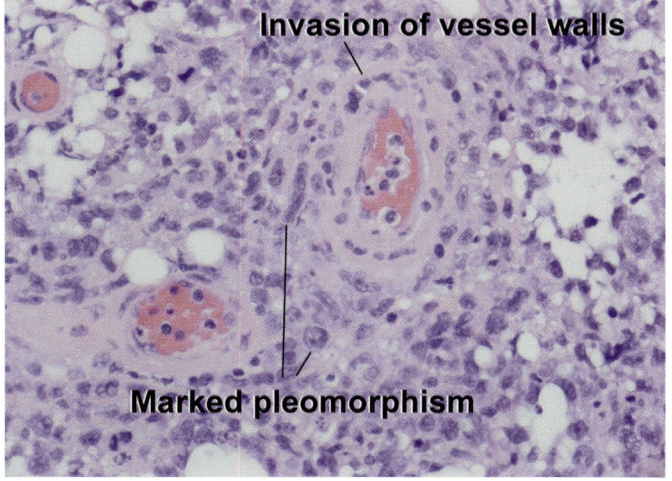

Fig 24-27 Extranodal NK/T-cell lymphoma, nasal type

patients. In most cases, no clonal rearrangement of the T-cell receptor can be demonstrated. The oncogenic role of *Epstein–Barr virus* is an important feature of this lymphoma.

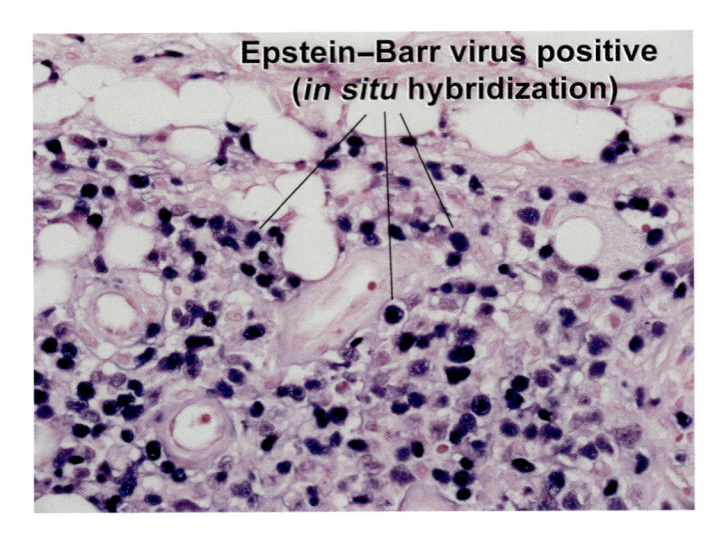

Fig 24-28 Extranodal NK/T-cell lymphoma, nasal type

Primary cutaneous peripheral T-cell lymphoma

Peripheral T-cell lymphoma is a heterogeneous category of lymphomas. Several distinctive, rare cutaneous variants are recognized:

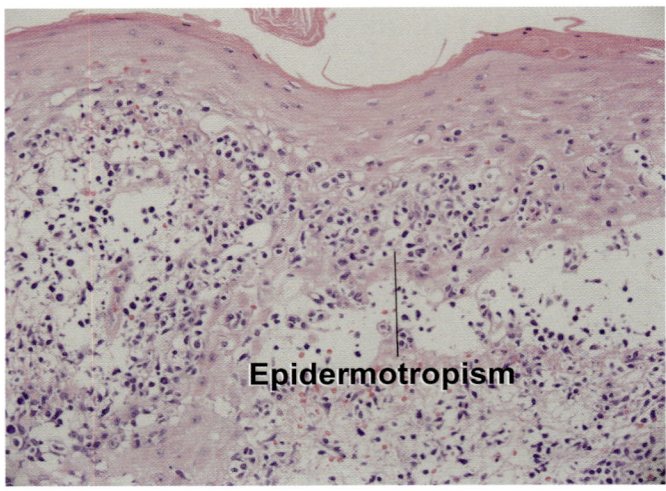

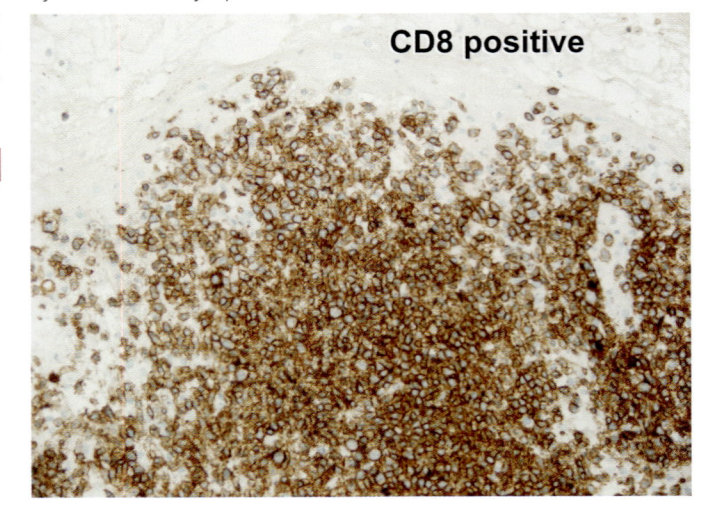

Primary cutaneous aggressive epidermotropic CD8+ cytotoxic T-cell lymphoma (provisional entity)

Key features
- Band-like, lichenoid lymphoid infiltrate with marked epidermotropism
- Beta F1+ CD3+ CD8+
- Cytotoxic phenotype: granzyme B+ TIA-1+ perforin+

Primary cutaneous aggressive epidermotropic CD8+ T-cell lymphoma presents with patches, papules, nodules, or tumors. Ulceration and hemorrhage are frequent. As the name implies, the clinical course is rapidly progressive.

Differential Diagnosis

Distinguished from the rare CD8+ variant of mycosis fungoides, Pagetoid reticulosis, and type D LyP by the clinical features (especially the aggressive clinical course).

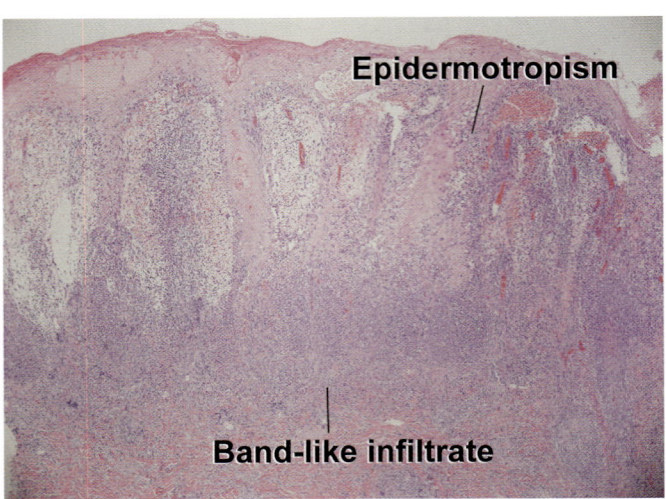

Fig 24-29 Primary cutaneous aggressive epidermotropic CD8+ cytotoxic T-cell lymphoma

Fig 24-30 Primary cutaneous aggressive epidermotropic CD8+ cytotoxic T-cell lymphoma

Fig 24-31 Primary cutaneous aggressive epidermotropic CD8+ cytotoxic T-cell lymphoma

Cutaneous gamma–delta T-cell lymphoma

Key features

- Location of infiltrate: subcutaneous, dermal, epidermal
- TCR gamma–delta+ Beta F1– CD3+ CD56+ CD4–
- Cytotoxic phenotype: granzyme B+ TIA-1+ perforin+
- Clonal rearrangement of T-cell receptor genes

Patients with cutaneous gamma/delta T-cell lymphoma develop plaques, ulcerated nodules, and tumors, most frequently involving the extremities. This lymphoma is sometimes associated with hemophagocytic syndrome. The clinical course is usually rapidly progressive.

PEARL

Subcutaneous cases of gamma–delta T-cell lymphoma may be histologically similar to subcutaneous panniculitis-like T-cell lymphoma, but the gamma–delta lymphomas have a much worse prognosis. Distinguishing the two entities is important. In contrast to SPTCL, gamma–delta lymphomas often extend into the dermis and sometimes into the epidermis. By immunohistochemistry, SPTCL is Beta F1 positive and TCR gamma–delta negative. Gamma–delta lymphoma is Beta F1 negative and TCR gamma–delta positive.

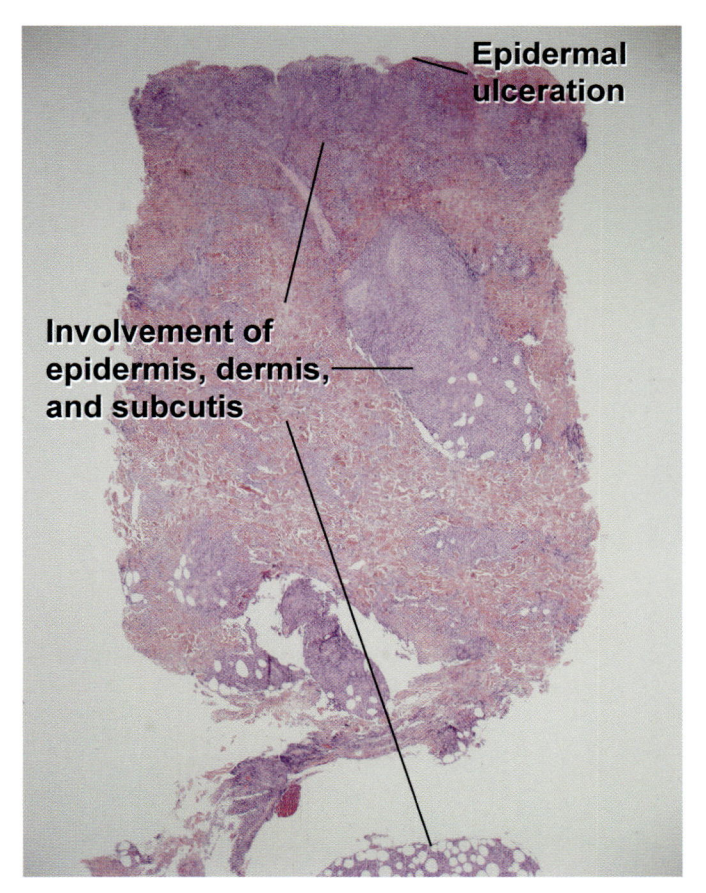

Fig 24-32 Primary cutaneous gamma–delta T-cell lymphoma

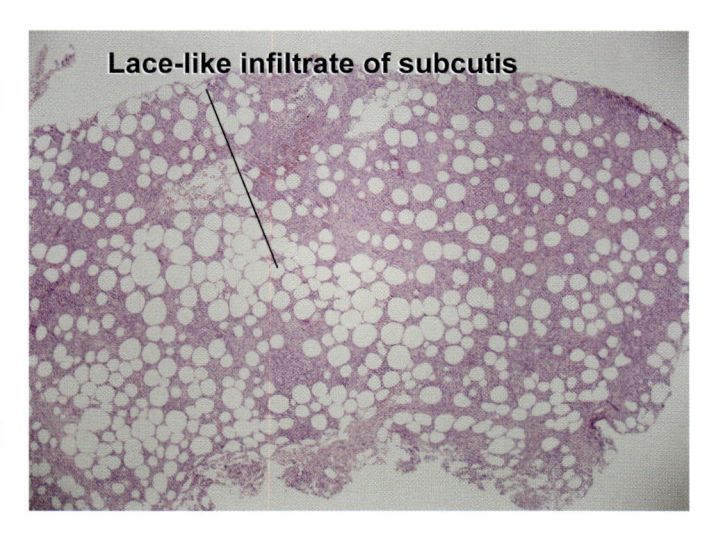

Fig 24-33 Primary cutaneous gamma–delta T-cell lymphoma

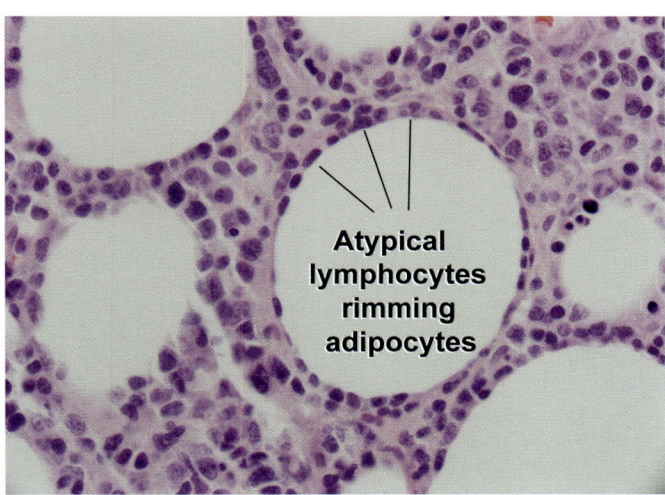

Fig 24-34 Primary cutaneous gamma–delta T-cell lymphoma

Primary cutaneous CD4+ small/medium T-cell lymphoma (provisional entity)

Key features

- Dermal infiltrate ± involvement of subcutaneous fat and epidermis
- CD3+ CD4+ CD8– CD30–
- Aberrant immunophenotype with loss of some T-cell markers
- Clonal rearrangement of T-cell receptor genes

Primary cutaneous CD4+ small/medium T-cell lymphoma is a provisional entity in the 2008 WHO classification. The lymphoma is remarkable for its localized distribution and relatively good prognosis. Patients usually present with a solitary plaque, nodule, or tumor. Diagnosis requires clinical correlation to exclude mycosis fungoides. In contrast to mycosis fungoides, no preceding patches are noted by history. By histology, epidermotropism is less conspicuous than that seen in early mycosis fungoides.

Some reports suggest that this provisional category may represent a heterogeneous group of lymphomas. A recently described entity termed *primary cutaneous follicular helper T-cell lymphoma* may partially overlap with primary cutaneous CD4+ small/medium T-cell lymphoma. Follicular helper T cells commonly express CD10, BCL-6, and CXCL-13. Expression of these markers has been variable in reported cases of primary cutaneous CD4+ small/medium T-cell lymphoma.

- Hypersensitivity to mosquito bites
- Angiocentric infiltrates of small or medium-sized lymphocytes
- Epstein–Barr virus detected within tumor cells by *in situ* hybridization
- TIA-1+, CD2+, CD8 variable, CD56 variable

Hydroa vacciniforme-like lymphoma is an Epstein–Barr virus-associated lymphoproliferative disease of childhood. Early in the course, the clinical presentation mimics hydroa vacciniforme, although the disease activity is often independent of sun exposure. Disordered immune regulation confers severe sensitivity to mosquito bites. Over a period of years, the lymphoma progresses to systemic involvement. Systemic associations include fever, lymphadenopathy, and organomegaly. When systemic involvement occurs, the clinical course is aggressive.

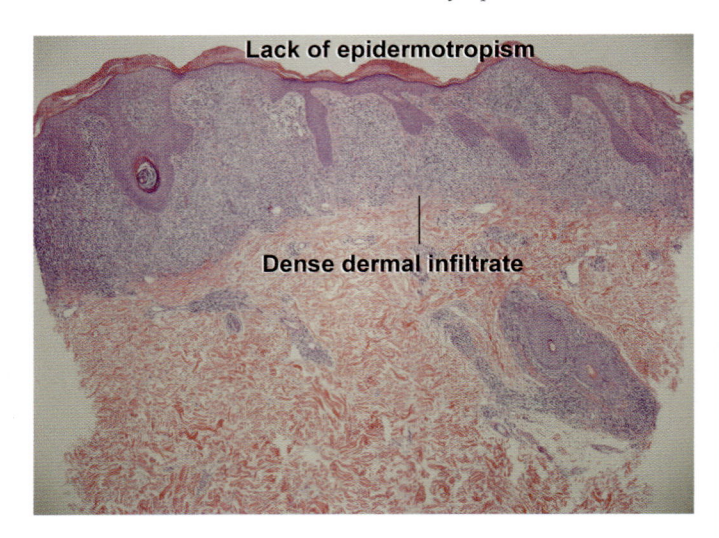

Fig 24-35 Primary cutaneous CD4+ small/medium T-cell lymphoma

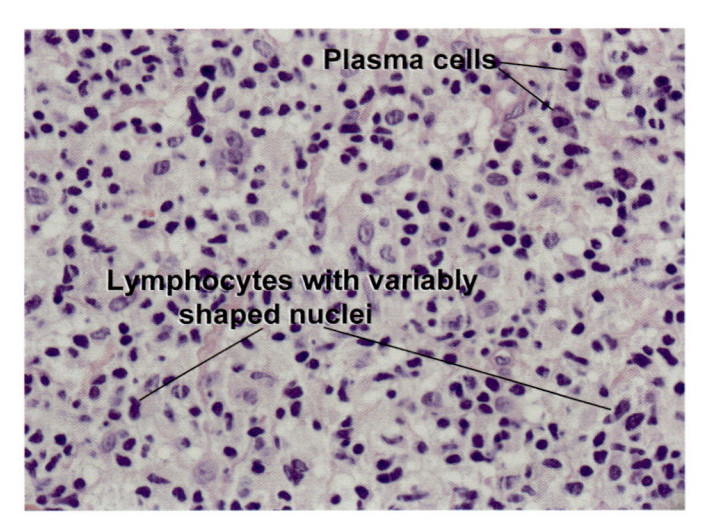

Fig 24-36 Primary cutaneous CD4+ small/medium T-cell lymphoma

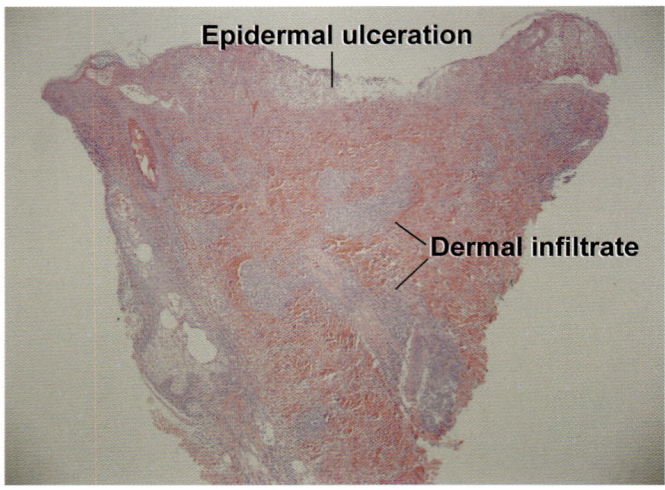

Fig 24-37 Hydroa vacciniforme-like lymphoma

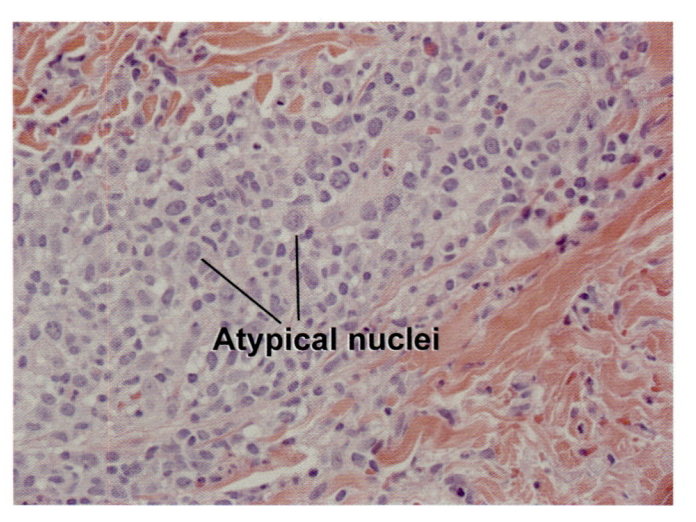

Fig 24-38 Hydroa vacciniforme-like lymphoma

Hydroa vacciniforme-like lymphoma

Key features

- Asian, Mexican, Central and South American children
- Ulcerative papulovesicles with scarring
- Face and extremities

Cutaneous T-cell lymphoma, NK-cell lymphoma, and myeloid leukemia

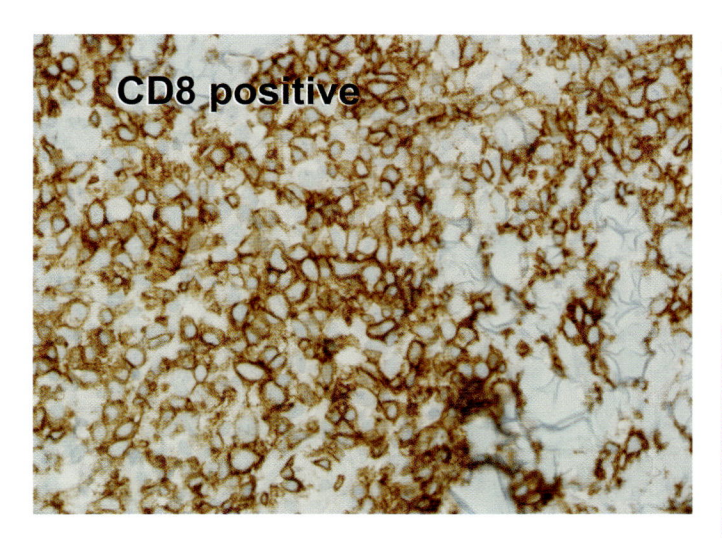

Fig 24-39 Hydroa vacciniforme-like lymphoma

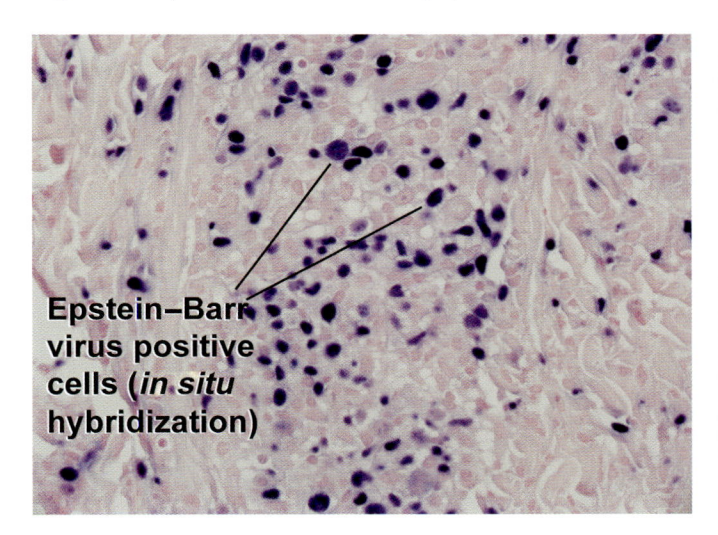

Fig 24-40 Hydroa vacciniforme-like lymphoma

Precursor hematologic neoplasm

Blastic plasmacytoid dendritic cell neoplasm

Key features

- Monomorphous or polymorphous infiltrate in the dermis and subcutis
- No epidermotropism
- No angioinvasion or necrosis
- CD4+ CD56+ CD123+ CD3– myeloperoxidase–
- Cytotoxic markers negative
- No clonal rearrangement of the T-cell receptor genes
- Negative *in situ* hybridization for Epstein–Barr virus

Previous names for this entity include CD4+/CD56+ hematodermic neoplasm and blastic NK-cell lymphoma. The cell of origin is a precursor of CD123-positive plasmacytoid dendritic cells. Patients present with solitary or multiple nodules or tumors. Tumor cells rapidly disseminate to the lymph nodes, bone marrow, and blood. The prognosis is poor. T-cell markers are negative, and there is no clonal rearrangement of the T-cell receptor genes. In the 2008 WHO classification, this tumor is classified as a precursor neoplasm related to acute myeloid leukemia (AML). An association with AML occurs in about 10–20% of patients.

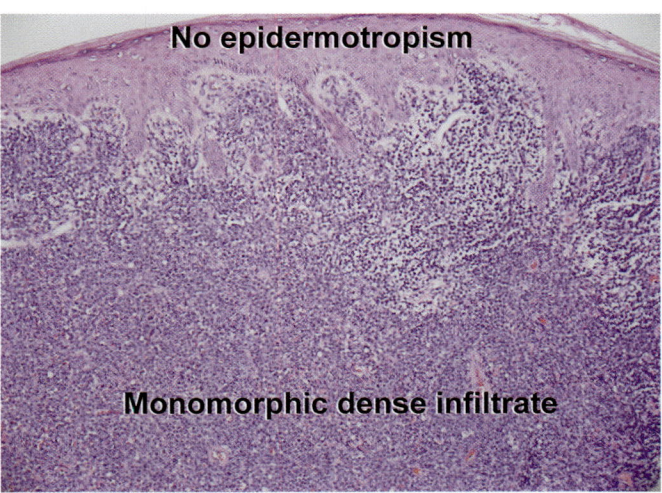

Fig 24-41 Blastic plasmacytoid dendritic cell neoplasm

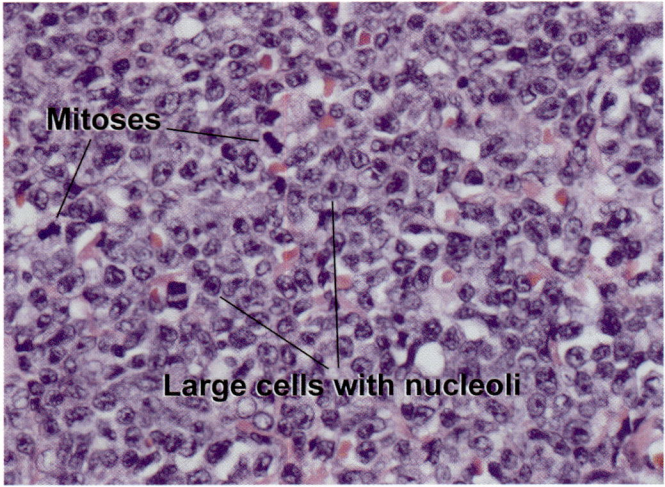

Fig 24-42 Blastic plasmacytoid dendritic cell neoplasm

Myeloid leukemia

Key features

- Diffuse interstitial, perivascular, and periadnexal infiltrate in dermis and subcutis
- No epidermotropism
- Grenz zone separates the infiltrate from the epidermis
- Single filing of cells splaying dermal collagen
- Mononuclear cells (blasts) ranging from large to small
- Prominent nucleoli (variable)
- Eosinophilic cytoplasm (variable)
- Scattered bilobed cells resembling neutrophilic "bands" sometimes present
- CD3– CD20– CD43+
- Lysozyme+ myeloperoxidase+ chloroacetate esterase+

Cutaneous infiltrates of leukemic cells occur commonly in acute myeloid leukemia and rarely in chronic myelogenous leukemia. Direct involvement of the skin is particularly common in M5 (acute monocytic) and M4 (acute myelomonocytic) leukemia. Infiltration of the gingivae is also common in these two subtypes. Patients present with papules, nodules, plaques, purpura, or ulcers. Unusual presentations include a generalized maculopapular eruption clinically resembling an allergic drug eruption or viral exanthem. In skin biopsy specimens, acute myeloid leukemia and chronic myelogenous leukemia may have similar morphologic features. Some types of acute leukemia are associated with specific chromosomal translocations, such as t(15;17) in promyelocytic leukemia (M3).

PEARL

Myeloid leukemia may be indistinguishable from lymphoma in H&E sections. CD43 is commonly used as a T-cell marker but is also expressed in myeloid cells. Myeloid leukemia should be considered when a CD43-positive infiltrate does not express the T-cell marker CD3 or the B-cell marker CD20. Lysozyme, myeloperoxidase, and chloroacetate esterase (Leder stain) may then be performed to confirm myeloid lineage.

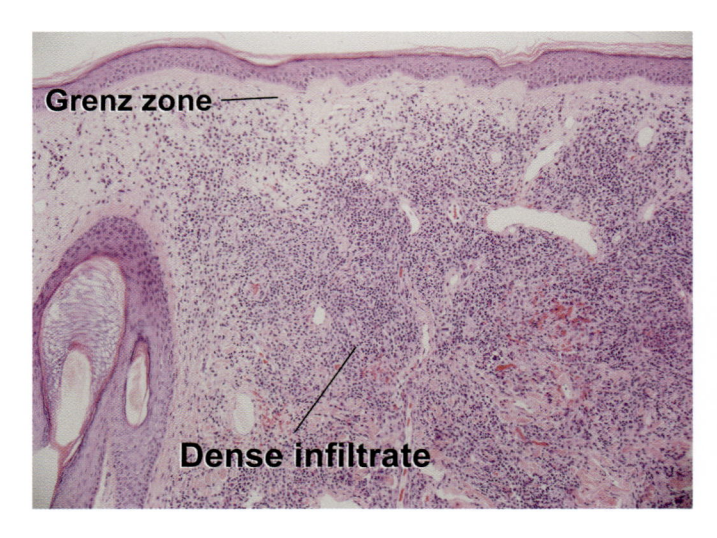

Fig 24-43 Acute myeloid leukemia

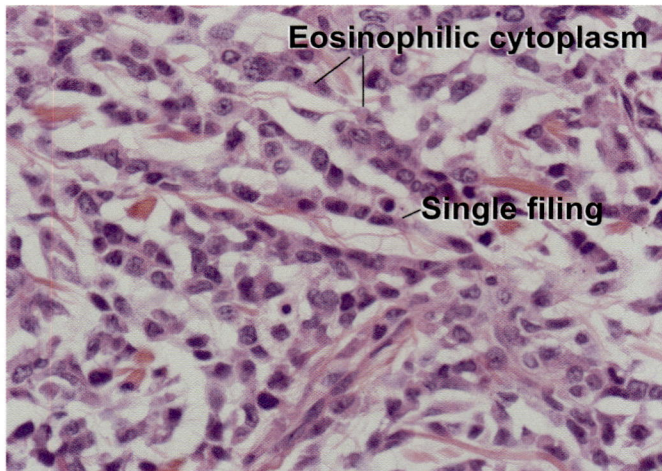

Fig 24-45 Acute myeloid leukemia

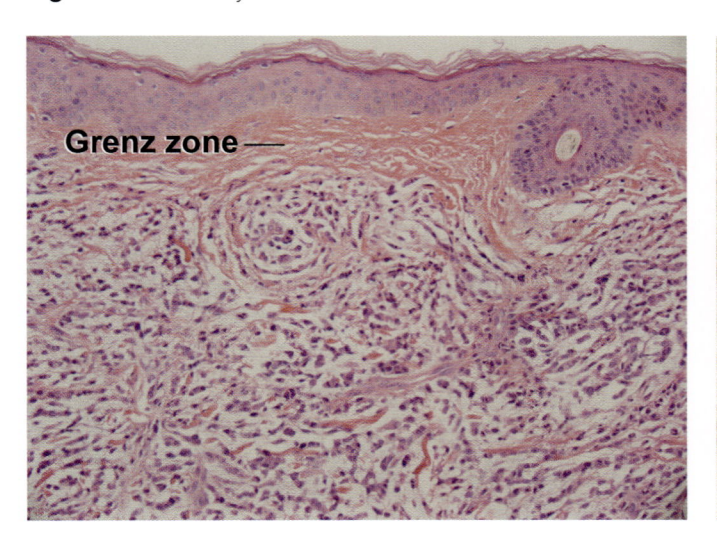

Fig 24-44 Acute myeloid leukemia

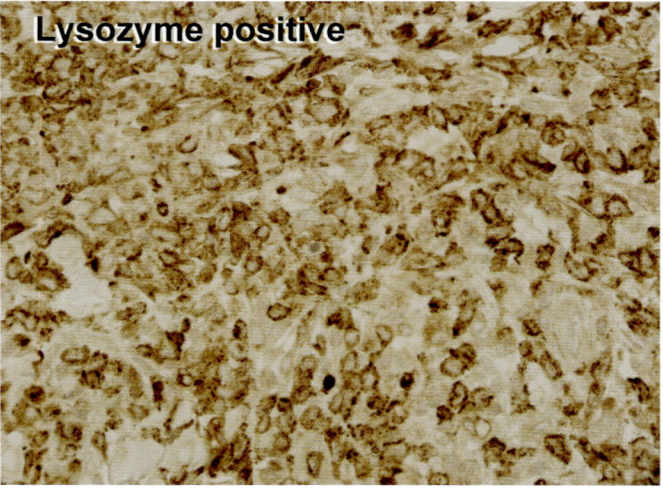

Fig 24-46 Acute myeloid leukemia

Further Reading

Battistella M, Beylot-Barry M, Bachelez H, et al. Primary cutaneous follicular helper T-cell lymphoma. Arch Dermatol 2012;148:832–839.

Beltraminelli H, Leinweber B, Kerl H, et al. Primary cutaneous CD4+ small-/medium-sized pleomorphic T-cell lymphoma: a cutaneous nodular proliferation of pleomorphic T lymphocytes of undetermined significance? A study of 136 cases. Am J Dermatopathol 2009;31:317–322.

Bittencourt AL, Barbosa HS, Vieira MD, et al. Adult T-cell leukemia/lymphoma (ATL) presenting in the skin: clinical, histological and immunohistochemical features of 52 cases. Acta Oncol 2009;48:598–604.

Campbell JJ, Clark RA, Watanabe R, et al. Sezary syndrome and mycosis fungoides arise from distinct T-cell subsets: a biologic rationale for their distinct clinical behaviors. Blood 2010;116:767–771.

Cota C, Vale E, Viana I, et al. Cutaneous manifestations of blastic plasmacytoid dendritic cell neoplasm – morphologic and phenotypic variability in a series of 33 patients. Am J Surg Pathol 2010;34:75–87.

El Shabrawi-Caelen L, Kerl H, Cerroni L. Lymphomatoid papulosis: reappraisal of clinicopathologic presentation and classification into subtypes A, B, and C. Arch Dermatol 2004;140:441–447.

Fernandez-Flores A. Comments on cutaneous lymphomas: since the WHO-2008 classification to present. Am J Dermatopathol 2012;34:274–284.

Gerami P, Guitart J. The spectrum of histopathologic and immunohistochemical findings in folliculotropic mycosis fungoides. Am J Surg Pathol 2007;31:1430–1438.

Kaddu S, Zenahlik P, Beham-Schmid C, et al. Specific cutaneous infiltrates in patients with myelogenous leukemia: a clinicopathologic study of 26 patients with assessment of diagnostic criteria. J Am Acad Dermatol 1999;40:966–978.

Kempf W, Kazakov DV, Schärer L, et al. Angioinvasive lymphomatoid papulosis: a new variant simulating aggressive lymphomas. Am J Surg Pathol 2013;37:1–13.

Kempf W, Ostheeren-Michaelis S, Paulli M, et al. Granulomatous mycosis fungoides and granulomatous slack skin. Arch Dermatol 2008;144:1609–1617.

Kempf W, Sander CA. Classification of cutaneous lymphomas – an update. Histopathology 2010;56:57–70.

Lee J, Viakhireva N, Cesca C, et al. Clinicopathologic features and treatment outcomes in Woringer-Kolopp disease. J Am Acad Dermatol 2008;59:706–712.

Massone C, El-Shabrawi-Caelen L, Kerl H, et al. The morphologic spectrum of primary cutaneous anaplastic large T-cell lymphoma: a histopathologic study on 66 biopsy specimens from 47 patients with report of rare variants. J Cutan Pathol 2008;35:46–53.

Nofal A, Abdel-Mawla MY, Assaf M, et al. Primary cutaneous aggressive epidermotropic CD8+ T-cell lymphoma: proposed diagnostic criteria and therapeutic evaluation. J Am Acad Dermatol 2012;67:48–59.

Rodríguez-Pinilla SM, Barrionuevo C, Garcia J, et al. EBV-associated cutaneous NK/T-cell lymphoma: review of a series of 14 cases from Peru in children and young adults. Am J Surg Pathol 2010;34:1773–1782.

Saggini A, Gulia A, Argenyi Z, et al. A variant of lymphomatoid papulosis simulating primary cutaneous aggressive epidermotropic CD8+ cytotoxic T-cell lymphoma. Description of 9 cases. Am J Surg Pathol 2010;34:1168–1175.

Swerdlow SH, Campo E, Harris NL, et al., eds. WHO Classification of Tumours of Haematopoietic and Lymphoid Tissues, 4th edn. Lyon: IARC, 2008.

Willemze R, Jaffe ES, Burg G, et al. WHO-EORTC classification for cutaneous lymphomas. Blood 2005;105:3768–3785.

Willemze R, Jansen PM, Cerroni L, et al. Subcutaneous panniculitis-like T-cell lymphoma: definition, classification, and prognostic factors: an EORTC cutaneous lymphoma group study of 83 cases. Blood 2008;111:838–845.

Xu Z, Lian S. Epstein-Barr virus-associated hydroa vacciniforme-like cutaneous lymphoma in seven Chinese children. Pediatr Dermatol 2010;27:463–469.

Chapter 25

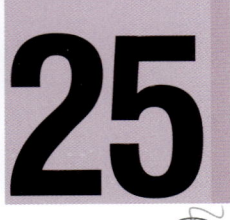

B-cell lymphoma and lymphocytic leukemia

Steven Peckham

A summary table on 'WHO Classification of B-cell Tumors of Hematopoietic and Lymphoid Tissues' and a lymphoma atlas can be found in the on-line content for this book.

Cutaneous B-cell lymphoproliferative disorders

The primary cutaneous B-cell lymphomas share some histologic features with their nodal counterparts, but in many cases represent distinct clinicopathologic entities with significant clinical, immunophenotypic, molecular, and prognostic differences from their extracutaneous counterparts. In general, primary cutaneous B-cell lymphomas have a better prognosis than their nodal-based counterparts, and treatment strategies for them may be different. The classification system used in this chapter reflects the 2005 World Health Organization/European Organisation for Research and Treatment of Cancer combined consensus conference classification for lymphoproliferative diseases of the skin. Note that not all entities included here are necessarily of primary cutaneous origin (e.g. chronic lymphocytic leukemia/small lymphocytic lymphoma, mantle cell lymphoma, Burkitt lymphoma, intravascular large B-cell lymphoma, lymphomatoid granulomatosis) but may frequently involve the skin.

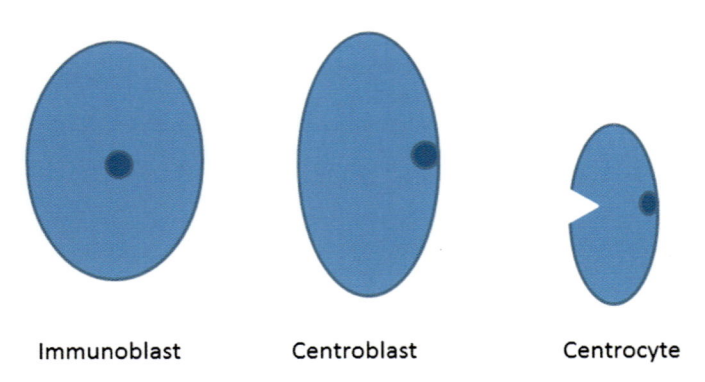

Fig 25-1 Nuclear features of an immunoblast, centroblast and centrocyte

Primary cutaneous marginal zone lymphoma

Key features

- Patchy, nodular, or diffuse infiltrate of lymphoid cells in the dermis and superficial panniculus
- Characteristic "inverse" pattern of central darker benign reactive lymphocytes with surrounding neoplastic cells with paler abundant cytoplasm (marginal zone cells)
- Lack of epidermotropism
- Small lymphocytes may surround or invade eccrine coils
- Surrounding benign reactive follicles may be colonized by neoplastic cells
- Neoplastic marginal zone cells often comprise only a minority of lymphoid cells in the lesions
- CD20+, CD79+, CD5–, CD10–, CD43–, BCL-6–, BCL-2+
- Clonal rearrangement of immunoglobulin (Ig) H gene in >70% of cases
- t(14;18)(q32;q21) present in a minority of cases
- Intracytoplasmic monoclonal immunoglobulin (kappa or lambda) restriction

Primary cutaneous marginal zone B-cell lymphoma is an indolent lymphoma of small lymphocytes of B-cell origin, including centrocyte (marginal zone)-like cells with small to medium-sized slightly irregular nuclei with inconspicuous nucleoli, admixed with plasmacytoid lymphocytes and occasional centroblast-like cells. Marginal zone lymphoma is one of the most common types of cutaneous B-cell lymphoma. The prognosis is excellent, with 5-year survival rates approaching 100%. The lesions usually present as violaceous nodules or plaques preferentially on the trunk and extremities, with upper extremities more commonly involved than lower extremities. The lesions have a nodular or diffuse architecture, often with a characteristic "inverse" pattern relative to benign reactive lymphoid follicles, i.e. they show a dense, darker-staining central nodular portion of benign reactive lymphocytes, which may contain germinal centers, surrounded by neoplastic lymphoid cells with slightly irregular nuclei and more abundant paler cytoplasm (monocytoid or marginal zone B cells). Often, the neoplastic lymphoid population only represents a minority of the cells in the lesion. The epidermis is spared, without epidermotropism of lymphocytes. Surrounding benign reactive germinal centers may be present, and are often colonized by tumor cells. In some cases, the neoplastic cells may surround and infiltrate eccrine coils, similar to the lymphoepithelial lesions seen in extranodal marginal zone lymphomas of the gastrointestinal tract (MALTomas). Primary cutaneous marginal zone B-cell lymphoma includes cases designated primary cutaneous immunocytoma in earlier classification systems. Primary cutaneous immunocytomas are often associated with *Borrelia* and demonstrate high numbers of monotypic (i.e. they demonstrate monoclonal intracytoplasmic immunoglobulin) plasma cells and lymphoplasmacytoid lymphocytes, some of which may contain intranuclear immunoglobulin deposits (Dutcher bodies).

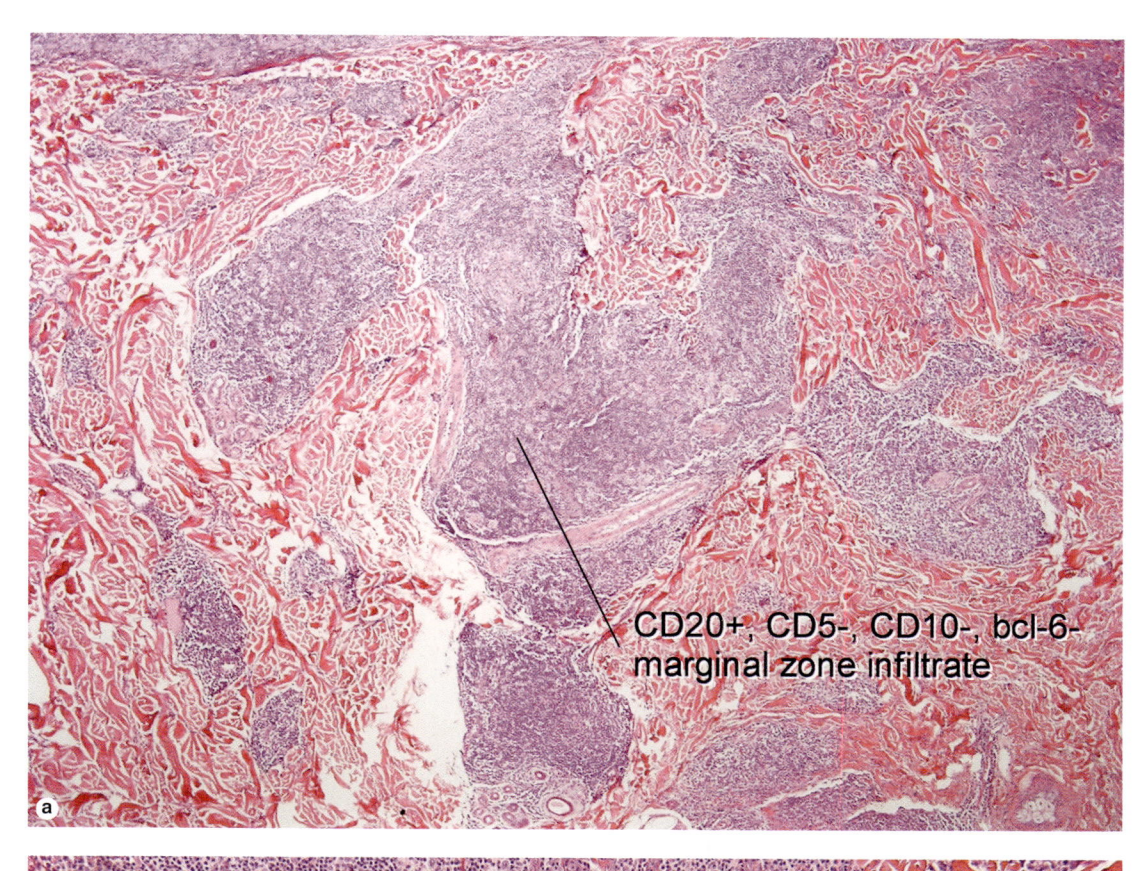

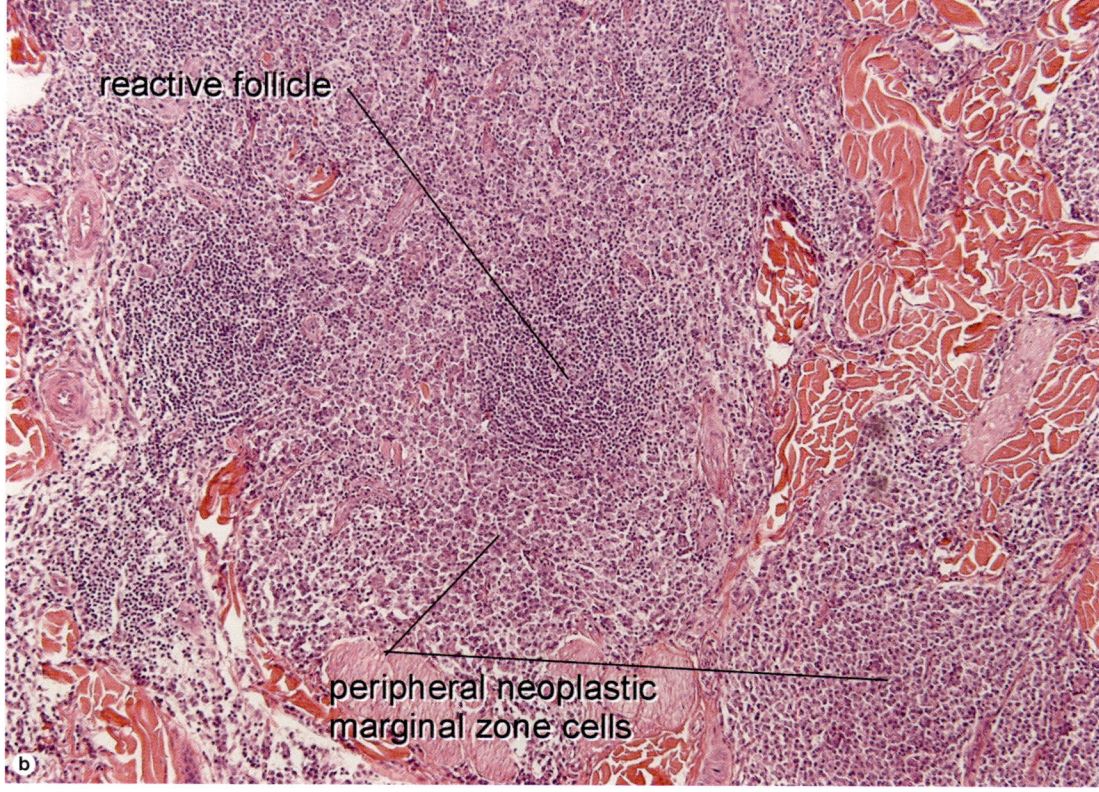

B-cell lymphoma and lymphocytic leukemia | Chapter 25 | 405

Fig 25-2 Primary cutaneous marginal zone lymphoma

Primary cutaneous follicle center cell lymphoma

Key features

- Diffuse, nodular and diffuse, or nodular lymphoid proliferation
- If mixed architecture, lesions tend to have neoplastic follicles at the periphery of a central diffuse neoplastic infiltrate
- Follicles have reduced or absent mantle zones
- Follicles have decreased to absent tingible body macrophages
- Lack of polarity of follicles (i.e. absent light and darker zones of polarity in follicle germinal centers)
- CD20+, CD79+
- CD10+ (follicular pattern, most cases) or CD10− (diffuse pattern, most cases)
- BCL-6+, BCL-2−, CD5−, CD43−
- Reduced proliferative fraction by MIB-1 compared to benign reactive germinal centers
- Monoclonal rearrangement of immunoglobulin heavy chain J gene
- t(14;18) translocation is very uncommon in primary cutaneous follicle center cell lymphoma lesions

Primary cutaneous follicle center cell lymphoma is also an indolent mature B-cell lymphoma, which exhibits a predilection for the head and trunk. In contrast to its nodal counterpart (primary nodal follicle center cell lymphoma), primary cutaneous follicle center cell lymphoma has a more favorable prognosis, with 5-year survival rates >90%. As with their nodal counterparts, these lesions may have a follicular, follicular and diffuse, or diffuse architecture, most commonly diffuse. However, it must be emphasized again that, despite similar appearances by hematoxylin and eosin, these lesions have different immunohistochemical, genetic, and prognostic features from primary nodal follicle center cell lymphomas. Histology shows a nodular or diffuse proliferation of centrocyte-like lymphocytes with small, slightly irregular nuclei, and variable numbers of larger centroblast-like cells with larger, rounded vesicular nuclei and one or a few prominent nucleoli. In nodular lesions, the follicles appear monomorphous, with a loss of the normal polarity of light and dark zones of the germinal centers, an attenuated mantle zone around germinal centers, and lack of tingible body macrophages in the germinal centers. In larger lesions, the center may show a diffuse architecture, with residual monomorphous neoplastic follicles at the periphery.

PEARL

In primary cutaneous follicle center cell lymphoma, the BCL-6-positive cells typically stray outside of the follicle. BCL-2 expression is characteristic of follicle center cell lymphoma in lymph nodes, but is rare in the primary cutaneous variety. At cutaneous sites, BCL-2 positivity in a follicle center cell lymphoma should raise suspicion for a nodal primary with secondary involvement of the skin.

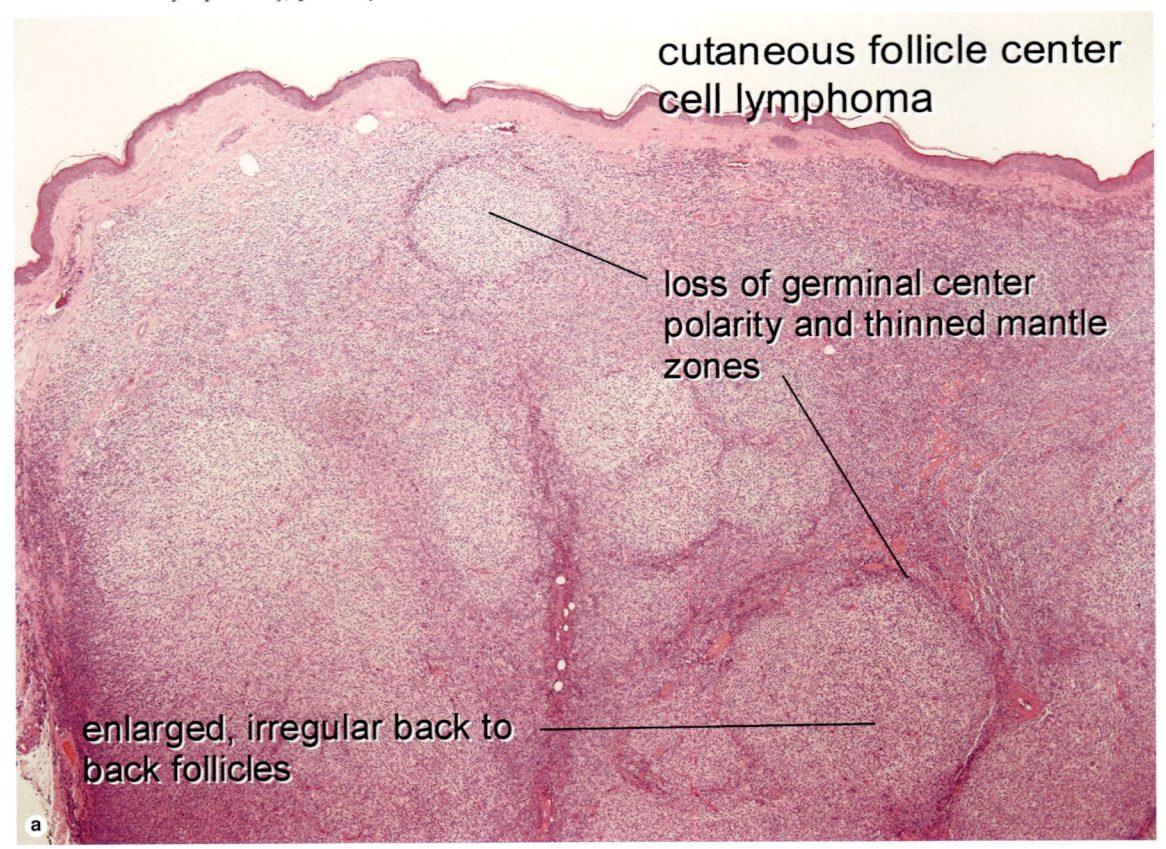

Fig 25-3 Primary cutaneous follicle center cell lymphoma

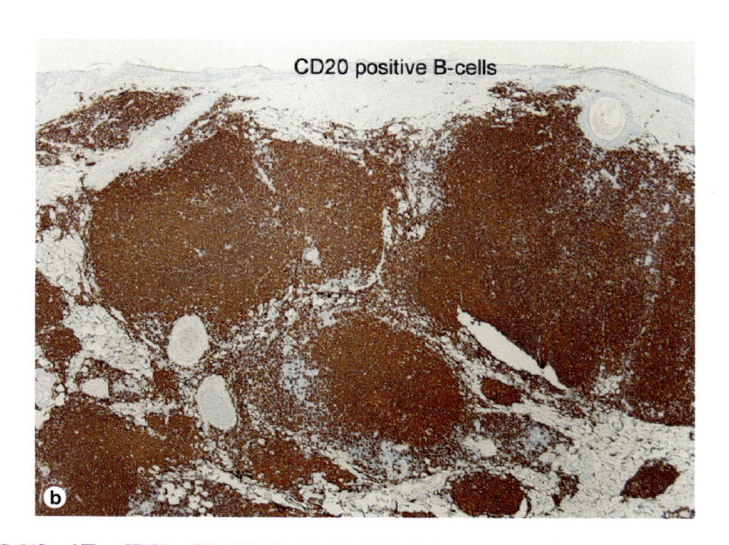

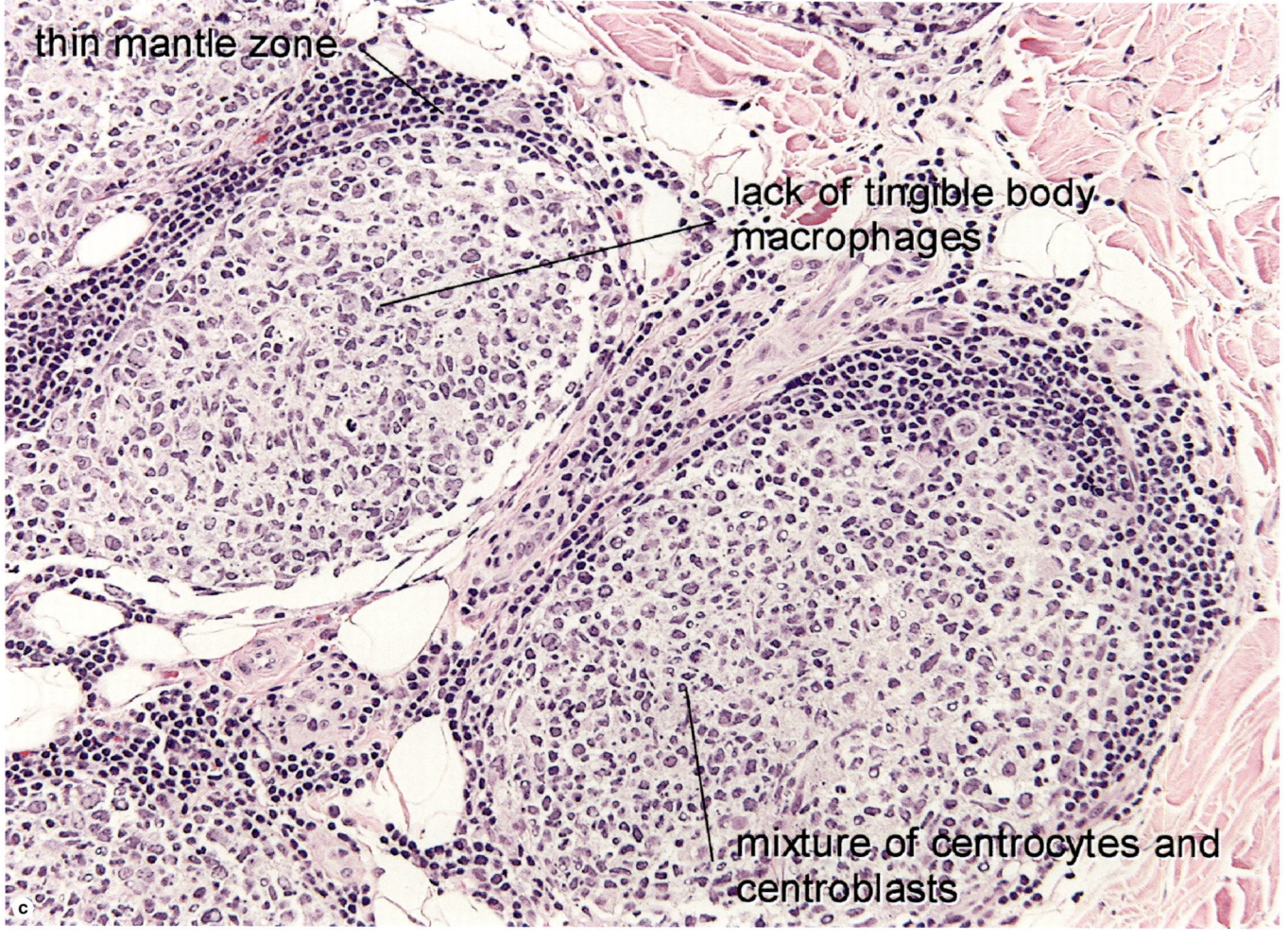

Fig 25-3, cont'd

Continued

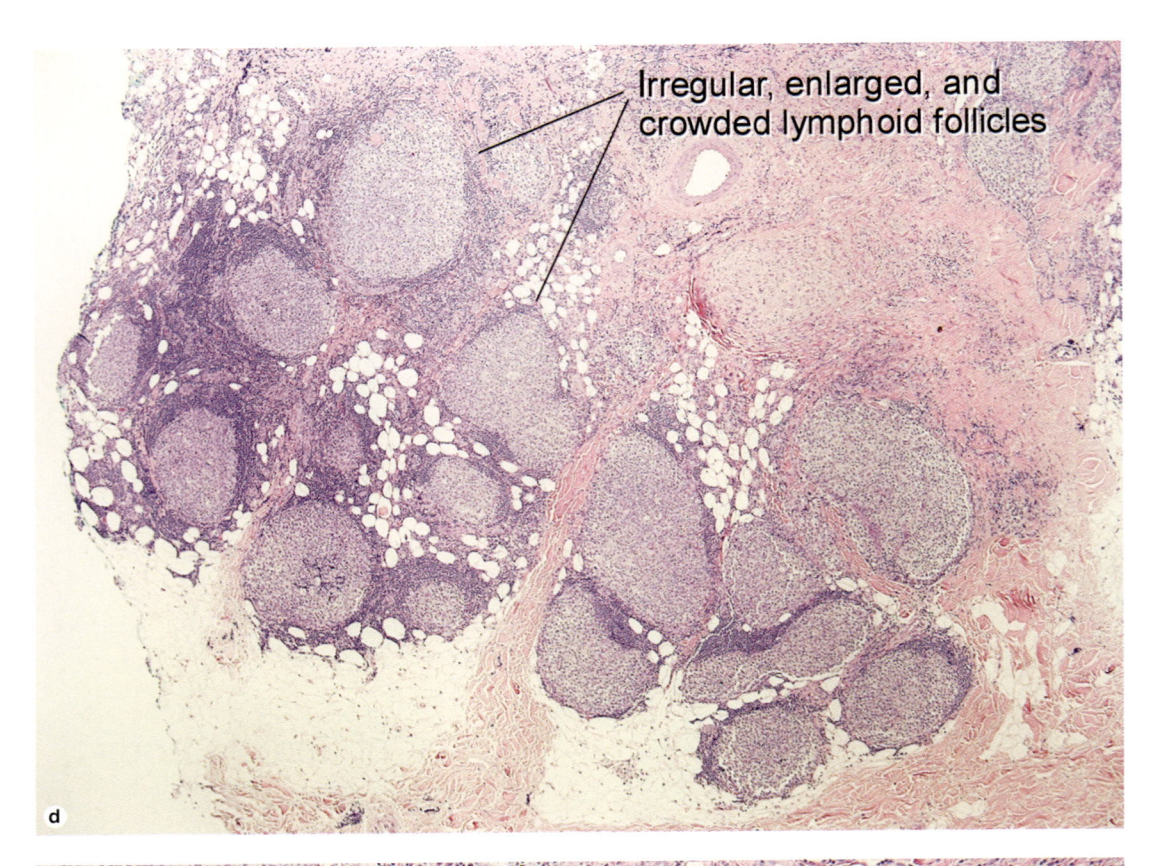

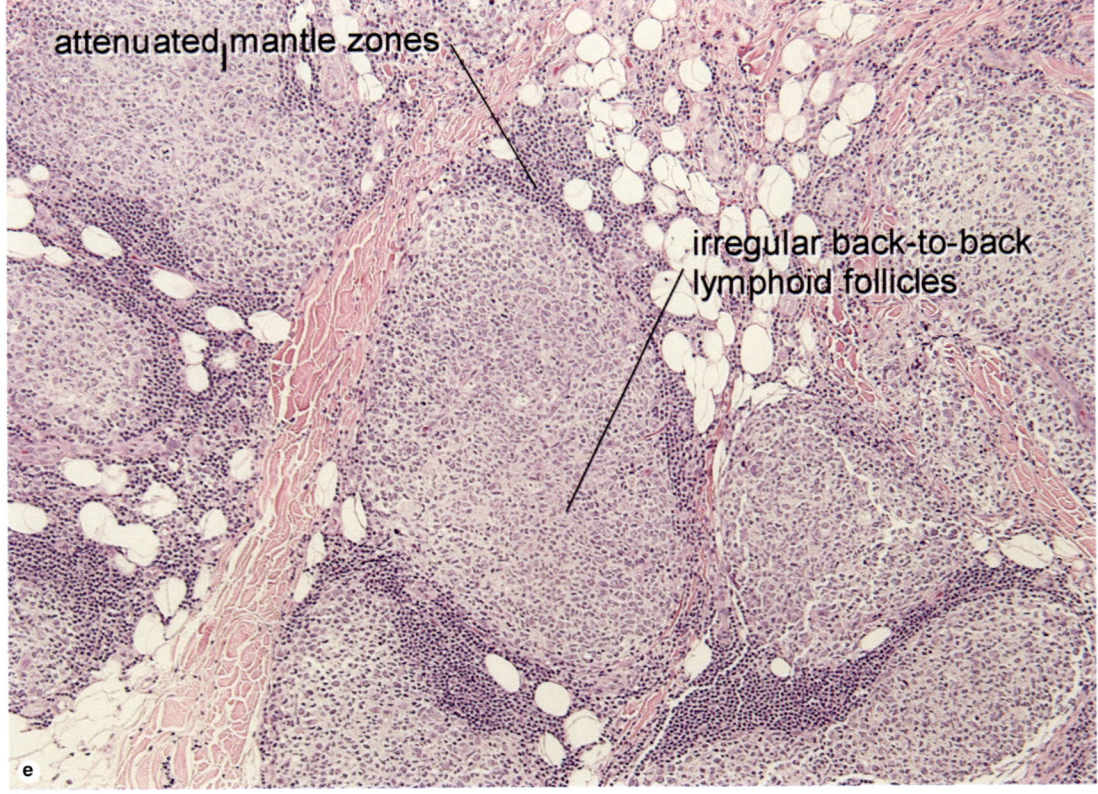

Fig 25-3, cont'd

Cutaneous diffuse large B-cell lymphoma, leg type

Key features

- Predominantly affects older patients (>70), with a predilection for females
- Usual location is one or more red to brown nodules on one distal extremity, although lesions can present as multiple nodules and at other sites
- 5-year survival of approximately 50%
- Histology reveals a dense diffuse infiltrate of predominantly large round immunoblast-type cells with prominent nucleoli; occasional large cleaved, multilobated, or anaplastic cells may also be seen
- Centrocytes are largely absent
- Grenz zone may be present, and adnexal structures are often destroyed
- Epidermotropism of neoplastic lymphoid cells may closely simulate the epidermotropism characteristic of T-cell lymphomas
- CD20+, CD79a+, BCL-2+ in great majority; most cases also express BCL-6 and/or CD10
- MUM-1/IRF4 strong positive staining is very important to distinguish from diffuse form of follicle center cell lymphoma (MUM-1−), which may look similar by routine hematoxylin and eosin staining
- Rare variant is positive for CD30 and must not be mistaken for anaplastic large cell lymphoma
- Monoclonal rearrangement of J heavy gene is present; no specific chromosomal alterations

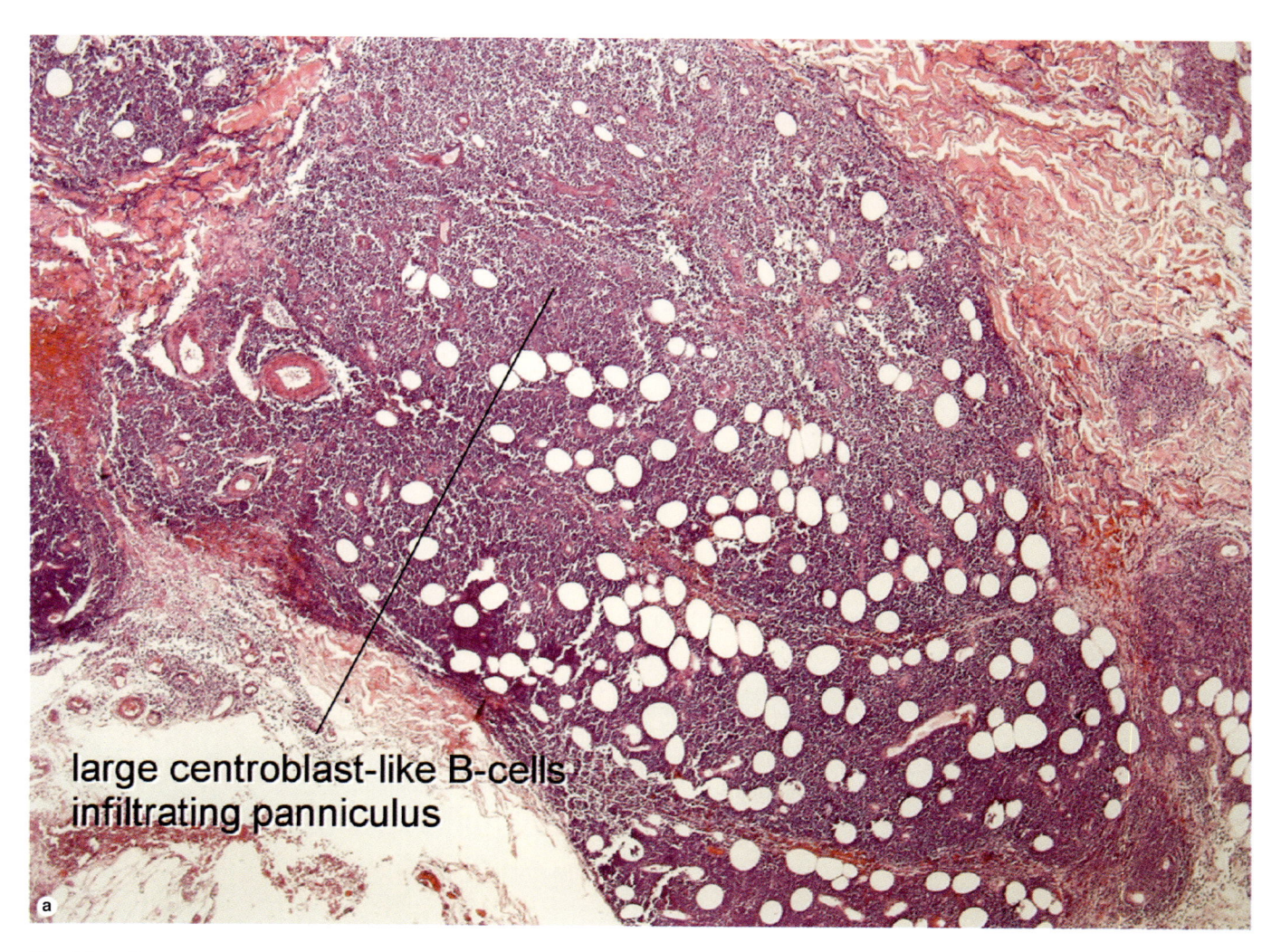

large centroblast-like B-cells infiltrating panniculus

Fig 25-4 Cutaneous diffuse large B-cell lymphoma, leg type

Continued

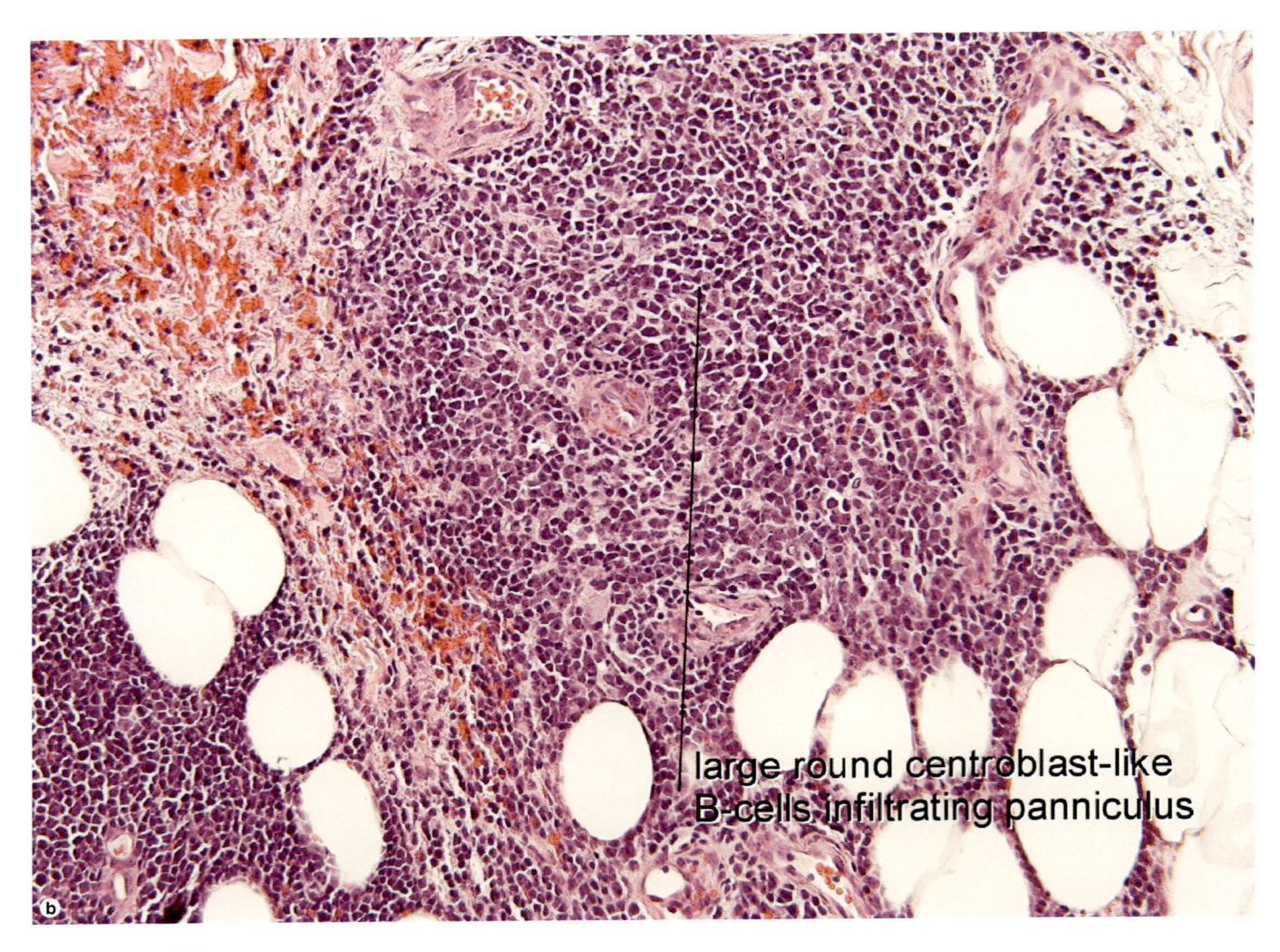

Fig 25-4, cont'd

Cutaneous diffuse large B-cell lymphoma, other than leg type

Key features

- Very rare
- May involve head, trunk, or extremities
- B-cell lymphoma showing a diffuse growth pattern composed of large transformed B cells, which lack the typical features of the previously described diffuse large B-cell lymphoma of leg type or the diffuse pattern of follicle center cell lymphoma
- Histology shows a monomorphous population of centroblast-like cells with a benign mixed background of lymphoid cells
- Usually BCL-6+, may be BCL-2–; otherwise express typical pan B-cell markers

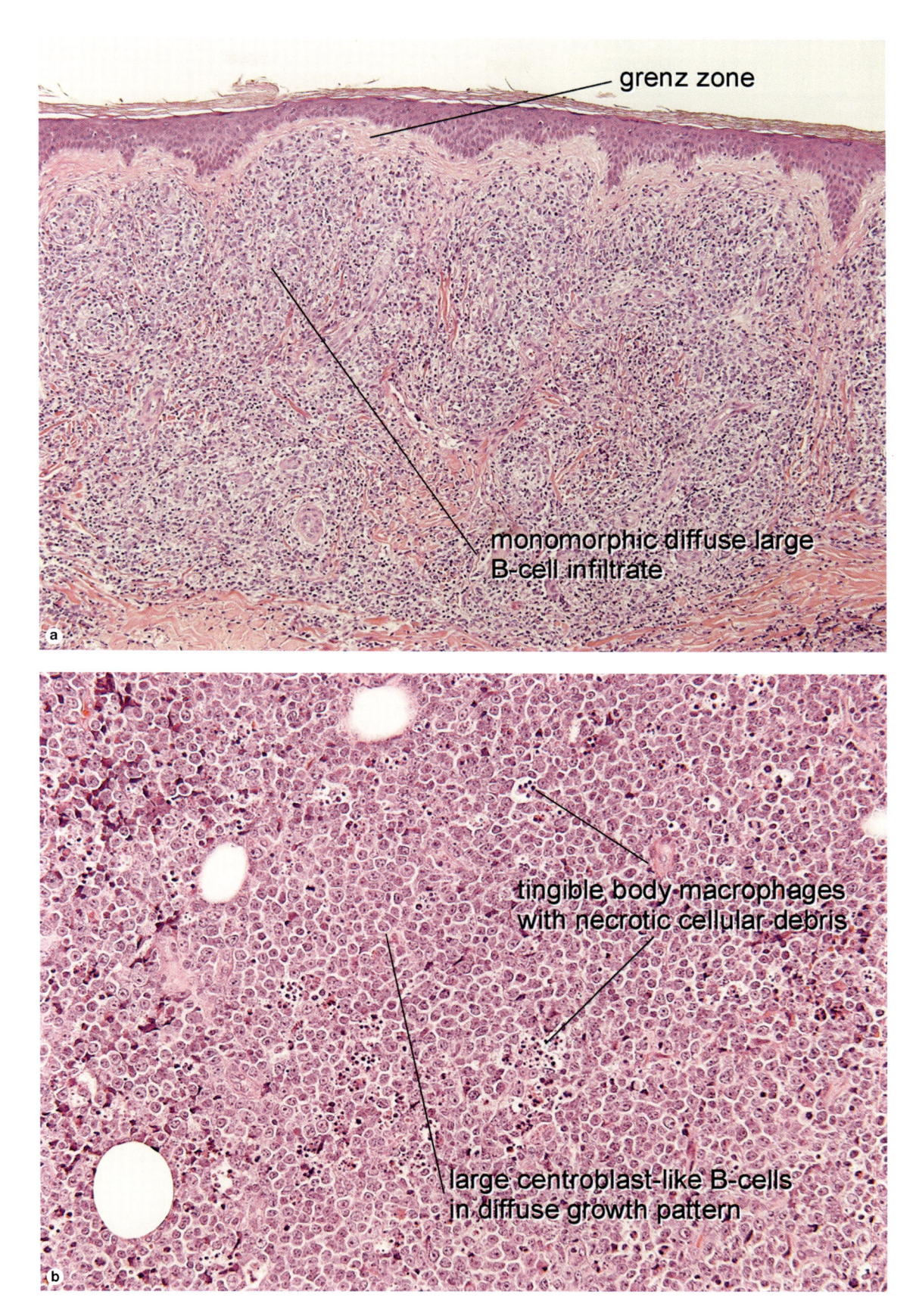

Fig 25-5 Cutaneous diffuse large B-cell lymphoma, other than leg type

Intravascular large B-cell lymphoma

Key features

- Highly malignant, rare neoplasm of large atypical B cells, which presents within the lumens of small vessels, particularly capillaries and venules
- May produce neurologic deficits through involvement of central nervous system
- Neoplastic cells are large with round or oval vesicular nuclei, prominent nucleoli, and frequent mitoses
- Tumor cells may appear to be attached to endothelium, giving a hobnail appearance
- Partial occlusion of vessels by tumor cells and fibrin causes a pattern of reticular erythema seen clinically
- Extravascular involvement may be present
- Must distinguish from reactive angioendotheliomatosis and intravascular lymphomas of other lineages
- Cells express CD20, CD79a, and may aberrantly coexpress CD5, CD10, CD11a

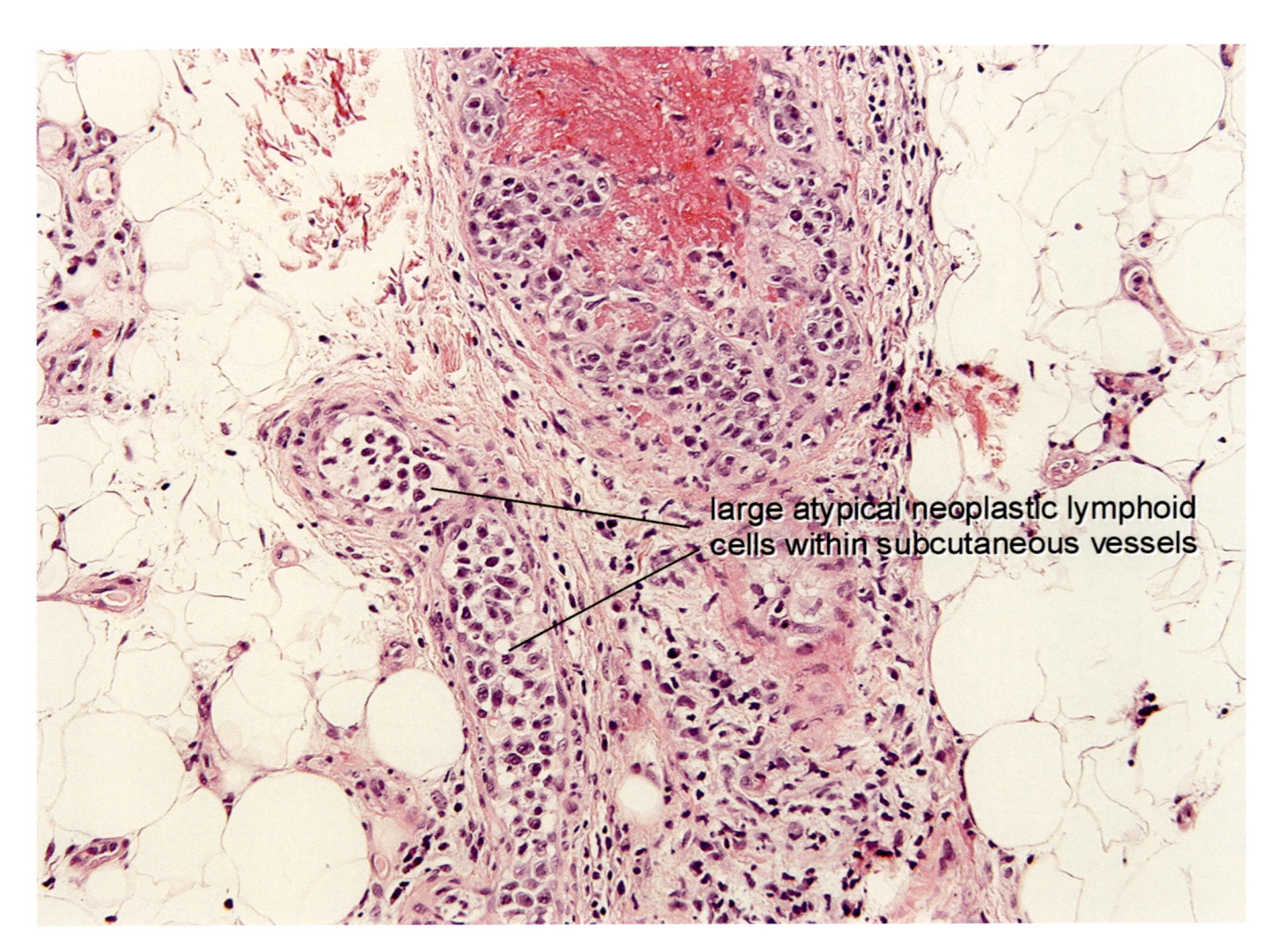

Fig 25-6 Intravascular large B-cell lymphoma

Lymphomatoid granulomatosis

Key features

- B-cell lymphoproliferative disorder associated with Epstein–Barr virus (EBV) infection
- Involves lungs and skin most often; histology shows a variable infiltrate of large atypical perivascular lymphoid cells and areas of necrosis
- Presence of an angiocentric and angiodestructive infiltrate with variable numbers of large EBV+ lymphocytes; granulomatous inflammation may also be present
- Lesions are graded histologically from 1 to 3, based upon the increasing proportion of EBV+ cells relative to the population of background reactive mixed infiltrate
- CD20+, EBV+ large B lymphocytes in a background of reactive T cells
- Important to recognize benign reactive T cells constitute the majority of cells of the lesions

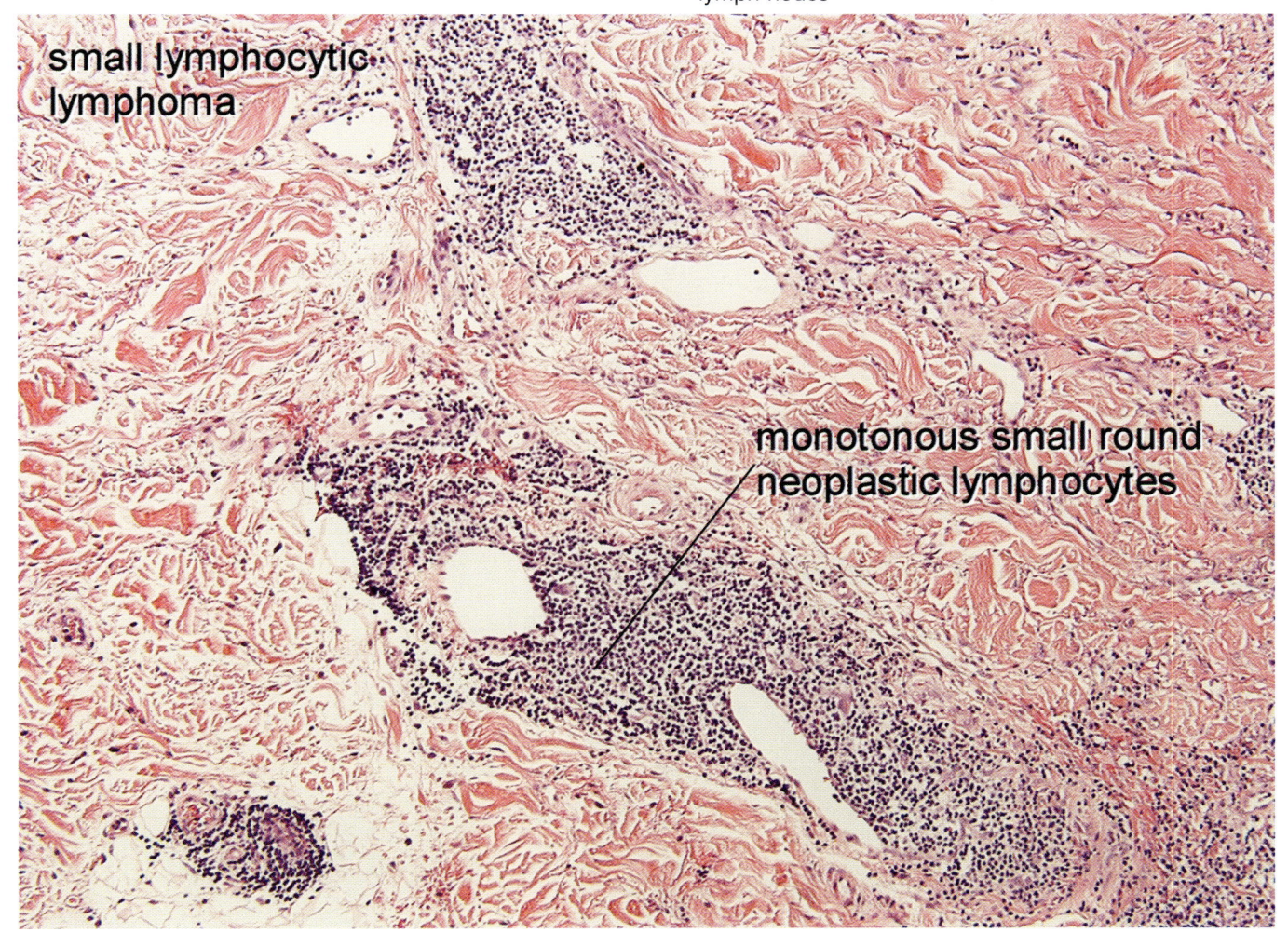

Chronic lymphocytic leukemia/small lymphocytic lymphoma

Key features

- Most common leukemia in adults in the Western hemisphere
- Proliferation of mature round lymphocytes of B-cell origin
- Same disease process as small lymphocytic lymphoma; difference is determined by the presence of tumor in blood/bone marrow for chronic lymphocytic leukemia versus malignant lymphoid cells in other tissues/organs for small lymphocytic lymphoma (without evidence of leukemia)
- Nodular and/or diffuse infiltration of the dermis with dark small round mature-appearing lymphoid cells
- May have occasional larger cells with vesicular nuclei with a single nucleolus (prolymphocytes)
- Grenz zone is often present
- CD19+, CD20+ (usually weak), CD5+, CD23+, CD43+, CD10–, cyclin D1–
- Proliferation centers are not seen as commonly as in lymph nodes

Fig 25-7 Chronic lymphocytic leukemia/small lymphocytic lymphoma

Mantle cell lymphoma

Key features

- Rare B-cell lymphoma that resembles mantle zone of lymphoid follicle
- Usually the result of nodal-based lymphoma with skin involvement; rare cases of putative primary cutaneous mantle cell lymphoma are of doubtful validity
- Histology shows diffuse monomorphous infiltrates of intermediate-sized lymphocytes with irregular nuclei and nucleoli frequently
- CD20+, CD5+, CD43+, BCL-2+, CD23–
- Cyclin D1+ is important marker; results from overexpression of gene product due to t(11;14) translocation

Burkitt lymphoma

Key features

- Not a primary cutaneous entity but infrequently shows cutaneous involvement
- Various clinical forms recognized (endemic form in Africa and sporadic in other regions)
- Most common in first two decades, but can occur at any age
- Monomorphic, diffuse growth of medium-sized cells with round (non-cleaved) vesicular nuclei, multiple nucleoli, moderate amount of basophilic cytoplasm which often contains multiple clear (lipid-filled) vacuoles
- "Starry-sky" pattern due to abundant benign macrophages within tumor phagocytizing necrotic tumor cells/debris
- Extremely high proliferative/mitotic index, nearly 100% observed with MIB-1
- CD19+, CD20+, CD79a+, CD22+, CD10+, CD5–, CD23–, BCL-2–, terminal deoxyribonucleotidyl transferase (TdT)–
- Atypical variant (Burkitt-like lymphoma) shows greater cellular pleomorphism and heterogeneity than classic Burkitt lymphoma

B-cell lymphoblastic lymphoma/leukemia

Key features

- A small proportion of patients with precursor B-cell lymphoblastic lymphoma/leukemia may present with solid tumors, most often in skin, bone, and lymph nodes
- Composed of lymphoblasts slightly larger than mature lymphocytes, but smaller than cells of large B-cell lymphoma
- Blasts contain round or convoluted nuclei and fine chromatin (paler and finer than normal mature lymphocytes), with inconspicuous nucleoli and scant basophilic cytoplasm
- Diffuse pattern with frequent mitoses and tingible body macrophages ("starry-sky" pattern)
- TdT+ (90%), CD34+ (75%), CD79a+, CD19+, CD22+, CD10+ (80–85%), CD20± (may be dim or negative), surface Ig–

Table 25-1 WHO classification of primary cutaneous B-cell lymphoma

Primary cutaneous follicle center lymphoma

- Most common anatomic site is head/neck (often scalp), followed by trunk
- Composed of neoplastic follicle center cells; i.e. centrocytes and centroblasts in various proportions
- Centrocytes are small with cleaved nuclei
- Centroblasts are larger, with non-cleaved nuclei and 1–3 nucleoli attached to inside of nuclear membrane
- If diffuse growth pattern with sheets of centroblasts, is classified as diffuse large B-cell rather than follicular lymphoma
- Otherwise, numbers of centrocytes and centroblasts do not matter as primary FCL is NOT graded
- Immunophenotype:
  - Follicular pattern
    - CD20+ CD79a+, BCL-6+ and CD10+
  - Diffuse pattern
    - CD20+ CD79a+, BCL-6+ and CD10–

Primary cutaneous marginal zone lymphoma (Cutaneous MALT-type lymphoma)

- Includes entities previously classified as:
- Primary cutaneous plasmacytoma without underlying myeloma
- Primary cutaneous immunocytoma
- Erythematous to purple nodules/tumors most often on trunk and extremities, often single or few lesions
- Proliferation of small marginal zone centrocyte-like B cells, usually surrounding benign reactive germinal centers
- Immunophenotype: CD20+, CD79a+, BCL-2+, CD5–, CD10–, BCL-6–
- Approximately 70% show evidence of monoclonal light chain restriction

Primary cutaneous diffuse large B-cell lymphoma, leg type

- 80% of cases occur in patients ≥70 years
- Poorer prognosis
- Diffuse proliferation of monotonous large transformed B cells
- Activated B-cell immunophenotype, with strong BCL-2+ cells which are MUM-1/IRF4+, CD19+, CD20+, CD79a+, BCL-6 variable

Primary cutaneous diffuse large B-cell lymphoma, other

- Includes intravascular/angiotropic B-cell lymphoma and other non-leg type diffuse large B-cell lymphomas with only skin involvement

Adapted from World Health Organisation Classification of Tumours of Haematopoietic and Lymphoid Tissues, 4th edition, 2008.

Further reading

Baldassano MF, Bailey EM, Ferry JA, et al. Cutaneous lymphoid hyperplasia and cutaneous marginal zone lymphoma: comparison of morphologic and immunophenotypic features. Am J Surg Pathol 1999;23(1):88–96.

Bradford PT, Devessa SS, Anderson WF, et al. Cutaneous lymphoma incidence patterns in the United States: a population based study of 3884 cases. Blood 2009;113:5064–5073.

Caro W, Helwig E. Cutaneous lymphoid hyperplasia. Cancer 1969;24:487–502.

De Laval L, Harris NL, Longtine J, et al. Cutaneous B-cell lymphomas of follicular and marginal zone types. Am J Surg Pathol 2001;25(6):732–741.

Demierre M, Kerl H, Willemze R. Primary cutaneous B cell lymphomas: a practical approach. Hematol Oncol Clin North Am 2003;17:1333–1350.

Kiyohara T, Kumakiri M, Kobayashi H, et al. Cutaneous marginal zone B cell lymphoma: a case accompanied by massive plasmacytoid cells. J Am Acad Dermatol 2003;48:S82–S85.

LeBoit PE, McNutt NS, Reed JA, et al. Primary cutaneous immunocytoma: a B cell lymphoma that can easily be mistaken for cutaneous lymphoid hyperplasia. Am J Surg Pathol 1994;18:969–978.

Ritter J, Adesokan P, Fitzgibbon J, et al. Paraffin section immunohistochemistry as an adjunct to morphologic analysis in the diagnosis of cutaneous lymphoid infiltrates. J Cutan Pathol 1994;21:481–493.

Roglin J, Boer A. Skin manifestations of intravascular lymphoma mimic inflammatory diseases of the skin. Br J Dermatol 2007;157:16–25.

Sander C, Kaudewitz P, Schirren C, et al. Immunocytoma and marginal zone B cell lymphoma (MALT lymphoma) presenting in skin-different entities or a spectrum of disease? J Cutan Pathol 1996;23:59a.

Sokol L, Naghashpour M, Glass F. Primary cutaneous B-cell lymphomas: recent advances in diagnosis and management. Cancer Control 2012;19(3):236–244.

Swerdlow SH, Campo E, Harris NL, et al. World Health Organization (WHO) Classification of Tumors of Hematopoietic and Lymphoid Tissues. Lyon: World Health Organization, 2008.

Van Maldegem F, van Dijk R, Wormhoudt TA, et al. The majority of cutaneous marginal zone B cell lymphomas express class-switched immunoglobulins and develop in a T-helper type 2 inflammatory environment. Blood 2008;112:3355–3361.

Willemze R, Jaffe ES, Burg G, et al. WHO-EORTC Classification for cutaneous lymphomas. Blood 2005;105:3768–3785.

Chapter 26

Metastatic tumors and simulators

Christine J. Ko

It is important to distinguish cutaneous metastases from primary adnexal tumors of the skin. Adenocarcinoma metastatic to the skin is commonly of breast or lung origin. Focal areas of glandular differentiation may be highlighted with a mucicarmine stain. Metastases are most often situated in the mid to deep dermis. Epidermotropic metastases form intraepidermal nests.

> **PEARL**
>
> Positivity with both cytokeratin 5/6 and p63 is suggestive of a primary cutaneous adnexal tumor over adenocarcinoma metastatic to the skin.

Breast carcinoma

> **Key features**
>
> - Poorly differentiated adenocarcinoma
> - Various patterns: single cells infiltrating through collagen, cords, and tubules of atypical cells, collections of cells with glandular formation, clusters of cells in pools of mucin, dense sheets of atypical cells
> - Occasionally, there is epidermotropism
> - Gross cystic disease fluid protein (GCDFP)-15 positive, estrogen receptor+, and cytokeratin (CK) 7+

Breast carcinoma is the most common cause of cutaneous metastatic disease in women. In general, metastases are seen on the chest wall, sometimes as a result of direct extension of the tumor. Various clinical and histologic presentations are possible. Distinct subtypes are discussed below.

Carcinoma en cuirasse

> **Key features**
>
> - Rectangular punch
> - Busy dermis
> - Dense collagen
> - Single files of hyperchromatic cells with nuclear molding (black box cars)

A cuirasse is a suit of armor made of leather. Carcinoma en cuirasse presents with woody induration of the skin. The skin is infiltrated by single files of hyperchromatic nuclei with prominent nuclear molding. Dense collagen is laid down between the tumor cells. Because the dermis is sclerotic, the punch is rectangular rather than tapered.

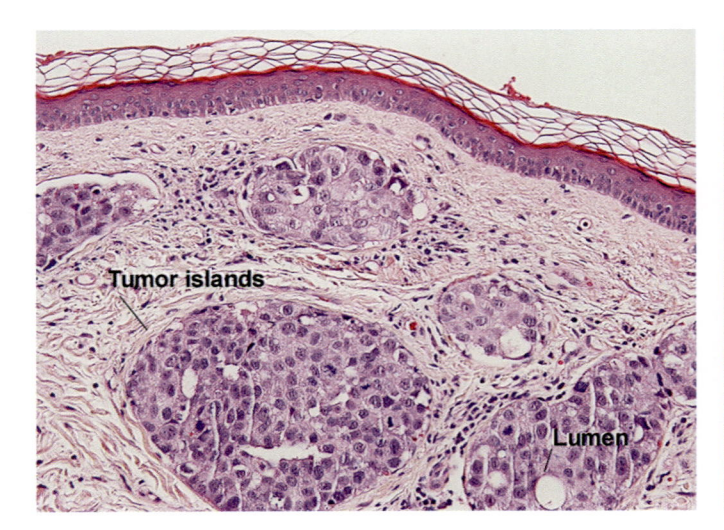

Fig 26.1 Breast carcinoma

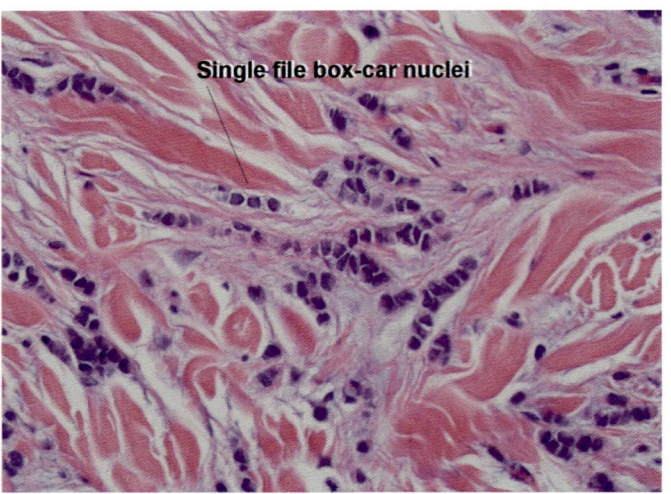

Fig 26.2 Carcinoma en cuirasse

Inflammatory carcinoma (carcinoma erysipeloides)

Key features

- Tumor cells within dilated lymphatic vessels
- Congested capillaries

Clinically, the lesions present with skin erythema that ranges from faint macular erythema to an erysipelas-like presentation. Inflammation is usually absent histologically, and the erythema is likely secondary to blood vessel congestion.

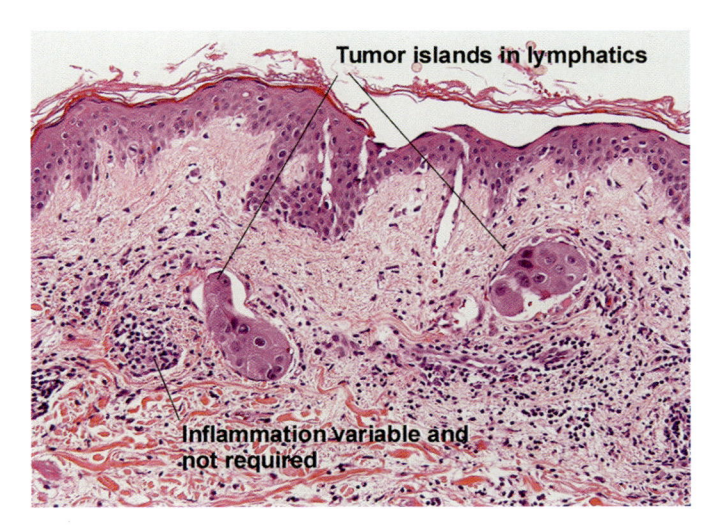

Fig 26.3 Inflammatory carcinoma

Alopecia neoplastica

Key features

- Sclerotic dermis
- Infiltrative cords of atypical cells
- Loss of hair follicles

Occasionally, metastatic breast carcinoma presents as skin-colored to slightly erythematous patches of alopecia on the scalp. Clinically, it is often mistaken for alopecia areata. A biopsy is performed when hair fails to regrow in response to intralesional injection of corticosteroid.

Lung carcinoma

Key features

- Metastases from the lung may be of the small cell-type, adenocarcinoma, squamous cell carcinoma, or undifferentiated
- Most are thyroid transcription factor (TTF)-1+

Lung carcinoma is the most common cause of cutaneous metastases in men. Generally, the metastases present on the trunk as a single nodule or cluster of papules.

Small cell lung carcinoma

Key features

- Sheets of uniform round blue nuclei with little cytoplasm
- Crush artifact may be prominent
- Nuclear molding may be seen
- TTF-1 positivity distinguishes this from Merkel cell carcinoma of the skin

Renal carcinoma

Key features

- Tubules of clear glycogenated cells
- Prominent vascular component with hemosiderin and extravasated erythrocytes
- CD10+
- Periodic acid–Schiff (PAS)+
- RCC+

The scalp is a common site for metastatic renal cell carcinoma (RCC). The lesion is typically nodular. The vessels have a "chicken wire" pattern.

418 Dermatopathology

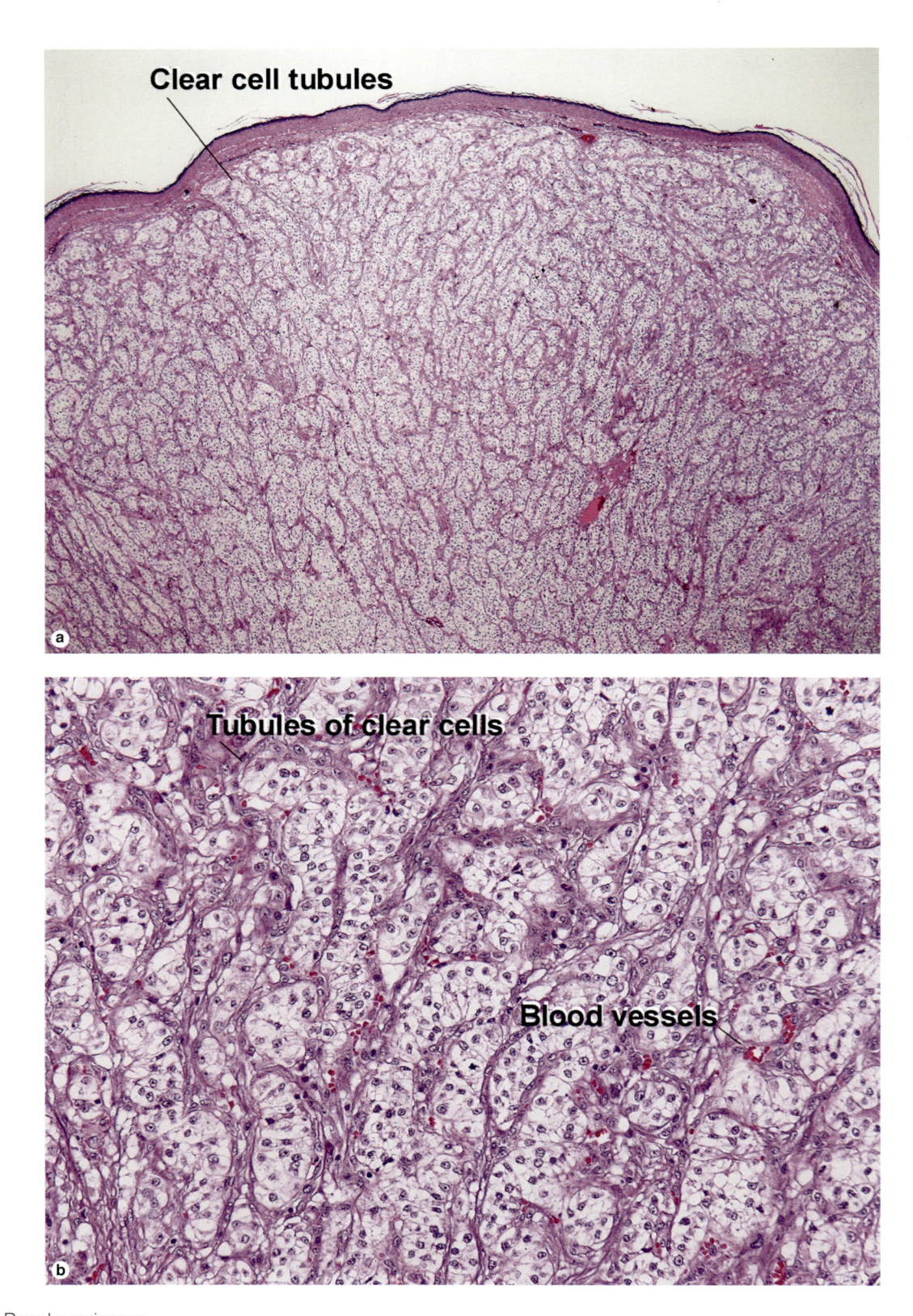

Fig 26.4 Renal carcinoma

Metastatic tumors and simulators

Colon carcinoma

Key features

- Well- to moderately differentiated adenocarcinoma
- May mimic mucinous carcinoma of the skin, with clusters of blue cells floating in pools of mucin
- Typically CK20+
- CDX2+

Colon carcinoma is typically CK20 positive and CK7 negative. Rectal carcinoma may stain with both, or with CK7 only. Figures 26.5c, d demonstrate this paradoxical immunostaining pattern in a rectal adenocarcinoma.

Ovarian carcinoma

Key features

- Well-differentiated adenocarcinoma
- Sometimes the tumor demonstrates papillary fronding
- Psammoma bodies (concentric calcifications) may be seen
- CK7+, CA125+

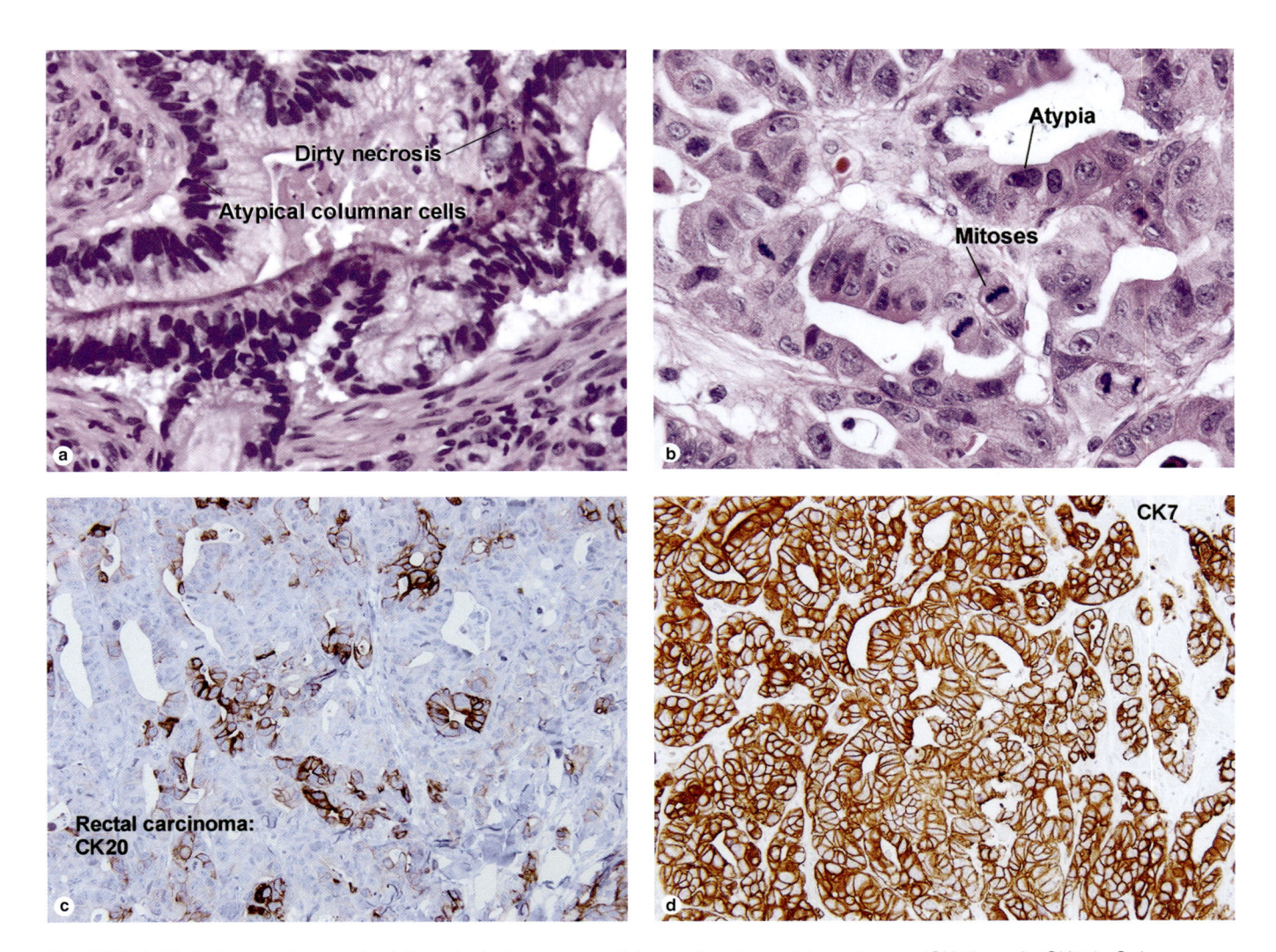

Fig 26.5 (a,b) Colon carcinoma. (c,d) Paradoxical immunostaining pattern in rectal carcinoma (CK20 weak, CK7+). Colon cancer is usually CK20+, CK7–

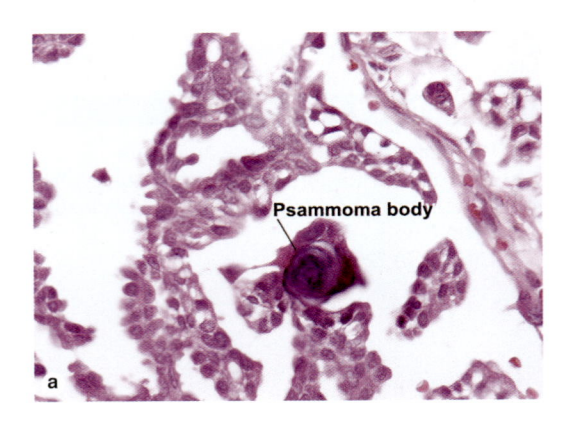

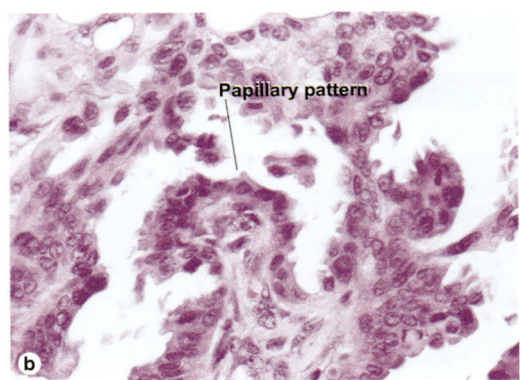

Fig 26.6 Ovarian carcinoma

Signet-ring carcinoma

Key features

- Atypical cells with central pale area (mucin) that compresses the nucleus to the periphery
- Loose stroma

The site of origin is most commonly gastric, although they may arise from other parts of the gastrointestinal tract or breast.

Thyroid carcinoma

Key features

- Papillary is most common, followed by follicular
- Psammoma bodies may be seen, especially in papillary carcinoma
- "Orphan Annie" nuclei (large nuclei, a pale center) and nuclear pseudoinclusions are typical of papillary carcinoma
- Medullary carcinoma stains with calcitonin
- Thyroglobulin+ and TTF-1+

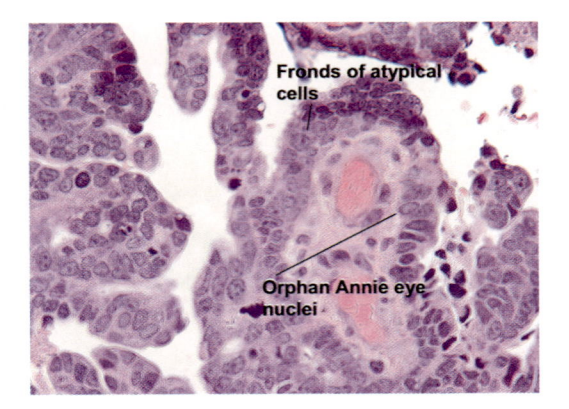

Metastases from the thyroid often spread hematogenously, allowing thyroid carcinoma to present at a variety of body sites. The scalp is a common site. Papillary thyroid carcinoma displays fronds of cells with occasional psammoma bodies and "Orphan Annie" eye nuclei. A follicular variant exists, but retains the characteristic "Orphan Annie" eye nuclei and pseudoinclusions. Follicular thyroid carcinoma is composed of thyroid follicles with colloid. Medullary thyroid carcinomas generally consist of sheets of atypical cells with amyloid; they may be sporadic but occasionally are markers for multiple endocrine neoplasia syndromes IIA (Sipple syndrome) and IIB.

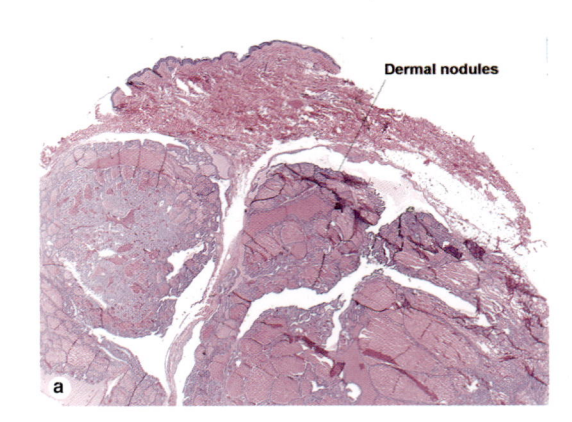

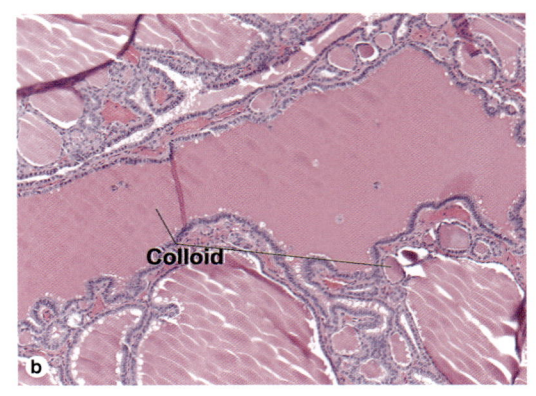

Fig 26.7 Papillary thyroid carcinoma

Fig 26.8 Follicular thyroid carcinoma

Prostate carcinoma

Key features

- Poorly differentiated adenocarcinoma
- Atypical cells infiltrating through collagen
- Prostate-specific antigen (PSA)+

Metastatic prostate carcinoma generally presents on the thighs/groin area, although it has been reported at other sites.

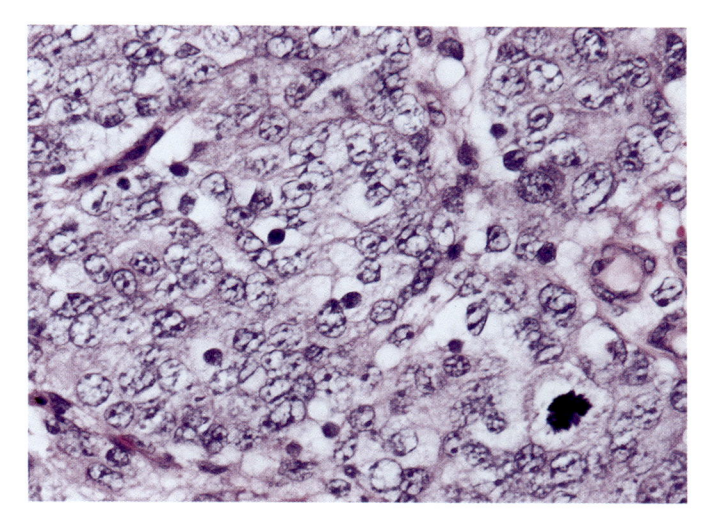

Fig 26.9 Prostate carcinoma

Metastatic squamous carcinoma

Key features

- Tumor in deeper dermis
- Generally lacks an epidermal connection
- Occasional squamous pearls present
- May be poorly differentiated; helpful positive stains include epithelial membrane antigen (EMA) and cytokeratins

Metastatic squamous cell carcinoma most commonly originates from the oral cavity, lung, or esophagus. Other rare primary sites include the cervix and the male genitalia. Epidermotropic metastases may simulate primary cutaneous squamous cell carcinoma.

Cytokeratin AE1/AE3 does not always stain squamous cell carcinoma. Pankeratin cocktails are commonly more reliable.

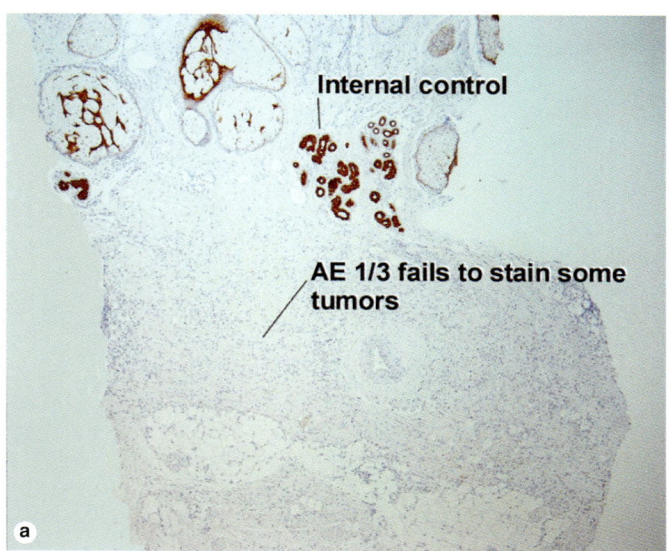

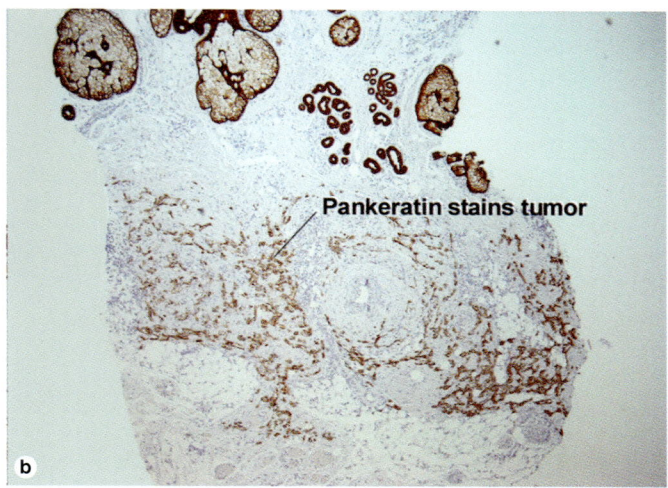

Fig 26.10 Squamous cell carcinoma

Meningioma

Key features

- Spindled to ovoid cells in whorls or groups
- Fibrocollagenous to loose stroma
- Cells may be in sheet-like syncytia
- Psammoma bodies may be seen
- EMA+

The cutaneous presentation of an intracranial meningioma may be secondary to direct extension of the intracranial tumor or true metastatic spread. Lesions are generally seen on the scalp.

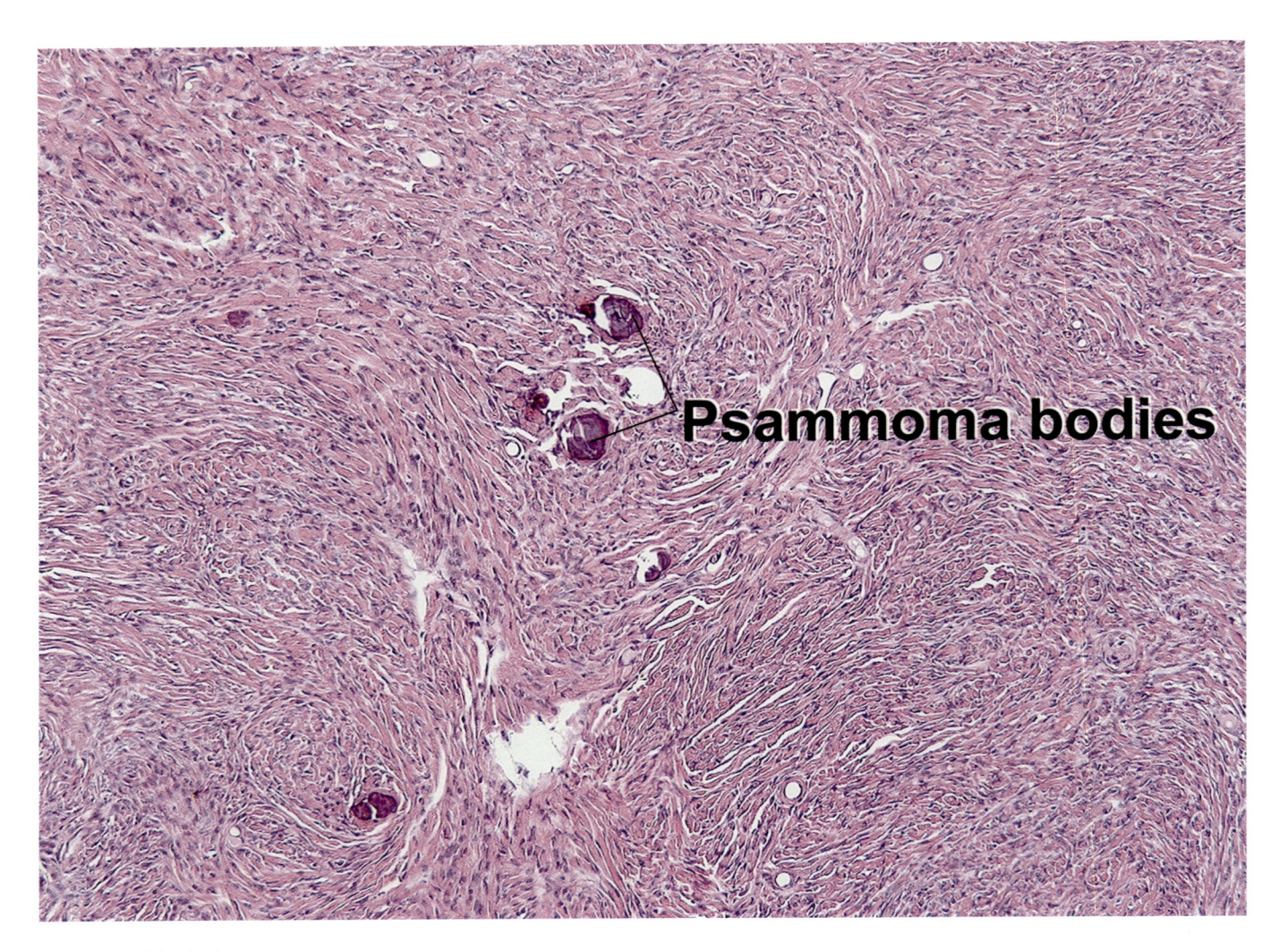

Fig 26.11 Meningioma

Table 26-1 Keratin immunostains for metastatic adenocarcinoma

	Breast	Colon	Lung	Urinary tract	Pancreas/biliary
Cytokeratin 7	+	–	+	+	+
Cytokeratin 20	–	+	–	+	+

Table 26-2 Immunostains for metastatic carcinoma

Adenocarcinoma	Immunostain
Breast	GCDFP-15+ (more common by 100:1), CEA+, CK7+, EMA+
Gastrointestinal	CEA+, CK20+, CDX2+
Lung	TTF-1+, CEA+
Ovarian	CA125+
	(mucinous subtype is CK7 and CK20+)
Prostate	PSA+
Renal	CD10+
	RCC+
Thyroid	TTF-1+, thyroglobulin+, calcitonin+ (medullary type)

CEA, carcinoembryonic antigen.

Metastatic tumors and simulators

Lesions that mimic metastatic carcinoma

Endometriosis

Key features

- Glandular spaces
- Loose concentric fibromyxoid stroma
- RBCs ± hemosiderin in stroma
- Decidualized endometriosis has large polygonal decidual cells in the stroma

Omphalomesenteric duct polyp

Key features

- Polypoid tumor in umbilical area
- Surface squamous epithelium adjacent to mucosal epithelium
- Columnar epithelium with goblet cells
- Smooth muscle may be present underlying the mucosal epithelium

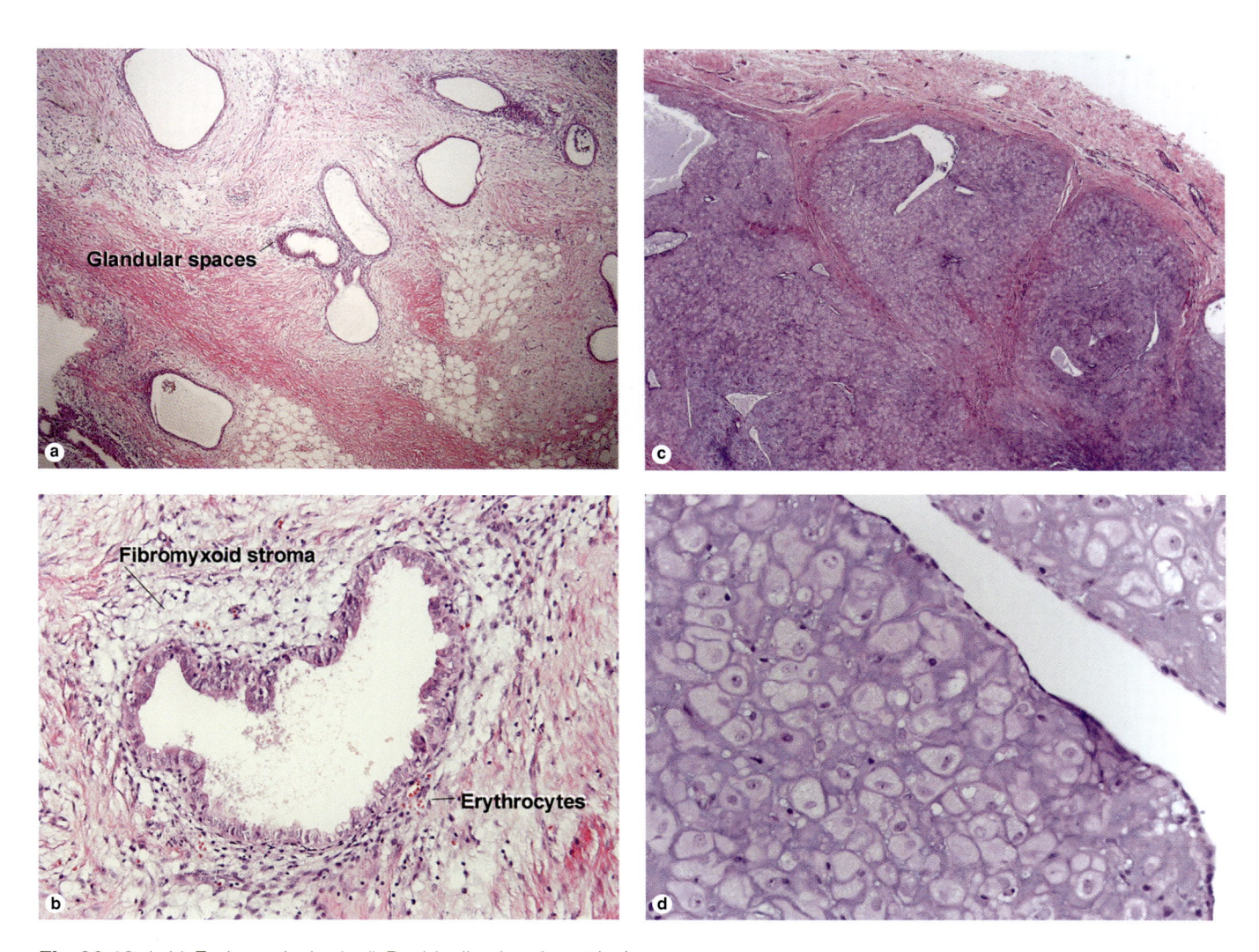

Fig 26.12 (a,b) Endometriosis. (c,d) Decidualized endometriosis

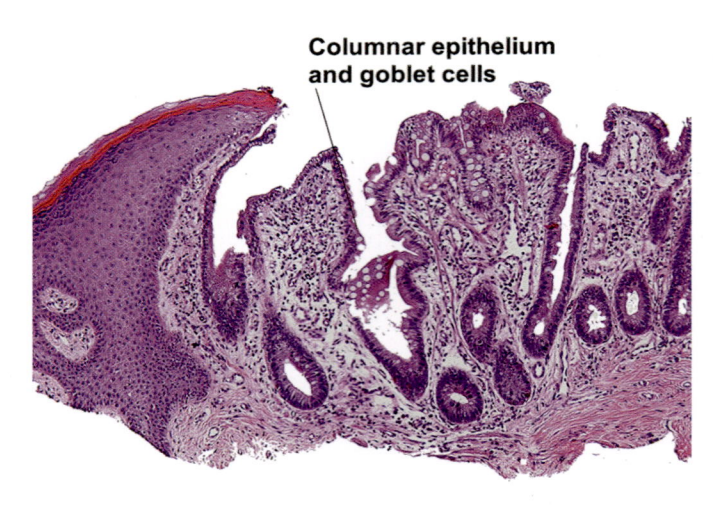

Fig 26.13 Omphalomesenteric duct polyp

Further reading

Abrol N, Seth A, Chattergee P. Cutaneous metastasis of prostate carcinoma to neck and upper chest. Indian J Pathol Microbiol 2011;54(2):394–395.

Marcoval J, Penín RM, Llatjós R, et al. Cutaneous metastasis from lung cancer: retrospective analysis of 30 patients. Australas J Dermatol 2012;53(4):288–290.

Relles D, Fong Z, Burkhart R, et al. Facial cutaneous metastasis of colon adenocarcinoma. Am Surg 2012;78(11):E454–E456.

Rollins-Raval M, Chivukula M, Tseng GC, et al. An immunohistochemical panel to differentiate metastatic breast carcinoma to skin from primary sweat gland carcinomas with a review of the literature. Arch Pathol Lab Med 2011;135(8):975–983.

Somoza AD, Bui H, Samaan S, et al. Cutaneous metastasis as the presenting sign of papillary thyroid carcinoma. J Cutan Pathol 2013;40(2):274–278.

Appendix 1

Dermatopathology mnemonics

Additional Mnemonics can be found in the on-line content for this book.

"Neuts in the horn" = PTICSS	Eosinophilic spongiosis = HAAPPIE	PEH with pus = "Here come big green leafy veggies"
Psoriasis **T**inea **I**mpetigo **C**andida **S**eborrheic dermatitis **S**yphilis	**H**erpes gestationis **A**rthropod bite **A**llergic contact **P**emphigus **P**emphigoid **I**ncontinentia pigmenti **E**rythema toxicum (spongiosis adjacent to a follicle)	**H**alogenoderma **C**hromomycosis **B**lastomycosis **G**ranuloma inguinale **L**eishmaniasis Pemphigus **v**egetans
Neuts stuffed in the dermal papillae = PLAID	Subcorneal pustule = CAT SIPS	Lichenoid DDX
Bullous **p**emphigoid **L**upus (bullous) EB**A** Linear **i**mmunoglobulin A **D**H	**C**andida **A**cropustulosis of infancy **T**ransient neonatal pustular melanosis **S**neddon – Wilkinson **I**mpetigo **P**ustular psoriasis **S**taphylococcal-scalded skin syndrome	LP LPLK (BLK) Lichenoid drug Lichenoid regression of melanocytic lesion Lichenoid graft-versus-host disease Lupus (acral – "lips and tips")
Stellate abscess (palisaded granuloma with neuts) = Stella has the "CLATS"	Parasitized histiocytes = "pH GIRL"	Busy dermis = "Busy dermis can kill grandma's sweet niece"
Cat-scratch **L**GV **A**typical mycobacterial **T**ularemia **S**porotrichosis (melioidosis, *Nocardia*)	**P**enicillium marneffei **H**istoplasmosis **G**ranuloma **i**nguinale **R**hinoscleroma **L**eishmaniasis/**l**eprosy	**B**lue nevus **D**F/**d**ermal Spitz **C**utaneous metastasis **K**aposi's (plaque) **G**ranuloma annulare **S**cleromyxedema **N**eurofibroma
	Lymph in every hole	
	MF LPLK (BLK) PLEVA PLC	
Vasculitis	Spindle cells "slam"med against the epidermis	Buckshot scatter

Vasculitis		Spindle cells "slam"med against the epidermis	Buckshot scatter
Big 5	Little 5	**S**pindle cell SCC **L**eiomyosarcoma **A**FX **M**elanoma (spindle cell)	Paget's Bowen's Melanoma Center of acral nevus Center of Spitz Sebaceous carcinoma
Wegener's Churg–Strauss Rheumatoid Septic Polyarteritis nodosa	HSP Cryos Drug CTD Serum sickness		

AFX, atypical fibroxanthoma; BLK, benign lichenoid keratosis; Cryos, mixed cryoglobulinemia; CTD, connective tissue disease; DDX, differential diagnosis; DF, dermatofibroma; DH, dermatitis herpetiformis; EBA, epidermolysis bullosa acquisita; HSP, Henoch–Schönlein purpura; LGV, lymphogranuloma venereum; LP, lichen planus; LPLK, lichen planus-like keratosis; MF, mycosis fungoides; PLC, pityriasis lichenoides chronica; PLEVA, pityriasis lichenoides et varioliformis acuta; SCC, squamous cell carcinoma.

Appendix 2

Skin ultrastructure
Sunita Bhuta

1. Desmosome

A classic desmosome showing the following features: (1) uniform gap of 20–30 nm between the apposed trilaminar plasma membranes with an intermediate line (arrow) in this gap; and (2) sharply delineated dense plaques into which tonofibrils (F) converge.

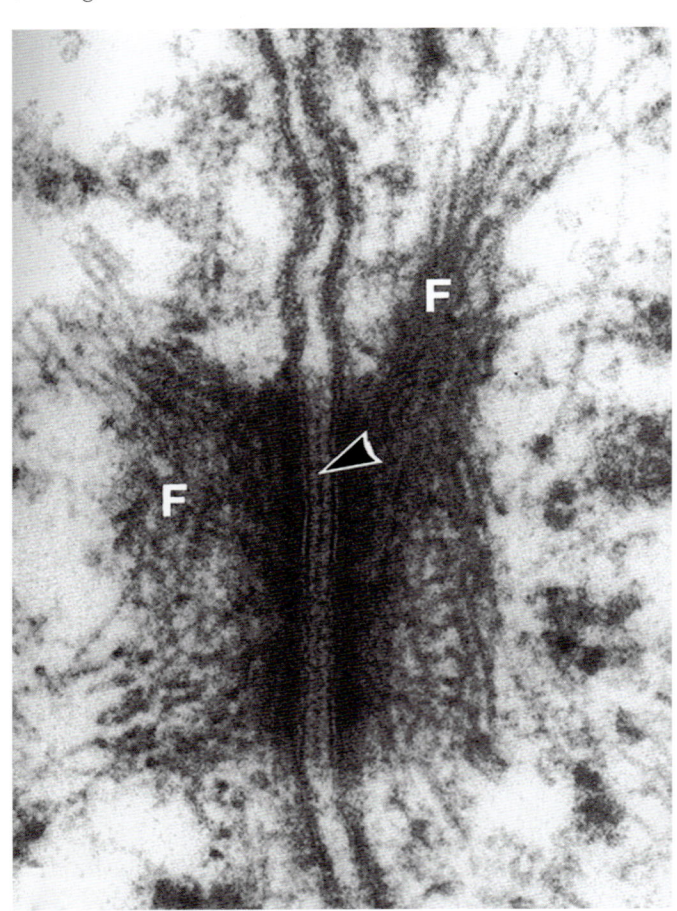

2. Langerhans cell (with Birbeck granules)

This electronmicrograph shows characteristic racket-shaped profiles of the granules in the cytoplasm (inset with higher magnification of the Birbeck granule).

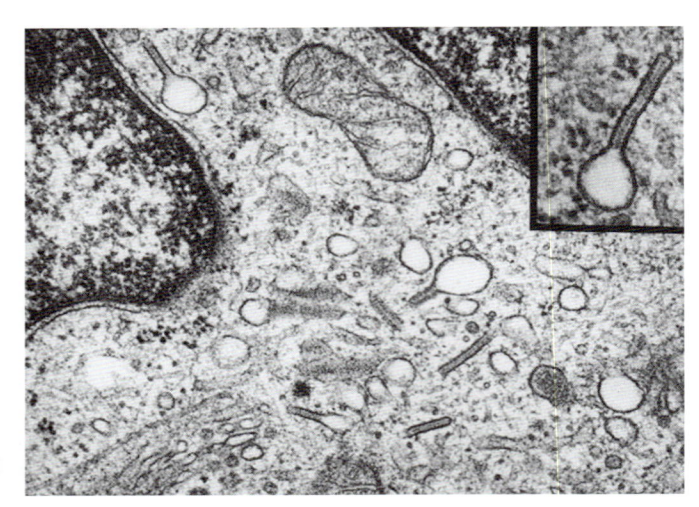

3. Premelanosome

Solitary melanosome with characteristic internal striated structure.

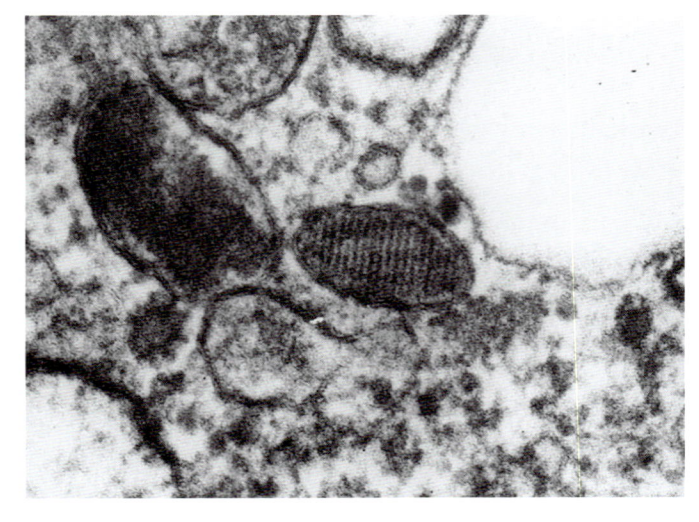

4. Tonofibrils

Tonofibrils (intermediate filaments) lying free in the cytoplasm of a squamous cell.

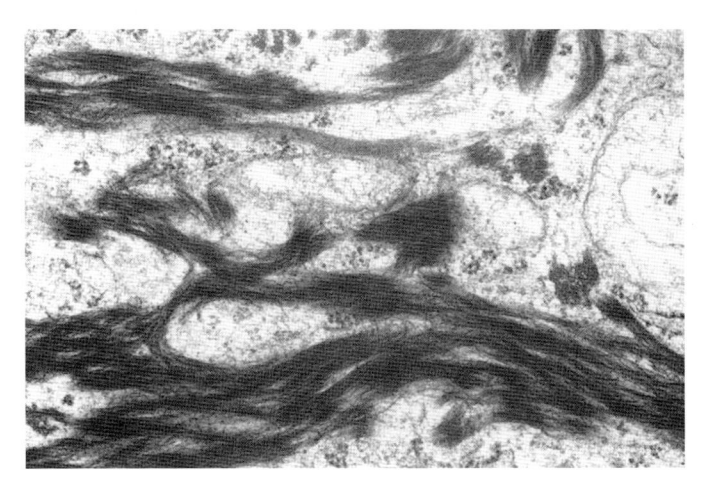

5. Eosinophil

(A) Binucleate (N) with intracytoplasmic specific granules.
(B) Specific granules have a finely granular matrix and a crystalline (Cr) core.

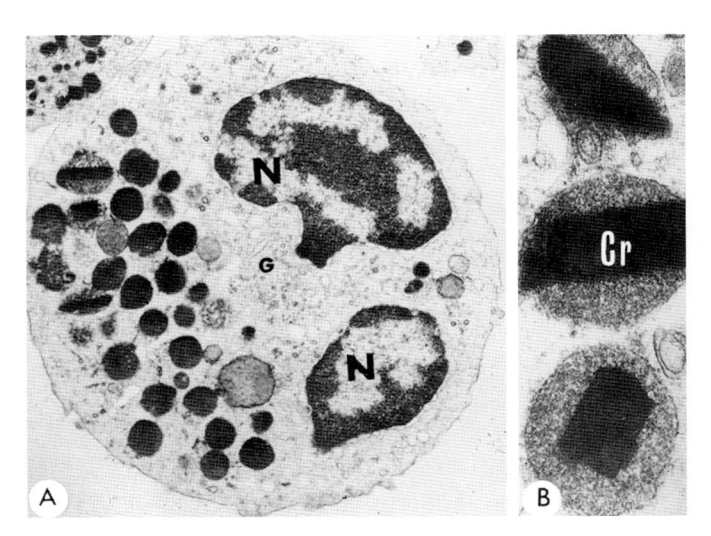

6. Mast cell

Mast cell with numerous electron-dense granules. Inset shows internal structure of granules with membranous whorls (scrolls).

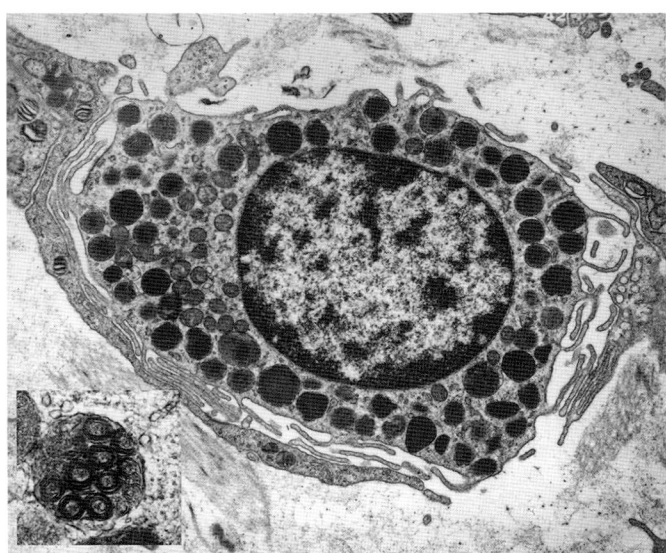

7. Merkel cell

Merkel cell with intracytoplasmic membrane-bound electron-dense round granules with a halo (neurosecretory granules).

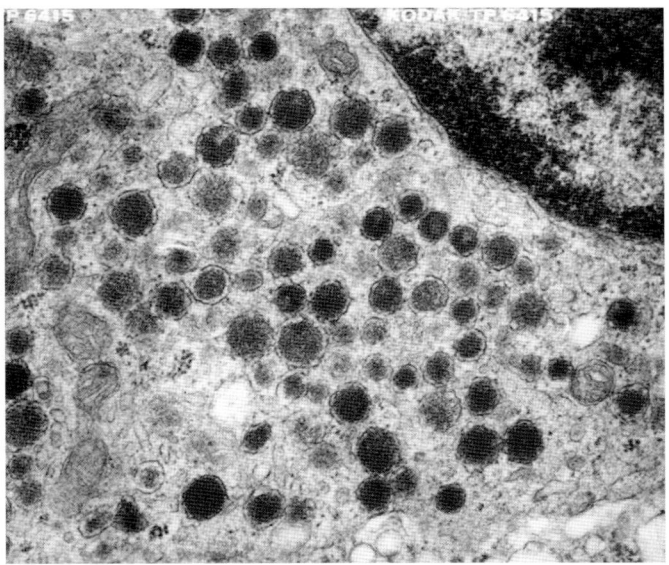

Appendix 3

External agents and artifacts

Tammie Ferringer

1. Electrocautery

- Keratinocytes show marked parallel vertical elongation
- Homogenization of the collagen

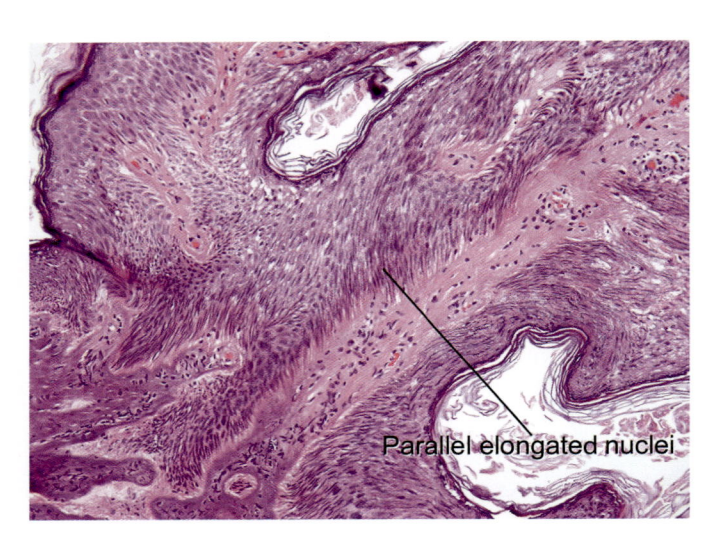

Figure Ap3.1 Electrocautery artifact.

2. Gelfoam®

- Blue-purple arabesque net-like pattern with surrounding granulomatous reaction

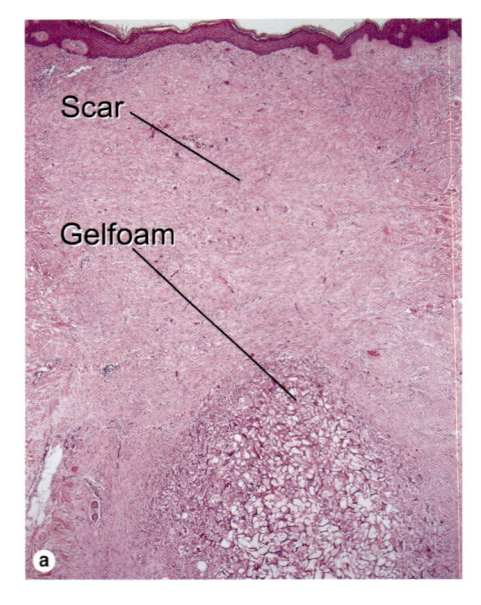

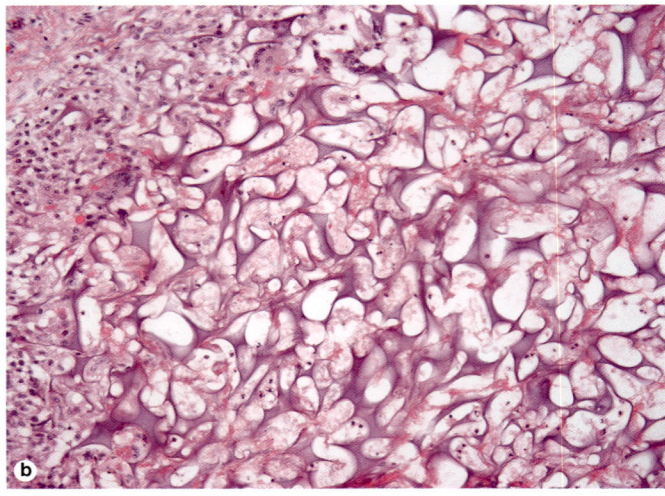

Figure Ap3.2 (a,b) Gelfoam®.

External agents and artifacts   Appendix 3   429

3. Aluminum chloride

- Epidermal effacement and horizontal fibrosis consistent with scar and underlying light gray-blue granules, often in histiocytes, with focal calcification

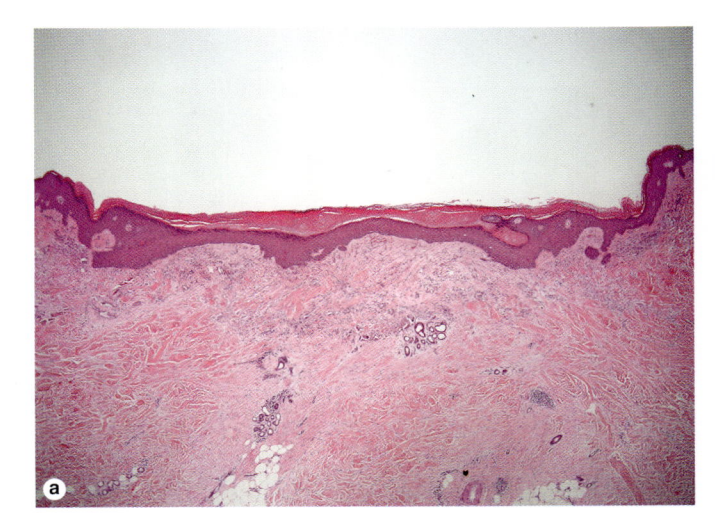

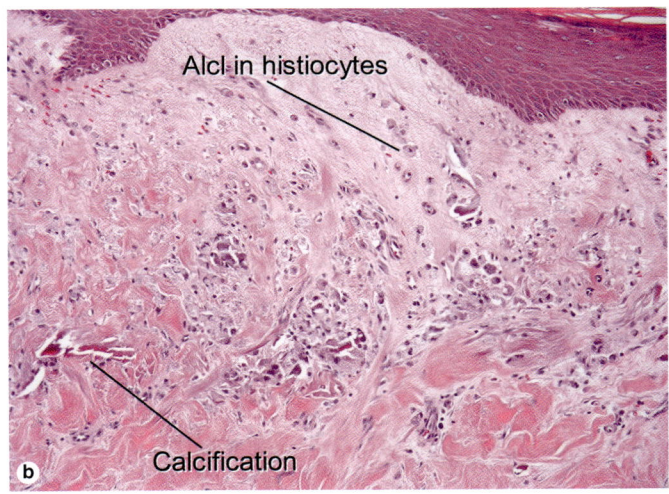

Figure Ap3.3 (a,b) Aluminum chloride at base of biopsy site.

4. Monsel's solution (ferric subsulfate)

- Epidermal effacement and horizontal fibrosis with collagen necrosis and chunky golden, refractile pigment in macrophages
- Perls' iron stain is strongly positive, distinguishing the pigment from melanin

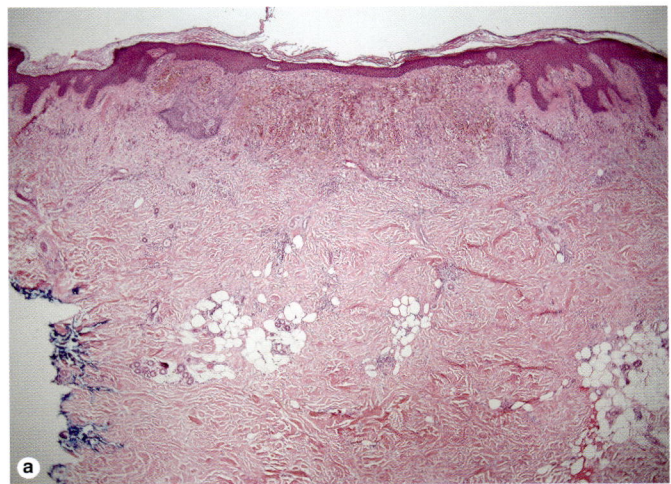

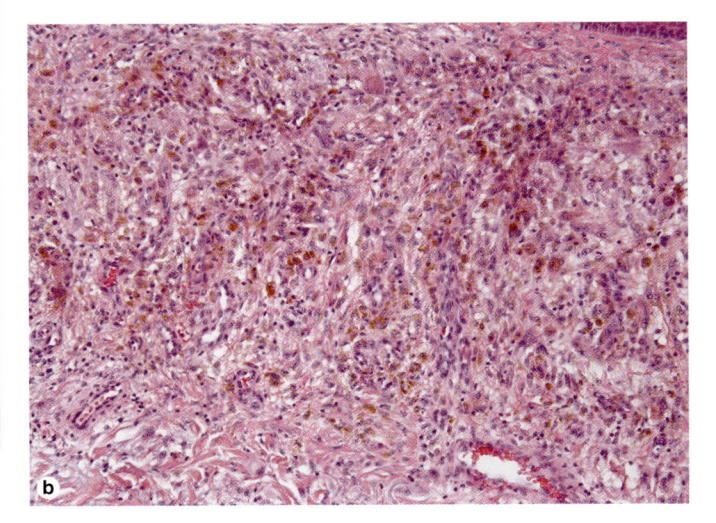

Figure Ap3.4 Monsel's solution tattoo.

5. Triamcinolone

- Lake of bluish granular to amorphous material, at times surrounded by histiocytic response

Triamcinolone is often seen localized within keloid or hypertrophic scar, where it is iatrogenically injected. It superficially resembles mucin but is negative with mucin stains

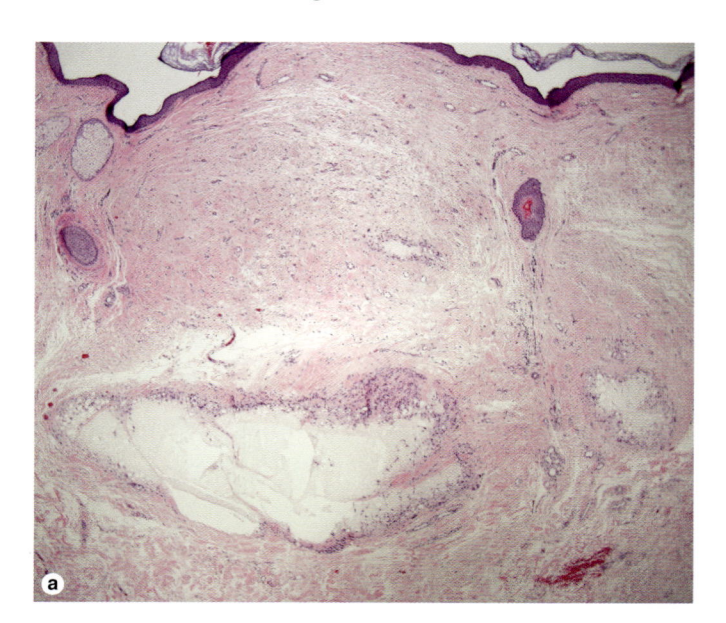

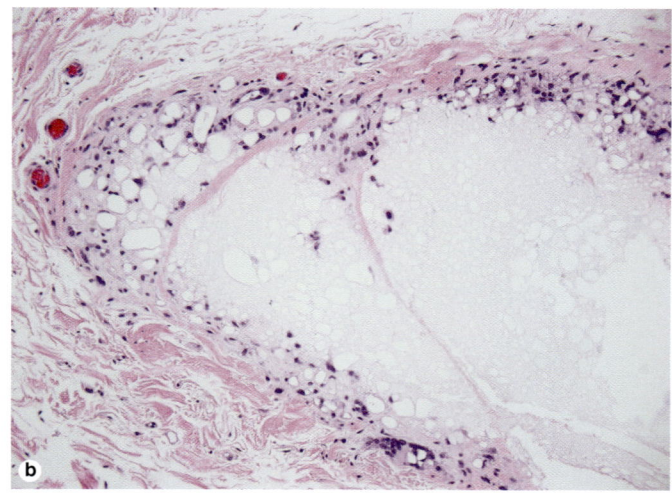

Figure Ap3.5 (a,b) Triamcinolone in scar.

6. Splinter

- Often brown fragment with honeycomb pattern of cell walls

When plant material is identified in the dermis it is prudent to perform stains for bacteria and fungi to exclude contaminating organisms

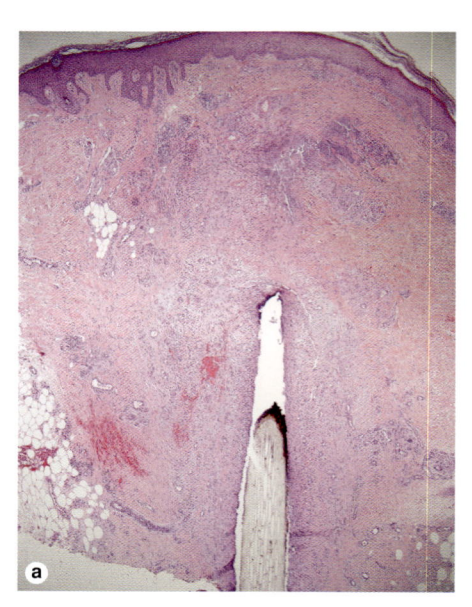

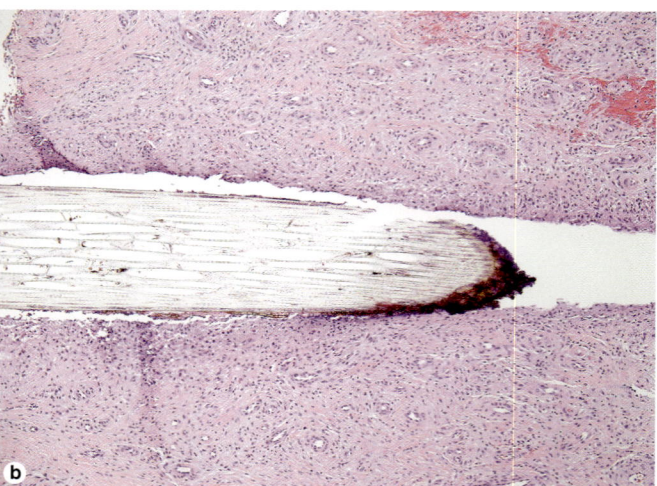

Figure Ap3.6 Splinter.

7. Suture

- Birefringent braided filaments
- Granulomatous foreign body reaction

8. Amalgam

- Golden or brown-black fragments and granules free in the dermis or deposited on connective tissue fibers

Amalgam tattoos consist of silver, mercury, and tin and likely occur following accidental implantation during dental procedures. The buccal, gingival, and alveolar mucosa are most commonly affected by these gray-blue macules.

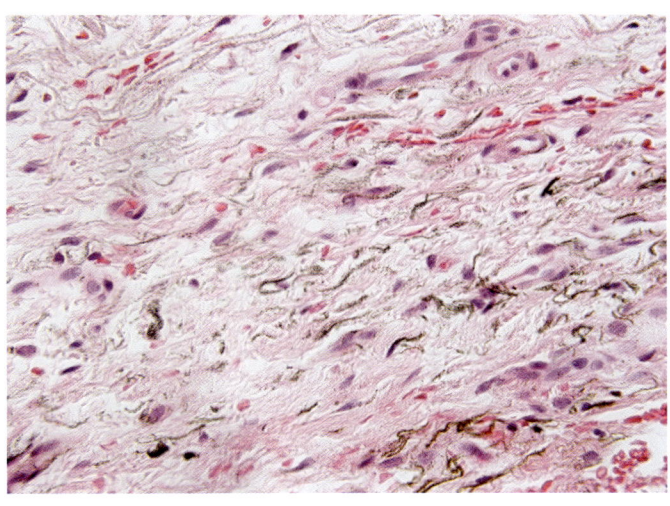

Figure Ap3.8 Amalgam tattoo.

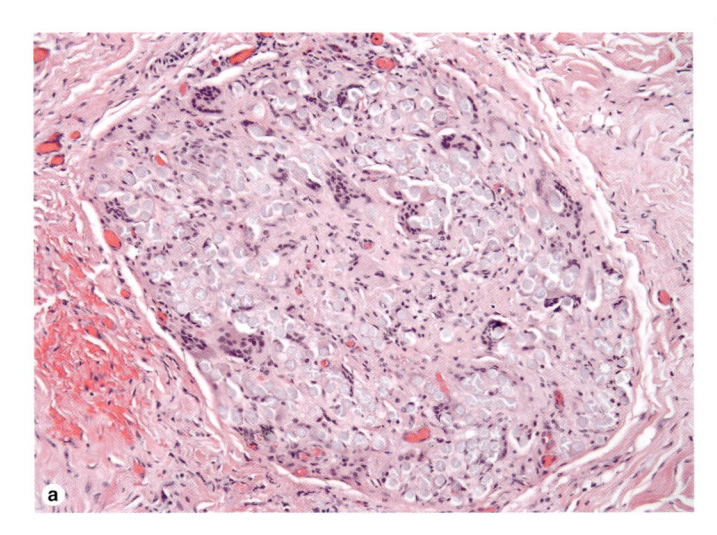

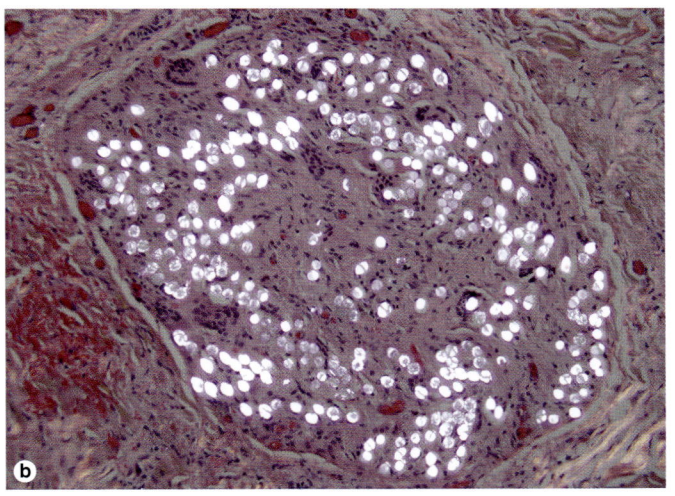

Figure Ap3.7 (a) Suture. (b) Suture (polarized microscopy).

Index

Page numbers followed by "f" indicate figures and "t" indicate tables.

Notes
    vs. indicates a comparison or differential diagnosis

A

ABCC6 transporter gene, pseudoxanthoma elasticum, 208
Absidia infection, 282
Acanthamoeba infection, 269, 269f
acantholysis
    definition, 1
    pemphigus vulgaris, 1f
acantholytic acanthoma, 48, 48f
acantholytic actinic keratosis, 57, 57f
acantholytic dermatosis, transient *see* transient acantholytic dermatosis (Grover's disease)
acanthoma(s), 37–49
    acantholytic, 48, 48f
    clear cell, 45, 45f
    epidermal nevi, 48–49
    epidermolytic, 48, 48f
    inverted follicular keratosis, 46, 46f
    large cell, 45–46, 46f
    melanoacanthoma, 45, 45f
    pale cell, 45
    pilar sheath, 80, 80f
    seborrheic keratoses *see* seborrheic keratoses
    warty dyskeratoma, 46, 47f
acanthosis
    definition, 1
    psoriasis, 1f
acanthotic seborrheic keratoses, 37, 37f–39f
    inflamed, 39f
    irritated, 38f–39f
accessory tragus (cartilaginous rest), 350, 350f
acne agminata, 175, 175f
acne keloidalis nuchae, 220, 220f, 244f
acne vulgaris, 239, 240f
acquired digital fibrokeratoma, 327, 359
ACR *see* American College of Rheumatology (ACR)
acral lentiginous melanoma, 127t
acral nevus, 114–116, 116f
acral skin, 11
acrodermatitis chronica atrophicans, 221, 221f, 268, 268f
acrodermatitis enteropathica, 232
acrospiromas, 97–100, 98f
    malignant, 101, 101f
actinic granulomas, 173, 174f
actinic keratosis, 56–57, 56f
    acantholytic, 57, 57f
    Bowenoid, 57, 57f
    hypertrophic, 57, 57f
    lichenoid, 57, 57f
actinic purpura, 206
actinomycetomas, 279, 279f, 279t
acute febrile neutrophilic dermatoses, 197, 198f
acute generalized exanthematous pustulosis, 162, 162f
acute Langerhans cell histiocytosis (histiocytosis X), 245, 245f
acute lupus erythematosus, 142f
acute myeloid leukemia (AML), 402, 402f
acute spongiform dermatitis, 155, 155f
acute urticaria (wheal), 199f
adamantinoid trichoblastoma, 77, 77f
Adamson's fringe, hair anatomy, 13
adenocarcinoma
    aggressive digital papillary, 89, 90f
    thyroid transcription factor, 25f
adenoid basal cell carcinoma, 68, 68f
adenoid cystic carcinoma, 103, 103f
adenomas
    papillary "eccrine", 102, 102f
    tubular apocrine, 102, 102f
adipocytes, lipoma, 341
adipophilin, 25
adult myofibroma, 311–312, 312f
adult T-cell leukemia/lymphoma (ATCLL), 393–394, 393f–394f
AE1, 23, 24f
    spindle cell neoplasms, 34t
AE3, 23, 24f
    spindle cell neoplasms, 34t
AFL *see* atypical fibroxanthoma (AFX)
African histoplasmosis, 277, 277f
aggressive digital papillary adenocarcinoma, 89, 90f
aggressive fibromatosis, 331, 331f
Alcian blue stain, 19
Alizarin red stain, 21
ALK-1, 32
alkaptonuria, 221
alopecia
    cicatricial *see* cicatricial alopecia
    inflammatory nonscarring *see below*
    pattern *see* pattern alopecia (androgenetic balding)
    syphilitic, 238
    traction, 237
alopecia areata, 237, 237f–238f, 237t
alopecia, inflammatory nonscarring, 237–239
    acne vulgaris, 239, 240f
    alopecia areata, 237, 237f–238f, 237t
    alopecia mucinosa, 238, 238f
    central cictricial alopecia, 244
    dissecting cellulitis, 244
    folliculitis decalvans, 244, 244f
    folliculotropic mycosis fungoides, 239, 239f
    idiopathic pseudopelade, 243, 243f
    lichen planopilaris, 241, 241t, 242f
    Majocchi's fungal folliculitis, 239, 240f
    syphilitic alopecia, 238, 238f
    tinea capitis, 239
alopecia mucinosa, 238, 238f
    follicular mucinosis, 5f

alopecia neoplastica, breast carcinoma metastases, 417
alopecia, non-inflammatory, 234–237
    pattern alopecia, 234–235, 234f
    telogen effluvium, 235, 235f
    traction alopecia, 237
    trichotillomania, 235, 235f–236f, 237t
alpha$_1$-antitrypsin deficiency, 253, 254f
American College of Rheumatology (ACR)
    Churg–Strauss syndrome, 190
    drug induced leukocytoclastic vasculitis, 193
    giant cell arteritis, 184
    Henoch–Schönlein purpura, 191
    idiopathic leukocytoclastic vasculitis, 193
    polyarteritis nodosa, 186
    Takayasu arteritis, 186
    thromboangiitis obliterans, 187
    vasculitis classification, 183
    Wegener's granulomatosis, 188
AML (acute myeloid leukemia), 402, 402f
amyloid, macular, 228, 228f
amyloidosis, 227–228
    epidermal-derived, 227
    keratin-derived, 227
    lichen *see* lichen amyloid
    nodular, 227, 228f
    systemic, 227
        see also specific diseases/disorders
amyloid stain, 20
    colloid milium, 231
anagen hairs, 13
anaplasia
    Bowen's disease, 1f
    definition, 1
    large cell lymphoma, 31f
anaplastic large cell lymphoma, CD30, 31f
"ancient" nevus, 117
ancient Schwannoma (neurilemmoma), 356, 356f
androgenetic balding *see* pattern alopecia (androgenetic balding)
anetoderma, 222, 222f
    Jadassohn–Pellizzari, 222
aneurysmal dermatofibroma, 310, 310f
angioblastomas (tufted angioma), 377, 377f–378f
angiofibromas, 325–327
    acquired digital fibrokeratoma, 327, 327f
    benign fibrous papule, solitary, 326–327, 326f
    fibrous papule of the face, 326–327, 326f
angiokeratoma, 366, 366f
angioleiomyoma, 348, 348f
angiolipoma, 342, 342f–343f
angiolymphoid hyperplasia with eosinophilia, 371, 372f
angioma
    cherry, 369, 370f
    serpiginosum, 367, 367f
    tufted, 377, 377f–378f
angiomatosis, bacillary, 369, 370f
angiomatous hamartoma, eccrine, 103, 375, 376f
angiomyolipoma, 345, 345f
angiosarcoma, 383–385, 384f–386f
    CD31, 27f
annular granuloma annulare, 173, 174f
Antoni A tissue, Schwannoma, 355
Antoni B tissue, Schwannoma, 355
aplasia cutis congenita, 223, 223f
apocrine adenoma, tubular, 102, 102f
aponeurotic fibroma, calcifying, 329, 330f
Apophysomyces infection, 282

apoptosis
    catagen follicle, 2f
    definition, 1
arborizing, 1
areolar skin, 11, 11f
arteries, 183f
arteriovenous hemangioma, 373, 374f
arteriovenous malformation, 373, 374f
arteritis
    giant cell, 183–184, 184f–185f
    Takayasu, 185–186, 185f–186f
    temporal, 183–184, 184f–185f
arthropods (insects), 304–307
    bites, 203, 203f, 304f, 306
    mydriasis, 307, 308f
    scabies, 303f–304f, 304–306
    spider bite, 307
    stings, 306
    tick bite, 305f–306f, 306–307
    tungiasis, 307, 308f
aspergillosis, 283, 283f
Aspergillus, 22f
asteroid bodies
    definition, 1
    sarcoidosis, 2f, 175, 176f
ATCLL (adult T-cell leukemia/lymphoma), 393–394, 393f–394f
ATP2A2 gene, keratosis follicularis, 165
ATP2C1 gene, familial benign chronic pemphigus, 164
atrophic papulosis, malignant, 202, 203f
atrophoderma, 222
atrophy, 2
atypical fibroxanthoma (AFX), 337, 337f
    CD10, 30f
    cell markers, 34t
    S100A6, 28f
atypical necrobiosis lipoidica of the face and scalp, 173, 174f
auramine–rhodamine stain, 23, 23f
auricle, pseudocyst of, 351, 351f

B

bacillary angiomatosis, 369, 370f
bacterial diseases, 257–266
    botryomycosis, 258, 258f
    bullous impetigo, 258, 258f
    chancroid, 260, 260f
    ecthyma granulosum, 259, 259f
    erythrasma, 259, 259f
    granuloma inguinale, 260, 260f
    impetigo, 257, 257f
    leprosy *see* leprosy
    pitted keratolysis, 258, 258f
    rhinoscleroderma, 260, 260f
    suppurative folliculitis, 258
    tuberculosis, 266, 266f
bacterial histochemical stains, 21, 22f
    see also specific stains
balanitis, Zoon's, 158, 159f
balding
    androgenetic *see* pattern alopecia (androgenetic balding)
    see alopecia
balloon cell nevus, 109, 110f
ballooning degeneration
    definition, 2
    herpes simplex virus infection, 2f
BANGLE mnemonic, 88, 342
Bannayan–Zonana syndrome, 341

basal cell carcinoma (BCC), 64–68, 73t, 74f
    adenoid, 68, 68f
    Ber-EP4, 26f
    differential diagnosis, 67
    fibroepithelioma of Pinkus, 68, 68f
    infiltrative, 67, 67f
    infundibulocystic, 67, 67f
    micronodular, 65, 65f
    morpheaform, 66–67, 66f, 75t, 77f, 94t
    nodular, 65, 65f
    superficial multifocal, 64, 64f
Bateman's purpura, 206
Bazin, erythema induratum of, 253, 253f
BCC see basal cell carcinoma (BCC)
B cell(s), 17
B-cell lymphoblastic lymphoma/leukemia, 414
B-cell lymphoma, 404–415
    cutaneous diffuse large, leg type, 409, 409f–410f
    cutaneous diffuse large, other than leg type, 410, 411f
    cutaneous disorders see cutaneous B-cell lymphoproliferative disorders
    lymphomatoid granulomatosis see lymphomatoid granulomatosis
BCL2, 33, 33t
    cutaneous diffuse large B-cell lymphoma leg type, 409
    seborrheic keratoses, 37
BCL6, 33t
Becker's nevi, 347
Bedlar tumor, 334f
benign acanthomas see acanthoma(s)
benign fibrous papule, solitary angiofibroma, 326–327, 326f
benign lichenoid keratosis, 137, 137f, 141–144, 142f
benign melanocytic nevus, 105–124, 106f–107f, 109t
benign symmetric lipomatosis, 341
Ber-EP4, 25
    basal cell carcinoma, 26f
BerH2 see CD30 (Kl-1, BerH2)
BetaF1, 34
"big 5" pattern, 425
    Churg–Strauss syndrome, 189
    medium vessel vasculitis, 187, 187f
Birbeck granules, 179
Birt–Hogg–Dubé syndrome, 78
bites
    insects, 203, 203f
    spiders, 307
    ticks, 305f–306f, 306–307
Blashkoid epidermolytic hyperkeratosis, 49
blastic plasmacytoid dendritic cell neoplasm, 397f, 401
blastomycosis, 274, 275f
    keloidal, 277, 277f
    South American, 276, 276f
bleomycin reactions, 215
blistering diseases see vesiculobullous disorders
Bloch–Sulzberger syndrome see incontinentia pigmenti (Bloch–Sulzberger syndrome)
blue nevus, 120, 120f
    cellular, 120, 121f
    common, 120
    epithelioid, 120, 122f
    HMB-45, 28f
bone tumors, 341–353
    accessory tragus, 350, 350f
    chondroma, 350, 350f
    chordoma, 351, 351f
    osteoma cutis, 349, 349f
    pseudocyst of the auricle, 351, 351f
    relapsing polychondritis, 349–353, 350f
    subungual exostosis, 352, 353f
Borrelia burgdorferi infection, 221
botryomycosis, 258, 258f
Bowenoid actinic keratosis, 57, 57f
Bowenoid papulosis, 289, 289f
Bowen's disease, 42, 42f, 58, 58f–60f
    anaplasia, 1f
    cell markers, 34t
    clear cell change, 60f
    clonal, 42f
    Paget's disease vs., 69
branchial cleft cyst, 52, 53f
branching alveolar mixed tumor, 96, 97f
breast carcinoma metastases, 416–417, 416f
    alopecia neoplastica, 417
    carcinoma en cuirasse, 416, 416f
    cell markers, 422t
    CK7, 24f
    inflammatory carcinoma, 417, 417f
bronchogenic cysts, 53, 53f
Brown–Hopps stain, 21
Buerger's disease, 187, 187f
bulb, hair anatomy, 13, 14f
bullous congenital ichthyosiform erythroderma, 211–212, 212f
bullous dermatosis, linear IgA, 170, 170f
bullous impetigo, 258, 258f
bullous lupus erythematosus, 171, 171f
bullous pemphigoid, 168–169, 169f
bullous pemphigoid antigen I
    bullous pemphigoid, 169
    paraneoplastic pemphigus, 166
bullous pemphigoid antigen II, 169
bullous tinea, 271, 271f
Burkitt lymphoma, 414
Buschke–Ollendorf syndrome, 222
Buschke, scleroderma of, 224, 224f

C

calcification
    cutaneous, 229–230
        see also specific diseases/disorders
    metastatic, 229
    subepidermal nodules, 229, 229f
calcifying aponeurotic fibroma, 329, 330f
calcifying epithelioma of Malherbe see pilomatricoma (calcifying epithelioma of Malherbe)
calcinosis, scrotal, 229–230, 230f
calciphylaxis, 229, 229f
calcium, histochemical stains, 21
calcyclin see S100A6 (calcyclin)
CALLA see CD10 (CALLA)
CAM5.2, 24
candidiasis, 272, 272f
carbohydrate stains, 19–20
carcinoembryonic antigen (CEA), 25, 34t
    Paget's disease, 25f, 58
carcinoma
    adenoid cystic, 103, 103f
    basal cell see basal cell carcinoma (BCC)
    follicular thyroid, 420f
    lung metastases see lung carcinoma metastases
    lymphoepithelioma-like, 70, 70f
    microcystic adnexal, 75t, 93–94, 93f, 94t
    mucinous, 91, 91f
    pancreatic, 422t
    papillary thyroid, 420f

pilomatrical, 72, 72f
primary neuroendocrine *see* Merkel cell carcinoma
renal cells, 25
signet-ring, 420
trabecular *see* Merkel cell carcinoma
urinary tract, 422t
verrucous, 61, 62f
carcinoma en cuirasse, 416, 416f
carcinoma erysipelatoides, 417, 417f
cartilaginous rest, 350, 350f
Castleman's disease, 376
catagen follicle, apoptosis, 2f
caterpillar bodies
definition, 2
porphyria cutanea tarda, 167f
CCCA (central cictricial alopecia), 244
CD1a, 33
Langerhans cell histiocytosis, 33f
CD2, 397
CD3, 31
adult T-cell leukemia/lymphoma, 393
patch stage mycosis fungoides, 390
subcutaneous T-cell lymphoma, 31f
CD4, 31
adult T-cell leukemia/lymphoma, 393
blastic plasmacytoid dendritic cell neoplasm, 401
mycosis fungoides, 31f
patch stage mycosis fungoides, 390
CD5, 31
chronic lymphocytic leukemia/small lymphocytic leukemia, 413
CD7, 32
mycosis fungoides, 32f
CD8, 31
CD10 (CALLA), 30, 33t
atypical fibroxanthoma, 30f
primary cutaneous follicle center cell lymphoma, 406
spindle cell neoplasms, 34t
CD19, 413
CD20, 30
chronic lymphocytic leukemia/small lymphocytic leukemia, 413
cutaneous diffuse large B-cell lymphoma leg type, 409
intravascular large B-cell lymphoma, 412
intravascular lymphoma, 30f
lymphomatoid granulomatosis, 413
primary cutaneous follicle center cell lymphoma, 406
CD21, 34
CD23, 413
CD25, 393
CD30 (Kl-1, BerH2), 31
anaplastic large cell lymphoma, 31f
tumor stage mycosis fungoides, 391
CD31, 27
angiosarcoma, 27f, 383
CD34, 26
angiosarcoma, 383
dermatofibroma, 309
dermatofibrosarcoma protuberans, 26f
interstitial dermis of morphea, 27f
morphea/scleroderma, 216f
CD43 (Leu-22), 33
chronic lymphocytic leukemia/small lymphocytic leukemia, 413
myeloid leukemia, 402
CD45Ra *see* LCA (CD45Ra)
CD45Ro (UCHL-1), 30
CD56, 32
blastic plasmacytoid dendritic cell neoplasm, 401
extranodal NK/T-cell lymphoma, nasal-type, 397

CD68 (KP-1), 32
granuloma annulare, 32f
CD79a, 31
cutaneous diffuse large B-cell lymphoma leg type, 409
intravascular large B-cell lymphoma, 412
primary cutaneous follicle center cell lymphoma, 406
CD117 (c-Kit), 32
mastocytosis, 210
urticaria pigmentosa, 33f
CD123, 32
blastic plasmacytoid dendritic cell neoplasm, 401
CD138 (syndecan-1), 31
plasmacytoma, 31f
CD163, 32
CD207 (langerin), 33
CDX2, 25
metastatic colon carcinoma, 25f
CEA *see* carcinoembryonic antigen (CEA)
cellular blue nevus, 120, 121f
cellular neurothekeoma, 362, 362f
cellulitis
dissecting, 244
eosinophilic, 199–200, 200f
central cictricial alopecia (CCCA), 244
chancroid, 260
Chapel Hill criteria
Churg–Strauss syndrome, 190
drug induced leukocytoclastic vasculitis, 193
giant cell arteritis, 184
Henoch–Schönlein purpura, 191
idiopathic leukocytoclastic vasculitis, 193
Kawasaki disease, 196
microscopic polyangiitis, 190
mixed cryoglobulin disease, 193
polyarteritis nodosa, 186
Takayasu arteritis, 185
Wegener's granulomatosis, 188
cherry angioma, 369, 370f
chicken pox, 292
cholesterol embolization, 204, 204f
chondrodermatitis nodularis helicis, 221, 221f, 245
chondroid syringoma, 96, 96f–97f
malignant, 97, 97f
chondroma, 350, 350f
chordoma, 351, 351f
chromoblastomycosis *see* chromomycosis
chromogranin, 30
chromomycosis, 282, 282f
Medlar body, 7f
chronic dermatitis, 157, 157f
pityriasis rosea, 157, 157f
radiation dermatitis, 213, 214f, 214t
spongiotic dermatitis with intraepidermal eosinophils, 158
spongiotic pigmented purpuric eruption, 157, 157f
stasis dermatitis, 157, 158f
Zoon's balanitis, 158, 159f
chronic discoid lupus erythematosus, 143f
chronic lymphocytic leukemia (CLL), 413, 413f
chronic urticaria, 199f
Churg–Strauss syndrome, 188–190, 189f
medium vessel vasculitis, 187
cicatricial alopecia, 239–244
lupus erythematosus, 239–241, 240f
cicatricial pemphigoid, 169, 169f
ciliated cyst, cutaneous, 54, 54f

Civatte bodies
　　definition, 2
　　lichenoid interface dermatitis, 134
　　lichen planus, 2f
CK7, 24, 24t, 34t
　　metastatic breast carcinoma, 24f
CK20, 24, 24t
　　Merkel cell carcinoma, 24f
　　small blue cell tumors, 34t
c-KIT see CD117 (c-Kit)
CK polyclonal keratin (pankeratin), 24
CLATS mnemonic, 277, 425
claudin-1, 364
clear cell acanthoma, 45
clear cell changes, Bowen's disease, 60f
clear cell hidradenoma, 100, 100f
clear cell sarcoma, 132, 132f
clear cell syringoma, 91, 92f
CLL (chronic lymphocytic leukemia), 413, 413f
clonal Bowen's disease, 42f
clonal seborrheic keratoses, 41–42, 41f–42f
　　inflamed, 42f
　　irritated, 41f–42f
coagulopathy
　　Kasabach–Merritt, 378
　　occlusive vascular disease, 206
coccidiomycosis, 273, 273f
Cokeromyces infection, 282
collagen, alterations in, 213–223
　　see also specific diseases/disorders
collagen entrapment
　　definition, 3
　　dermatofibroma, 3f
collagenoma, 222, 223f
collagenosis, reactive perforating, 218, 218f
colloidal iron, 19
　　focal mucinosis, 19f, 227f
colloid bodies see Civatte bodies
colloid milium, 222, 222f, 231, 231f
colon carcinoma metastases, 419, 419f
　　CDX2, 25f
　　cell markers, 422t
combined nevus, 123
common blue nevus, 120
common epidermal nevus, 48
condyloma acuminatum, 288, 288f
congenital nevus, 111, 111f
Congo red, 20
　　nodular amyloidosis, 228f
　　salivary gland, 20f
Conidiobolus coronatus infection, 282
connective tissue nevus, 222
connective tissue stains, 18
coronoid lamellae
　　definition, 3
　　porokeratosis, 3f
corps rond
　　Darier's disease, 3f
　　definition, 3
Corynebacterium infection, 258
Cowden's syndrome, 341
Cowdry A bodies, 3
Cowdry B bodies, 3
cranial fasciitis, 329
crust, 3
cryoglobulinemia type I, 204, 204f
cryptococcosis, 274, 274f

Cryptococcus, 20f
crystal violet, 20
　　amyloidosis, 227
Cunninghamella infection, 282
cutaneous B-cell lymphoproliferative disorders, 404–412
　　classification, 404
　　cutaneous diffuse large B-cell lymphoma leg type, 409, 409f–410f
　　cutaneous diffuse large B-cell lymphoma, other than leg type, 410, 411f
　　intravascular large B-cell lymphoma, 412, 412f
　　primary cutaneous follicle center cell lymphoma, 406, 406f–408f
　　primary cutaneous marginal zone lymphoma, 404, 405f
　　see also specific diseases/disorders
cutaneous calcification, 229–230
　　see also specific diseases/disorders
cutaneous ciliated cyst, 54, 54f
cutaneous diffuse large B-cell lymphoma leg type, 409, 409f–410f
cutaneous diffuse large B-cell lymphoma, other than leg type, 410, 411f
cutaneous gamma/delta T-cell lymphoma, 399, 399f
cutaneous ganglioneuroma, 363, 363f
cutaneous primary lymphomas see under primary
cutaneous T-cell lymphoma, 239, 239f, 390–403, 392f
　　adult T-cell leukemia/lymphoma, 393–394, 393f–394f
　　blastic plasmacytoid dendritic cell neoplasm, 397f, 401
　　cutaneous gamma/delta T-cell lymphoma, 399, 399f
　　extranodal NK/T-cell lymphoma, nasal-type, 397–398, 397f–398f
　　hydroa vacciniforme-like T-cell lymphoma, 400, 400f–401f
　　mycosis fungoides see mycosis fungoides
　　precursor hematologic neoplasms, 401
　　primary cutaneous aggressive epidermotropic CD8+ cytotoxic T-cell lymphoma, 398, 398f
　　primary cutaneous CD4+ small/medium T-cell lymphoma, 399–400, 400f
　　primary cutaneous CD30+ lymphoproliferative disorders see primary cutaneous CD30+ lymphoproliferative disorders
　　Sézary syndrome, 393, 393f
　　subcutaneous panniculitis-like T-cell lymphoma, 396, 397f
cuticle, nail anatomy, 15
cylindroma, 86, 86f, 88t
cyst(s), 49–55
　　branchial cleft cyst, 52, 53f
　　bronchogenic cysts, 53, 53f
　　cutaneous ciliated cyst, 54, 54f
　　dermoid cysts, 50, 50f
　　digital myxoid cyst, 227f
　　epidermoid cysts see epidermoid cysts
　　median raphe cyst, 54, 54f
　　pilar cysts see pilar cysts
　　proliferating pilar, 51–52, 51f–52f
　　pseudohorn see pseudohorn cyst
　　steatocystoma, 53, 54f
　　thyroglossal duct cyst, 55, 55f
　　thyroglossal ducts, 55
　　vellus hair cysts, 50, 50f
　　verrucous, 290, 291f
cysticercosis, 301f
cystic papilloma, 290, 291f
cytokeratin 7, 422t
cytokeratin 20, 422t
cytomegalovirus infection, 295, 295f
cytophagic histiocytic panniculitis, 254, 255f

D

D2–40 (podoplanin), 27
　　angiosarcoma, 383
　　melanoma, 27f

Darier's disease (keratosis follicularis), 165, 165f
    corps rond, 3f
    grains, 3f
Darier's sign, 210
deep penetrating nevus, 120, 122f
Degos disease, 202, 203f
dendritic "equine-type" melanomas, 120
dendrocytes, dermal, 16
Dercum's disease, 341
dermal dendrocytes, 16
dermal duct tumor, 99, 99f
dermal hypoplasia, focal, 353, 353f
dermal leiomyosarcoma, 348
dermatitis
    acute spongiform, 155, 155f
    chronic radiation, 213, 214f, 214t
    interface *see* interface dermatitis
    lichenoid interface *see* lichenoid interface dermatitis
    patch stage mycosis fungoides *vs.*, 391
    seborrheic, 156
    spongiotic *see* spongiotic dermatitis
    stasis, 157, 158f
    vacuolar interface, 134–135, 139
dermatitis herpetiformis, 170, 170f
dermatofibroma, 309–311, 310f
    adult myofibroma, 311–312, 312f
    aneurysmal, 310, 310f
    CD34, 309
    collagen entrapment, 3f
    dermatomyofibroma, 312, 313f–314f
    factor VIIIa, 27f, 309
    fibromatosis, 315
    fibrous histiocytoma, 310, 311f
    immunostaining, 309
    infantile myofibromatosis, 316, 317f
    juvenile hyaline fibromatosis, 318, 318f
    lipidized siderophages, 309
    monster cells, 311, 311f
dermatofibrosarcoma protuberans, 332–334, 333f
    CD34, 26f
    diffuse neurofibroma, 354
dermatomyofibroma, 312, 313f–314f
dermatomyositis, 145
    lupus erythematosus *vs.*, 144
dermatoses
    acute febrile neutrophilic, 197, 198f
    neutrophilic, 197–199
    nutritional, 232, 232f
    subcorneal pustular, 162, 162f
    transient acantholytic *see* transient acantholytic dermatosis (Grover's disease)
    see also specific diseases/disorders
dermoid cysts, 50
desmin, 26
    piloleiomyoma, 26f
    spindle cell neoplasms, 34t
desmoglein 1
    paraneoplastic pemphigus, 166
    pemphigus foliaceus, 161
desmoglein 3
    paraneoplastic pemphigus, 166
    pemphigus vulgaris, 163
desmoid tumors, 331, 331f
desmoplakin, 166
desmoplastic melanoma, 123, 127t, 129
    P75, 29f
    Sox-10, 29f

desmoplastic trichilemmoma, 81, 81f
desmoplastic trichoepithelioma, 75, 75t, 76f, 94t
desmosome, 426, 426f
diabetes mellitus type 2, 224
Dieterle stain, 23
diffuse neurofibroma, 354
digital fibrokeratoma, acquired, 327, 359
digital myxoid cyst, 227f
dilated pore of Winer, 79, 79f
direct immunofluorescence
    bullous pemphigoid, 169f
    dermatitis herpetiformis, 170f
    pemphigus vulgaris, 163f
dirofilariasis, 303–304
discoid lupus erythematosus, 241t
    chronic, 143f
dissecting cellulitis, 244
Donovan body, 3
Dowling–Degos disease, 41, 41f
drug eruptions
    lupus erythematosus *vs.*, 144
    morbiliform, 202
drug induced leukocytoclastic vasculitis, 193
Dupuytren's contracture, 315, 315f
Dutcher bodies, 404
    definition, 3
dyskeratosis, 3
dysplastic nevus, 123, 124f

E

ear, skin, 11f
early-patch stage Kaposi's sarcoma, 385, 386f–387f
EBA (epidermolysis bullosa acquisita), 168, 168f
EBV *see* Epstein–Barr virus (EBV)
eccrine angiomatous hamartoma, 103, 375, 376f
eccrine glands, 12f
eccrine hidradenitis, neutrophilic, 246, 246f
eczematous purpura, 200
EDV (epidermodysplasia verruciformis), 287
EED (erythema elevatum diutinum), 194, 195f–196f
effacement, 3
EI (erythema induratum) of Bazin, 253, 253f
elastic tapping, pseudoepitheliomatous hyperplasia, 8f
elastin, alterations in, 213–223
    see also specific diseases/disorders
elastofibroma dorsi, 322, 323f
    Verhoeff–Van Gieson stain, 18f
elastoma, 222
elastosis perforans serpiginosa, 217–218, 217f
electron microscopy, transport media, 35
elephantiasis, 302, 302f
EMA *see* epithelial membrane antigen (EMA)
encapsulated fat necrosis, 352
endometriosis, metastatic tumors *vs.*, 423, 423f
endoplakin, 166
entomophthorales infection (entomophthoromycosis), 282
entomophthoromycosis, 282
EORTC (European Organisation for Research and Treatment of Cancer), cutaneous B-cell lymphoproliferative disorder classification, 404
eosinophil(s), 17, 427, 427f
    hypersensitivity, 17f
eosinophilic cellulitis, 199–200, 200f
eosinophilic fasciitis, 216–217, 216f–217f
eosinophilic granuloma, 179
eosinophilic panniculitis, 252, 252f

eosinophilic spongiosis
    definition, 3
    incontinentia pigmenti, 3f
epidermal (keratin)-derived amyloidosis, 227
epidermal hyperplasia, lentiginous, 6
epidermal inclusion cysts *see* epidermoid cysts
epidermal nevus, 48–49
    common, 48
    inflammatory linear verrucous, 48–49, 49f, 152, 152f
epidermal transglutaminase-3, 170
epidermis
    benign tumors, 37–55
    cysts, 37–55
    malignant tumors, 56–70
        see also actinic keratosis; basal cell carcinoma (BCC); Bowen's disease; keratoacanthoma; squamous cell carcinoma (SCC)
epidermodysplasia verruciformis (EDV), 287
epidermoid cysts, 49, 49f
    with pilomatrical differentiation, 50, 50f
epidermoid keratinization, nail, 16
epidermolysis bullosa acquisita (EBA), 168, 168f
epidermolytic acanthoma, 48, 48f
epidermolytic hyperkeratosis, 4f
    Blashkoid, 49
    definition, 4
epidermolytic ichthyosis, 211–212, 212f
epidermotropism
    definition, 4
    mycosis fungoides, 4f
epithelial markers, 23–25
    see also specific markers
epithelial membrane antigen (EMA), 25, 364
    epithelioma, 25f
epithelioid blue nevus, 120, 122f
epithelioid hemangioendothelioma, 382f
epithelioid sarcoma, 338, 338f–339f
epithelioma
    calcifying of Malherbe *see* pilomatricoma (calcifying epithelioma of Malherbe)
    epithelial membrane antigen, 25f
EPP (erythropoietic protoporphyria), 231, 231f
Epstein–Barr virus (EBV)
    extranodal NK/T-cell lymphoma, nasal-type, 397
    hydroa vacciniforme-like T-cell lymphoma, 400
    lymphomatoid granulomatosis, 413
    lymphomatoid papulosis type E, 395
erosion, 4
eruptive xanthoma, 181, 181f
erythema
    gyrate, 201, 201f
    necrolysing migratory, 154f, 232
erythema annulare centrifugum, 201, 201f
erythema elevatum diutinum (EED), 194, 195f–196f
erythema induratum (EI) of Bazin, 253, 253f
erythema marginatum, 201
erythema migrans, 268
erythema multiforme, 146, 146f
erythema nodosum, 249, 250f
erythema nodosum leprosum, 262, 263f
erythrasma, 259, 259f
erythropoietic protoporphyria (EPP), 231, 231f
eumycetomas, 278–279, 279f, 279t
European Organisation for Research and Treatment of Cancer (EORTC), cutaneous B-cell lymphoproliferative disorder classification, 404
exanthematous pustulosis, acute generalized, 162, 162f
exocytosis, 4

exostosis, subungual, 352, 353f
extranodal NK/T-cell lymphoma, nasal-type, 397–398, 397f–398f
eyelid, skin, 10f–11f

F

face
    anatomy, 10
    fibrous papule, 326–327, 326f
    sun-damaged skin, 10f
factor VIIIa, 27
    angiosarcoma, 383
    dermatofibroma, 27f, 309
familial benign chronic pemphigus (Hailey–Hailey disease), 164, 164f
familial multiple lipomatosis, 341
fasciitis
    cranial, 329
    eosinophilic, 216–217, 216f–217f
    nodular, 327–329, 327f–328f
    proliferative, 329, 329f
fat necrosis
    encapsulated, 352
    newborn subcutaneous, 251, 252f
    nodular-cystic, 352
fat tumors, 341–353
    focal dermal hypoplasia, 353, 353f
    hibernoma, 346, 346f
    mobile encapsulated lipoma, 352, 352f
    nevus lipomatosis superficialis of Hoffmann and Zurhelle, 347
Favre–Racouchot syndrome, 220, 220f
febrile neutrophilic dermatoses, acute, 197, 198f
festooning, 4
fetus, skin anatomy, 12, 12f–13f
fibroblastoma, giant cell, 334, 334f–335f
fibroepithelioma, Pinkus', 68, 68f
fibroepithelioma of Pinkus, 68, 68f
fibrofolliculoma, 78, 78f
fibrokeratoma, acquired digital, 327, 359
fibrolipoma, 344, 344f
fibroma
    calcifying aponeurotic, 329, 330f
    inclusion body, 321, 321f
    infantile digital, 321, 321f
    pleomorphic, 325, 325f
    sclerotic, 323, 324f
    of the tendon sheath, 322, 322f
fibromatosis, 315
    aggressive, 331, 331f
    juvenile hyaline, 318, 318f
    plantar, 315
fibrosarcoma, 335
fibrous hamartoma of infancy, 319, 320f
fibrous histiocytoma, 310, 311f
fibrous papule of the face, 326–327, 326f
fibrous tumors, 309–340
    angiofibromas *see* angiofibromas
    borderline tumors, 331–332
        see also specific diseases/disorders
    calcifying aponeurotic fibroma, 329, 330f
    dermatofibroma *see* dermatofibroma
    desmoid tumors, 331, 331f
    elastofibroma dorsi, 322, 323f
    fibroma of the tendon sheath, 322, 322f
    fibrous hamartoma of infancy, 319, 320f
    giant cell tumor of the tendon sheath, 321–322, 321f
    infantile digital fibroma, 321, 321f
    malignant *see below*
    nodular fasciitis, 327–329, 327f–328f

pleomorphic fibroma, 325, 325f
plexiform fibrohistiocytic tumor, 331–332, 331f–332f
scars *see* scars
sclerosing perineurioma, 325, 325f
sclerotic fibroma, 323, 324f
fibrous tumors, malignant, 332–338
    atypical fibroxanthoma, 337, 337f
    dermatofibrosarcoma protuberans, 332–334, 333f
    epithelioid sarcoma, 338, 338f–339f
    fibrosarcoma, 335, 335f–336f
    giant cell fibroblastoma, 334, 334f–335f
    pleomorphic undifferentiated sarcoma, 338
fibroxanthoma, atypical *see* atypical fibroxanthoma (AFX)
Fite acid-fast stain
    mycobacteria, 22
    Nocardia, 22f
fixed drug eruption, interface dermatitis, 147, 148f
flag sign, actinic keratosis, 56
flame figure, 4
flat warts, 287, 287f
fluke infections, 299–304
    see also specific diseases/disorders
foam cells
    definition, 5
    verruciform xanthoma, 5f
focal dermal hypoplasia, 353, 353f
focal mucinosis, 227, 227f
    colloidal iron, 19f
follicular keratosis, inverted, 46, 46f
follicular mucinosis
    alopecia mucinosis, 5f
    definition, 5
follicular thyroid carcinoma, 420f
folliculitis
    Majocchi's fungal, 239, 240f
    suppurative, 258
folliculitis decalvans, 244, 244f
folliculotropic mycosis fungoides, 239, 239f, 392, 392f
Fontane–Masson melanin stain, 21
    phaeohyphomycosis, 280
    vitiligo, 21f
fungal histochemical stains, 22
fungal infections, 270–285
    actinomycetomas, 279, 279f, 279t
    African histoplasmosis, 277, 277f
    aspergillosis, 283, 283f
    blastomycosis, 274, 275f
    candidiasis, 272, 272f
    chromomycosis, 282, 282f
    coccidiomycosis, 273, 273f
    cryptococcosis, 274, 274f
    entomophthorales infection, 282
    eumycetomas, 278–279, 279f, 279t
    fusariosis, 283, 283f
    histoplasmosis, 276–277, 276f
    hyalohyphomycosis, 283
    lobomycosis, 277, 277f
    Majocchi's folliculitis, 239, 240f
    mucorales, 282
    mycetomas, 278–279
    onychomycosis, 271, 271f
    paracoccidioides infection, 276, 276f
    phaeohyphomycosis, 280, 281f
    protothecosis, 284, 284f
    rhinosporidiosis, 284–285, 285f
    sporotrichosis, 277–278, 278f
    tinea, 270–271, 270f
    tinea nigra, 280, 280f
    tinea versicolor, 271f
    zygomycosis, 282
fusariosis, 283, 283f

G

ganglioneuroma, cutaneous, 363, 363f
Gardner's syndrome, 341
gastrointestinal tumors, cell markers, 422t
generalized exanthematous pustulosis, acute, 162, 162f
genital nevus, 116f
genodermatoses, 208–212
    pseudoxanthoma elasticum, 208, 208f
GFAP, 364
Gianotti–Crosti syndrome, 299
giant cell(s), 16, 16f
    osteoclast-like, 16f
    Touton giant, 176
giant cell arteritis, 183–184, 184f–185f
giant cell fibroblastoma, 334, 334f–335f
giant cell tumor of the tendon sheath, 321–322, 321f
Giemsa stain, 23
    mastocytosis, 210
    urticaria pigmentosa, 23f
glial heterotropia, 364, 364f
glioma, nasal, 364, 364f
glomangioma, 367, 368f–369f
glomeruloid hemangioma, 376, 376f
glomus tumor, 367, 368f
    glomangioma, 367, 368f–369f
glossary, 1–10
glucagonoma syndrome, 232
GLUT1, 27
    infantile hemangioma, 28f, 371
    perineurioma, 364
GMS (Grocott's methenamine silver), 22
    Aspergillus, 22f
Goltz syndrome, 353, 353f
    nevus lipomatosis superficialis of Hoffmann and Zurhelle, 347
Gougerot–Blum purpura, 200
gout, 230, 230f
    palisading, 7f
graft-versus-host disease
    interface dermatitis, 147, 148f
    lichenoid, 137, 137f
grains
    Darier's disease, 3f
    definition, 3
granular cell tumor, 360–361, 360f–361f
    S100, 28f
granular parakeratosis, 154, 154f
granuloma(s)
    actinic, 173, 174f
    annulare *see* granuloma annulare
    categorization, 172
    definition, 172
    eosinophilic, 179
    pyogenic, 369, 369f
    reticulohistiocytic, 177–178, 178f
    sarcoid, 5f
granuloma annulare, 172–173, 172t
    differential diagnosis, 172–173
    interstitial, 172, 173f
    palisading, 172, 173f
    subcutaneous tissue, 172
granuloma faciale, 193–194, 194f
granuloma inguinale, 260, 260f

granulomatosis
    lymphomatoid *see* lymphomatoid granulomatosis
    Wegener's *see* Wegener's granulomatosis
granulomatous, 5
granulomatous diseases, 172–182
    see also specific diseases/disorders
granulomatous panniculitis, 253
granulomatous slack skin, mycosis fungoides, 392–393, 392f–393f
Grenz zone
    cutaneous diffuse large B-cell lymphoma leg type, 409
    definition, 5
Grocott's methenamine silver *see* GMS (Grocott's methenamine silver)
Grover's disease *see* transient acantholytic dermatosis (Grover's disease)
Guarnieri body, 5
guttate psoriasis, 150, 152f
gyrate erythema, 201, 201f

H

HAAPPIE mnemonic, 210
Hailey–Hailey disease, 164, 164f
hair anatomy, 12–13, 14f–15f
    Adamson's fringe, 13
    bulb, 13, 14f
    infundibulum, 12
    isthmus, 13
    stem, 13
halo nevus, 117, 118f
    Mart-1, 29f
hamartoma
    basaloid follicular, 79, 79f
    eccrine angiomatous, 103, 375, 376f
    fibrous hamartoma of infancy, 319, 320f
    smooth muscle *see* smooth muscle hamartoma
Hame figure, Wells' syndrome, 4f
hand, foot and mouth syndrome, 299, 299f
Hand–Schüller–Christian disease, 179
HAP (hidradenoma papilliferum), 89, 89f
Heck's disease, 290, 290f
helminth infections
    flatworms, 300
    roundworms, 299–304
hemangioendothelioma
    epithelioid, 382f
    Kaposiform, 378, 378f–379f
    retiform, 383, 383f
    spindle cell, 380, 381f
hemangioma
    arteriovenous, 373, 374f
    glomeruloid, 376, 376f
    hobnail, 374, 374f–375f
    infantile *see* infantile hemangioma
    microvenular, 377, 377f
    sclerosing, 310, 310f
    spindle cell, 380, 381f
    targetoid hemosiderotic, 374, 374f–375f
hemangiopericytoma, 380, 380f
hematopoietic markers, 30–34
hemosiderotic hemangioma, targetoid, 374, 374f–375f
Henderson–Paterson body, 5
Henoch–Schönlein purpura, 191, 192f–193f
"Here comes the big green leafy veggies" mnemonic, 260, 274
herpes gestationis, 169
herpes simplex virus infection, 292, 292f
    ballooning degeneration, 2f

herpes zoster, 292, 293f–294f
herpetic infections, 292–295
    chicken pox, 292
    herpes simplex virus infection *see* herpes simplex virus infection
    herpes zoster, 292, 293f–294f
    verrucous VZV infections, 294, 294f
    see also specific diseases/disorders
HHV8 (human herpesvirus-8), 34f
hibernoma, 346, 346f
hidradenitis suppurativa, 247, 247f
hidradenoma
    clear cell, 100, 100f
    nodular, 100, 100f
hidradenoma papilliferum (HAP), 89, 89f
hidroacanthoma simplex, 42, 42f, 99, 99f
hidrocystoma, 95, 95f
histiocytes, 16
    diseases of, 172–182
        see also specific diseases/disorders
    see also granuloma(s)
histiocytic panniculitis, cytophagic, 254, 255f
histiocytoma, fibrous, 310, 311f
histiocytosis X *see* Langerhans cell histiocytosis (histiocytosis X)
histochemical stains, 18–23
    amyloid, 20
    bacteria, 21, 22f
    calcium, 21
    carbohydrate stains, 19–20
    connective tissue stains, 18
    fungi, 22
    iron, 20
    lipids, 21
    mast cell stains, 18–19
    melanin, 21
    mycobacteria, 22–23
    spirochetes, 23
    see also specific stains
histoid leprosy, 262, 262f
histoplasmosis, 276–277, 276f
    African, 277, 277f
HIV infection, verrucous VZV infections, 294
HMB-45, 28
    benign melanocytic nevus, 105–109
    blue nevus, 28f
    Spitz nevus, 113f
hobnail hemangioma, 374, 374f–375f
Hoffmann, nevus lipomatosis superficialis of, 347
homogentistic oxidase deficiency, 221
HPV-1 (human papillomavirus 1), myrmecia, 287
HPV-13, 290
HPV-32, 290
HTLV-1 (human T-cell leukemia virus type 1), adult T-cell leukemia/lymphoma, 393
human herpesvirus-8 (HHV8), 34f
human papillomavirus(es), 290
human papillomavirus 1 (HPV-1), myrmecia, 287
human T-cell leukemia virus type 1 (HTLV-1), adult T-cell leukemia/lymphoma, 393
hyaline fibromatosis, juvenile, 318, 318f
hyalinosis cutis et mucosae, 212, 212f, 231, 231f–232f
hyalohyphomycosis, 283
hydroa vacciniforme-like T-cell lymphoma, 400, 400f–401f
hypergranulosis
    definition, 5
    keratoacanthoma, 62
    lichen planus, 5f

hyperkeratosis
    Blashkoid epidermolytic, 49
    epidermolytic *see* epidermolytic hyperkeratosis
    seborrheic keratoses, 39, 39f–40f
hyperkeratotic seborrheic keratoses, inflamed, 40f
hyperpigmentation, 6
hyperplasia
    lentiginous epidermal, 6
    sebaceous, 82, 82f
hypersensitivity, eosinophils, 17f
hypertrophic actinic keratosis, 57, 57f
hypertrophic lupus erythematosus, 138, 138f
hypertrophic scars, 219, 219f, 319, 319f
hypogranulosis
    definition, 5
    lichen planus, 5f
hyponychium, nail anatomy, 15
hypopigmentation, 6
hypoplasia, focal dermal, 353, 353f

I

ichthyosis, epidermolytic, 211–212, 212f
ichthyosis vulgaris, 208–209, 209f
idiopathic leukocytoclastic vasculitis, 193
idiopathic pseudopelade, 243, 243f
IFK (inverted follicular keratosis), 46, 46f
IgA bullous dermatosis, linear, 170, 170f
immunofluorescence
    direct *see* direct immunofluorescence
    transport media, 35
immunoglobulin G lambda gammopathy, scleromyxedema, 225
immunohistochemical stains, 23
    dermatofibroma, 309
    epithelial markers, 23–25
    hematopoietic markers, 30–34
    infectious disease markers, 34
    mesenchymal markers, 26–28
    neuroectodermal markers, 28–29
    neuroendocrine markers, 29–30
    proliferation markers, 35
    Spitz nevus, 113f
        see also specific stains
impetigo, 257
    bullous, 258, 258f
inclusion body fibroma, 321, 321f
incontinentia pigmenti (Bloch–Sulzberger syndrome), 209–210
    eosinophilic spongiosis, 3f
    pigmented, 209, 210f
    verrucous, 209, 210f
    vesicular, 209, 209f
infantile digital fibroma, 321, 321f
infantile hemangioma, 371, 371f
    GLUT1, 28f
infantile myofibromatosis, 316, 317f
infectious disease markers, 34
infiltrative basal cell carcinoma, 67, 67f
inflamed acanthotic seborrheic keratoses, 39f
inflamed clonal seborrheic keratoses, 42f
inflamed hyperkeratotic seborrheic keratoses, 40f
inflamed seborrheic keratoses, 43–44, 43f–44f
inflammatory carcinoma, 417, 417f
inflammatory cells, 16–17
inflammatory linear verrucous epidermal nevus (IVEN), 48–49, 49f, 152, 152f
inflammatory nonscarring alopecia *see* alopecia, inflammatory nonscarring

inflammatory subepidermal vesiculobullous disorders, 168–171
    see also specific diseases/disorders
inflammatory vascular diseases, 183–207
    lymphoid vasculitis, 202–203
    non-inflammatory purpura, 206
    occlusive vascular disease, 204–206
    perivascular lymphoid infiltrates, 200–202
    see also specific diseases/disorders
infundibular cysts *see* epidermoid cysts
infundibulocystic basal cell carcinoma, 67, 67f
infundibulum, hair anatomy, 12
insects *see* arthropods (insects)
interface, 6
interface dermatitis, 134–149
    benign lichenoid keratosis, 137, 137f, 141–144, 142f
    dermatomyositis, 145, 145f
    erythema multiforme, 146, 146f
    fixed drug eruption, 147, 148f
    graft-versus-host disease, 147, 148f
    hypertrophic lupus erythematosus, 138, 138f
    late-phase, 135, 136f
    lichenoid *see* lichenoid interface dermatitis
    lichenoid drug eruption, 137, 137f
    lichenoid graft-versus-host disease, 137, 137f
    lichenoid regression of lentigo maligna, 138, 138f
    lichen planus *see* lichen planus
    lichen striatus, 144, 144f
    lupus erythematosus *see* lupus erythematosus
    mycosis fungoides, 139, 140f
    paraneoplastic pemphigus, 147, 147f
    pityriasis lichenoides chronica, 141, 142f
    pityriasis lichenoides et varioformis acuta, 141, 141f
    polymorphous light eruption, 144, 144f
    porokeratosis, 139, 139f
    spongiotic, lichenoid *vs.*, 134–135
    syphilis, 145, 145f
    toxic epidermal necrolysis, 147, 147f
    vacuolar, 134–135
    vacuolar interface dermatitis, 139
interstitial dermis of morphea, CD34, 27f
interstitial granuloma annulare, 172, 173f
intertriginous xanthomas, 180
intradermal Spitz nevus, 114f
intraepidermal porocarcinoma
    Bowen's disease *vs.*, 58
    Paget's disease *vs.*, 69
intraepidermal vesiculobullous disorders, 163–166
    see also specific diseases/disorders
intravascular large B-cell lymphoma, 412, 412f
intravascular lymphoma, CD20, 30f
intravascular papillary endothelial hyperplasia of Masson (IPEH), 373, 373f
inverted follicular keratosis (IFK), 46, 46f
IPEH (intravascular papillary endothelial hyperplasia of Masson), 373, 373f
iron, colloidal *see* colloidal iron
iron stains, 20
irritated acanthotic seborrheic keratoses, 38f–39f
irritated clonal seborrheic keratoses, 41f–42f
irritated seborrheic keratoses, 42–43, 43f
    squamous eddies, 9f
isthmus, hair anatomy, 13
isthmus catagen cysts *see* pilar cysts
Ito, nevus of, 124
"I vacuum dog pus" mnemonic, 228
IVEN (inflammatory linear verrucous epidermal nevus), 48–49, 49f, 152, 152f

J

Jadassohn, nevus sebaceus of, 81–82
Jadassohn–Pellizzari anetoderma, 222
Jadassohn, postpubertal nevus sebaceus of, 81–82, 81f
Jadassohn, prepubertal nevus sebaceus of, 82, 82f
junctional lentiginous nevus, 124, 124f
juvenile hyaline fibromatosis, 318, 318f

K

Kamino body
    definition, 6
    Spitz nevus, 6f
    trichome stain, 113f
Kaposiform hemangioendothelioma, 378, 378f–379f
Kaposi's sarcoma, 385–387
    early-patch stage, 385, 386f–387f
    late-patch/plaque, 387, 387f
    nodular, 366f, 387
    plaque, 387, 387f
Kappa, 32
karyorrhexis
    definition, 6
    leukocytoclastic vasculitis, 6f
Kasabach–Merritt coagulopathy, 378
Kawasaki disease, 196
keloid, 219–220, 219f, 319, 319f
keloidal blastomycosis, 277, 277f
keratin-derived amyloidosis, 227
keratinization
    epidermoid, 16
    nail anatomy, 16
    onchyolemmal, 16
keratoacanthoma, 62–63, 63f, 63t
    regressing, 63, 64f
keratolysis, pitted, 258, 258f
keratoses
    benign lichenoid, 137, 137f, 141–144, 142f
    inflamed acanthotic seborrheic, 39f
    inverted follicular, 46, 46f
    seborrheic *see* seborrheic keratoses
keratosis follicularis *see* Darier's disease (keratosis follicularis)
KI-1 *see* CD30 (KI-1, BerH2)
Kimura's disease, 371, 372f
Kinyoun's acid-fast stain, 22
Klebsiella rhinoscleromatis infection, 260
Kogoj, spongiform pustule of, 9
koilocytes, 6
KP-1 *see* CD68 (KP-1)
Kytococcus sedentarius infection, 258

L

Lambda, 32
Langerhans cell(s), 16, 16f, 426, 426f
Langerhans cell histiocytosis (histiocytosis X), 179, 179f
    acute, 245, 245f
    CD1a, 33f
langerin (CD207), 33
large B-cell lymphoma, 33f
large cell acanthoma, 45–46, 46f
large vessel vasculitis, 183–187
late-patch/plaque Kaposi's sarcoma, 387, 387f
late-phase (burnt-out) interface dermatitis, 135, 136f
LCA (CD45Ra), 30
    small blue cell tumors, 34t
Lederhose disease, 315, 316f
Leder stain (naphthol ASD chloroacetate esterase), 19
    mastocytosis, 210
    urticaria pigmentosa, 19f
leiomyoma, 347–348
    angioleiomyoma, 348, 348f
    leiomyosarcoma, 348, 348f–349f
    piloleiomyoma, 347, 347f
leiomyosarcoma, 348, 348f–349f
    cell markers, 34t
    dermal, 348
    subcutaneous, 348
    superficial, 348
Leishman–Donovan body
    definition, 6
    leishmaniasis, 6f
leishmaniasis, 268, 269f
    Leishman–Donovan body, 6f
LEMONS mnemonic, 360
lentiginous epidermal hyperplasia, 6
lentiginous melanocytic growth pattern, 6
lentigo maligna, 127t, 128, 128f
    lichenoid regression, 138, 138f
lentigo maligna melanoma, 127t, 129
lepromatous leprosy, 261, 261f
leprosy, 261–264
    erythema nodosum leprosum, 262, 263f
    histoid, 262, 262f
    lepromatous, 261, 261f
    Lucio's reaction, 264, 264f–265f
    reactions, 262–264, 262f
    tuberculoid, 262, 262f
Letterer–Siwe disease, 179
Leu-22 *see* CD43 (Leu-22)
leukemia
    acute myeloid, 402, 402f
    adult T-cell, 393–394, 393f–394f
    B-cell lymphoblastic l, 414
    chronic lymphocytic, 413, 413f
    myeloid, 402
    small lymphocytic3, 413, 413f
leukemia cutis, myeloperoxidase, 32f
leukocytoclasia, 6
leukocytoclastic vasculitis, 183–200, 183f
    classification, 183
    drug induced, 193
    idiopathic, 193
    karyorrhexis, 6f
    large vessel vasculitis, 183–187
    medium vessel vasculitis, 187–190
    small vessel vasculitis, 190–193
    unique forms, 193–196
        see also specific diseases/disorders
lichen amyloid, 228, 229f
    thioflavin T, 20f
lichenoid actinic keratosis, 57, 57f
lichenoid dermatitis, 6
lichenoid drug eruption, 137, 137f
    patch stage mycosis fungoides *vs.*, 391
lichenoid graft-versus-host disease, 137, 137f
lichenoid infiltrate, 6
lichenoid interface dermatitis, 134–135, 135f
    benign, 137, 137f, 141–144, 142f
    inflamed seborrheic keratoses with, 44f
    spongiotic *vs.*, 134–135
lichenoid keratosis, benign, 137, 137f, 141–144, 142f
lichenoid regression of lentigo maligna, 138, 138f
lichen planopilaris (LPP), 241, 241t, 242f

lichen planus, 136, 136f
  civatte/colloid bodies, 2f
  hypergranulosis, 5f
  hypogranulosis, 5f
lichen sclerosus (et atrophicus), 213, 213f, 214t
  morphea/scleroderma relationship, 214
lichen simplex chronicus *see* chronic dermatitis
lichen striatus, 144
  lupus erythematosus *vs.*, 144
linear IgA bullous dermatosis, 170, 170f
linear verrucous epidermal nevus, inflammatory, 48–49, 49f, 152, 152f
lipidized siderophages, dermatofibroma, 309
lipid stains, 21
lipoblasts, signet-ring, 344
lipodermatosclerosis, 254, 254f
lipoid proteinosis (hyalinosis cutis et mucosae, Urbach–Wiethe disease), 212, 212f, 231, 231f–232f
lipoma, 341–345, 341f
  angiolipoma, 342, 342f–343f
  angiomyolipoma, 345, 345f
  fibrolipoma, 344, 344f
  mobile encapsulated, 255, 352
  pleomorphic, 344, 344f
  spindle cell, 343, 343f
lipomatosis, familial multiple, 341
liposarcoma, pleomorphic, 344f
"little 5" pattern, 425
  Henoch–Schönlein purpura, 191
  leukocytoclastic vasculitis, 191f
livedoid vasculopathy, 204, 205f
LMDF (lupus miliaris disseminatus faciei), 175, 175f
lobomycosis, 277, 277f
lobular panniculitis, 249f, 250–254
  see also specific diseases/disorders
LPP (lichen planopilaris), 241, 241t, 242f
Lucio's reaction, leprosy, 264, 264f–265f
lung carcinoma metastases, 417
  cell markers, 422t
  small cell lung carcinoma, 417
lunula, nail anatomy, 16
lupus erythematosus, 141–144
  acute, 142f
  bullous, 171, 171f
  chronic discoid, 143f
  cictricial alopecia, 239–241, 240f
  differential diagnosis, 144
  hypertrophic, 138, 138f
  subacute, 142f
lupus miliaris disseminatus faciei, 175, 175f
lupus panniculitis (lupus profundus), 250, 250f
  subcutaneous panniculitis-like T-cell lymphoma *vs.*, 396
lupus profundus *see* lupus panniculitis (lupus profundus)
Lyme disease, 268
lymphadenoma, 77, 77f
lymphadenopathy, massive with sinus histiocytosis, 178, 178f–179f
lymphangioma, 366, 366f
lymphocytes, 17
  exocytosis, 4f
lymphoepithelioma-like carcinoma, 70, 70f
lymphoid vasculitis, 202–203
  see also specific diseases/disorders
lymphoma
  B cell *see* B-cell lymphoma
  cell markers, 34t
  intravascular, 30f, 412, 412f
  mantle cell, 414
  T cell *see* T-cell lymphoma

lymphomatoid drug eruption, patch stage mycosis fungoides *vs.*, 391
lymphomatoid granulomatosis, 413–414
  B-cell lymphoblastic lymphoma/leukemia, 414
  Burkitt lymphoma, 414
  chronic lymphocytic leukemia/small lymophocytic leukemia, 413, 413f
  mantle cell lymphoma, 414
lymphomatoid papulosis, 394–395, 394f–395f
  type A, 394, 394f
  type B, 394–395, 395f
  type C, 394–395, 395f
  type D, 394–395
  type E, 394–395

M

MAC (microcystic adnexal carcinoma), 75t, 93–94, 93f, 94t
macular amyloid, 228, 228f
Madelung's disease, 341
Majocchi's fungal folliculitis, 239, 240f
Majocchi's purpura, 200
Malherbe, calcifying epithelioma of *see* pilomatricoma (calcifying epithelioma of Malherbe)
malignant acrospiroma, 101, 101f
malignant atrophic papulosis, 202, 203f
malignant chondroid syringoma, 97, 97f
malignant melanoma *see* melanoma, malignant
malignant mixed tumor, 97, 97f
malignant peripheral nerve sheath tumors (MPNST), 356, 362–364, 362f
  cutaneous ganglioneuroma, 363, 363f
  glial heterotropia, 364, 364f
  meningeal heterotopia, 364, 364f
  perineurioma, 364
malignant poroma, 101, 101f
malignant Schwannoma *see* malignant peripheral nerve sheath tumors (MPNST)
malignant tumors
  acrospiroma, 101, 101f
  atrophic papulosis, 202, 203f
  chondroid syringoma, 97, 97f
  epidermis, 56–70
    see also actinic keratosis; basal cell carcinoma (BCC); Bowen's disease; keratoacanthoma; squamous cell carcinoma (SCC)
  fibrous *see* fibrous tumors, malignant
  melanoma *see* melanoma, malignant
  mixed tumor, 97, 97f
  peripheral nerve sheath *see* malignant peripheral nerve sheath tumors (MPNST)
  poroma, 101, 101f
  Schwannoma *see* malignant peripheral nerve sheath tumors (MPNST)
MALTomas, 404
mantle cell lymphoma, 414
Mart-1, 29
  halo nevus, 29f
Mascaro, syringofibroadenoma of, 101, 101f
massive lymphadenopathy with sinus histiocytosis, 178, 178f–179f
Masson's intravascular papillary endothelial hyperplasia, 373, 373f
Masson's trichrome stain, 18, 18f
mast cells, 17, 211f, 427, 427f
mastocytoma, 17f
mastocytosis, 210–211, 210f–211f
matrix, nail anatomy, 15
median raphe cyst, 54, 54f
medium vessel vasculitis, 187–190

Medlar body
    chromomycosis, 7f
    definition, 6
melan A, 29
melanin stains, 21
melanoacanthoma, 45, 45f
melanocytic neoplasms, 105–133
    acral nevus, 114–116, 116f
    "ancient" nevus, 117, 117f
    balloon cell nevus, 109, 110f
    benign melanocytic nevus, 105–124, 106f–107f, 109t
    blue nevus *see* blue nevus
    clear cell sarcoma, 132, 132f
    combined nevus, 123, 123f
    congenital nevus, 111, 111f
    desmoplastic melanoma *see* desmoplastic melanoma
    dysplastic nevus, 123, 124f
    genital nevus, 116f
    halo nevus, 117, 118f
    junctional lentiginous nevus, 124, 124f
    lentigo maligna, 127t, 128, 128f
    lentigo maligna melanoma, 127t, 129
    melanotic macule, 105, 105f
    metastatic melanoma, 132, 132f
    Mongolian spot, 126f, 127
    neutral nevus, 111, 111f
    nevus of Ito, 124
    nevus of Ota, 124, 125f
    nodular melanoma, 127t, 129, 131f
    pigmented spindle cell nevus of Reed, 114, 114t, 115f
    recurrent nevus, 124, 124f
    regressing melanoma, 132, 132f
    solar lentigo, 105, 105f
    "special site" nevus, 114
    spindle cell melanoma, 129, 129f
    Spitz nevus, 112–114, 112f, 114t
    superficial spreading malignant melanoma, 127–132, 128f
melanocytic nevus, benign, 105–124, 106f–107f, 109t
melanoma, malignant, 107f–108f
    cell markers, 34t
    D2-40, 27f
    dendritic "equine-type", 120
    desmoplastic *see* desmoplastic melanoma
    differential diagnosis
        benign melanocytic nevus *vs.*, 109t
        Bowen's disease *vs.*, 58
        Paget's disease *vs.*, 69
    halo nevus *vs.*, 119f
    lentigo maligna, 127t, 129
    metastatic, 132
    MIB-1, 35f
    microphthalmia-associated transcription factor, 29f
    mucosal, 127t
    nodular, 127t, 129, 131f
    pHH3, 35f
    regressing, 132, 132f
    spindle cell, 129, 129f
    superficial spreading, 127–132, 127t, 128f
melanotic macule, 105, 105f
melanotic Schwannoma, psammomatous, 355f
meningeal heterotopia, 364, 364f
meningioma, metastatic tumors, 421, 422f
meningocele, rudimentary, 364, 364f
Merkel cell carcinoma, 359–360, 360f
    cell markers, 34t
    neuron-specific enolase, 30f
Merkel cells, 427, 427f

mesenchymal markers, 26–28
metabolic disorders, 224–233
    amyloidosis, 227–228
    cutaneous calcification, 229–230
    mucinoses, 224–227
    mucocele, 232, 232f
    nutritional dermatoses, 232, 232f
    oxalosis, 233, 233f
    see also specific diseases/disorders
metachromasia, 7
metaplasia, syringosquamous, 8f
metastatic calcifications, 229
metastatic carcinoma, 416–424
    breast carcinoma *see* breast carcinoma metastases
    colon carcinoma, 25f, 419, 419f
    differential diagnosis, 423
    lung carcinoma *see* lung carcinoma metastases
    melanoma, 132
    meningioma, 421, 422f
    ovarian cancer *see* ovarian carcinoma metastases
    prostate cancer *see* prostate carcinoma metastases
    renal carcinoma *see* renal cell carcinoma metastases
    signet-ring carcinoma, 420
    small cell carcinoma of the lung, 34t
    squamous carcinoma, 421, 421f
    thyroid carcinoma, 420, 420f
MIB-1 (Ki-67), 35
    benign melanocytic nevus, 105–109
    malignant melanoma, 35f
Michaelis–Gutman body, 7
microabscesses, Pautrier's, 390
microcystic adnexal carcinoma (MAC), 75t, 93–94, 93f, 94t
micronodular basal cell carcinoma, 65, 65f
microphthalmia-associated transcription factor (MITF), 29
    melanoma, 29f
microscopic polyangiitis, 190
    medium vessel vasculitis, 187
microvenular hemangioma, 377, 377f
Miescher's facial granuloma, 173, 174f
migratory erythema, necrolysing, 154f, 232
milker's nodules, 298
MITF *see* microphthalmia-associated transcription factor (MITF)
mixed cryoglobulin disease, 193
mixed tumor (chondroid syringoma), 96
MLH-1, sebaceoma, 82
mnemonics
    BANGLE mnemonic, 88
    CLATS mnemonic, 277, 425
    HAAPPIE mnemonic, 210
    "Here come the big green leafy veggies" mnemonic, 260, 274
    "I vacuum dog pus" mnemonic, 228
    LEMONS mnemonic, 360
    PEPSI LiTe mnemonic, 208
    PLAID mnemonic, 425
    PTICSS mnemonic, 425
    RAP MOPED mnemonic, 218
mobile encapsulated lipoma, 255, 352
modified Dieterle stain, 23, 23f
molluscum contagiosum, 297, 297f
Mongolian spot, 126f, 127
monkey pox, 296
monster cells, dermatofibroma, 311, 311f
morbiliform drug eruptions, 202
morphea, 214–215, 215f–216f
    interstitial dermis of, 27f
morpheaform basal cell carcinoma, 66–67, 66f, 75t, 77f, 94t
Mortierella infection, 282

Index

MPNST *see* malignant peripheral nerve sheath tumors (MPNST)
MSH-2, sebaceoma, 82
MSH-6, sebaceoma, 82
mucicarmine, 20
   Cryptococcus, 20f
mucinoses, 224–227
   focal *see* focal mucinosis
   follicular *see* follicular mucinosis
      see also specific diseases/disorders
mucinous carcinoma, 91, 91f
mucocele, 232, 232f, 248, 248f
mucorales, 282
Mucor infection, 282
mucormycosis, 282
mucosa, skin anatomy, 12, 12f
mucosal melanoma, 127t
Muir–Torre syndrome, 82
mulberry lipoblasts, 344
multiple lipomatosis, familial, 341
multiple myeloma oncogene-1 (MUM-1), 33, 33t
   cutaneous diffuse large B-cell lymphoma leg type, 409
   large B-cell lymphoma, 33f
MUM-1 *see* multiple myeloma oncogene-1 (MUM-1)
Munro microabscess
   definition, 7
   psoriasis, 7f
muscle tumors, 341–353
   leiomyoma *see* leiomyoma
   smooth muscle hamartoma, 352, 352f
mycetomas, 278–279
mycobacterial stains, 22–23
Mycobacterium leprae infection *see* leprosy
mycosis fungoides, 139, 140f, 152, 390–393
   CD4, 31f
   CD7, 32f
   epidermotropism, 4f
   folliculotropic variant, 239, 239f, 392, 392f
   granulomatous slack skin, 392–393, 392f–393f
   pagetoid reticulosis variant, 392, 392f
   patch stage, 390–391, 390f
   plaque stage, 391, 391f
   tumor stage, 391, 391f
mydriasis, 307, 308f
myeloid leukemia, 402
myeloperoxidase, 32
   leukemia cutis, 32f
myofibroma, adult, 311–312, 312f
myofibromatosis, infantile, 316, 317f
myrmecia, 287, 287f
myxedema, pretibial, 224–225, 225f
myxoid neurothekeoma, 361, 361f
myxoma, nerve sheath, 361, 361f

N

nail anatomy, 15–16
   cuticle, 15
   hyponychium, 15
   keratinization, 16
   lunula, 16
   matrix, 15
   solehorn, 15
naphthol ASD chloroacetate esterase *see* Leder stain (naphthol ASD chloroacetate esterase)
nasal glioma, 364, 364f
nasal turbinate, skin anatomy, 12, 12f

natural killer (NK) cell(s), 17
   lymphoma *see* cutaneous T-cell lymphoma
   nasal-type extranodal NK lymphoma, 397–398, 397f–398f
necrobiosis, 7f
   definition, 7
necrobiosis lipoidica, 7f, 172t, 174, 174f–175f
   atypical of the face and scalp, 173, 174f
necrobiotic xanthogranuloma, 176–177, 176f–177f
necrolysing migratory erythema, 154f, 232
Negri body, 7
NEMO gene, incontinentia pigmenti, 209
neoplasms
   pilar *see* pilar neoplasms
      see tumors/neoplasms
nephrogenic cystemic fibrosis, 226f
nerve growth factor receptor *see* P75 (nerve growth factor receptor)
nerve sheath myxoma, 361, 361f
neural tumors, 354–365
   granular cell tumor, 360–361, 360f–361f
   malignant peripheral nerve sheath tumors *see* malignant peripheral nerve sheath tumors (MPNST)
   Merkel cell carcinoma, 359–360, 359f–360f
   neurofibroma *see* neurofibroma
   neuromas *see* neuromas
   neurothekeoma *see* neurothekeoma
   Schwannoma *see* Schwannoma (neurilemmoma)
   supernumerary digit, 359, 359f
      see also specific diseases/disorders
neurilemmoma *see* Schwannoma (neurilemmoma)
neuroectodermal markers, 28–29
neuroendocrine markers, 29–30
neurofibroma, 354–355, 354f
   diffuse, 354
   plexiform, 354, 354f–355f
neurofibrosarcoma *see* malignant peripheral nerve sheath tumors (MPNST)
neuromas, 357–358
   palisaded encapsulated, 357–358, 358f
   traumatic, 357, 357f
neuron-specific enolase (NSE), 29
   Merkel cell carcinoma, 30f
neurothekeoma, 361–362
   cellular, 362, 362f
   myxoid, 361, 361f
neutral nevus, 111, 111f
neutrophil(s), 17
   Sweet syndrome, 17f
neutrophilic dermatoses, 197–199
   acute febrile, 197, 198f
      see also specific diseases/disorders
neutrophilic eccrine hidradenitis, 246, 246f
nevus
   "ancient", 117
   balloon cell, 109, 110f
   benign melanocytic, 105–124, 106f–107f, 109t
   blue *see* blue nevus
   combined, 123
   common epidermal, 48
   congenital, 111, 111f
   connective tissue, 222
   deep penetrating, 120, 122f
   dysplastic, 123, 124f
   epidermal *see* epidermal nevus
   genital, 116f
   halo *see* halo nevus
   inflammatory linear verrucous epidermal, 48–49, 49f, 152, 152f
   of Ito, 124

nevus *(Continued)*
    junctional lentiginous, 124, 124f
    neutral, 111, 111f
    organoid, 81–82
    of Ota, 124, 125f
    persistent, 124, 124f
    recurrent, 124, 124f
    "special site", 114
    Spitz *see* Spitz nevus
nevus flammeus, 367, 367f
nevus lipomatosis superficialis of Hoffmann and Zurhelle, 347
nevus sebaceus of Jadassohn (organoid nevus), 81–82
Nikolsky sign, 163
nipples, supernumerary, 351, 352f
NK1/C3, 362
Nocardia, 22f
nodular amyloidosis, 227, 228f
nodular basal cell carcinoma, 65, 65f
nodular-cystic fat necrosis, 352
nodular elastosis with cysts and comedones, 220, 220f
nodular fasciitis, 327–329, 327f–328f
nodular hidradenoma, 100, 100f
nodular Kaposi's sarcoma, 366f, 387
nodular melanoma, 127t, 129, 131f
nodular vasculitis, 253
nodules
    milker's, 298
    rheumatoid, 175, 175f
    subepidermal calcified, 229, 229f
non-inflammatory nonscarring alopecia *see* alopecia, non-inflammatory
non-inflammatory purpura, 206
    see also specific diseases/disorders
NSE *see* neuron-specific enolase (NSE)
nutritional dermatoses, 232, 232f
    see also specific diseases/disorders

O

occlusive vascular disease, 204–206
    see also specific diseases/disorders
ochronosis, 221, 221f
oil red O stain, 21
onchocerca microfilaria, 303
onchocerciasis, 302–303, 303f
onchocercoma, 302–303, 302f
onchokeratinization, nail, 16
onchyolemmal keratinization, nail, 16
onychomycosis, 271, 271f
ophthalomesenteric duct polyp, metastatic tumors *vs.*, 423, 424f
orf, 298, 298f
organoid nevus, 81–82
orthokeratosis, 7
osmium tetroxide, 21
osteoclast-like giant cells, 16f
osteoma cutis, 349, 349f
Ota, nevus of, 124, 125f
ovarian carcinoma metastases, 419, 420f
    cell markers, 422t
oxalosis, 233, 233f

P

p63, 24
    spindle cell squamous cell carcinoma, 24f
P75 (nerve growth factor receptor), 29
    desmoplastic melanoma, 29f
Pacinian corpuscles, 12f

Pagetoid cells
    definition, 7
    Paget's disease, 7f
pagetoid reticulosis mycosis fungoides, 392, 392f
Pagetoid scatter
    definition, 7
    Paget's disease, 7f
Paget's disease, 69, 69f
    carcinoembryonic antigen, 25f, 58
    cell markers, 34t
    differential diagnosis, 69
    Pagetoid cells, 7f
    Pagetoid scatter, 7f
    PAS, 58
pagoda red, amyloidosis, 227
paisley-tie tumors, 75
pale cell acanthoma, 45
palisading
    definition, 7
    encapsulated neuromas, 357–358, 358f
    gout, 7f
    granuloma annulare, 172, 173f
pancreatic carcinoma, 422t
pancreatic panniculitis, 251, 251f
pankeratin, 24
panniculitis, 249–256
    cytophagic histiocytic, 254, 255f
    eosinophilic, 252, 252f
    granulomatous, 253
    lobular, 249f, 250–254
        see also specific diseases/disorders
    pancreatic, 251, 251f
    septal, 249, 249f
    suppurative, 253
papillary digital carcinoma, 89, 90f
papillary "eccrine" adenoma, 102, 102f
papillary mesenchymal body
    definition, 8
    trichoepithelioma, 8f
papillary thyroid carcinoma, 420f
papillomatosis, 8
papulosis
    Bowenoid, 289, 289f
    lymphomatoid *see* lymphomatoid papulosis
paracoccidioides infection, 276, 276f
parakeratosis
    definition, 8
    granular, 154, 154f
paraneoplastic pemphigus, 147, 147f, 166, 167f
PAS (periodic acid–Schiff), 19, 19f
    fungi, 22, 22f
    Paget's disease, 58
patch stage mycosis fungoides, 390–391, 390f
pattern alopecia (androgenetic balding), 234–235, 234f, 237t
    differential diagnosis, 237
Pautrier's microabscesses, 390
PCT (porphyria cutanea tarda), 167, 167f, 215
PEH *see* pseudoepitheliomatous hyperplasia (PEH)
pellagra, 232
pemphigoid, 158f
    bullous, 168–169, 169f
    cicatricial, 169, 169f
    urticarial, 169f
pemphigus
    familial benign chronic, 164, 164f
    paraneoplastic, 147, 147f, 166, 167f
pemphigus erythematosus, 161

pemphigus foliaceus, 161, 161f
pemphigus gestationis, 169
pemphigus vegetans, 163
    pseudoepitheliomatous hyperplasia, 163f–164f
pemphigus vulgaris, 163, 163f
    acantholysis, 1f
    direct immunofluorescence, 163f
    familial benign chronic pemphigus vs., 164
penicillamine-induced altered elastic, 218f
PEPSI LiTe mnemonic, 208
perforating collagenosis, reactive, 218, 218f
perineurioma, 364
    sclerosing, 325, 325f
periodic acid–Schiff see PAS (periodic acid–Schiff)
periplakin, paraneoplastic pemphigus, 166
perivascular lymphoid infiltrates, 200–202
    see also specific diseases/disorders
Perls stain (Prussian blue), 20, 21f
perniosis, 203, 203f
persistent nevus, 124, 124f
Peyronie's disease, 315
PGP9.5, 362
phaeohyphomycosis, 280, 281f
"pH girl," histoplasmosis, 276
pHH3, 35
    malignant melanoma, 35f
phototoxic eruptions, lupus erythematosus vs., 144
pigmentation
    acanthotic seborrheic keratoses, 38f
    clonal seborrheic keratoses, 41f
    incontinentia pigmenti, 209, 210f
    purpura of Doucas and Kapetanakis, 200
    purpuric eruption, 200–201, 200f
    seborrheic keratoses, 42
    spindle cell nevus of Reed, 114, 114t, 115f
pigment incontinence, 8
pilar cysts, 50–51, 51f
    proliferating, 51–52, 51f–52f
pilar neoplasms, 71–81
    basaloid follicular hamartoma, 79, 79f
    desmoplastic trichilemmoma, 81, 81f
    dilated pore of Winer, 79, 79f
    fibrofolliculoma, 78, 78f
    lymphadenoma, 77, 77f
    pilar sheath acanthoma, 80, 80f
    pilomatrical carcinoma, 72, 72f
    pilomatricoma, 71
    trichilemmoma, 80, 80f
    trichoadenoma, 79, 79f
    trichoblastoma, 72–73, 72f
    trichoepithelioma see trichoepithelioma
    trichofolliculoma, 78, 78f
pilar sheath acanthoma, 80, 80f
piloleiomyoma, 347, 347f
    desmin, 26f
    smooth muscle actin, 26f
pilomatrical carcinoma, 72, 72f
pilomatricoma (calcifying epithelioma of Malherbe), 52, 52f, 71
    shadow cells, 9f
Pinkus' fibroepithelioma, 68, 68f
pitted keratolysis, 258, 258f
pityriasis lichenoides chronica, 141, 142f
pityriasis lichenoides et varioformis acuta (PLEVA), 141, 141f
pityriasis rosea, 157, 157f
pityriasis rubra pilaris, 160f
PLAID mnemonic, 425
planar xanthomas, 180

plantar fibromatosis, 315
plaque Kaposi's sarcoma, 387, 387f
plaque psoriasis, 150, 151f
plaque stage mycosis fungoides, 391, 391f
plasma cells, 17, 18f
plasmacytoma, CD138, 31f
pleomorphic fibroma, 325, 325f
pleomorphic lipoma, 344, 344f
pleomorphic liposarcoma, 344f
pleomorphic undifferentiated sarcoma, 338
pleomorphism, 8
PLEVA (pityriasis lichenoides et varioformis acuta), 141, 141f
plexiform fibrohistiocytic tumor, 331–332, 331f–332f
plexiform neurofibroma, 354, 354f–355f
PMS, sebaceoma, 82
podoplanin see D2–40 (podoplanin)
POEMS syndrome
    glomeruloid hemangioma, 376
    microvenular hemangioma, 377
polyangiitis, microscopic see microscopic polyangiitis
polyarteritis nodosa, 186, 186f
polychondritis, relapsing, 349–353, 350f
polydactyly, rudimentary, 359, 359f
polymorphous light eruption, 144, 144f, 202, 202f
polythelia, 351, 352f
porocarcinoma, 101, 101f
porokeratosis, 139, 139f, 155, 155f
    coronoid lamellae, 3f
poroma, 98, 99f
    malignant, 101, 101f
porphyria cutanea tarda (PCT), 167, 167f, 215
postpubertal nevus sebaceus of Jadassohn, 81–82, 81f
pox virus infections, 295–299
    Gianotti–Crosti syndrome, 299, 299f
    hand, foot and mouth syndrome, 299, 299f
    milker's nodules, 298
    molluscum contagiosum, 297, 297f
    monkey pox, 296f
    orf, 298, 298f
    smallpox, 295, 295f
precursor hematologic neoplasms, 401
premelanosome, 426, 426f
prepubertal nevus sebaceus of Jadassohn, 82, 82f
pretibial myxedema, 224–225, 225f
primary cutaneous CD30+ lymphoproliferative disorders, 394–396
    lymphomatoid papulosis see lymphomatoid papulosis
    primary cutaneous anaplastic large cell lymphoma, 396, 396f
primary cutaneous lymphoma
    anaplastic large cell, 396, 396f
    B-cell see B-cell lymphoma
    follicle cell, 406, 406f–408f, 414t
    marginal zone, 404, 405f, 414t
    T-cell see T-cell lymphoma
primary neuroendocrine carcinoma of the skin see Merkel cell carcinoma
proliferating pilar cysts, 51–52, 51f–52f
proliferation markers, 35
proliferative fasciitis, 329, 329f
prostate carcinoma metastases, 421
    cell markers, 422t
Proteus syndrome, 341
protothecosis, 284, 284f
protozoan diseases, 268–269
    Acanthamoeba, 269, 269f
    leishmaniasis, 268, 269f
Prussian blue (Perls stain), 20, 21f
psammoma body, 8

psammomatous melanotic Schwannoma, 355f
pseudocyst of the auricle, 351, 351f
pseudoepitheliomatous hyperplasia (PEH)
    definition, 8
    elastic tapping, 8f
    keratoacanthoma, 62
    syringosquamous metaplasia, 8f
pseudohorn cyst
    definition, 8
    seborrheic keratosis, 8f
pseudomelanoma, 124, 124f
Pseudomonas, ecthyma granulosum, 259
pseudopelade, idiopathic, 243, 243f
pseudoporphyria, 167
pseudoxanthoma elasticum, 208, 208f–209f
psoriasis, 150
    acanthosis, 1f
    guttate, 150, 152f
    Munro microabscess, 7f
    plaque, 150, 151f
    pustular, 150, 151f
PTICSS mnemonic, 425
purpura
    actinic, 206
    Bateman's, 206
    eczematous, 200
    Gougerot–Blum, 200
    Henoch–Schönlein, 191, 192f–193f
    Majocchi's, 200
    non-inflammatory, 206
        see also specific diseases/disorders
    senile, 206
    solar, 206
pustular dermatosis, subcorneal, 162, 162f
pustular psoriasis, 150, 151f
pyogenic granuloma, 369, 369f

R

radiation dermatitis, chronic, 213, 214f, 214t
radiation therapy, angiosarcoma, 383
RAP MOPED mnemonic, 218
Raynaud's phenomenon, 214
RCC (renal cell carcinoma), 25
reactive perforating collagenosis, 218, 218f
recurrent nevus, 124, 124f
regressing keratoacanthoma, 63, 64f
regressing melanoma, 132, 132f
relapsing polychondritis, 349–353, 350f
renal cell carcinoma (RCC), 25
renal cell carcinoma metastases, 417, 418f
    cell markers, 422t
reticular degeneration
    definition, 8
    variola, 9f
reticulated, 8
reticulated pigmented anomaly of the flexures, 41, 41f
reticulated seborrheic keratoses, 40–41, 40f
reticulohistiocytic granuloma, 177–178, 178f
reticulohistiocytoma, solitary, 177–178, 178f
reticulohistiocytosis, 179
retiform hemangioendothelioma, 383, 383f
RET proto-oncogene, 357
RF4, 409
rheumatoid nodules, 175, 175f
rheumatoid vasculitis, 190
    medium vessel vasculitis, 187
rhinoscleroderma, 260, 260f

rhinoscleroma, 9f
rhinosporidiosis, 284–285, 285f
Rhizomucor infection, 282
Rhizopus infection, 282, 282f
ringed lipidized siderophages, 16f
Rosai–Dorfman disease, 178, 178f–179f
roundworm infections, 299–304
    see also specific diseases/disorders
routine transport media, 35
rudimentary meningocele, 364, 364f
rudimentary polydactyly, 359, 359f
Russell body
    definition, 8
    rhinoscleroma, 9f

S

S100, 28, 34t
    cellular neurothekeoma, 362
    glial heterotropia, 364
    granular cell tumor, 28f
    small blue cell tumors, 34t
    spindle cell neoplasms, 34t
    Spitz nevus, 113f
S100A6 (calcyclin), 28
    atypical fibroxanthoma, 28f
salivary gland, Congo red, 20f
sarcoid, granulomas, 5f
sarcoidosis, 175–176, 176f
    asteroid body, 2f
sarcoma
    clear cell, 132, 132f
    epithelioid, 338, 338f–339f
    Kaposi *see* Kaposi's sarcoma
    pleomorphic undifferentiated, 338
Saskenaea infection, 282
scabies, 303f–304f, 304–306
scalp, skin anatomy, 10, 10f
scars, 219, 219f, 318–319, 318f
    hypertrophic, 219, 219f, 319, 319f
SCC *see* squamous cell carcinoma (SCC)
Schamberg's disease, 200
Schaumann bodies
    definition, 9
    sarcoidosis, 175
Schistosoma haematobium, 299–300, 300f
Schistosoma japonicum, 300, 300f
Schistosoma mansoni, 300, 300f
schistosomiasis, 299–300, 299f–300f
Schwannoma (neurilemmoma), 355–356, 355f
    ancient, 356, 356f
    malignant *see* malignant peripheral nerve sheath tumors (MPNST)
    psammomatous melanotic, 355f
    Verocay bodies, 355, 355f
    Verocay body, 9f
Schweninger–Buzzi anetoderma, 222
scleroderma, 214–215, 215f–216f
scleroderma of Buschke, 224, 224f
sclerodermoid graft-versus-host disease, 215–216, 216f
scleromyxedema, 225, 225f
sclerosing hemangioma, 310, 310f
sclerosing perineurioma, 325, 325f
sclerosing sweat duct carcinoma, 94, 95f
sclerotic fibroma, 323, 324f
scrotal calcinosis, 229–230, 230f
scurvy, 206, 206f
sebaceoma, 82, 83f

sebaceous carcinoma, 83f–85f
    Bowen's disease vs., 58
sebaceous hyperplasia, 82, 82f
sebaceous neoplasms, 81–83
    nevus sebaceus of Jadassohn, 81–82
    sebaceoma, 82, 83f
    sebaceous carcinoma, 83, 83f–85f
    sebaceous hyperplasia, 82, 82f
seborrheic dermatitis, 156
seborrheic keratoses, 37–44
    acanthotic see acanthotic seborrheic keratoses
    BCL-2, 37
    clonal see clonal seborrheic keratoses
    hyperkeratotic, 39, 39f–40f
    inflamed, 39f, 43–44, 43f–44f
    inflamed clonal, 42f
    inflamed hyperkeratotic, 40f
    irritated, 38f–39f, 42–43, 43f
    irritated clonal, 41f–42f
    pigmented, 42, 42f
    pseudohorn cyst, 8f
    reticulated, 40–41, 40f
    stratum corneum, 37
secondary syphilis, 267, 267f
senile purpura, 206
septal panniculitis, 249, 249f
septic vasculitis, 190, 190f
    medium vessel vasculitis, 187
Sézary syndrome, 393, 393f
shadow cells
    definition, 9
    pilomatricoma, 9f
Shulman's disease, 216–217, 216f–217f
siderophages
    lipidized dermatofibroma, 309
    ringed lipidized, 16f
signet-ring carcinoma, 420
signet-ring lipoblasts, 344
simple sebaceous duct cyst, 53, 54f
sinus histiocytosis with massive lymphadenopathy, 178, 178f–179f
skin anatomy, 10–17
    acral skin, 11
    areolar skin, 11, 11f
    face, 10
    fetus, 12, 12f–13f
    mucosa, 12, 12f
    nasal turbinate, 12, 12f
    scalp, 10, 10f
    trunk, 10
    volar skin, 11, 11f–12f
skin appendage disorders, 234–248
    acute Langerhans cell histiocytosis, 245, 245f
    chondrodermatitis nodularis helicis, 245, 246f
    cictricial alopecia see cicatricial alopecia
    hidradenitis suppurativa, 247, 247f
    inflammatory nonscarring alopecia see alopecia, inflammatory nonscarring
    mucocele, 248, 248f
    neutrophilic eccrine hidradenitis, 246, 246f
    non-inflammatory alopecia see alopecia, non-inflammatory
    see also specific diseases/disorders
SMA see smooth muscle actin (SMA)
small blue cell tumors, 34t
small cell lung carcinoma, 417
    metastatic, 34t
small lymphocytic leukemia, 413, 413f
smallpox (variola) see variola (smallpox)

small tubular mixed tumor, 96, 96f
small vessel vasculitis, 190–193
smooth muscle, submucosa, 12f
smooth muscle actin (SMA), 26
    piloleiomyoma, 26f
smooth muscle hamartoma, 352, 352f
    differential diagnosis, 347
Sneddon–Wilkinson disease, 162, 162f
solar lentigo, 40f, 105, 105f
    seborrheic keratosis vs., 40
solar purpura, 206
solehorn, nail anatomy, 15
solitary reticulohistiocytoma, 177–178, 178f
South American blastomycosis, 276, 276f
Sox-10, 29
    desmoplastic melanoma, 29f
    spindle cell neoplasms, 34t
Sparganum proliferum, 300, 300f–301f
SPCTL (subcutaneous panniculitis-like T-cell lymphoma), 255, 255f
"special site" nevus, 114
spider bite, 307
spindle cell hemangioendothelioma, 380, 381f
spindle cell hemangioma, 380, 381f
spindle cell lipoma, 343, 343f
spindle cell melanoma, 129, 129f
spindle cell neoplasms, 34t
spindle cell squamous carcinoma, 62, 62f
    p63, 24f
spiradenocarcinoma, 88, 88f
spiradenoma, 87–88, 87f, 88t
spirochete-mediated disease, 267–268
    acrodermatitis chronica atrophicans, 268, 268f
    Lyme disease, 268
    syphilis see syphilis
Spitz nevus, 112–114, 112f, 114t
    immunostaining, 113f
    intradermal, 114f
    Kamino body, 6f
spongiform pustule of Kogoj, 9
spongiosis
    definition, 9
    eosinophilic see eosinophilic spongiosis
spongiotic dermatitis, 150–160
    acute, 155, 155f
    with intraepidermal eosinophils, 158
    subacute see subacute spongiotic dermatitis
spongiotic pigmented purpuric eruption (PPE), 157, 157f
sporotrichosis, 277–278, 278f
SPTCL (subcutaneous panniculitis-like T-cell lymphoma), 396, 397f
squamatization, 9
squamotization, 9
squamous cell carcinoma (SCC), 60–62, 61f, 63t
    cell markers, 34t
    metastatic tumors, 421, 421f
    spindle, 62, 62f
    verrucous carcinoma, 61, 62f
squamous eddies
    definition, 9
    irritated seborrheic keratosis, 9f
stasis change, occlusive vascular disease, 204, 205f
stasis dermatitis, 157, 158f
steatocystoma, 53, 54f
Steiner stain, 23, 23f
stem, hair anatomy, 13
Stevens–Johnson syndrome, 168, 168f
storiform, 9
stratum corneum, seborrheic keratoses, 37

stratum lucidum, volar skin, 11f
subacute lupus erythematosus, 142f
subacute spongiotic dermatitis, 156, 156f
  lymphocyte exocytosis, 4f
subcorneal pustular dermatosis, 162, 162f
subcorneal vesiculobullous disorders, 161–162
  see also specific diseases/disorders
subcutaneous fat necrosis of the newborn, 251, 252f
subcutaneous leiomyosarcoma, 348
subcutaneous panniculitis-like T-cell lymphoma (SPTCL), 255, 255f, 396, 397f
subcutaneous T-cell lymphoma, CD3, 31f
subcutaneous tissue, granuloma annulare, 172
subepidermal calcified nodules, 229, 229f
subepidermal vesiculobullous disorders, 167–168
  inflammatory, 168–171
  see also specific diseases/disorders
submucosa, smooth muscle, 12f
subungual exostosis, 352, 353f
Sudan black, 21
sun-damage, facial skin, 10f
superficial leiomyosarcoma, 348
superficial multifocal basal cell carcinoma, 64, 64f
superficial spreading malignant melanoma, 127–132, 127t, 128f
supernumerary digits, 359, 359f
supernumerary nipples, 351, 352f
suppurative folliculitis, 258
suppurative panniculitis, 253
sweat duct carcinoma, sclerosing, 94, 95f
sweat gland neoplasms, 86–104
  acrospiromas, 97–100, 98f
  adenoid cystic carcinoma, 103, 103f
  clear cell hidradenoma, 100, 100f
  cylindroma, 86, 86f, 88t
  dermal duct tumor, 99, 99f
  eccrine angiomatous hamartoma, 103, 103f
  hidradenoma papilliferum, 89, 89f
  hidroacanthoma simplex, 99, 99f
  hidrocystoma, 95, 95f
  malignant acrospiroma, 101, 101f
  malignant mixed tumor, 97, 97f
  microcystic adnexal carcinoma, 93–94, 93f, 94t
  mixed tumor, 96
  mucinous carcinoma, 91, 91f
  nodular hidradenoma, 100, 100f
  papillary digital carcinoma, 89, 90f
  papillary "eccrine" adenoma, 102, 102f
  poroma, 98, 99f
  sclerosing sweat duct carcinoma, 94, 95f
  spiradenocarcinoma, 88, 88f
  spiradenoma, 87–88, 87f, 88t
  syringocystadenoma papilliferum, 88, 89f
  syringofibroadenoma of Mascaro, 101, 101f
  syringoma, 91, 91f, 94t
Sweet's syndrome, 17f, 197, 198f
synaptophysin, 30
  small blue cell tumors, 34t
syndecan-1 see CD138 (syndecan-1)
syphilis, 152–154, 153f
  chancre, 267
  interface dermatitis, 145, 145f
  secondary, 267, 267f
  tertiary, 268, 268f
syphilitic alopecia, 238
syringocystadenoma papilliferum, 88, 89f
syringofibroadenoma of Mascaro, 101, 101f

syringoma, 75t, 91, 94t
  chondroid, 96, 97f
  clear cell, 91, 92f
syringosquamous metaplasia, 8f
systemic amyloidosis, 227

T

Takayasu arteritis, 185–186, 185f–186f
tapeworms, 299–304
  see also specific diseases/disorders
targetoid hemosiderotic hemangioma, 374, 374f–375f
T-cell(s), 17
  cutaneous lymphoma see cutaneous T-cell lymphoma
T-cell lymphoma
  cutaneous see cutaneous T-cell lymphoma
  subcutaneous, 31f
  subcutaneous panniculitis-like, 255, 255f
T-cells type 1 (TH1), 17
T-cells type 2 (TH2), 17
telangiectasia maculans eruptiva perstans (TMEP), 210, 211f
telogen effluvium, 235, 235f
telogen hairs, 13, 15f
temporal arteritis, 183–184, 184f–185f
tendon sheath, giant cell tumor, 321–322, 321f
tertiary syphilis, 268, 268f
thioflavin T, 20
  amyloidosis, 227
  lichen amyloid, 20f
thromboangiitis obliterans, 187, 187f
thrombophlebitis, 187
thyroglossal duct cyst, 55
thyroid gland carcinoma
  follicular carcinoma, 420f
  papillary, 420f
thyroid gland carcinoma metastases, 420, 420f
  cell markers, 422t
thyroid transcription factor (TTF-1), 25
  adenocarcinoma, 25f
  Merkel cell carcinoma, 359
  small blue cell tumors, 34t
tick bite, 305f–306f, 306–307
tinea, 270–271, 270f
tinea capitis, 239
tinea nigra, 280, 280f
tinea versicolor, 271
TMEP (telangiectasia maculans eruptiva perstans), 210, 211f
toludine blue, 18, 20
  urticaria pigmentosa, 18f
tonofibrils, 427, 427f
toxic epidermal necrolysis, 147, 168, 168f
trabecular carcinoma see Merkel cell carcinoma
traction alopecia, 237
transglutaminase-3, 170
transient acantholytic dermatosis (Grover's disease), 166
  Darier's type, 165, 166f
  Hailey–Hailey variant, 164
transport media, 35
traumatic fat necrosis, 255
traumatic neuromas, 357, 357f
Treponema palladium
  immunochemical stains, 34f
  infection see syphilis
trichilemmal cyst see pilar cysts
trichilemmoma, 80, 80f
  desmoplastic, 81, 81f
trichoadenoma, 79, 79f

trichoblastoma, 72–73
    adamantinoid, 77, 77f
trichoepithelioma, 73, 73f–74f, 103
    basal cell carcinoma vs., 73t
    desmoplastic, 75, 75t, 76f, 94t
    papillary mesenchymal body, 8f
trichofolliculoma, 78, 78f
trichome stain, Kamino body, 113f
trichoptilosis see trichotillomania
trichotillomania, 235, 235f–236f, 237t
    differential diagnosis, 237
trunk, skin anatomy, 10
TTF-1 see thyroid transcription factor (TTF-1)
tuberculoid leprosy, 262, 262f
tuberculosis, 266, 266f
tuberous xanthelasma, 180, 180f
tubular apocrine adenoma, 102, 102f
tufted angioma, 377, 377f–378f
tufted angiomas (angioblastomas), 377, 377f–378f
tumid lupus erythematosus, 202, 202f, 226, 226f
tumors/neoplasms
    benign epidermal, 37–55
        see also specific tumors
    bone see bone tumors
    branching alveolar mixed tumor, 96, 97f
    cylindroma (turban tumor), 86, 86f, 88t
    dermal duct, 99, 99f
    fat see fat tumors
    fibrous see fibrous tumors
    gastrointestinal tumors, 422t
    giant cell tumor of the tendon sheath, 321–322, 321f
    glomus see glomus tumor
    granular cell see granular cell tumor
    malignant see malignant tumors
    melanocytic see melanocytic neoplasms
    muscle see muscle tumors
    neural tumors see neural tumors
    supernumerary nipple, 351, 352f
    vasculature see vascular tumors
tumor stage mycosis fungoides, 391, 391f
tungiasis, 307, 308f
turban tumor, 86, 86f, 88t

U

UCHL-1 (CD45Ro), 30
UEA-1 (Ulex europeus agglutinin), 27
Ulex europeus agglutinin (UEA-1), 27
Ulex europus lectin, angiosarcoma, 383
undifferentiated sarcoma, pleomorphic, 338
Urbach–Wiethe disease, 212, 212f, 231, 231f–232f
urinary tract carcinoma, cell markers, 422t
urticaria (wheal), 198–199, 199f
    acute, 199f
    chronic, 199f
urticarial pemphigoid, 169f
urticaria pigmentosa
    CD117, 33f
    Giemsa stain, 23f
    Leder stain, 19f
    toludine blue, 18f

V

vacuolar change, 9
vacuolar interface dermatitis, 134–135, 139
    benign lichenoid keratosis, 137, 137f, 141–144, 142f
    dermatomyositis see dermatomyositis
    erythema multiforme, 146, 146f
    fixed drug eruption, 147, 148f
    graft-versus-host disease, 147, 148f
    lichenoid see lichenoid interface dermatitis
    mycosis fungoides see mycosis fungoides
    paraneoplastic pemphigus, 147, 147f, 166, 167f
    pityriasis lichenoides chronica, 141, 142f
    pityriasis lichenoides et varioformis acuta, 141, 141f
    syphilis see syphilis
    toxic epidermal necrolysis, 147, 168, 168f
varicella zoster virus (VZV), 292, 293f–294f
    immunochemical stains, 34f
variola (smallpox), 295, 295f
    reticular degeneration, 9f
vascular disease
    inflammatory see inflammatory vascular diseases
    occlusive, 204–206
        see also specific diseases/disorders
vascular tumors, 366–389
    angiokeratoma, 366, 366f
    angiolymphoid hyperplasia with eosinophilia, 371, 372f
    angioma serpiginosum, 367, 367f
    angiosarcoma, 383–385, 384f–386f
    arteriovenous malformation, 373, 374f
    bacillary angiomatosis, 369, 370f
    cherry angioma, 369, 370f
    eccrine angiomatous hamartoma, 375, 376f
    epithelioid hemangioendothelioma, 380, 382f
    glomeruloid hemangioma, 376, 376f
    glomus tumor see glomus tumor
    hemangiopericytoma, 380, 380f
    infantile hemangioma, 371, 371f
    intravascular papillary endothelial hyperplasia of Masson, 373, 373f
    Kaposiform hemangioendothelioma, 378, 378f–379f
    Kaposi's sarcoma see Kaposi's sarcoma
    Kimura's disease, 371, 372f
    lymphangioma, 366, 366f
    microvenular hemangioma, 377, 377f
    nevus flammeus, 367, 367f
    pyogenic granuloma, 369, 369f
    retiform hemangioendothelioma, 383, 383f
    spindle cell hemangioma, 380, 381f
    targetoid hemosiderotic hemangioma, 374, 374f–375f
    tufted angioma, 377, 377f–378f
    venous lake, 367, 367f
vasculitis
    drug induced leukocytoclastic, 193
    idiopathic leukocytoclastic, 193
    large vessel, 183–187
    leukocytoclastic see leukocytoclastic vasculitis
    lymphoid, 202–203
    medium vessel, 187–190
    nodular, 253
    rheumatoid see rheumatoid vasculitis
    septic see septic vasculitis
    small vessel, 190–193
        see also specific diseases/disorders
vasculopathy, livedoid, 204, 205f
veins, 184f
vellus hair cysts, 50, 50f
venous lake, 367, 367f
Verhoeff–Van Gieson stain, 18
    anetoderma, 222, 222f
    elastofibroma dorsi, 18f
    normal elastic pattern, 234f

Verocay bodies
	definition, 9
	Schwannoma, 355, 355f
	schwannoma, 9f
verruca plana, 287, 287f
verruca vulgaris, 286, 286f
verruciform xanthoma, 181, 181f–182f
	foam cells, 5f
verrucous carcinoma, 61, 62f
verrucous cyst, 290, 291f
verrucous epidermal nevus, inflammatory linear, 48–49, 49f, 152, 152f
verrucous incontinentia pigmenti, 209, 210f
verrucous VZV infections, 294, 294f
vesicular incontinentia pigmenti, 209, 209f
vesiculobullous disorders, 161–171
	inflammatory subepidermal, 168–171
	intraepidermal, 163–166
	subcorneal, 161–162
		see also specific diseases/disorders
villus
	definition, 10
	warty dyskeratoma, 10f
vimentin, 28
vinyl chloride exposure, 215
viral exanthem, lupus erythematosus vs., 144
viral infections, 286–299
	cytomegalovirus, 295, 295f
	herpetic infections, 292–295
	pox infections see pox virus infections
	warts see warts
		see also specific viral infections
vitiligo, Fontane–Masson stain, 21f
volar skin, 11, 11f–12f
	stratum lucidum, 11f
Von Kossa stain, 21, 21f
VZV see varicella zoster virus (VZV)

W

Warthin–Starry stain, 23
warts, 286–290
	Bowenoid papulosis, 289, 289f
	condyloma acuminatum, 288, 288f
	epidermodysplasia verruciformis, 287
	Heck's disease, 290, 290f
	myrmecia, 287, 287f
	verruca plana, 287, 287f
	verruca vulgaris, 286f
	verrucous cyst, 290, 291f
warty dyskeratoma, 46, 47f
villus, 10f
Wegener's granulomatosis, 188, 188f
	medium vessel vasculitis, 187
Wells' syndrome, 4f
Well's syndrome, 199–200, 200f
wheal see urticaria (wheal)
Winer's dilated pore, 79, 79f
Woringer–Kolopp mycosis fungoides, 392
World Health Organization (WHO), cutaneous B-cell lymphoproliferative disorder classification, 404

X

xanthelasma, 180, 180f
	tuberous, 180, 180f
xanthogranuloma, 177, 177f
	necrobiotic, 176–177, 176f–177f
xanthomas, 179–181
	eruptive, 181, 181f
	intertriginous, 180
	planar, 180
	verruciform see verruciform xanthoma

Z

Ziehl–Neelsen acid-fast stain, 22
Zoon's balanitis, 158, 159f
Zurhelle, nevus lipomatosis superficialis of, 347
zygomycosis, 282